Maggie Kearney
(360) 983-8479
P.O. Box 249
Morton, WA 98356

Evaluation and Treatment of Chronic Pain

Third Edition

Evaluation and Treatment of Chronic Pain

Third Edition

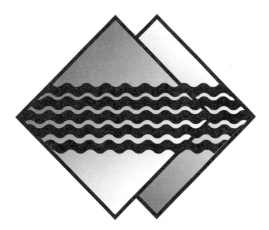

Gerald M. Aronoff, MD

Medical Director
Presbyterian Center for Pain Medicine
Presbyterian Orthopaedic Hospital
Charlotte, North Carolina

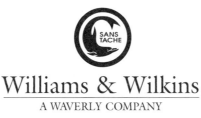

Williams & Wilkins
A WAVERLY COMPANY

BALTIMORE • PHILADELPHIA • LONDON • PARIS • BANGKOK
BUENOS AIRES • HONG KONG • MUNICH • SYDNEY • TOKYO • WROCLAW

Editor: Charles W. Mitchell

Managing Editor: Marjorie Kidd Keating

Marketing Manager: Peter Darcy

Project Editor: Peter J. Carley

Designer: Mario Fernandez

Copyright © 1999 Williams & Wilkins

351 West Camden Street

Baltimore, Maryland 21201–2436 USA

Rose Tree Corporate Center

1400 North Providence Road

Building II, Suite 5025

Media, Pennsylvania 19063–2043 USA

Printed in the United States of America

First Edition, 1985

Second Edition, 1992

Library of Congress Cataloging-in-Publication Data

Evaluation and treatment of chronic pain / [edited by] Gerald M.
   Aronoff. -- 3rd ed.
      p.   cm.
   Includes bibliographical references and index.
   ISBN 0–683–30149–7
   1. Chronic pain.   I. Aronoff, Gerald M.
   [DNLM: 1. Pain--diagnosis.   2. Pain--therapy.   3. Chronic Disease.
WL 704 E92 1998]
RB127.E85   1998
616'.0472--dc21
DNLM/DLC
for Library of Congress   98-22557
                                                              CIP

The publishers have made every effort to trace the copyright holders for borrowed material. If they have inadvertently overlooked any, they will be pleased to make the necessary arrangements at the first opportunity.

To purchase additional copies of this book, call our customer service department at (800) 638-0672 or fax orders to (800) 447–8438. For other book services, including chapter reprints and large quantity sales, ask for the Special Sales department.

Canadian customers should call (800) 665–1148, or fax (800) 665–0103. For all other calls originating outside of the United States, please call (410) 528–4223 or fax us at (410) 528-8550.

Visit Williams & Wilkins on the Internet: http://www.wwilkins.com or contact our customer service department at custserv@wwilkins.com. Williams & Wilkins customer service representatives are available from 8:30 am to 6:00 pm, EST, Monday through Friday, for telephone access.

99   100   101   102   103
1   2   3   4   5   6   7   8   9   10

Dedication

This book is dedicated to
my father
Solomon Aronoff, MD,

whose medical career and empathic approach to patient care
were exemplary. His commitment to a high standard of medical
ethics has remained with me as a driving force and has helped me
to become a healer in addition to being a physician.

It is also dedicated to my patients, whose sufferings have shown
me courage and helped me meet the challenge of algology—to
better serve those in chronic pain.

And most of all to my wife, Minna, whose encouragement, support,
love and friendship have added a new dimension to my life.

Gerald M. Aronoff, MD

Forewords

To the First Edition

The conceptualization of pain has undergone radical change in the past 2 decades. Previously, in the main, pain was thought of as a sensory experience that occurred as a response to some form of body damage or nociceptive stimulation. If, for any reason, the body damage or physical findings factor did not account for the indications by patient behavior or the report by the patient of pain, the accepted alternative explanation was some form of mental or emotional disturbance. Such terms as conversion reaction, hysteria, or hypochondriasis were invoked. As is well recognized now, that kind of conceptual approach represented a form of mind-body dualism; the problem was either in the mind or in the body. With the appearance of Melzack and Wall's monumental paper proposing the gate control theory of pain, the systematic synthesis of mental and physical processes in relation to pain was begun. Subsequently, the rapidly advancing field of behavioral science spawned analyses of pain in behavioral terms. Pain was conceptualized as behavior. As such, pain could be seen as subject to the same laws or influences as any other form of behavior. The so-called operant or contingency management approaches to the evaluation and treatment of pain appeared in the professional literature, pointing the way to treating pain problems without recourse specifically to medically or surgically based interventions or to interventions aimed at trying to change mental states or personality. Instead, the patient underwent a reactivation program. At the same time, systematic efforts were made to change such contingencies as analgesic delivery patterns and the social feedback from others to sick and well behavior.

A second and related, although different, approach to dealing with pain then emerged in the form of so-called cognitive-behavioral methods. Whereas in "pure" and isolated form, operant approaches tended to view the patient as a somewhat passive recipient of learning—conditioning effects, cognitive—behavioral approaches identified more active contributions from the mental processes of the person. It was recognized that the perception of a stimulus or a sensation and, most importantly, the label assigned to it could have profound effects on pain and ensuing behavior. It might be said about the cognitive-behavioral perspective that behavior is in important degree a function of the label attached to the stimulus initiating that behavior. In effect, "If I think what I just experienced or perceived as a stimulus was 'pain,' I will draw from my pain behavior repertoire to behave. If, however, I perceive the stimulus not as 'pain,' I will behave differently; i.e., in the way appropriate to whatever label I may assign."

The most important part of these historical comments is the recognition that body or physical and mind or mental (learning-conditioning and cognitive labeling) interact in systematic ways. These complex interactions take on special significance in regard to chronic pain.

The distinction between acute and chronic pain is basic to an understanding of clinical pain. The distinction can be thought about from several perspectives. First, of course, it is a time statement. Chronicity ensures that time will have passed, time during which a host of effects both within and without the body will have had opportunity to exert influence.

The distinction between acute and chronic can also be viewed from a systems analysis perspective. That a given pain problem persists into chronicity means, by definition, that the health care system has failed to solve the problem. It could be that the problem is unsolvable. On the other hand, it could mean that the understanding of the problem and the methods used to do something about it have somehow missed the mark. It is this point that forms the basis for the need to assimilate and integrate behavioral with neurophysiological approaches to pain. That is one of the major aims of this book and the reason why it is needed.

We must bring these new concepts to first-line care. This book has that objective. It provides a broad review of up-to-date information about virtually all of the clinical pain problems encountered in practice. In addition, however, and of special importance, the book integrates the neurophysiological with the mental, emotional, and psychological. As such, it will provide a reference book of great value to a wide range of health care practitioners concerned with persons burdened with pain.

Wilbert E. Fordyce, PhD
1985

To the Second Edition

In the ensuing years since publication of the first edition of Evaluation and Treatment of Chronic Pain, our knowledge about and understanding of chronic pain has continued to grow. I want to add one thought to the foreword I wrote to the 1985 edition. It is increasingly clear that the unifying thing about chronic pain patients is that they are suffering, even though that suffering may have only an incidental or historically contiguous relationship to tissue injury. The health care system, generally, seems not yet to understand well enough that the suffering chronic pain patient is not necessarily suffering from significant ongoing nociception. Better recognition of this fact would diminish markedly the need for specialized chronic pain treatment facilities. In the meantime, this book addresses those concerns.

Wilbert E. Fordyce, PhD
1992

Forward to the Third Edition

I welcome the opportunity to contribute a foreword to the third edition, both for its own sake and because it provides a chance to reflect on changes in my own thinking since the 1985 and 1992 editions.

Dr. Aronoff has expanded into new territory wisely with this latest edition, as well as updating and revising chapters from earlier editions. These modifications engage well with evolving perspectives on pain. There have also been important changes in the format and procedures of health care delivery, particularly as pertains to chronic pain. These have important implications for management of chronic pain. It is about some of these changes that I wish to comment.

The domain of pain is composed of inter-locking dimensions. One of the frequently under-appreciated dimensions is the influence of environmental factors in determining and shaping how we experience pain and what we do about it. We have long been aware of the power of contingent reinforcement on pain behaviors, of how those contingencies may intensify or ameliorate experienced pain. Indeed, as Romano and colleagues (1) have shown, contingent reinforcement of pain behaviors may cause those behaviors to persist even when peripheral nociceptive stimulation seems no longer to be present. Contingent reinforcement of pain behaviors and their alternative, well behaviors, reflect a specific linkage between environmental consequences and actions of the person. But there are broader linkages between patient behavior and extant or anticipated environmental consequences. These have, I believe, under-appreciated implications. I refer now to effects of anticipated consequences or, stated another way, of environmental cues indicating probable forthcoming consequences—immediately or in the foreseeable future—that can and do evoke behavior.

This focus centers not in the person—his or her biomedical status—nor on personality or motivation. Rather, it considers functional relations between patterns of behavior and environmental cues and consequences. One cannot understand a behavior, or in the domain of pain, a symptom or complaint, in isolation from the contextual influences with which it interacts. Mostly "symptoms" of pain are linked to pathoanatomical factors within the person. However, not all symptoms of pain are so linked, and of those that have such a linkage, contextual forces are also likely to exert influence.

This is not the place to develop fully a treatise on contextual influences on pain behaviors. Here I wish to consider the pain clinician—patient interaction, for that is also a contextual influence or environmental cue. Many clinicians implicitly or explicitly proceed from the perspective that biomedical factors are the certain, likely, or "first-choice" explanations for the person's suffering. In recent-onset pain problems that is a good bet, though not a certain one. It is one thing for a clinician to conceptualize the diagnostic mission as one of seeking to identify causation and to start with examining biomedical factors. It is quite another thing for that clinician to adopt a posture with a patient that conveys by word or deed that the solution to the problem is to be found in biomedical considerations. Such a posture will certainly influence anticipated consequences and thereby patient behavior toward the diagnostic and treatment process. The clinician risks conveying: "The problem you—the patient—present is one that I (hopefully) can 'fix' *and* that you cannot." To do that is to suggest implicitly a scenario for the patient in which he or she passively awaits a solution. If, then, biomedical factors and their medical management are not the answer to the pain problem—or are only partially so—what are we to expect from the patient? There may be anger or dissatisfaction at the failure to receive a solution. There may be insistence on further biomedically-rooted diagnostic or treatment procedures even when those have not led to a solution. The patient may come to anticipate enduring limitation from the dysfunction that led him or her to seek care-: a giving-up, or a seeking of the social and economic shelter of disability status.

To hold somewhat exclusively to a biomedical perspective on the complex set of factors that make up pain problems—most particularly when they are chronic—ensures underestimation of contextual influence on suffering. This error is, I believe, a significant source of iatrogenic pain and of unneeded disability problems, and it leads to policy defects in managed care decision-making.

The diagnosing clinician needs to see himself or herself as a coach and not a repair mechanic. The clinician is a powerful part of the patient's world, one who inevitably influences patient anticipations. That must be recognized in setting the tone of the diagnostic process. The patient needs to be helped to recognize that simple solutions arrived at and delivered by the clinician are unlikely.

There are also broader implications to the difficulties arising out of our tendency to fix our thinking too much on a biomedical perspective, one that implicates decision-making processes in managed care. Non-professionals and conceptually unsophisticated professionals are at risk to perceive acute pain as biomedically -rooted, which, as noted earlier, sometimes raises a problem. However, if the pain persists into chronicity, it is often attributed solely to psychiatric or psychological problems. There are two errors in that. One is that chronic pain isn't one or the other, biomedical or psychiatric–psychological. It isn't a dichotomy and it isn't limited to those two choices. Contextual influences shaping pain behaviors and their persistence are not being appreciated. The second error is that managed care programs are prone to discourage comprehensive (i.e., psychosocial) management of chronic pain under the mistaken notion that to provide such care is to undertake management of something perceived as different from the pain problems they accept as part of their mandate. Clearly, waste of effort and resources occur when chronic pain is too readily over-simplified as biomedical or psychiatric–psychologic. But human suffering, family stability, and economic productivity are also lost when managed care relegates chronic pain to an unenfranchised status. Moreover, in doing so, it violates its mandate.

The composition of Dr. Aronoff's book shows us that pain is a complex phenomenon that requires a broad, an interdisciplinary, and a multidimensional perspective, one that responds to both patient and context. People are complex. Their pain problems are complex. They—patient and clinician—exist in a complex world. This book helps us to deal with that.

1. Romano J, et al. Observational assessment of chronic pain patient-spouse behavioral interactions. Behav Res Ther 1991;22:549–567.

Wilbert E. Fordyce, PhD
University of Washington
Seattle, Washington
1998

Preface

To the Third Edition

This book is meant to meet the needs of physicians and other clinicians engaged in the management of patients with chronic pain. It is meant to be practical rather than esoteric, research oriented, or concentrated on the basic sciences. It is comprehensive, so as to be useful as a resource for the diagnosis and treatment of chronic pain. Because of the many changes in the diagnosis and treatment of pain since the second edition was published in 1992, the chapters retained from that edition have been updated. Some chapters have been deleted; many have been added to reflect current clinical practice and research as of 1998.

One of the major criticisms of modern medical practice arises out of what might also be perceived as one of its major strengths. As technology flourishes, physicians become more highly specialized. With specialization has come the tendency for physicians to treat organ systems rather than the whole patient. Whether this is a common occurrence I can only speculate; however, having now consulted on more than 11,000 pain patients through the Boston Pain Center and more recently the Presbyterian Center for Pain Medicine, I can say that this is frequently the patient's perception. It is unfortunate that as highly trained as most physicians are, they so often overuse sophisticated diagnostic equipment and invasive procedures in treating chronic pain syndrome patients. These procedures have not made an appreciable improvement in most chronic pain syndromes or alleviated the suffering of most such patients. On the contrary, there is evidence that in the United States for many years we have performed per capita far more invasive procedures, especially nerve blocks and back surgeries, than have clinicians in other industrialized countries for similar conditions, without evidence that our results are significantly better. There is evidence that this trend is changing and that interventional approaches are being used with greater specificity and with better-defined selection criteria. This is gratifying to witness and is discussed in more detail throughout the book.

As discussed in greater detail in other sections of this book, chronic pain has become a major public health problem in the United States—a problem that I believe is inadequately addressed in terms of funding for both basic research and clinical studies. Dr. John Bonica, who wrote the introduction to the second edition of this text, did a superb job in trying to improve this situation. He died in 1995 but left a legacy for all who knew him and for the entire field of pain medicine. His leadership is missed, and certainly much more work is needed for organized medicine to recognize the importance of pain medicine as a discipline. Some of this, I anticipate, will come from the regional, national, and international pain societies and some from the American Academy of Pain Medicine with its specific goal of improving the clinical management of chronic pain patients.

The driving force, however, should come from physicians and other clinicians primarily engaged in the clinical management of chronic pain patients. We are dealing with an extremely difficult subgroup of the medical population. For the most part, the intractable chronic nonmalignant pain syndromes concern individuals who not only have persistent pain but who have extreme life disruption and enmeshment with physicians and hospitals because of their pain. The conceptual model of treatment that has made the most sense to me philosophically is that initially discussed by Crue and modified by Loeser, Hollister, Seres, Rosomoff, Addison, Paul, and others, who emphasized the importance of physical and emotional rehabilitation, evaluating and modifying dysfunctional pain behaviors, and improving the quality of life for our patients. Pain medicine owes an enormous debt of gratitude to the pioneering work on pain behavior done by Sternbach, Fordyce, Wolfe, Turk, and others who have shaped the treatment programs of most major pain centers.

As a group, we need to sharpen our clinical acumen and perhaps rely less on sophisticated diagnostic studies. We must learn to take a firm stand with our patients and not perpetuate their careers as patients. We must recognize that they are often stuck in the organic medical model: the worse they feel, the more they request testing and procedures to undo how they feel. We must not allow ourselves to make the same errors they do in their endless quest for a cure. This is a population very prone to iatrogenic complications. Perhaps a shingle should be hung outside our offices saying, "Caution: Too many visits to this office may be hazardous to your health." We should recognize that many of the patients we see will not be "fixed"; we must be honest with them, helping them to recognize that they can lead full and productive lives in spite of pain.

We must not be hypocrites. If we are committed to improving the health care of our patients, I believe our treatments should reflect this philosophy. We should not allow ourselves to be intimidated into compromising our practice of medicine. With nonemergency medical treatment, the patient's motivation and attitude are critical determinants of response to treatment. Patient selection is as important for physicians as the selection of a physician is for patients. We cannot make patients give up their pain if they choose not to. If a patient stands to gain more by staying in pain than by relinquishing it, successful treatment is unlikely unless we can modify the reinforcement contingencies. As physicians, we can help patients appreciate the difference between living with a handicap and being disabled.

The traditional medical model is one in which physicians are in an authoritarian position, actively evaluating symptoms of patients who are passive recipients of health care, undergoing tests, submitting to procedures, seeking prescriptions for medication after medication. John Loeser has stated that "many of the patients we see with chronic pain are manifesting symptoms whose genesis does not lie in structural or functional abnormality of the body part which hurts." Quoting Oliver Wendell Holmes, Loeser says, "I firmly believe that if the whole materia medica, as now used, could be sunk to the bottom of the sea, it would be all the better for mankind—and all the worse for the fishes."

We live in an era in which patients themselves are rarely responsible for most of the financial aspects of their own health care. Many patients are, however, being asked to contribute more financially than ever before and are expressing discontent about services for which they are not covered and to which they are being denied access. This is true specifically in the area of chronic pain management. Although their anger is meant to be directed at their health care insurer, in fact it is often displaced to the health care provider. Often we have the tools to alleviate their suffering, but frequently insurers are unwilling to reimburse for those services, and patients may be unable to afford them.

Managed care is now deeply entrenched in American medicine along with private insurers and state and federal health care programs. As third parties pay more of the bills, big business becomes more integrated into the health care delivery system. Because big business exists to be profitable, the health care system may be more influenced by socioeconomic and perhaps political decisions than by medical need. As physicians, we should be incensed at this reality. Only through such organizations as the existing pain societies and the American Medical Association with its local chapters do we have even the remotest possibility of improving a system that appears to be steadily veering away from sound medical practice. Physicians should not stand idly by while bureaucrats practice medicine. Businessmen cannot dictate for our patients what treatments should be available and with what frequency they may be used. The bureaucracy should not test the quality of a treatment program only on the basis of cost factors. I am not suggesting that cost containment and cost effectiveness should not be among the goals of any good program or treatment. Certainly, we have only finite resources and therefore must make certain decisions as to which treatments are in the patient's best interest. However, we must not lose sight of our goals as physicians and healers, which are to alleviate suffering and improve the quality of our patients' lives. We must never forget the golden rule of medicine: "Above all, do no harm."

Although this book is meant to be comprehensive and to assist physicians and other clinicians primarily of nonpsychiatric specialties in the diagnosis and management of pain, it emphasizes psychiatric and psychological issues as being integral in the evaluation and treatment process. Such was my intention. Dr. Benjamin Crue has stated to many audiences of medical and surgical colleagues that the treatment of chronic pain is basically psychotherapeutic. He and I have discussed this on numerous occasions. Certainly it is not his intent to imply that the chronic pain patient should be treated only by psychologists and psychiatrists; rather, in addition to addressing relevant medical or surgical needs, any clinician involved in the management of chronic pain patients should approach the patient in a caring and psychotherapeutic manner, rather than futilely pursuing only a source of nociception.

Each of the contributing authors was carefully selected because of demonstrated expertise in a specific area of chronic pain management. My hope is that you will learn from them, as I have, and that your continued involvement with chronic pain patients will give you the personal gratification that comes from helping these patients with their suffering and resumption of a better quality of life.

Gerald M. Aronoff, MD
1998

Acknowledgments

Thanking all the individuals who have contributed to this volume is a difficult task because many gave so much encouragement and support. Let me begin by thanking my family, who have been and continue to be a source of inspiration for me. I would like to express my appreciation to the participating authors for their contributions, to the publisher, Williams & Wilkins, for its confidence in me and in this project, and to Margie Keating, managing editor, for her many suggestions. I am especially grateful to the members of the staff at the Presbyterian Center for Pain Medicine for their support since my relocation from Boston, for their dedication to patient care, and for their willingness to take the time to make the interdisciplinary concept work. Special thanks go to Jeffrey Feldman, PhD, program director, who reviewed several of the chapters and offered constructive comments that improved the final product.

Many of us choose a career path as a result of special individuals who share their vast knowledge with us and do it with such a sense of caring that they become mentors. I have been fortunate to have had several such individuals touch my life; this volume would not have emerged were it not for them. There is also a good chance that without them, I would not have entered the field of pain medicine.

As a psychiatric resident I was ambivalent about remaining in the field. It was Dr. Dietrich Blumer, a neuropsychiatrist, who helped educate me about the psychodynamics of the pain-prone personality, a constellation of early-life traumas that put certain persons at risk for developing chronic pain syndromes. He shared with me his fascination for working with this difficult population of pain sufferers. It was contagious.

Dr. Nathaniel Hollister, psychiatrist and neurosurgeon, in 1972 founded the pain unit that later became the Boston Pain Center. He and I spent approximately a year working closely together, and during that year he was my guru. His wisdom and compassion helped me better understand the art of medicine. He remains a dear friend.

Dr. Stephen Freidberg, past president of the New England Neurosurgical Society and chief of neurosurgery at Lahey Clinical Medical Center, helped me to appreciate the importance of careful patient selection for surgical as well as pain center treatment. His ability to make difficult therapeutic decisions based on his assessment of what would best benefit the patient, rather than primarily on what the patient wanted, made him a valued consultant to the Boston Pain Center and to me.

My first contact with Dr. William Sweet came during my neurology rotation at the Massachusetts General Hospital. He is a neurosurgical pioneer who has dedicated his life to the study of pain, and he became an important figure in my professional development. As much as I have learned from him about the workings of the nervous system and the mechanisms of pain in various disorders, it is his sense of dedication, his ethics, and his willingness to stand by his principles that have guided my career. He has been one of my greatest inspirations.

Dr. Philipp Lippe, retired neurosurgeon and dedicated executive medical director to the American Academy of Pain Medicine (AAPM), has worked closely with me this past year in my presidency of the AAPM. I have learned a great deal from him about the politics of organized medicine and its influence on our field and on our patients.

Finally, Dr. Benjamin Crue, neurosurgeon, pioneer in the field of pain medicine, founder and first president of the American Academy of Algology (now American Academy of Pain Medicine), my colleague and friend, has taught me more about the behavioral workings of the nervous system and treatment of chronic pain syndromes than any other individual.

To all of you, my deepest appreciation.

Gerald M. Aronoff, MD

Contributors

Adewunmi A. Akande, MD
Department of Anesthesiology
New Jersey Medical School
Newark, New Jersey

Charles E. Argoff, MD
Assistant Professor, Department of Neurology
Codirector, Pain Management Center
North Shore University Hospital
New York University School of Medicine
Manhasset, New York

Gerald M. Aronoff, MD
Medical Director, Presbyterian Center for Pain Medicine
Presbyterian Orthopaedic Hospital
Charlotte, North Carolina
Immediate Past President, American Academy of Pain
   Medicine
President, North Carolina Pain Society
Assistant Clinical Professor
Tufts University School of Medicine
Boston, Massachusetts

William K. Baker, EdD
Director, Multidisciplinary Pain Center
HealthSouth Rehabilitation Hospital of Sarasota
Sarasota, Florida

Dhirendra S. Bana, MD, FACP
Director, John R. Graham Headache Center
The Faulkner Hospital
Boston, Massachusetts

William T. Beaver, MD
Professor of Pharmacology and Anesthesia
Georgetown University School of Medicine
Washington, D.C.

Gary J. Bennett, PhD
Professor, Department of Neurology
Allegheny University of Health Sciences
Philadelphia, Pennsylvania

Donald F. Booth, DMD
Professor and Chairman
Department of Oral and Maxillofacial Surgery
Boston University Medical Center
Boston, Massachusetts

Allen W. Burton, MD
Assistant Professor, Department of Anesthesiology
University of Texas Medical Branch at Galveston
Galveston, Texas

Daniel B. Carr, MD
Saltonstall Professor of Pain Research
Department of Anesthesia
New England Medical Center
Professor of Anesthesiology and Medicine
Tufts University School of Medicine
Boston, Massachusetts

Margaret A. Caudill, MD, PhD
Codirector, Arnold Pain Center
Beth Israel Deaconess Medical Center
Boston, Massachusetts
Director, Pain Management
Lahey Hitchcock Clinic
Nashua, New Hampshire

Nathan Cherny, MD
Cancer Pain and Palliative Medicine Services
Medical Oncology
Shaare Zedek Medical Center
Jerusalem, Israel

Liane M. Clamen, BA
Harvard Medical School
Boston, Massachusetts

Nessa Coyle, RN, MS, FAAN
Director, Supportive Care Program, Pain
Palliative Care Service
Department of Neurology
Memorial Sloan-Kettering Cancer Center
New York, New York

R. Brian Cutler, PhD
Assistant Professor, Department of Psychiatry
University of Miami School of Medicine
Miami Beach, Florida

Marshall Devor, PhD
Professor, Department of Cell and Animal Biology
Life Sciences Institute
Hebrew University of Jerusalem
Jerusalem, Israel

David N. Dupuy, MD
Mid-Atlantic Center for Pain Medicine
Presbyterian Orthopaedic Hospital
Charlotte, North Carolina

Neil Ellison, MD
Associate Professor
Department of Oncology and Hematology
Geisinger Medical Center
Danville, Pennsylvania

Serdar Erdine, MD
Chairman, Department of Algology
Istanbul University
Istanbul, Turkey

Charles A. Fager, MD
Department of Neurosurgery
Lahey Hitchcock Medical Center
Burlington, Massachusetts

Jeffrey B. Feldman, PhD
Program Director
Mid-Atlantic Center for Pain Medicine
Presbyterian Orthopaedic Hospital
Charlotte, North Carolina

David A. Fishbain, MD, FAPA
Professor of Psychiatry, Neurological Surgery, and
  Anesthesiology
University of Miami School of Medicine
Comprehensive Pain and Rehabilitation Center
Miami Beach, Florida

Wilbert E. Fordyce, PhD
Professor Emeritus, Rehabilitation Medicine
University of Washington
Seattle, Washington

Bradley S. Galer, MD
Assistant Professor
Departments of Neurology and Anesthesiology
Attending Neurologist, Multidisciplinary Pain Center
Director, Pain Clinical Research Center
University of Washington School of Medicine
Seattle, Washington

Rollin M. Gallagher, MD, MPH
Director of Pain Medicine
MCP/Hahnemann School of Medicine
Director, Comprehensive Pain and Rehabilitation Center
Allegheny University of the Health Sciences
Philadelphia, Pennsylvania

Paul A. Glazer, MD
Clinical Instructor
Department of Orthopaedic Surgery
Harvard University
Beth Israel Deaconess Medical Center
Boston, Massachusetts

F. Michael Gloth III, MD
Chief, Division of Geriatrics
Union Memorial Hospital
Assistant Professor of Medicine
Johns Hopkins University School of Medicine
Clinical Assistant Professor of Medicine
University of Maryland School of Medicine
Medical Director, Carroll Hospice
Baltimore, Maryland

Don L. Goldenberg, MD
Chief of Rheumatology
Newton-Wellesley Hospital
Newton, Massachusetts
Professor of Medicine
Tufts University School of Medicine
Boston, Massachusetts

J. David Haddox, DDS, MD
Southeastern Pain & Rehabilitation Institute
Atlanta, Georgia

Samuel J. Hassenbusch, MD, PhD
Department of Neurosurgery
University of Texas MD Anderson Cancer Center
Houston, Texas

James E. Heaver, DVM, PhD
Professor, Anesthesiology and Physiology
Director, Anesthesia Research
Texas Tech University Health Sciences Center
Lubbock, Texas

Michael J. Hunter, DMD
Assistant Professor
Department of Oral and Maxillofacial Surgery
Boston University Medical Center
Boston, Massachusetts

Jonathan Kleefield, MD
Director of Neuroradiology
Beth Israel-Deaconess Medical Center
Boston, Massachusetts
Associate Professor of Radiology
Harvard Medical School
Cambridge, Massachusetts

Richard M. Kream, PhD
Professor of Anesthesiology, Pharmacology,
and Experimental Therapeutics
Department of Pharmacology
New England Medical Center
Tufts University School of Medicine
Boston, Massachusetts

Ronald J. Kulich, PhD
Clinical Director, Pain Management Program
New England Medical Center
Assistant Professor of Anesthesia
Tufts University School of Medicine
Boston, Massachusetts

Philipp M. Lippe, MD
Executive Medical Director
American Academy of Pain Medicine
Executive Vice President
American Board of Pain Medicine
Glenview, Illinois
Clinical Professor, Neurological Surgery
Stanford University
Stanford, California

John D. Loeser, MD
Professor of Neurological Surgery
  and Anesthesiology Director
Multidisciplinary Pain Center
University of Washington
Seattle, Washington

Edward Lor, PharMD
Assistant Clinical Professor of Pharmacy
San Francisco General Hospital
San Francisco, California

Henry U. Lu, MD
Fellow, Department of Neurology
Pain and Palliative Care Service
Memorial Sloan-Kettering Cancer Center
New York, New York

Angela Mailis, MD, MSc
Director, Pain Investigation Unit
Head of Physical Medicine and Rehabilitation
Departments of Medicine and Surgery
The Toronto Hospital
Associate Professor
Department of Medicine
University of Toronto
Toronto, Ontario

Theresa Hoskins Michel, MS PT, CCS
Assistant Professor of Physical Therapy
Graduate Program in Physical Therapy
MGH Institute of Health Professions
Physical Therapist Clinical Associate
Physical Therapy Services
Massachusetts General Hospital
Boston, Massachusetts

David Niv, MD
Director, Pain Control Unit
Tel-Aviv Sourasky Medical Center
Tel-Aviv, Israel

Akiko Okifuji, PhD
Research Assistant Professor
Department of Anesthesiology
University of Washington
Seattle, Washington

Martin T. Orne, MD, PhD
Professor Emeritus of Psychiatry
University of Pennsylvania School of Medicine
Director, Unit for Experimental Psychiatry
Senior Attending Psychiatrist
The Institute of Pennsylvania Hospital
Philadelphia, Pennsylvania

William N. Pachas, MD
Clinical Assistant Professor
Department of Medicine
Harvard Medical School
Director of Rheumatology
Spaulding Rehabilitation Hospital
Rheumatology Associates
Massachusetts General Hospital
Boston, Massachusetts

Steven D. Passik, PhD
Department of Psychiatry
Memorial Sloan-Kettering Cancer Center
New York, New York
Director
Oncology Symptom Control Research
Community Cancer Care, Inc.
Indiana, Indianapolis

Richard B. Patt, MD
Associate Professor
Departments of Anesthesiology and Neuro-oncology
Director, Anesthesia Pain Services
University of Texas MD Anderson Cancer Center
Houston, Texas

Richard Payne, MD
Professor of Medicine (Neurology)
Chief, Section of Pain and Symptom Management
Department of Neuro-oncology
University of Texas MD Anderson Cancer Center
Houston, Texas

Leslie M. Phillips, PhD
Presbyterian Orthopaedic Hospital
Mid-Atlantic Center for Pain Medicine
Charlotte, North Carolina

Russell K. Portenoy, MD
Chairman, Department of Pain Medicine
  and Palliative Care
Beth Israel Medical Center
New York, New York

Gabor B. Racz, MD, DABPM
Professor and Chairman
Director of Pain Services
Department of Anesthesiology
Texas Tech University Health Sciences Center
Lubbock, Texas

P. Prithvi Raj, MB
Department of Anesthesiology
Texas Tech University Health Sciences Center
Lubbock, Texas

Hubert L. Rosomoff, MD, DMedSc
Professor and Chairman
Department of Neurological Surgery
Medical Director
Comprehensive Pain and Rehabilitation Center
South Shore Hospital and Medical Center
University of Miami
Miami Beach, Florida

Renee Steele Rosomoff, RN, BSN, MBA
Programs Director
Comprehensive Pain and Rehabilitation Center
University of Miami School of Medicine
Nursing Adjunct Associate Professor
Department of Neurological Surgery
Miami Beach, Florida

Karen S. Rucker, MD
Chairman and Herman J. Flax, MD, Professor
Department of Physical Medicine and Rehabilitation
Virginia Commonwealth University
Medical College of Virginia
Richmond, Virginia

Ricardo Ruiz-López, MD
Medical Director
Clínica del Dolor de Barcelona
Barcelona, Spain

Grannum R. Sant, MD
Professor and Acting Chair
Department of Urology
Tufts University School of Medicine
Boston, Massachusetts

Joel R. Saper, MD
Director
Michigan Head Pain and Neurological Institute
Ann Arbor, Michigan

John Stansell, MD
Medical Director, AIDS Program
San Francisco General Hospital
San Francisco, California

Michael D. Stanton-Hicks, MBBS, DrMed
Director, Pain Management Center
The Cleveland Clinic Foundation
Cleveland, Ohio

Andrew W. Sukiennik, MD
Director, Pain Management
Department of Anesthesia
New England Medical Center
Boston, Massachusetts

Ronald R. Tasker, MD
Professor, Division of Neurosurgery
Department of Surgery
University of Toronto
The Toronto Hospital (Western Division)
Toronto, Ontario, Canada

Edwin M. Todd, MD, JD, PhD
Arcadia, California

Dennis C. Turk, PhD
John and Emma Bonica Professor of Anesthesiology
  and Pain Research
Department of Anesthesiology
University of Washington School of Medicine
Seattle, Washington

Ursula Wesselmann, MD
Assistant Professor of Neurology, Neurological Surgery,
  and Biomedical Engineering
Blaustein Pain Treatment Center
Johns Hopkins University School of Medicine
Baltimore, Maryland

Michael D. West, PhD
Research Associate
Department of Physical Medicine and Rehabilitation
Rehabilitation Research and Training Center
  on Supported Employment
Virginia Commonwealth University
Medical College of Virginia
Richmond, Virginia

Wayne G. Whitehouse, PhD
Research Associate, Department
  of Psychology
Temple University
Philadelphia, Pennsylvania

Harriet Wittink, PhD, PT, OCS
Clinical Specialist
Pain Management
New England Medical Center
Boston, Massachusetts

Wen-Hsien Wu, MD
Director, Pain Management Center
Professor of Anesthesiology
New Jersey Medical School
Newark, New Jersey

Laurie Zoloth-Dorfman, PhD
Associate Professor, Social Ethics
  and Jewish Philosophy
College of Humanities
San Francisco State University

Contents

Part VIII: Special Topics

Introduction

John D. Loeser, MD
University of Washington
School of Medicine
Seattle, Washington

Pain management as a specialty of medicine was first proposed by John Bonica about 50 years ago. This was an idea whose time had come. Today, physicians, nurses, and other health care providers specialize in the treatment of pain throughout the world. The Bonica-induced momentum has accelerated in the past 20 years, and now there are pain clinics and pain centers in every developed country. Regional, national, and international professional societies have been established and are educating scientists, clinicians, and the public about pain research and management. Professional journals and hundreds of books address a variety of topics in pain management. There also have been major advances in the sciences basic to the management of pain, none more important than the development of animal models for chronic pain states. New technologies, such as positron emission tomography (PET) and magnetic resonance imaging (MRI), have opened windows into the anatomy and physiology of pain. Psychological and psychosocial studies have opened new vistas into the significance of the complaint of pain. Public awareness of issues in pain management, particularly in the debates about end-of-life health care and the reasonable use of opiates, has heightened concern about effective pain management.

The movement toward outcomes-based medical practice is likely to alter all aspects of health care, including pain management. In addition, the high costs of both the technology and the time of health care providers have come to the attention of those who pay the bills. Managed care is changing the moral and clinical foundations of health care delivery. If pain management specialists and pain clinics are to survive, they will have to demonstrate both their efficacy and their relative value compared with other forms of health care. The discipline of pain management must achieve the status of other medical specialties. This implies the need for rigorous training programs and a practitioner certification process as well as accreditation of treatment programs.

A profound change is occurring in medical practice throughout the developed world. No longer are professorial statements accepted as gospel. Epidemiological studies are beginning to reveal the true incidence and prevalence of painful illnesses, and population-based statistics are becoming available. Health services research has identified the allocation of resources for the treatment of various painful conditions; wide variations between countries, portions of a country, and small areas within one state have been demonstrated (3,12). This is true, of course, for painless afflictions, as well. The natural history of chronic diseases is being studied; in chronic diseases the patient's symptoms are often not stable and the phenomena of regression to the mean and spontaneous remission now have been recognized.

Finally, outcomes research is gaining momentum. Payers want to know if the treatment alters the patient's complaints. They also want to know whether anything besides what the patient says is changed. Does the treatment reduce future health care consumption? Are there measurable functional improvements? Does the patient return to work? These are new questions for physicians to answer, and many of us are not prepared to deal with these challenges (5). We had best learn how, for those who control the pursestrings may not permit us to continue to deliver expensive health care in the absence of evidence that we make a difference, both to the patient's well-being and to health care and compensation costs.

This may be the wave of the future, but it ignores the most ancient and important role of the physician: to provide education, guidance, prognostication, support, and sympathy. These are not driven by technology, and they have a much longer heritage in medicine. Such tasks are very hard to quantify, and they do not show up in anyone's cost-benefit study. Because we are the pain management specialists, we must fight to keep this aspect of what we do from being eclipsed by those who look only at measurable outcomes and costs. This is the conflict that will determine whether or not physicians are going to become technicians exclusively and thereby leave the human side of their endeavors to other types of health care providers.

So much of our professional activities is governed by the concepts that we use to explain the phenomena of pain. The International Association for the Study of Pain (IASP) definition of pain, which is the most serviceable to date, is "an unpleasant sensory and emotional experience associated with actual or potential tissue damage or described in terms of such damage" (8). For more than 400 years, Western thought has been plagued by cartesian dualism: the division of a human being into mind and body. We now know that this is not a valid distinction when one looks at the phenomena of chronic pain. A person's experience, fears, anxieties, and the anticipated consequences are all capable of modulating the response to physical events. Environmental factors can exert strong influences upon the individual. The mind and the body are really inseparable insofar as pain is concerned. Concepts determine how physicians ask about their patients' illnesses and what types of therapies are considered. The continued development of the field of pain management depends upon concepts that work, not the outmoded legacy of the Enlightenment: dualism and reductionism (6).

There certainly is a tissue-damage detection system in the somatic tissues of all animals. Activation of this system is nociception. Studies during the past 20 years have dramatically increased our understanding of this component of pain. We now know that the nociceptors can be biased by both local tissue changes, such as those seen with injury or inflammation, and by neural messages from the central nervous system. Activity in nociceptive axons enters the spinal cord or brainstem in the dorsal horn, where plasticity, not the hard wiring of circuits, seems to be the rule. Line labeling just does not exist within the central nervous system. The dorsal horn is the site of the transformation of nociception into "pain," but this process is influenced both by other segmental afferent activity and by downstream activity from the brain. Nerve injury can also lead to the activation of cells in the dorsal horn or more rostral nuclei so that pain is reported in the absence of the tissue damage that normally leads to nociception. At this level, our understanding of the painful processes becomes murky, for we do not understand the genesis of the affective component of pain, which is best known as suffering. Our understanding of the neural substrates of suffering and its linkage to peripheral events, as well as memory, anticipation, and cognition is limited to the recognition that the limbic system is required. Suffering is caused not only by pain but also by loss of loved objects, anxiety, fear, and isolation; yet the language of pain is used for suffering, regardless of why the patient suffers. The clinician can only infer the existence of nociception, pain, and suffering, for these are personal, private events in the patient. We depend upon the patient's "pain behaviors" for any insight into what he or she is feeling. Pain behaviors are exquisitely linked to the patient's environment, experiences, fears, and anticipated consequences. Human beings do not exist independent of their environments, so the assessment of pain in our patients must include the recognition that environmental factors may play a significant role. Of course, the patient's brain is interposed between the environment and the noxious stimulus. Ultimately, it will be the understanding of how the brain functions that will complete the understanding of painful neurophysiologic processes. With this concept of pain we can see clearly that there are several issues that continue to threaten modern pain management.

The most important debate can be summarized by the question "what is chronic pain?" The argument that it is per-

sistent noxious stimulation certainly applies to some conditions, such as cancer pain and untreated osteomyelitis; this explanation falls down with pains that follow central nervous system injury or those that persist long after the apparent healing of an injury. New knowledge of the abilities of noxious information to effect long-lasting changes in the spinal cord and brain make it possible that chronic pain states reflect permanent changes in the nervous system after an acute, massive noxious input. Finally, experimental data clearly show that some chronic pain patients are manifesting learned responses that are the result of environmental and affective factors. Then there is the possible role of genetic factors in the nervous system response to injury. It is obvious that all of these factors may be operative in an individual patient.

Another contentious issue is the relation between caring for a patient and participating in the administrative processes that determine what benefits that patient may get from the government or an insurance company. When workers compensation systems were being established in the first half of the 20th century, organized medicine was strongly opposed to the physician being the gatekeeper in the compensation process. This has long since been forgotten, and we now have expert witnesses purporting to testify on the basis of medical facts but somehow expressing viewpoints favorable to the litigant who is paying the expert witness fee. We have political decisions about who is eligible for benefits that are tied to medical evaluations. To some degree this reflects the medicalization of our society in the past 50 years, but it also directly derives from the physician's concepts of what pain is and how it may be remedied.

There are real tensions within the group of us who consider ourselves pain management specialists. Everyone would like to believe that his or her way of making a diagnosis or treating a specific ailment is the best or even the only method of helping the patient. Should we intervene at the level of nociception or pain, or should we address pain behaviors by environmental manipulation? There are no properly conducted trials that can tell us which therapy is optimal for even the common painful afflictions. This is critically important when there are wide differences in cost between alternative treatment methods. So each of us does what we best know how to do. Surgeons leave scars, anesthesiologists small round holes; others make the patient physically fit, and still others stretch the mind (or shrink it). Duration of treatment, costs, and complications vary widely. Rarely does the patient get to make the decisions about what type of care to receive for his or her painful condition. There are few if any standard or tested algorithms for the diagnosis or treatment of any painful conditions. Standards or guidelines for health care delivery are always both scientific and political, for we lack the absolute knowledge about natural history of diseases or treatment outcomes; the gaps are filled in nonscientific fashions (7). As long as we remain in the dark about the natural history of the conditions we treat or the effects of our treatments upon the patient's illness, we remain in great peril of being left out of the health care delivery of the future, for those who control the health care funding will demand proof of efficacy.

Health care is not and never has been driven by science. It is instead an integral part of the culture of any society, and that culture determines the roles physicians play and the types of treatments that are considered health care. Nowhere is this more apparent than in the history of industrial accidents and their compensation (1, 4). It is social convention, not medical science, that has made repetitive strain injury and low-back pain compensable conditions. A social problem has been medicalized, or as others would argue, a medical problem has been turned into a social welfare system. Furthermore, in the United States we are fascinated by technology and by things from the mysterious Orient. As people lose faith or funding in traditional medicine, they have turned even more to nonscientific remedies outside the pale of rational behavior.

Patients come seeking a "laser treatment" in hopes that they have some disease that is amenable to treatment by the magical light. The "gamma knife" sounds much more effective than "physical and psychological rehabilitation"; how does one make a rational decision when both are offered in the treatment of chronic low back pain? Performing surgery and using injections have an aura of magical power; they must be more effective than something the patient can do for himself or herself. The technology we have legitimizes the doctor-patient interaction, but that does not mean that the benefit the patient describes is a specific effect of the treatment. Nonspecific effects are likely to be very potent in health care, and we do not begin to know how to assess them or use them to our patients' benefit (11). This must be the reason taking potions, sitting under a pyramid, or applying snake oil have been around for so long and have so many proponents. In fact, nonspecific effects are much more potent than physicians would like to believe. A placebo responder may or may not have significant disease and may or may not have a useful response to a specific therapy.

Further research on what we do not know about diseases and injuries will be useful; but what we really need now are studies that look directly at treatment outcomes for common painful conditions. For example, the Quebec study (10) addressed the treatments for low-back pain, and the researchers came to the conclusion that almost nothing that was done by any type of health care provider for people with low-back pain had any demonstrated efficacy. Similar findings were generated by the AHCPR Report in the United States(2) and by the United Kingdom report (9). Low-back pain is very common; more than 80% of the U.S. population will have it at some time. Vast sums of money are spent on health care for low back pain; yet we have a larger fraction of our population claiming disability due to low-back pain than most countries. There are good reasons to suggest that the administrative polices and practices of most compensation systems prolong disability and lead to excessive claims submission. Does all of this health care add to or reduce disability?

This poses some interesting policy issues. For example, if we are dealing with a common condition, such as low-back pain, should we continue to allow unproven treatments to be offered outside of a clinical trial format designed to collect information on outcomes? Millions of epidural steroid injections and facet joint blocks continue to be performed each year in the absence of data on efficacy. For how long should this be tolerated? Yes, conducting clinical research trials is time consuming and expensive. That is why the U.S. Congress mandated that such studies should be done and established the Agency for Health Care Policy and Research. Alas, politics has virtually killed that organization, for it was unwise enough to fund research on low-back pain treatments that recommended that the excess of surgery for low-back pain in our country be controlled; some orthopaedic surgeons promptly lobbied Congress to abolish the agency. Funding for similar research was drastically reduced by Congress. Health care is political as well as medical. Yet, if we were to abolish all unproven treatments, patients would not be able to find physicians to help them through the natural history of their disease or offer advice, guidance, and solace. Unproven treatments may be beneficial, for the absence of proof is not the same as proof of absence. Since physicians have two distinct roles, that of technician and that of teacher, consoler, and prognosticator, we should not allow the absence of proven efficacy to eliminate the role of physician.

Health care in the Western world is entering a new phase. Disease processes are being studied to determine the natural history of chronic illnesses. Health services research is identifying varieties, costs and outcomes of treatments. It will no longer suffice to treat symptoms without data as to the efficacy of one treatment compared with that of others. The high cost of our technological solutions to symptom and disease diagnosis and treatment has carried medicine out of a private cottage industry into a public, politically sensitive megabusiness. Those who provide pain management services will have to learn about the illness they treat, to determine treatment outcomes, and to assemble data on their treatments in a meaningful and scientifically valid way. This is a costly process, and no one has come forward to provide the necessary funds. The burden falls squarely upon our shoulders. If we do not arm ourselves with facts and participate in the political process, we are at peril of being eliminated from the health care delivery system. It is to be hoped that the debate will center not only on cost-benefit ratios but also on moral benefit concepts that remain largely unarticulated in the market place of medicine. "After all, it is only pain" remains a common theme. We must get the public to understand the need for and agree to pay for our services. Children and the aged are most at risk to suffer unnecessary pain if we do not establish the legitimacy of pain management. This will be an interesting challenge. The permanence of the pain movement is not at all assured at this time. Forceful spokespersons, such as John Bonica, are few; we also need to establish a mechanism to support those who are willing to devote their resources to public education and political change. Only by building a corpus of knowledge and a professional group with a shared knowledge base and treatment goals can we move forward and exert increasing influence upon decision making in health care. Dr. Aronoff has selected authors for this book who will address the current issues in pain management. This volume is certain to be one of the stepping-stones in the journey to reduce pain and suffering in our patients and to perpetuate pain medicine as an important medical specialty.

References

1. Allen DB, Waddell G. An historical perspective on low back pain and disability. Acta Orthop Scand 1989;60(Suppl 234):1–23.
2. Bigos A, Bauger O, Braen G, et al. Acute low back problems in adults. Clinical practice guideline 14. AHCPR Publication 95–0642. Rockville, MD: Agency for Health Care Policy and Research, 1994.
3. Cherkin DC, Deyo R A, Loeser J D, et al. An international comparison of back surgery rates. Spine 1994;19:1201–1206.
4. Denbe AE. Occupation and disease. New Haven: Yale University Press, 1996.
5. Deyo RA. Practice variations, treatment fads and rising disability. Spine 1993,12:2153–2162.
6. Loeser JD. Unlocking the secrets of pain. The treatment: a new era. In: 1988 Medical and Health Annual, Encyclopedia Britannica, Chicago. 1987;120–131.
7. Loeser JD. Mitigating the dangers of pursuing cure. In: Campbell JN, Cohen MJ, eds. Pain treatment at a crossroads: a practical and conceptual reappraisal. Progress in pain research and management, vol. 7. Seattle: IASP Press, 1996;101–108.
8. Merskey H, ed. Classification of chronic pain: description of chronic pain syndromes and definition of pain terms. Pain 1986;Suppl 3:S1.
9. Rosen M, ed. Back pain: report of a CSAG committee on back pain. London: HMSO, 1994.
10. Spitzer WO, LeBlanc F E, Dupuis M, et al. Scientific approach to the assessment and management of activity-related spinal disorders: a monograph for physicians. Report of the Quebec Task Force on Spinal Disorders. Spine 1987;12(Suppl):S1–S59.
11. Turner JA, Deyo R A, Loeser J D, et al. Placebo effects: their importance in chronic pain treatment and research. JAMA. 1994;271:1609–1614.
12. Volinn E, Mayer J, Diehr P, et al. Small area analysis of surgery for low-back pain. Spine 1992;17:575–581.

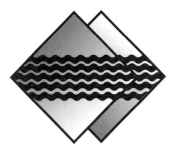

PART I

Basic Principles

CHAPTER 1

Pain: Historical Pespectives[1.1]

Edwin M. Todd

Pain is timeless, ineluctable, and disconcertingly indefinable. The anguished cry of the newborn infant is a reverberating echo of our primordial roots in pain. In the listener, it strikes the deepest reaches of the sensibilities, where it is perceived as a paradox of curse and blessing imposed ineradicably upon the human trinity of birth, existence, and death. Humans are put in awe by the wonder of creation, and the awe is conditioned in the first instance by the shattering impact of this release from the womb. It is the pervading essence that marks and mocks his journey from cradle to grave, discoloring his thinking and evoking groping heuristic efforts to express its influence on evolving and passing civilizations.

When man began to think, preeminent among the perplexities and problems that weighed upon him was the irksome nature of pain, and this concern has traveled with him through time. He must have sensed that it was his protector, but even as it happened, he could hardly have recognized it as the central core of his feelings of compassion, sympathy, and forgiveness that served to bond his fellowship with other creatures in the humblest origins of social intercourse. Without it, life could have been nothing for human beings but a flat complacency, and the species would not have survived. But man did survive, and he must have puzzled over the nature of this noxious benefactor even as we speculate on its historical associations, courteously respectful in the awareness of our own interpretive inadequacies.

Somewhere within us, say the pundits, there is a sensorium commune, an undetermined site wherein the nature of pain is revealed. More elusive than the Holy Grail for which medieval man sought widely and in vain, the quest for the sensorium commune has preoccupied and frustrated thinking man since time immemorial. To find it, and define it, may resolve the problem of dealing with it; but, so far, biopsychosocial research has only given new insights into the complexity of the quest. Its epistemological orientations are only vaguely perceived in

anthropological suggestions, and its ontological essences are shrouded in confused psychological inferences.

In all ages, pain has been a very real and immediate concern; but, always, humans' attitudes and beliefs have been shaped by magical, demonological, theological, philosophical, and practical influences in varying degrees and with shifting emphases. It is our purpose to capture and examine some of these changing patterns of thought in our spotty passage through time.

PRIMITIVE SOCIETY

Man took a giant step forward seven thousand years ago, when he emerged from obscurity with the discovery of a written means of recording his activities. Beyond this curtain lay many thousands of years of intelligent existence about which we can only speculate; but, there is evidence in his fossil remains, in his surviving tools, in his paintings and carvings, and in the study of his primitive counterparts throughout the modern world from which we can form reasonable hypothetical constructs of his behavior and beliefs.

It is reasonable to suppose that early humans found rational means of dealing with minor ills and obvious wounds, just as we see modern primitives, untouched by civilization, utilizing heat and cold, mud packs and poultices, intoxicants and analgesics, simple foreign body extraction techniques, and bone-setting procedures. Trephinations and ceremonial mutilations such as circumcisions, castrations, and piercing operations bear witness to very old surgical skills (1). In contrast, internal pain most certainly had supernatural connotations. Causation was steeped in superstition, as life itself was a

[1.1]Reprinted with permission from Todd EM. Pain: Hostorical Perspectives. In: Crue BL Jr, ed. Chronic pain: further observations from City of Hope National Medical Center. Jamaica, NY: Spectrum Publications, 1978:39–56.

strange and magical process, and management necessarily entailed supernatural means. The source of the pain was external, something magical and insidious acting upon the body by "intrusion" of objects and spirits or by life-sapping "withdrawal" of vital substance. Active pain states were instances of intrusion, such as the "ghost shot" of medicine men in New Guinea tribal relics of the Stone Age, whereas wasting and death were extraction processes manipulated by sinister outside forces. The concept of intrusion reaches through time, and it is preserved in Welsh superstition as the "shot of the elf" and in the German *Hexenschuss* or "witches' shot" for lumbago (2). This remote, external cause of pain in primitive human thought found its site in mysterious hovering spirits seeking a body to inhabit. Treatment was directed toward extracorporeal flights of fancy, and physiology had not yet awakened in the Stone Age mentality (3).

ANCIENT KINGDOMS

As man became more civilized, he settled in fertile valleys at the mouths of great waterways and founded thriving communities where his sophistication increased. Under the growing stimulus of accumulating knowledge and technology, medicine flourished in early settlements along the Nile, the Indus, the Yangtze and Hwang Ho, and in the fertile crescent between the Euphrates and the Tigris.

Egypt

Owing to a combination of fortuitous circumstances, including a dry climate, an ideal reed growing abundantly in the deltas, and a talent for concocting stable dyes and inks, some notion of the lost art of ancient Egyptian medicine has come down to us through the Ebers, Berlin, and Edwin Smith papyri (4). It is only a fragmented glimpse, but it is quite revealing in many respects where it establishes precedents and preserves precious little cameos of medical practice. A surprisingly rational empiricism is exhibited in the therapeutic decisions of the Edwin Smith papyrus, copied by scribes in the sixteenth century A.D. from earlier medical writings ascribed to the era of Imhotep of the Third Dynasty. It was Imhotep, builder of pyramids, architect, astronomer, and blameless physician, whose apotheosis later served as the prototype for the Greek deification of Asclepios (5).

Unfortunately, the high level of clinical competence of the Smith papyrus and the amazing spectrum of pharmaceutical knowledge of the Ebers manuscript were not sustained in later periods as Egyptian medicine declined under the growing influences of religious mysticism and demonology.

A priceless legacy of Egyptian civilization is the fact that there were no proscriptions against human dissection. Consequently, we have a wealth of surviving material for study in mummies and in descriptive accounts of anatomical dissection. Regrettably, the art reached its highest expression in the masterful works of morticians rather than physicians, and the former were a secretive lot who never broadcasted their mar-

velous techniques but left only their products for our edification. Nevertheless, there are numerous references in the papyri from which we may draw reasonable assumptions. It is clear that their anatomical knowledge was poorly organized and their physiology crude and inconsistent. Their concepts of pain were muddied by magicoreligious influences differing little from primitive beliefs except in imaginative complexity. Anthropomorphic spirits of the dead with sinister intent to cause pain were dispatched by the gods and other forces of darkness into their orifices or through their pores to wreck havoc within them. The left nostril was a favorite portal of entry for sinister purposes. Yet for all the mystical aberrations there was a groping effort to provide rational explanations in anatomical and physiological terms. The brain was totally ignored as a vital organ, although paresis of the opposite side of the body due to head injury is described in the Smith papyrus (4). It was the one organ destroyed or discarded in the embalming process, which more or less signifies the esteem it engendered. The Egyptians elevated the heart to a status of preeminence over all organs, and with its vessels reaching out into all areas it became the seat of all motor and sensory activity. There was no knowledge of a nervous system. Instead they believed that the heart and its vessels served all these functions. This included the appreciation of pain from obvious causes such as gross injury, although the anatomical references are often intermingled with confusing mystical associations (6). With the passage of centuries the rational practices and astute clinical observations of the early Egyptians were replaced by sorcery and incantation, offering nothing of value to medicine or our review of pain concepts; but the influences of the early physicians were to have profound and enduring effects on subsequent civilizations (3).

India

Unlike other ancient civilizations that rose to enjoy a lusty moment in history and then faded back into obscurity, those that crystallized along the murky waters of the Indus and the lazy river valleys of China endured and projected their ancient medical practices almost intact into the living present. In both countries, drugs to relieve pain and anesthetic techniques were old when civilization was new.

The oldest of the sacred books of India, the *Rig-Veda,* allegedly written as far back as 4000 years B.C., describes hundreds of remedies deriving from mineral, plant, and animal sources, including anesthetics and analgesics still in use. Practical healing and vigorous therapeutic measures ranging through a versatile surgical repertory culminated in Susruta, the great physician and surgeon, who lived about 500 A.D. It was a time when disease had a locus in anatomy, and physiological explanations aided in the diagnosis of disturbed function. A crude nervous system centered on the heart, from which ducts radiated to all sensory organs and all excitable parts. Susruta's writings reflect some awareness of pain pathways connected with this misconceived center (7). The advent of Buddhism in the fifth century A.D. cast a pall over scientific discovery and directed medical thinking into spiritual channels, where the sensorium commune became illusory. Physiological phenomena were unreal, and pain was denied existence. The slow, steady crawl of scientific progress in anatomical matters was abruptly arrested by religious dogma just as it seemed poised on the threshold of new adventure, and the creative energies of Indian medicine were diverted to other interests (8).

Mesopotamia

No place on earth holds deeper significance for the history of human progress than the fertile crescent of land lying between the Euphrates and the Tigris rivers, aptly designated as the Cradle of Civilization. It was here that a practical system of writing was first invented to initiate a cultural and intellectual metamorphosis in human relationships. A stable and well-organized society is portrayed in the Code of Hammurabi, but medical practice failed to achieve the high standard of the legal system. Rational practitioners competed at a disadvantage with exorcist-priests who dealt in omens, divination, astrology, and magic arts. It was eminently safer to diagnose and treat in accordance with revelations conjured out of livers and other entrails of sacrificed animals than to rely on surgical skills, for it was expressly stated in the Code: "If a surgeon has opened an eye infection with a bronze instrument and so saved the man's eye, he shall take 10 shekels. If a surgeon has opened an eye infection with a bronze instrument and thereby destroyed the man's eye, they shall cut off his hand." Scientific medicine at best was a descriptive art, singularly unencumbered by physiological considerations that might conflict with dominant magic-religious dictates, designating the heart as the seat of intelligence, the liver of emotion, the uterus of compassion, and the stomach, curiously, of cunning (9). Little stimulus was afforded for rational investigation of painful afflictions where disease was regarded as a punishment for sin and the gods demanded homage in the form of sacrifice and prayer for these transgressions (8). The pregnant promises of early ingenuity in writing, art, architecture, law, and astronomy never quite extended into the medical arts, which remained unexceptional and uninspiring to future scientific interests.

China

From very early times the inscrutable Chinese viewed the human predicament as a microcosm of the harmonious universe. Harmony prevailed in life when the polarity of Yang and Yin was in proper balance. *Nei Ching,* the Chinese canon of medicine, reflects the very ancient concern with maintaining a state of equilibrium between opposing forces. There is no clear distinction between mythology and historical reality in these writings, and mystical numerology, remindful of Pythagorean precepts, strongly influences an oversystematized medical taxonomy (10). Yang represents maleness, light, heat, aggressiveness, and strength, while Yin exemplifies femaleness, darkness, cold, passivity, and weakness. There are five elements in nature (earth, water, fire, wood, and metal), five organs in the body (heart, lungs, liver, spleen, and kidneys), five winds that inhabit the arteries, and natural laws regulating the universe also participate in the functioning of human physiology as reflected in the forces of Yang and Yin. The brain is simply the marrow of the skull, playing no part in vital activities. The heart is the majordomo of organs as the storehouse of the blood and airs, which contain the vital energy and intelligence that circulates to all areas, announcing the state of health of the body in a variety of pulses. Clinical practice depends on an astute appreciation of subtle messages conveyed in these pulsations. There are 365 parts of the body, and each has a precise focal representation so important to the therapeutic arts of acupuncture and moxibustion (2). The arcane bases of these distinguished oriental practices remain largely incomprehensible to the occidental mind, but each has enjoyed fitful vogues in Western medicine over the centuries.

Pain has no particular center; but, disturbance in Yang or Yin, especially excesses of heat or cold, usually relate to the heart and vessels. Emotional overindulgence upsets Yang or Yin and begets pain in the particular organ allotted the psychological function involved. Rage upsets Yin in the liver, and violent joy is hurtful to Yang in the heart; excessive grief disturbs the lung, and evil thoughts provoke the spleen. Obviously, moderation in all things was as important to Yang and Yin as it was to healthy coexistence of mind and body in Hellenic Greece (6). The anatomy of pain had multifocal, situational orientation for ancient China, evoking therapeutic responses that still prevail but remain uniquely oriental.

HELLENIC GREECE

The miracle of the Greek achievement is exemplified, rather than explained, by the enduring enchantment it continues to exert over the imaginations of men. Greek ideas in medicine, as in art, architecture, astronomy, literature, and philosophy, still excite and exalt us. Pain-relieving drugs and healing arts are woven into the fabric of Homeric legend and Greek mythology, from which their medicine originated. Mythology and legend provided a strong base for early medical practice in other ancient societies as well, but Greek emphasis on individual achievement allowed the creative thinkers to emerge from anonymity, and the line between mythology and history is more distinct with biographical knowledge of their great figures (6).

We know little about the birth of Greek science in the sixth century A.D. in Ionia, but we all share the wealth of the intellectual revolution that was fostered when the veils of myth and religious dogma were swept aside to reveal a wondrous world operating in an orderly manner in accordance with rational, ascertainable natural laws. The legacy of Thales (624–545 B.C.) and his philosophical colleagues was a new open-minded worldview that filtered down from philosophy to science and ignited an intellectual explosion that ricocheted through time and space into every aspect of human inquiry. The first great medical figure to surface was Alcmaeon (circa 500 A.D.) of

Croton. Alcmaeon was a student and disciple of Pythagoras (566–497 B.C.), the mystic numerologist and patron saint of theoretical science. Pythagoras had already established a brotherhood and center for the arts and sciences in this ancient Greek colony at the southern tip of the Italian peninsula when Alcmaeon added his medical school. Relying upon the findings of animal dissection, Alcmaeon elaborated a theory of sensory appreciation that comprehended the brain as the center for sensation. He postulated a mechanism of consciousness dependent on variations in cerebral circulation for sleep and wakefulness. His nervous system consisted of a network of ducts and vessels carrying sensation in the form of particles of elements that invaded the body through various sensory organs to the sensorium in the brain (8). The views of Alcmaeon, the lonely empiricist, fell on the deaf ears of a rationalist society that eschewed vulgar dissection for more noble mental gymnastics in physiological matters.

Democritus (460–362 B.C.), who taught that all matter was composed of ever-changing atoms of the elements of fire, air, earth, and water, applied his atomic theory to sensation and pain. Sensation was a state of awareness in the soul atoms, occasioned when elementary particles invaded the bodies' pores and ducts. The size, shape, and movement of particles determined the nature of the perception. Thus, pain was an intrusion of sharp hooked particles in a state of agitated motion disturbing the normal calm of the soul atoms. Democritus scattered his body and soul atoms over a universe in which life and death did not exist, where everything was always changing and only the total quantity of matter remained constant; but he did make reluctant concessions to materialism by placing the center of consciousness and reason in the brain, emotions in the heart, and lust in the liver (2).

The Hippocratic Corpus reflects the medical spirit and methods of the venerated physician Hippocrates (circa 460–360 B.C.) of Cos. Hippocratic medicine was practical and rational, stressing an expectant attitude while trusting in the marvelous healing power of nature (9). Anatomy was rudimentary, and physiology was based on a proper balance of the four elements, the four qualities (hot, cold, moist, and dry), and the four humors present in every body. Pain was a manifestation of conditions disturbing the natural state of equilibrium in a healthy body. The brain was regarded as a gland of sorts, excreting mucous matter that played a part in regulating body heat. With his disciples, Hippocrates paid considerable attention to the problems of pain, ever seeking effective measures for easing human suffering at the clinical level. They experimented with drugs, including opium, mandrake, and hemlock, actively employed cooling techniques and physiotherapy, and, to ease the pain of surgery, sometimes produced unconsciousness by compressing the carotid arteries, the name carotid deriving from karoun, the Greek word for deep sleep. Always stressing moderation, Hippocrates cautioned his students and colleagues to observe carefully, proceed slowly, and exercise restraint in treatment, a philosophy admirably expounded in his aphorism, "First, do no harm" (6, 11, 12).

That the Greeks were independent and original thinkers we can have no doubt. The magnitude of their minds stunned subsequent generations of men to the extent that the gross errors of the Greeks became indistinguishable from their magnificent triumphs, sharing the same slavish acceptance as irrefutable law. The astonishing physiological inaccuracies of Plato and Aristotle stem from a common ignorance of human anatomy. We can only admire the fanciful flights of their richly speculative minds where they strayed; and, if we must condemn, place the blame where it belongs, that is, in gullible, locked-in lesser minds that bought the packages sight unseen.

The speculative physiology of Plato (427–347 B.C.), lacking the necessary substratum of anatomy, as with all Greeks since Alcmaeon, frequently becomes unintelligible to the modern reader. In Timaeus, Plato aspires to present a comprehensive account of the nature of man. The fundamental blending of mortal body with immortal soul entails a rather complicated commotion of atoms and elements in relation to a percipient soul scattered among a multiplicity of organs (6). Pain is perceived by the soul in its various sites from the intrusion of the four elements, streaming into the body from without, in disharmonious and violent motions. The heart became the receiving and distribution center for sensory input. In deference to Alcmaeon, perhaps, the brain was allotted memory and reasoning. The liver harbored lust and other lower level appetites. Sensations, entering the body as atoms in motion, were conveyed to the heart and somehow distributed in accordance with protocol to the souls residing in the various organs. So to the brain went those sensations affecting mental processes, to the liver those likely to stir baser instincts, and retained in the heart were those related to love, pleasure, and nobler emotions. The size and shape of particles and violence of the intruding motion graded the level of awareness by which they were perceived in the respective souls as pleasure or pain (2).

Aristotle (384–322 B.C.), son of a physician, was surprisingly uninterested in medicine, but in biological matters he was superbly knowledgeable. The astonishing wealth of detail in his writings never restricts the broadness and complexity of his outlook. There is no reference to human dissection in his works, which deal exclusively with animal comparative anatomy. A teleological point of view permeates his thinking on structure and function. De Partibus Animalius, his major physiological treatise, reiterates the premise that everything has a design or purpose, as "nature never makes anything that is superfluous." It is sometimes difficult to reconcile the exquisitely detailed differentiations of form and function in his comparative anatomy with his completely erroneous ideas concerning the brain and heart. For Aristotle the heart was the seat of intelligence, emotion, and sensation, and the brain was relegated to the specious role of thermostatic sponge for cooling the heart to prevent overheating. Vital heat in the heart's blood controlled sensitivity to pain. Flesh was the end organ from which pain sensation was conveyed by blood vessels to the heart, where it was perceived and dealt with in accordance with the heart's enormous proclivities for regulating receipt and response. The irony of mistaken identification is compounded by the fact that it was Aristotle who coined the term *sensorium commune,* and the powerful effects of his prodigious output in all fields of knowledge gave his works a force of dogma that misdirected physiological research for 2000 years (2, 6, 8).

With the death of Alexander in 323 B.C. and of his tutor Aristotle the following year, the glorious era of Hellenic Greece quietly faded from the center stage of history. The spotlight casually shifted across the Mediterranean Sea to a new and vigorously creative scientific community rising like a phoenix from the germinal ashes of a reawakening ancient culture.

ALEXANDRIAN INTERLUDE

For a brief moment in history the restraints imposed by dogma and tabu on scientific investigation were lifted to allow an unprecedented breath of fresh air for intellectual debate and expansion. This exciting interlude occurred in Alexandria, fertile cultural center and thriving crossroad for international commerce and learning. Under the enlightened suzerainty of General Ptolemy, following the fragmentation of the Greek empire, a free spirit of inquiry acted as a magnet to attract bright young minds to long-dormant problems in anatomy and physiology. Greek disdain for work with the hands was temporarily abandoned, as mind and technical skills were united for intensive study of the human body in health and disease. Inchoate dabbling at human dissection in pre-Confucian China and pre-Buddhist India had never really progressed to a level of fruitful revelation. Meaningful study of pain and discovery of a functioning nervous system were now possible under conducive circumstances.

Irresistibly drawn to Alexandria by the inviting intellectual climate, Herophilus (315–280 B.C.) of Chalcedon was the first great talent to address these problems. His extensive anatomical dissections on human cadavers identified the brain as the seat of motor and sensory function. He clearly distinguished between nerves and arteries and traced the course of nerves to and from the brain and spinal cord. Moreover, he recognized the function of these nerves in motor and sensory activities. From his laboratory findings he was led to speculate on the site of the soul and placed it in the fourth ventricle (12–14). These original observations were first challenged, then brilliantly expanded a generation later by Erasistratus (310–250 B.C.) of Cheos. Erasistratus went into great detail describing and differentiating between the cerebrum and cerebellum with their deep-lying system of ventricles and connecting foramina. Curiously, he chose to differ with Herophilus on the proper dwelling for the soul, ensconcing it somewhere in the cerebellum. He commented on the rich convolutional development of the human brain and hypothesized an association with intellectual capacity. He noted the constant tripartite company of artery, vein, and nerve along pathways subserving organs and other discrete anatomical parts. The heart was identified as a central pump propelling blood and air to all parts of the body and discredited as a sensory

organ. All the original texts of these great contributions have disappeared in the quagmire of wasteful wars, fires, and cultural dissolutions, but medical historians have pieced together enough fragmentary accounts from Galen and other diverse sources to amply justify our recognition of Herophilus as the father of human anatomy and of Erasistratus as the founder of experimental physiology (2, 8, 14). Celsus, the elegant translator and encyclopedic compiler of first century A.D. Rome, for reasons not disclosed, chose to ignore their work on the nervous system. However, in *De Re Medicina,* he establishes their lofty status in other areas and specifically recounts their important practical interests in pain. "Moreover, as pain and also various kinds of disease arise in the internal parts, they hold that no one can apply remedies for these who are ignorant of the parts themselves: hence it becomes necessary to lay open bodies of the dead to scrutinize their viscera and intestines, for when pain occurs internally, it is not possible for one to learn what hurts the patient unless he has acquainted himself with the position of each organ or intestine; nor can a diseased portion of the body be treated by one who does not know what that part is" (2, 8).

Centuries would pass before the fickle vehicle of human progress could renegotiate the brightly lighted pathways consummately laid out for us by our distant Alexandrian colleagues.

ROME

During the years that Rome evolved from a scattered assortment of tribal colonies to an orderly society, these sober, practical people remained remarkably unimpressed by the development of medical science in other parts of the world. Pain was something to be borne with magnanimity and stoic indifference, as is usually characteristic of the warrior mentality. For hundreds of years, ancient herbal lore and prayers or incantations to a variety of household gods served their unpretentious medical requirements. As waves of Roman legions spread out over the known world, the culture and finer representations of the conquered were preserved and absorbed. Greek medical arts were part of the bounty, and while the Romans never exhibited an enthusiasm to participate, they often did encourage and actively patronize some of the more gifted Greek practitioners. In a long poem, *De Rerum Natura,* Lucretius (97–54 B.C.), an Epicurean disciple, brought a wide spectrum of Greek science to the attention of literate Romans. His pain physiology, based on the atomic theories of Democritus, stimulated considerable interest, but the Romans were doers, with an innate distrust for fanciful theorizing (14). They were content with compilation and commentary, as was so admirably demonstrated by the works of Celsus (first century A.D.) and Pliny the elder (23–79 A.D.). It remained for Galen (130–200 A.D.), a Greek physician from Pergamon, to rescue the great achievements of the Alexandrians and to restore the theory of a central nervous system to explain the physiology of sensation. Animal dissection supplemented by practical observations in his role as surgeon to the gladiators led Galen to much personal theorizing about physiological mechanisms. It is not possible to fractionate his own opinions from the knowledge he acquired of Herophilus and Erasistratus, but his systematized organization of data had a compelling ring of authority that appealed to the church fathers, who later attached the stamp of dogma to his work. Galen's experiments on the spinal cord and peripheral nerves were richly rewarding in providing new information about motor and sensory enervation. He concluded that pain was the lowest form of conscious sensation, caused by either dissolution of continuity in tissues (e.g., cuts, burns, and overdistention of hollow viscera) or by sudden violent commotion in the humors (e.g., pressure and tension). Unfortunately, Galen's physiology was contaminated by Aristotelian teleological influences. Instead of attempting to ascertain how the organs and systems functioned, he sought to determine why, and this led his reasoning off on bizarre tangents at times. His doctrine of vitalism, his transmission of blood from right to left heart through invisible pores, and his concept of suppuration as an essential part of healing sent medical theory off on senseless wild goose chases for centuries, yet his fruitful experimental physiology, his excellent anatomical descriptions, and his encyclopedic records of the knowledge of his time far outweigh his errors. Roman medicine died with Galen (11, 14, 15).

DARK AGES

The Dark Ages between the fall of Rome and the Renaissance were truly dark, sterile, and regressive years for medicine. Crushed and devastated beneath succeeding ravages of war, famine, plagues, and economic chaos, the human spirit sank to unaccustomed depths of despair, mirroring the desolation of the European civilization (16). Christianity was the rallying force that restored some promise of salvation, but its triumph was a defeat for science. Physiological experimentation was dead under the oppressive weight of Church dogma that brooked no threat of challenge or contradiction. Pain was to be perceived in the light of Christian doctrine as a means of purification and redemption, for had not the sufferings of Christ endowed it with a touch of divinity? Mystical attitudes toward pain promoted martyrdom and gave voluntary suffering an exalted aura of spiritual beauty. Nature could never be questioned for her secrets. Medieval thinkers were restricted under the ban of authority to seek truth through logical deduction. The library replaced the laboratory as the source of discovery. It was a tedious period of scientific and intellectual decadence when Western medicine and pain concepts deteriorated to primitive levels (17–20).

ISLAMIC BRIDGE OF CULTURE

As the imperial majesty of Rome crumbled and Western European civilization sank into the obscurity of the Dark Ages, a fresh spring of intellectual inspiration was flooding the arid lands of distant Persia. To Jundishapur and other Persian centers fled refugee scholars attracted by an unprejudiced climate for learning and generous patronage of the ruling class. Hindu, Chinese, and native Persian influences blended with surviving vestiges of ancient Near Eastern cultures gathered by Jewish and Syrian scholars. This selective corpus of knowledge was richly expanded by Greek and Roman remnants brought by the Nestorians after their expulsion from Edessa in 489. In 529, the year of the founding of Monte Cassino, the Greek Academy was closed by Justinian because of its perverse pagan teachings. Many of its teachers escaped to Persia with priceless treasures of Greek learning that otherwise most certainly would have been destroyed. Far from the chaos and desolation of decadent Europe, a desert oasis had collected a colony of learned exiles who, with meager baggage but retentive minds, had preserved the major sources of our visions of the ancient worlds. Most of what we know about the anatomy and physiology of pain we owe to the miraculous coincidences of time and place that made such a magnificent reservoir possible. The wonder is awesomely compounded by the subsequent course of events.

Following the death of Muhammed, Arab prophet and founder of Islam, in 632, Muslim hordes poured out of the Saudi Arabian desert, conquering all before them and proclaiming that "there is no god but God, and Muhammed is the messenger of God." These fanatical warriors carried their message triumphantly into Persia and India, and in one of the great paradoxes of all history, exhibited a tender and merciful regard for preserving the culture and properties of the conquered in deference to the veneration for knowledge and learning preached by their prophet. The true greatness of Muhammed is best exemplified in the Islamic doctrine, "Science lights the path to paradise. Take ye knowledge even from the lips of the infidel. The ink of the scholar is more holy than the blood of the martyr." For this we are profoundly grateful—it was the guiding precept in the preservation of antiquity. Islamic centers of learning gathered scholars of all faiths and ethnic backgrounds. The school of medicine founded by the Nestorians in Jundishapur was the first of many spread out over the Arab world, and science flourished. Ancient Greek and Latin texts were translated by Jewish and Syrian philologists into Syriac and Hebrew and later into Arabic. Persian centers dominated in the early years of Islam with new developments in chemistry and pharmacology and with the emergence of great medical writers. Al Rhazi (860–932) wrote extensively, elaborating on ancient ideas and contributing new ones. The most influential physician was another Persian, Avicenna or Ibn Sina (980–1063). His medical textbook, the *Canon,* exercised a persuasive influence over medical practice for centuries. Avicenna's notions of pain were drawn from his encyclopedic knowledge of Hippocrates, Aristotle, Galen, and Nemesius, a fourth-century Syrian. He recognized 15 varieties of pain produced by humoral changes that disturbed the natural state of things in the body. Not satisfied with the vague cerebral sensory centers of Galen, he followed the lead of Herophilus, who advocated a fourth ventricle localization, but distributed the sites more generously through the ventricles, as suggested by Nemesius. From extensive Arab pharmaceutical lore he extracted three groups of medicinals for relief of pain: those contrary to the cause, those that exert a soothing effect, and those that have anesthetic properties. Opium, henbane, and mandrake were liberally prescribed. By the eleventh century the scientific and medical leadership had shifted westward to the Moorish capitals on the Iberian peninsula, largely dominated by Jewish scholars who reached great heights in medicine and philosophy under Islam. Jewish medicine, and pain treatment in particular, was basically rational, practical, and highly effective. Their creative energies exhausted, the decline of Islam coincided with a corresponding reawakening of long-slumbering cultural interests in Western Europe (2, 8, 21, 22).

The priceless treasures of ancient learning, incubated in Persia and assiduously nurtured with loving care by their serendipitous conservators, had been borne across the Islamic bridge of culture to a revitalized Europe, anxious to reclaim its lost heritage.

RENAISSANCE

In a growing spirit of confidence the minds of Renaissance men were awakened with a sense of excitement to two great discoveries: classical antiquity and themselves. These newfound interests produced an explosion of creativity and achievement in which medicine and science were bountiful participants. It was all made possible by a fruitful chemistry of unrelated but extraordinary interacting events, strategically centered and affecting Western civilization at this particular point in time. The invention of printing most advantageously facilitated communication, as navigation broadened geographical perspectives, and the idea of a heliocentric universe awesomely exposed a new universe. Gunpowder demolished the last strongholds of feudalism, and following the fall of Constantinople in 1453, a wave of fleeing Greek scholars fanned out over Europe to give the humanist movement the necessary impetus. A closer intermingling of the arts and sciences provided mutual benefits. Interest of the legal profession in autopsies spurred the revival of human dissection, which in turn was raised to a higher plane by the involvement of physicians in art and artists in dissection. Berengarius, Vesalius, and Eustachius were notable anatomists with uncommon artistic skills, and of course, the sublime Leonardo da Vinci was a skilled dissector whose great original anatomical discoveries and physiological speculations were mislaid for centuries (17, 20, 23, 24). Da Vinci's extensive dissections on cadavers were conducted in secrecy for a very practical reason-survival. It was not selfishness or the need for further experimental proofs that led da Vinci to devise mirror image note-taking, nor devious purposes that caused him to conceal his findings. The specter of heresy still muted the creative urge. Church dogma and stultifying tradition dictated an attitude of caution for those adventurous souls who would peek beyond the curtain of authority

to view the unknown. Da Vinci's dissections focused on the ventricles, brainstem, and spinal cord, but there are voluminous notes on peripheral nerves and their functions. He described but did not recognize the significance of the sympathetic nervous system or the reflex arc. Experimenting with frogs, he found persisting sensation and motion after decerebration but almost instant death when he pithed the medulla. He concluded that this must be the site of the soul. He regarded pain as a component or particularly intense aspect of the sensation of touch. His animal experiments included sensory mapping of anesthetic areas produced by cutting specific nerves. From these investigations he was motivated to speculate on the selective protectiveness of pain in vital areas for man's preservation (2, 20).

A more open and audacious anatomist was Vesalius, a Belgian lured to Padua by the superior facilities and academic opportunities, whose masterful technique and original inquiring mind unmasked the absurdities of Galenic animal dissections. His great work, *De Humani Corporis Fabrica* (1543), brilliantly illustrated by woodcuts of Von Kalcar and possibly Titian and superbly printed by Oporinus at Basle, is one of the priceless treasures of the Renaissance. He brazenly refuted many established anatomical misconceptions and paid the price in character assassination and exile (15, 17, 23). No less beautiful in design or accurate in detail are the exquisite copperplates of Eustachius, which, possibly because of the fate of Vesalius, remained unprinted until recovered from the Vatican library 162 years later (18).

Religious proscriptions put an effective damper on the employment of pain-relieving drugs, although sporadic accounts of their use appear in the literature. Paracelsus rediscovered ether, the "sweet vitriol" of Ramon Lullus, when he mixed sulfuric acid and alcohol, and he was aware of its sleep-inducing qualities. Surgeons were known to use soporific sponges and physicians were well acquainted with the narcotic effects of opium; but these were dangerous times, when pain was considered an instance of God's will, and the stake loomed as a threat to those who would ally themselves with the devil's work. Kings could "lay hands on" to accomplish miraculous cures; the lowly practitioner had to avoid the inquisitors of witchcraft and heresy. Nevertheless, carotid compression anesthesia was utilized by Ambroise Paré. Snow packs and other cold applications were used for local anesthesia, and a small body of rebellious free spirits, taking courage from the writings and example of Paracelsus, used atropine, belladonna, mandrake, and a host of other medicinals for pain, as described in the splendid pharmaceutical books of Cordus and others (2, 8).

The inexorable march of progress gradually eroded the shackles of dogma and blind authority, but the process was slow and the course quite dangerous for those enlightened physicians and scientists who persisted in the struggle to conquer pain. Fortunately, the Renaissance had its share of courageous men to accept the challenges, and we are ever in their debt.

EARLY MODERN

In the seventeenth century the chain of events initiated by Copernicus and substantially implemented by Kepler and Galileo culminated in the synthesis of Newton to complete the scientific revolution. This brought forth a rash of attempts to systematize all fields of knowledge. Efforts to demonstrate a system of medicine reflecting the same order as Newton's universe approached the ludicrous. While fanciful preoccupation with systems orientation diverted some of the better minds, and the mysteries of the central nervous system remained unresolved, random individual contributions of enormous consequence were made in anatomy and physiology. However, it was not until 1800, when Bell and Magendie defined the roles of the anterior and posterior nerve roots, that pain physiology could step beyond the advances made by the ancient Alexandrians. Meanwhile, scientific discovery was furnishing patchy pieces for the puzzle of pain as certain developments, such as the birth of scientific societies and journals, the invention of the microscope, and a technological explosion, were helping to organize and consolidate a solid foundation from which modern biological concepts could evolve (22). Publication of William Harvey's (1578–1657) *De Motu Cordis* in 1628 did for physiology what the *Fabrica* had done for anatomy. Not only was the circulation of the blood proved by morphological, experimental, and mathematical arguments, but physiology itself was elevated on the strength of this discovery to the status of a dynamic science. Harvey's genius for inductive reasoning did not sustain him when he ventured into the realm of sensation, where his Aristotelian indoctrination misled him to see the circulating blood as the abode of the soul and the heart as the center of sensation and the seat of all natural emotion.

Medieval mysticism continued to exert a crippling influence on scientific thought well into the nineteenth century. Iatrochemists made notable contributions to physiology and added to our comprehension of pain, while introducing considerable confusion with their mysterious "archeus," or spirit forces that governed bodily functions. Von Helmont (1577–1649), follower of Paracelsus, was so fascinated by the stomach in his original studies on digestion that he made it the dominant organ of the body and resting place of the soul, holding dominion over consciousness, emotion, and pain. Despite the confusing superimposition of circulating spirits on physiological systems, the iatrochemists were the first to introduce the idea of a physical transmission of nerve impulses in motor and sensory processes (2).

In contrast to the carefully documented experimentation and inductive proofs of Harvey, the Frenchman René Descartes (1596–1650) developed his concepts of man as a machine out of pure deductive reasoning. Man functioned as any other machine, differing only in sensitivity and reasoning capacity. He derived his physiology from Galen. Impressed by the delicately poised central position of the pineal gland, he imbued it with a soul and imagined a sensory-motor response mechanism operating from the pineal gland that fits our concept of the reflex arc (*De Homine,* 1662).

With the passage of time, piece by piece, the knowledge of pain and effective means for its alleviation increased quantitatively in a somewhat amorphous mass of seemingly unrelated data that awaited unscrambling and reorganization into a coherent theoretical structure for modern debate and methodological application to the problems of our times. Other chapters in this book will deal with these problems, standing on the shoulders of the past to recapitulate the great progress that science has made to achieve our present sophistication in these matters; however, the puzzle is far from solved. The enigma of pain is still with us. To cast a retrospective glance back to the remote past is a pause that refreshes and assures us that we are not alone in our frustration. The task has always been arduous, and we must press on in the noble tradition of the great minds that have laid the groundwork for us.

References

1. Gurdjian ES. Head injury from antiquity to the present with special reference to penetrating head wounds. Springfield, IL: Charles C Thomas, 1973.
2. Keele KD. Anatomies of pain. Springfield, IL: Charles C Thomas, 1957.
3. Margotta R. The story of medicine. In: Lewis P, ed. The Golden Book of Life Sciences. New York: Golden Press, 1968.
4. Breasted JH. The Edwin Smith Surgical Papyrus. Chicago: University of Chicago Press, 1930.
5. Camac CNB. From Imhotep to Harvey. New York: Paul B. Hoeber, 1931.
6. Sarton G. A history of science: ancient science through the golden age of Greece. New York: Norton, 1952.
7. Methu DC. The antiquity of Hindu medicine and civilization. New York: Paul B. Hoeber, 1931.
8. Seeman B. Man against pain. New York: Chilton, 1962.
9. Agnew LRC. Medicine (history of). In: The new Catholic encyclopedia. New York: McGraw-Hill, 1967.
10. Morse WR. Chinese medicine. New York: Paul B. Hoeber, 1929.
11. Gordon BL. Medicine throughout antiquity. Philadelphia: FA Davis, 1949.
12. Singer CJ. Greek biology and Greek medicine. London: Oxford University Press, 1922.
13. Asimov I. A short history of biology. Garden City, NY: Natural History Press, 1964.
14. Sarton G. A history of science: Hellenistic science and culture in the last three centuries B.C. New York: Norton, 1959.
15. Cumston CG. An introduction to the history of medicine. London: Dawsons of Pall Mall, 1968.
16. Clark K. Civilization: a personal view. New York: Harper & Row, 1969.
17. Ackerknecht EH. A short history of medicine. New York: Ronald Press, 1968.
18. Garrison FH. An introduction to the history of medicine, 4th ed. Philadelphia: Saunders, 1929.
19. Reisman D. The story of medicine in the middle ages. New York: Paul B. Hoeber, 1935.
20. Todd EM. The neuroanatomy of Leonardo da Vinci. Santa Barbara, CA: Capra Press, 1983.
21. Browne EG. Arabian medicine. Cambridge, UK: Cambridge University Press, 1921.
22. Simpson MWH. Arab medicine and surgery. London: Oxford University Press, 1922.
23. Boas M. The scientific renaissance 1450–1630. New York: Harper & Row, 1962.
24. Castiglione A. The renaissance of medicine in Italy. Baltimore: Johns Hopkins Press, 1934.

CHAPTER 2

Neurobiology of Normal and Pathophysiological Pain[1]

Marshall Devor

INTRODUCTION

There is a growing consensus that classical textbook descriptions of the pain system are incomplete, notably for their failure to account for a range of often bizarre pain phenomena seen in patients. Clinical management of pain, particularly chronic pain, is often correspondingly unsatisfactory. This failure of theory and practice has prompted a good deal of basic research on the subject, work that has begun to yield a new conceptual synthesis concerning the neural mechanisms of subacute and chronic pain (1). The new synthesis attempts to address physiological and pathophysiological modifications of normal pain processes in a way that is clinically relevant. It can be expected to change pain management in the future. In this chapter I outline the new synthesis, emphasizing pain processes involving trauma or disease in the peripheral nervous system (PNS).

THE PAIN SYSTEM

The role of the pain system is to process information on the intensity, location, and dynamics of strong tissue-threatening stimuli. Traditionally it is presented as a serial bottom-up system in which afferent (sensory) impulses generated by noxious stimuli are encoded in the periphery, propagated centrally, processed, and perceived. While retaining this basic layout, the new synthesis adds powerful modulatory (gating) influences among the adjacent system modules. Abnormal and chronic pain states are understood in terms of the functioning of these modulatory processes as much as by variations in the primary noxious input. Figure 2.1 indicates the major components of the pain system and the modulatory relations among them.

This chapter discusses a number of types of modulation. An important example is injury-triggered central sensitization. Sensory input generated in nociceptive $A\delta$ and C affer-

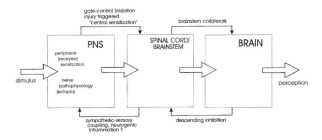

Figure 2.1. The major components of the pain system and modulatory relations among them. This review stresses the left-hand side of the diagram. For a review of the topics on the right, see Basbaum and Fields (18).

ent neurons normally signals pain. However, such input may also have a second, modulatory, effect. It triggers a transient spinal hyperexcitability state called central sensitization. In the presence of central sensitization, nociceptor input is amplified, yielding more pain than would otherwise be expected (hyperalgesia). Moreover, low-threshold $A\beta$ touch inputs are amplified too, so that light touch comes to evoke pain (allodynia). The fact that $A\beta$ touch input can trigger pain sensation is nothing short of revolutionary in light of the long-held dogma that $A\beta$ input subserves touch and vibration sense, while $A\delta$ and C-input signals pain and temperature.

In most discussions of pain and pain syndromes, a sharp line is drawn between the two major classes of pain: normal, or nociceptive, pain (which includes acute, subacute, and inflammatory pain), and pathophysiological pain (neuropathic, radiculopathic, deafferentation, and central pain).

[1]Adapted from Devor M. Pain mechanisms. Neuroscientist 1996:2:233–244

Nociceptive pain results from noxious stimuli and inflammation in otherwise *intact* tissue. The pain system is functioning as nature intended it to. Pathophysiological pain is associated with frank injury to neural tissue, and it reflects *abnormal* functioning of the pain system. The difference between normal and pathophysiological pain encompasses precipitating factors, symptoms, underlying mechanisms, and effective treatments. In this chapter I will use the terms pathophysiological pain and neuropathic pain interchangeably.

The distinction between the two is not the same as the distinction between acute and chronic pain. Both nociceptive and pathophysiological pain can come on instantaneously, and both may be long lasting. Rheumatoid arthritis is an example of chronic nociceptive pain; acute sciatica is an example of acute pathophysiological pain. It is true, however, that nociceptive pain states tend to be self-limiting, while pathophysiological pain states tend not to be. Thus, when pains persist for months and years, it is prudent at least to consider a neuropathic origin.

A striking implication of the new synthesis is the realization that pain following tissue injury, with or without inflammation, and pain following nerve or spinal root injury (peripheral neuropathic pain), are alike in many ways. In both, pain results from nerve impulses arising in the periphery, normally or ectopically, and from central amplification triggered and maintained by the peripheral afferent input.

Sensory Input: Normal Operation of the Pain System

Sensory Reception

How are sensory signals initially generated in skin, muscle, tendons, viscera, and so on? Primary sensory neurons reside in the paraspinal dorsal root ganglia (DRGs). They extend one branch through peripheral nerves to their peripheral target tissue. A second branch in the dorsal root extends from the DRG to enter the central nervous system (CNS) (Fig. 2.2). Transduction of noxious energies (force, temperature, irritant chemicals) occurs at the terminal membrane of the peripheral axon branch (Fig. 2.3). There are no known examples of peripheral nonneural sensory transduction cells that drive primary afferents as do, say, hair cells in the auditory and vestibular systems; the Merkel cell remains the one possible exception (2). The mechanisms of sensory reception remain poorly understood, mostly because of the difficulty of studying the very fine axonal endings where the sensory signal is generated. However, two distinct processes are clearly involved: signal transduction and stimulus encoding (3, 4) (Fig. 3A).

Transduction

Stimuli generate an inward transmembrane electrical current in the sensory axon ending (generator current, Fig. 2.3) and hence a depolarizing sensory generator potential. The electrical current consists of a flow of ions (e.g., Na^+, K^+, Cl^-), not electrons, as in copper wire. For mechanical stimuli the

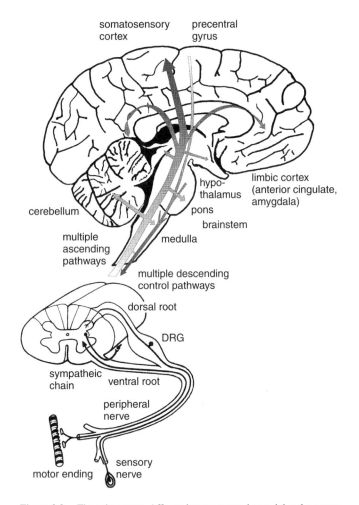

Figure 2.2.   The pain system. Afferent input generated at peripheral sensory endings converges on first-order central neurons of the spinal cord gray matter and in the dorsal column nuclei. The responsiveness of these cell networks is modulated by descending control pathways that originate directly and indirectly in the diencephalon, midbrain, pons, medulla, and cerebral cortex. Ascending pathways convey the already partly processed sensory signals to numerous locations in the brainstem and cerebellum, cortical and subcortical divisions of the limbic system, and via thalamic relays to somatosensory areas of the cerebral cortex.

generator current is due to ions flowing through unique transmembrane channels that are normally closed but that open momentarily when the axon terminal membrane has been stretched by a mechanical stimulus. Mechanosensitive (MS), or stretch-activated (SA), channels are large membrane-bound proteins found in virtually all cells, including bacteria, but presumably enriched in mechanoreceptive sensory endings (5–7). Amino acid sequence information is available for a few MS channel types, but little is known about structure-function relations or about the particular MS channel type or types in mechanosensitive afferents. It is possible, for example, that mechanonociceptors and low-threshold mechanoreceptors have different sensitivities because they use different types of MS channels. We do not yet have any drugs that effectively block the functioning on MS channels in nociceptive afferents. If we did, they might prove good analgesics.

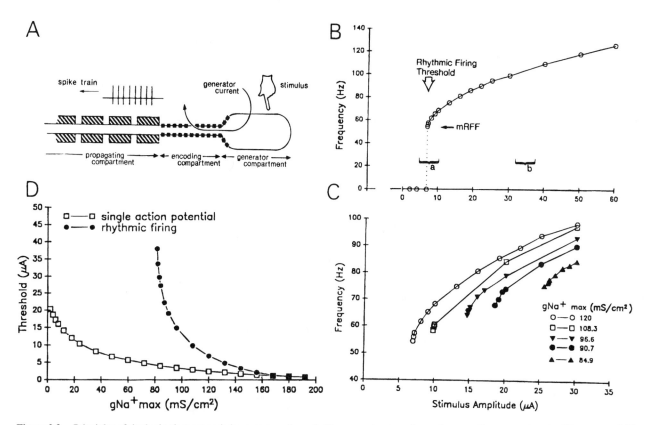

Figure 2.3. Principles of rhythmic electrogenesis in sensory endings. **A.** The generator, encoding and propagating compartments of the axon end. The generator compartment is sometimes embedded in a special sheath of nonneural cells, as in the pacinian corpuscle. At nerve injury sites the generator and encoding compartments may be coterminous. **B-D.** Computer simulation of repetitive firing in response to a prolonged depolarizing generator current, based on the Hodgkin-Huxley equations for the squid giant axon (9). **B.** Frequency-current (f-I) relation (encoding function). At threshold, firing rate increases stepwise from zero to the fiber's minimum rhythmic firing frequency (mRFF). A small change in stimulus strength around threshold (region a) has a much larger effect on firing frequency than the same change in region b. **C.** A family of f-I curves using gradually increasing Na^+ channel density (gNa^+_{max}). As Na^+ channels are added, repetitive firing threshold decreases, as does the mRFF. **D.** The change in rhythmic firing threshold and the threshold for evoking a single spike as functions of Na^+ channel density. Note that below about 80 mS/cm^2 repetitive firing cannot be elicited no matter how strong the stimulus, using the parameters adopted (9).

The mechanism of thermal transduction, hence warm and cold sensation, is not yet known. It presumably involves either transmembrane proteins or intracellular effector molecules with a high thermal sensitivity (Q_{10}). Chemoreception (in polymodal C fibers) is presumed to be based on specific receptor-effector molecules analogous to neurotransmitter and olfactory receptors. There are probably many types. A few are exteroceptors of pH and certain plant and animal toxins (e.g., vanilloid receptors for capsaicin, the "hot" in hot peppers). Evolutionarily the mucous membranes of the oral cavity are the probable biological target tissue, but cutaneous and deep afferents are also responsive. Most chemoresponsive nociceptive afferents are interoceptors that detect intrinsic mediators of inflammation (discussed later).

Stimulus Encoding

The generator potential decays to zero in the distal few hundred micrometers of the axon end. This signal does not reach the CNS. For sensory stimuli to be felt, the generator potential must be translated into a train of propagating electrical impulses (spikes, Fig.2.3A). This is the encoding process. Encoding of the generator potential into an impulse train is accomplished by a specialized patch of axonal membrane near the sensory axon end. This special part of the axon, which is rich in voltage-sensitive Na^+ channels, functions like the axon hillock-initial segment zone of CNS projection neurons. In contrast to transduction, encoding is sensitive to local anesthetics and related drugs.

Encoding is a fundamentally nonlinear process. There is always a threshold stimulus below which no spikes are generated (single-spike threshold). Many afferent types also have a second higher threshold for repetitive firing (8, 9) (Fig. 2.3B). The threshold for repetitive firing may be as important as the size of the generator potential in determining the sensitivity of afferent endings, that is, whether an afferent ending responds like a nociceptor or like a low-threshold touch ending. A generator potential of a given size may trigger no impulses in one sensory ending and a prolonged impulse train in another, all because of the properties of encoding. Correspondingly, any factor that shifts the threshold for spike encoding toward lower stimulus values would sensitize the sensory ending much like an increase in generator potential (Fig. 2.3, C and D). Chemical mediators of inflammation have long been known to contribute to pain by sensitizing nociceptor endings so that they respond to weak stimuli and not just to noxious ones. It is possible that inflammatory mediators act on the transduction process, the encoding process, or both (10–13). In the case of nerve injury an important cause of pain appears to be the creation of an abnormal encoding capability at the nerve injury site (discussed later).

In addition to sensory modality (mechanical, thermal, chemical) and response threshold, sensory endings differ from one another in their dynamic characteristics. For example, some afferent types show frequency adaptation; impulse firing rate declines with time even when the stimulus is maintained. Adaptation is caused by intrinsic factors such as inactivation of MS channels or activation of activity-dependent K^+ conductances, as well as by extrinsic ones, notably viscoelastic relaxation in the tissue in which the sensory ending is embedded. Other afferent types, such as slowly adapting touch endings, and many C nociceptors, fire repetitively without adaptation (14). The unique sensations evoked by normal sensory stimuli, such as the feel of a piece of cloth, the touch of someone's hand, or the sting of a firm slap, derive from the coactivation of many types of sensory afferents, each with its own transduction and encoding characteristics and each with its own dynamics. Sensation is a symphony. Abnormalities in the transduction and/or encoding characteristics of afferents can alter sensation in bizarre ways.

Pain Processing in the Central Nervous System

The ways sensory signals are integrated in the CNS to generate action and conscious perception are highly complex, largely unknown, and beyond the scope of this chapter. However, a few organizing principles should be noted. First and foremost, the old notions of a specific pain pathway and a specific CNS pain center are a fairy tale that few sophisticated investigators still believe. Rather, numerous pathways and brain structures are involved in pain processing. Beginning at the first central synapse in the dorsal horn of the spinal cord, information on noxious stimulus events is mostly combined with information on nonnoxious events. Noxious input becomes just a part of the sensory symphony. Correspondingly, noxious stimuli affect neural activity in large portions of the brain (15–17) (Fig. 2.2). Areas involved in pain perception include the classical lemniscal and nonlemniscal somatosensory pathways, certain classical motor structures (e.g., cerebellum), and limbic structures of the midbrain, diencephalon, and cortex. Among the latter structures, the anterior part of the cingulate gyrus has attracted particular attention.

Second, CNS pain signaling is not a serial process in which messages are passed progressively from lower to higher centers until they reach consciousness. Modulation from higher to lower structures and laterally among discriminative, emotional, and cognitive areas is clearly a major part of the process. The brain is an active player in perception. Memory, expectation, and anticipation—brain states that *precede* the arrival of afferent signals from the periphery—play an essential role in decoding the ascending pain signal.

Finally, there is almost certainly no central "narrator" of conscious perception of pain that sits at "headquarters" and waits passively for reports of noxious peripheral events to arrive. We still lack even a framework for thinking about how mental and emotional events are represented by neural activity in the CNS. It would be astounding, however, if what we call pain perception did not involve complex patterns of activity in numerous neural structures simultaneously. Pain, with its meaning for the organism, is the most primitive of percepts. Evolutionarily pain may well have set down the initial architecture of awareness that other sensory systems later adopted.

INFLAMMATORY AND NEUROPATHIC PAIN

Sensory Input: Sensitization Following Tissue Injury and Inflammation

Tissue injury with inflammation typically evokes both spontaneous pain and hyperresponsiveness to applied stimuli and to movement. The activation of normal nociceptors is a satisfactory account of the pain we feel during the initial noxious event, be it a cut, a scrape, or a burn. However, tenderness beyond the first few minutes must be understood in terms of processes that temporarily increase the sensitivity of the pain system itself. Such sensitization is thought to include both PNS and CNS components: peripheral and central sensitization. Both are design functions of the pain system, not reflections of disease. They presumably evolved to minimize use of injured and fragile tissue. In this sense they are analogous to the central descending pain control pathways (descending inhibition in Fig. 2.1) (18) that suppress pain responses at times of stress and emergency.

Peripheral Sensitization

Within a few minutes of tissue injury the classical inflammatory triple response of vasodilation (reddening and heat), swelling, and pain set in. Tissue inflammation increases the sensitivity of nociceptive endings in peripheral tissues by means of a complex soup of inflammatory mediator molecules (13). The list of these inflammatory mediators has grown rapidly in recent years. Some derive from the enzymatic breakdown of circulating precursors (e.g., bradykinin from kininogen). Others are released by resident cells (e.g., histamine and 5-hydroxytryptamine [5-HT] by mast cells; prostaglandins [PGs], by fibroblasts and sympathetic varicosities). Still others are released by glial cells and invasive cells of the immune system (e.g., cytokines, neutrophils, and tumor necrosis factor [TNF] by macrophages).

Inflammatory mediators are thought to act either directly on afferent membrane receptors (e.g., histamine, 5-HT, and some PGs), or indirectly by inducing release of direct-acting mediators from other cells. Macrophages, for example, activate fibroblasts by means of interleukin 1 (IL-1) and TNF. Products of arachidonic acid metabolism by cyclo-oxygenase and lipoxygenase include a profusion of direct and indirect mediators (e.g., PGs, leukotrienes). These are the targets of corticosteroids and aspirinlike nonsteroidal anti-inflammatory drugs (NSAIDs). Interestingly, many of the mediators of peripheral sensitization also play a central role in the immune and repair response to tissue injury as vasodilators, cytokines, and growth factors. This is part of our reason for believing that increased pain sensitivity is an integral part of the organism's adaptive response to everyday tissue injury, not a form of disease.

Inflammatory mediators activate nociceptor endings and also sensitize them, that is, make them more prone to activation by weak touch and thermal stimuli and during movement. These two effects may be independent. Some mediators, for example, do not induce ongoing pain but do sensitize, yielding allodynia and hyperalgesia. Sensitization and excitation often interact, however. Mediator A may sensitize to mediator B, which is present in the tissue at previously subthreshold concentrations. The result is apparent excitation by A. As many as one third of nociceptors in skin, joints, viscera, and so on cannot normally be activated by even strong noxious stimuli. These silent nociceptors are engaged only in the presence of inflammation (19).

Despite the dearth of direct evidence, it is usually assumed that inflammatory mediators sensitize by activating membrane receptors, depolarizing the nociceptor ending and hence bringing it closer to firing threshold (13). Another possibility is that they cause a shift in the encoding function (9, 11, 12, 20) (Fig. 2.3). For example, the threshold for repetitive firing may move to the left by modulation of the gating properties of voltage-sensitive Na^+ or K^+ channels in the encoder patch (e.g., by channel phosphorylation).

By lowering the response threshold of nociceptor endings in inflamed tissue, peripheral sensitization evokes both the direct nociceptive barrage that is felt as ongoing pain (burning, stinging), and also touch-, movement-, and temperature-evoked pain. This is primary hyperalgesia. The resulting sustained nociceptive input in turn is capable of triggering and maintaining central sensitization, the spinal hyperexcitability state that permits $A\beta$ touch-evoked input to be felt as pain (discussed later). In this way $A\beta$ afferents contribute to inflammatory pain even though they are not in general directly affected by inflammatory mediators.

Sensory Input: Effects of Nerve Injury and Neuropathic Pain

Burns and bruises evoke pain and tenderness that are familiar to everyone. In contrast, damage to peripheral nerves and spinal roots often triggers bizarre, chronic, and intractable pain states. Examples are phantom limb pain, trigeminal neuralgia, carpal tunnel syndrome, causalgia (CRPS2), diabetic neuropathy, sciatica, and many instances of cancer pain, to name just a few. With the impulse-conducting pathway compromised, sensation should be dulled, not amplified. Why, then, is nerve injury so often a direct cause of intense and prolonged neuropathic pain? The new synthesis has begun to resolve this paradox.

Nerve Injury: Pathophysiology and Ectopia

Tissue inflammation may alter the transduction and encoding properties of sensory endings, but the endings themselves remain intact. In injured nerves the receptor endings of afferent axons are either physically severed from the cell body or functionally disconnected by segmental demyelination block. This should silence the affected afferent and block any contribution it might make to sensation. In fact, however, many injured afferents develop hyperexcitability during the hours and days following axotomy or demyelination (20). This is reflected in ongoing discharge and stimulus-evoked activity arising at ectopic midnerve sites (Fig. 2.4).

Ectopic discharge (ectopia) originates mostly in the region of nerve injury and/or in the axotomized parent neuron in the DRG. There may also be a contribution from regenerating sprouts, especially ones trapped distal to the lesion site (disseminated microneuromas), and perhaps even from collateral sprouts of neighboring afferents that were not injured at all. Microneurographic recording in patients with a variety of neuropathic pain conditions has revealed a direct relation between ectopic discharge and felt paresthesias, dysesthesias, and pain (21–23).

Ectopic firing may develop in both low-threshold $A\beta$ afferents and in $A\delta$ and C nociceptors. When *only* $A\beta$ fibers are active, the result is painless paresthesias (23, 24). However, as with nociceptive or inflammatory pain, ectopic firing in nociceptors contributes to pain in two ways. First, it evokes pain directly. Second, it evokes central sensitization, hence (*a*) initiating allodynia in skin and deep tissue areas with residual $A\beta$ innervation and (*b*) augmenting spontaneous and movement-evoked pain from ectopically active $A\beta$ and nociceptive afferents.

The dual role of nociceptor ectopia is best illustrated under conditions in which a well-localized ectopic focus can be identified. Sheen and Chung (25), for example, severed the spinal nerve just peripheral to the L5 and L6 DRGs in rats, creating a focus of ectopic discharge in the L5 and L6 spinal nerve neuromas and DRGs. The result was behavioral signs of ongoing pain and allodynia in the hind limb skin served by the neighboring intact afferents of the L4 segment (Fig. 2.5). Blocking central propagation of the ectopia by secondarily cutting the L5 and L6 dorsal roots eliminated the ongoing pain as expected. Remarkably, it also normalized sensation in the previously tender L4 territory, presumably by eliminating the central sensitization triggered by the L5 and L6 ectopia. Gracely et al. (26) demonstrated similar events in man. One of their neuropathic pain patients, for example, had a focally painful scar near the knee and allodynia extending up the thigh and down the calf. Local anesthetic block of the scar eliminated the extended allodynia, as well as the scar pain, for the duration of the block.

Mechanisms of Ectopia

The development of ectopic hyperexcitability in the hours and days following axonal injury and demyelination is thought to be due to remodeling of the axon membrane's local

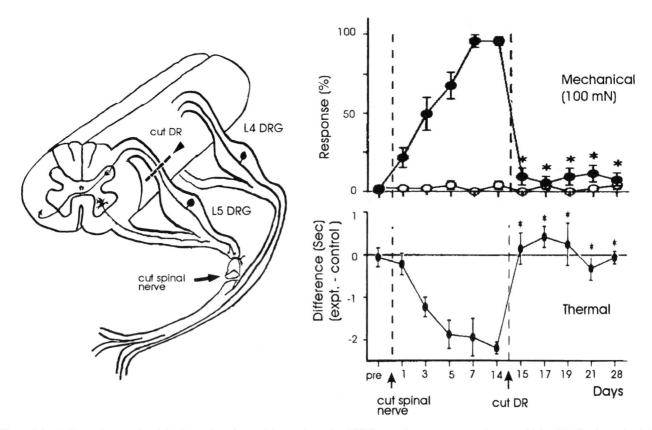

Figure 2.4. Evidence that ectopia originating at sites of nerve injury and associated DRGs contributes to cutaneous hypersensitivity (25). Graphs on the right plot withdrawal responses of rats to mechanical probing and to radiant heat projected onto the plantar surface of the foot. **Upper graph.** Percent of trials on which there was a withdrawal response. *Open circles,* intact side; *solid circles,* operated side. **Lower graph.** Response latency calculated as operated side minus control side. Negative values reflect excess sensitivity on the operated side. Preoperatively (pre) the feet are symmetrical. After transection of the L5 and L6 spinal nerve, mechanical and thermal allodynia emerge. The afferent input from the foot enters the spinal cord along the residual intact L4 dorsal root (DR). After the 14th postoperative day the L5 and L6 DRs were cut, blocking the barrage of ectopic L5 and L6 activity from reaching the spinal cord. Although the afferent route from the foot (L4) was not touched, the mechanical and thermal hypersensitivity of the foot disappeared.

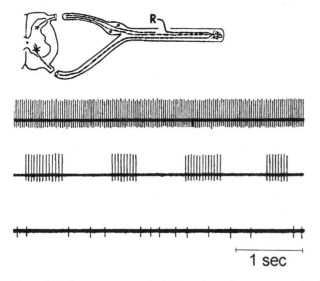

Figure 2.5. Spontaneous ectopic discharge from afferent axons ending in an experimental nerve-end neuroma. Typically, fine axon bundles (microfilaments) are teased from the nerve upstream of the injury and placed on a single recording electrode (R) referenced to a nearby indifferent electrode. Examples of tonic, bursty, and irregular firing patterns are shown (20).

electrical properties (11, 20, 27). The principal underlying mechanism appears to be the accumulation of excess voltage sensitive Na^+ channels in terminal swellings (neuroma end bulbs) and sprouts in the region of injury and in patches of demyelination (11, 28, 29) (Fig. 2.6). Na^+ channels, like other integral membrane proteins, are synthesized in the cell soma in the DRG, transported down the axon by anterograde axoplasmic flow, and incorporated into the axolemma by exocytotic vesicle fusion.

At midnerve sites in intact axons Na^+ channel density is too low to support the generation of repetitive firing in response to natural stimuli, which yield slowly depolarizing generator potentials. Press on your median nerve as it runs along the forearm, for example. The pressure is felt locally, but not in the distribution of the median nerve (medial hand). Blunt pressure does not induce impulse activity when applied to healthy nerves. However, had the median nerve been chronically injured where you pressed, paresthesias and pain would probably be felt in the medial part of your hand because pressure stimuli do evoke impulses at nerve injury sites. Na^+ channel accumulation following axonal injury apparently results from

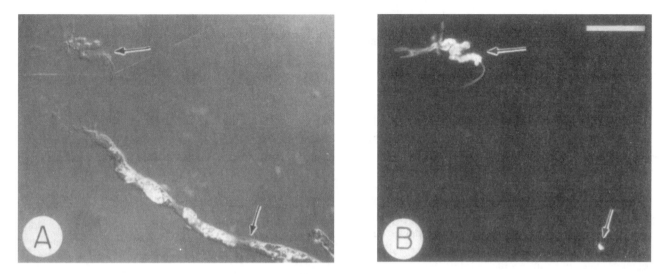

Figure 2.6.   Na⁺ channel accumulation in chronically injured axons. Nomarski (**A**) and immunofluorescence (**B**) images of a myelinated afferent axon teased from an 11-day experimental neuroma. Arrows show heavy Na⁺ channel immunolabeling on the terminal end bulb and sprouts and at a proximal node of Ranvier (arrow). The S-shaped demyelinated segment just proximal to the end bulb is also labeled, but the adjacent segment that still has compact myelin is not. Scale bars, 100 μm. (Reprinted with permission from Devor M, Keller CH, Deerinck TJ, et al. Na⁺ channel accumulation on axolemma of afferent endings in nerve-end neuromas in Apteronotus. Neurosci Lett 1989;102:149–154.)

elimination of factors that normally exclude Na⁺ channels from the midaxon membrane, particularly myelin, and from damming up of channels originally destined for downstream targets (11, 28). In addition, axonal injury appears to trigger up-regulation (increase) of synthesis of key channels in the cell soma in the DRG and even to induce the expression of previously absent Na⁺ channel types (30, 31). Nerve injury sites are rich in nerve growth factor (NGF) released by local nonneural cells (32). In vitro exposure to NGF has been shown to trigger up-regulation of Na⁺ channel synthesis in DRG neurons (33). Therefore, it is possible that altered neurotrophin concentration ultimately leads to altered regulation of the cellular proteins responsible for neural excitability.

The accumulation of excess Na⁺ channels at neuroma end bulbs and at patches of demyelination confers on these sites the characteristics of a sensory encoder. Still, to generate ectopic discharge there must be an adequate generator current. This appears to be provided by passive membrane leak (i.e., ion channels that are open at rest) or by transducer receptors and channels, as in normal sensory endings (e.g., MS channels). Like Na⁺ channels, these are synthesized in the DRG neuron and transported distally (34). Thus, they too may accumulate at sites of axotomy and demyelination. Their presence is indicated by the fact that ectopic firing sites respond in a specific manner to mechanical displacement, temperature changes, and relevant chemical mediators, including inflammatory mediators and adrenergic agonists (20, 35). Indeed, there is evidence that individual axons recapitulate the specific sensitivities and adaptation characteristics that they possessed at their normal transducer ending before axotomy (36, 37). An appreciation of the role of Na⁺ channel-dependent spike initiation in the origin of neuro-

pathic pain has prompted the increased use of systemically administered Na⁺ channel blockers (e.g., systemic lidocaine, mexiletine, carbamazepine, and lamotrigine) in the clinical management of a broad range of neuropathic pain states (38).

Spinal Modulation and Central Sensitization

Afferent Convergence

Individual primary sensory neurons encode specific stimuli within a narrow range of stimulus intensities. This fact shaped the classical notion that each somatosensory modality, including pain, follows a separate and specific pathway all the way to consciousness. This specificity theory was only partly shaken by the discovery that most second-order spinal cord neurons that receive noxious input also receive low threshold input (i.e., they have a wide dynamic range [WDR]). There does exist a small proportion of spinal neurons that normally respond selectively to noxious stimuli. However, most of these send their ascending axon through a restricted part of the dorsolateral spinal white matter, and cutting this tract does not eliminate pain sensation (39). On the other hand, pain *is* eliminated, at least for a time, by cutting the ascending pathways that carry the axons of WDR neurons (mainly the spinal anterolateral column). How WDR neurons code highly specific touch and pain sensations is still an open question. A likely possibility is that as in the periphery, progressively stronger stimuli recruit WDR neurons that have sequentially overlapping encoding functions. Thus, if a significant proportion of WDR neurons were to become sensitized, a weak stimulus would generate the same population activity formerly produced by a stronger one.

Modulation at the First Central Synapse

The idea of central modulation was brought to center stage by Melzack and Wall (40) in their gate control theory of pain. This theory was based on the observation that input along low-threshold Aβ afferents inhibits the response of postsynaptic WDR neurons to nociceptive input, hence "closing a gate" on pain. An everyday example is the relief obtained from gently rubbing bruised skin. Melzack and Wall attributed this effect primarily to presynaptic inhibition of nociceptive primary afferent terminals by spinal interneurons activated by low-threshold Aβ afferents. The main evidence was that Aβ input, in contrast to Aδ or C input, generates subthreshold depolarization of the central terminals of neighboring afferents. This so-called primary afferent depolarization (PAD) reduces the amount of neurotransmitter released from the neighbors and thus inhibits their ability to drive postsynaptic neurons.

Over the years the gate control theory has been revised. For example, it is now known that low-threshold input generates *postsynaptic* inhibition in addition to presynaptic inhibition. Likewise, there remains controversy concerning the theory's proposal that nociceptor input selectively disinhibits PAD, hence generating primary afferent hyperpolarization and *opening* spinal gates. Such details aside, the fundamental concept of signal modulation introduced by the theory has been vindicated by the richness of modulatory processes that form the basis of the new synthesis.

Central Sensitization and Secondary Hyperalgesia

Following localized trauma, tenderness (mechanical but not thermal allodynia) spreads a considerable distance beyond the area of injury, including into areas where there is no detectable inflammation. Pain in this extended area is secondary hyperalgesia. An important historical debate centered on whether secondary hyperalgesia is due to nociceptors sensitized by diffusion of algogenic substances or by axon reflex activity or is due to altered processing of impulses entering the CNS along low-threshold Aβ touch afferents (41, 42). Data sufficient to tilt the scale toward the latter hypothesis have been obtained only recently.

There are four main lines of evidence that argue for a contribution of low-threshold Aβ afferent neurons to pain sensation (43–47). First, using cuff and anesthetic procedures that block A and C fibers (relatively) selectively, secondary hyperalgesia fades with block of A-fiber conduction and returns only when A-fiber conduction is restored. Second, the stimulus-to-response latency of touch-evoked pain corresponds to conduction at A-fiber velocity. Third, intraneural and transcutaneous electrical stimulation of Aβ axons, bypassing their sensory ending, elicits pain in the zone of secondary hyperalgesia and in the zone of primary hyperalgesia but not in intact skin. Finally, recording experiments have failed to yield evidence of nociceptor sensitization away from the area of obvious inflammation. The same types of evidence indicate that in many cases of neuropathy, allodynic pain is evoked by activity in Aβ afferents (26, 44). Aβ-evoked pain appears to be due to central sensitization triggered by C fiber input generated alternatively by noxious stimulation of intact skin or deep tissue, stimulation of sensitized C nociceptors in inflamed tissue, or ectopic firing of C afferents at sites of nerve injury and associated DRGs.

Neural Mechanism of Central Sensitization

Central sensitization as manifested behaviorally and psychophysically has its counterpart in spinal cord electrophysiology. Within a few minutes of delivering a brief (seconds) noxious conditioning stimulus to afferent C fibers in acute experiments in rats and in monkeys, a transient hyperexcitability state develops in postsynaptic neurons in the dorsal horn representation of the corresponding body part. The indicators of emerging hyperexcitability include (*a*) windup, a stimulus-to-stimulus augmentation in response magnitude when afferent C fibers are stimulated once every second or two; (*b*) expansion of cutaneous receptive fields; and (*c*) the acquisition by nociceptive-selective neurons of WDR properties (48–51). The latter two phenomena are illustrated in Figure 2.7. In each case Aβ afferents come to drive postsynaptic neurons they were previously ineffective at driving. The exaggerated postsynaptic responses persist for tens of minutes, up to more than an hour in the case of conditioning on a muscle nerve. Correspondingly, awake animals show the expected behavioral allodynia (43).

The mechanism thought to account for central sensitization (Fig. 2.8) is similar to that involved in another short-term memory process, cortical long-term potentiation (LTP). Briefly, spinal terminals of Aβ touch afferents normally activate WDR neurons by releasing glutamate. This drives the neurons modestly, via postsynaptic non-N-methyl-D-aspartate (non-NMDA) glutamate receptors. NMDA glutamate receptors, which are blocked at normal membrane potentials by Mg^{2+} ions, are not activated. Impulse activity in C nociceptors releases glutamate and also peptide neurotransmitters, notably substance P (SP). Adequately intense C input produces prolonged (tens of seconds) SP-evoked depolarization. This displaces the Mg^{2+} block, enabling the NMDA receptors and rendering them responsive to the glutamate released from Aβ touch afferents. Since the Aβ fibers now act via NMDA as well as non-NMDA receptors, they drive WDR neurons more effectively than before and hence elicit a stronger postsynaptic response and allodynia. The persistence of sensitization beyond the duration of the SP-evoked depolarization is thought to be due to Ca^{2+} entry through the NMDA receptor channels. This may activate a specific Ca^{2+}-dependent protein kinase and phosphorylate ion channels, sustaining the sensitized state (51).

Time-Constant (Persistence of) Central Sensitization

Central sensitization can apparently be sustained indefinitely if the noxious conditioning input is maintained, as in chronic inflammatory diseases or sustained ectopic firing in neuropathy. On the other hand, when the sustaining noxious

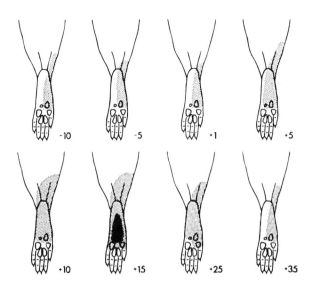

Figure 2.7. Two manifestations of central sensitization from Cook et al. (48). This neuron, recorded in the dorsal horn of the spinal cord, initially responded to pinch stimuli on the medial hind limb (stippled area at time −10 and −5 minutes). By 5 minutes after delivery of 20 C-fiber strength-conditioning shocks (1 per second) to the gastrocnemius-soleus nerve, the receptive field had begun to expand. A few minutes later this initially nociceptive-selective neuron began to respond to innocuous touch stimuli (black area at time +15 minutes) and thus acquired the characteristics of a WDR neuron. Subsequently the receptive field returned to its initial size and sensitivity.

input is eliminated, such as by cooling or use of local anesthetics, Aβ pain disappears rapidly, usually within minutes (26, 44). For this reason, the primary noxious focus is said both to trigger and to maintain central sensitization. It is possible that amplification due to central sensitization may be prevented with pharmacological antagonists to NMDA receptors. Many clinical trials of this approach are in progress. Another strategy being tested in an attempt to lessen postoperative nociceptive pain is preemptive analgesia (52, 53). The idea is to prevent the central sensitizing effects of noxious input during surgery by supplementing general anesthetics with regional anesthetic block or with systemic opiates. Preemptive analgesia is discussed in detail in Chapter 3.

Long-term Central Nervous System Plasticity

There is a venerable belief in the clinical literature that persistent pain can burn its way into the CNS, becoming independent of peripheral input and nearly impossible to treat (centralization of pain). In fact, injury to peripheral nerves triggers a spectrum of long-term changes in central somatosensory circuitry that are not related in any obvious way to the nociceptor-driven central sensitization mechanism just discussed (54–56). In principle, these could form a basis for the transition of pain from a labile, acute form to a centralized, intractable form. The recent discovery that peripheral injury and injury-related sensory signals can alter gene expression in CNS neurons has given renewed impetus to the idea of centralization (57). However, the reality of this transition is uncertain. Persistent pain may be hard to treat simply

because it results from an intractable process from the very beginning. There may in fact be no change in mechanism, no centralization (Chapter 3).

Centrifugal Modulation of Afferent Input

In several sensory modalities the actual responsiveness of sensory receptor endings is directly or indirectly controlled by the CNS. Examples are the olivocochlear bundle in audition, gamma efferent control in proprioception and motor control, and the isthmo-optic system in vision (in some species). Centrifugal control of this sort is not known to occur in the resting pain system, although sympathetic activation may subtly affect the response of normal pacinian corpuscles and some other cutaneous endings (59, 60). In the event of tissue or nerve injury, however, prominent adrenosensitivity develops in a considerable proportion of low-threshold mechanoreceptors and nociceptors. Likewise, the tissue milieu of sensory endings is affected by antidromic impulses in nociceptive afferents. These effects appear to play an important role in chronic inflammatory and pathophysiological pain states (59, 61–63).

Sympathetic-Sensory Coupling

In inflamed skin and joints and in injured nerves, many afferents show accelerated firing in response to systemic adrenaline and to sympathetic efferent stimulation (64–70). This sympathetic-sensory coupling is thought to contribute to allodynia, hyperalgesia, and ongoing pain in inflamed tissue, in chronic sympathetic-dependent pain states such as CRPS2

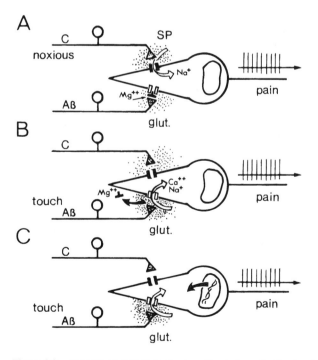

Figure 2.8. The proposed neural mechanism of central sensitization (see text for an explanation). The idea (**C**) that Ca++ entry through NMDA receptors may alter gene expression in a way that makes central sensitization permanent and independent of ongoing nociceptor drive remains highly speculative.

and reflex sympathetic dystrophy (RSD, or CRPS1), and in some cases of phantom limb pain. The evidence for this includes the exacerbation of pain by natural and pharmacological sympathetic stimulation and pain relief by diagnostic sympathetic block and sympatholysis (62, 63). In the presence of central sensitization sympathetic activation of normal low-threshold afferents may also contribute to pain (71), as may sympathetic activation of ectopic firing in Aβ afferents.

Sympathetic-sensory coupling is mediated predominantly by α_2-adrenoreceptors, with a lesser contribution by α_1-adrenoreceptors (69, 72). The most likely coupling mechanism is a direct action of neurally released noradrenaline and of circulating adrenaline on adrenoreceptors in the afferent membrane. α_2-Adrenoreceptor mRNA and protein are present in intact afferent neurons, and sympathetic efferents are present in the vicinity of the afferent endings. The primary change that initiates sympathetic-sensory coupling remains uncertain. The most obvious possibility is that afferent hyperexcitability, due to peripheral sensitization and/or Na^+ channel accumulation, reveals a latent adrenosensitivity in afferent neurons. In the case of nerve injury, there may also be adrenoreceptor up-regulation (67).

Recently the DRG has been identified as a potentially important site of sympathetic-sensory coupling. Nerve injury triggers sprouting of perivascular sympathetic endings in the ganglion, some of which form distinctive basketlike webs around neuronal somata in the DRG (73, 74). Sympathetic stimulation is then able to drive afferent discharge originating in the DRG.

Neurogenic Inflammation

A second mode of centrifugal influence on afferent endings is by means of antidromic impulses in the afferents themselves. Antidromic stimulation of afferent C fibers evokes the release of peptide neurotransmitters such as SP, neurokinin A (NKA) and calcitonin gene-related peptide (CGRP) from their peripheral endings, both in normal and inflamed tissues and at sites of nerve injury. This triggers plasma extravasation from postcapillary venules, resulting in neurogenic edema and the appearance of inflammatory mediators such as histamine and bradykinin in the affected tissue. Some neuropeptides may sensitize nociceptor endings directly. This mechanism may contribute to pain in chronic inflammatory disease and in RSD (13, 19, 61). But what could be the source of centrifugal antidromic drive? Possibilities include axon reflex, ectopic firing originating from in-continuity axons and DRG cells, and dorsal root reflexes.

SOME EXAMPLES: PHANTOM LIMB PAIN, SCIATICA, AND TRIGEMINAL NEURALGIA

We will now consider some specific chronic pain syndromes in light of the principles embodied in the new synthesis (Fig. 2.1). For this purpose I have chosen three chronic pain

syndromes that on the face of it have little in common. It should become obvious that in light of the new synthesis they may have a good deal in common. I hasten to point out that this discussion is an intellectual exercise, an attempt to apply evolving basic science ideas to clinical observations. It should by no means be taken as the last word on these pain syndromes or even as a consensus view. Some of these conditions are discussed from other perspectives elsewhere in this volume.

Phantom Limb Pain

I begin with phantom limb pain, a most mysterious pain state on which so many words have been written with so little closure. Phantom limb pain, of course, is felt to originate in an absent (amputated) body part. Amputees always continue to feel their missing arm or leg. Although the sensation is usually benign, in most individuals (about 80%) it is painful some of the time, and in some it is painful most of the time (75). The sensation is related to neural injury, not to loss of the limb per se. Painful phantoms can occur when the limb is still present but deafferented, such as following brachial plexus avulsion. Phantom pain must be distinguished from pain felt in the stump. Stump pain is felt locally and is akin to other persistent scar pains; phantom pain is felt in (referred into) the missing or insensate body part.

The origin of phantom limb sensation, including pain, is believed by various authors to be alternatively (a) the residual parts of the peripheral sensory neuron, (b) the CNS, and (c) the psyche, as a sort of unconsummated mourning for the lost but not forgotten body part (76–79). I do not propose to resolve this dispute here but rather to consider the consequences for the pain system when a limb is severed. What kinds of pain processes may be engaged?

The Peripheral Nerve

Amputation entails severing the sensory and motor axons in the nerves that used to serve the tissue that was cut away. One must remember that the primary sensory neurons to which these severed axons belong are not themselves in the limb. They reside far central to the amputation site, near the spine in the DRGs. The sensory neurons of the amputated limb are wounded by the amputation, but they remain alive and still connected to the stump and to the spinal cord (Fig. 2.2).

As noted earlier, there is a wealth of evidence showing that such wounded primary sensory neurons change their biology, for example by generating abnormal impulse discharge both in the region of the axonal injury itself and within the DRG. This ectopic signal is conducted centrally into the spinal cord, where it activates spinal sensory neurons. From there the sensory signal is conducted to the brain. Thus, whatever part the psyche may play in the generation of phantoms, an abnormal peripheral signal is generated in the neurons that used to innervate the now absent limb. This signal is expected to be perceived as the limb because it arrives in the brain along nerve fibers that used to be connected to the limb. The quality of the sensation evoked by ectopic peripheral afferent input may be distorted by the abnormal circumstances under which this signal is generated and processed.

Among the primary afferent neurons wounded by amputation are nociceptors. When these become active, they can cause phantom pain directly and by triggering central sensitization. In the presence of central sensitization Aβ touch input can contribute to pain sensation. This includes ectopic Aβ input generated in the injured peripheral axons and in the DRG.

Adding to the logic of a peripheral contribution to phantom limb sensation is the fact that there is often a moment-to-moment correlation between the degree of ectopic firing and the intensity of the phantom sensation. For example, mechanical pressure applied to stump neuromas and increased sympathetic efferent activity exacerbate both the ectopia and the phantom sensation. Direct injection of excitatory drugs into neuromas evokes intense phantom pain. Likewise, blocking stump nerves usually diminishes or eliminates phantom limb pain for the duration of the block (76). In amputees in whom nerve block has no obvious effect on phantom limb pain the possibility remains that the block was not performed satisfactorily or that a major portion of the pain signal arises in the DRG. When the nerve block wears off, of course, the phantom is expected to return. There is no logic to the myth that failure of a single block or a series of blocks to eliminate phantom limb pain permanently indicates an origin in the CNS.

The Central Nervous System

The existence of an obvious peripheral signal associated with the nerves of the amputated limb does not rule out the possibility of a genuine CNS contribution as well. The idea of pain centralization was noted earlier. For example, there are numerous reports of phantom limbs featuring rings, bunions, focal pains, and other preamputation detail (80). Similarly, the position of the phantom is thought often to reflect the last position of the limb prior to amputation. Unfortunately, it is difficult to know whether these anecdotes reflect current specific sensations or are simply memories, anchored by paresthesias associated with stump neuromas or ectopic DRG activity. The same problem holds for phantoms that persist despite dorsal rhizotomy or spinal cord transection. These events trigger (new) deafferentation and central pains that may be rationalized by the patient and physician as continuation of an old pain that is in fact gone.

Controlled prospective studies are needed. Jensen et al. (81) made the first effort in this direction. In their cohort virtually all of the patients had limb pain prior to amputation. Immediately after amputation phantom pain was reported to bear some resemblance to the preamputation pain in location and character in only a third of the patients, and after 2 years in only 10%. Sudden traumatic amputation of previously healthy limbs does not appear to yield results very different from amputation after extended periods of pain (75).

Low-Back Pain and Sciatica

Low-back pain and sciatica (pain felt in the leg along the sciatic nerve distribution) are often associated with bulging or herniation of the intervertebral disc, narrowing of the vertebral or nerve root canal (spinal or lateral stenosis), vertebral dislocation, and other forms of spinal injury and disease. This is a very common problem encountered by most adults at one time or another. Sometimes it is crippling in intensity and duration. What kind of pain is it?

Inflammatory versus Neuropathic Pain

The most widely held view is that low back pain and sciatica are primarily due to tissue (including facet joint) inflammation (82). A key idea is that the changes associated with aging weaken the otherwise tough annular ring of fibrous tissue that gives the disc its strength. Eventually there is a moment, while picking up a heavy object or bending over the wrong way, when too much force is applied to the weakened disk and as a result the annular ring bulges out and tears, releasing a soup of inflammatory chemicals from the disc interior into the tissue of the lower back. This sensitizes local nociceptive endings, making them more responsive than normal to mechanical stimuli, for example on movement. Radiation of pain into the leg is blamed on sensitization of the axons in the passing nerve root, although as discussed above, inflammatory mediators act on sensory endings, not on mid-nerve axons.

Imaging of the lower back often shows at least some disc herniation (82, 83). Nonetheless, relatively little attention is normally paid to the direct impact of the disc on nerve tissue unless the lesion is severe enough to cause negative neurological signs such as numbness or weakness in the leg. One only rarely hears talk of back pain in the context of neuropathy. The reason is probably that most of us still think of nerve fibers as electrical wires that either conduct or fail to conduct nerve impulses. However, disc herniation and spinal or root stenosis are very likely preludes to ectopia, both spontaneous and mechanically evoked during movement.

As noted earlier, the DRG has been identified as an important source of ectopic afferent discharge in the event of nerve injury, and this is likely so also in low back pain and sciatica. The herniated intervertebral disc may compress the DRG directly, and tension in the impacted spinal nerve may pull on the DRG, distorting it mechanically and disrupting its vascular supply. Most patients with low back pain find straight leg lifting intensely painful. This maneuver applies tension to the sciatic nerve and hence to the lower lumbar DRGs. Correspondingly, in experiments in which the deep spinal tissues were surgically exposed in awake patients, direct mechanical stimulation of the traumatized region of nerve root or its DRG or traction on the dural sleeve reproduced the patients' sciatica pain (84). Pressure on the intact part of the nerve or other tissues in the low back never evoked sciatica. Finally, microneurographic recording in patients during painful straight leg lifting has revealed intense ectopic impulse activity that is closely correlated with the provoked sensation (21). As in other neuropathic pain conditions, the effects of ectopia may be amplified by central sensitization.

Trigeminal Neuralgia (Tic Douloureux)

Some chronic pain conditions have a paroxysmal shocklike quality. In fact, this is sometimes held to be the sine qua non of neuropathic pain, although certain unequivocally neuropathic pain states may lack it. Pain in diabetic neuropathy, for example, often has a steady, burning quality. We shall consider the possible origins of shocklike pain sensations in the context of trigeminal neuralgia.

Tic Pain

Although relatively rare, trigeminal neuralgia stands out among chronic pain syndromes both for its dramatic symptoms and for the relatively high frequency with which it responds to therapy (85). The disease presents as an intermittent paroxysmal pain felt unilaterally in one or more divisions of the trigeminal nerve. The pain is brief but excruciating. It usually appears spontaneously, with no obvious precipitating events.

A peculiarity shared with only a few other conditions is triggering. There is usually one but occasionally more trigger points at which light touch, hair movement, wind puffs, chewing, talking, and so on fire off the pain. Amazingly, noxious stimuli such as pressure, pinch, or intense heat are generally ineffective. Pain paroxysms may also occur spontaneously. In most patients pain is paroxysmal, with a sudden, shocklike onset. In others it comes on more gradually, building up to a crescendo over several seconds. It rarely lasts more than a few seconds, although episodes of rapidly recurring attacks lasting hours can occur. Pain is usually described as shooting, cutting or like an electric shock. Attacks typically come in clusters separated by remissions lasting for months or even years. Individual paroxysms are followed by an interval lasting a minute or two during which the ability to trigger an attack is reduced (postattack refractory period).

Central versus Peripheral Causation

Since there is no obvious inflammation or tenderness in the skin, no precipitating trauma, and little if any numbness on the face, trigeminal neuralgia has traditionally been considered an example of central pain. This impression is strengthened by the fact that it responds well to certain anticonvulsant drugs. Routine computed tomography (CT) and magnetic resonance imaging (MRI) usually indicate no PNS or CNS abnormality except in cases of tic associated with multiple sclerosis or space-occupying lesions. However, at surgical exploration a small blood vessel is frequently found to be lying against the trigeminal root between the trigeminal ganglion and the brainstem. This microvascular compression is often sufficient to leave a groove in the root when the vessel is lifted off and a grayish discoloration that on pathological examination shows segmental demyelination and microneuroma formation. This hidden neural trauma suggests that the disease may in fact have a peripheral neuropathic origin. However, as similar anomalies occur in many autopsy specimens of individuals who do not have symptoms of trigeminal neuralgia, the relation of microvascular compression to the lightning pain is a subject of controversy (86).

More than 80% of patients with trigeminal neuralgia respond to anticonvulsant medication, particularly carbamazepine. The anticonvulsant valproate and barbiturates are ineffective. Eventually, nearly half of tic patients stop responding at tolerable drug doses and become candidates for either percutaneous (partial) damage to the trigeminal ganglion or root or open surgical microvascular decompression. Both techniques are highly effective, with initial success on the order of 80 to 90% of patients, although there are recurrences as time goes by.

Electric Shock-Like Sensation

How can we understand the peculiar paroxysmal nature of pain attacks in trigeminal neuralgia, and why does the sensation often feel like an electric shock? The experiential quality of evoked or spontaneous sensations is a powerful hint at their underlying cause. If pain is described as burning, for example, it is likely to be associated with normal or abnormal neural activity in heat-sensitive primary afferents or the CNS cells that they preferentially drive. It is for this reason that pain descriptors (pain words) are such a useful item in diagnostic tools such as the McGill Pain Questionnaire. By this logic shocklike pain should be a result of neural activity similar to that evoked by an electric shock.

The thing that distinguishes electric shock stimuli from natural ones such as touch, heat, and cold is that electrical currents activate all of the different types of afferents simultaneously, without much selectivity. Hence we would expect the shocklike pain of trigeminal neuralgia to result from simultaneous firing of many different types of sensory neurons. But what can cause this, particularly in the wake of a local light touch (triggering) stimulus?

One proposed answer it that the trigger stimulus sets off a virtual explosion of neural activity, not unlike a chemical or nuclear chain reaction (87). The idea is based on the discovery of mutual cross-excitation among neighboring sensory cells. Imagine a trigger stimulus exciting a small number of sensory cells that are coupled to neighbors. Soon the neighbors start firing. But these are coupled to still more neighbors that in turn are coupled to still more. If there is nothing to damp down the excitation, such a positive-feedback chain reaction can build up rapidly, soon involving large numbers of neurons of all types. The result is an electric shock-like pain paroxysm.

The classical idea of trigeminal neuralgia being a kind of epileptic seizure in the trigeminal brainstem fits this pattern well. However, cross-excitation among primary afferents in the periphery, either in the zone of trigeminal root compression or in the trigeminal ganglion, is no less likely. It is true that there are no synapses in the periphery to mediate cross-excitation. However, two other viable processes have been discovered in recent years. One is ephaptic (electrical) cross-talk; the second is a novel form of neurotransmitter and K^+ ion-mediated interaction called neural cross-excitation (88). Both types of coupling are known to occur at sites of nerve injury, including demyelination sites, as well as in sensory ganglia, especially after nerve injury (20). Together they constitute an epileptic seizure, so to speak, of the peripheral nerve.

Interestingly, abnormal firing in injured nerves and their DRGs is suppressed by the same Na^+ channel blocking (membrane stabilizing) anticonvulsant agents that suppress pain attacks in trigeminal neuralgia (e.g., carbamazepine). It is not suppressed by synaptic-acting anticonvulsants, like barbiturates, that suppress CNS seizure activity but are not effective in trigeminal neuralgia. Putting together the observation of trigeminal root injury caused by microvascular compression, the process of neural cross excitation, and the response of hyperexcitable primary afferents to membrane stabilizing anticonvulsant drugs, the idea that trigeminal neuralgia is a peripheral neuropathic pain state becomes an attractive possibility.

CONCLUSIONS

The days are gone when the pain system could be rationally viewed as a simple labeled-line switchboard designed to propagate a specific pain signal from peripheral Aδ and C nociceptors to pain perception centers in the CNS. The contemporary scheme stresses ongoing and injury-provoked modulation. In the presence of central sensitization pain can be signaled by large- as well as by small-diameter afferents. Both nociceptive and low-threshold inputs play two roles: they signal sensory events and they participate in the setting of central excitability states. Finally, impulses originating from ectopic sources make major contributions to both processes. This new perspective holds out an abundance of potentially exploitable opportunities for the improvement of clinical pain management.

Acknowledgment

The author's work on pain mechanisms is supported primarily by the U.S.-Israel Binational Science Foundation, the German-Israel Foundation for Research and Development, the Israel Science Foundation, and the Hebrew University Center for Research on Pain.

References

1. Devor M, Basbaum AI, Bennett GJ, et al. Mechanisms of neuropathic pain following peripheral injury. In: Basbaum A, Besson JM, eds. Towards a new pharmacology of pain. Chichester: Dahlem Konferenzen, Wiley, 1991;417–440.

2. Diamond J, Mills LR, Mearow KM. Evidence that the Merkel cell is not the transducer in the mechanosensory Merkel cell-neurite complex. In: Hamann W, Iggo A, eds. Progress in Brain Research, vol 74. Amsterdam: Elsevier 1988;51–56.

3. Hille B. Ionic channels of excitable membranes. 2nd ed. Sunderland, MA: Sinauer, 1992.

4. Loewenstein WR. Mechano-electric transduction in Pacinian corpuscle: initiation of sensory impulses in mechanoreceptors. In: Iggo A, ed. Handbook of sensory physiology, vol 1. New York: Springer, 1971;267–290.

5. Erxleben C. Stretch-activated current through single ion channels in the abdominal stretch receptor organ of the crayfish. J Gen Physiol 1989;94:1071–1083.

6. Hamill OP, McBride DW Jr. The cloning of a mechano-gated membrane ion channel. Trends Neurosci 1994;17:439–443.

7. Sachs F. Biophysics of mechanoreception. Membrane Biochem 1986;6:173–192.

8. Jack JJB, Noble D, Tiens RW. Electric current flow in excitable cells. Oxford, UK: Clarendon, 1983.

9. Matzner O, Devor M. Na^+ conductance and the threshold for repetitive neuronal firing. Brain Res 1992;597:92–98.

10. Devor M, White DM, Goetzl EJ, Levine JD. Eicosanoids, but not tachykinins, excite C-fiber endings in rat sciatic nerve-end neuromas. Neuroreport 1992;3:21–24.

11. Devor M, Lomazov P, Matzner O. Na^+ channel accumulation in injured axons as a substrate for neuropathic pain. In: Boivie J, Hansson P, Lindblom U, eds. Touch, temperature and pain in health and disease. Wenner-Gren Center Foundation Symposia. Seattle: IASP Press, 1994;207–230.

12. Gold MS, Reichling DB, Shuster MJ, Levine JD. Hyperalgesic agents increase a tetrodotoxin-resistant Na+ current in nociceptors. Proc Natl Acad Sci U S A 1996;93:1108–1112.

13. Levine J, Taiwo Y. Inflammatory pain. In: Wall PD, Melzack R, eds. Textbook of pain. 3rd ed. London: Churchill-Livingston, 1994;45–56.

14. Vallbo AB, Hagbarth KE, Torebjork HE, Wallin BG. Somatosensory, proprioceptive, and sympathetic activity in human peripheral nerves. Physiol Rev 1979;59:919–957.

15. Apkarian AV. Functional imaging of pain: new insights regarding the role of the cerebral cortex in human pain perception. Semin Neurosci 1995;7:279–293.

16. Guilbaud G, Bernard JF, Besson JM. Brain areas involved in nociception and pain. In: Wall PD, Melzack R, eds. Textbook of pain. 3rd ed. London: Churchill Livingstone, 1994;113–128.

17. Hsieh JC, Belfrage M, Stone-Elander S, et al. Central representation of chronic ongoing neuropathic pain studied by positron emission tomography. Pain 1995;63:225–236.

18. Basbaum A, Fields HL. Endogenous pain control systems: brain-stem spinal pathways and endorphin circuitry. Ann Rev Neurosci 1984;7:309–338.

19. Schmidt RF, Schaible HG, Meslinger K, et al. Silent and active nociceptors: structure, function, and clinical implications. In: Gebhart GF, Hammond DL, Jensen TS, eds. Progress in pain research and management, vol 2. Seattle: IASP Press 1994;213–250.

20. Devor M. The pathophysiology of damaged peripheral nerve. In: Wall PD, Melzack R, eds. Textbook of pain. 3rd ed. London: Churchill Livingstone, 1994;79–100.

21. Nordin M, Nystrom B, Wallin U, Hagbarth KE. Ectopic sensory discharges and paresthesiae in patients with disorders of peripheral nerves, dorsal roots and dorsal columns. Pain 1984;20:231–245.

22. Nystrom B, Hagbarth KE. Microelectrode recordings from transected nerves in amputees with phantom limb pain. Neurosci Lett 1981;27:211–216.

23. Ochoa J, Torebjork HE. Paraesthesiae from ectopic impulse generation in human sensory nerves. Brain 1980;103:835–854.

24. Torebjork HE, Vallbo AB, Ochoa JL. Intraneural microstimulation in man: its relation to specificity of tactile sensations. Brain 1987;110:1509–1529.

25. Sheen K, Chung JM. Signs of neuropathic pain depend on signals from injured fibers in a rat model. Brain Res 1993;610:62–68.

26. Gracely RH, Lynch SA, Bennett GJ. Painful neuropathy: altered central processing, maintained dynamically by peripheral input. Pain 1992;51:175–194.

27. Rasminsky M. Hyperexcitability of pathologically myelinated axons and positive symptoms in multiple sclerosis. In: Waxman SG, Ritchie JM, eds. Demyelinating diseases: basic and clinical electrophysiology. New York: Raven Press, 1981;289–297.

28. England JD, Happel LT, Kline DG, et al. Sodium channel accumulation in humans with painful neuromas. Neurology 1996;47:272–276.

29. Matzner O, Devor M. Hyperexcitability at sites of nerve injury depends on voltage-sensitive Na$^+$ channels. J Neurophysiol 1994;72:349–357.

30. Rizzo MA, Kocsis JD, Waxman SG. Selective loss of slow and enhancement of fast Na$^+$ currents in cutaneous afferent DRG neurons following axotomy. Neurobiol Dis 1995;2:87–96.

31. Waxman SG, Kocsis JD, Black JA. Type III sodium channel mRNA is expressed in embryonic but not in adult spinal sensory neurons, and is reexpressed following axotomy. J Neurophysiol 1994;72:466–470.

32. Heumann R, Lindholm D, Bandtlow C, et al. Differential regulation of mRNA encoding nerve growth factor and its receptor in rat sciatic nerve during development, degeneration and regeneration: role of macrophages. Proc Natl Acad Sci U S A 1987;84:8735–8739.

33. Zur KB, Oh Y, Waxman SG, Black JA. Differential up-regulation of sodium channel α- and α$_1$-subunit mRNAs in cultured embryonic DRG neurons following exposure to NGF. Brain Res Mol Brain Res 1995;30:97–103.

34. Laduron PM. Axonal transport of presynaptic receptors. In: Smith RS, Bisby M, eds. Axonal transport. New York: Liss, 1987;347–363.

35. Welk E, Leah JD, Zimmerman M. Characteristics of A- and C-fibers ending in a sensory nerve neuroma in the rat. J Neurophysiol 1990;63:759–766.

36. Devor M, Keller CH, Ellisman MH. Spontaneous discharge of afferents in a neuroma reflects original receptor tuning. Brain Res 1990;517:245–250.

37. Koschorke GM, Meyer RA, Tillman DB, Campbell JN. Ectopic excitability of injured nerves in monkey: entrained responses to vibratory stimuli. J Neurophysiol 1991;65:693–701.

38. Fields HL, Rowbotham MC, Devor M. Excitability blockers: anticonvulsants and low concentration local anesthetics in the treatment of chronic pain. In: Dickenson AH, Besson JM, eds. Handbook of experimental pharmacology, vol 130. The pharmacology of pain. Heidelberg: Springer Verlag, 1997;93–116.

39. Vierck CJ Jr, Hamilton DM, Thornby JI. Pain reactivity of monkeys after lesions to the dorsal and lateral columns of the spinal cord. Exp Br Res 1971;13:140–158.

40. Melzack R, Wall PD. Pain mechanisms: a new theory. Science 1965;150:971–979.

41. Hardy JD, Wolf HG, Goodell H. Pain sensations and reactions. New York: Williams & Wilkins, 1952.

42. Lewis T. Pain. New York: Macmillan, 1942.

43. Coderre TJ, Katz J, Vaccarino AL, Melzack R. Contribution of central neuroplasticity to pathological pain: review of clinical and experimental evidence. Pain 1993;52:259–285.

44. Koltzenburg M, Torebjork HE, Wahren LK. Nociceptor modulated central sensitization causes mechanical hyperalgesia in acute chemogenic and chronic neuropathic pain. Brain 1994;117:579–591.

45. LaMotte RH, Shain D, Simone DA, Tsai EF. Neurogenic hyperalgesia: psychophysical studies of underlying mechanisms. J Neurophysiol 1991;66:190–211.

46. Meyer RA, Campbell JN, Raja SN. Peripheral neural mechanisms of nociception. In: Wall PD, Melzack R, eds. Textbook of pain. 3rd ed. London: Churchill Livingstone, 1994;13–44.

47. Torebjork HE, Lundberg LER, LaMotte RH. Central changes in processing of mechanoreceptive input in capsaicin-induced secondary hyperalgesia in humans. J Physiol 1992;448:765–780.

48. Cook AJ, Woolf CJ, Wall PD, et al. Dynamic receptive field plasticity in rat spinal dorsal horn following C-primary afferent input. Nature 1987;325:151–153.

49. Willis W, ed. Hyperalgesia and allodynia. New York: Raven Press, 1992;1–400.

50. Woolf CJ. Excitability changes in central neurons following peripheral damage, In: Willis WD Jr , ed. Hyperalgesia and allodynia. New York: Raven Press, 1991;221–243.

51. Woolf CJ, Thompson SWN. The induction and maintenance of central sensitization is dependent on N-methyl D-aspartic acid receptor activation: implications for the treatment of postinjury pain hypersensitivity states. Pain 1991;44:293–299.

52. Niv D, Devor M. Does preemptive analgesia work, and why? Pain Rev 1996;3:79–90.

53. Woolf CJ, Chong MS. Preemptive analgesia: treating postoperative pain by preventing the establishment of central sensitization. Anesth Analg 1993;77:362–379.

54. Devor M. Central changes mediating neuropathic pain. In: Dubner R, Gebhart GF, Bond MR, eds. Pain research and clinical management, vol 3. Amsterdam: Elsevier, 1988;114–128.

55. Kaas JH, Merzenich MM, Killackey HP. The reorganization of somatosensory cortex following peripheral nerve damage in adult and developing mammals. Ann Rev Neurosci 1983;6:325–356.

56. Katz J, Vaccarino AL, Coderre TJ, Melzack R. Injury prior to neurectomy alters the pattern of autotomy in rats: behavioral evidence of central neural plasticity. Anaesthesiology 1991;75:876–883.

57. Dubner R, Ruda M. Activity-dependent neuronal plasticity following tissue injury and inflammation. Trends Neurosci 1992;15:96–103.

58. Deleted.

59. Janig W, Koltzenburg M. What is the interaction between the sympathetic terminal and the primary afferent fiber? In: Basbaum AI, Besson JM, eds. Towards a new pharmacotherapy of pain: Dahlem workshop reports. Chichester: John Wiley & Sons, 1991;331–352.

60. Santini M. Towards a theory of sympathetic-sensory coupling: the primary sensory neuron as a feedback target of the sympathetic terminal. In: Zotterman Y, ed. Sensory function of the skin in primates with special reference to man, Oxford, UK:Pergamon Press, 1976;15–35.

61. Blumberg H, Janig W. Clinical manifestations of reflex sympathetic dystrophy and sympathetically maintained pain. In: Wall PD, Melzack R, eds. Textbook of pain. 3rd ed. London: Churchill Livingstone, 1994;685–697.

62. Bonica JJ. Causalgia and other reflex sympathetic dystrophies. In: Bonica JJ, ed. The management of pain. 2nd ed. Philadelphia: Lea & Febiger, 1990;220–243.

63. Janig W, Schmidt RF, eds. Reflex sympathetic dystrophy: pathophysiological mechanisms and clinical implications. Weinheim, New York: VCH Verlagsgesellschaft, 1992.

64. Burchiel KJ. Spontaneous impulse generation in normal and denervated dorsal root ganglia: sensitivity to alpha-adrenergic stimulation and hypoxia. Exp Neurol 1984;85:257–272.

65. Devor M, Janig W. Activation of myelinated afferents ending in a neuroma by stimulation of the sympathetic supply in the rat. Neurosci Lett 1981;24:43–47.

66. Habler HJ, Janig W, Koltzenburg M. Activation of unmyelinated afferents in chronically lesioned nerves by adrenaline and excitation of sympathetic efferents in the cat. Neurosci Lett 1987;82:35–40.

67. Perl ER. A reevaluation of mechanisms leading to sympathetically related pain. In: Fields HI, Liebeskind JC, eds. Pharmacological approaches to the treatment of chronic pain: new concepts and critical issues. Seattle: IASP Press, 1994;129–150.

68. Sato J, Perl ER. Adrenergic excitation of cutaneous pain receptors induced by peripheral nerve injury. Science 1991;608–1610.

69. Sato J, Suzuki S, Iseki T, Kumazawa T. Adrenergic excitation of cutaneous nociceptors in chronically inflamed rats. Neurosci Lett 1993;164:225–228.

70. Xie Y, Zhang J, Petersen M, Lamotte RH. Functional changes in dorsal root ganglion cells after chronic nerve constriction in the rat. J Neurophysiol 1995;73:1811–1820.

71. Roberts WJ. A hypothesis on the physiological basis for causalgia and related pains. Pain 1986;24:297–311.

72. Chen Y, Michaelis M, Janig W, Devor M. Adrenoreceptor subtype mediating sympathetic-sensory coupling in injured sensory neurons. J Neurophysiol 1996;76:3721–3730.

73. Devor M, Janig W, Michaelis M. Modulation of activity in dorsal root ganglion (DRG) neurons by sympathetic activation in nerve-injured rats. J Neurophysiol 1994;71:38–47.

74. McLachlan EM, Janig W, Devor M, Michaelis M. Peripheral nerve injury triggers noradrenergic sprouting within dorsal root ganglia. Nature 1993;363:543–546.

75. Sherman RA, Sherman CJ, Parker L. Chronic phantom and stump pain among American veterans: results of a survey. Pain 1984;18:83–95.

76. Devor M. Phantom pain as an expression of referred neuropathic pain. In: Sherman RA, Devor M, Casey Jones DE, et al., eds. Phantom pain. New York: Plenum, 1996;33–57.

77. Haber WB. Reactions to loss of limb: physiological and psychological aspects. Ann N Y Acad Sci 1956;75:624–636.

78. Melzack R. Phantom limbs, the self and the brain. Can Psychol 1989;30:1–16.

79. Szasz TS. Pain and pleasure: a study of bodily feeling. New York: Basic Books, 1957.

80. Katz J, Melzack R. Pain "memories" in phantom limbs: review and clinical observations. Pain 1990;43:319–336.

81. Jensen TS, Krebs B, Nielsen J, Rasmussen P. Immediate and long-term phantom pain in amputees: incidence, clinical characteristics and relationship to pre-amputation pain. Pain 1985;21:268–278.

82. Weinstein J, Gordon S, eds. Low back pain: a scientific and clinical overview. Rosemont, IL: American Academy of Orthopaedic Surgeons, 1996.

83. Nowicki BH, Haughton VM, Schmidt TA, et al. Occult lumbar lateral spinal stenosis in neural foramen subjected to physiologic loading. Am J Neuroradiol 1996;17:1605–1614.

84. Kuslich SD, Ulstro CL, Michael CJ. The tissue origin of low back pain and sciatica. Orthop Clin North Am 1991;22:181–187.

85. Fromm GH, Sessle BJ, eds. Trigeminal neuralgia: current concepts regarding pathogenesis and treatment. Boston: Butterworth-Heinemann, 1991.

86. Adams CBT. Microvascular compression: an alternative view and hypothesis. J Neurosurg 1989;57:1–12.

87. Rappaport ZH, Devor M. Trigeminal neuralgia: the role of self-sustaining discharge in the trigeminal ganglion (TRG). Pain 1994;56:127–138.

88. Amir R, Devor M. Chemically-mediated cross-excitation in rat dorsal root ganglia. J Neurosci 1996;16:4733–4741.

CHAPTER 3

Transition from Acute to Chronic Pain

David Niv and Marshall Devor

INTRODUCTION

The acute pain that is felt at the moment of an impact or injury results from the activation of nociceptive sensory endings in the affected skin or deep tissue. Often this is the end of the story. Pain hits and is gone in minutes. This chapter addresses pains that persist and with events that occur *after* the moment of acute impact. Prolonged pains, the ones that have real effects on the lives of people, cannot be understood strictly in terms of acute pain processes that last. Rather, real-life pains, particularly in chronic pain patients, reflect a series of transitions in which ever more complex physiological and psychosocial processes come into play in sculpting the pain experience.

We discuss two such transitions. The first is the transition of pain from the moment of the acute noxious event to a subacute state that may last for hours, days, or weeks. This includes pain from everyday injuries such as muscle sprains, minor burns, and infections, as well as more serious events, such as pain from frank wounds and surgery. The second transition is from subacute to chronic pain. The individual begins with a short-term, supposedly self-limiting pain and a well-founded expectation that he or she will soon be out of the woods. Only gradually does the person become aware that things are not as they should be and that pain is likely to become a major player in his or her life. For both of these transitions we consider the physiological processes that may be involved, as well as the experiential ones faced by the pain patient.

THE TRANSITION FROM ACUTE TO SUBACUTE PAIN

Two Types of Sensitization

The transition from acute to subacute pain involves the initiation of two distinct types of sensitization: peripheral, or inflammatory, and central. The term peripheral sensitization describes events that play out within the injured tissue itself beginning shortly following the injury. Specifically, a complex array of chemical and cellular mediators of inflammation is mobilized from within the tissue and from the circulatory system (1, 2). The inflammatory mediators sensitize nociceptor endings in the skin and deep tissue and cause them to generate sensory impulses in response to stimuli that would otherwise be too weak. The results are the familiar tenderness of the skin on light touch (allodynia and hyperalgesia) and soreness and aching of deep tissue (muscles, tendons, joints, and so on), particularly on movement. The role of peripheral sensitization in subacute pain has been appreciated for many years. A good deal is known about the underlying biology (1–5), and a wide array of effective anti-inflammatory agents, most notably nonsteroidal anti-inflammatory drugs (NSAIDs), are available to combat it.

The second type, central sensitization, has only recently become widely accepted as a major factor in subacute pain (6–8). Central sensitization is an abnormal degree of amplification of the incoming sensory signal in the central nervous system (CNS), particularly in the spinal cord. Think of the pain system as a public address facility, with a microphone, an amplifier, and loudspeakers. Your voice is the sensory stimulus; the sound coming out of the loudspeakers is the level of pain perception. Peripheral sensitization would occur if the microphone were damaged and put out a bigger signal than usual. Central sensitization would occur if someone turned up the volume on the amplifier. Both result in more sound (pain) for a given stimulus. The two types of sensitization usually occur together.

The neurophysiological mechanism of central sensitization is understood today with a fair degree of confidence. Briefly, conditions that trigger central sensitization cause a temporary increase in the synaptic strength of preexisting but previously subliminal spinal synaptic terminals. This yields more effective drive, that is, amplification, of postsynaptic spinal neurons, which signal pain to a conscious brain (9–11). Some of the details are given in Chapter 2. A key aspect of the central sensitization mechanism is the involvement of a specific type of receptor for the spinal cord neurotransmitter glutamate. This glutamate receptor, the NMDA (*N*-methyl-D-aspartate) receptor, is a potential target for the development of novel analgesic drugs.

The sensory amplification brought about by central sensitization differs in many ways from that brought about by peripheral sensitization. The most important difference is that peripheral sensitization acts almost exclusively on nociceptor endings in peripheral tissue, mostly C fibers (1, 2). Even before injury and inflammation, the activation of these sensory endings evokes pain sensation. Peripheral sensitization simply renders them more responsive. Central sensitization amplifies the signal of nociceptors, but it also amplifies the signal of low-threshold A β sensory fibers (touch-sensitive fibers). In particular, it causes A β touch input to be felt as pain (12–20). For example, there is now abundant evidence that mechanical allodynia (tenderness) felt when stroking sunburned or bruised skin comes not just from sensitized nociceptors but also from activity in A β fibers. In light of the classical dogma that A β fibers mediate touch and vibration sense, while C and A δ nociceptors mediate pain sensation, the discovery of A β-evoked pain is nothing short of a revolution in thinking. What causes central sensitization?

Central Sensitization Triggered by Noxious Stimuli

A large series of experiments in animals and in humans have shown that a brief (seconds) noxious conditioning stimulus to afferent C fibers is capable of igniting spinal central sensitization that lasts a few tens of minutes or even longer. A simple example is when a small burn is made on the forearm or a patch of irritant chemical, usually mustard oil or capsaicin, is injected under the skin or applied topically. This noxious conditioning stimulus produces tenderness in the area directly affected by the burn or the irritant, the area of primary hyperalgesia, but also in a substantial zone of intact *surrounding* skin, the area of secondary hyperalgesia (13–15).

Tenderness in the area of primary hyperalgesia is due largely to the activation of sensitized nociceptors. In contrast, in the surrounding area, tenderness is due to spinal amplification of otherwise normal touch input (mechanical allodynia). That is, it is due to central sensitization. The conclusion that allodynia in the surrounding area (the area of secondary hyperalgesia) is signaled by impulses in low-threshold A axons, not by peripherally sensitized nociceptors, is based on experiments using selective nerve block, reaction time measurement, and intraneural and transcutaneous recording and stimulation (13–19).

Secondary hyperalgesia is a dynamic phenomenon that fades away when the noxious stimulus that triggers it ceases (8, 19). Once ignited, it can probably persist indefinitely if maintained by an ongoing noxious barrage. For example, it

persists for as long as nociceptor impulses continue to arise in the area of primary hyperalgesia. But when this maintaining barrage falls silent, as when skin that was directly affected by the noxious stimulus is locally anesthetized, central sensitization and hence secondary hyperalgesia fade within a few minutes, at most a few hours (15–20).

The Experience of Subacute Pain

Subacute pain involves a variable degree of unpleasantness and suffering and a greater or lesser degree of physical incapacitation. The physical incapacitation is partly due to the fact that movement usually activates sensitized nociceptors and centrally sensitized A β afferents, evoking stabs of pain with each breath or each step. A second factor in the incapacitation is the feeling of weakness, somnolence, exhaustion, and general illness that typically accompanies subacute pain to a greater or lesser extend. Wall (21) has argued that these suppressive symptoms are part of an adaptive mechanism designed by evolution to get animals in the wild (and people) away from their normal activities and back to their lairs (homes). The aim is to facilitate tissue repair. The physiological mechanisms of feeling ill have only begun to be explored in earnest. Early evidence suggests that this feeling is a systemic effect brought about by the release of specific neuroimmune mediators into the bloodstream (22–25).

The transition from acute to subacute pain is also accompanied by a range of emotional reactions. These often include fear, anxiety, anger, and helplessness, natural reactions to suddenly finding oneself a patient in a strange and sometimes threatening medical environment. There may also be feelings of embarrassment, sheepishness, or remorse: "How could I have been so irresponsible/unlucky/selfish/stupid as to get into this situation?" Whatever the emotional response in the subacute stage, it is likely to be grounded in apparent reality and to be seen that way by family, friends, and caretakers. There has been unequivocal injury, and therefore there is no special reason to doubt the fundamental veracity of the pain report, be the patient a stolid stoic or a flighty hysteric. The patient, family, friends, and caretakers are in an emergency mode, with every expectation that the storm will soon pass and that in short order things will get back to normal.

Preventing or Preempting the Transition from Acute to Subacute Pain

The mainstay drug treatments for acute and subacute pain are (*a*) NSAIDs, which act to reduce levels of inflammatory mediators in the tissue, and (*b*) opiates, which activate an endogenous CNS pain control mechanism. A number of clinical trials are testing the efficacy of NMDA receptor antagonists as a means of suppressing pain amplification due to central sensitization. However, the discovery that central sensitization is triggered by nociceptor input from the periphery suggested an alternative approach to overcoming or, more precisely, avoiding the effects of central sensitization. The idea is to prevent the induction of central sensitization in the first place by blocking the arrival of nociceptive input to the spinal cord. Of course, this strategy, preemptive analgesia, is applicable only when one knows in advance that an intensely noxious input is about to arrive. As a practical matter, this means that preemptive analgesia is a potential strategy for minimizing the subacute pain felt in the hours and days following surgery.

For those scheduled to undergo surgery, one knows in advance that the CNS is about to be bombarded with an intense nociceptive impulse barrage originating in the region of the operation. This is just the sort of signal that is likely to trigger central sensitization. Animal experiments have shown that conscious awareness of the noxious input is not required for the development of central sensitization. The process occurs at the spinal level and is not thought to be prevented by general anesthesia (discussed in more detail later). Thus, even though the noxious C fiber input generated during surgery is not felt by the anesthetized patient, it may nonetheless trigger central sensitization in the spinal cord that may persist well into the postoperative period when the patient is awake. Central sensitization may therefore be a major contributor to postoperative pain. To prevent (preempt) the initiation of central sensitization, one must prevent the noxious signal generated during the surgery from reaching the spinal cord. In principle, this could be accomplished with regional analgesia (e.g., nerve blocks, epidural opiates) or systemic analgesia (e.g., opiates) as a supplement to general anesthesia before the first surgical incision is made (26).

Experiments in animals suggest that preemptive analgesia may also work in man. For example, injection of formalin into the skin of the paw increases the electrophysiological responsiveness of spinal dorsal horn neurons, a measure of central sensitization. Intrathecal μ-opiate agonists given before the injection of formalin into the skin of the paw inhibits the sensitization, while the same opiates given just after the formalin (i.e., after entry of the conditioning C volley into the spinal cord) have much less effect. Corresponding results have been obtained in a number of behavioral studies. For example, preemptive local anesthetic block of the acute phase of pain evoked by intracutaneous formalin injection (the conditioning stimulus) reduces the late phase of hyperalgesia otherwise evoked by the formalin. These studies have been reviewed by Coderre et al. (8).

Clinical Trials of Preemptive Analgesia

The animal data continue to prompt a considerable number of clinical trials designed to evaluate the effect of intraoperative analgesia on postoperative pain. There were antecedents to this type of clinical research. Long before the idea of preemptive analgesia caught on, there was considerable clinical expe-

rience comparing postoperative pain following surgery done under regional block versus under general anesthesia. This experience is reflected in the common dictum of veteran anesthesiologists that patients do better with regional anesthesia with regard to both postsurgical discomfort and general recovery. The idea of preemptive analgesia, however, says something more. Specifically, it predicts that antinociceptive measures taken *prior* to surgery under general anesthesia should reduce postoperative pain more than the same measures taken *after* the surgery. Timing is the essence. Counterintuitive as it may seem, the proposal is to provide analgesic cover for the surgical field even though the patient is fully anesthetized and totally unresponsive to even intense noxious stimuli.

The modern clinical trials fall into two groups (27, 28). Virtually all of those carried out before the hypothesis of preemptive analgesia was put forward, and many of those carried out since, compare postoperative pain in patients who were operated (*a*) under general versus regional anesthesia, (*b*) under general anesthesia with versus without the addition of preincisional local anesthesia, or (*c*) under general anesthesia with versus without the addition of opioids or NSAIDs. This literature, which is summarized in Tables 3.1–3.5 and in the section in this chapter on anesthesia supplemented by analgesia (29–66), contributes to the knowledge of postoperative pain relief provided by different intraoperative analgesic techniques. However, it does not test the idea of preemptive analgesia, and in particular, it does not illuminate the role of central sensitization in the transition from acute to subacute pain.

The second group of studies *does* constitute a test of the essence of preemptive analgesia. Unlike the first group of studies, in the second group the *identical* analgesic technique was applied to experimental and control patients, with the only difference being timing: presurgical analgesia in experimental group patients and postsurgical analgesia in control group patients. Only in this way can the effect of preemption be separated from the multitude of pharmacological and pharmacokinetic differences that distinguish, say, regional from general anesthesia. This literature is summarized in Tables 3.6–3.12 and in the section in this chapter on anesthesia supplemented by presurgery versus postsurgery analgesia (67–96).

Anesthesia Supplemented by Analgesia

Representatives of the first group trials are summarized in Tables 3.1 to 3.5. The general picture supports the efficacy of supplementing anesthesia with analgesia. The studies are grouped as follows:

Surgery under General or Regional Anesthesia with and without Infiltration of the Wound with Local Anesthetics (Table 3.1)

These studies almost uniformly report that in the patients who received supplemental local anesthetic infiltration, postoperative pain scores and/or postoperative use of analgesics

Table 3.1.   Surgery under General or Regional Anesthesia with and without Wound Infiltration with Local Anesthetics

Investigator Procedure	Patients Trial Type	Treatment Drug, Route	Premedication	Anesthetic	Postoperative Pain Relief?
Patel et al. (29) Cholecystectomy	40 DB/R	Bupivacaine, local infiltration at closure of wound	Not stated	General anesthesia	Yes
Ringrose and Cross (30) Knee joint surgery	100 NB	Bupivacaine, nerve block	Omnopon	Nitrous oxide, fentanyl	Yes
Moss et al. (31) Cholecystectomy	149 RS	Bupivacaine, local infiltration at closure of wound	Not stated	General anesthetics	Yes
McQuay et al. (32) Orthopedic procedures	631 RS	Local anesthestics block, regional or spinal	No opioid premedication	General anesthetics	Yes
Tuffin et al. (33) Molar tooth extraction	84 DB/R	Bupivacaine or prilocaine plus fenylpressing, local infiltration	Temazepam, droperidol	Nitrous oxide, enflurane	Yes
Tverskoy et al. (34) Inguinal hernia repair	24 DB/R	Bupivacaine, infiltration	Promethazine	Nitrous oxide, halothane	Yes
Fisher and Meller (35) Limb amputation	31 NB	Bupivacaine, convous nerve sheath block	Not stated	General anesthesia	Yes
Rademaker et al. (36) Cholecystectomy	30 DB/R	Bupivacaine, nerve block	Diazepam	Halothane	Yes
Mogensen et al. (37) Upper abdominal surgery	50 DB/R	Bupivacaine, infiltration	Not stated	Nitrous oxide, enflurane, thoracic epidural analgesia	Yes
Jebeles et al. (38) Tonsillectomy	14 DB/R	Bupivacaine, local infiltration	Not stated	Nitrous oxide, isofluran	Yes
Christie and Chen (39) Cesarean section	28 OC	Half wound, bupivacaine, infiltration, 2nd half saline	None	Epidural bupivacinae and sulfentanil	Yes
Milligan et al. (40) Lumbar discectomy	60 DB/R	Bupivacaine, wound infiltration	Temazepam	Morphine, nitrous oxide, isoflurane	Yes
Dierking et al. (41) Herniorraphy	28 DB/R	Bupivacaine, infiltration at closure of wound	Diazepam	Nitrous oxide, alfentanil	Yes
Johansson et al. (42) Cholecystectomy	66 DB/R	Ropivacaine, infiltration	Meperidine	Fentanyl, thiopental, nitrous oxide, isiflurane	No
Ganta et al. (43) Cesarean section	62 DB/R	Bupivacaine, ilioinguinal block, wound infiltration	None	Nitrous oxide, isoflurane	Yes
Shenfeld et al. (44) Inguinoscrotal surgery	90 DB/R	Bupivacaine, wound irrigation	Chloralhydrate	Halothane, nitrous oxide	Yes

NB,not blinded; RS, Retrospective; OC, patients served as their own controls; DB, Double blind; R, randomized.

are reduced 4 to 12 hours into the postoperative period. Although in many of the studies the authors discuss the results in terms of preemptive analgesia, this is unwarranted. In fact, in several cases, local anesthetic infiltration was performed at the end of the surgery, just before wound closure (29, 31, 39–41). This surely would not have blocked noxious peripheral input. Yet in these studies too, the treatment group had less postoperative pain than the controls.

It is true that the nerve-blocking effects of the local anesthetics are likely to have worn off before the postoperative pain evaluation was carried out. However, local anesthetic drugs infiltrating local tissues and carried into the systemic circulation are known to have analgesic effects at much lower concentrations than those required to block nerve conduction, and these effects persist far longer than nerve block (97–99). Thus, at the time of assessment, the treatment group had an analgesic drug on board (regional and systemic local anesthetic) that the control group did not have. In addition to the analgesic effects of low concentrations of regional and systemic local anesthetics, it has been suggested that these drugs may have anti-inflammatory effects, either by a direct or an indirect action on cells that release chemical mediators of inflammation. Finally, local anesthetics may affect axoplasmic transport mechanisms (97, 100). All three of these factors may contribute to a carry-over of analgesia well into in the postoperative period.

Surgery under General Anesthesia with and without Preincisional Administration of Spinal or Epidural Local Anesthetics (Table 3.2)

Only one of five studies in this group (47) failed to show improved postoperative pain control in patients in whom general anesthesia was supplemented with epidural analgesia. The authors of this study considered that no difference was found because of incomplete blockade of nociceptive afferents by the epidural bupivacaine. To test this, in a separate group they used a higher dose of epidural bupivacaine. In this group they did obtain superior pain relief and reduced opioid requirement in the postoperative period. As in the trials summarized in Table 3.1, the direct analgesic effect of the systemic dose of

Table 3.2.   Surgery under General Anesthesia with and without Preincisional Administration of Spinal or Epidural Local Anesthetics

Investigator Procedure	Patients Trial Type	Treatment Drug, Route	Premedication	Anesthetic	Postoperative Pain Relief?
Cullen et al. (45)	30	Bupivacaine, epidural	Diazepam	General anesthesia	Yes
Major abdominal operations	DB/R				
Tverskoy et al. (34)	24	Bupivacaine, spinal anesthesia	Promethazine	Nitrous oxide, halothane	Yes
Inguinal hernia repair	DB/R				
Heard et al. (46)	137	Lidocaine, spinal	Midazolam	Nitrous oxide, isofluran	Yes
Knee surgery	DB				
Shir et al. (47)	62	Bupivacaine, epidural	Morphine	Nitrous oxide, morphine, isoflurane	No
Prostatectomy	DB/R				
Wang et al. (48)	90	Bupivacaine, epidural or spinal	None	Nitrous oxide, halothane	Yes
Cesarean section	DB/R				

DB, double blind; R, randomized.

local anesthetic undermines any conclusion with respect to preemptive analgesia.

Surgery under General Anesthesia with and without Preincisional Administration of Systemic Opioids (Table 3.3)

Again, four of five trials showed favorable effects. In these studies the experimental group had the preoperative dose of opiates and the control group did not. Unlike the case of systemic local anesthetics, with which quite long-lasting analgesic effects occur, it could be argued that this preoperative opioid dose was no longer in effect during the postoperative period. This argument has some merit, and it supports the belief that maximizing intraoperative antinociception minimizes postoperative pain.

Surgery under General or Regional Anesthesia with and without Preincisional Administration of Systemic NSAIDs (Table 3.4)

All seven of the studies advocate the addition of NSAIDs to general or regional anesthesia to achieve better postoperative pain relief. It is likely that the improved analgesic effects obtained in the treated groups compared with the placebo control groups resulted mostly from the anti-inflammatory effect of the drug at the wound site.

Multimodal Analgesia before Surgery versus None (Table 3.5)

The large majority of these studies obtained superior pain control in the treatment group. Again, by maximizing intraoperative antinociception, better postoperative pain relief can be obtained. However, it is not possible to draw reliable inferences concerning preemptive analgesia.

The results of the first group of studies affirm the common clinical experience that presurgical analgesia yields the benefit of reduced postoperative pain. The studies, however, are not able to establish whether this result is due to analgesic drug carryover into the postoperative period, reduced need for

and use of general anesthetic agents, or prevention of central sensitization. As far back as 1913, Crile (101) warned of the "stressful stimuli" associated with surgery and recommended regional anesthesia as a means of protecting the CNS against the metabolic consequences of noxious input. Is there merit to this belief?

Anesthesia Supplemented by Presurgery versus Postsurgery Analgesia: The Idea of Preemptive Analgesia

Tables 3.5 to 3.12 summarize the second group of trials, which compare presurgical with postsurgical analgesia as a supplement to anesthesia. Reduced postsurgical pain in patients receiving analgesia before the first incision would support the idea that central sensitization plays an important role in postsurgical pain. No difference would favor the conclusion that drug carryover or reduced anesthetic use is the primary reason for the success of the first group of trials. Unfortunately, neither outcome is a clear winner. Although many studies found no difference between the experimental and control group patients, some found a modest but statistically significant benefit to preincisional analgesia.

Comparison of the Effect of Presurgical versus Postsurgical Local Anesthetic Blockade on Postoperative Pain (Table 3.6)

Ringrose et al. (30) used femoral nerve block in patients undergoing knee surgery under general anesthesia with nitrous oxide and fentanyl. The patients who had preemptive block received less opiate analgesia postoperatively. However, the study was not run blind, and the evaluation of how much opiate to give was at the discretion of the nursing staff. Two other studies with similar protocols obtained contradictory results (67, 68). Ejlersen et al. (67) found in patients having herniorrhaphy that preoperative local infiltration with lidocaine increased the time to first request for analgesics. On the other hand, Dierking et al. (68) found no significant difference in

Table 3.3. Surgery under General Anesthesia with and without Preincisional Administration of Systemic Opioids

Investigator Procedure	Patients Trial Type	Studied Drug, Route	Premedication	Anesthetic	Postoperative Pain Relief?
McQuay et al. (32) Orthopaedic procedures	830 Retrospective	Opioids	None	General anesthetics	Yes
Campbell and Kendrick (49) Molar tooth extraction	160 DB/R	Fentanyl, intravenous or diclofenac, IM or IV	Diazepam halothane	Nitrous oxide	No
Kiss and Killian (50) Lumbar disc surgery	98 prospective	Pethidine, IM with triflupromazine or flunitrazepam, oral	Studied drugs given as premedication	Nitrous oxide, Fentanyl, halothane or enflurane or isoflurane	Yes
Tverskoy et al. (51) Hysterectomy	27 DB/R	Fentanyl, IV or ketamine, IV	Midazolam	Isoflurane alone or with fentanyl or with ketamine	Yes
Katz et al. (52) Hysterectomy	45 DB/R	Alfentanil, intravenous	Diazepam	Nitrous oxide, isoflurane	Yes

DB, double blind; IM, intramuscular; IV, intravenous; R, randomized.

Table 3.4. Surgery under General or Regional Anesthesia with and without Preincisional Administration of Systemic NSAIDs

Investigator Procedure	Patients Trial Type	Treatment Drug, Route	Premedication	Anesthetic	Postoperative Pain Relief?
Dueholm et al. (53) Femoral in inguinal herniotomy	60 DB/R	Naproxen, suppository	Diazepam	Nitrous oxide, halothane	Yes
Hutchison et al. (54) Molar tooth extraction	50 DB/R	Piroxicam, oral	None	Nitrous oxide, enflurane	Yes
Campbell and Kendrick (49) Molar tooth extraction	120 DB/R	Diclofenac, IM or IV	Diazepam	Nitrous oxide, halothane	Yes
McGlew et al. (55) Spine surgery	10 DB/R	Indomethacin, suppository	Pethidine Diazepam Metoclopramide	Nitrous oxide, halothane, orenflurane	Yes
Bianchi et al. (56) Prostatectomy	15 DB/R	Ketorolac, IM	None	Spinal anesthesia	Yes
Kokki et al. (57) Lower abdomen	81 DB/R	Ibuprofen, rectal	Flunitrazepam;	Spinal anesthesia	Yes

DB, double blind; NSAIDs, nonsteroidal anti-inflammatory drugs; R, randomized.

postoperative pain in patients having an inguinal field block before versus after herniorrhaphy under general anesthesia.

Turner and Chalkiadis (69) tested lidocaine infiltration of the surgical wound site before and after surgical appendectomy. They did not find any difference in postoperative pethidine requirements in the two groups. However, before surgery the patients had acute pain for which they were given opioids, a possibly confounding factor (discussed later). Two studies compared the effect of subcutaneous infiltration of bupivacaine before and after abdominal hysterectomy (71) or hernioplasty in children (72). There was no difference in either study.

The effect of local anesthetic infiltration was also tested in patients undergoing tonsillectomy under general anesthesia. In a trial of pretonsillectomy infiltration versus no infiltration, Jebeles et al. (38) found a favorable effect of the local anesthetic, although this study does not speak to the efficacy of preemptive analgesia. Orntoft et al. (70) repeated this study using pretonsillectomy versus posttonsillectomy infiltration. They concluded

that there was no difference in postoperative pain between the two groups and thus in their study no evidence of a preemptive analgesic effect. A novel approach for postcholecystectomy pain relief was recently studied by Pasqualucci et al. (73). Bupivacaine sprayed into the peritoneal cavity at the beginning of surgery induced significantly more postoperative pain relief than did use of the bupivacaine spray at the end of surgery.

Presurgery versus Postsurgery Epidural Analgesia Using Local Anesthetics (Table 3.7)

Three studies (74, 75, 77) examined the effect of caudal epidural block with local anesthetics in children undergoing ambulatory operations under general anesthesia (hypospadias, herniorrhaphy, hydrocele repair, orchiopexy, circumcision). There was no significant difference in pain or use of analgesics postoperatively between caudal block given before surgery and that given at the end of surgery. Three other studies in the

Table 3.5.   Multimodal Analgesia before Surgery versus None

Investigator Procedure	Patients Trial Type	Treatment Drug, Route	Premedication	Anesthetic	Postoperative Pain Relief?
Hill et al. (58) Molar tooth extraction	114 DB/R	Ibuprofen with or without codeine, oral and local anesthetics, local infiltration	—	Local anesthetics	Yes
Dupuis et al. (59) Molar tooth extraction	20 DB/crossover	Flurbiprofen, oral	—	Carbocaine	Yes
McQuay et al. (32) Orthopaedic procedures	596 Retrospective	Opioid, oral with local anesthetics, nerve block	—	General anesthetics	Yes
Bugedo et al. (60) Inguinal hernia repair	45 DB/R	Bupivacaine, Local infiltration Lignocaine, spinal	Diazepam	Lignocaine, spinal	Yes
Smith and Brook (61) Molar tooth extraction	38 DB/R	Fenbufen, oral and local anesthetics	—	Local anesthetics	No
Mogensen et al. (37) Upper abdominal surgery	50 DB/R	Bupivacaine, Local Infiltration	Not stated	Nitrous oxide enflurane with morphine, bupivacaine epidural	Yes
Kavanagh et al. (62) Thoracotomy	7 DB/R	Morphine, IV Indomethacin, PR Bupivacaine, Nerve block	Midazolam	Nitrous oxide, isofluran, fentanyl	Yes
Cade and Ashley (63) Vaginal termination of pregnancy	834 DB/R	Parcetamol, oral	—	Nitrous oxide, enflurane	No
Atallah et al. (64) Hypospadias repair	30 DB/R	Bupivacaine, morphine, epidural and subpubic block	Diazepam	Nitrous oxide, halothane	Yes
Kavanagh et al. (65) Thoracic surgery	30 DB/R	Morphine, IM perphenazine, IM indomethazine, supp. bupivacaine, intercostal block	Midazolam	Nitrous oxide, isoflurane, fentanyl	No
Bartholdy et al. (66) Abdominal surgery	20 DB/R	bupicacaine and morphine, thoracic epidural; local anesthetics, infiltration of surgical area	Diazepam	Nitrous oxide, enflurane	Yes

DB, double blind; IM, intramuscular; IV, intravenous; PR, rectally; R, randomized.

Table 3.6.   Surgery under General Anesthesia with Presurgical versus Postsurgical Local Infiltration with Local Anesthetics

Investigator Procedure	Patients Trial Type	Treatment Drug, Route	Premedication	General Anesthetic	Preemptive Analgesia?
Ringrose and Cross (30) Knee joint surgery	20 NB	Bupivacaine, nerve block	Omnopon	Nitrous oxide, fentanyl	Yes
Ejlersen et al. (67) Inguinal hernia repair	37 DB/R	Lidocaine, local infiltration	Diazepam	Nitrous oxide, isoflurane	Yes
Dierking et al. (68) Inguinal hernia repair	32 DB/R	Lidocaine, local infiltration	Diazepam	Nitrous oxide, alfentanil	No
Turner and Chalkiadis (69) Appendectomy	90 DB/R	Lidocaine, local infiltration	Opioids or other analgesics	Nitrous oxide, "volatile agent," fentanyl	No
Orntoft et al. (70) Tonsillectomy	35 DB/R	Bupivacaine, local infiltration	Diazepam	Nitrous oxide, isoflurane	No
Victory et al. (71) Hysterectomy	56 DB/R	Bupivacaine, local infiltration	Diazepam sufentanil	Nitrous oxide, sufentanil	No
Dahl et al. (72) Hernioplasty in children	50 DB/R	Bupivacaine, local infiltration	—	Nitrous oxide, halothane, paracetamol	No
Pasqualucci et al. (73) Cholecystectomy	120 DB/R	Bupivacaine, intraperitoneal	Diazepam	Fentanyl, nitrous oxide, isoflurane	Yes

DB, double blind; NB, not blinded; R, randomized.

Table 3.7.   Surgery under General Anesthesia with Presurgical versus Postsurgical Administration of Epidural Local Anesthetics

Investigator Procedure	Patients Trial Type	Treatment Drug, Route	Premedication	General Anesthetic	Preemptive Analgesia?
Rice et al. (74) Herniotomy, orchiopexy, hydrocelectomy	40 DB/R	Bupivacaine, caudal	Not stated	Nitrous oxide, halothane	No
Gunter et al. (75) Hypospadias repair	24 DB/R	Bupivacaine, caudal block	Not stated	Nitrous oxide, halothane	No
Pryle et la. (76) Abdominal hysterectomy, myomectomy	36 DB/R	Bupivacaine, epidural	Morphine	Nitrous oxide, enflurane	No
Holthusen et al. (77) Circumcision	25 DB/R	Lidocaine, caudal block	Midazolam	Nitrous oxide, halothane	No
Katz et al. (78) Lower abdominal surgery	42 DB/R	Bupivacaine, epidural	Midazolam	Nitrous oxide, isoflurane	Yes
Nakamura et al. (79) Hysterectomy	90 DB/R	Mepivacaine, Epidural	Diazepam	Nitrous oxide, sevoflurane	Yes
Dakin et al. (80) Hysterectomy	38 DB/R	Bupivacaine, spinal	Morphine	Nitrous oxide, enflurane	No

DB, double blind; R, randomized.

epidural local anesthetics group tested the effect of presurgical versus postsurgical treatment in adults undergoing lower abdominal operations (76, 78, 79). All were performed under general anesthesia using nitrous oxide and a gas anesthetic (enflurane, isoflurane, and sevoflurane). In two of the studies (78, 79), the use of epidural local anesthetics (bupivacaine and mepivacaine respectively) before surgery significantly reduced postoperative pain and analgesic requests compared with use of the same drugs at the end of surgery. In the third study (76), however, no such preemptive effect was observed.

Presurgery versus Postsurgery Epidural Analgesia Using Local Anesthetics and Opioids (Table 3.8)

In two separate studies using epidural morphine plus bupivacaine in patients undergoing major abdominal surgery or total knee arthroplasty, Dahl et al. (81, 82) did not find a significant benefit of preemptive analgesia. They concluded that the timing of perioperative analgesia using a conventional epidural regimen has no major clinical importance for postoperative pain.

Presurgery versus postsurgery epidural analgesia using opioids (Table 3.9)

The one trial of epidural opioids without local anesthetics found evidence of preemptive analgesia. Katz et al. (83) gave epidural fentanyl either prior to thoracotomy or 15 minutes after the incision. The group with preemptive treatment had significantly lower pain intensity as measured with the Visual Analog Scale (VAS) 6 hours postoperatively. At 12 to 24 hours the pain scores equalized, but only because of the somewhat larger amounts of morphine drawn from the patient-controlled analgesia (PCA) units by the group that received fentanyl postincisionally.

Presurgery versus Postsurgery Systemic Opioids (Table 3.10)

Richmond et al. (84) reported that intravenous morphine given before versus just after surgery for abdominal hysterectomy yielded a 27% reduction in the consumption of opiates (PCA) during the first 24 hours postoperatively and a reduction in the tenderness of skin near the scar. This experimental design was later repeated by Collis et al. (87), using a higher dose of morphine (20 mg versus 10 mg in the initial study). Slightly better (preemptive) analgesia was obtained, but at the cost of an unacceptable level of nausea. A dose ceiling appears to have been encountered.

These positive results encouraged additional studies on abdominal hysterectomy using other opioids. Wilson et al. (85) and Mansfield et al. (86) tested the effect of intravenous alfentanil administered before versus after making the incision in patients about to undergo hysterectomy. Unfortunately, neither found a significant group difference that would have indicated preemptive analgesia. A possible caveat is that alfentanil is a shorter-acting opiate than morphine. Also, in both studies opiate cover was present in both experimental and control groups during the bulk of the surgical procedure.

Another potentially important factor is that the alfentanil dose may have been too low. Wilson et al. (85) used 40 $\mu g/kg$ alfentanil and Mansfield et al. (86) used only 15 $\mu g/kg$. For comparison, Katz et al. (52, 102) studied the effects of presurgically administered alfentanil 30 versus 100 $\mu g/kg$. The surgery was again hysterectomy. Pain reports and morphine consumption (PCA) using the 30-μ/kg dose were no different from those of a third group that received no opiates at all. The higher dose was only marginally more effective, although it produced sufficient sedation to permit the surgery to be carried out using nitrous oxide alone, without a gas anesthetic. These observations, together with the dose-response study of Collis et al. (87), indicate that if there is an effective dose window for

Table 3.8.   Surgery under General Anesthesia with Presurgical versus Postsurgical Administration of Epidural Local Anesthetics plus Opioids

Investigator Procedure	Patients Trial Type	Treatment Drug, Route	Premedication	General Anesthetic	Preemptive Analgesic?
Dahl et al. (81) Colonic surgery	32 DB/R	Bupivacaine with morphine, epidural	Diazepam	Nitrous oxide, enflurane, fentanyl	No
Dahl et al. (82) Knee Joint Surgery	32 DB/R	Bupivacaine with morphine, epidural	Diazepam	Nitrous oxide, enflurane, fentanyl	No

DB, double blind; randomized

Table 3.9.   Surgery under General Anesthesia with Presurgical versus Postsurgical Administration of Epidural Opioids

Investigator Procedure	Patients Trial Type	Treatment Drug, Route	Premedication	General Anesthetic	Preemptive Analgesic?
Katz et al. (83) Thoractomy	30 DB/R	Fentanyl, epidural	Diazepam	Nitrous oxide, isoflurane	Yes

DB, double blind; R, randomized.

Table 3.10.   Surgery under General Anesthesia with Presurgical versus Postsurgical Administration of Systemic Opioids

Investigator Procedure	Patients Trial Type	Treatment Drug, Route	Premedication	General Anesthetic	Pre emptive Analgesic?
Richmond et al. (84) Hysterectomy	60 DB/R	Morphine, intravenous	Morphine	Nitrous oxide, enflurane	Yes
Wilson et al. (85) Skin incision	40 DB/R	Alfentanil, intravenous	Temazepam	Nitrous oxide, enflurane	No
Mansfield et al. (86) Skin incision	60 SB/R	Alfentanil, intravenous	Temazepam	Nitrous oxide, enflurane	No
Collins et al. (87) Hysterectomy	60 DB/R	Morphine, intravenous	Temazepam	Nitrous oxide, enflurane	Yes
Sarantopoulos and Fassoulaki (88) Hysterectomy	39 DB/R	Sufentanil, intravenous	Midazolam	Nitrous oxide, isoflurane	No

DB, double blind; R, randomized; SB, single blind.

systemic opiates, it is quite narrow. Unfortunately, none of the patients studied by Katz et al. (52, 102) received 100 µg/kg alfentanil postsurgically, so no conclusions can be drawn from this study concerning preemptive analgesia itself. Recently Sarantopoulus and Fassoulaki (88) conducted a similar study on hysterectomies using sufentanil. They found that presurgery sufentanil was not more beneficial for postoperative pain control than postsurgery administration.

Presurgery versus postsurgery systemic NSAIDs (Table 3.11)

Flath et al. (89) administered the NSAID flurbiprofen before versus 3 hours after tooth pulpectomy. There was no difference between pain scores of the two groups 7 and 24 hours later. Similar results were obtained by Sisk et al. (90) and Sisk and Grover (91) using an NSAID, either diflunisal or naproxen,

given before versus 30 minutes after third molar extraction. In all three studies, surgery was performed under local anesthetic block. This in itself would have preempted the development of central sensitization due to the surgery per se. Nonetheless, the groups that received the NSAID presurgically might have had some benefit from being spared noxious input associated with nonincisional manipulations in the oral cavity and from earlier protection from postsurgical inflammation.

Different results with NSAID were obtained in two orthopaedic studies. Bünemann et al. (92) tested the effect of naproxen in patients undergoing short orthopaedic procedures under fentanyl-propofol anesthesia. A significant difference in pain scores was found only in the first postoperative hour in favor of the group receiving naproxen before surgery. Fletcher et al. (93) obtained longer pain relief in patients undergoing total hip replacement under general anesthesia

Table 3.11.   Surgery under General or Regional Anesthesia with Presurgical versus Postsurgical Administration of Systemic NSAIDs

Investigator Procedure	Patients Trial Type	Treatment Drug, Route	Premedication	General Anesthetic	Preemptive Analgesic?
Flath et al. (89) Pulpectomy	120 DB/R	Flurbiprofen, oral	None	Local anesthesia, block	No
Sisk et al. (90) Removal of impacted molar	20 WS	Diflunisal, oral	None	Local anesthesia, block, midazolam IV	No
Sisk and Grover (91) Impacted molar	36 WS	Naproxen, oral	None	Local anesthesia, block, midazolam IV	No
Bünemann et al. (92) Outpatient orthopaedic surgery	180 DB/R	Naproxen, not stated	None	O_2 in air, fentanyl, propofol	Yes (1st h)
Fletcher et al. (93) Hip replacement	60 DB/R	Ketorolac, intravenous	Hydroxyzine	Nitrous oxide, Fentanyl, Isoflurane	Yes
Vanlersberghe et al. (94) Minor orthopaedic surgery	60 DB/R	Ketorolac, intravenous	Diazepam	Nitrous oxide, halothane	No

DB, double blind; R, randomized; SB, single blind; WS, within subject design; NSAIDs, nonsteroidal anti-inflammatory drugs.

with fentanyl and nitrous oxide. In the first 6 postoperative hours patients who received intravenous ketorolac prior to surgery had less pain than those receiving ketorolac after the operation. However, Vanlersberghe et al. (94) failed to replicate these findings using intravenous ketorolac.

Presurgery versus Postsurgery Multimodal Analgesic Approach (Table 3.12)

One final set of trials deserves special mention. In two groups of patients undergoing major surgery, a combination of different types of analgesics with different mechanisms of action were tested before versus after surgery (95, 96). Both groups of authors found that a preemptive effect can be obtained if maximal blockade of nociception is practiced.

Lessons on the Transition from Acute to Subacute Pain

The effectiveness of supplemental antinociceptive measures taken while the patient is anesthestized is most conservatively interpreted as persistence of action of the analgesics into the postoperative period. Whether there is also a benefit from preemption can be determined only through the second group of trials, and here the answer is equivocal. Does this mean that the development of central sensitization is not an important factor in the transition from acute to subacute pain? Why are the benefits of preemptive analgesia not more striking?

Triggering of Central Sensitization Postoperatively

In their original animal studies, Woolf (6), Cook et al. (9), Woolf and Thompson (10), Woolf and Wall (103), and Woolf et al. (104) stressed that it is sufficient to provide a minimal conditioning C volley to evoke central sensitization. Likewise, in the human psychophysical studies noted earlier, secondary hyperalgesia is evoked by a fairly modest chemical or thermal burn. The tissue-wrenching stimuli associated with surgery are

not a necessary condition. Even modest noxious input in the postoperative period may kindle full-blown central sensitization. All of the clinical trials of preemptive analgesia involved invasive, tissue-injuring surgical procedures. Even skillfully applied regional anesthesia probably does not totally block input associated with surgery. But even if it did, what happens when the block begins to wear off? In every case a surgical wound, a sure source of C fiber input, is present. We (27) call this the Hydra problem after the many-headed mythological monster who, when one head was severed, instantly grew another one in its place. Central sensitization is expected to appear with the first hint of postoperative pain.

Niv et al. (105) used a novel research protocol that permits administration of controlled doses of noxious input in a clinical surgical setting. They examined two groups of patients who underwent childbirth with analgesia provided by epidural bupivacaine. One group was given 2 mg morphine epidurally on completion of episiotomy and prior to the onset of pain; the second group was given saline. Later, if and when a predetermined amount ("dose") of pain occurred in the area of the episiotomy, the second group was given 2 mg morphine epidurally and the first saline. The group that received morphine preemptively reported considerably better pain control overall, even though part of their morphine dose had been "wasted" on a period when bupivacaine cover was present. The group not given preemptive epidural morphine needed much more than 2 mg of morphine to control pain. It appears to be easier to prevent pain than to eliminate it once it has developed. The only way to avoid inducing central sensitization postoperatively, that is, to avoid the Hydra problem, may be to block all pain originating in the surgical field from the time of initial incision until final wound healing.

Routine Anesthetic Protocols May Already Incorporate Preemptive Analgesia

A second reason for the somewhat disappointing results of the second group of clinical trials is that many of the benefits of preemptive analgesia may already be captured in con-

Table 3.12.   Surgery under General Anesthesia with Presurgical versus Postsurgical Multimodal Analgesic Approaches

Investigator Procedure	Patients Trial Type	Treatment Drug, Route	Premedication	General Anesthetic	Preemptive Analgesic?
Richardson et al. (95) Thoracotomy	56 DB/R	Diclofenac/PR morphine/IM bupivacaine/paravertebral continuous intercostal block	Fentanyl propofol	Nitrous oxide isoflurane	Yes
Rockmann et al., (96) Major abdominal surgery	142 DB/R	Diclofenac/IM metamizole/IV mepivacaine and morphine/epidural	Fentanyl thiopental	Nitrous oxide enflurane	Yes

DB, double blind; IM, intramuscular; IV, intravenous; PR, rectally; R, randomized.

ventional protocols of surgery under general anesthesia. In the studies reviewed, various supplemental analgesics, often fentanyl or alfentanil and always nitrous oxide, were used before and during the surgery. Pain ratings were relatively low in all groups, including the controls. These analgesics may well have blunted the central sensitization that might otherwise have developed in the patients from whom regional block was withheld until after surgery. In this way they may have masked an advantage that would otherwise have accrued in the group given preemptive analgesia. The trials that showed the most prominent effect of preemptive analgesia (83, 84, 87) scrupulously avoided the use of preoperative opiates in the control (postincisional) group. This is appropriate for the research. However, routine anesthetic practice almost always includes supplemental analgesics (106, 107).

In fact, some of the agents routinely used in general anesthesia may themselves obtund central sensitization and hence deliver preemptive analgesia. In the state of surgical anesthetic unconsciousness, pain is not felt. However, it cannot be taken for granted that noxious inputs reaching the spinal cord during all types of anesthesia are able to trigger central sensitization. In their animal experiments Woolf (6), Cook et al. (9), Woolf and Thompson (10), Woolf and Wall (103), and Woolf et al. (104) took specific precautions to avoid general anesthetics during the time that noxious conditioning stimuli were delivered and electrophysiological recordings were made. They frequently point out, for example, that the central sensitizing effects of noxious inputs are much less dramatic when experiments are carried out in animals under barbiturate anesthesia.

The mechanisms whereby general anesthetic agents act on neural circuitry and the regional differences in these effects are largely unknown. Some agents, however, clearly have a profound suppressive effect on spinal cord excitability (108–110). Suppression of spinal responses to nociceptive input from the periphery is expected to block central sensitization in the same way that opiates do, although this prediction should be checked experimentally for each agent. The most commonly used inhalation anesthetics, isoflurane and halothane, apparently do not themselves block central sensitization at the spinal level (111).

Remarkably, there is experimental evidence in rats that 75% nitrous oxide does block central sensitization (112), perhaps by the same mechanism as opiates (113). If this finding is reliable and extends to man, all surgery carried out today using nitrous oxide, which includes virtually all surgeries under gas anesthesia including the work listed in Tables 3.6–3.12, already captures much of what preemptive analgesia has to offer. In the few positive trials this masking effect may have been only partial. One caveat, however, must be noted. While Goto et al. (112) showed that nitrous oxide itself induces preemptive analgesia, their results indicate that the addition of halothane partly antagonizes this effect (111). This antagonism is both unexpected and unexplained, but if true, it tends to temper the conclusion that nitrous oxide provides preemptive analgesia. More research on this point is needed.

One final factor should be considered in evaluating the clinical trials of preemptive analgesia and hence the role of central sensitization in subacute pain. The central aim of general anesthesia is to make surgery pain free. General anesthetic agents, however, vary in their intrinsic analgesic effect. When supplemental analgesic drugs are used, a surgical plane of anesthesia can usually be obtained using lower doses of general anesthetics. This benefit, of course, is obtained only when the supplemental analgesics are given before the surgery, not when given afterward. It is possible that what is taken as preemptive analgesia is in fact a reflection of reduced use of general anesthetic agents.

The Role of Central Sensitization in Subacute Pain

Despite the equivocal results of the trials of preemptive analgesia, it cannot be concluded that central sensitization plays no role in postoperative pain or in the transition from acute to subacute pain in general. The reasons are that the clinical trials probably failed to prevent postoperative triggering of central sensitization (the Hydra problem) and that the anesthetic protocols used in many of the studies may have inadvertently preempted the development of central sensitization in the control as well as the experimental arms of the study. Evaluation of the true importance of central sensitization in subacute pain, that is, evaluation of the *degree* of amplification caused by central versus peripheral sensitization, will have to depend on other types of clinical evidence.

THE TRANSITION FROM SUBACUTE TO CHRONIC PAIN

Persistence of Subacute Pain

In a substantial number of patients with subacute pain, relief is not obtained and the pain becomes chronic. The transition to chronicity is not a sudden definable event, but rather a drawn-out process. It involves a characteristic set of changes in the outlook of the patient and on the way he or she is viewed and treated by the family, caretakers, and society. It may also reflect a specific set of changes in the underlying neural mechanism. If so, the transition may have crucial consequences for prognosis and treatment options. This possibility is discussed later in the chapter. We stress at the outset, however, that the human experience of the transition to chronicity is unlikely to be related in any direct fashion to late neurophysiological changes triggered by the injury or disease.

After how long can a pain be said to be chronic? If there were a defined change in underlying neural mechanism, this change could serve as a yardstick of transition to chronicity. However, no such indicator is available at present. Rather, the transition to chronicity reflects a gradual realization by the patient and physician that the pain isn't going away in the time frame that was hoped for. That is, whether a pain lasting 3 weeks can be defined as chronic or one has to wait 3 months or 3 years must be determined with reference to the prior expectations of the individuals involved. Ideally, these expectations are based on epidemiological knowledge of the natural history of pain in the particular condition and risk category involved. The time at which a prolonged pain can be called chronic is an actuarial matter, the tail of a statistical distribution.

The likelihood that pain will become chronic varies greatly with the specific condition and according to the physical status and the age of the patient. For example, the likelihood of pain lasting more than a few weeks after a simple appendectomy is very low. In contrast, it has been estimated that nearly half of patients who undergo thoracotomy are left with a burning or aching scar pain a year and more after the surgery (114). Likewise, painful eruptions of herpes zoster usually resolve within about 2 to 3 weeks, but in some patients an intense burning or stabbing pain lasts much longer. This is postherpetic neuralgia (PHN). PHN lasting more than 1 year can be expected in about 4% of patients 10 to 20 years of age, in about 18% of patients 50 to 60 years of age, and in about 48% of patients older than 70 years (115) (see Chapter 7).

Behavioral Changes Induced by Subacute Pain May Contribute to or Even Cause Transition to Chronicity

Whether or not the transition to chronicity involves a specific change in the underlying pain mechanism, this transition may be accelerated or exacerbated by behavioral responses of the patient. For example, a patient may respond to subacute pain by prolonged and exaggerated inactivity or by adopting an abnormal posture or gait. Such secondary behavioral changes, if maintained over time, can actually trigger painful disorders of the spine; osteoporosis; degenerative changes of joints, bones, and connective tissue; and even fractures and skeletal deformation.

Another facet of pain behavior that often contributes to a transition to chronicity is the emotional and cognitive responses of the patient and his or her associates. These are partly due to the pain itself and partly due to disability and its significance to the patient. Prolonged pain almost always imposes severe emotional, physical, economic, and social stresses on the patient, family, and society (116, 117). Unfortunately, these very real stresses have a tendency to be self-reinforcing. A patient whose response to pain is extreme, for whatever reason, is likely to suffer from depression; anger; feelings of helplessness and hopelessness; preoccupation with the pain problem; dependency on medication, caretakers, and the health care system; and generally impaired interpersonal functioning. Likewise, the people around him or her may come to feel abused and resentful, especially if the patient's response appears to them to be out of proportion to the physical disorder. The veracity of the patient's pain report comes into question, leading to the suspicion, sometimes justified, of exploitation for secondary gains. This may plunge the patient still deeper into isolation and despair.

All of these responses reinforce one another in a vicious circle leading to ever-increasing disability, depression, and suffering. The underlying pain, in the meantime, may have remained stable or even subsided somewhat. Pain behavior and associated emotional and psychological dysfunction can become the crux of the problem (116–118). An important part of the art of pain management is to disentangle pain from the complex psychosocial responses to it. This theme is taken up in considerable detail in later chapters in this volume.

During the acute and subacute phases a manifest lesion is often present, and the psychosocial picture is at baseline. But as time goes by and the psychosocial terrain surrounding the patient begins to change, it becomes increasingly difficult to know how much of the pain picture is sensory and how much reactive. This is partly because of the fundamental subjectivity, the privateness, of pain experience. An additional factor, however, is our still-fuzzy understanding of neural mechanisms in chronic pain conditions and our lack of tools capable of providing objective evidence. In some patients the main sensory burden of the pain may have faded, leaving a condition of suffering and disability that is framed around pain but that is in fact largely a psychosocial residue. In other patients, the pain processes may be irreversible from the beginning because of the nature of the underlying neurophysiology. Psychosocial changes in such patients are an added burden to an already sad plight. In still others, the pain condition may have been treatable or self-limiting at the beginning but changed with time, becoming intractable. If such patients actually exist, and if they could be reliably identified, their transition to chronicity might in principle be prevented.

Centralization of Pain

There is a venerable belief in the clinical literature that intense pain left untreated eventually "burns its way into the CNS." This process is called centralization. The presumption is that there is a fundamental change in the mechanism of pain such that treatments that may have been effective earlier on cease to be effective. The belief in pain centralization has had considerable influence on pain theory and practice for many years (discussed later). In the past decade it has received a strong boost from the observation of central sensitization triggered by noxious stimuli. The logic is simple. If a minor, brief noxious stimulus induces transient central sensitization, surely an intense, prolonged pain must produce persistent central sensitization. This logic is further supported by the observation that noxious inputs and nerve injuries rapidly (hours) induce regulatory immediate early genes such as c-fos and c-jun and after a somewhat longer latency (days) affect the expression of genes with a likely effector role (e.g., dynorphin [119]). Changes in gene expression could lead to persistent structural changes in synapses, hence in relevant neural networks. Indeed, there are numerous examples of long-lasting change in CNS anatomy and physiology following chronic nerve injury (120), although not yet following prolonged pain without nerve injury. But is there evidence to justify the extrapolation from transient central sensitization to pain centralization? Let us examine two of the classic examples in which centralization of pain is widely believed to be the firmly established.

Early Aggressive Treatment in Type 1 Complex Regional Pain Syndrome

The first example is reflex sympathetic dystrophy (RSD), recently renamed type 1 complex regional pain syndrome (CRPS1) (121). In CRPS1 common wisdom holds that if pain is not successfully treated early, it is much more likely to become chronic and hence untreatable (e.g., Bonica [122]). The reason usually offered is that pain eventually becomes centralized, rendering the condition intractable. The belief that untreated CRPS1 is likely to become chronic if not treated aggressively at an early stage is an example of a clinical belief with clear, practical implications for clinical management. Unfortunately, it has never been tested in a controlled prospective study. Rather, it is based on the clinical observation that in CRPS1 patients whose pain does not respond to treatment and does not resolve spontaneously, the pain persists for years and is refractory to treatment. Does the conclusion follow from the observation?

The clinical observation that chronic CRPS1 responds poorly to treatment is undoubtedly accurate. However, the astute reader will catch the circular, self-fulfilling nature of the argument. Imagine that some CRPS1 cases are refractory from the beginning, perhaps because of a particularly grim underlying mechanism. These cases do not resolve spontaneously, nor are they likely to respond to early treatment. Therefore, they persist and eventually are called chronic and intractable. This interpretation of the clinical observations does not require a change in the underlying mechanism. Moreover, it predicts no unique early time window in which standard treatment might have been effective but no longer is. Has the belief in centralization of CRPS1 saved patients from never-ending chronic pain or has it subjected them to ineffective and futile sympathectomies? We are unlikely to know until the appropriate prospective controlled trials are carried out.

Pain Memories in Amputees

A second classic case of presumed centralization of pain is pain memories in amputees (123). Typical examples of pain memories are the many anecdotes of amputees feeling in their phantom limb rings, bunions, sores, and other long-standing preamputation sensations (123–127). Similarly, the position of the phantom is thought often to reflect the last position of the limb prior to amputation. As in CRPS1, it is easy to imagine these persistent inputs inducing a permanent state of central sensitization, hence stamping pain into the nervous system. Unfortunately, it is difficult to know whether these anecdotes, however honestly reported, indeed reflect actual, specific sensations. The alternative possibility is that they represent vivid memories conjured up in suggestible individuals, perhaps with prompting by the attending physician, by qualitatively similar dysesthesias generated by ectopic discharge in injured sensory neurons ("anchoring"). The same problem holds for phantoms that persist despite dorsal rhizotomy or spinal transection. These injuries also trigger (new) deafferentation and central pains that could be rationalized by the patient and his physician as continuation of an old pain that is in fact gone. Controlled, prospective studies are needed.

Jensen et al. (128) made the first prospective effort to relate pains before amputation to the sensory qualities of the phantom limb. In their cohort virtually all of the patients had prolonged limb pain prior to amputation. Immediately after amputation, phantom pain resembled the preamputation pain in location and character in only a third, and after 2 years, in only 10%. Sudden traumatic amputation of previously healthy limbs does not appear to yield many fewer instances of painful phantoms than amputation after extended periods of pain (129, 130), an observation that is inconsistent with the idea of phantom pain being a consequence of centralization. However, this issue has not been studied in a sufficiently systematic manner.

A striking prediction of the idea that phantom limb pain is a result of pain centralization is that preemptive block of limb pain prior to and during amputation should prevent the later development of chronic phantom pain. There is some suggestive evidence to this effect in animal preparations (8, 131–135). In addition, there are three relevant studies of human amputees (136–138). In these, extensive and prolonged analgesic block of the painful limb was carried out before a scheduled therapeutic amputation. The reported result, as predicted, was a lower than expected incidence of phantom pain on follow-up 6 months and 1 year post amputation. Unfortunately, however, the development of phantom limb pain is a notoriously variable and unpredictable event, and we still have too small a sample size and too short a follow-up time to draw definitive conclusions.

The mere fact that in most amputees nerve or spinal block transiently suppresses phantom pain indicates that the generator does not become independent of the periphery even when the pain has lasted for years. A similar conclusion can be drawn from studies of chronic nonphantom pain in patients and in animals. For example, a patient described by Gracely et al. (139) had a localized scar that proved to be the primary source of a long-standing neuropathic pain. This source triggered A β touch-mediated allodynia over a large part of the limb, presumably as a result of central sensitization. Within seconds or minutes of local anesthetic block of the primary ectopic source, the widespread tenderness disappeared, and it returned immediately as the block wore off.

Certainly the vast majority of even very severe and/or prolonged pains, when ultimately relieved, do not leave an indelible trace. Consider the passage of kidney stones, total hip replacement, and childbirth. None of these leave pain memories. The problem is particularly acute with respect to pain memories of events that are only moderately painful or not painful at all. For example, pain memories are said to include the feeling of a heavy plaster cast, an odd but non-painful posture, or a distinctive ring. Noncritical acceptance of the idea that phantom memories reflect pain centralization leads to the clearly mistaken conclusion that almost any pain ever felt should be felt forever. The same conclusion can be drawn for the idea of pain centralization in general. In our opinion, there is no convincing evidence at present that pain per se, however severe and prolonged, can trigger a permanent state of central sensitization.

Long-Term Changes Following Nerve Injury

Injury to peripheral nerves, as distinct from pain per se, triggers a spectrum of long-term changes not related in any obvious way to the nociceptor-driven central sensitization mechanism discussed earlier (120). Changes in the electrical excitability of injured primary afferent neurons in the periphery is a prime example. There is abundant evidence that ectopic firing originating at the nerve injury site and in the associated dorsal root ganglia, among other locations, makes an important contribution to spontaneous neuropathic pain, neuropathic allodynia, and hyperalgesia (Chapter 2). Such peripheral changes may evolve gradually in time and result in chronic pain.

Nerve injury also triggers persistent and slowly evolving changes in the spinal cord and brain. In principle, such CNS changes may form the basis for true centralization in the case of neuropathic pain. For example, when nerves of the foot are cut acutely, dorsal horn neurons in the spinal foot representation cease to respond to peripheral stimuli. However, within a few days (for rats) or weeks (for cats) these cells acquire *new* receptive fields on the nearest adjacent innervated skin, thigh, or lower back. This somatotopic remapping reflects synaptic changes in the CNS and not aberrant regeneration in the periphery (140). As expected, spinal cord and brainstem remapping projects corresponding patterns of remapping onto the cerebral cortex (141), yielding the predicted perceptual correlates in man. For example, upper limb amputees often feel stimuli to the shoulder or cheek as originating in their phantom hand (125, 142). If such functional remapping occurs in the modality domain as it does in the spatial domain, one consequence might be persistent pain in response to light touch. Indeed, it has recently been reported that the extent of cortical remapping in amputees correlates well with phantom pain sensation (143). The cortical change is most likely a simple reflection of spinal central sensitization due to intense ectopic neural activity in the periphery. On the other hand, it may be causal.

Somatotopic remapping almost certainly involves adjustments in synaptic efficacy rather than the formation of new long-distance connections, although short-range sprouting may play a role (120, 144). The trigger may be altered trophic relations between CNS and periphery, perhaps mediated by altered gene expression. A particularly pregnant alternative is that remapping reflects sustained changes in the intensity and pattern of sensory input from the periphery because of ectopic firing, modified patterns of limb use, or both. For example, Clark et al. (145) and Jenkins et al. (146) showed that enhanced nonnoxious sensory input in intact animals can lead to an expansion of the cortical representation of the corresponding body part. This implies that throughout life somatosensory processing circuits adjust dynamically to sensory experience, if with a long time constant, much as in the visual cortex during the critical period of early development.

A number of other centralization mechanisms have been proposed in relation to neuropathic pain. A few examples: (*a*) Nerve injury is known to induce persistent up-regulation of a number of peptide neurotransmitters in dorsal root ganglion (DRG) neurons. Since these play a role in nociceptor-induced central sensitization, they may underlie pain centralization (147, 148). (*b*) Injury discharge triggered by acute nerve injury or ongoing noxious firing may induce excitotoxic damage to spinal inhibitory interneurons, yielding spinal hyperexcitability (119, 134). (*c*) Surround inhibition, as reflected in primary afferent depolarization (PAD), collapses a few days after nerve injury (149), perhaps because of depletion of γ-aminobutyric acid-A (GABA-A) receptors on primary afferent terminals in the spinal cord (150). The resulting disinhibition may yield pain. (*d*) Following nerve injury afferent spikes may invade a higher proportion of collaterals in the preterminal spinal branching network, amplifying residual inputs (151). (*e*) Finally, we should mention the possibility of chronic changes in descending modulation of spinal pain-processing networks. Each of these processes, and others, may yield persistent nerve injury-induced CNS sensitization quite different from the transient nociceptor-driven central sensitization discussed earlier.

Prognostic Indicators of Transition to Chronicity

In nearly all of the subacute pain conditions that sometimes become chronic it is notoriously difficult, often impossible, to predict whose pain will resolve in reasonable time and in whom it will become chronic. The apparent capriciousness of the eventual outcome is a particular source of frustration in conditions in which there is a belief, sound or unsound, that aggressive treatment may prevent the transition to chronicity. The discovery of prognostic indicators would be extremely valuable. For example, if one knew in advance that subacute pain in a particular patient was likely to become chronic, one could apply extreme therapeutic measures, such as the use of costly implantable devices, early in the process. At a minimum, the patient and family could be offered counseling before the agonizing psychosocial consequences of chronic pain set in.

There is evidence from animal studies that the likelihood of developing chronic neuropathic pain following major nerve transection is a heritable trait controlled by one or a small number of autosomal recessive Mendelian genes (152). If this proves to be true in humans as well, it may be possible in the future to develop prognostic tests based on genetic markers. In the meantime, careful clinical observation may provide useful predictive indicators. For example, Katz et al. (153) reported that in postthoracotomy patients, the more severe the pain in the subacute stage, the more likely was it to become a long-term problem. Their conclusion was that early postthoracotomy pain is likely to become centralized and that therefore aggressive early management is indicated. This conclusion, of course, suffers from the logical error discussed above with respect to CRPS1: confusion of a statistical correlation with a causal relation.

SUMMARY AND CONCLUSIONS

The sort of pain that brings people to seek help cannot be understood in terms of the activation of nociceptive sensory endings alone. Rather, shortly after the moment of acute impact, a series of transitions begin to shape the pain experience. In this chapter we discuss the two major transitions that sometimes unfold: the transition from acute to subacute pain and the transition from subacute to chronic pain. The first of these transitions is dominated by a change in the underlying pain neurophysiology. Most notably, pain ceases to be determined strictly by the activity of normal tissue nociceptors and becomes dominated by two sensitization processes: peripheral (inflammatory) sensitization and central sensitization. The hope that one may easily prevent postoperative pain by preventing central sensitization has not been fulfilled, although research on such preemptive analgesia continues.

There is no mistaking that in the presence of subacute pain the patient and caretakers are dealing with real suffering and all its attendant emotional burden. However, for the most part, they are operating on the rational premise that the problem is temporary and will soon pass. The transition from subacute to chronic pain often brings about a qualitative change in the pain experience. With the gradual realization that pain has become a major player in one's life comes a range of complex and not necessarily rational or adaptive psychosocial reactions. These can affect the well-being of the patient as much as the pain itself. There is often an apparent mismatch between the patient's report of pain and the physical evidence of injury or disability. This can drive a wedge of mistrust between the patient and the people around him or her, magnifying the evolving psychosocial distress.

The neural substrates of transition to chronicity are not well understood. The widespread belief that prolonged unrelieved pain can burn its way into the nervous system, becoming intractable because of a fundamental change in mechanism, rests on shaky foundations. It may not be true. In contrast to pain per se, nerve injury is known to trigger a broad range of peripheral and central nervous system changes with the potential for causing chronic pain. A better understanding of the neural mechanisms of chronic pain could benefit patients in many ways: lifting the stigma of mistrust, perhaps providing novel treatment options, and perhaps providing an opportunity to prevent the transition to chronicity in the first place.

Acknowledgment

Our work on pain mechanisms is supported primarily by the U.S.-Israel Binational Science Foundation (BSF), the German-Israel Foundation for Research and Development (GIF), the Israel Science Foundation, the Fritz Thyssen Stiftung, the Hebrew University Center for Research on Pain (M.D.), and the Pain Foundation of the Tel-Aviv Sourasky Medical Center (D.N.).

References

1. Lewis T. Pain. New York: Macmillan, 1942.
2. Levine J, Taiwo Y. Inflammatory pain. In: Wall PD, Melzack R, eds. Textbook of pain. 3rd ed. London: Churchill Livingstone, 1994;45–56.
3. Meyer RA, Campbell JN, Raja SN. Peripheral neural mechanisms of nociception. In: Wall PD, Melzack R, eds. Textbook of pain. 3rd ed. London: Churchill Livingstone, 1994;13–44.
4. Thalhammer JG, LaMotte RH. Spatial properties of nociceptor sensitization following heat injury of the skin. Brain Res 1982;231:257–265.
5. Raja S, Meyer JN, Meyer RA. Peripheral mechanisms of somatic pain. Anesthesiology 1988;68:571–590.
6. Woolf CJ. Evidence for a central component of postinjury pain hypersensitivity. Nature 1983;308:686–688.
7. Willis W, ed. Hyperalgesia and allodynia. New York: Raven, 1992;1–400.
8. Coderre TJ, Katz J, Vaccarino AL, Melzack R. Contribution of central neuroplasticity to pathological pain: review of clinical and experimental evidence. Pain 1993;52:259–285.
9. Cook AJ, Woolf CJ, Wall PD, McMahon SB. Dynamic receptive field plasticity in rat spinal cord dorsal horn following C-primary afferent inputs. Nature 1987;325:151–153.

10. Woolf CJ, Thompson SWN. The induction and maintenance of central sensitization is dependent on N-methyl-D-aspartic acid receptor activation: implications for treatment of post-injury pain hypersensitivity states. Pain 1991;44:293–299.

11. Woolf CJ. Excitability changes in central neurons following peripheral damage: role of central sensitization in the pathogenesis of pain. In: Willis W, ed. Hyperalgesia and allodynia. New York: Raven, 1992:221–244.

12. Hardy JD, Wolf HG, Goodell H. Pain sensations and reactions. New York: Williams & Wilkins, 1952.

13. Raja SN, Campbell JN, Meyer RA. Evidence for the different mechanisms of primary and secondary hyperalgesia following heat injury to the glabrous skin. Brain 1984;107:1179–1188.

14. Campbell JN, Raja SN, Meyer RA, MacKinnon SE. Myelinated afferents signal the hyperalgesia associated with nerve injury. Pain 1988;32:89–94.

15. Torebjörk HE, Lundberg LER, LaMotte RH. Central changes in processing of mechanoreceptive input in capsaicin-induced secondary hyperalgesia in humans. J Physiol 1992;448:765–780.

16. LaMotte RH, Shaine CN, Simone DA, Tsai EFP. Neurogenic hyperalgesia: psychophysical studies of underlying mechanisms. J Neurophysiol 1991;66:190–211.

17. Koltzenburg M, Lundberg LER, Torebjörk HE. Dynamic and static components of mechanical hyperalgesia in human hairy skin. Pain 1992; 51: 207–219.

18. Treede RD, Meyer RA, Raja SN, Campbell JN. Peripheral and central mechanisms of cutaneous hyperalgesia. Prog Neurobiol 1992;38:397–421.

19. Koltzenburg M, Torebjörk HE, Wahren LK. Nociceptor modulated central sensitization causes mechanical hyperalgesia in acute chemogenic and chronic neuropathic pain. Brain 1994;117:579–591.

20. LaMotte RH, Lundberg LER, Torebjörk HE. Pain, hyperalgesia and activity in nociceptive C units in humans after intradermal injection of capsaicin. J Physiol 1992;448:749–764.

21. Wall PD. On the relation of injury to pain. Pain 1979;6:253–264.

22. Frayn KN. Hormonal control of metabolism in trauma and sepsis. Clin Endocrinol 1986;24:577–599.

23. Watkins LR, Maier SF, Goehler LE. Immune activation: the role of proinflammatory cytokines in inflammation, illness responses and pathological pain states. Pain 1995;63:289–302.

24. Yirmiya, R. Endotoxin produces a depressive-like episode in rats. Brain Res 1996;711:163–174.

25. Yirmiya R, Barak O, Avitsur R, et al. Intracerebral administration of Mycoplasma fermentans in rats produces sickness behavior: involvement of prostaglandins. Brain Res 1997;749: 71–81,.

26. Wall PD. The prevention of postoperative pain. Pain 1988;33:289–290.

27. Niv D, Devor M. Does the blockade of surgical pain pre-empt postoperative pain and prevent its transition to chronicity? IASP Newslett 1993;6:2–7.

28. Niv D, Devor M. Pre-emptive analgesia in the relief of postoperative pain. Curr Rev Pain 1996;1:79–92.

29. Patel JM, Lanzafama RJ, Williams JS, et al. The effect of incisional infiltration of bupivacaine hydrochloride upon pulmonary functions, atelectasis and narcotic need following elective cholecystectomy. Surg Gyn Obstetr 1983;157:338–340.

30. Ringrose NH, Cross MJ. Femoral nerve block in knee joint surgery. Am J Sports Med 1984;12:398–402.

31. Moss G, Regal ME, Lichtig L. Reducing postoperative pain, narcotics and length of hospitalization. Surgery 1986;99:206–210.

32. McQuay HJ, Carrol D, Moore RA. Postoperative orthopedic pain: the effect of opiate premedication and local anaesthetic blocks. Pain 1988;33:291–295.

33. Tuffin JR, Cunliffe DR, Shaw SR. Do local analgesics injected at the time of third molar removal under general anaesthesia reduce significantly post operative analgesic requirements? A double-blind controlled trial. Br J Oral Maxillofac Surg 1989;27:27–32.

34. Tverskoy M, Cozacov C, Ayache M, et al. Postoperative pain after inguinal herniorrhaphy with different types of anaesthesia. Anesth Analg 1990;70:29–35.

35. Fisher A, Meller Y. Continuous postoperative regional analgesia by nerve sheath block for amputation surgery: a pilot study. Anesth Analg 1991;72:300–303.

36. Rademaker BMP, Sih IL, Kalkman CJ, et al. Effects of intrapleurally administered bupivacaine 0.5% on opioid analgesic requirements and endocrine response during and after cholecystectomy: a randomized double-blind controlled study. Acta Anaesthesiol Scand 1991;35:108–112.

37. Mogensen T, Bartholdy J, Sperling K, et al. Preoperative infiltration of the incisional area enhances postoperative analgesia to a combined low-dose epidural bupivacaine and morphine regime after upper abdominal surgery. Reg Anesth 1992;17(Suppl 35):74.

38. Jebeles JA, Reilly JS, Gutierrez JF, et al. The effect of preincisional infiltration of tonsils with bupivacaine on the pain following tonsillectomy under general anaesthesia. Pain 1991;47:305–308.

39. Christie JM, Chen GW. Secondary hyperalgesia is not affected by wound infiltration with bupivacaine. Can Anaesth 1993;40:1034–1037.

40. Milligan KR, Macafee AL, Fogarty DJ, et al. Intraoperative bupivacaine diminishes pain after lumbar discectomy: a randomized double-blind study. J Bone Joint Surg 1993;75:769–771.

41. Dierking GW, Ostergaard E, Ostergaard HT, Dahl JB. The effects of wound infiltration with bupivacaine versus saline on postoperative pain and opioid requirements after herniorrhaphy. Acta Anaesthesiol Scand 1994;38:289–292.

42. Johansson BO, Gilse H, Hallaerback B, et al. Preoperative local infiltration with ropivacaine for postoperative pain relief after cholecystectomy. Anesth Analg 1994;78:210–214.

43. Ganta R, Samra SK, Maddineni VR, Furness G. Comparison of the effectiveness of bilateral ilioinguinal nerve block and wound infiltration for postoperative analgesia after cesarean section. Br J Anaesth 1994;72:229–230.

44. Shenfeld O, Eldar I, Lotan G, et al. Intraoperative irrigation with bupivacaine for analgesia after orchiopexy and herniorrhaphy in children. J Urol 1995;153:185–187.

45. Cullen ML, Staren ED, El-Ganzouri A, et al. Contiunous epidural infusion for analgesia after major abdominal operations: a randomized, prospective, double-blind study. Surgery 1985;98:718–728.

46. Heard SO, Edwards WT, Ferari D, et al. Analgesic effects of intraarticular bupivacaine or morphine after arthroscopic knee surgery: a randomized, prospective, double-blind study. Anesth Analg 1992;74:822–826.

47. Shir Y, Raja SN, Frank SM. The effect of epidural versus general anesthesia on postoperative pain and analgesics requirements in patients undergoing radical prostatectomy. Anesthesiology 1994;80: 49–56.

48. Wang JJ, Ho ST, Liu HS, et al. The preemptive effect of regional anesthesia on post-cesarean section pain. Acta Anesthesiol Sin 1995;33:211–216.

49. Campbell WI, Kendrick R. Intravenous diclofenac sodium: does its administration before operation suppress postoperative pain? Anaesthesia 1990;45:763–766.

50. Kiss I, Killian M. Does opiate premedication influence postoperative analgesia? A prospective study. Pain 1992;48:157–158.

51. Tverskoy M, Oz Y, Isakson A, et al. Pre-emptive effect of fentanyl and ketamine on postoperative pain and wound hyperalgesia. Anesth Analg 1994;78:205–209.

52. Katz J, Clairoux M, Redahan C, et al. High dose alfentanil pre-empts pain after abdominal hysterectomy. Pain 1996;68:109–118.

53. Dueholm S, Forrest M, Hjortso NC, Lemvigh E. Pain relief following herniotomy: a double-blind randomized comparison between naproxen and placebo. Acta Anaesthesiol Scand 1989;33:391–394.

54. Hutchison GL, Crofts SL, Gray IG. Preoperative piroxicam for postoperative analgesia in dental surgery. Br J Anaesth 1990;65:500–503.

55. McGlew IC, Angliss DB, Gee GJ, et al. A comparison of rectal indomethacin with placebo for pain relief following spinal surgery. Anesth Intens Care 1991;19:40–45.

56. Bianchi M, Allora A, Panerai AE. A randomized placebo-controlled study on the efficacy of ketorolac tromethamine in the prevention of postoperative pain. Eur J Pain 1993;14:10–13.

57. Kokki H, Hendolin H, Maunuksela EL, et al. Ibuprofen in the treatment of postoperative pain in small children: a randomized double-blind placebo-controlled parallel group study. Acta Anaesth Scand 1994;38:467–472.

58. Hill CM, Carroll MJ, Giles AD, Pickvance N. Ibuprofen given pre- and postoperatively for the relief of pain. Int J Oral Maxillofac Surg 1978;16:420–424.

59. Dupuis R, Lemay H, Bushnetter MC, Dung GH. Preoperative flurbiprofen in oral surgery: a method of choice in controlling postoperative pain. Pharmacotherapy 1988;8:193–200.

60. Bugedo GJ, Carcamo CR, Mertens RA, et al. Preoperative percutaneous ilioinguinal and iliohypogastric nerve block with 0.5% bupivacaine for postherniorrhaphy pain management in adults. Reg Anaesth 1990;15:130–133.

61. Smith AC, Brook IM. Inhibition of tissue prostaglandin synthesis during third molar surgery: use of preoperative fenbufen. Br J Oral Maxillofac Surg 1990;28:251–253.

62. Kavanagh B, Katz J, Sandler A, et al. Is postoperative pain reduced by preoperative multi-modal nociceptive blockade? A randomized, double-blind, placebo-controlled study. Can J Anesth 1992;39:A76.

63. Cade L, Ashley J. Prophylactic paracetamol for analgesia after vaginal termination of pregnancy. Anaesth Intens 1993;21:93–96.

64. Atallah MM, Saied MA, Yahya R, Ghaly AM. Presurgical analgesia in children subjected to hypospadias repair. Br J Anaesth 1993;71:418–421.

65. Kavanagh BP, Katz J, Sandler AN, et al. Multimodal analgesia before thoracic surgery does not reduce postoperative pain. Br J Anaesth 1994;73:184–189.

66. Bartholdy J, Sperling K, Ibsen M, et al. Preoperative infiltration of surgical area enhances postoperative analgesia of a combined low-dose epidural bupivacaine and morphine regimen after upper abdominal surgery. Acta Anaesthesiol Scand 1994;38:262–265.

67. Ejlersen E, Andersen HB, Eliasen K, Mogensen T. A comparison between preincisional and postincisional lidocaine infiltration and postoperative pain. Anesth Analg 1992;74:495–498.

68. Dierking GW, Dahl JB, Kanstrup J, et al. Effect of pre- vs postoperative inguinal field block on postoperative pain after herniorrhaphy. Br J Anaesth 1992;68:344–348.

69. Turner GA, Chalkiadis G. Comparison of preoperative with postoperative lignocaine infiltration on postoperative analgesic requirements. Br J Anaesth 1994;72:541–543.

70. Orntoft S, Longreen A, Moiniche S, Dhal JB. A comparison of pre- and postoperative tonsillar infiltration with bupivacaine on pain after tonsillectomy: a pre-emptive effect? Anaesthesia 1994;94:151–154.

71. Victory RA, Gajarj NM, Elstraete AV, et al. Effect of preincision versus postincision infiltration with bupivacaine on postoperative pain. J Clin Anesth 1995;7:192–196.

72. Dahl V, Raeder JC, Erno PE, Kovdal A. Preemptive effect of preincisional versus post-incisional infiltration of local anesthesia on children undergoing hernioplasty. Acta Anesthesiol Scand 1996;40:847–851.

73. Pasqualucci A, De Angelis V, Contardo R, et al. Preemptive analgesia: intraperitoneal local anesthetic in laparoscopic cholecystectomy. Anesthesiology 1996;85:11–20.

74. Rice LJ, Pudimant MA, Hannallah RS. Timing of caudal block placement in relation to surgery does not affect duration of postoperative analgesia in pediatric ambulatory patients. Can J Anaesth 1990;37:429–431.

75. Gunter JB, Forestner JE, Manley CB. Caudal epidural anesthesia reduces blood loss during hypospadias repair. J Urol 1990;144:517–519.

76. Pryle BJ, Vanner RG, Enriquez N, Reynolds F. Can pre-emptive lumbar epidural blockade reduce postoperative pain following lower abdominal surgery? Anaesthesia 1993;48:120–123.

77. Holthusen H, Eichwede F, Stevens M, et al. Pre-emptive analgesia: comparison of preoperative with postoperative caudal block on postoperative pain in children. Br J Anaesth 1994;73:440–442.

78. Katz J, Clairoux M, Kavanagh BP, et al. Pre-emptive lumbar epidural anaesthesia reduces postoperative pain and patient-controlled morphine consumption after lower abdominal surgery. Pain 1994;59:395–403.

79. Nakamura T, Yokoo H, Hamakawa T, Takasaki M. Pre-emptive analgesia produced with epidural analgesia administered prior to surgery. Masui 1994;43:1024–1028.

80. Dakin MJ, Osinubi OYO, Carli F. Preoperative spinal bupivacaine requirement in women undergoing total abdominal hysterectomy. Reg Anesth 1996;21:99–102.

81. Dahl JB, Hansen BL, Hjorsto NC, et al. Influence of timing on the effect of continuous extradural analgesia with bupivacaine and morphine after major abdominal surgery. Br J Anesth 1992;69:4–8.

82. Dahl JB, Daugaard JJ, Rasmussen B, et al. Immediate and prolonged effects of pre- versus postoperative epidural analgesia with bupivacaine and morphine on pain at rest and during mobilisation after total knee arthroplasty. Acta Anaesthesiol Scand 1994;38:557–561.

83. Katz J, Kavanagh BP, Sandler AN, et al. Pre-emptive analgesia: clinical evidence of neuroplasticity contributing to postoperative pain. Anesthesiology 1992;77:439–446.

84. Richmond CE, Bromley LM, Woolf CJ. Preoperative morphine pre-empts postoperative pain. Lancet 1993;342:73–75.

85. Wilson RJT, Leith S, Jackson IJB, Hunter D. Pre-emptive analgesia from intravenous administration of opioids. Anaesthesia 1994;49:591–593.

86. Mansfield M, Meikle R, Miller C. A trial of pre-emptive analgesia: influence of timing of preoperative alfentanil on postoperative pain and analgesic requirements. Anaesthesia 1994;49:1091–1093.

87. Collis R, Brandner B, Bromley LM, Woolf CJ. Is there any clinical advantage of increasing the pre-emptive dose of morphine or combining pre-incisional with postoperative morphine administration? Br J Anaesth 1995;74:396–399.

88. Sarantopoulos C, Fassoulaki A. Sufentanil does not preempt pain after abdominal hysterectomy. Pain 1996;65:273–276.

89. Flath RK, Lamar Hicks M, Dionne RA, Pelleu GB. Pain suppression after pulpectomy with preoperative flurbiprofen. J Endodont 1987;13:339–347.

90. Sisk AL, Mosley RO, Martin RP. Comparison of preoperative and postoperative diflunisal for suppression of postoperative pain. J Oral Maxillofac Surg 1989;47:464–468.

91. Sisk AL, Grover BJ. A comparison of preoperative and postoperative naproxen sodium for suppression of postoperative pain. J Oral Maxillofac Surg 1990;48:674–678.

92. Bünemann L, Thorshauge H, Herlevsen P, et al. Analgesia for outpatient surgery: placebo versus naproxen sodium (a non steroidal anti-inflammatory drug) given before or after surgery. Eur J Anaesth 1994;11:461–464.

93. Fletcher D, Zetlaoui P, Monin S, et al. Influence of timing on the analgesic effect of intravenous ketorolac after orthopedic surgery. Pain 1995;61:291–297.

94. Vanlersberghe, Lauwers MH, Camu F. Preoperative ketorolac administration has no preemptive analgesic effect for minor orthopedic surgery. Acta Anaesthesiol Scand 1996;40:948–952.

95. Richardson J, Sabaratnam S, Mearns AJ, et al. Efficacy of pre-emptive analgesia and continuous extrapleural intercostal nerve block on postthoracotomy pain and pulmonary mechanics. J Cardiovasc Surg 1994;35:219–228.

96. Rockmann MG, Seeling W, Bischof C, et al. Prophylactic use of epidural mepivacaine/morphine, systemic diclofenac, and methimazole reduces postoperative morphine consumption after major abdominal surgery. Anesthesiology 1996;84:1027–1034.

97. Byers MR, Fink BR, Kennedy RD, et al. Effects of lidocaine on axonal morphology, microtubules, and rapid transport in rabbit vagus nerve in vitro. J Neurobiol 1973;4:125–143.

98. Fields HL, Rowbotham MC, Devor M. Excitability blockers: anticonvulsants and low concentration local anesthetics in the treatment of chronic pain. In: Dickenson AH, Besson JM, eds. Handbook of experimental pharmacology: the pharmacology of pain. Heidelberg: Springer Verlag, 1997; 93–116.

99. Tanelian DL, Victory RA. Sodium channel-blocking agents: their use in neuropathic pain conditions. Pain Forum 1995;4:75–80.

100. Arner S, Lindblom U, Meyerson BA, et al. Prolonged relief of neuralgia after regional anesthetics blocks: a call for further experimental and systemic clinical studies. Pain 1990;43:287–297.

101. Crile GW. The kinetic theory for shock and its prevention through anoci-associated (shockless) operation. Lancet 1913;2:7.

102. Katz J, Redahan C, Clairoux M, et al. High-dose systemic alfentanil pre-empts pain after abdominal hysterectomy: a randomized double-blind study. Can Pain Soc Abstr 1995;A17:58–59.

103. Woolf CJ, Wall PD. Morphine-sensitive and morphine-insensitive actions of c-fibre input on the rat spinal cord. Neurosci Lett 1986;64:221–225.

104. Woolf CJ, Thompson SWN, King AE. Prolonged primary afferent induced alterations in dorsal horn neurones, an interacellular analysis in vivo and in vitro. J Physiol (Paris) 1989;88:255–266.

105. Niv D, Wolman I, Yashar T, et al. Epidural morphine pre-treatment for postepisiotomy pain. Clin J Pain 1994;10:319–323.

106. Miller RD, ed. Anesthesia, vol 1. 4th ed. New York: Churchill Livingstone, 1993.

107. Niv D, Varrassi G. Blockade of nociception during surgery in relation to postoperative pain. Pain Digest 1992;2:189–192.

108. Goodchild CS, Gent JP. Spinal cord effects of drugs used in anaesthesia. Gen Pharmacol 1992;23:937–944.

109. Borges M, Antognini JFA. Does the brain influence somatic responses to noxious stimuli during isoflurane anesthesia. Anesthesiology 1994;81:1511–1515.

110. Collins JG, Kendig JJ, Mason P. Anesthetic actions within the spinal cord: contributions to the state of general anesthesia. Trends Neurosci 1995;18:549–554.

111. Abram SE, Yaksh TL. Morphine, but not inhalation anesthesia, blocks post-injury facilitation: the role of pre-emptive suppression of afferent transmission. Anesthesiology 1993;78:713–721.

112. Goto T, Marota JJ, Crosby G. Nitrous oxide induces pre-emptive analgesia in the rat that is antagonized by halothane. Anesthesiology 1994;80:409–416.

113. Berkowitz BA, Ngai SH, Fink AD. Nitrous oxide "analgesia": resemblance to opiate action. Science 1976;194:967–968.

114. Dajczman E, Gordon A, Kreisman H, Wolkove N. Long-term post-thoracotomy pain. Chest 1991;99:270–274.

115. Morgas JM, Kierland RR. The outcome of patients with herpes zoster. Arch Dermatol 1957;75:193–196.

116. Bonica JJ. Importance of the problem. In: Aronoff GM, ed. Evaluation and treatment of chronic pain. Baltimore: Urban and Schwarzenberg, 1985.

117. Pilowsky I. Pain and illness behaviour: assessment and management. In: Wall PD, Melzack R, eds. Textbook of pain. 3rd ed. London: Churchill Livingstone, 1994;1309–1319.

118. Cailliet R. Chronic pain: is it necessary? Arch Phys Med Rehabil 1979;60:4–7.

119. Dubner R, Ruda M. Activity-dependent neuronal plasticity following tissue injury and inflammation. Trends Neurosci 1992;15:96–103.

120. Devor M. Central changes mediating neuropathic pain. In: Dubner R, Gebhart GF, Bond MR, eds. Pain research and clinical management, vol 3. Amsterdam: Elsevier, 1988;114–128.

121. Complex regional pain syndromes (CRPS). In: Merskey H, Bogduk N, eds. Classification of chronic pain. 2nd ed. Seattle: IASP, 1994;40–43.

122. Bonica JJ, Buckley FP. Regional analgesia with local anesthesia. In: Bonica JJ, ed. The management of Pain. Philadelphia: Lea & Febiger, 1990;1883–1965.

123. Katz J, Melzack R. Pain "memories" in phantom limbs: review and clinical observations. Pain 1990;43:319–336.

124. Henderson WR, Smyth GE. Phantom limbs. J Neurol Neurosurg Psychiatry 1948;11:88–112.

125. Cronholm B. Phantom limb in amputees: study of changes in integration of centripetal impulses with special reference to referred sensations. Acta Psychiatr Neurol 1951;72(Suppl):1–85.

126. Haber WB. Reactions to loss of limb: physiological and psychological aspects. Ann N Y Acad Sci 1956;75:624–636.

127. Parkes CM. Factors determining the persistence of phantom pain in the amputee. J Psychosom Res 1973;17:97–108.

128. Jensen TS, Krebs B, Nielsen J, Ramussen P. Immediate and long-term phantom limb pain amputees: incidence, clinical characteristics and relationships to preamputation limb pain. Pain 1985;21:267–278.

129. Carlen PL, Wall PD, Nadvorna H, Steinbach T. Phantom limbs and related phenomena in recent traumatic amputations. Neurology 1978;39:89–93.

130. Sherman RA, Sherman CJ. A comparison of phantom sensations among amputees whose amputations were of civilian and military origin. Pain 1985;21:91–97.

131. Dennis SG, Melzack R. Self-mutilation after dorsal rhizotomy in rats: effects of prior pain and pattern of root lesions. Exp Neurol 1979;65:412–421.

132. Gonzales-Darder JM, Barbera J, Abellan J. Effect of prior anaesthesia on autotomy following sciatic transection in rats. Pain 1986;24:87–91.

133. Coderre TJ, Melzack R. Cutaneous hyperalgesia: contributions of peripheral and central nervous systems to the increase in pain sensitivity after injury. Brain Res 1987;404:95–106.

134. Seltzer Z, Beilin BZ, Ginzburg R et al. The role of injury discharge in the induction of neuropathic pain behavior in rats. Pain 1991;46:327–336.

135. Katz J, Vaccarino AL, Coderre TJ, Melzack R. Injury prior to neurectomy alters the pattern of autotomy in rats. Anesthesiology 1991;75:876–883.

136. Bach S, Noreng MF, Tjellden NU. Phantom limb pain in amputees during the first 21 months following limb amputation, after preoperative lumbar epidural blockade. Pain 1988;33:291–301.

137. Jahangiri M, Jayatunga AP, Bradley JW, Dark CH. Prevention of phantom pain after major lower limb amputation by epidural infusion of diamorphine, clonidine and bupivacaine. Ann R Coll Surg Engl 1994;76:324–326.

138. Schug SA, Burrell R, Payne J, Tester P. Pre-emptive epidural analgesia may prevent phantom limb pain. Reg Anesth 1995;20:256 (letter).

139. Gracely RH, Lynch SA, Bennett GJ. Painful neuropathy: altered central processing, maintained dynamically by peripheral input. Pain 1992;51:175–194.

140. Devor M, Wall PD. The effect of peripheral nerve injury on receptive fields of cells in the cat spinal cord. J Comp Neurol 1981;199:277–291.

141. Kaas JH, Merzenich MM, Killackey HP. The reorganization of somatosensory cortex following peripheral nerve damage in adult and developing mammals. Ann Rev Neurosci 1983;6:325–356.

142. Ramachandran VS, Stewart M, Rogers-Ramachandran DC. Perceptual correlates of massive cortical reorganization. Neuroreport 1992;3:583–586.

143. Flor H, Elbert T, Knecht S, et al. Phantom-limb pain as a perceptual correlate of cortical reorganization following arm amputation. Nature 1995;375:482–484.

144. Woolf CJ, Shortland P, Coggeshall RE. Peripheral nerve injury triggers central sprouting of myelinated afferents. Nature 1992;355:75–78.

145. Clark SA, Allard T, Jenkins WM, Merzenich MM. Syndactyly results in the emergence of double digit receptive fields in somatosensory cortex in adult owl monkeys. Nature 1988;332:444–445.

146. Jenkins WM, Merzenich MM, Ochs MT, et al. Functional reorganization of primary somatosensory cortex in adult owl monkeys after behaviorally controlled tactile stimulation. J Neurophysiol 1990;63:82–104.

147. Lewin GR, Mendell LM. Nerve growth factor and nociception. Trends Neurosci 1993;16:353–359.

148. Hokfelt T, Zhang X, Wiesenfeld-Hallin Z. Messenger plasticity in primary sensory neurons following axotomy and its functional implications. Trends Neurosci 1994;17:22–30.

149. Wall PD, Devor M. The effect of peripheral nerve injury on dorsal root potentials and on the transmission of afferent signals into the spinal cord. Brain Res 1981;209:95–111.

150. Kingery WS, Fields RD, Kocsis JD. Diminished dorsal root GABA sensitivity following chronic peripheral nerve injury. Exp Neurol 1988;100:478–490.

151. Wall PD. Do nerve impulses penetrate terminal arborizations? A pre-presynaptic control mechanism. Trends Neurosci 1995;18:99–103.

152. Devor M, Raber P. Heritability of symptoms in an animal model of neuropathic pain. Pain 1990;42:51–67.

153. Katz J, Jackson M, Kavanagh BP, Sandler AN. Acute pain after thoracic surgery predicts long-term post-thoracotomy pain. Clin J Pain 1996;12:50–55.

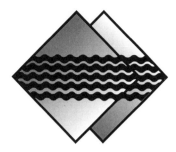

PART II

Clinical Aspects

CHAPTER 4

Neuropsychiatric Physical Examination

J. David Haddox

INTRODUCTION

Pain medicine is a maturing specialty. Many of its practitioners derive from primary specialty training backgrounds such as anesthesiology, neurological surgery, neurology, psychiatry, physiatry, and primary care specialties. As practitioners are called on to consult in the management of patients presenting with pain complaints, they must be able to perform a basic neurological and psychiatric evaluation to avoid missed diagnoses, to provide a sound opinion on the appropriateness of interventional procedures, and to put together a comprehensive multidisciplinary treatment plan that provides optimal opportunity to rehabilitate the person in pain. Most surveys indicate that most patients seen by practitioners of pain medicine have low back and leg pain, neck and arm pain, headache, and muscle pain. Therefore, pain medicine practitioners must be able to perform a screening neuropsychiatric and a detailed peripheral neurological examination to localize lesions and to rule out other conditions.

To facilitate this process, this chapter describes the elements of such an examination. It reviews the basic approach one practitioner takes with new patients, with emphasis on diagnoses that are frequently seen in a large pain medicine practice and maneuvers to detect them. The complete mental status examination, orthopaedic evaluation, and neurological examination are beyond the scope of this chapter. Rather, this chapter provides some general review and describes a basic schema that any pain physician should be able to perform. Obviously, the approach to a given patient varies with the presentation of the patient, the background of the evaluating physician, and the presumed differential diagnosis. However, certain aspects of the evaluation of the patient with pain are germane to most initial clinical encounters.

The pain-directed neuropsychiatric examination can be divided into three parts. The first is general observation. This can begin even before the formal encounter has begun, such as observing the patient walking down the hall to the examination room. Too often, especially in today's environment, little time or thought is given to this valuable first step in the examination, in which the first clues to the diagnosis can often be discerned. The second part of the process is the screening examination, which consists of tests of cerebellar function, cranial nerve examination, and a brief mental status examination. The third part of the examination is designed to review in some detail the functional status of the neuromuscular system, including looking for some nonneurologic phenomena that may mimic neurological findings or may present with a history that sounds "neurological."

OBSERVATION

The clinician should notice pain behaviors and other behaviors, coordination, habitus, amount and fluidity of movement, body mechanics, and posture. During the observation period pain behaviors may fluctuate, especially if the observation is continued as the patient leaves the examining area. Thus careful observation may provide a surprising amount of information, all of which can be factored into the comprehensive formulation of a treatment approach to the patient's problems.

The first impression generally is based on dress, appearance, and gait. The initial observation should include the appropriateness of dress for a medical evaluation, which usually consists of casual clothes. The general state of grooming and condition of clothes (stained, torn, disheveled) should be noted. If, for example, a man appears for evaluation wearing a three-piece suit or a woman appears wearing a dress with pantyhose, one may infer that the patient is not expecting or is unwilling to submit to a detailed physical examination. Obviously, this is not the only reason to dress for a physician appointment this way, as the visit may be immediately before or after work, so inferences should be made with caution. Still, the astute observer should be attuned to these issues.

General appearance beyond dress should also be noted. The facial expression, eye contact, nutritional status, habitus, and skin should be observed. Facial expression can provide valuable clues to the emotional state of the patient, which is discussed later. The mask facies can indicate Parkinson's disease or a drug-induced parkinsonian state, often from use of neuroleptics or antiemetics. Facial appearance can suggest Cushing's syndrome from epidural or intramuscular (trigger point) steroid injections. A facial expression can often reveal information about emotional state. Reacting to the anxious patient with a calm demeanor often has a very important role in establishing good rapport, for example. It is useful to notice the nares in particular. Opioid withdrawal is typified by clear rhinorrhea and resultant sniffling.

Eye contact can provide clues to affective state, culture, and veracity. Depressed patients often make little eye contact with anyone, looking at the floor instead. Latino and African-American patients are often taught to avoid direct eye contact with authority figures as a show of respect, and this can easily be misinterpreted by the examiner as averting the gaze for other reasons. Patients who are being less than honest may avoid eye contact when answering direct questions. The color or injection of the sclera may provide a clue to drug use in the chronic pain patient.

Nutritional status and habitus can give information regarding general well-being, health consciousness, and disease. Cachectic patients may have temporomandibular disorders, trigeminal neuralgia, or a life-threatening disease such as cancer or AIDS. Obese patients may have little interest in adopting and maintaining healthful lifestyle changes, have Cushing's disease, or have unrecognized hypothyroidism.

The skin of the patient should be observed before and after disrobing for the examination. Special notice should be made of lesions, bruises, or injection sites as evidence of trauma or self-injected medication. Repeated injections can give rise to atrophy of the subcutaneous tissues with dimpling scars or in severe cases, muscle contractures. Tattoos sometimes reveal an individual's background and social status. Especially important is the home-made five-spoked figure with dots at the end of some or all of the spokes, as this is often used in prison populations as a mark of daring, in that when each spoke is dotted, it represents completion of a particular felony, such as rape or murder. Changes in skin tone, color, and texture may indicate vascular problems, complex regional pain syndromes, or other conditions relevant to the presenting complaint. An unexpected temperature difference between feet in a patient with low-back pain can indicate pressure or traction on the lumbar sympathetic chain from a retroperitoneal tumor. Piloerection is typical in opioid withdrawal and occasionally is observed in the absence of other signs and symptoms such as rhinorrhea, irritability, crampy abdominal pain, diarrhea, diffuse myalgias, and deep pain ("my bones hurt").

Gait is often revealing. The most commonly observed gait in most practices can be described as antalgic, or pain avoiding. This may manifest in numerous ways, such as a slow gait with a short stride, a limp, the use of an assistive device, or unusual posture during walking. Waddling can be seen in weakness of the glutei muscles. A festinating gait, or walking in short but fast strides, may suggest Parkinson's disease, especially in the absence of arm swinging. A steppage gait, or raising the feet higher than necessary, is seen in cases of impaired proprioception caused by vitamin B_{12} deficiency, in other peripheral sensory neuropathies and tabes dorsalis, and in peroneal neuropathy leading to foot drop (1). Trendelenberg's sign is noted when the iliac crest dips as the ipsilateral leg is being flexed and indicates weakness in the contralateral gluteal medius muscle (2). A simian or apelike posture, with the lumbar spine flexed such that the center of gravity of the body is forward of normal, can be seen with spinal stenosis or ankylosing spondylitis.

Walking engages a significant portion of the neurological system and is a good general screen for serious neurological disease. When observing walking, watch the fluidity, the length of stride, the swinging of the arms, the balance, and the general ease with which it is accomplished. It is often useful to have the patient pace back and forth to observe the ease with which he or she can change directions, as this is more complex than simply walking in one direction and may reveal deficits that are otherwise compensated. Pain behaviors often influence walking when the patient is aware of being observed. These behaviors may include unsteadiness, more apparent concentration than necessary, inconsistencies such as varying length of stride, weaving to one side on one occasion and to the other side later, and variable base (distance feet are held apart during walking and standing). Instruct the patient to walk backward (difficult to do with femoral nerve injuries), to walk on toes (testing plantar flexion providing insight into the function of the S1 root and associated muscles), to walk on heels (testing dorsiflexion and providing insight into the function of L5 and associated muscles), and to tandem-walk, or walk with one foot placed directly in front of the other down a straight line, which places the patient on a narrow base and tests both dorsal column function and coordination.

INTERVIEW

Before one undertakes to examine a pain patient, a detailed history must be obtained. The nuances of this skill are beyond the scope of this presentation but should be mastered before the examination, simply because without a history, the physical examination may be unrewarding, misleading, or misdirected. As Clark Sleeth, a skilled family practitioner and former dean of West Virginia University School of Medicine, told me on many occasions, "If you listen to the patient long enough, they'll tell you the diagnosis."

After the initial observations, the interview begins. It is vitally important to allow the patient to develop his or her story with minimal interruption for several minutes. Rather than interject questions, let the patient speak. Make notations about things that require clarification or chronological ordering and ask them after a few minutes have elapsed. This allows a number of thing to occur: (*a*) The patient feels that the examiner values the patient's input. (*b*) The patient becomes more at ease. (*c*) Valuable inferences can be made by listening to the things the patient says, as patients tend to talk about the most important things first. The mental status examination has already begun by this point. The way the patient phrases things often reveals significant emotional content, for instance anger at previous physicians, distrust of an insurer or employer, or hopelessness at his or her predicament. After the patient has had some time to expound on his or her problem, with the observations made to this point, one can develop an efficient directed interview strategy.

SCREENING EXAMINATION

Cerebellar Function

At this point in the encounter the astute clinician has already noted any gross deficit in cerebellar function. By observing gait, sitting, buttoning, talking, and gestures, one can rule out most significant dysfunctions in the domain of cerebellar functions. More sensitive tests, all of which can be influenced by emotional state, degree of cooperation and pain behaviors, include checking rapid alternating movements (diadochokinesia is the ability to perform these tasks), finger-to-nose tests, heel-to-shin tests, and having the patient alternately touch his or her nose and the examiner's finger. In this last test, if the examiner's finger is moved to various areas of the visual fields and the patient is instructed to keep the head still, one is also checking gross visual acuity and the function of cranial nerves III, IV, and VI via the innervation of the extraocular muscles. Looking for Romberg's sign by having the patient stand with feet together, is often done as a confirming test. A patient who has been able to perform tandem walking, however, is unlikely to show Romberg's sign, since tandem walking also involves a narrow base and cannot be performed well in the presence of significant dorsal column or cerebellar dysfunction.

Cranial Nerve Examination

Likewise, by this time in the examination most cranial nerve functions have been observed. Specific testing takes very little time (3). Cranial nerve I (olfactory) is usually not tested but should be considered in selected cases, as anosmia (loss of sense of smell) can be present with frontal lobe tumors compressing the olfactory bulbs or tracts.

Cranial Nerve II: The Optic Nerve

Confrontational visual field testing is generally adequate for clinical screening, although funduscopic examination of the optic disc is needed for a more complete evaluation of the optic nerve. The limitations of direct ophthalmoscopy without the use of pupillary dilation must be recognized, however. At a minimum, the characteristics of the optic disc, major vessels, and eye grounds must be observed.

Cranial Nerves III, IV, and VI: The Oculomotor, Trochlear, and Abducens Nerves

As noted earlier, the somatic motor component of the oculomotor nerve (III) may have already been tested. The visceral motor component is tested by reaction to light (direct and consensual responses) and the presence of pupillary constriction and convergence of the eyes upon presentation of a stimulus requiring near vision (accommodation). The antimuscarinic effects of many drugs commonly taken by pain patients may interfere with the pupillary constriction component of accommodation, which is a parasympathetic cholinergically mediated phenomenon. Such drugs include tricyclic antidepressants, antispasmodics prescribed for irritable bowel syndrome or diarrhea, and antihistamines.

Cranial nerve IV (trochlear) supplies the superior oblique muscle, which enables one to look down and out. Deficit of this nerve causes extortion (outward rotation) of the globe due to the unopposed action of the inferior oblique muscle. Cranial nerve VI (abducens) supplies the lateral rectus muscle, which abducts the globe to facilitate lateral gaze. The course of the abducens nerve across the petrous ridge of the temporal bone makes it vulnerable to changes in intracranial pressure. Thus, in a low CSF pressure headache, such as after dural puncture, paralysis of lateral gaze with resultant diplopia can be seen.

Cranial Nerve V: The Trigeminal Nerve

The fifth cranial nerve, or trigeminal, is complex in function and anatomy. It supplies cutaneous and mucosal sensation to the face and oral cavity. The first (ophthalmic) division of the trigeminal nerve supplies the skin to the forehead, the orbit, the eye (including cornea) and the frontal and ethmoid sinuses. Testing of sensation to light touch, pinprick, and temperature is easily accomplished by applying these stimuli to the forehead. The corneal reflex is elicited by slowly approaching the cornea from the side with a fine cotton wisp. The afferent limb is mediated by the ophthalmic division of cranial nerve V and the efferent limb is via cranial nerve VII to the orbicularis oculi muscle. If the patient is able to see the wisp coming, the reflex elicited may actually be the blink reflex, which does not test the integrity of the fifth nerve. Occasionally a pain patient is too nervous to allow adequate testing of the corneal reflex. Obviously, contact lenses generally preclude testing of this reflex. The miosis and ptosis seen as part of Horner's syndrome following cervicothoracic sympathetic blockade with local anesthetics (stellate ganglion block) are due to paralysis of cervical sympathetic preganglionic fibers that synapse in the superior cervical ganglion. The postganglionic fibers travel along the internal carotid artery to the ophthalmic division of the fifth nerve, thence to the dilator pupillae muscle via the long ciliary nerve (miosis) and to the superior tarsal muscle (ptosis) (4). The second division of cranial nerve V is the maxillary division, which supplies the skin of the midface, where it terminates as the infraorbital nerve; the maxillary sinus; the nasal cavity, the palate, and upper teeth.

Only the third (mandibular) division has any motor innervation, supplying the muscles of mastication (internal and external pterygoids, masseter and temporalis), mylohyoid, tensor veli palatini and the anterior belly of the digastric. The muscles of mastication are tested by having the patient clench the teeth and observing the contraction of the temporalis and masseters (the internal pterygoid is also a jaw-closing muscle but cannot be seen). Opening the mouth gently involves the external pterygoid. Opening against force or maximal opening recruits the anterior strap muscles of the neck. This division also supplies the skin on the lower third of the face, with the mental nerve being the cutaneous termination. It supplies sensation to the anterior two thirds of the tongue, the mandibular teeth, and the floor of the mouth.

The most common disease condition of the fifth nerve is trigeminal neuralgia, or tic douloureux. This is characterized by brief, severe, lancinating pain in one or more dermatomes of the trigeminal nerve. It is usually bilateral; its prevalence increases with age; and generally it has trigger zones (not to be confused with muscular trigger points), stimulation of which initiate pain paroxysms. Most textbooks indicate that the clinical examination is entirely normal in this disease, but I have noted subtle areas of abnormal sensation in several patients with trigeminal neuralgia who have not had surgical interventions. In younger people, trigeminal neuralgia may be the first symptom of multiple sclerosis. The trigeminal territories are also the second most common location for herpes zoster, after the thoracic region.

Cranial Nerve VII: The Facial Nerve

The facial nerve supplies the muscles of facial expression, taste to the anterior two thirds of the tongue, and sensation to the concha of the ear and a small area behind the ear. The innervation of the facial motor nucleus is contralateral for the lower muscles and bilateral for the upper muscles. Therefore, a lower motor neuron lesion (e.g., Bell's palsy) results in loss of control and tone of all of the muscles (upper and lower) on the same side of the face as the lesion. A stroke involving the internal capsule containing axons from the cortex (upper motor neurons), however, results in loss of voluntary control of muscles in the lower part of the face contralateral to the stroke. In this circumstance some action of facial muscles that are no longer under voluntary control can still be seen with emotional reactions. Weakness of facial muscles is apparent on attempts to smile widely, purse the lips, raise the eyebrows, or close the eyes. Many patients with facial nerve palsy lose skin folds, so the forehead is smooth and the nasolabial fold is less promi-

nent. The corner of the mouth droops, and the lower eyelid falls away from the globe such that the punctum is no longer in approximation to the globe, leading to tearing onto the cheek.

Cranial Nerve VIII: The Vestibulocochlear Nerve

The vestibulocochlear nerve subserves hearing and balance. Hearing may be tested by lightly rubbing the examiner's fingers together on alternating sides while the patient's eyes are closed. Lesions of cranial nerve VIII can cause tinnitus, vertigo, or decreased hearing. Acoustic neuromas can cause vertigo and tinnitus followed by deafness. Ipsilateral facial paralysis can also occur (lower motor neuron facial palsy), as can trigeminal symptoms such as pain. Eventually signs of increased intracranial pressure and cerebellar signs can occur. This constellation of signs and symptoms is cerebellopontine angle syndrome.

Cranial Nerve IX: The Glossopharyngeal Nerve

The glossopharyngeal nerve predominantly provides sensation and taste to the posterior third of the tongue. The gag reflex is mediated by this nerve. A rare condition without clear causation, glossopharyngeal neuralgia, is characterized by brief, severe paroxysms of pain in the throat, side of the neck in front of the ear, and back of the mandible. It can be triggered by swallowing or talking. It is said to be similar to the well-known ice cream headache.

Cranial Nerve X: The Vagus Nerve

The vagus nerve, whose name means wanderer, is aptly named. In addition to supplying smooth muscle in abdominal and thoracic viscera, it supplies most of the muscles of the pharynx, including the levator palatini, which is the one most commonly tested by having the patient say ah. In the normal situation the posterior soft palate and uvula elevate in the midline. With a lower motor neuron lesion, the denervated side is slack, causing the uvula to deviate to the side opposite the lesion. Hoarseness often accompanies lesions of cranial nerve X. Hoarseness with normal uvular movements, which suggests involvement of the recurrent laryngeal nerve, can be seen after stellate ganglion block, with aortic aneurysms (due to stretching of the nerve), and with enlarged paratracheal nodes due to metastases.

Cranial nerve XI: The Spinal Accessory Nerve

Cranial nerve XI, also known as the spinal accessory nerve, supplies innervation to the sternocleidomastoid and trapezius muscles. It is so named because the lower motor neurons actually reside in the spinal cord. It is important to remember that the upper motor neurons travel from the motor cortex through the pyramidal decussation to the spinal cord; that is, they cross the midline. The fibers from the lower motor neurons travel with the cord up through foramen magnum and then leave the cranium via the jugular foramen. To test the integrity of the part of this nerve to the trapezius, the examiner asks the patient to shrug the shoulders without the use of the arms to help push the shoulders up. The sternocleidomastoid is tested by having the patient rotate the head to one side against resistance. The left sternocleidomastoid muscle rotates the head to the right because it originates posterior to the axis of rotation of the cervical spine and inserts anterior to it. Radical neck dissection can injure the nerve, causing drooping of the shoulder and weakened head rotation.

Cranial Nerve XII: The Hypoglossal Nerve

The hypoglossal nerve innervates almost all of the muscles of the tongue. Since the upper motor neurons cross the midline, lesions can be localized with some certainty. A lower motor neuron lesion causes the tongue to deviate to the affected side, since protrusion of the tongue requires both genioglossus muscles to pull the tongue out, not push it out. Conversely, an upper motor neuron causes the tongue to deviate to the contralateral side.

Mental Status Examination

All too frequently valuable information is not recorded in the chart because of oversight or the inability to describe a clinical encounter accurately. The purpose of this review is to refresh the pain physician's observational, diagnostic, and descriptive skills in regard to the mental status of the patient in pain.

Physicians with little formal training in psychiatry and behavioral sciences should ensure that they review the skills necessary to perform a basic mental status examination so they can provide a comprehensive evaluation of the pain patient. One should think of the mental status examination as merely the portion of the physical examination that deals with the higher functions of the brain. Behaviors, both motoric and verbal, can be important clues to the clinical problem, as can thought content, perceptions, and other mental functions.

A major problem with clinical assessment of the mental status examination is the notion that it has to be done separately from the rest of the examination. In fact, good mental health professionals often conduct a perfectly reliable mental status examination during what seems like the course of a normal conversation. One should endeavor to work the mental status examination into the rest of the examination, making mental or written notes about things to assess with more formal testing when something seems amiss. What follows is the bare bones of a complete mental status examination. There may be many other things that should be assayed in the pain patient, according to the particulars of the presentation.

The best way to think about the reporting of the mental status examination findings is to record it in a systematic fashion. To help remember the essential features, I have created an acronym, **A SAD COMB.** This stands for **a**ppearance, **s**uicide, **a**lcohol, **d**rug use, **c**ognitive functions, **o**rientation, **m**ood and affect, and **b**ehaviors. While there are more com-

plete examination schemata, including formal assessment of memory, intellect, judgment, and so on, this abbreviated examination of mental status suffices for most of the situations encountered in the clinical evaluation of chronic pain. Each of these areas is discussed in turn.

Appearance

A brief statement about the patient's physical appearance should begin the physical examination. As mentioned previously, this can include the habitus, dress, neatness, makeup, tattoos, and any discrepancy between chronological and apparent age. It is customary to follow with a statement about how the patient related to the examiner (e.g., cooperative, resistant) insofar as the evaluation is concerned.

Suicide

The risk of suicide is quite real in some pain patients (5). It is a well-described sequela of tic douloureux and postherpetic neuralgia. It is usually thought of as being associated with affective disorders but can occur in personality disorders (revenge, punishment, anger) or thought disorders (delusional, command auditory hallucinations).

In assessing risk of suicide, it is best to start with an opening statement that grants permission to discuss the issue such as, "Have you ever thought about just going to sleep and not waking up?" Then one can ask more direct questions as the clinical situation dictates. One should use the terms the patient uses and always demonstrate concern and compassion. Virtually everyone has contemplated suicide to some degree at one time, and most patients fear that a physician will think they are crazy or have them committed if they discuss it. Suicidal ideation that is voiced during the encounter is physical examination data and is recorded as such in the written record, not as history. A statement in the examination section such as "the patient voices no current suicidal ideation" or "the patient is not suicidal at present" is sufficient documentation. Note that these statements do not imply prediction about future suicidal ideation or attempts, but merely indicate that at the time of the evaluation no evidence of suicidal intent was forthcoming.

In contrast to the rest of the history and physical, the history of suicidal thoughts usually does not emerge until the issue of current suicidal ideation has been broached. The suicide history (placed under history of present illness [HPI] or review of systems [ROS] in the written report) is the best predictor of future outcome. Ask about GAP-gestures (feigned attempts with low intended lethality), attempts (bona fide efforts to end life) and plans (pistol, pills, having a note already written, knowing their significant other's travel plans, giving away personal items, and so on). Because of inadequate knowledge on the part of the patient, gestures occasionally have inadvertently high lethal probability (e.g., acetaminophen overdosage). This is still classified as a gesture, however, because the *intent* was nonlethal.

If a clinician believes that a person is suicidal, a no-harm contract can often be useful to get a person by temporarily. It is advisable to remember that tricyclic antidepressants, which are often quite useful in the management of chronic pain, are very effective tools for suicide. Serotonin-specific reuptake inhibitors (SSRIs), however, have a very high therapeutic index.

Suicidal thoughts should be taken seriously. Learn the laws in your state or nation that apply to this situation and do not hesitate to consult a mental health professional for advice or to arrange hospital admission. Every patient must be handled differently, because suicidal ideation does not necessarily represent a wish to die. As mentioned earlier, the statement that one is suicidal can derive from any of numerous motivations, such as a wish to end suffering (as opposed to ending life), an attempt to make the examiner take the patient seriously, an attempt to get back at someone in anger, or an attempt to manipulate the situation. Clinical experience does show that not only depressed patients but also patients in chronic pain and those who are very angry are at risk for attempting suicide.

Alcohol

It should be a routine part of the assessment of chronic pain to inquire about alcohol consumption. This drug is commonly overlooked as a cause of problems in the management of chronic pain. Many patients attempt to self-medicate with alcohol to treat pain, sleep disruption, depression, anxiety, or panic disorders. This topic should be approached in a nonaccusatory, matter-of-fact manner to put the patient at ease and to obtain the best information. The disease of addiction, however, is typified by lying. This is generally not done on a totally conscious level, as it is merely a manifestation of denial, so one should not personalize it if it occurs. It is not uncommon to find successively more accurate historical information about drinking and associated behaviors with subsequent clinical encounters. A clinically useful screen is the CAGE question set (6). CAGE is an acronym for (need to) **c**ut down, (being) **a**nnoyed (by others' criticism of drinking), (feeling) **g**uilty (about drinking), (having an) **e**ye-opener. Developed for ease of use and utility in identifying individuals who may be suffering from alcoholism, it is outlined in Table 4.1.

Drug Use

Drug use is an area of much confusion in the assessment of the patient suffering from chronic pain. Many clinicians seem to be confused about drug use terminology. The *Diagnostic and Statistical Manual of Mental Disorders,* ed. 4 (DSM-IV) of the American Psychiatric Association, to the cursory reader, only adds to the confusion (7). Looking only at the numbered criteria, one could erroneously make a diagnosis of substance dependence in many chronic pain patients by counting tolerance, withdrawal syndrome, and a great deal of time spent to obtain the substance (e.g., visiting multiple

Table 4.1.   The CAGE Questions

Have you ever felt you ought to cut down on your drinking?
Have people annoyed you by criticizing your drinking?
Have you ever felt bad or guilty about your drinking?
Have you ever had a drink first thing in the morning to steady your nerves or get rid of a hangover (eye-opener)?
Scoring: Two "yes" answers indicate likely alcoholism. Three or four indicate very high probability.

doctors or driving long distances), as the three criteria sufficient to establish the diagnosis. This constellation is often seen in the setting of chronic pain: (*a*) Underprescribing leads to more frequent requests for medication that can be misinterpreted as tolerance. (*b*) Underdosing leads to withdrawal syndromes when a patient, in an effort to achieve comfort, uses a prescription faster than intended and is required to wait for more medication; when a patient is treated with infrequent doses of a short-acting agent; or when a patient is dismissed from a practice for any of a number of reasons (commonly, the practitioner's discomfort with the amount of medication required). (*c*) Patients who benefit from the use of opioids drive long distances to keep regular appointments with a physician who is willing to treat them when they cannot find anyone nearby who will treat them. More careful reading of the DSM-IV diagnostic criteria, however, indicate that pain patients who have this constellation do *not* meet the criteria for diagnosis of substance dependence. The diagnosis substance dependence, which is a euphemism for addiction, requires the demonstration of "a *maladaptive* pattern of substance use, leading to clinically significant impairment or distress, as manifested by three (or more) of the following, occurring at any time in the same 12-month period . . ." (emphasis added). This group of diagnostic criteria requires strict adherence for clinical accuracy, and the constellation described here is not necessarily maladaptive.

When evaluating drug use, one must be familiar with terminology and phenomenology. Probably the greatest confusion comes with the distinction between physical dependence, which is a pharmacological feature of many drugs, and addiction, which is a biobehavioral syndrome manifested by an individual's interaction with a drug. Desperation in the patient seeking relief and poor understanding of drug actions can often lead to improper drug use or *drug misuse* in the chronic pain patient. Cultural factors also figure in this. In some regions, such as Appalachia, it is a commonly held belief that one aspirin tablet is a hypnotic. Most physicians would consider this drug misuse rather than abuse. It is imperative, therefore, to take a thoughtful history to analyze the patient's drug use correctly.

Cognitive Functions

The assessment of cognitive (thinking) functions can be done formally with tests of concentration but is generally discernible by attention to the patient during a typical evaluation. Speech offers the best view of cognition in the examination setting, since thoughts cannot be directly observed. Fluency of speech, cadence, prosody, and variety of speech are all elements that can be observed. Pressured speech (loud and rapid) is typical of mania and some drug intoxications. Circumstantial speech is littered with parenthetical comments and purposeless speech, but it does eventually get to the point. This can be seen in early dementia and brain injuries or may simply be due to anxiety or wanting to make sure the examiner gets the entire history as seen by the patient. Tangential speech starts out on task but deviates from the topic and never gets back on track. This can be seen with mania, dementia, or intoxication.

Thought content and perceptual aberrations can be inferred by speech content as well. *Delusions* are fixed false beliefs not shared within the patient's culture that persist despite obvious evidence that they are wrong. In the pain patient, fears about what is wrong with himself or herself, despite having seen so many doctors, often approaches delusional proportions. *Obsessions* are intrusive, unwanted (egodystonic) thoughts that pervade the waking state.

Perceptual disturbances, such as hallucinations, can occur as a result of drug withdrawal or toxicity. *Hallucinations* are perceptions without any antecedent sensory stimuli. They may be visual (almost always drug-related), auditory (usually due to a psychiatric disorder), olfactory (tumor, temporal lobe epilepsy), gustatory (temporal lobe epilepsy, vitamin deficiency), or tactile (delusional disorders, withdrawal). It is always important to take hallucinations seriously. A benign type of hallucination that may people experience occurs just as they are falling asleep (hypnagogic) or as they are awakening (hypnopompic). These may be auditory, such as hearing someone call their name; or visual, which probably represents the early onset of rapid eye movement (REM) sleep, frequently reported by pain patients because of disrupted sleep cycles, underdosing, or abrupt cessation of sedating antidepressants (REM rebound). *Illusions* (misperceptions of actual sensory stimuli), though generally not so serious, can still signal significant problems according to their severity and persistence.

Orientation

Orientation is the ability to process environmental cues along with short-term memory skills. It is most frequently described in terms of person, place, time, and situation. If a person who has been hospitalized for a few days misses the day of the week by one day, this is generally not cause for concern. If, however, that individual has a bedside calendar that has been marked off each day, missing by one day suggests some deficit in processing environmental cues. Orientation in the outpatient setting is usually inferred during the interview. Many patients try to compensate for perceived deficits in orientation by such maneuvers as looking at a digital watch when asked the date.

Mood and Affect

Mood is the pervasive emotional state experienced by the patient. It can be assessed by direct report, either spontaneously or in response to a question (subjective mood). It can also be assessed by observing behavioral clues to the underlying emotional state (so-called objective mood). One should think of mood as being like climate, while affect is like weather. Mood can be described many ways, but some accepted terms form the mnemonic SHAAA-sad, happy, angry, anxious, and apathetic.

Affect is the immediate observable expression of emotion. It has four parameters: range, amplitude (or intensity), stability, and appropriateness. Range is the repertoire of the person. It can be full, constricted, or severely constricted. Amplitude is the degree of expression of a particular emotion and is usually described as excessive, normal, decreased, blunted, or flat. By convention, "flat affect" is generally used only to describe schizophrenics. Stable affect doesn't change without a change in conversation topic or tone, whereas labile affect changes abruptly during an evaluation, often within a sentence. Appropriateness of affect is determined by the degree of match between content of thought (speech) and affect.

Behaviors

Behaviors are the observable aspects of the patient's interaction with the environment. If everyone had the same capacity to observe and describe patients, there would be complete concurrence about behaviors during a specific clinical encounter, since these are objective events.

In many pain patients, pain or pain-avoiding behaviors are frequently observed yet rarely commented upon. If possible, observe some of these behaviors without the patient's knowledge to gauge how the presence of an examiner influences the execution of some behaviors and suppresses others. Antalgic gait, as noted previously, is frequently observed in the patient complaining of low-back pain. Grimacing, sighing, moaning (a verbal behavior), verbalizing pain, splinting, guarding, cautious movement, difficulty getting onto the examination table, and breakaway weakness when testing muscle strength are frequently observed. Symptom amplification, a common nonspecific finding among chronic pain patients, is often detected by responses that are in excess of those expected with diagnostic maneuvers or are inconsistent throughout the examination. A specific set of illness behaviors observed in patients complaining of low-back pain have been described by Gordon Waddell, an orthopaedic surgeon practicing in Glasgow. Called Waddell's signs, they are discussed separately later in the chapter.

Certain terms are useful to define specific behaviors. For example, *agitation* is often used incorrectly to describe an emotional state, when in fact it has nothing directly to do with emotions but rather describes excessive purposeless motor behavior (e.g., fidgeting, toe tapping, finger drumming). *Hyperactivity* is an excess of goal-directed behaviors, such as opening a door, untying shoes, or taking a pen from one's pocket, as might be observed in an individual with attention deficit hyperactivity disorder. *Tics* are quick, repetitive movements that are usually confined to small muscle groups, such as a facial twitch. They often increase with anxiety. *Stereotypies* are more complex repetitive movements involving larger muscle groups; often they are an acquired habit that served a function at one time, such as tossing one's hair out the face by flipping the head to one side rapidly or tugging at one's collar. *Dystonia* is used to describe abnormally increased muscle tone, often with a limb held in a relatively fixed, nonfunctional position. *Psychomotor retardation* implies an overall picture of paucity of movement and slow movement, especially when an affective state is presumed to be the cause. *Bradykinesia* means slow movements, such as seen with Parkinson's disease. *Akinesia,* sometimes also used to describe patients with parkinsonian presentations, is rare, as it means no movement at all. *Compulsions* are behaviors repeated habitually to relieve a specific anxiety, as Lady Macbeth constantly wrung her hands to "wash" the imagined blood from the murder away.

Such behaviors as smiling, crying, and interruption of the examiner are all valid subjects of observation.

COMMONLY ENCOUNTERED PSYCHIATRIC CONDITIONS

Depression, anxiety and panic disorders, and posttraumatic stress disorder are discussed in other chapters in detail. There are, however, some discrete syndromes or phenomena that bear comment.

Akathisia, which is seen most commonly in young individuals, is one type of extra-pyramidal side effect (EPSE) caused by dopamine antagonists. It is characterized by intense restlessness, a sense that something serious is wrong without the ability to describe what is amiss, and an intense desire to move about. It can be treated acutely with antimuscarinics and more permanently by discontinuing the offending drug.

Acute dystonic reactions to dopamine antagonists are also commonly observed in the younger population. These can range from orobuccolingual dystonias to "oculogyric crisis," a misnamed syndrome, as there is no crisis that cannot be treated with reassurance and antimuscarinics. A respiratory muscle variant, with decreased pulmonary function, has been described.

Drug-induced parkinsonism occurs most frequently in the elderly and on examination may be indistinguishable from Parkinson's disease. It may be characterized by festinating gait; bradykinesia; inability to initiate movement, such as getting out of a chair or climbing stairs; mask facies; pill-rolling tremor; and cogwheel rigidity.

Delayed-onset movement disorders caused in part by exposure to dopamine antagonists are called *tardive* (late) *dyskinesias.* They commonly affect the orobuccal muscles but can involve any muscles. About one third of cases resolve after the drug is removed; one third improve after drug cessation; and one third of cases are permanent.

Delirium is an alteration in sensorium. It is usually transient and often fluctuates. The main deficit is a waxing and waning of alertness and attentiveness, with consequent impairment in orientation. Hallucinations may or may not be present or suspected. In the pain population it is usually due to drug effects, either from toxicity or withdrawal. Metabolic causes are frequently implicated in the general medical population.

Dementia is used to describe a long-standing decrement from previously normal intellectual functioning. The dementias are not generally reversible and do not tend to fluctuate, but rather have a slow downward course. Contrast this term, de-(downward, less) and -mentia (thinking) with mental retardation, which is used to describe individuals who never achieve an expected norm of intellectual function. Dementia and other organic brain diseases, such as medication toxicity, can be rapidly assessed in a quantifiable manner with the Mini Mental State Examination (Table 4.2) (8). This rapid screen for mental status changes can be used daily on hospitalized patients to monitor progress. It is not, in and of itself, a diagnostic test (8).

Transference is one of the most important concepts in psychoanalytical theory. It means the unconscious assignment to others of feelings and attitudes that were originally associated with important figures in one's early life. Freud coined the term because he thought that these emotional sets were transferred from one object (person) to another. The phenomenon occurs every day in the doctor–patient relationship and must be recognized. If a patient responds to a physician in an emotional way that is not apparent from the context of the examination, consider the possibility that there is a transference reaction occurring. The examiner may represent some other authority figure, such as the father, and the patient may be relating to the physician as if to that other authority figure.

Countertransference is the same phenomenon with the opposite vector, that is, the physician's emotional reaction to the patient. Failure to recognize transference and countertransference is a common cause of stress in the practice of pain medicine. It is in the practitioner's interest to endeavor to understand his or her own strong negative or positive reactions to a particular patient or type of patient.

As a specific example, it is important not to personalize transference reactions, as many pain patients are quite angry and often focus that anger poorly. Personalization of anger leads to a defensive posture on the part of the health care provider that can escalate a situation. This can result in a countertherapeutic encounter and does not facilitate optimal care for the patient in pain. There are several options for dealing with angry patients, but they must be thought out ahead of time. The first option entails listening to the patient. It is a common litany among pain patients that they have not been heard by health care providers.

Many chronic pain patients are angry for good reason. Many have suffered loss of income, social status, job role, family role, and self-esteem. Compounding these losses are the specters of improper diagnoses and treatments, with unabated suffering looming for the future. Many of these patients, per-

Table 4.2.   Mini Mental State Examination (MMSE)

Score	Items Tested
5	Season, day, date, month, year
5	State, county, town, hospital, floor (or similar items)
3	Repeat the names of three objects (registration)
5	Spell "world" backward *or* serial 7s × 5 (93, 86, 79, 72, 65)
2	Name two objects (e.g., pencil, watch, tie)
1	Repeat: "no ifs, ands, or buts"
1	"Read this and do what it says." (Give patient a paper on which is written the following).
3	"Take this paper, fold it in half and put it on the bed"
1	"Write a complete sentence" (subject and verb, grammatically correct)
3	Recall the three objects from above (short-term memory)
1	Copy a design (such as square and a triangle that intersect)
	Scoring
	26–30, normal
	20–25, mild cognitive impairment
	12–20, significant cognitive impairment
	09–12, probably demented

Adapted from Folstein MF, Folstein S, McHugh PR. Minimental state: a practical method for grading the cognitive state of patients for the clinician. J Psychiatr Res 1975;12:189.

haps rightfully so, have the impression that they have been lied to by their employer, their insurer, and their doctors. Validation of these feelings can often calm an angry patient.

Another response to the inappropriately directed outburst of anger is to assume a nonthreatening and passive attitude until the storm blows over. This is accomplished by remaining at or below the patient's eye level (preferably sitting), respecting the patient's space, assuming a relaxed posture, and remaining attentive to the patient.

In summary, the mental status examination of the pain patient should become second nature when practiced regularly. By being attuned to the dynamics of the interaction during the evaluation, one can glean a great deal of useful information to assist in formulation of a comprehensive treatment plan.

SENSORY TESTING

Sensation should be tested with the patient resting as comfortably as possible. It should begin with a directed history to clarify where the patient believes there are sensory disturbances, so that attention can be directed to those areas on examination. It should begin with nonnoxious modalities, such as light touch. The modalities that should be tested are light touch (LT), pinprick (PP) and vibration (Vib) with a 128-Hz tuning fork, especially in the lower extremities. Depending on the nature of the examination, it may include testing to cold (alcohol wipe, vapocoolant spray, ice, or water-filled glass syringe kept in a refrigerator) or heat (glass syringe filled with hot water).

To map out an area suspected of having decreased feeling, begin from the center of the region and work outward while the patient keeps the eyes closed. It is much easier to perceive an increased sensation than one that is gradually decreasing. Likewise, if examining an area suspected of increased sensitivity, begin on normal skin and progress to the border of the abnormal area. The rule is always progress from an area of decreased or absent sensation to an area with more or increased sensation. Terms to describe altered sensation include the following: (9)

allodynia: pain due to a stimulus that does not normally cause pain (see also hyperalgesia).

dysesthesia: an unpleasant abnormal sensation, whether spontaneous or evoked (specify).

hyperesthesia: increased sensitivity to painless stimuli.

hyperalgesia: increased response to a stimulus that is normally painful. For example, heat hyperalgesia is used to describe the feeling one gets when putting sunburned shoulders under shower water that feels comfortably warm to the hand. (Note: This term can be confusing, because many respected researchers use this term to mean a painful response to normally painless stimuli, as well as a heightened painful response to normally mildly painful stimuli).

hyperpathia: a painful *syndrome* characterized by increased reaction to a stimulus, especially a repetitive stimulus, as well as an *increased* threshold.

hypalgesia (hypoalgesia): diminished sensitivity to stimuli that are normally considered noxious.

hypesthesia (hypoesthesia): diminished sensitivity to stimulation, generally used with nonnoxious stimuli.

neuralgia: pain in the territory of a nerve or nerves.

neuropathy: a disturbance in function or a pathological change in a nerve: If confined to one nerve, it is called mononeuropathy; if it involves several, mononeuropathy multiplex; if symmetrical and bilateral, polyneuropathy.

pain threshold: the minimum stimulus required to cause a perception of pain.

pain tolerance level: the greatest level of pain that a subject is prepared to tolerate. This can vary over time and with gender, culture, and situation.

paresthesia: an abnormal painless sensation, whether spontaneous or evoked (specify).

radiculopathy: a disturbance of function or pathological change in one or more nerve roots.

tender point: an area of the body that when palpated with a force of 4 kg/cm², causes a complaint of pain. A group of 18 consistent tender points have been described in the American College of Rheumatology's (ACR) clinical case definition of fibromyalgia syndrome. Some of the ACR tender points are muscular and some are osseous or cartilaginous (10).

trigger point: a hypersensitive fusiform or nodular area or site in muscle or connective tissue, usually associated with myofascial pain syndrome.

trigger zone: an area that when stimulated, causes a paroxysm of pain in trigeminal neuralgia.

When testing sensory function, both peripheral nerve territories and dermatomes are being assayed, as peripheral nerves derive from spinal nerve roots. All too often clinicians rely on a standard peripheral nerve or dermatome chart as if the anatomy were irrefutable. As with most things in medicine, few things are absolute. There is a considerable variation in the population regarding dermatomal and peripheral innervation. Generally the published charts cover the average case; however, significant individual variation occurs. It is useful to consider how dermatome charts were derived. Techniques have included actual dissection of nerve fibers of one single root to the periphery, analyzing patterns of herpetic eruptions, tracing cutaneous hyperesthesia associated with visceral disease, injecting individual spinal nerves with anesthetics or cutting single roots, and studying war injuries of nerves and the spinal cord (11–13). Obviously, this variation in methods, as well as the variation in humans, suggests that charts should be used as a rough guide only (Figs. 4.1 to 4.3).

Study of numerous charts yields some consistencies that can be used clinically. Listed in Table 4.3 are some useful landmarks.

It is important to approach the sensory examination with a view to the presenting situation. For example, in the case of a thoracic epidural infusion of local anesthetic that migrates cephalad and causes numbness of the little fingers, one would correctly assume that the source of the problem was anesthetic agent reaching the C8 roots, as opposed to the ulnar nerve, even though the presentation and sensory examination would be about the same, since the little fingers are innervated by the ulnar nerve with fibers arising from the C8 dorsal root ganglia. Conversely, numbness arising after an elbow contusion would likely be due to ulnar nerve injury and would not represent a C8 sensory neuropathy.

REFLEX TESTING

Reflex testing can be very useful in determining a level of involvement of a spinal process, such as a herniated nucleus pulposis. There are also caveats with this part of the examination, however. A certain percentage of the population demonstrate reflex abnormalities or "pathological" reflexes that for the purposes of a pain examination are meaningless. It is, for instance, not uncommon to permanently lose a triceps surae tendon (ankle jerk) reflex after a herniated L5-S1 disc, even if the herniation is successfully treated surgically. This may persist as an "abnormal" finding in the absence of any other findings and may have no clinical significance. Likewise, certain signs thought of as pathological are seen in the absence of disease and injury (discussed later).

Reflexes usually elicited on routine clinical examination are of the muscle stretch and cutaneous types. Muscle stretch reflexes are often imprecisely called deep tendon reflexes. The afferent limb of the reflex arc arises from muscle spindles that are sensitive to stretch. It is convenient to stretch the muscle abruptly by percussing its tendon. This sends a volley of impulses, usually across only one synapse, to the associated

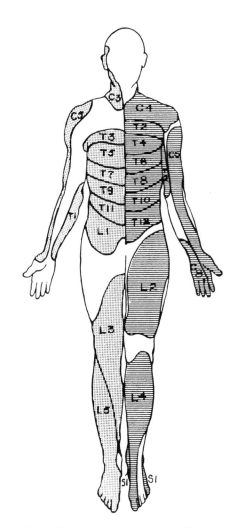

Figure 4.1. Dermatomes according to Foerster. These data were derived by examining remaining sensibility on humans with known nerve lesions. (Reprinted with permission from Foerster O. The dermatomes in man. Brain 1933;56:1.)

anterior horn cells, which constitute the efferent limb. The action potentials from the anterior horn cells cause a protective tightening of the muscle to prevent overstretching. Cutaneous reflexes, which are in the class of superficial reflexes, have an arc composed of skin (afferent) to muscle (efferent). Reflexes can be graded for purposes of reporting findings. Asymmetry is especially important. An accepted system is presented in Table 4.4.

Plantar stimulation, a superficial reflex often tested and recorded at the same time as the muscle stretch reflexes, is often recorded as flexor (indicated by a downward arrow) in the normal condition, absent (indicated by a 0), or abnormal (indicated by an upward arrow). Babinski's sign is upward movement of the great toe accompanied by fanning of the small toes.

Comments on the speed of the reflexes, such as "the right patellar reflex was 2+ and brisk" are also relevant. Hypothyroidism may, for example, slow the recovery phase of a reflex without necessarily affecting its presence or absence. Remember that muscle stretch reflexes are inhibited from

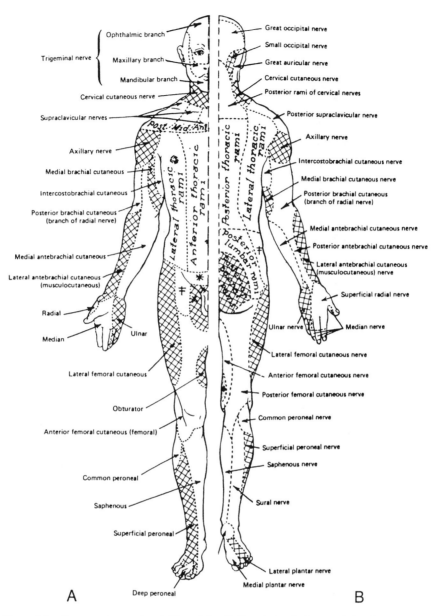

Figure 4.2.   Cutaneous innervation. **A.** Ventral view. **B.** Dorsal view. In the ventral view the nerves represented by symbols are iliohypogastric (*), ilioinguinal (x), and genitofemoral (‡). (Reprinted with permission from Chusid JG. Functional neurology and correlative neuroanatomy. 18th ed. Los Altos: Lange Medical Publishers, 1982;208–209.)

higher centers, such that a lesion more rostral in the central nervous system (CNS) than the level tested usually causes a *loss of tonic inhibition,* making the reflex hyperactive. In withdrawal from CNS depressants (alcohol, barbiturates, benzodiazepines) all reflexes may be hyperactive.

Two abnormal reflexes generally indicate upper motor neuron lesions. These are Babinski's sign and Hoffmann's sign. They are assessed as follows:

Babinski's Sign

Babinski's sign is elicited by lightly stroking the lateral aspect of the sole, from the heel to the ball of the foot, stopping at the metatarsal heads. The normal person demonstrates a rapid flexion of the toes, with the small toes flexing more than the great toe. The abnormal response has two parts, extension of the great toe and fanning of the small toes. There may also be ankle dorsiflexion, knee and hip flexion, and slight abduction of the thigh. It is best elicited with the patient recumbent with the lower extremities extended and the heels resting on the examining table. It may be enhanced by having the patient turn the head to the opposite side. In the anxious patient or patient with hyperalgesia of the plantar surface of the foot, an exaggerated withdrawal may impair the ability to evaluate for Babinski's sign.

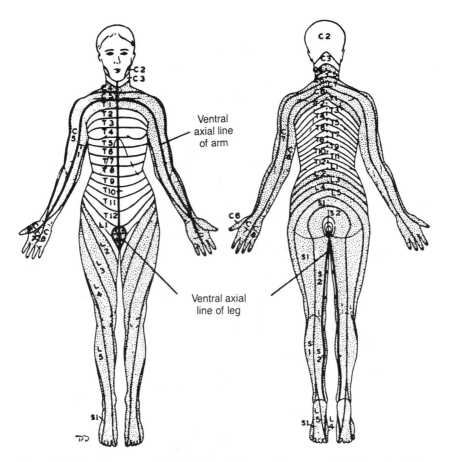

Figure 4.3. Dermatomes according to Keegan and Garrett. These were derived from hypalgesia due to compression of single nerve roots. Compare with Figure 4.1. (Reprinted with permission from Keegan JJ, Garrett FD. The segmental distribution of the cutaneous nerves in the limbs of man. Anat Rec 1943;102:409.)

Table 4.3.   Landmarks for Testing Sensation

Dermatome	Territory	Peripheral Nerve
C5	Shoulder patch	Axillary
C6	Six shooter	Radial (thumb), median (index)
C7	Long finger	Median
C8	Small finger	Ulnar
T1	Medial arm	Medial brachial cutaneous
T2	Sternal notch	Intercostal
T4	Nipples	Intercostal
T6	Xiphoid process	Intercostal
T10	Umbilicus	Intercostal
L1	Inguinal ligament	Ilioinguinal
L2	Anterolateral thigh	Anterior and later femoral cutaneous
L3	Medial knee	Obturator
L4	Anteromedial shin	Saphenous
L5	Dorsum of foot (esp. 1st web space)	Deep peroneal
S1	Lateral aspect of foot	Sural

Table 4.4.   Reflex Grading System

0	Absent
1+	Trace (brought out with Jendrassik's maneuver or other reinforcement)
2+	Elicited without reinforcement
3+	Increased but not to a pathological degree, unsustained clonus, hyperactive, may spread to other muscles
4+	Sustained clonus, often involves other muscles, abnormal

Hoffmann's Sign

Hoffmann's sign can, *with the caveats mentioned earlier,* be thought of as the upper extremity equivalent of the sign of Babinski. It is elicited by holding the patient's hand with the wrist slightly more extended than neutral, then grasping the distal phalanx of the middle finger, extending the digit in the process. The nail of the extended finger is then snapped by a sharp flick of the examiner's thumb, such that a quick forced flexion of the of the distal phalanx is followed by a sudden release. The response is flexion of the index finger and flexion and adduction of the thumb. However, this sign is commonly found in the general population in its incomplete form (only one digit moves or both move slightly), or when a person exhibits an increase in all muscle stretch reflexes. When present bilaterally in the setting of generally hyperactive reflexes, it is considered a normal finding. Since anxiety is one reason for hyperactive reflexes, it is commonly seen, especially in the incomplete form, in the pain patient. When present in its full form, it usually indicates a pyramidal tract lesion above the sixth cervical segment.

Conditions such as cervical myelopathy from an osteophytic bar can cause Hoffmann's or Babinski's sign or both. General anesthesia, intravenous sedation, and coma can also cause these signs via cerebral depression with loss of tonic inhibition.

Confounding the interpretation of reflex testing is the fact that there is only general agreement about which roots innervate each muscle stretch reflex and the relative contribution of each root when multiple roots are known to be involved. A summary of what are thought to be the most commonly accepted levels appears as Table 4.5.

One must examine reflexes with an idea of the underlying disease to gain the most information. For example, if the C6 root is suspected of being compressed by herniation of the C5-C6 disc, one might expect to see depression of the biceps brachii, the brachioradialis, and the finger flexor reflexes with relative preservation of the triceps reflex. If, on the other hand, a radial nerve injury was suspected on account of the history, one might only see diminishment of the brachioradialis and the triceps reflexes.

Some reflexes are called inverted when an antagonistic response is elicited. This can be caused by disease of the normal efferent limb of the reflex, such that the afferent stimulus causes a contraction of antagonist muscle groups. Examples include testing the brachioradialis (radial, radial periosteal, or supinator) reflex in the presence of a lesion involving the C5 root. This may give rise to contraction of the flexors of the wrist and fingers with no supination, due to denervation of the supinators and unopposed contraction of the wrist flexors, causing inversion of the radial reflex. This may also be seen in testing the triceps in the face of damage to the C7 and C8 roots, in which one sees unopposed contraction of the biceps brachii, brachioradialis, and brachialis, causing flexion of the elbow instead of the expected extension. This is also called the paradoxical triceps reflex.

Cutaneous reflexes are less consistently present, respond more slowly, and fatigue more quickly than muscle stretch reflexes, but they may still have utility in locating a disorder. Some useful cutaneous reflexes are listed in Table 4.6.

MUSCLE TESTING

Muscle strength testing is subject to volition and can be very difficult to assess in the uncooperative patient. A well-accepted grading system is outlined in Table 4.7. Note should be made of muscle mass asymmetry. A tape measure can be employed to document differences in limb circumference due to atrophy of muscles or edema. The character of muscle contraction should be observed. Patterns commonly seen in pain

Table 4.5.   Muscle Stretch Reflexes

Reflex	Roots	Peripheral Nerves
Deltoid	**C5** (C6)	axillary
Biceps brachii	**C6** (C5)	musculocutaneous
Brachioradialis	**C6** (C5)	radial
Finger flexor	**C6** (C7-T1)	median and ulnar
Triceps:	**C7** (C6–8)	radial
Patellar (quadriceps)	**L4** (L2–4)	femoral
Medial hamstring Semimembranosus Semitendinosus	**L5** (L4-S2)	tibial portion of sciatic
Achilles (triceps surae)	**S1** (L5-S2)	posterior tibial

Dominant root is in boldface, followed by less dominant in parentheses. The third column is the peripheral nerve(s) involved in the reflex arc.

Table 4.6.   Cutaneous Reflexes

Reflex	Roots	Nerves
Superficial abdominal	T6-T12	Intercostals
Cremasteric	L1-L2	Ilioinguinal, genitofemoral
Plantar	L4-S2	Tibial
Superficial anal (wink)	S2-S5	Inferior hemorrhoidal

Table 4.7.   Muscle Strength Grading System

Grade	Description
0	No contraction visible
1	Flicker or trace of contraction
2	Complete range of motion with gravity eliminated
3	Complete range of motion against gravity
4	Complete range of motion against gravity, with some resistance
5	Complete range of motion against gravity, with full resistance

patients include breakaway weakness, incomplete effort, and cogwheel rigidity. Cogwheel rigidity is usually caused by dopamine blocking drugs (antipsychotics, some antiemetics) and is characterized by a ratchety or bumpy feel to flexor muscles when a joint is passively extended against slight resistance. Hoover's sign is demonstrated by placing the examiner's hand under the supine patient's heel and instructing the patient to lift the opposite lower extremity off the examining table. When genuine effort is expended by the attempt to raise the leg, definite downward pressure is felt on the examiner's hand as that leg comes into play to stabilize the pelvis to allow the other to rise. If effort to raise the other leg is not significant, no pressure will be appreciated. This can occur in a number of contexts, such as feigning weakness, excessive illness behaviors, and malingering, and it must be interpreted correctly. Key upper extremity muscles to test are listed in Table 4.8.

Table 4.8.   Upper Extremity Muscles

Muscle	Action	Dominant Root	Peripheral Nerve
Deltoid	Shoulder abduction	**C5** (C6)	Axillary
Biceps, brachialis	Elbow flexion	**C6** (C5)	Musculocutaneous
Flexor carpi radialis	Wrist flexion, radial deviation	**C6–C7**	Median
Triceps	Forearm extension	**C7** (C6–C8)	Radial
Extensors carpi	Wrist extension	**C7** (C5–C8)	Radial
Flexor dig. superficialis	Flexion of PIP joint	**C8** (C7–T1)	Median
Flexor carpi ulnaris	Wrist flexion, ulnar deviation	**C8** (C7–T1)	Ulnar
Abductor digiti minimi	Abduction of fifth digit	**C8–T1**	Ulnar
First dorsal interosseous	Abduction of second digit	**T1** (C8)	Ulnar

Froment's sign is an indication of ulnar neuropathy. It is seen during testing of ulnar adduction of the thumb (adduction of the thumb in an ulnar direction), as one might hold a key or hold a piece of paper with the thumb and the head of the second metacarpal bone. The muscle responsible for this action is the adductor pollicis, which is innervated by the ulnar nerve. If there is ulnar neuropathy, the adductor pollicis will be weak, and in an attempt to hold the paper, the patient will flex the interphalangeal joint of the thumb by engaging the flexor pollicis longus muscle, which is innervated by the median nerve.

Muscles that can be useful in localization of lesions affecting the lower extremities are listed in Table 4.9.

MODIFIED SCHOBER'S MEASUREMENT

Schober's measurement is helpful in assessing the range of motion of the lumbar spine in flexion. It is not as accurate as inclinometry but is performed without equipment beyond a tape measure and generally suffices for clinical purposes, although not for impairment evaluation (15). When a person bends forward at the waist, most of the motion occurs in the hips, not the spine. In a effort to isolate the spinal motion component, Schober described a test that has been modified by others as follows (16, 17): Make a line between the posterior superior iliac spines (dimples of Venus) crossing the midline of the lumbar spine. Measure up 10 cm and down 5 cm and make a mark at leach level on the midline. Have the patient flex as far as possible and measure the distance between the cephalad and caudad marks. In a normal range of lumbar motion, this should increase from 15 to 20 cm. It can be more accurate with repetition.

NERVE TENSION AND IMPINGEMENT MANEUVERS

Nerve tension and impingement maneuvers can be useful guides in the clinical evaluation of low-back or cervical pain. The best-known is the straight leg raising test (SLR), which is generally performed *incorrectly*. For this test, which tenses the sciatic nerve, to have any clinical usefulness as a test for nerve root involvement, it must be done passively. All of the effort must be on the part of the examiner, not the patient. With chronic pain patients, this degree of relaxation and cooperation is frequently difficult to achieve. Many have been exposed to this test by numerous other practitioners, so they know what to expect. A patient who has been hurt by this maneuver before will logically expect to be hurt again and will guard, making the maneuver unreliable as a means of assessing sciatica. If the patient cannot relax or assists you in raising the extremity despite encouragement not to help, a false-positive result can often be due to tightening of lower back and extremity muscles. This can be diagnosed by holding the extremity steadily at the least angle that causes pain and coaxing the patient to relax. If muscles are contributing to the result, the pain will significantly diminish or vanish as the patient relaxes.

At levels below 30° there is little tension on the nerve, although there is some motion that can result in positive findings in an acutely irritated nerve root. At levels beyond 70°, little tension is added; therefore the reasonable range of observation is between these values (18). A positive SLR (Lasègue's sign) is a reproduction of the patient's sciatica (*not* back or hip pain and *not* popliteal tightness) when the lower extremity is *passively* flexed at the hip with the knee fully extended. Additional information may be obtained by dorsiflexion of the foot (Bragard's sign), which increases nerve tension. This must, as with all diagnostic maneuvers in chronic pain patients, be done with no cues as to the expected results. Grasp the foot of the leg that has been lifted to the maximum allowable angle and first plantar flex the foot, which releases tension on the sciatic nerve by slacking the tibial portion. Then ask the patient, "Does this change your pain?" This is a nondirected question. Then dorsiflex the foot (Bragard's maneuver) and ask the same question. This provides more valid information than doing Bragard's maneuver and asking, "Does this make your pain worse?" which implies a positive response.

A variation of the SLR is passively raising the sound limb, causing distally radiating pain in the extremity that is not being raised, the so-called crossed SLR. This is thought by many clinicians to indicate root pathology.

A somewhat analogous sign for the cervical region is Spurling's maneuver, but its results rest on *impingement* rather

Table 4.9.   Lower Extremity Muscles

Muscle	Action	Dominant Root	Peripheral Nerve
Thigh adductors	Adduction	**L2–L3** (L4)	Obturator, some sciatic contribution
Iliacus, psoas	Flexion of hip	**L2** (L1–L3)	Nerve to psoas and femoral (iliacus)
Quadriceps femoris	Knee extension	**L4** (L2–L4)	Femoral
Tibialis anterior	Foot inversion	**L5** (L4-S1)	Deep peroneal
Gluteus medius	Hip abduction	**L4-L5** (S1)	Superior gluteal
Extensor hallucis longus	Great toe extension	**L5** (S1)	Deep peroneal
Gastrocnemius/soleus	Plantar flexion	**S1-S2**	Tibial
Peroneus longus	Foot eversion	**S1** (L4-S1)	Superficial peroneal

than tension. To perform the maneuver, the patient's head is laterally flexed to the affected side and extended and compressed with some force. A positive result causes radiation of pain along a cervical root dermatome that is due to narrowing of the cervical neuroforamina on that side. False-positive results frequently occur with myofascial pain syndromes aggravated by anticipatory tensioning of affected muscles.

SCREENING FOR OTHER CONDITIONS

Muscle Pain Syndromes

Several muscle pain syndromes mimic neurogenic pain, as can facet arthropathy and hip disease. Myofascial pain syndrome, a common presentation in the pain medicine practice, frequently seems to be triggered by the abrupt, often unexpected, application of significant force to a muscle (impact loading). It can be confined to a single muscle but is frequently found to be regional, involving the muscles originally injured and their antagonists. It is exacerbated by sleep disturbance, which almost invariably accompanies the condition. It is made more severe by the deconditioning usually seen in chronic pain patients.

The diagnosis is made on the basis of a number of factors, including a decreased range of motion of joints moved by affected muscles. Taut bands within muscles that have a rope-like character are also appreciated. Trigger points are palpable, often fusiform nodular areas within taut bands that are tender to touch. Palpation of them often gives rise to referred pain. Snapping or flipping a trigger point under one's fingers often elicits the local twitch response, a local contraction that occurs a few seconds after the palpation. Travell and Simons argue that this feature is pathognomonic for myofascial pain syndrome (19).

A somewhat similar condition called fibromyalgia syndrome has tender points, some of which are myofascial trigger points and some of which are not. In 1990 the ACR codified fibromyalgia syndrome as having three diagnostic criteria. The first is at least a 3-month history of widespread pain. Pain is considered widespread when it affects all of the following areas: the left and right sides of the body, above and below the waist, and the axial skeleton (cervical spine, low back, anterior chest, thoracic spine). The second criterion is pain in 11 of 18 tender point sites (Table 4.10) on digital palpation, which must be performed with approximately 4 kg/cm^2 force. To have a

Table 4.10   ACR Fibromyalgia Tender Points

Name	Location
Occiput	Bilateral, at suboccipital muscle insertions
Low cervical	Bilateral, at anterior aspects of intertransverse spaces C5-C7
Trapezius	Bilateral, at midpoint of upper border
Supraspinatus	Bilateral, at origins, above scapular spine near medial border
Second rib	Bilateral, near second costochondral junctions, just lateral to junctions on upper surfaces
Lateral epicondyle	Bilateral, 2 cm distal to epicondyles
Gluteal	Bilateral, in upper outer quadrants of buttocks in anterior fold of muscle
Greater trochanter	Bilateral, posterior to trochanteric prominence
Knee	Bilateral, at medial fat pad proximal to joint line

positive finding, the subject must state that the palpation was painful, not merely tender. The third criterion is that the presence of a second disorder does not preclude the diagnosis of fibromyalgia (10). These patients often present with sleep disturbance and fatigue.

A particular myofascial syndrome that is frequently misattributed to spinal disease is the piriformis muscle syndrome. This deep muscle originates from the sacrum and forms a tendon that inserts in the intertrochanteric groove of the femur. It is an external rotator of the femur and is often the culprit when a person habitually sits cross-legged and has pain deep in the buttock and down the posterior aspect of the thigh. Because of its close approximation with the sciatic nerve, it occasionally causes sciatica (pain along the tract of the nerve). In the supine position the entire extremity may be externally rotated (piriformis sign). To examine a patient for the piriformis syndrome, place him or her in a lateral decubitus position with the painful side up. Flex the hip and knee of the affected extremity to 90° as though performing a sciatic nerve block. Draw a line from the greater trochanter to the posterior superior iliac spine. Bisect the line and drop down about 3 to 5 cm, depending on the size of the buttock. Using these landmarks, palpate deeply with one finger. The muscle may be felt through the gluteus maximus as a tight band extending from the sacrum at its widest point, to the trochanter, where it narrows to the tendon. A local twitch response is often seen in the muscle.

Facet Syndrome and Hip Disease

Facet syndromes can be suggested by lateral flexion, rotation, and extension of the spine. However, the very existence of facet joint-induced symptoms has been called into question. It is quite popular to inject facet joints. One must be aware, however, that a needle traverses muscles and ligaments to get to the joint, calling into question the specificity of the facet injection.

Patrick's Sign

Patrick's sign is useful in implicating hip disease as a cause of complaint. It is performed by placing the heel on the opposite knee with the patient recumbent and pressing the knee down toward the table. If this reproduces pain, it is worth evaluating the hip radiographically. This will also cause groin and medial thigh pain if the thigh adductors are tight. Since this involves **f**lexion, **ab**duction and **e**xternal **r**otation, followed by lightly forced **e**xtension, is sometimes called the Fabere test (there is, alas, no Dr. Fabere who devised this test, so the possessive form is incorrect).

Waddell's Signs

In 1979, in an attempt to standardize part of the examination of patients complaining of low-back pain, Waddell (20) described a set of nonorganic physical signs. These have are commonly called Waddell's signs. He classified them into five groups, as listed in Table 4.11.

It is unfortunate that Waddell's interpretations have been altered with time. All too often a physician asserts that because a patient had some of Waddell's signs on examination, there is nothing wrong with the patient. This is seen in general medical practice, compensation cases, and impairment evaluations. I have routinely observed university and community physicians who determine an impairment value of zero when Waddell's signs are present, ignoring all other findings. This was not the intent by Waddell and colleagues. Rather, the original article was written to assist physicians in the avoidance of unnecessary surgery and to identify patients with clear surgical indications who would likely benefit from a formal psychosocial evaluation of their complaints prior to surgery. It is invalid to use this constellation of signs as prima facie evidence of malingering or secondary gain.

In scoring the evaluation of Waddell's signs, any positive sign is credited as a positive type (i.e., either superficial or nonanatomical tenderness counts as tenderness; both are not required). His research indicated that a finding of three or more positive groups or types is significant. It is important that he asserted that isolated positive signs should be ignored. Too often physicians use these signs in isolation or are apparently so focused on "revealing" the patient's true motivation for complaints that attempts to elicit the signs are performed incorrectly or the examiner's bias is given the benefit of the doubt and the patient is incorrectly labeled. In his original description, Wad-

Table 4.11   Nonorganic Physical Signs in Low Back Pain

Tenderness
   Superficial
   Nonanatomic
Simulation
   Axial loading
   Rotation
Distraction
   Straight leg raising
Regional
   Sensory
   Weakness
Overreaction

Reprinted with permission from Waddell G, McCulloch JA, Kummel E, et al. Nonorganic physical signs in low-back pain. Spine 1980;5:117–125.

dell called attention to incorrect interpretation and false positives that should be considered. Some conditions in which Waddell's signs are often erroneously attributed are discussed next.

Tenderness

Superficial skin roll tenderness is frequently seen in fibromyalgia syndrome and may easily present a false-positive if taken out of context. Waddell's signs have been validated in the complaint of low-back pain, not diffuse pain as seen in fibromyalgia syndrome. In the 1979 article he stated that an isolated band of tenderness can be seen in the territory of a posterior primary ramus due to radiculitis and that this does not count as a positive sign. Nonanatomical tenderness, originally described as deep tenderness over a wide area, can often be seen in patients with myofascial pain and fibromyalgia syndromes. Such tenderness generally does not indicate surgically correctable diseases of the spine. It does not imply, however, that there is nothing wrong with the patient.

Simulation Tests

Waddell cautions that suggestion is to be minimized when giving the patient the idea that an examination maneuver to stress the spine is being carried out. I have observed physicians performing simulation tests while asking the patient, "Does this make your back pain worse?" Clearly, the vector of expected answer is implied. Both simulated axial spine loading and truncal rotation can elicit positive responses in the individual who has a muscle pain syndrome and who is guarded (tensing affected muscles) while performing these maneuvers. Again, these instances do not indicate operable disease but should not be interpreted improperly.

Distraction Tests

As a method of verification of an organic basis for a positive physical sign elicited on examination, the finding can be sought again when the patient is distracted from what the examiner is actually testing. Waddell admonishes that the distraction should not be painful, emotional, or surprising to the patient. He states that the best way to perform this is as described early in this chapter: simple attentive observation of the patient. If findings are consistently present, they likely have an anatomical or physiological basis. If they are intermittent, especially present only on formal examination, he allows that they *may* have a nonorganic component. Perhaps the most common distraction device is the SLR done with the patient sitting and the examiner ostensibly evaluating the strength of ankle dorsiflexion or checking the sole for plantar warts, compared with the SLR done with the patient recumbent (the so-called flip test). However, the pelvis is not in the same position relative to the spine when sitting and recumbent. Also, all of the errors previously mentioned about the SLR apply here.

Regional Disturbances

Under regional disturbances Waddell describes giving way of muscles and cogwheeling. Reasons for cogwheeling, on a purely neurochemical basis, have already been described. Pain is often a reason for giving way of strength on testing muscles. Sensory disturbances are described as stocking patterns rather than dermatomal ones. While a stocking pattern of diminished sensation is not generally caused by surgically correctable spine disease, it can be seen in patients with low-back pain, such as a paraneoplastic neuropathy, concurrent diabetic neuropathy, or multiple root involvement in spinal stenosis or from arachnoiditis, especially with prior surgeries.

Overreaction

Waddell noted that overreaction was the one sign that was most sensitive to observer bias, so caution should be exercised in recording and interpreting this sign. It is very common for patients with long-standing suffering to display excessive pain behaviors. One can think of this as merely a nonverbal communication of the seriousness of the problem to the patient. Its presence is not useful for the purposes of determining disease that is amenable to surgery. It does not indicate absence of a problem, however.

Further research has been done by Waddell and others into this facet of the examination. They concluded that overt pain behaviors provided additional information about illness behavior in low-back pain patients (21). Work by Werneke and colleagues suggests that failure of overt behaviors to diminish over the course of a work-oriented physical rehabilitation program correlated with failure to return to work and may be seen as a reason for referral to a program with a more psychological focus (22). In the setting of a more comprehensive approach to pain rehabilitation, however, Waddell's signs did not predict success at 1-year follow-up (23). The program that was studied attempted to address all barriers to reintegration into the work force and to manage somatization complaints effectively in all participants.

In summary, Waddell's signs, properly assessed and scored, can be an efficient adjunct to the clinical evaluation of the patient presenting with low back pain, especially in determining which patients may benefit from a formal psychosocial assessment as opposed to further workup for surgical interventions. Performed incorrectly or interpreted improperly, they detract from the evaluation process.

SUMMARY

While it is impractical for pain physicians to complete residencies in neurology, psychiatry, and spine surgery, it is possible to perform an efficient, thoughtful evaluation of the patient with the complaint of unremitting pain. It is hoped that review of the information presented in this chapter will enable the pain physician to combine skills and knowledge from various other specialties to assist in the formulation of a comprehensive plan of care for pain patients.

References

1. Aminoff MJ, Greenberg DA, Simon RP. Clinical Neurology. 3rd ed. Stamford, CT: Appleton & Lange, 1996;153.
2. Cipriano JJ. Photographic manual of regional orthopaedic and neurological tests. Baltimore: Williams & Wilkins, 1991.
3. Wilson-Pauwels L, Akesson EJ, Stewart PA. Cranial nerves: anatomy and clinical comments. Toronto: BC Decker, 1988.
4. Haerer AF. DeJong's Neurological Examination. 5th ed. Philadelphia: Lippincott, 1992.
5. Fishbain DA, Cutler R, Rosomoff HL, Rosomoff RS. Chronic pain-associated depression: antecedent or consequence of chronic pain? A review. Clin J Pain 1997;13:116–137.
6. Ewing JA. Detecting alcoholism: the CAGE questionnaire. JAMA 1984;252:1905 –1907.
7. First MB, ed. Quick reference to the diagnostic criteria from DSM-IV. Washington: American Psychiatric Association 1994;108–112.
8. Folstein MF, Folstein S, McHugh PR. Minimental state: a practical method for grading the cognitive state of patients for the clinician. J Psychiatr Res 1975;12:189.
9. Merskey H., Bogduk N. Classification of chronic pain: descriptions of chronic pain syndromes and definitions of pain terms. 2nd ed. Seattle: International Association for the Study of Pain, 1994;210–213.
10. Wolfe F, Smythe HA, et al. American College of Rheumatology 1990 criteria for the classification of fibromyalgia: report of the Multicenter Criteria Committee. Arthritis Rheum 1990;33: 60–172.
11. Foerster O. The dermatomes in man. Brain 1933;56:1–39.
12. Keegan JJ, Garrett FD. The segmental distribution of the cutaneous nerves in the limbs of man. Anat Rec 1943;102:409.
13. Young JH. The revision of the dermatomes. Aust N Z J Surg 1949;18:171.
14. Reference deleted.
15. Hyytianinen K, Salminen JJ, Suvitie T, et al. Reproducibility of nine tests to measure spinal mobility and trunk muscle strength. Scand J Rehab Med 1991;23:3–10.
16. Schober P. Lendenwirblesaule und Kreuzschmerzen. Munchn Med Wschr 1937;84:336–338.
17. Macraw IF, Wright V. Measurement of back movement. Ann Rheum Dis 1969;28:584.
18. Deyo RA, Rainville J, Kent DL. What can the history and physical examination tell us about low back pain? JAMA 1992;268:760–765.
19. Travell JG, Simons DG. Myofascial pain and dysfunction the trigger point manual. Baltimore: Williams & Wilkins, 1983;60–62.

20. Waddell G, McCulloch JA, Kummel E, et al. Nonorganic physical signs in low-back pain. Spine 1980;5:117–125.
21. Waddell G, Richardson J. Observation of overt pain behaviour by physicians during routine clinical examination of patients with low back pain. J Psychosom Res 1992;36:77–87.
22. Werneke MW, Harris DE, Lichter RL. Clinical effectiveness of behavioral signs for screening chronic low-back pain patients in a work-oriented physical rehabilitation program. Spine 1993;18:2412–2418.
23. Polatin PB, Cox B, Gatchel RJ, et al. A prospective study of Waddell signs in patients with chronic low back pain when they may not be predictive. Spine 1997;22:1618–1621.

Suggested Readings

Deyo RA, Rainville J, Kent DL. What can the history and physical examination tell us about low back pain? JAMA 1992;268:760–765.

Haerer AF, ed. DeJong's Neurologic Examination. ed 5. Philadelphia: Lippincott, 1992.

Hoppenfeld S. Orthopedic neurology: a diagnostic guide to neurologic levels. Philadelphia: Lippincott, 1977.

Van Allen MW, Rodnitzky RL, eds. Pictorial manual of neurologic tests. 2nd ed. Chicago: Yearbook Medical, 1981.

APPENDIX

EVALUATIONS OF PATIENTS PRESENTING WITH LOW BACK OR LEG PAIN AND NECK OR UPPER EXTREMITIES PAIN

Low-Back and Leg Pain

Observe gait and station. Note antalgic behaviors during history and physical examination (e.g., moving, climbing onto examination table). Note overreaction behaviors (e.g., sighing, moaning, grimacing.)

Have patient walk forward, backward and tandem, toe walk and heel walk, squat on both legs, and on each in turn. This provides a quick assessment of lower extremity strength.

Check Schober's measurement and other range of motion (lateral flexion, extension and rotation). Check skin roll tenderness and do simulated truncal rotation and axial loading.

Have patient sit. Check pulses and temperature of feet. Check sensation, noting pattern and abnormalities by sensory modality. Check proprioception. Check muscle strength, noting character and location of any deviation from normal. Check for plantar warts and calluses by extending each leg in turn (sitting version of the SLR, the flip test).

Check reflexes, including looking for Babinski's sign.

Have patient recline. Observe the fluidity of this movement and behaviors emitted during it. Recheck SLR, observe for piriformis sign, and check for Patrick's sign.

Turn to one side; check for piriformis pain. Hyperextend femur to assess sacroiliac joint pain and upper lumbar root pain (femoral nerve stretch).

Turn prone. Examine paraspinous muscles for trigger points. Turn to the other side and check for piriformis and sacroiliac.

Neck and Upper Extremity Pain

Observe gait and station. Note antalgic behaviors during history and physical examination (e.g., moving, climbing onto examination table). Note overreaction behaviors (e.g., sighing, moaning, grimacing).

Have patient walk forward, backward and tandem, toe walk and heel walk, squat on both legs and on each in turn. This provides a quick assessment of lower extremity strength.

Test sensation, muscle strength and range of motion of neck and upper extremities. Test reflexes in all four extremities, including Babinski's and Hoffmann's signs. Check proprioception.

Perform Spurling's maneuver. Examine posterior and anterior cervical muscles while upright.

Recline the patient and reexamine the muscles by palpation.

CHAPTER 5

Medical Evaluation and Management of Chronic Pain from a Primary Care Perspective

Margaret A. Caudill

INTRODUCTION

The symptom pain demands an explanation. As human beings, we are driven to find the cause of our physical and emotional pain. It is the very nature of pain, to warn the organism of danger and harm, that fuels the search. Many times this involves presenting to the health care provider with pain as the main complaint or as one of several symptoms in need of explanation and treatment. In the majority of cases, the discovery and treatment of the underlying disease or disorder that stimulated the pain system generally calms the pain as well. The residual pain that may persist while healing is taking place is usually responsive to nonsteroidal anti-inflammatory agents or opioid pain medication. But what happens when the disease is incurable and is associated with pain and/or the pain persists even though laboratory or radiological evidence of causal factors is not apparent? What can the health care provider do?

GOALS OF THIS CHAPTER

This chapter addresses the issues of chronic pain evaluation and management from a primary health care perspective. Implicit assumptions are that primary health care providers are not expert in all chronic pain-producing diseases and disorders, that they are serving a patient population with diverse physical and emotional needs, and that they are under time and cost constraints. These modern-day practice realities make the identification and treatment of chronic pain, including the psychosocial sequelae, particularly problematic and frustrating for both patient and health care provider. There is, however, a growing literature that helps to elucidate the pathology and physiological principles involved in chronic pain. Applying this rudimentary understanding to the treatment of chronic pain and addressing the psychosocial management of pain can bring an improved quality of life to the sufferer. The intent of this chapter is to describe the physiology of chronic pain, the treatments that address the biopsychosocial needs of this population, and the resources available for more complex pain management evaluation and treatment.

WHY THE PRIMARY CARE PROVIDER IS OPTIMALLY POSITIONED TO HELP

There are three compelling reasons for the primary health care provider to aggressively identify and treat persistent pain. The first reason is that the primary care provider usually sees the patient at the onset of the pain and ideally has a relationship with the patient that can give context to the complaint. The primary care provider is well positioned to coordinate the recommendations from multiple specialty consultants who may have been asked to assist with identifying and resolving the underlying problem. This established relationship between patient and provider may ensure compliance with treatment recommendations and offer validation and understanding during the many months it may take to establish a diagnosis and satisfactory treatment regimen.

The second reason is that early intervention to stop the pain signal may be critical to preventing chronic pain. It is becoming increasingly apparent that certain mechanisms may permanently establish the pain signal in the central nervous system, where it is much more difficult to turn off, if the pain is allowed to persist for an indeterminate period. Therefore, early recognition and treatment of pain in a disease, trauma, or illness appear to be critical.

The third reason for identification and aggressive treatment of persistent pain is to maintain function and minimize the effect of pain, from whatever the source, on quality of life. Pain and its associated disability have a societal effect of major proportion. The disruption of employment, family and societal interactions, and individual integrity is enormous and costs billions of dollars annually (1).

CHALLENGES TO EFFECTIVE AND COMPREHENSIVE TREATMENT

The first challenge to treating chronic pain effectively is overcoming the myth that persistent pain is a psychological disorder without physiological mechanisms. This assumption tends to devalue the complaint and places on the patient the sole responsibility for failure to improve or cope effectively. In our experience, the complexity of the pain experience makes it impossible to distinguish the contribution of mind from that of body. Evaluation and treatment goals should be to identify and treat the underlying cause of the pain signal, and while that is being done, if nothing alters the pain signal, the patient must be assisted in managing his or her life in spite of the pain.

The second challenge is to acquire the information needed to assist in the diagnosis and treatment of chronic pain. Since the education of health care providers traditionally has not included pain treatment, much of what providers have at their disposal is outdated and incomplete. This is slowly being corrected. As guidelines are established and recommendations adopted by institutions and regulatory bodies, there is a concomitant improvement in access to pain medicine information for health professionals and the public.

In October 1995, a National Institutes of Health (NIH) consensus panel met and concluded that incorporation of relaxation and cognitive behavioral therapies into the biomedical treatment of chronic pain was effective, practical, and necessary (2). Two of the barriers preventing adoption of such therapies into chronic pain treatment were identified in this report. One was lack of physician support in recommending such treatments, and the other was lack of patient compliance with skills practice. Physician support depends on understanding the rationale of biopsychosocial treatment and identifying local resources for providing such interventions. Patient compliance also requires understanding of the need to incorporate many biopsychosocial therapies into their comprehensive treatment of chronic pain.

BENEFITS TO PATIENTS AND HEALTH CARE PROVIDERS

Chronic pain is one of the richest biopsychosocial experiences, challenging the skills of the health care provider and the resourcefulness of the patient. There is no reliable treatment to turn off the pain signal that has been established in chronic pain. Early intervention to prevent activation of the central nervous mechanisms that perpetuate the pain signal may be our only hope in the near future. However, addressing the biopsychosocial needs of those with persistent pain and acknowledging that the subjective experience of pain cannot be totally appreciated from our external perspective can go along way in providing a framework for treatment and living with chronic pain.

There are three benefits to the patient and health care provider who address the biopsychosocial experience of pain. One is the reduction in suffering and reported improvement in self-efficacy and function associated with decreasing pain and/or providing information, stress management skills, and support (3). A second benefit is the decrease in clinic visits that arise from the patients' need for reassurance and/or feelings of frustration (4). This directly translates into cost savings for the health care system. The third benefit is the personal satisfaction derived from supporting and managing one of the most difficult medical problems and the opportunity to observe the resiliency of the human organism faced with a very difficult symptom.

DIFFERENCES BETWEEN CHRONIC PAIN AND ACUTE PAIN

To provide adequate understanding, evaluation, and treatment of the patient with persistent pain, it is important to understand that the mechanisms thought to play a role in chronic pain are not exactly those involved in acute pain. The pain system is a critical survival mechanism. It lies in wait for the organism to be injured or for injurious processes such as inflammation or excessive heat or cold to occur and then rallies a complex process that engages physical, emotional, and behavioral responses. Once the organism responds to the emergency, it takes certain steps, such as the inflammatory process and sickness behavior, that begin the healing (5).

Pain accompanying chronic diseases such as rheumatoid or lupus arthritis is presumably the result of mechanisms associated with an aberrant inflammatory or autoimmune process. Such mechanisms may be conceptualized as causing chronic pain by the persistence of chemical irritants released in inflammation that cause the nociceptors to fire. However, some conditions, such as endometriosis, clearly point to other mechanisms playing a role in chronic pain production. For example, the number of endometrial implants does not appear to correlate with the amount of pain a woman has (6). Over the past 2 decades there has been a growing literature describing mechanisms that may account for the persistence of pain in the apparent absence of persistent disease or injury. These observations implicate the spontaneous firing during recovery of injured small unmyelinated pain nerves called C fibers, the lowering of the firing threshold of pain fibers, the recruitment of mechanical sensory fibers into the pain process, and the perpetuation and amplification of the pain signal through central nervous system mechanisms (7, 8). More recently immune system mechanisms that may also contribute to the development of chronic pain and explain the complex "sickness" response associated with these conditions have been identified (5). These observations appear to implicate a mechanism involving the breakdown of the normal checks and balances in the pain system resulting in the pain signal persisting long after the noxious stimulus has disappeared (9). Furthermore, there may be neurotoxic mechanisms that fix this abnormal state of the injured pain system by destroying inhibitory interneurons. If that happens, the pain signal amplification becomes irreversible. It is from such observations that there arises a growing sense of urgency for timely evaluation and treatment of pain before it becomes fixed into a chronic process (10). The length of time it takes in humans, if indeed this process does occur, has not been determined. Given the resistance of chronic pain to "usually effective" interventions and the neuroplasticity thought to thwart many of the potential treatments, it appears that our best hope of a cure is in preventing establishment of the chronic pain mechanisms (11). In terms of concrete recommendations, however, this concept is in its infancy. For now, biopsychosocial assessment and treatment of chronic pain, once established, remains a viable alternative to cure or prevention.

PSYCHOLOGICAL AND SOCIAL CONSEQUENCES OF CHRONIC PAIN

Research has also demonstrated rich connections between the pain input through the dorsal roots and the brain. These connections involve pathways leading directly to the phylogenetically "old" centers of the brain, such as the limbic system, and the "newer" centers, which include cortex (12). The emotional response to pain when it is serving as a warning system is immediate and generally described as fear or anxiety. Behaviorally it drives an organism to seek treatment and/or elicits sickness behavior, which is thought to help the organism to rest and recuperate. Both acute and long-term pain show a complex response composed of learned responses, cultural nuances, genetics, gender, and socioeconomic factors. This rich psychosocial response is generally not a conscious one and may be subject to misinterpretation from someone not in pain. Pain, once experienced, is stored as an aversive circumstance, such as touching fire, to be avoided. However, in memory the quality of the stimulus appears to be blunted, perhaps so that we can react freshly the next time we feel ourselves burning.

It is hard to relate to someone who reports a continuing pain stimulus. While there is considerable controversy among pain specialists about whether chronic pain can be said to be a disability, the tendency to stop functioning when in pain is a strong biological one. Furthermore, having a constant symptom that from all previous experiences means "danger!" and "warning!" can be very stressful to the affected person, who has also been told that nothing can be done about it. The necessity for consideration of chronic pain as a complex biopsychosocial experience is further emphasized when pain management (not cure) is proposed.

BIOPSYCHOSOCIAL MEDICAL EVALUATION

The goals of evaluation of the patient with persistent pain are to identify reversible or occult processes (diabetes, human immunodeficiency virus [HIV], cancer), identify contributing factors that may increase the pain complaint (insomnia, deconditioning, poor diet, posttraumatic stress disorder), identify coping strategies and beliefs about the pain (denial, idea that it is cancer) assess psychological dysfunction (depression, anxiety) and physical dysfunction (activities of daily living, sex, work). The value of a thorough history and physical examination of the patient complaining of persistent pain (Table 5.1) cannot be underestimated. Although the definition

Table 5.1.   History and Physical Examination

	Acute	Chronic
Time	Limited (10–14 days)	>3 months
Quality	Sharp, tingling, searing	Aching, burning, throbbing
Signs	Local injury, edema, erythema, reflexive spasm of muscles	Sensory, autonomic, motor changes
Other symptoms	Increased pulse, blood pressure, respiratory rate	Insomnia, fatigue, muscle tension
		Change in appetite
		Body aches
		Poor concentration and memory
Distribution	Localized, dermatomal	Spreading, somatotopic
Emotion	Anxiety, fear	Depression, anger, hostility
Behaviors	Verbal complaints, moans, grimaces	Sleep disturbance
	Protects area, increased motor activity	Inactive, physical deconditioning
	Rubbing	Social isolation
		Decreased function
		Hypervigilance
Cognitive	Worried, concern, urgency	Despair, hopelessness, helplessness
		Feeling misunderstood, a failure, guilty
		Out of control

of chronic pain has been described in terms of a duration exceeding 3 to 6 months, there is no restriction to considering reevaluation as early as 4 weeks if the pain is out of clinical context. Failure of the pain to respond to time and usually effective treatments are red flags, and they must be attended to. From here, of course, it immediately becomes difficult to talk in generalities. There is clear evidence demonstrating that most patients with acute back pain feel better by 2 weeks (13), but some complex surgical procedures, such as knee replacements, are associated with weeks of pain. In many chronic diseases, such as Crohn's disease, associated with pain, treatment is usually aimed at the underlying pathophysiology and only the "intolerable" pain treated at times of acute exacerbations. However, in general the persistence of pain beyond an expected time of resolution should not be ignored.

History

Additional information that may prove helpful is a description by the patient of the quality of pain, noting words such as stabbing (lancinating), burning, aching, throbbing, dull, and so on. It is thought that nerve damage pain elicits such descriptions. The traditional questions—how, when, where, what makes it better or worse, what have you done for the symptom, and what were the results—are all appropriate for persistent pain as well.

The assessment should include questions about function with activities of daily living, work, socialization, and sexual activities. Inquire into sleep disturbance, whether the patient feels rested upon awakening, number of hours of sleep, presence of anxiety, dysphoria, appetite, and significant life events and/or stressors. It is important to ask what the patient has been doing to reduce the pain, including therapies that may not have been prescribed by you. It is crucial to inquire from the patient what he or she feels or fears may be going on. Designing a plan, whether it be further testing or waiting for a little more time to pass, must be done with the patient's understanding.

Early teaching of the patient to use pain scales and descriptors can be valuable for long-term follow-up and treatment assessment. The use of a diary (Fig. 5.1) to elicit patterns may also prove helpful. There are a variety of pain scales that can be useful depending on the age and cognitive abilities of the person (14). A verbal or visual analogue scale from 0 (no pain) to 10 (worst pain) can easily be used by most people once they are taught its relevance and how to do it.

Helping the patient to describe the quality of sensation may also help to objectify the experience and make it less terrifying. Persistent use of emotional descriptors of the pain may be a clue that the patient is in need of emotional reassurance as well as physical help with the pain. Developing an awareness of both the emotional and sensory components of pain can help validate the patient's mind and body experience. We recommend that during the initial evaluation period and during any flare-ups, the patient keep a diary of pain sensation and associated distress on a scale of 0 to 10, recording three times a day at the same time each day. We have found this to be helpful in determining the contribution of physical and emotional sensations to the total pain experience. In addition, over time the patient's assessment of pain with a diary can provide information as to whether treatment is effective.

The periodic use of questionnaires to assess function, as with the SF36[1], or mood, as with the SCL90R[2], Center for Epidemiological Study Depression scale (17), or Beck Depression Index (18), may help you watch for improvement or deterioration in a patient's response to treatment. In addition, they can provide important documentation of other important parameters that may change even if the pain continues.

Discussion of past and present stressors and any previous chronic pain can be helpful. Significant physical or emotional trauma or sexual abuse history can lead to considerable coping difficulties. The presence of a chronically ill person in the home necessitating lifting or bending may exacerbate a chronic pain problem as well as exhaust a person's coping reserves. A history of prolonged pain following a previous injury may indicate a genetic predisposition or other unknown factors contributing to delayed recovery. Multiple surgeries at the same site can also predispose to nerve injury and nerve compression from scar tissue.

---

[1] For use of the SF36, contact the Medical Outcomes Trust, Box 1917, Boston, MA 02205.
[2] For information on the SCL90, contact National Computer Systems, Box 1416, Minneapolis, MN 55140; 800-627-7271.

Physical Examination

The goal of the physical examination by the primary care provider is to elucidate any previously unidentified treatable medical problems that may have pain as a primary complaint. The most common of these are diabetes, thyroid disease, HIV or other occult infection, neoplasm, rheumatological disorders such as rheumatoid arthritis and ankylosing spondylitis, neurological disorders such as trigeminal neuralgia and postherpetic neuropathy, and musculoskeletal disorders such as disc or facet disease.

The physical evaluation begins at the first contact with the patient. It is very helpful to observe the patient coming from the waiting room into the examination room or office. Speed of movement, gait, use of assistive devices, grimacing, and rubbing all help to create a picture of what the patient wants to communicate to you about his or her pain. Caution should be used in judging "appropriateness" of behaviors out of context of the entire history and physical examination, since such judgment may get in the way of empathically and objectively developing a treatment or diagnostic strategy. The initial examination should be done with the patient in an examination gown. Vital signs, weight, and height if not previously determined may be helpful as the patient is followed over time. It may be quite valuable to examine the patient on several occasions. This is beneficial because many patients find that the examination can exacerbate the pain, and the stability of findings can also be better assessed over time.

In addition to the general physical examination, the system involving the pain complaints should be assessed in detail. Generally, special emphasis is placed on the musculoskeletal and neurological system (Chapter 4). Spreading of pain complaints, such as "my neck was really sore after the accident, but now I ache all over my upper back" and poor sleep quality may be associated with tender points identified as being related to fibrositis (Chapter 13). Persistent back pain when all x-rays, computed tomography (CT), and/or magnetic resonance imaging (MRI) show little in the way of disease or injury may be associated with musculoskeletal imbalances that perpetuate the pain because of asymmetrical musculoskeletal weaknesses. Hypersensitivity of the skin over the painful site (hyperpathia) or the reporting of burning upon light touch of the skin by the examiner (allodynia) may indicate nerve damage and a variant of complex regional pain syndrome (Chapter 11). Low skin temperature, sweating, and swelling may indicate sympathetically maintained pain.

Diagnostic Testing

The discovery or suspicion raised from the history and physical examination should guide the health care provider in the selection of further diagnostic tests. Caution should be used in depending entirely on diagnostic test results if they do not confirm or deny a patient's complaint of persistent pain. Even nerve conduction studies may not reveal the damage in

Sample Pain Diary

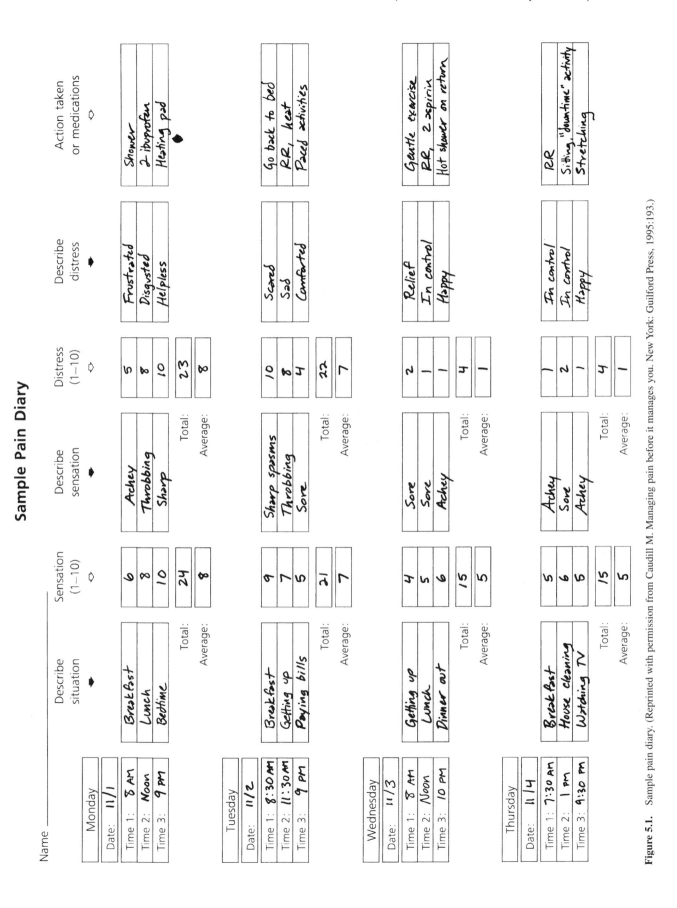

Figure 5.1. Sample pain diary. (Reprinted with permission from Caudill M. Managing pain before it manages you. New York: Guilford Press, 1995:193.)

small C fiber sensory pain nerves that are firing spontaneously. Conversely, too much dependence on abnormal findings that are not consistent with the physical examination or complaints, such as disc bulging or degenerative changes on CT scan or MRI, may also produce ineffective results.

WHEN TO REFER TO A PAIN SPECIALIST

A constant apprehension that you are missing something may be present during the initial identification, diagnosis, and treatment regimen of the patient with persistent pain. The availability of a multidisciplinary pain clinic, pain specialist, or a medical-surgical consultant in the immediate locale must be determined. If the patient has unremitting pain and the treatment is not effective, the cause is unresolved, and/or the patient is finding the experience to be intolerable as reflected in poor functioning and increased depression or anxiety, referral to a pain specialist is highly recommended. Multidisciplinary pain clinics can provide a comprehensive evaluation and treatment strategy for the patient who must live with chronic pain. Pain medicine expertise and experience may also allow these clinics to offer other interventions to help reduce the pain and suffering of the patient. The American Pain Society, American Academy of Pain Medicine, or International Association for the Study of Pain (Appendix) can provide names of physicians and other health care providers specializing in pain medicine.

TREATMENT OF PERSISTENT PAIN

Many patients' pain cannot be resolved. The underlying disease is chronic, the damage to the pain system irreversible, or both. In these cases the goals of treatment are aimed at functional restoration, symptom reduction (including pain and other constitutional symptoms), and self-management of symptoms. This shift from curing (elimination of a disease) to healing (used here as maximizing the person's physical, emotional, social, and spiritual coping) is critical to the treatment and management of chronic pain (Table 5.2). Addressing the biopsychosocial therapy issues is essential for therapeutic success. As future research elucidates the physiological mechanisms that perpetuate chronic pain, there is hope that pharmacological products or procedures will control if not eliminate the alterations that occur in the central nervous system. For now, treatment is directed at supporting the patient in managing the symptoms and living a life with quality and purpose.

Components of Biological Treatment

The pharmacological agents used in chronic pain are primarily targeted at the proposed underlying pain system aberration or central nervous system control mechanisms theorized to modulate pain under normal circumstances. Medications used for reducing chronic pain symptoms include the tricyclic antidepressants, muscle relaxants, anti-inflammatory drugs, antiseizure medications, oral nerve anesthetics, and opioids.

Nonsteroidal anti-inflammatory drugs are used extensively by patients with chronic pain, and they may potentiate opioid medications (19). However, many patients report that anti-inflammatory agents do little to control or decrease their pain. Demonstration of the potential for asymptomatic gastrointestinal bleeding and renal toxicity make careful monitoring in long-term use mandatory.

Low-dose *tricyclic antidepressants,* such as amitriptyline, desipramine, and imipramine, are used to enhance sleep and are thought to facilitate the central pain inhibitory pathways (20). Dosing can be started low, 10 to 25 mg at bedtime, and these drugs may be effective without increasing to 150 mg (as recommended in older texts). The most common side effect is daytime sedation, which may be alleviated by reducing the dose or taking the medication earlier in the evening. Many women report weight gain in spite of a stable diet and exercise program, particularly with amitriptyline. Sometimes stopping the medication is the only way they can reduce their weight. Time should be taken to explain to the patient that these medications are indeed antidepressants but at these low doses are not being used to treat depression. Many a patient who has not learned the rationale from the prescribing health care provider refuses to take these potentially beneficial medications after finding out from the pharmacist or friends what class of medication has been prescribed. The concern of being taken seriously, that the physician may think it is "all in the patient's head," should be respected.

The use of *anticonvulsant medications,* such as carbamazepine, clonazepam, and phenytoin, has a long tradition in conditions such as trigeminal neuralgia and postherpetic neuralgia (20, 21). It is thought that the mechanism of action is the inhibition of abnormal nerve conduction in the damaged pain nerve. The recent appearance of newer anticonvulsants, such as gabapentin, may also be beneficial. While these and most medications used for chronic pain are considered off-label indications, there is enough preliminary research and anecdotal success to try them in some of the neuropathic syndromes that fail to respond to conservative therapies or time. Anticonvulsant doses are generally prescribed for phenytoin (300 mg/day) and carbamazepine (500 to 1000 mg/day), and toxicity is followed with serum drug levels. Gabapentin may be pushed to higher doses than used for seizure control, up to 3600 mg per day, but many patients get benefit from lower doses, between 600 and 1800 mg/day, in three divided doses. The most common complaints, dizziness, fatigue, and nausea, may be helped by prescribing low doses and gradually increasing the dose over several weeks. It is important to advise the patient of the rationale for the use of anticonvulsants in chronic pain and to recommend that they obtain the package insert or the list of possible side effects from the pharmacist for these and any prescription medication.

Other medications used for the treatment of neuropathy include baclofen, mexiletine, and capsaicin. Baclofen, which

Table 5.2.   Treatment

	Acute	Chronic
Medications	Drugs targeting underlying disease, NSAIDs, narcotics	NSAIDs, tricyclic antidepressants Antiseizure medications, baclofen Oral anesthetics, NMDA blockers Narcotics
Other Treatments	Physical, occupational therapy Manipulation therapy	Physical therapy for conditioning Vocational assessment/retraining Complementary alternative medicine therapies Bracing
Procedures	Surgery, preemptive analgesia, nerve blocks, epidural blocks	Nerve blocks, epidural blocks Spinal cord stimulator, intrathecal pumps
Psychosocial	Reassurance, diagnosis with prognosis	Information, social support Antidepressants, pain diary Relaxation skills, pacing activities Cognitive therapy skills, family therapy

acts on GABA-B receptors, has been used as an antispasmodic for muscle hyperspasticity (20). At 30 to 60 mg per day in three divided doses it may be beneficial in reducing both burning and muscle cramping in select patients. Mexiletine is an oral antiarrhythmic that has been used to treat diabetic neuropathy and postherpetic neuralgia (22). The dose is 200 mg two to three times a day. Some practitioners challenge the patient with an IV lidocaine infusion to toxic side effect levels before prescribing mexiletine. A cardiology evaluation may be helpful to assess cardiac vulnerability when using such agents, particularly in the diabetic patient.

Capsaicin is the active ingredient in hot chili peppers. It is known to deplete substance P, a pain neurotransmitter, from nerve terminals in some animal pain models. The clinical results have been variable, although benefits in diabetic neuropathy and postherpetic neuralgia (23) have been reported. Patients must be advised that a temporary increase in pain is an important indication of activity, but it may not be tolerated by some. Patients who use the over-the-counter ointment need to be instructed that application must be at least five to six times a day and that they are to treat the ointment as if they were handling hot chili peppers, avoiding contact with eyes and mucous membranes and washing their hands thoroughly after application.

Although the use of *opioids* in chronic pain is controversial, some persons definitely benefit from their use. Pain intensity has been found to be directly related to disability (24). Theoretically, a decrease in pain intensity through the use of opioids can increase function and decrease disability. This outcome has yet to be confirmed. Recently the American Academy of Pain Medicine and the American Pain Society issued a consensus statement in favor of using opioids in chronic pain (25). The decision to use opioids in chronic pain is challenging for many providers because of the concerns about behavioral addiction and the scrutiny of drug regulatory boards. There is considerable ignorance and confusion among some state regulatory boards, health care practitioners, and

the public regarding addiction and the goals of using opioids in chronic pain. However, the fact remains that anecdotally, some persons remain functional and/or report a higher quality of life with the use of opioids for pain management (Chapters 30 and 32). While physiological dependence can occur as soon as 10 days after regular administration, the development into behavioral addiction and substance abuse is in fact quite the exception (26). Probably the biggest disappointment for the patient with chronic pain is that the opioid doesn't stop the pain. It may take the edge off or reduce the intensity below 5 on a scale of 0 to 10, but it does not usually have the same results as taking it for a toothache, a fractured bone, or postoperative pain. Therefore it is important for the patient who will be prescribed the opioid medication to understand that it is ideally used with a variety of pain management therapies and skills, including heat and ice, exercise, pacing activities, relaxation techniques, and other medications mentioned previously. The use of opioids for sleep disorders, anxiety in anticipation of pain, or escape from pain, while understandable, only adds to abusive behaviors and considerable frustration because of its general ineffectiveness.

When a person reports that his or her functioning is quite impaired because of pain or that he or she is feeling significant distress from pain, a trial of opioids may be warranted. Many providers feel more comfortable in using opioids to treat pain associated with an identifiable process such as rheumatoid arthritis, but this approach may significantly undertreat those with complex pain syndromes that can be identified only by their historical factors. It is important to heed the wisdom given to practitioners 2 centuries ago by Samuel Johnson, M.D., who said, "Those who do not feel pain seldom think that it is felt." We must trust our patients and help them to help us understand their pain and the effectiveness of our therapies. The use of a long-acting opioid, such as morphine, oxycodone, fentanyl, or methadone, can sometimes avoid the erratic peaks and valleys associated with short-acting opioids. This however, is not a hard and fast rule.

Some patients report that having a short-acting opioid available for use as needed is more beneficial to them. Establishing a long-term relationship with the patient, using contracts to clarify expectations, and teaching them accurate reporting of their pain can demonstrate the benefits of using opioids. Use of measures of function such as the SF36 or family input is also very helpful in assessing therapeutic effectiveness and problems. While relief of pain from the opioid may be important to the person, the lack of total pain relief necessitates the development of other coping skills. Furthermore, the incorporation of cognitive behavioral skills makes the additional use of opioids for sleep, anticipation of pain increases, and stress less likely. Regular periodic reassessment of benefit is helpful with careful documentation to comply with drug enforcement regulations. If opioids are to be stopped, reduction of the total daily dose by 20% per day is generally satisfactory. Clonidine can be prescribed for any uncomfortable withdrawal symptoms. Switching to a different kind or class of opioid according to an equianalgesic chart such as that found in the Agency for Health Care Policy Research Guidelines for cancer pain therapy may be useful. Keep in mind that the potentiation or synergy from using anti-inflammatory agents and tricyclic antidepressants with opioids has been well documented in the treatment of cancer pain. Another precaution is to be aware of acetaminophen content in many oral opioid agents. Regular doses above 4000 mg/day are toxic, and the safety or unsafety of long-term exposure is not known. Likewise, discussion of a bowel program with regular use of sennosides, docusate sodium, and bisacodyl can prevent additional exacerbations of pain from constipation and impaction (27).

When depression or an anxiety disorder is identified in addition to the pain problem, the use of the newer antidepressants, such as selective serotonin uptake inhibitors and anxiolytic medications, may be helpful. The antidepressants may also be helpful in potentiating serotonin-mediated inhibitory pathways thought to be modulating pain signals. Psychotherapy can also provide benefit.

Physical therapy and *occupational therapy* can address mechanical imbalances, physical deconditioning, and compensation for functional deficits. The extended use of passive modalities (heat, ultrasound, or electrical stimulation) for months to years is rarely warranted and can contribute to dependency, which can contribute to feeling out of control. An exercise program that stretches tight limbs and trunk, strengthens muscles, and conditions heart, lungs, and muscles can be helpful both for the pain process and for the general health of the patient. While massage can help reduce tension in muscles and tightness in soft tissue structures and can relax the person in chronic pain, it is important to supplement it with skills and therapies that maximize self-management.

Nerve blocks, such as sympathetic or facet blocks and epidurals, are probably most effective in the earlier stages of postinjury treatment, presumably before the alterations in the central nervous system become fixed. *Spinal cord stimulation* may, in selected persons, provide pain control, although the effectiveness does seem to decrease with time (28). *Intrathecal* or *epidural catheters* and subcutaneous pumps for delivery of opioids are, in addition to being very expensive to maintain, associated with considerable side effects and should not be considered in the absence of an adequate trial by the oral or membranous delivery systems.

Nutritional recommendations are best kept to focusing on weight control and avoidance of excesses of caffeine, alcohol, preservatives, over-the-counter vitamins, and fats. The use of a food diary with pain syndromes such as headaches and migraines may prove helpful in eliminating food triggers (29). There has been some suggestion that central nervous system serotonin levels may be increased and therefore pain may be decreased by eating certain foods such as tryptophan-rich foods (turkey, cottage cheese, sardines) with complex carbohydrate–vegetarian types of diets (30). However this has not been widely accepted or reproduced. Following the nutritional guidelines associated with the food pyramid and an emphasis on fruits, vegetables, and grains is still the most widely supported recommendation.

Sleep complaints of restlessness, insomnia, or early morning awakening are common in patients with chronic pain. Sleep deprivation can lead to depression, daytime fatigue, poor concentration, and irritability. In addition to the tricyclic antidepressant medications, attention to sleep hygiene is important. The following recommendations to patients can be helpful. Going to bed and rising each morning at the same time are critical. If naps are necessary, they should be limited to 30 to 45 minutes so that the biological clock is not reset, disrupting nighttime sleep. A hot shower or bath or exercise 2 hours before sleep will raise the body temperature; the cooling down afterward can help trigger sleep onset. A light carbohydrate snack before bed can induce sleep. If sleep onset is delayed for more than 30 minutes, advise the patient to get up and do some activity until he or she is sleepy again. Lying in bed for hours with eyes wide open only increases the anxiety of not going to sleep, which in turn perpetuates sleeplessness. Using a relaxation tape or practicing diaphragmatic breathing can be helpful in sleep preparation and unwinding from the day's activities (31).

PSYCHOSOCIAL THERAPIES

Learning and applying pain management skills is an important but not necessarily well-received recommendation. Understandably, most patients do not want to manage pain, they want it to go away. However, pain management can provide the person with a means of living a life of quality in spite of the pain. Many self-help organizations and resources can assist the patient as well (Appendix). The multidisciplinary treatment of chronic pain has long been accepted as the most effective approach. The primary care provider will find local resources to teach yoga, self-massage, relaxation response, stress management, pool exercises, and support groups to be invaluable adjuncts to treatment.

Relaxation response techniques can be quite beneficial in balancing the stressful effects of long-term pain, and specific techniques, such as self-hypnosis and visualization, can be used for temporarily altering pain perception. There are several techniques and resources from which to choose. The basic instructions are (*a*) to choose a repetitive focus point, a word, phrase, or just the in and out of the breath and (*b*) when the mind wanders, nonjudgmentally guide it back to the focus point. Practice 10 to 20 minutes once a day (2, 31).

Introducing the patient to the quieting effects of *diaphragmatic breathing* and the relation between breath and tension can also be very helpful. Ask the patient to make a fist and then to observe what happens to the breath. The usual observation is that the breath is held. Then ask the patient to make a fist and keep breathing. During that time ask him or her to observe what happens to the tension in the fist. Usually the fist tension is difficult to maintain while breathing. Then point out that most people hold their breath or pant when they feel pain or are anxious, depressed, or angry. Awareness of these habits and taking deep, diaphragmatic breaths can be helpful in reducing tension and pain and can contribute to altering moods. This exercise, which can be demonstrated in the office in 5 minutes, can be very helpful to the patient in making the mind-body connection (31).

Pacing activities so that the pain level is kept from escalating to levels associated with dysfunction and distress is very valuable. This can be done by alternating a series of activities that involve changing positions and function so that a person stays busy but does not remain in any one position or posture that might be associated with increased pain. For example, a person with low back pain may find that standing at the sink doing dishes is associated with increasing pain after 10 minutes. Once this is determined, it is recommended that after 10 minutes, using a timer if necessary, the person stops doing dishes and sits down, perhaps paying bills, writing letters, or calling a friend, until the pain is reduced. Pacing activities makes the continuation of a full and productive schedule, albeit done differently, both possible and rewarding (31).

Assisting a person with the *emotional distress* associated with pain is quite challenging for most health care providers (Part 4 [Chapters 20–24]). The challenge for both patient and provider is that there is an inherent misunderstanding of the role that emotions may play in coping with pain. While there is considerable discussion of the causal role of psychological issues in pain perception, there is no doubt that the pain experience is greatly altered by a person's level of anxiety, depression, and anger. These common emotional responses can produce their own stress and disruption of function if left unchecked and unbalanced. Like a filter through which the pain signal passes, the emotional context can focus or diminish the signal. It is important when discussing the emotional content of the pain experience that support and validation of the difficulties be acknowledged and respected. Early introduction of assessing mind and body in a chronic pain syndrome assists in the proper acknowledgment of these impor-

tant interactions. Waiting to discuss these mind-body interactions after all testing and therapies have failed to take the pain away only mistakenly emphasizes the physical symptoms as "real" and the emotional symptoms as irrelevant. It is critical to identify and treat significant depression and anxiety, which may hinder the ability to carry out a pain management plan. Professional assessment by mental health providers and/or the use of depression screening tools may help. Exploration of factors predisposing to posttraumatic stress disorder may also identify persons who may benefit from assistance with differentiating the suffering associated with physical, emotional, or sexual abuse from the pain experience.

Cognitive therapy skills used to examine the thoughts associated with pain and dysfunction are very helpful (Chapter 23). For example, a person gets up in the morning with a plan for a picnic, only to become aware that the pain is increased; he or she is having a flare-up. The person might say, "This is the worst thing that could have happened," "It always happens when I try to make plans," "It's not fair," and so on. The anger and frustration, while understandable, will more than likely contribute to body tension and other stress-related symptoms that compound the feeling of being out of control. Through a series of exercises called reframing, persons can acknowledge the frustration but identify the options by asking themselves, "What can I do? What do I need?" In so doing they may be able to alter their emotional filter and regain control by saying something like this: "I'm having a flare-up, and the timing couldn't be worse, but I will take my medicine and use my other pain management strategies. I will call my friends and let them know. Maybe we can rent a movie and stay here or have our picnic in the backyard" (31).

Once again, it is important to acknowledge that there is no objective measure of a person's pain or suffering and that our own cultural, gender, and experience bias may make it difficult to empathize with the person who continues to complain of pain. For example, there is evidence that some of the barriers to appropriate medication use even in acute or cancer pain are associated with gender and cultural biases. In one study of patient-controlled analgesia orders, it was demonstrated that orders were written with a hierarchy in the amount of medication prescribed. Men received more pain medication in their orders than women, whites were ordered more than Hispanics, and blacks were ordered more than Asian or Hispanic patients (32). This was in spite of the fact that when the actual amount of medication taken by patients was calculated, there did not appear to be any difference in use among the various cultures or genders represented. These biases are insidious and generally unconscious, and they must be considered when there is a failure to take the pain at the person's word.

CHRONIC PAIN SYNDROMES

At this time, as the discipline of pain medicine is in its infancy, there is much to be discovered in prevention and diagnostic guidelines for conditions associated with chronic pain. As the physiological mechanisms are elaborated, therapeutic agents for the relief of pain, a basic tenet of medical practice, will also evolve. The following syndromes, many of which are discussed in whole chapters to come, have been included here because they seem to be the more common ones seen in a primary care setting. Early recognition of these syndromes or symptom complexes may prevent unnecessary surgery or repetition of inappropriate therapies. Early identification also benefits the patient and provider by identifying the immediate need to develop a biopsychosocial approach of assessment and treatment to the problem.

Musculoskeletal Disorders

Fibromyalgia

Numerous disorders of the musculoskeletal system are related to inflammatory and autoimmune abnormalities. Many are confirmed by rheumatological testing and respond to both nonsteroidal and steroidal medications. Attention to the treatment of osteoporosis is directed more toward identifying and prophylactically treating the woman who is at risk for developing compression and long bone fractures. Probably the most controversial rheumatological disorder is fibromyalgia. This syndrome of diffuse pain, poor sleep quality, fatigue, tender points (33), and a myriad of other ill-defined symptoms arising either spontaneously or in the presence of a history of physical or emotional trauma or chronic illness has generated considerable theory as to its cause. It appears that it is not a peripheral process, even though considerable "muscle and joint" symptoms are reported. Poor sleep quality and intolerance to physical exercise "because it hurts" provide the clues for directing therapy. Consider this diagnosis in any patient who complains of increasing symptoms that wax and wane and migrate for no apparent reason. It can develop in the presence of another pain syndrome, such as chronic back pain, endometriosis, or irritable bowel syndrome, presumably as a result of poor sleep quality and decreased exercise tolerance in genetically susceptible women. For example, in a patient still complaining of neck pain that is spreading to her upper back and arms months to years after a motor vehicle accident and with a negative radiological and neurological evaluation, you may find the additional complaints of fatigue, poor sleep, and a reduction in activities because of pain. Check for tender points in the areas defined by the American College of Rheumatology (33). The use of antidepressants for sleep and depression commonly associated with the disorder can be very therapeutic, as can exercising in warm water. It can be very reassuring to talk to the patient, who reports that it feels as if something is terribly wrong and life threatening. Knowing that there is a name associated with the symptoms and that it is generally not associated with progressive degeneration or is not a serious or life-threatening illness is validating and reassuring.

There are support groups sponsored by the Arthritis Foundation and a very active Fibromyalgia Network Association (Appendix). The latter organization can provide patients with more information about the disorder and the latest research efforts on diagnosis and treatment. However, fibromyalgia is a diagnosis of exclusion, so it is important to evaluate the complaints and periodically reassess if the complaints increase or change significantly (Chapter 10).

Chronic Back Pain

Treatment of "failed back syndromes" (persistent back pain post surgery) or nonspecific back pain can be frustrating for both the patient and health care provider. It is also a major socioeconomic problem given the rising health care costs. Indeed, 7.5% of the persons with chronic low back pain consume 75% of all treatment and disability-related costs (34). The number of problems that can involve the back anatomy or function is beyond the scope of this discussion (Chapters 14–16). It has become increasingly apparent that multiple structures (e.g., facets, spinal ligaments, disc disease) as well as abnormal mechanics can give rise to persistent pain, so that a careful examination and history are an essential beginning point. However, many postoperative patients may have the physiology demonstrated in animal models of neuropathy secondary to trauma (ligation, compression) of peripheral nerves. In this population, maintaining function and considering treatment with medications aimed at central nervous system mechanisms may be beneficial. In addition, job modification and addressing the complex psychosocial complications are critical factors.

Chest Pain

Atypical chest pain can present a difficult diagnostic challenge because of the necessity to consider cardiac disease. Further challenging the health care provider are the facts that cardiac pain may not involve only the chest or left arm, presenting instead as jaw or neck pain, and that esophageal pain may mimic cardiac pain (squeezing chest discomfort with radiation into the throat). Research directed at identifying the incidence of cardiac events in patients with atypical chest pain has demonstrated that in patients with normal coronary arteries the incidence of myocardial infarction or death is low, 0 to 0.6% (35). Esophageal disorders (reflux, spasm, motility dysfunction) are estimated to cause atypical chest pain in one third of patients with normal coronary arteries. There has been a growing appreciation among gastrointestinal specialists that many of the eosphageal motility disorders have a significant association with anxiety, depression, and ineffective coping strategies (35). The use of provocative tests for esophageal dysfunction and the exclusion of coronary artery disease through an arteriogram are essential before reassuring the patient with recurrent chest pain. In addition, the biopsychosocial assessment and treatment of persons, no matter what causes their symptoms, is essential.

Musculoskeletal disorders associated with chest pain can involve the small costochondral joints usually associated with pinpoint tenderness on examination. Anti-inflammatory agents and examination of the patient for tender points associated with fibromyalgia may be useful. Chest wall pain can arise from impingement of small thoracic nerves as they exit the vertebral column. Pain in these situations can be reproduced by palpation over the spinous processes, commonly from T4 to T7, and of the paraspinous muscles along the medial scapular edge. Trigger point injections and manipulative therapies may be beneficial in such cases.

Appreciation that intercostal nerves can be traumatized and give rise to persistent pain is an important consideration. Postherpetic neuralgia, thoracic surgical disruption of musculoskeletal tissue, instrument traction trauma, and radiation treatment to chest structures can all give rise to persistent pain. Nerve blocks, medication therapy, such as anticonvulsants and tricyclic antidepressants, transcutaneous nerve stimulation (TENS), and additional psychosocial support all may be beneficial.

Visceral Hyperalgesia

Disorders of the visceral organs are perhaps the most challenging of chronic pain syndromes. The symptoms are generally diffuse and difficult to localize by the patient. Relief is difficult to achieve. Pelvic and abdominal pain, for example irritable bowel complaints, are most commonly found in women. Some diseases associated with pain must be considered when persistent abdominal or pelvic pain is present. Endometriosis, interstitial cystitis, colitis, and pancreatitis have all been associated with acute intermittent pain as well as constant persistent pain. Surgical procedures for lysis of adhesions and removal of organs have many times failed to relieve such constant persistent pain. The persistent pain that can develop in spite of total abdominal hysterectomy for endometriosis, in the face of normal pancreatic enzymes in chronic pancreatitis, or after a cystectomy in interstitial cystitis is thought to be related to visceral hyperalgesia. It is has been proposed that the visceral sensory pain pathways are prone to trauma just as are the somatic pain sensory nerves (36). When they become irritated or traumatized, they begin to fire spontaneously and/or at pressures that normally would not stimulate them; that is, they exhibit a lower threshold for firing. This sensitization of bowel to increased pressures can develop in normal subjects over minutes in acute pain research. Since the visceral afferent nerves synapse on the same dorsal horn cells as the somatic pain afferents, the patient may also feel somatic "referred" pain as well as visceral pain. In general the treatment of patients with visceral hyperalgesia is quite inadequate. Addressing the possible central nervous system mechanisms, avoiding unnecessary surgical trauma, and addressing the psychosocial needs are key. Special attention to the inevitable sexual dysfunction and consequences with relationships as well as to any history of sexual abuse is critical. The emotional distress attendant to these issues, in addition to the pelvic and/or abdominal pain, may make emphasis on physical treatment less than optimal if maximal results are to be obtained.

Interstitial Cystitis (37)

Dysuria, frequency, and urgency of urination may develop over months to years in interstitial cystitis (Chapter 17). The clean voided specimen is generally sterile, although many women receive antibiotics because of the complaints. The disease is diagnosed with a cystoscopy that stretches the bladder and causes pinpoint hemorrhages in the bladder wall. Biopsy reveals mast cells. The cause is unknown, and the treatments are empirical and variable in results. They include dimethyl sulfoxide (DMSO) and Chlorpactin (bleach) bladder instillation, pentosan polysulfate sodium (Elmiron) therapy, dietary manipulation, various electrical stimulation techniques, and so on. Many patients go on to develop shrunken bladders with such small capacities that they must urinate 50 to 70 times, day and night. In these patients bladder reconstruction or cystectomy has been performed to alter voiding frequency. However, many times the pain persists, suggesting a possible mechanism involving visceral hyperalgesia.

The use of opioids in this population can relieve pain and reduce distress. In addition, the use of medications, including anticonvulsant medications such as gabapentin and tricyclic antidepressants, to address central nervous system mechanisms thought to perpetuate chronic pain may provide additional relief.

Endometriosis

Endometriosis is hormonally responsive endometrial tissue outside the uterine cavity. It has a prevalence rate of 5 to 10% in the general population of the United States (6). The original explanation of causation was that there was retrograde dispelling of endometrial tissue outside the uterus and into the pelvic cavity. This is apparently a common observation, up to 90% in one study (39). Why this tissue begins to implant and invade surrounding tissue in some women is not known. Recent studies suggest immunological factors and a genetic propensity in some women. It has been theorized that the shedding of this displaced tissue in response to monthly hormonal cycling causes an inflammatory response, hence the pain. The unsuspected presence of endometrial implants found in an asymptomatic patient or the presence of just a few implants in a patient complaining of incapacitating pain only highlights the incongruity between presence of endometrial implants and the cause of pain in this disorder. Many hormonal treatments can bring the pain under control in some patients. However, multiple surgical procedures and even removal of all reproductive organs have been met in some patients with persistent pain. Again, early addressing of ongoing psychosocial coping issues as well as medication that may alter the central nervous system mechanisms is worth considering, particularly if the patient has not responded to laser surgery, hormonal manipulation, or ablative surgery.

Neurological Disorders

Headaches

Headaches are the seventh leading reason for outpatient visits in the United States. In the United States 17.6% of women and 6% of men have headaches meeting the International Headache Society (IHS) criteria (40). The development of the IHS diagnostic criteria in 1988 (41) has helped to guide therapeutic rationale and alert the clinician to circumstances requiring further investigation. The treatment of migraines and muscle tension headaches, which has become quite extensive (Chapter 9), is targeting the pathophysiology thought to be responsible for headaches, such as serotonin inhibitory receptors and inhibition of parameningeal inflammation. Headache specialists are available for intractable headaches. Knowledge of drugs associated with rebound headaches, for example over-the-counter aspirin, acetaminophen, and ibuprofen; butalbital mixtures, ergotamine, and opioids; and antihistamines and decongestants, is important for the primary care provider. The insidious nature of rebound headaches because of self-treatment and inaccurate reporting by patients as to frequency of dosing makes specific inquiry into self-medication or dosing frequency important. The benefit of relaxation, self-hypnosis, and biofeedback therapies should not be forgotten (2).

Complex Regional Pain Syndrome (42)

After minor or major trauma to an extremity some patients develop increased pain characterized by complaints of burning and sensitivity to even light touch. Physical examination findings in the type 1 syndrome, formerly known as reflex sympathetic dystrophy, reveals hyperpathia, allodynia, and if there is a sympathetically maintained component to the pain, swelling of the limb, with cyanosis, cold, pale skin, and increased sweating. Treatment strategies stress (*a*) prompt identification and treatment of any previously unidentified source of continuous pain stimuli in the area of injury, such as neuromas, nerve entrapment, and bone infection; (*b*) nerve blocks targeting the sympathetic nervous system or peripheral nerves to the area involved; and (*c*) aggressive physical and functional restoration. For the primary care provider, early recognition of the syndrome may assist in timely referral for treatment by a pain specialist and/or multidisciplinary pain clinic.

The terminology of complex regional pain syndrome was in part devised to challenge pain researchers and clinicians to reexamine the pathophysiology and clinical presentation of a wide spectrum of patients who present with puzzling pain that seems to exceed the injury or the diagnostic capabilities of our current laboratory tests, imaging devices, or nerve studies. The diagnostic guidelines and available treatments are still empirical.

Acquired Immunodeficiency Syndrome

Pain is the second most common reason for hospitalization of acquired immunodeficiency syndrome (AIDS) patients (43). The pain may arise from any of a variety of systems, including neurological, musculoskeletal, and gastrointestinal. Patients with AIDS are as susceptible to the common diseases associated with pain, such as peptic ulcer disease, disc herniation, and tension headaches, as uninfected persons, but because of their compromised immune system, they can develop a multitude of pain-producing complications, including metastatic disease, vasculitis, thrombophlebitis, esophageal herpetic infections, inflammatory polyneuropathy, and infectious cholecystitis. The challenge of caring for patients with HIV is to be aware that they are susceptible to many of the usual and unusual pain-producing diseases and that careful evaluation and treatment of the underlying cause, including pain-relieving medications, is mandatory for compassionate care.

SUMMARY

The evaluation and treatment of chronic pain poses a significant challenge to the health care provider. A growing literature points to the wisdom of prevention and early treatment of pain, but as yet there are few guidelines. At present it is recommended that a careful evaluation, including a thorough history and physical examination, be performed and that appropriate diagnostic tests be obtained. Treatment should address the physical, emotional, behavioral, and cognitive components of the pain. If a diagnosis or physiological explanation is not forthcoming, referral to a pain specialist or pain clinic for assistance is warranted. If the pain persists, the development of a long-term relationship between the primary care provider and the patient with chronic pain can be very rewarding if it is conducted in a biopsychosocial model of care. In this context the patient is ultimately responsible for managing the stress of the symptoms and maintaining maximal functioning, and the health care provider is responsible for recommending and directing the treatment and support needed by the patient and family. The healing effects of having someone listen to and validate the difficulty of living with pain should not be underestimated. At this point in the application of the principles of pain medicine, the pain may be mandatory, but the suffering is definitely optional.

References

1. Bonica JJ. Pain research and therapy: past and current status and future needs. In: Ng LKY, Bonica JJ, eds. Pain, discomfort and humanitarian care. New York: Elsevier, 1980:1–46.
2. NIH Technology Assessment Panel. Integration of behavioral and relaxation approaches into the treatment of chronic pain and insomnia. JAMA 1996;276:313–318.
3. Lorig KR, Mazonson PD, Holson HR. Evidence suggesting that health education for self management in patients with chronic arthritis has sustained health benefits while reducing health care costs. Arthritis Rheum 1993;36:439–446.

4. Caudill M, Schnable R, Zuttermeister P, et al. Decreased clinic use by chronic pain patients: response to behavioral medicine intervention. Clin J Pain 1991;7:305–310.

5. Watkins LR, Maier SF, Goehler LE. Immune activation: the role of proinflammatory cytokines in inflammation, illness responses and pathological states. Pain 1995;63:289–302.

6. Lu PY, Ory SJ. Endometriosis: current management. Mayo Clinic Proc 1995;70:453–463.

7. Fields HL. Pain. New York: McGraw-Hill, 1987.

8. Devor M. Neuropathic pain and injured nerve: peripheral mechanisms. Br Med Bull 1991;47:619–630.

9. Malmberg AB, Yaksh TL. Hyperalgesia mediated by spinal glutamate or substance P receptor blocked by spinal cyclooxygenase inhibition. Science 1992;257:1276–1279.

10. McQuay HJ, Dickenson AH. Implications of nervous system plasticity for pain management. Anesthesia 1990;45:101–102.

11. Woolf CJ, Chong MS. Preemptive analgesia: treating postoperative pain by preventing the establishment of central sensitization. Anesth Analg 1993;77:362–379.

12. Fields HL, Basbaum AI. Central nervous system mechanisms of pain modulation. In: Wall PD, Melzack R, eds. Textbook of pain. 3rd ed. New York: Churchill Livingstone, 1994;243–257.

13. Roland M, Morris R. A study of the natural history of back pain. Spine 1983;2:145–150.

14. White P. Pain measurement. In: Warfield C, ed. Principles and practice of pain management. New York: McGraw-Hill, 1993:27–41.

15. Deleted.

16. Deleted.

17. Radloff LS, Teri L. Use of the Center for Epidemiological Study Depression scale with older adults. Clin Gerontol 1986;5:119–134.

18. Beck AT, Ward CH, Mendelson M, et al. An inventory for measuring depression. Arch Gen Psychiatry 1961;4:561–571.

19. Katz JA. Opioids and nonsteroidal antiinflammatory analgesics. In: Raj PP, ed. Pain medicine: a comprehensive review. St Louis: Mosby, 1996;126–140.

20. Haddox JD. Coanalgesic agents. In: Raj PP, ed. Pain medicine: a comprehensive review. St Louis: Mosby, 1996:142–151.

21. Swerdlow M. Anticonvulsant drugs and chronic pain. Clin Neuropharmacol 1984;7:51–82.

22. Tanelian DL, Brose WG. Neuropathic pain can be relieved by drugs that are use-dependent sodium channel blockers: lidocaine, carbamazepine, and mexiletine. Anesthesiology 1991;74:949–951.

23. Watson CP, Evans RJ, Watt VR. Postherpetic neuralgia and topical capsaicin. Pain 1988;33–36.

24. Burton AK, Tillotson KM, Main CJ, Hollis S. Psychosocial predictors of outcome in acute and subchronic low back trouble. Spine 1995;20:722–728.

25. Consensus statement from the American Academy of Pain Medicine and the American Pain Society. The use of opioids for the treatment of chronic pain. Clin J Pain 1997;13:6–8.

26. Marks RM, Sachar EJ. Undertreatment of medical inpatients with narcotic analgesics. Ann Intern Med 1973;78:173–181.

27. Levy MH. Pharmacologic treatment of cancer pain. N Engl J Med 1996;335:1124–1130.

28. North RB. Neural stimulation techniques for chronic pain. In: Tollison CD, ed. Handbook of pain management. 2nd ed. Baltimore: Williams & Wilkins, 1994;74–84.

29. Radnitz C. Food-triggered migraine: a critical review. Ann Behav Med 1990;12:51–64.

30. Seltzer S, Stoch R, Marcus R, Jackson E. Alteration of human pain thresholds by nutritional manipulation and L-tryptophan supplementation. Pain 1982;13:385–393.

31. Caudill MA. Managing pain before it manages you. New York: Guilford Press, 1995.

32. Ng B, Dimsdale JE, Rollnik JD, Shapiro H. The effect of ethnicity on prescriptions for patient-controlled analgesia for post-operative pain. Pain 1996;66:9–12.

33. Wolfe F, Smythe HA, Yunus MB, et al. American College of Rheumatology 1990 criteria for the classification of fibromyalgia. Arthritis Rheum 1990;33:160–172.

34. Quebec Task Force on Spinal Disorders. Scientific approach to the assessment and management of activity-related spinal disorders. Spine 1987;12:S16.

35. Castell DO, ed. Proceedings of a symposium: chest pain of undetermined origin. Newton, MA: Cahners, 1992.

36. Ness TJ, Gebhart GF. Visceral pain: a review of experimental studies. Pain 1990;41;167–234.

37. Hanno PM, ed. Interstitial cystitis. Philadelphia: Saunders, 1994.

38. Deleted.

39. Halme J, Hammond MG, Hulka JF, et al. Retrograde menstruation in healthy women and in patients with endometriosis. Obstet Gynecol 1984;64:151–154.

40. Tepper SJ. A primary care approach to migraine and chronic headache. Prim Care Rep 1996;2:150–159.

41. Headache Classification Committee of the International Headache Society. Classification and diagnostic criteria for headache disorders, cranial neuralgias, and facial pain. Cephalgia 1988;9(Suppl 7); 120–196.

42. Jänig W, Stanton-Hicks MD, eds. Reflex sympathetic dystrophy: a reappraisal. Progress in pain research and management, vol 6. Seattle: IASP Press, 1996.

43. Warfield CA. Management of pain in AIDS. Hosp Pract 1990;25:51–54.

CHAPTER 6

Painful Neurological Disorders: From Animals to Humans

Angela Mailis and Gary J. Bennett

Pain arising from the abnormal operation of the nervous system requires a basic understanding of the underlying pathophysiologic mechanisms in order to apply rational treatments. This chapter reviews the status of knowledge regarding underlying physiology and pathophysiology of painful neurological conditions in animals and humans.

INTRODUCTION

Nociceptive pain is pain "arising from nociception, i.e., the normal operation of the pain sensory system" (1). **Neuropathic pain** results from "abnormal operation of the nervous system after damage" (1). It is defined formally by the International Association for the Study of Pain (IASP) as "pain initiated or caused by a primary lesion or dysfunction in the nervous system" (neuropathic or neurogenic pain) (2). Pain in these cases can occur and persist long after the completion of tissue damage and repair.

An example of nociceptive (i.e., "normal") pain is pain due to local tissue injury that is followed by increased sensitivity of primary afferent nociceptors at the site of injury. Even if there is evidence (3) that tissue injury is followed by changes in the responsiveness of central-pain processing neurons in the spinal cord and maybe other parts of the central nervous system (CNS), these phenomena are normal processes. Some but not all kinds of neuropathic pains may constitute abnormal expressions of these normal processes.

Phantom limb pain, poststroke and postspinal cord injury pain (all examples of central pain), causalgia after nerve damage, and so on are examples of neuropathic pain and are all discussed in detail in this chapter. The coexistence of nociceptive and neuropathic pain is a very common and very often forgotten phenomenon. For example, a herniated disc compressing a nerve or nerve root produces pain, motor and sensory phenomena, and reflex muscle spasm. Compression of the spinal root or nerve produces neuropathic pain as well as nerve nociceptive pain arising from activation of nociceptors innervating the neural sheath (4), while reflex muscle spasm generates nociceptive pain secondary to ischemic excitation of muscle nociceptors. A tumor invading skeletal and soft tissues or viscera activates nociceptors in those tissues and can also produce neuropathic pain if it affects peripheral or central neural structures (5).

It has been traditional to consider that inability to detect a "physical" or "organic" injury that adequately explains the patient's complaints of pain and disability constitutes evidence of **psychogenic pain.** In reality, there is no single definition of psychogenic pain. Various shades of meaning exist. However, implicit in any use of the term is that psychological variables in some way cause the pain. Much of the current psychological literature appears to be concerned with (effective or ineffective) coping reactions to presumably "real" pain and nociception. Nevertheless, the intensely diverse positions to the "coping" approach are best illustrated by the rather strong statement that "the search for a pain prone personality and psychogenic pain has been futile. The many variables that have been perceived to be part of a personality constellation related to psychogenic pain may actually be reactions to illness, independent of psychiatric illness" (6). This statement indeed contrasts with the literature supporting psychological vulnerability to develop chronic pain syndromes (7).

The highly influential *Diagnostic and Statistical Manual of Mental Disorders* (DSM-IV) in its fourth edition (1994) defines as pain disorder the disorder that fulfills five distinct criteria:

A. Pain in one or more anatomical sites is the predominant focus of clinical presentation . . .
B. The pain causes clinically significant distress or impairment in social, occupational, or other important areas of functioning.

C. Psychological factors are judged to have an important role in the onset, severity, exacerbation, or maintenance of the pain.
D. The symptom or deficit is not intentionally produced or feigned…
E. The pain is not better accounted for by a Mood, Anxiety, or Psychotic Disorder . . . (7a).

DSM-IV (7a) also states that while pain disorder associated with psychological factors only or with both psychological factors and a general medical condition is classified as mental disorder, pain disorder in the presence of a general medical condition (psychological factors if present are considered insignificant) is not.

We find the DSM-IV classification confusing. We believe that the distinction between "psychogenic factors" and "psychological reactions" is artificial and that the disposition to respond in a certain manner and the actual manner of coping may be two sides of the same coin. To many, the term psychogenic means that pain is all in the mind or brain. As a matter of fact, pain is indeed in the brain, as the end sensory organ of all pain perceptions. Our position regarding the relation of perceived pain, pain disability, and psychological factors is summarized by the following set of constructs:

1. *Expressed pain (and subsequent pain disability) may vary* with the "response bias" to report pain when nociceptive or neuropathic causes are present in variable degrees. The response bias may be exaggerated or blunted, based on a multiplicity of personality, cognitive, emotional, social, and environmental factors. Examples are as follows: Minor physical injuries may give rise to much more than expected pain in the presence of emotional disturbances, anxiety, or depression (8). Patients with hypochondriasis tend to focus excessively and amplify somatic symptoms that in the absence of their neurosis would go almost unnoticed (9–12).
2. *Behaviors or responses arising from psychological factors* may lead to secondary physiological processes generating more pain. Examples are (*a*) excessive fear of pain leading to guarding and immobility of an extremity, producing in turn alteration of blood flow, release of tissue-irritating substances and further pain; and (*b*) muscle contraction or tension pains (the common hypothesis holds that inadequate removal of waste products from the tissues evokes pain), as in the well-studied cases of muscle contraction headaches (13, 14).
3. *Pain perception in the absence of any noxious stimulus* ("imaginary" pain) may indeed exist, but it is seen only in certain psychiatric disorders as a product of delusions (rarely in schizophrenia) or thoughts (as part of a hysterical process). One of the best examples of the latter is the couvade syndrome, in which husbands experience labor pains similar to those felt by their wives

(15–20). However, the diagnosis of hysteria should be made very cautiously and not on the mere absence of physical evidence but on the basis of "positive" evidence, that is, that there are psychological factors and causes directly linked with the appearance and/or maintenance of the symptoms. While this may be easier in the presence of paralysis (when it can be shown that the patient is able to do things that are not consistent with the displayed paralysis), in the case of pain this may be difficult to prove. Furthermore, classic nonorganic signs (21) have been shown to have a physiological basis in several patients with neuropathic pain (discussed later), and even to be present in patients with acute organic disease of the nervous system (22).
4. Poor use or interpretation of diagnostic modalities or absence of appropriate diagnostic techniques or advances may *hinder the disclosure of nociceptive and/or neuropathic causes of pain* (with a tendency to label pain as psychogenic or at best idiopathic).

The distinction of **pain** (as a function of nociception, i.e., the primary sensory experience arising from a noxious stimulus) from **suffering** (as a reaction to this sensory experience) is very important. We perceive suffering as a form of response bias (i.e., superimposed on nociceptive or neuropathic abnormalities). Suffering, however, may indeed continue once the original tissue damage has been repaired. Then the question of a *central neurophysiological substrate* contributing to the initiation and/or maintenance of suffering is a challenging one. The presence and/or degree of actual psychophysiological or neurobiological correlates of any response bias at the CNS levels, either primary (causative) or secondary (as a consequence) to the primary sensory experience, remains an open issue. However, use of functional imaging techniques is accumulating evidence that patients with chronic pain (even when detectable—with current means—pathology cannot be seen) activate brain areas differentially (23), although the cause and effect relation of these differential responses has not been elucidated. Furthermore, in the more specific case of neuropathic pain, animal and human work (24–26) has clearly demonstrated a physiological basis for phenomena that until recently were considered evidence of psychogenic pain. The practicing clinician should be reminded that the truth is usually somewhere in the middle of the road: disorders considered originally psychogenic or even the product of malingering (simulation of disease process to obtain external secondary gains, usually in the form of compensation, drugs, and so on) have been found to have distinct (causally related) physiological substrates. Examples are facial pain with dyskinesias, thoracic outlet syndrome in the presence of physical signs, localized myofascial syndromes, and so on (27). On the other hand, the mind-body interaction (so frequently forgotten in the traditional medical model) is extremely important even in the generation of physiological responses to any kind of medical intervention in humans, as it occurs for example in placebo responses (28, 29).

Therefore, we have elected to adopt the **biopsychosocial model of disease** (30) as best expressing our approach to neuropathic pain (and for that matter to *any* kind of chronic pain). This approach allows for exploring the existence of any *physical impairment* generating pain as it relates to loss of organ or function; impairment is, therefore, an organ-based concept as per the 1980 World Health Organization definitions. In the presence of physical impairment, the reaction to it (based on psychological and socioenvironmental factors) shapes the expressed *disability* (disability is a task-based concept). It is apparent that in the case of absent or minimal "biological" factors, psychological and socioenvironmental factors acquire major significance in the expressed pain-disability. Ultimately, we adopt the **whole-person approach** with the aim of treating pain-disability according to the understanding of the *degree of contribution* of biological, psychological, and socioenvironmental factors.

HUMAN NEUROPATHIC PAIN: SYMPTOMS AND SIGNS

Neuropathic pain has been linked with a multiplicity of signs and symptoms. While multiple combinations of these signs and symptoms may be present in patients with injury or dysfunction of the nervous system, their incidence, specificity, and sensitivity are highly variable. A list of symptoms and signs associated with painful neurological disorders is outlined next.

Pain and Sensory Phenomena

Spontaneous Pain

Spontaneous neuropathic pain can be either ongoing and continuous (steady or fluctuating in intensity) or intermittent (paroxysmal or episodic). It refers as a rule to somatic structures and can be superficial (cutaneous) or deep (arising from muscles, bones, tendons, and so on). Continuous, spontaneous pain seems to be prominent in patients with central pain and in certain peripheral neuropathic disorders (complex regional pain syndromes [CRPS] types 1 and 2 [RSD and causalgia, respectively]). Paroxysmal pains may be superimposed on continuous pains or constitute the primary pain in some patients, for example those with tic douloureux (trigeminal neuralgia) or postherpetic neuralgia (31). Visceral neuropathic pain is reported rarely. There are few case reports of visceral phantom pain after removal of bladder or rectal structures (32).

Evoked Pains

Allodynia is "pain due to a stimulus which does not normally provoke pain" (3). Allodynia can be cutaneous or arise from deep tissues. It may be specific to the stimulus that induces it (e.g., cool, warming, or mechanical stimuli; movement). Mechanical (tactile) allodynia to light stroking of the skin (otherwise called *dynamic mechanical allodynia*) can be

tested by stroking the skin with a brush, gauze, or cotton applicator and by hair movement or vibration by something such as a tuning fork (1). Another form of cutaneous allodynia is elicited by applying firm pressure without movement or normally innocuous punctate stimuli (like von Frey hairs of moderate stiffness); it is known as *static allodynia* (33). Commercial pressure algometers have been used to test for static allodynia (34). In this case (depending on factors such as the site and rate of pressure application) stimulation of tissues other than skin (e.g. muscle, bone) occurs; therefore the term static allodynia may not be always appropriate. Algometric pressure thresholds have been used actually as a measure of "deep pain" arising primarily from periosteum when pressures are applied over bony prominences in upper and lower extremities (25, 35). Deep pain can be very characteristic of neuropathic pain syndromes (36). Nevertheless, while cutaneous (dynamic) allodynia is a very characteristic manifestation of neuropathic pain syndromes, it may not be exclusive to them (36). *Deep tissue allodynia* can be *static* (with pain produced upon firm, normally painless pressure over deep structures) or *kinesthetic* (with pain arising from normally painless range of movement). While this phenomenon is commonly seen in nociceptive pain from inflamed joints, it has also been reported in neuropathic pain patients (25, 35, 37). In neuropathic pain syndromes, cutaneous (dynamic) allodynia particularly may obscure other neuropathic abnormalities and even conceal nerve injury (25). From the practical point of view, cutaneous mechanical allodynia (manifested with cloth and/or hair movement intolerance) renders the examination of the patient difficult and constitutes one of the most debilitating neuropathic pain symptoms. Another form of allodynia, *cold allodynia,* is a very characteristic symptom of neuropathic pain (36). For example, patients with CRPS may complain that a cool draft or exposure to air conditioning is increasing their pain, and the appearance of such a patient with double gloves or socks on the involved limb is not unusual.

Hyperalgesia is "an increased response to a stimulus which is normally painful" (2). Again, this may be found with application of mechanical, heat, or cold stimuli, and while it is a very common symptom in neuropathic pain, it is not exclusive to it (36). Deep tissue hyperalgesia is also common in ordinary tissue injury. It should be stressed that there is confusion regarding the variable use of the terms allodynia and hyperalgesia, particularly in the older literature. Furthermore, confusion arises when the same stimulus modality can evoke both painful and painless sensations. The literature on sensory abnormalities contains both stimulus-defined descriptions (e.g., allodynia, brush-evoked pain) and mechanistic descriptions (like Aβ-mechanical allodynia). These terms are not equivalent, and they should not be used interchangeably. In this discussion we accept the position that "pain threshold to a stimulus in the pathological area is lower than the threshold in normal skin" as characteristic of both allodynia and hyperalgesia. We will also continue to be specific when using these terms by indicating stimulus or underlying mechanism generating these abnormalities.

The term **hyperpathia** is defined by the IASP (2) as "a painful syndrome characterized by abnormally painful reaction to a stimulus, especially a repetitive stimulus, as well as an increased threshold." This means that the pain is elicited in an area of decreased sensation, it characteristically radiates and persists after the removal of the stimulus, and it occurs with an unusual delay after the stimulus (38). It is unclear whether hyperpathia is a specialized kind of abnormality. It may make more sense to consider it as occurring in the context of reduced sensation with superimposed allodynia or hyperalgesia (31).

Paroxysmal evoked pains may be associated with a distinct focus (or foci) which if stimulated generates electric shock-like sensations. These pains may radiate throughout the length of the involved extremity. They may occur in certain posttraumatic neuropathies at the site of neuroma formation (39) or be generated in an area distal to and separate from the focus, as in tic douloureux (40).

The coexistence of two classes of evoked pain has been demonstrated (25) in patients with different types of neuropathic pathology (particularly those with CRPS 1 and 2 but not limited to CRPS): *cutaneous* (elicited by, e.g., tactile, pricking, cold stimuli applied to the skin), and *deep* (elicited by pressure over periosteum). Sodium amytal, a medium-action barbiturate, administered intravenously affects almost exclusively tactile allodynia while other (cutaneous) as well as deep pains remain unaffected (25). Characteristically, both cutaneous and deep evoked pains in this study (25) were shown to have borders well beyond the definable territories of a nerve or root and expand beyond the site of original tissue injury. While cutaneous tactile allodynia seems to depend specifically on deep pain (39), deep pain may be independent of cutaneous sensory abnormalities, and it has different temporal and physiological characteristics (25).

Special features of neuropathic stimulus-evoked pains may involve abnormalities in quality, duration, radiation, and spreading of the pain, as well as abnormal interplay and convergence between a visceral stimulus and its somatic expression. An example of the latter is the occurrence of CRPS 1 after a myocardial infarction. A significant characteristic of many neuropathic pain syndromes is the "extraterritorial" spreading of pain (i.e., pain experienced at and well beyond the site of original injury, even in glove-and-stocking distribution), which may be associated with similar and expanded sensory abnormalities outside the territory of a nerve or nerve root. Such an expansion beyond definable physiological territories has been a cornerstone of inorganic or psychogenic symptoms and signs (41). Nevertheless, there is evidence now (discussed later) both in humans (24) and in animals (26) that this phenomenon has a physiological basis in an abnormally functioning central nervous system.

We must make special mention of **negative sensory phenomena** expressed as hypoesthesia ("decreased sensitivity to stimulation, excluding the special senses" (2) and hypoalgesia ("diminished pain in response to a normally painful stimulus") (2) to various testing modalities. While "extraterritorial"

spreading of pain and positive sensory phenomena (allodynia, hyperalgesia) are well accepted in certain neuropathic pain syndromes (e.g. CRPS), the same is not equally acceptable for negative sensory phenomena. The exemption is the glove-and-stocking hypoesthesia of multiple peripheral nerve damage (as in the case of diabetic neuropathies), multisegmental root involvement (as in spinal arachnoiditis and plexopathies) or central nervous system lesions (e.g., stroke, spinal cord injury). An unexplainable (usually in glove-and-stocking distribution) sensory deficit not associated with detectable peripheral or central nervous system damage is often attributable to a conversion reaction. It is reasonable to assume that if the CNS possesses the capacity for widespread extraterritorial pain and diffuse positive sensory phenomena, it should be equally capable of negative sensory phenomena, even in the absence of clinically detectable peripheral or CNS lesions. Widespread negative phenomena are at least twice as common in patients with conversion disorders (as per DSM-IV criteria and after careful exclusion of possible underlying neurological disorders) (36). The characteristic of these conversion sensory phenomena is their normalization after application of various techniques operating via physiologically diverse mechanisms (e.g., normal saline and/or sodium amytal infusions, sham tourniquet blocks). Normalization involves *all* sensory negative abnormalities to different cutaneous and deep stimuli (41, 42). This response sharply contrasts with (a) the selective modality-related modulation seen in neuropathic positive phenomena (e.g., selective reduction of tactile allodynia with intravenous barbiturates) and (b) the persistence of negative sensory abnormalities after normal saline or sodium amytal infusions, sham blocks, and so on in the presence of structural peripheral or CNS injury (25). In a preliminary study Mailis and Nicholson (42) reported that these negative somatosensory abnormalities were associated strongly with an hysterical personality organization as demonstrated by multiple psychometric tests. The consistency and reproducibility of these currently unexplainable somatosensory phenomena in a select group of patients gives grounds to the suspicion that they arise from neuropsychiatric entities with psychophysiological and neurophysiological correlates within the CNS, associated with an hysterical personality organization (42).

Phenomena Other Than Pain

Many painful neurological disorders are associated with vasomotor, sudomotor, trophic and motor phenomena, as well as certain behaviors. **Vasomotor, sudomotor,** and **trophic** phenomena can be attributed to a multiplicity of either interrelated or independent but coexistent factors. Examples include the wasting and atrophy occurring in: (a) a central (brain or spinal cord) lesion or a peripheral plexus, root, or nerve lesion with both sensory abnormalities and motor weakness; (b) immobilization of a painful limb for fear of further injury or pain, and (c) CRPS 1, even in the absence of immobilization or distinct large nerve injury. While lack of movement and muscle-pumping action is a major known contributor to wasting of paralyzed limbs, lack of neurotrophic influences, primary or secondary changes within the sympathetic nervous system controlling vasomotor and sudomotor function, and abnormal neurovascular reflexes leading to bone rarefaction (43, 44) can be variably involved. Detailed review is beyond the scope of this chapter.

Motor phenomena occasionally occur in many painful neurological disorders, either primary (e.g., in Parkinson's disease and other neurodegenerative disorders associated with pain) or secondary (e.g., in CRPS patients with associated positive or negative motor phenomena) (45). Disorders of muscle tone generating spasticity (as in upper motor neuron injuries) or hypertonia (an example is stiff person syndrome with anti-GAD [glutamic acid decarboxylase] antibodies against skeletal muscles) are associated with intermittent pain. Occasionally motor and sensory painful phenomena coexist, as in the syndrome of painful legs, moving toes, and it is very difficult to ascertain the primary or secondary nature of those abnormalities.

Specific **complex behaviors** involving motor, sensory, cognitive, and affective phenomena (for example the self-injurious behavior seen rarely in neuropathic pain syndromes, with the patient attacking compulsively and exclusively the painful part) have been also reported in humans with neuropathic pain of various causes (46). The act of targeted self-injurious behavior in these patients seems to be the counterpart of animal autotomy after experimental injuries of the peripheral or central nervous system (46).

PATHOLOGICAL MECHANISMS UNDERLYING NEUROPATHIC PHENOMENA

Background: Normal Functions of Primary Afferent Neurons

To understand pathological phenomena at the level of the primary afferent neuron, one should be familiar with the **normal function** of both nociceptive and low-threshold mechanoreceptive primary afferents. Simultaneous Aδ and C fiber stimulation in the skin generates a "first" well-localized pain of sharp, pricking quality (attributable to Aδ nociceptors) followed by a poorly localized "second" pain of burning quality (due to the delayed arrival of C nociceptor input) (47). Muscle nociceptor stimulation produces aching or cramping pain even in the absence of muscle contraction (48, 49). Anatomically, both cutaneous and deep nociceptors terminate in different regions of the spinal gray matter (50–53). The distinct pain qualities produced by cutaneous and deep nociceptors, as well their different central terminations, raise the question of whether different neuropathic pain sensations are due to abnormalities of (a) different kinds of primary afferents, (b) their associated central encoding circuits or (c) both.

Low-intensity electrical shocks of the skin or a nerve produce a tapping tactile sensation. With higher stimulation frequency the taps merge into a buzzing or tingling sensation that is, however, painless. These sensations are due to Aβ fiber stimulation as it appears during simultaneous neurogra-

phy. When the stimulation increases further in intensity, activating Aδ fibers, a sharp, stabbing pain is added. Finally, the recruitment of C fibers generates additional burning pain with a distinct delay (31). The afferent volleys occurring under electrical stimulation, however, are unnatural, massive, and highly synchronized.

With application of a tourniquet to a limb at inflation pressures of 80 to 100 mm Hg above systolic blood pressure, differential ischemic blockade of primary afferents occurs. Large myelinated afferents (e.g., Aβ fibers subserving touch) are the most sensitive to ischemic conduction block. Therefore, the sensation of touch is the first one to be abolished, approximately 20 to 25 minutes after tourniquet application. Very soon afterward, Aδ (thinly myelinated) fibers subserving the sensation of both cold and first pain are blocked. The unmyelinated C nociceptive fibers are the most resistant to ischemia, and burning pain and pinprick sensation are the last to be blocked. Therefore, it is feasible to differentiate with simple clinical means the types of primary afferents that subserve different kinds of sensations in man.

Neuropathic Pain Phenomena and Abnormalities of the Primary Afferent Neurons

When one considers **abnormalities at the level of the primary afferent neuron** subserving nociception (C and Aδ fibers) and other sensations (large myelinated fibers like Aβ responsible for, e.g., tactile functions), multiple abnormalities are possible:

1. Following injury or in the presence of inflammation, primary afferent nociceptors that normally respond to potentially or clearly noxious stimuli become sensitized by release of multiple mediators (e.g., serotonin, histamine, bradykinin, purines, cytokines, substance P, calcitonin gene-related peptide [CGRP], eicosanoids, and various ions). Sensitized nociceptors acquire ongoing spontaneous discharges, a lowered threshold for activation, and an increased response to suprathreshold stimuli. This **peripheral nociceptor sensitization** may continue after healing of the original tissue injury (54, 55). In a very well studied case (54) this abnormality was associated with skin warmth (attributed to C nociceptor antidromic excitation, release of vasoactive substances, and vasodilation). Cutaneous vasodilation associated with C nociceptor sensitization may be, however, masked by the vasoconstriction produced by a pain-evoked sympathetic reflex (56).

2. Evidence from animal work suggests that there is some relation between C fiber terminal sensitization and the **sympathetic nervous system.** It has been shown that (a) sensitized C nociceptors acquire sensitivity to sympathetic stimulation and norepinephrine; (b) surviving C nociceptors after partial nerve injury also acquire adrenergic sensitivity (58); and (c) even

sympathetic nerve damage alone suffices to produce de novo sensitivity of C nociceptors to norepinephrine (59). In relation to human neuropathic pain, partial sympathetic nerve damage contributing to abnormal nociceptor sensitization may be responsible for the pain of CRPS 1 and CRPS 2 and for that of patients with diabetic neuropathy and postherpetic neuralgia (31).

3. **Continuous activation** of normal or sensitized nociceptors by occult, ongoing tissue injury or alteration of tissue environment and nociceptor milieu has been speculated to occur in cases of burning pain in both primary neuropathic disorders, such as diabetic neuropathy (60, 61), and in patients with neuropathic phenomena, for example erythromelalgia due to excessive platelet production and thrombi formation (62).

4. In many conditions, the distal portion of an injured nerve sprouts (**regenerative sprouting**). Examples include traumatic neuromas following nerve transection, diabetic and other dying-back neuropathies with degeneration and regeneration of the distal axons due to metabolic abnormalities, herpes zoster axonal damage after viral duplication and inflammation, and stretch and crush injuries without total nerve damage (31). Both the regenerating sprouts of primary afferent nociceptors and low-threshold mechanoreceptors acquire capacity to discharge either spontaneously or with subtle (mechanical, noradrenergic, thermal, and ionic) stimuli. Another form of sprouting occurs when a completely denervated area receives collateral innervation from neighboring intact primary afferents (**collateral sprouting**). Animal experiments (63–65) demonstrate allodynia and hyperalgesia to mechanical stimuli in skin innervated by collateral sprouts. Sometimes this may be the source of painful or dysesthetic sensations in humans (66). While collateral sprouting has not been shown to occur after partial nerve damage, this remains a possibility. Unnatural and highly synchronized afferent volleys (like those occurring with electrical stimulation) may be the basis of shocklike pains experienced by patients with traumatic neuromas, given the acquired capacity of sprouts to discharge spontaneously or with minimal stimulation (67).

5. These abnormalities in the sprouts of damaged primary afferents are also expressed at their cell bodies in the **dorsal root ganglia** (DRG) (68). Therefore, abnormal activity may be generated not only at the periphery but also at the DRG and more central sites beyond the DRG in the spinal cord and/or brain. It has been shown recently that the DRG ectopic generators are four to five times as sensitive to low doses of systemic local anesthetics as the peripheral sprouts themselves (69). It is, however, possible that CNS mechanisms are also very sensitive to low doses of systemic anesthetics.

6. While **ephapses** (abnormal electrical connections between demyelinated adjacent axons) have been shown in animal studies, (70), they have not been shown in humans. In only one case report in humans (71) abnormal stimulus mislocalizations that may be attributable to ephapses have been described.

Neuropathic Pain Phenomena and Abnormalities in CNS Neurons

CNS Changes after Peripheral Nerve Injury

Recent evidence suggests that primary afferent pathophysiology may in turn evoke central pathophysiology. Alternatively, some conditions arise exclusively from pathology within the CNS (e.g., as a result of a stroke). In the case of peripheral nerve injury multiple changes take place in the CNS: (*a*) Axotomized primary afferents sprout and invade new territories within the dorsal horn (72–74). (*b*) Normal neuropeptide production from the axotomized afferents (e.g., substance P and CGRP) is replaced by production of other neuropeptides (e.g., neuropeptide Y, galanin, vasoactive intestinal peptide [VIP]) (75, 76); and (*c*) Dramatic up-regulation of early immediate gene production (e.g. c-fos) affects input to second-order neurons (77). These anatomical and neurochemical changes clearly suggest that peripheral nerve damage has central consequences, even if the degree and significance of these central changes are not exactly known. Animals with chronic constriction of the sciatic nerve (78) develop behavioral signs of spontaneous pain, hyperalgesia, and allodynia. In these rats a subset of spinal neurons acquire abnormal responses (79, 80). Similar abnormal responses are seen in thalamic neurons (mostly contralaterally, but occasionally and unexpectedly, ipsilaterally) and cortical neurons (81, 82). Some rats with this nerve injury develop signs of neuropathic pain in the paw opposite the injury site (83). These mirror images, which have been noted in humans with CRPS, may be associated with the unexpected abnormalities seen in the rat ipsilateral thalamus. Expansion of the receptive field of spinal neurons has been seen after nerve injury (79, 80). Inflammatory agents or repeated tissue injury also lead to expansion of receptive fields of spinal dorsal neuron (84–88) and trigeminal brainstem nociceptive neurons (57). Clearly, local (peripheral) sensitization or changes in the physical environment of nociceptors that in turn generate nociceptor responses to mechanical stimuli applied in distal sites cannot be solely responsible for the observed expansion of receptive fields (90).

Large Fiber-Evoked Central Abnormalities

A large body of evidence shows that in neuropathic pain, activity in Aβ low-threshold mechanoreceptors (AβLTMs) is responsible for burning pain sensation generated by normally innocuous touch due to abnormal CNS processing (39, 90, 91). Touch-evoked pain (dynamic allodynia) disappears in many patients with neuropathic pain during a tourniquet block at the same time as normal tactile sensations (corresponding to the blockade of Aβ fibers in the neurogram). Static allodynia, in contrast, does not depend on activation of AβLTMs (33). In normal human volunteers, intradermal injection of capsaicin (the active ingredient of chili peppers) produces touch-evoked burning pain (dynamic allodynia) that is similar or identical to the touch-evoked pain experienced by some neuropathic pain patients. This pain seems also to be subserved by the activity of AβLTMs (92–94). Similarly, after capsaicin intradermal injection in normal humans, static allodynia appears (72, 93) with distinct temporal, spatial, and other characteristics. In summary, dynamic allodynia involves AβLTMs, while static allodynia involves Aδ and/or C nociceptors. These abnormalities can exist independently in patients or coexist (95). While a generalized central hyperexcitability mechanism has been hypothesized involving spinal wide dynamic range (WDR) neurons (96), the differential appearance of symptoms both in normal subjects after intradermal capsaicin injection and in patients with neuropathic pain points to the existence of multiple central mechanisms.

C-Nociceptive Fiber–Evoked Central Abnormalities, Including Central Sensitization

C nociceptive afferent volleys elicit changes in dorsal horn neurons of experimental animals (both nociceptive-specific and WDR types). These changes in excitability involve reduction in stimulation threshold, increase in general responsiveness, expansion of receptive fields, and alteration of temporal characteristics of the normal discharge patterns. Central hyperexcitability or "central sensitization" (as opposed to peripheral sensitization of nociceptors) is a normal process in nocireceptive dorsal horn neurons. While these changes are fleeting with small volleys, a large nociceptive barrage can produce long-lasting changes in the absence of ongoing nociceptive input (51, 74, 97). Many peripheral neuropathic syndromes are likely to be associated with C nociceptor barrages, as for example in partial or complete nerve transections accompanied by injury discharge or the neuritic and cutaneous inflammation of herpes zoster. In animal models Aδ nociceptor discharges seem to evoke only weak central hyperexcitability changes. Central sensitization, once initiated by peripheral inputs, may be maintained by continuous peripheral inputs (39). It has been further proposed (98) that initial sensitization, ongoing sensitization, and peripheral inputs contribute to the net activity of dorsal horn neurons, influencing the expression of persistent pain and hyperalgesic phenomena.

Some CRPS patients have abnormal summation of pain that has its counterpart in a physiological phenomenon known as windup. Increasing C fiber input at intervals of 3 seconds or less produces increasingly great discharges of spinal cord neurons receiving this C fiber input; therefore it is a central process (47). In these CRPS patients, however, burning sensations of increasing intensity occur when stimuli of Aβ fiber strength are presented at intervals of 3 seconds or less (91, 95). Therefore, a central mechanism that is normally accessed only by C nociceptor input seems now to be accessed by Aβ input in certain neuropathic pain patients.

The Neurochemical Basis of Central Sensitization

There is a growing body of evidence from animal work that central sensitization involves use of glutaminergic N-methyl-D-aspartate (NMDA) synapses for both its induction (initiation) and maintenance (74). High levels of activity at these NMDA synapses has been shown to produce an excitotoxic effect in certain CNS neurons in experimental animals. This "toxicity," which is the result of excessive glutamate release due to discharge of injured neurons, affects inhibitory interneurons, producing disinhibition. Electrophysiological evidence for such disinhibition has been obtained in animal models (100–102).

Pathophysiological Basis of Extraterritorial Spontaneous and Stimulus-Evoked Pain

A puzzling neuropathic phenomenon is the expansion of spontaneous and stimulus-evoked pains beyond the site of the injury in areas not defined by dermatomes or nerve territories. These phenomena are seen in patients with CRPS 1 and 2 and at times in patients with postherpetic neuralgia whose pain is outside the scarred areas. Experimental work in animals (26) and in humans (24) provides evidence for a central mechanism responsible for these changes. It seems that pain due partially or entirely to a central mechanism is thought to arise from body areas corresponding to the location of the receptive fields of abnormal central neurons (in the dorsal horns of the spinal cord, the thalamus, and the cortex). Nerve territory borders are invisible within the somatotopic maps because the receptive fields (for example of dorsal horn neurons) often include input from more than one nerve or root. Pain of nonanatomical distribution has been considered traditionally (and incorrectly) as one of the hallmarks of the so-called psychogenic or nonorganic pain (see Waddell signs [21]).

Central Changes Evoked by Primary Afferent Loss

The gate control theory of Melzack and Wall (102), by proposing that loss of AβLTM-inhibition alters sensory processing at the dorsal horn level, extended Noordenbos's (38) idea of the contribution of AβLTM loss to some peripheral neuropathies. Nevertheless, while nerve damage leads to loss of primary afferent-mediated inhibition, there is no evidence that this requires differential damage to Aβ fibers. However, there is evidence in humans that differential loss of Aδ cold-specific fibers may generate cold allodynia (103, 104). Cold pain in normal humans is produced by temperatures of 5 to 10° C and has an aching quality together with a sensation of cold. Normally Aδ input (a) produces the cold sensation and (b) centrally inhibits C nociceptor-evoked sensation (hot, burning pain). When Aδ axons are damaged and C fibers are spared, their central inhibition is lost; therefore the C fiber-evoked sensation is unmasked, and while the Aδ-mediated cold sensation is lacking, the pain is felt as burning. Such patients (103) (a) cannot detect cold stimuli (cold hypoesthesia), (b) have a cold pain threshold that is decreased to around 20° C (cold hyperalgesia), and (c) complain of hot and burning pain upon application of cold stimuli (CCC, or triple C syndrome). Some additional mechanisms for cold allodynia or hyperalgesia are further hypothesized; for example, since some AβLTMs discharge to cooling, they could produce burning pain in patients with AβLTM-mediated allodynia (105).

Central Changes Evoked by CNS Lesions

Patients with spontaneous and evoked as well as dysesthetic pain arising from injury to (a) dorsal spinal roots and/or (b) spinal cord, (c) brainstem, and (d) (rarely) cortex (106) are considered to suffer from central pain. Experimental evidence in animals and direct evidence in neuropathic pain patients shows that deafferentation directly from damage to the CNS can produce hyperresponsiveness and spontaneous discharges in CNS neurons (central deafferentation). There are some similarities with CNS changes evoked by peripheral deafferentation (i.e., the central effects of peripheral nerve damage), but there are also important differences (107).

Dorsal root injury, usually as the result of trauma or avulsion, deafferents spinal cord neurons, and some spinal cord damage is present. These neurons (in experimental animals) acquire abnormal spontaneous discharges (108, 109) in the form of (a) long trains of regular discharges and (b) paroxysmal discharges. Spontaneous discharges appear as early as 6 hours post root section but clearly increase for several weeks and thereafter decline over the course of several months. Loeser et al. (110) demonstrated high-frequency regular discharges and paroxysmal bursts (findings essentially identical to those seen in experimental animals) in a man with cauda equina injury to dorsal roots 19 months before. This patient had spontaneous burning pain in anesthetic regions. In deafferented cats, Basbaum and Wall (111) have shown formation of "new" receptive fields (one might better think of enlarged receptive fields with silent cores), encompassing skin along the borders innervated by the injured roots. Similar changes may occur in humans with dorsal root injuries.

Abnormal bursting discharges have been confirmed in somatosensory thalamus and cortex in experimental animals with multiple root transections (112–114). The thalamic abnormalities (a) are most intense in the areas of the somatotopic map deafferented by rhizotomies, (b) are also present in adjacent regions or the contralateral thalamus, and (c) appear considerably later than spinal phenomena. The poor outcome of spinal tract, hemicord, or complete cord transections in humans (with poor outcome in the treatment of root injury pain (106)) supports the hypothesis that after the initiation of important thalamocortical pathophysiology by root damage, these abnormalities become independent of spinal cord input, acquiring a life of their own.

Proposed explanations for this hyperresponsiveness of spinal neurons after root injury (with little direct supporting experimental evidence for the first, however) are (a) denervation supersensitivity to primary afferent transmitters (exaggerated effect of transmitter released by intact adjacent afferents), and (b) disturbance of the tonic descending inhibitory controls from the brainstem (115–117). The generally accepted conclusion is that there is a common feature to all patients with central pain: damage to some part of the classical spinothalamic system (118–120).

Our understanding of spontaneous and evoked pain pathophysiology after injury to parts of the spinothalamic system comes primarily from studies of awake humans with injuries to the CNS. Microelectrodes are used to confirm thalamic borders physiologically before therapeutic lesions (for movement disorders, epilepsy or major psychiatric disorders) are inflicted and to insert stimulating electrodes for treatment of chronic central pain or movement disorders. In patients with central pain, thalamic neurons in the somatotopic map representing anesthetic areas do not have detectable receptive fields. In contrast, neurons with receptive fields surrounding the anesthetic areas have enlarged receptive fields. Many of these thalamic neurons (with and without receptive fields) display spontaneous high-frequency burst discharges, a finding rarely seen in normal humans. Microstimulation around these neurons (with and without receptive fields) frequently elicits pain felt in the anesthetic area in central pain patients (contrasting the painless paraesthetic and dysesthetic sensations produced in normal humans when these areas are stimulated) (106, 121, 122).

Basal Ganglia, Nociception, and Pain

Chudler and Dong (123) reviewed the role of basal ganglia in nociception and pain. In summary, recent neurophysiological, clinical, and behavioral experiments indicate that the basal ganglia (striatum, globus pallidus, and substantia nigra) process painful and painless somatosensory information apart from their well-studied role in motor movements. With the exception of the primary somatosensory cortex (SI), the other areas of the brain (SII, area 7b, cingulate cortex, amygdala, intralaminar thalamic nuclei) that may transmit nociceptive information to the basal ganglia contain nociceptive and WDR neurons with large receptive fields, which may suggest that basal ganglia are not important in stimulus localization. Many of these neurons encode noxious stimulation intensity, which may play a role in the *sensory-discriminatory* dimensions of pain. Projections to substantia nigra and striatum from areas known to be engaged in emotional processes (cingulate cortex, amygdala, prefrontal cortex) may indicate that the basal ganglia play a role in *pain modulation*. Pathways in the form of a *gating mechanism* for sensory information to higher motor centers that may regulate the strength or form of a behavioral response (i.e., escape or attack) elicited by noxious stimuli may allow nociceptive information to be processed first in the basal ganglia before arriving to the intralaminar thalamic nuclei and premotor cortex. Collectively the basal ganglia may be involved in (a) motivational-affective, (b) cognitive, and (c) sensory-discriminative dimensions of pain, in (d) modulation of nociceptive information, and in (e) sensory gating of nociceptive information to higher motor areas. Modulation of nociceptive and behavioral responses at the basal ganglia seem to be mediated by opioid, dopaminergic, and GABAergic mechanisms. When pharmacological, electrostimulation, and lesional data are examined closely, it seems that most of this modulation takes place at supraspinal rather than spinal level. It has been hypothesized that dopamine, GABA, and opiates within the basal ganglia tonically inhibit thalamic activity. Pharmacological manipulations that increase or replenish the activity of these neurotransmitters within the basal ganglia (e.g., administration of dopaminergic agonists) may be expected to have analgesic effect. For a detailed review of the subject, see Chudler and Dong (123).

CONCLUSIONS

We have very good evidence from animal and human research that neural injury-evoked abnormalities in the peripheral and central nervous system may be significant for the production of human neuropathic pain syndromes. For the clinician, some principles have paramount importance in understanding the pathophysiology of neuropathic pain:

1. *Similar clinical abnormalities* may be produced by *different pathophysiologic mechanisms,* and more than one abnormality may *coexist* in any given patient. For example, allodynia to tactile stimuli (mechanoallodynia) may be the product of: (*a*) abnormal C nociceptor sensitization, (*b*) AβLTM-mediated ("dynamic") allodynia as the product of peripheral (C nociceptor-induced) sensitization, (*c*) Aδ/C fiber-mediated allodynia of the static type via another C nociceptor-evoked mechanism of central hyperexcitability, and (*d*) allodynia due to central deafferentation-evoked hyper-responsiveness (central pain). Another example is the cold extremity of a patient with a peripheral nerve injury. Coldness can be the result of an (*a*) an increase in sympathetic vasoconstrictor tone (sympathetic hyperactivity), (*b*) denervation supersensitivity (exaggerated response to norepinephrine released by adjacent intact sympathetic efferents despite the presence of sympathetic denervation), or (*c*) an "innocent somatosympathetic reflex" (124) as the result of tissue injury. Similarly, a warm extremity may be secondary to (*a*) sympathetic vasoparalysis, (*b*) antidromic C nociceptor activation and release of vasoactive mediators (neurogenic inflammation), or (*c*) release of inflammatory (tissue damage-induced) mediators. Two or more of these processes may be superimposed, and the presentation may be the dynamic sum of more than one process.
2. The initial tissue or nerve injury may produce one pathogenic mechanism, which in turn may generate others peripherally or centrally in a domino effect. While the original damage may heal, the secondary changes (again peripherally or centrally) may acquire a life of their own.

References

1. Gracely RH, Price DD, Roberts WJ, Bennett GJ. Quantitative sensory testing in patients with complex regional pain syndromes (CRPS) I and II. In: Janig W, Stanton-Hicks M, eds. Reflex sympathetic dystrophy: a reappraisal. Progress in Pain Research and Management, vol 6. Seattle: IASP Press, 1996;151.
2. Merskey H, Bogduk N, eds. Classification of Chronic Pain, 2nd ed. Seattle: IASP Press, 1994.
3. Dubner R, Basbaum AI. Spinal dorsal horn plasticity following tissue or nerve injury. In: Wall PD, Melzack R, eds. Textbook of pain. 3rd ed. Edinburgh: Churchill Livingstone, 1994;225.
4. Ashbury AK, Fields HL. Pain due to peripheral nerve damage: an hypothesis. Neurology 1984;34:1587.
5. Brose WG, Cousins MJ. Subcutaneous lidocaine for treatment of neuropathic cancer pain. Pain 1991;45:145.
6. Turk DC, Melzack R. The measurement of pain and the assessment of people experiencing pain. In: Turk DC, Melzack R. Handbook of pain assessment. New York: Guilford Press, 1992;3.
7. Grzesiak RC, Ciccone DS, eds. Psychological vulnerability to chronic pain. New York: Springer, 1994.
7a. American Psychiatric Association. Diagnostic and Statistical Manual of Mental Disorders. 4th ed. Washington: APA, 1994.
8. Walters A. Psychogenic regional pain alias hysterical pain. Brain 1961;84:1.
9. Barsky AJ, Klerman GL. Overview: hypochondriasis, bodily complaints and somatic styles. Am J Psychiatry 1983;140:273.
10. Barsky AJ, Wyshak G. Hypochondriasis and somatosensory amplification. Br J Psychiatry 1990;157:404.
11. Kellner R. Somatization and hypochondriasis. New York: Prager, 1986.
12. Pilowski I. Dimensions of hypochondriasis. Br J Psychiatry 1967;113:89.
13. Bakal DA, Kaganov JA. Muscle contraction and migraine headache: psychophysiologic comparison. Headache 1977;17:208.
14. Pozniak-Patewicz E. Cephalgic spasm of head and neck muscles. Headache 1976;15:261.
15. Bardhan PN. The couvade syndrome. Br J Psychiatry 1965;111:908.
16. Bardhan PN. The fathering syndrome. US Armed Forces Med J 1965;20:200.
17. Curtis JL. A psychiatric study of 55 expectant fathers. US Armed Forces Med J 1965;6:937.
18. Reik T. Ritual: psychoanalytical studies. London: Hogarth, 1914.
19. Trethowan WH. The couvade syndrome: some further observations. J Psychosomat Res 1968;12:107.
20. Trethowan WH, Conlon MF. The couvade syndrome. Br J Psychiatry 1965;3:57.
21. Waddell G, McCulloch JA, Kummel EG, Venner RM. Non-organic physical signs in low-back pain. Spine 1980;5;117.
22. Gould R, Miller BL, Goldberg MA, Benson DF. The validity of hysterical signs and symptoms. J Nervous Mental Dis 1986;174:593.
23. Derbyshire SWG, Jones AKP, Devani P, et al. Cerebral responses to pain in patients with atypical facial pain measured by positron emission tomography. Pain Med J Club J 1995;1:15.
24. Lacerenza M, Marchettini P, Formaglio F, et al. Extra-territorial mechanical hyperalgesia in patients with proven nerve damage involves adjacent undamaged nerves. IASP Abstr, VIII World Congress in Pain. 1996;37.
25. Mailis A, Amani N, Umana M, et al. Effect of intravenous sodium amytal on cutaneous sensory abnormalities, spontaneous pain and algometric pain pressure thresholds in neuropathic pain patients: a placebo-controlled study. II. Pain 1997;70:69.
26. Tal M, Bennett GJ. Extra-territorial pain in rats with a peripheral mononeuropathy: mechano-hyperalgesia and mechano-allodynia in the territory of an uninjured nerve. Pain 1994;57:375.
27. Merskey H. Pain and psychological medicine. In: Wall PD, Melzack R, eds. Textbook of Pain, 3rd ed. Edinburgh: Churchill Livingstone, 1994;903.

28. Roberts A, Kewman DG, Mercier L, Hovell M. The power of nonspecific effects in healing: implications for psychosocial and biological treatments. Clin Psychol Rev 1993;13:375.

29. Turner JA, Deyo RA, Loeser JD, et al. The importance of placebo effects in pain treatment and research. JAMA 1997;271;1609.

30. Waddell G. A new clinical model for the treatment of low-back pain. Spine 1987;12:632.

31. Bennett GJ. Neuropathic pain. In: Wall PD, Melzack R, eds. Textbook of pain. 3rd ed. Edinburgh: Churchill Livingstone, 1994;201.

32. Ovesen P, Kroner K, Ornsholt J, Bach L. Phantom-related phenomena after rectal amputation: prevalence and clinical characteristics. Pain 1991;44:289.

33. Ochoa JL, Roberts WJ, Cline MA, et al. Two mechanical hyperalgesia in human neuropathy. Soc Neurosci Abstr 1989;15:472.

34. Jensen K, Andersen H, Oleson J, Lindblom U. Pressure-pain threshold in human temporal region: evaluation of a new pressure algometer. Pain 1986;25:313.

35. Mailis A, Umana M, Roe S, Basur R. Algometric pain pressure threshold ratios in normal subjects and patients with limb pain: a novel clinical method for the assessment of deep pain. IASP Abstr. VIII World Congress in Pain, 1996;370.

36. Umana M, Mailis A, Roe S. Clinico-pathological diagnoses underlying neuropathic phenomenology: three-year experience. IASP Abstracts, VIII World Congress in Pain, 1996:370.

37. Beric A. Central pain: "New" syndromes and their evaluation. Muscle Nerve 1993;16:1017.

38. Noordenbos W. Pain. Amsterdam: Elsevier, 1959.

39. Gracely RH, Lynch SA, Bennett GJ. Painful neuropathy: altered central processing, maintained dynamically by peripheral input. Pain 1992;51:175.

40. Dubner R, Sharav Y, Gracely RH, Price DD. Idiopathic trigeminal neuralgia: sensory features and pain mechanisms. Pain 1987;31:23.

41. Mailis A. Mind, body and pain: are there any borders? Humane Med 1995a;11:152.

42. Mailis A, Nicholson K. Effect of normal saline controlled intravenous administration of sodium amytal in patients with pain and unexplainable widespread non-anatomical sensory deficits: a preliminary report. Submitted to American Pain Society 1997 (abstract).

43. Mailis A. Is diabetic autonomic neuropathy protective against reflex sympathetic dystrophy? Clin J Pain 1995b;11:77.

44. Mailis A, Meindok H, Papagapiou M, Pham D. Alterations of the three phase bone scan after sympathectomy. Clin J Pain 1994;10:146.

45. Schwartzman RJ, Kerrigan J. The movement disorder of reflex sympathetic dystrophy. Neurology 1990;40:57.

46. Mailis A. Compulsive targeted self-injurious behavior in humans with neuropathic pain: a counterpart of animal autotomy? Four case reports and literature review. Pain 1996;64:569.

47. Price DD. Psychological and neural mechanisms of pain. New York: Raven Press, 1988;76.

48. Simone DA, Caputi GM, Marchettini P, Ochoa JL. Cramping pain and deep hyperalgesia following intramuscular injection of capsaicin. Soc Neuroci Abstr 1992;18:34.

49. Torebjork HE, Ochoa JL, Schady W. Referred pain from intraneural stimulation of muscle fascicles in the median nerve. Pain 1984;18:145.

50. Cervero F, Connell LA. Distribution of somatic and visceral primary afferent fibers within the thoracic spinal cord of the cat. J Compar Neurol 1984;230:88.

51. Cervero F, Shouenborg J, Sjolund BH, Waddell PJ. Cutaneous inputs to dorsal horn neurons in adult rats treated at birth with capsaicin. Brain Res 1984;301:335.

52. Cervero F, Tattershall JE. Somatic and visceral inputs to the thoracic spinal cord of the cat: marginal zone (lamina I) of the dorsal horn. J Physiol (Lond) 1987;388:383.

53. Sugiura Y, Terui NM, Hosoya Y, Kohno K. Distribution of unmyelinated primary fibers in the dorsal horn. In: Cervero F, Bennett GJ, Headley PM, eds. Processing of sensory information in the superficial dorsal horn of the spinal cord. New York: Plenum, 1989;15.

54. Cline MA, Ochoa J, Torebjork HE. Chronic hyperalgesia and skin warming caused by sensitized C nociceptors. Brain 1989;112:621.

55. Ochoa J. The newly recognized painful ABC syndrome: thermographic aspects. Thermology 1986;2:65.

56. Ochoa JL, Yarnitsky D, Marchettini P, et al. Interaction between sympathetic vasoconstrictor outflow and C nociceptor induced antidromic vasodilatation. Pain 1993,54:191.

57. Reference deleted.

58. Sato J, Perl ER. Adrenergic excitation of cutaneous pain receptors induced by peripheral nerve injury. Science 1991;251:1608.

59. Bossut DF, Perl ER. Sympathectomy induces novel adrenergic excitation of cutaneous nociceptors. Soc Neurosci Abstr 1992;18:287.

60. Leriche R. The surgery of pain. Baltimore: Williams & Wilkins, 1939.

61. Livingston WK. Pain mechanisms: a physiological interpretation of causalgia and its related states. New York: Macmillan, 1943.

62. Kurzrock R, Cohen PR. Erythromelalgia and myeloproliferative disorders. Arch Intern Med 1989;149:105.

63. Kingery WS, Vallin JA. The development of chronic mechanical hyperalgesia, autotomy, and collateral sprouting following sciatic nerve section in rat. Pain 1989;38:321.

64. Markus H, Pomeranz B, Krushelnycky D. Spread of saphenous somatotopic projection map in spinal cord and hypersensitivity of the foot after chronic sciatic denervation in adult rat. Brain Res 1984;296:27.

65. Vallin HA, Kingery WS. Adjacent neuropathic hyperalgesia in rats: a model for sympathetic independent pain. Neurosci Lett 1991;133:241.

66. Inbal R, Rousso M, Ashur H, et al. Collateral sprouting in skin and sensory recovery after nerve injury in man. Pain 1987;28:141.

67. Chabal C, Jacobson L, Russell LC, Burchiel KJ. Pain responses to perineuromal injection of normal saline, gallamine, and lidocaine in humans. Pain 1992;49:9.

68. Devor M. The pathophysiology of damaged peripheral nerves. In: Wall PD, Melzack R, eds. Textbook of pain. 3rd ed. Edinburgh: Churchill Livingstone, 1994;79.

69. Devor M, Wall PD, Catalan N. Systemic lidocaine silences ectopic neuroma and DRG discharge without blocking nerve conduction. Pain 1992;48:261.

70. Jänig W. Pathophysiology of nerve following mechanical injury in man. In: Dubner R, Gebhart GF, Bond MR, eds. Pain research and clinical management, vol 3. Amsterdam: Elsevier, 1988;89.

71. Raymond SA, Rocco AG. Ephaptic coupling of large fibers as a clue to mechanisms in chronic neuropathic allodynia, following damage to dorsal roots. Pain 1990;(Suppl 5):S276.

72. LaMotte RH, Shain CN, Simone DA, Tsai EFP. Neurogenic hyperalgesia: psychophysical studies of underlying mechanisms. J Neurophysiol 1991;66:190.

73. Snow PJ, Wilson P. Denervation induced changes in somatotopic organization: the effective projections of afferent fibers and structural plasticity. In: Cervero F, Bennett GJ and Headley PM, eds. Processing of sensory information in the superficial dorsal horn of the spinal cord. New York: Plenum, 1989;285.

74. Woolf CJ, Thompson SWN. The induction and maintenance of central sensitization is dependent on N-methy-D-aspartic acid receptor activation: implications for the treatment of post injury pain hypersensitivity states. Pain 1992;44:293.

75. Bennett GJ, Kajander KC, Sahara Y, et al. Neurochemical and anatomical changes in the dorsal horn of rats with an experimental painful peripheral neuropathy. In: Cervero F, Bennett GJ, Headley PM, eds. Processing of sensory information in the superficial dorsal horn of the spinal cord. New York: Plenum, 1989;463.

76. Wakisaka S, Kajander KC, Bennett GJ. Effects of peripheral nerve injuries and tissue inflammation on the levels of neuropeptide Y-like immunoreactivity in rat primary afferent neurons. Brain Res 1992; 209: 95.

77. Basbaum AI, Chi SI, Levine JD. Peripheral and central contribution to the persistent expression of the c-fos protooncogene in spinal cord after peripheral nerve injury. In: Willis WD, ed. Hyperalgesia and allodynia. New York: Raven Press, 1992;295.

78. Bennett GJ, Xie YK. A peripheral mononeuropathy in rat that produces disorders of pain sensations like those seen in man. Pain 1988;33:87.

79. Laird JMA, Bennett GJ. An electrophysiological study of dorsal horn neurons in the spinal cord of rats with an experimental peripheral neuropathy. J Neurophysiol 1993;69:2072.

80. Palecek J, Paleckova V, Dougherty PM, et al. Responses of spinothalamic tract cells to mechanical and thermal stimulation of skin in rats with experimental peripheral neuropathy. J Neurophysiol 1992;67:1562.

81. Guilbaud G. Neuronal responsivity at supra-spinal levels (ventrobasal thalamus complex and SMI cortex) in a rat model of mononeuropathy. In: Besson JM, Guilbaud G, eds. Lesions of primary afferent fibers as a tool for the study of clinical pain. Amsterdam: Excerpta Medica, 1992;219.

82. Guilbaud G, Benoist JM, Jajat F, Gautron M. Neuronal responsivity in the ventrobasal thalamic complex of rats with an experimental peripheral mononeuropathy. J Neurophysiol 1990;64:1537.

83. Attal N, Jajat F, Kayser V, Guilbaud G. Further evidence for "pain-related" behaviors in a model of unilateral peripheral mononeuropathy. Pain 1990;41:235.

84. Hylden JLK, Nahin RL, Traub RJ, Dubner R. Expansion of receptive fields of spinal lamina I projection neurons in rats with unilateral adjuvant-induced inflammation: the contribution of dorsal horn mechanisms, Pain 1989;37:229.

85. Laird JMA, Cervero F. A comparative study of the changes in the receptive-field properties of multireceptive and nocireceptive rat dorsal horn neurons following noxious mechanical stimulation. J Neurophysiol 1989;62:854.

86. McMahon SB, Wall PD. Receptive fields of rat lamina I projection cells move to incorporate a nearby region of injury, Pain 1984;19:235.

87. Menetrey D, Besson JM. Electrophysiological characteristics of dorsal horn cells in rats with cutaneous inflammation resulting from chronic arthritis. Pain 1982;13:343.

88. Woolf CJ, King AE. Dynamic alterations in the cutaneous mechanoreceptive fields of dorsal horn neurons in the rat spinal cord. J Neurosci 1990;10:2717.

89. Dubner R. Hyperalgesia and expanded receptive fields. Pain 1992;48:3.

90. Campbell JN, Raja SN, Meyer RA. Painful sequelae of nerve injury. In: Dubner R, Gebhart GF, Bond MR, eds. Pain research and clinical management, vol 3. Amsterdam: Elsevier, 1988;135.

91. Price DD, Bennett GJ, Rafii A. Psychophysical observations on patients with neuropathic pain relieved by a sympathetic block. Pain 1989;36:273.

92. Gracely RA, Lynch SA, Bennett GJ. Evidence for Aβ low-threshold mechanoreceptor-mediated mechano-allodynia and cold hyperalgesia following intradermal injection of capsaicin in the foot dorsum. Abstracts VII World Congress on Pain, 1993:372.

93. Koltzenburg M, Lundberg LER, Torebjörk HE. Dynamic and static components of mechanical hyperalgesia in human hairy skin. Pain 1992;51:207.

94. Torebjörk HE, Lundberg LER, LaMotte RH. Central changes in procession of mechanoreceptive input in capsaicin-induced secondary hyperalgesia in humans. J Physiol 1992;448:765.

95. Price DD, Long S, Huitt C. Sensory testing of pathophysiological mechanisms of pain in patients with reflex sympathetic dystrophy. Pain 1992;49:163.

96. Roberts WJ. A hypothesis on the physiological basis for causalgia and related pain states. Science 1986;24:485.

97. Woolf CJ, Wall PD. Relative effectiveness of C primary afferent fibers of different origins in evoking a prolonged facilitation of the flexor reflex in the rat. J Neurosci 1986;6:1433.

98. Coderre TJ, Katz J. Peripheral and central hyperexcitability: differential signs and symptoms in persistent pain. Brain Behav Sciences 1997 (in press).

99. Reference deleted.

100. Wall PD, Devor M. The effects of peripheral nerve injury on dorsal root potentials and transmission of afferent signals into the spinal cord. Brain Res 1981; 209:95.

101. Woolf CJ, Wall PD. Chronic peripheral nerve section diminishes the primary A-fiber, mediated inhibition of rat dorsal horn neurons. Brain Res 1982; 424: 77.

102. Melzack R, Wall PD. Pain mechanisms: a new theory. Science 1965;150:971.

103. Ochoa JL, Yarnitsky D. Triple cold ("CCC") painful syndrome. Pain 1990(Suppl 5):S278.

104. Yarnitsky D, Ochoa JL. Release of cold-induced burning pain by block of cold-specific afferent input. Brian 1989;113:893.

105. Frost SA, Raja SN, Campbell JN, et al. Does hyperalgesia to cooling stimuli characterize patients with sympathetically maintained pain (reflex sympathetic dystrophy)? In: Dubner R, Gebhart GF, Bond MR, eds. Pain research and clinical management, vol 3. Amsterdam: Elsevier, 1988;151.

106. Tasker RR. Pain resulting from central nervous system pathology (central pain). In: Bonica JJ, ed. The management of pain. Philadelphia: Lea & Febiger, 1990;264–283.

107. Bonica JJ. Introduction: semantic, epidemiologic, and educational issues. In: Casey KL, ed. Pain and central nervous system disease: the central pain syndromes. New York: Raven Press, 1991;13.

108. Loeser JD, Ward AA. Some effects of deafferentation on neurons of the cat spinal cord. Arch Neurol 1967;17:629.

109. Lombard MC, Larabi Y. Electrophysiological study of cervical dorsal horn cells in partially deafferented rats. In: Bonica JJ, Lindblom U, Iggo A, eds. Advances in pain research and therapy, vol 5. New York: Raven Press, 1983;147.

110. Loeser JD, Ward AA, White LE. Chronic deafferentation of human spinal cord neurons. J Neurosurg 1968;29:48.

111. Basbaum AI, Wall PD. Chronic changes in the responses of cells in adult dorsal horn following partial deafferentation: the appearance of responding cells in a previously non-responding region. Brain Res 1976;116:181.

112. Albe-Fessard D, Lombard MC. Use of an animal model to evaluate the origin of and protection against deafferentation pain. In: Bonica JJ, Lindblom U, Iggo A, eds. Advances in pain therapy and research, vol 5. New York: Raven Press, 1983;691.

113. Albe-Fessard D, Rampin O. Neurophysical studies in rats deafferented by dorsal root sections. In: Dahsold BS, Ovelmen-Levitt J, eds. Deafferentation pain syndromes: pathophysiology and treatment, New York: Raven Press, 1991;125.

114. Lombard MC, Nashold BS, Albe-Fessard D, et al. Deafferentation hypersensitivity in the rat after dorsal rhizotomy: a possible animal model for chronic pain. Pain 1979;6:163.

115. Hodge CJ, Apkarian AV, Owen MP, Hanson BS. Changes in the effects of stimulation of locus coeruleus and nucleus raphe magnus following dorsal rhizotomy. Brain Res 1983;299:325.

116. Rampin O, Morain P. Cortical involvement in dorsal horn cell hyperactivity and abnormal behavior in rats with dorsal root section. Somatosens Mot Res 1987;4:237.

117. Zimmermann H. Central nervous mechanisms modulation pain-related information: do they become deficient after lesions of the peripheral or central nervous system? In: Casey KL, ed. Pain and central nervous system disease: the central pain syndromes. New York: Raven Press, 1991;183

118. Boivie J, Leijon G, Johansson I. Central post-stroke pain: a study of the mechanisms through analyses of the sensory abnormalities. Pain 1989;37:173.

119. Cassinari V, Pagni CA. Central pain: a neurological survey. Cambridge: Harvard University Press, 1969.

120. Leijon G, Boivie J, Johansson I. Central post-stroke pain: neurological symptoms and pain characteristics. Pain 1989;36:13.

121. Lenz FA. The thalamus and central pain syndromes: human and animal studies. In: Casey KL, ed. Pain and central nervous system disease: the central pain syndromes. New York: Raven Press, 1991;171.

122. Lenz FA, Rasker RR, Dostrovsky JO. Abnormal single unit activity recorded in the somatosensory thalamus of a quadriplegic patient with central pain. Pain 1987;31:225.

123. Chudler EH, Dong WK. The role of basal ganglia in nociception and pain, Pain 1995:60;3.

124. Ochoa JL, Verdugo RJ. Reflex sympathetic dystrophy. A common clinical avenue for somatoform expression. Malingering and conversion reactions. Neurol Clin 1995;13:353.

CHAPTER 7

Painful Neurological Disorders: Clinical Aspects

Angela Mailis and Gary J. Bennett

PAIN SYNDROMES: CENTRAL VERSUS PERIPHERAL

When one discounts pains attributed to central pain-generating mechanisms exclusively, there are very few neuropathic pain syndromes initially arising from peripheral nerve injury or dysfunction that will not activate ultimately central mechanisms as well. Therefore, we describe painful neuropathic disorders in a particular descending rank order: those with exclusive or primarily central origin will be described first and those with primarily peripheral origin, last. Effort is made to list central and peripheral contributions if they both exist.

Central pain (CP) is defined by the International Association for the Study of Pain as "pain caused by lesion or dysfunction of the central nervous system" (1). The concept of CP has been included recently as part of the broader concept of deafferentation pain (2), "based on the assumption that pain is due to decreased afferent input into various part of the nervous system with consequent sensitization" (3), but this clearly has not been universally accepted. The most representative CP syndromes discussed under this heading include central poststroke pain, pain after spinal cord lesions, and syringomyelia/syringobulbia. The list also includes pain in multiple sclerosis, epilepsy, and basal ganglia disorders.

It appears that all kinds of brain or spinal cord lesions can cause CP. The lesion can be right- and left-sided, thalamic and extrathalamic, supratentorial and infratentorial (4), involving brainstem and parietal cortex, as well as all levels of spinal cord. Vascular hemorrhagic or ischemic lesions, traumatic injuries, syringobulbia, multiple sclerosis, tumors, abscesses, viral encephalitis, and myelitis have all been reported (5, 6).

CENTRAL POSTSTROKE PAIN

Central poststroke pain is the best-studied form of CP. In 1906 Déjérine and Roussy (7) described a group of patients following a thalamic stroke with excruciating pain on the contralateral side of the body. It is only since the mid-1970s that the syndrome received significant attention. Poststroke pain is not as rare as was originally thought. There are large differences in the prevalence of CP (8), and no true epidemiological studies have been done. The exception is a recent prospective study of 267 stroke patients (4) that reported an 8% prevalence of CP in stroke victims; in more than half of these patients the pain was reported as moderate to severe. This same study showed that allodynia and/or dysesthesias to tactile and thermal stimuli occurred in the majority of patients with CP, almost all of whom had somatosensory dysfunction, but not in stroke patients with somatosensory dysfunction without pain. Partial sensory loss is a well-known feature of CP (5). While sensory loss alone is not sufficient for the development of CP, the development of sensory loss and hyperalgesia or allodynia in a body part deafferented by the stroke is considered by some a necessary and sufficient condition for poststroke pain (9). It is important to differentiate nociceptive pains that can also be found in stroke patients (relating to spasticity, persistent muscle spasms, and so on).

The location of the brain lesion determines the location of the pain. In terms of quality of pain, while burning is the most common descriptor, many other descriptors have also been applied (e.g., aching, lancinating, pricking, lacerating, pressing) (5). Most of these patients have more than one kind of pain quality, and they may suffer from a variety of spontaneous pains, usually continuous as well as paroxysmal, and stimulus-evoked pains, an example of which is proprioceptive or kinesthetic allodynia (10). The intensity may be constant or fluctuate. It may be higher in thalamic and low brainstem lesions (11). Tasker et al. (6) reviewed 73 personal cases. Pain appeared immediately post stroke in almost a third of the patients. In half of the patients the pain appeared within days or up to 12 months later. Delay of 2 years was shown in 9.5% of the patients, and in a minority (4.5%) the delay was longer than 2 years. A multiplicity of neurological signs are seen in these patients, including a large spectrum of motor and somatosensory abnormalities, such as hypoesthesia, hyperesthesia, paresthesias, and dysesthesias with radiation, prolonged response latencies, and aftersensations.

CP OF SPINAL CORD ORIGIN

The quoted incidence of spinal cord injury (SCI) pain varies from 7.5% to 94% (6). Trauma is the most frequent cause. The pain syndrome seems to be more complex than those arising from brain injury because it may involve variable peripheral contributions. Donovan et al. (12) recognized the following pain syndromes in SCI: (a) central dysesthetic pain at and caudad to the level of injury; (b) radicular pain from damaged roots at the level of injury; (c) musculoskeletal syndromes due to bone injuries, spinal malalignment, or muscle and ligamentous strain or overuse above the injury level; (d) visceral pains; and (e) pain primarily based on psychogenic factors in a minority of patients. Beric et al. (13) considered that lesions seemingly complete may indeed be incomplete at subclinical levels. We have observed (Mailis, unpublished data) that the sensation of pressure over deep tissues (muscle and periosteum) as measured by the use of sensitive pressure algometers may be preserved caudally in seemingly complete spinal cord injuries and in brain injuries (in some cases with complete hemibody deafferentation and loss of somatosensory functions as well as vibration and joint position sense). Preservation of pressure sensation below the level of seemingly complete SCI or in the presence of clinically complete deafferentation after stroke may indicate that pain from deep structures is conveyed through pathways that seem to be more resistant to the injury. In reality the mapping of the "sensory homunculus" at thalamic and cortical levels has always been based on detection of sensory cutaneous stimuli and not stimuli from deep tissues.

Tasker et al. (6) reviewed the essential features of 127 personal cases. Three quarters of the patients were men; more than half were below age 40; trauma was the most common cause by far; and most lesions were cervical (42%), followed by thoracolumbar lesions (37%). Of the lesions, 32% were clinically complete, and in 4% overall there was no detectable sensory loss. The onset of the pain was delayed up to 1 month in 18% of the cases and more than a year in 26%. Three types of pain were experienced: steady spontaneous pain (96%), spontaneous paroxysmal lancinating pain (31%), and stimulus-evoked pain (47%). The ongoing spontaneous pain was described as burning in 75% of the patients and numb or tingling in 26%. Nevertheless, it is unclear whether patients with clinically incomplete injuries have different pain characteristics from those with complete injuries.

Special reference is made to patients with syringomyelia (cavitary lesions in the spinal cord) and syringobulbia (cavitation in the lower brainstem). While these are rare diseases, they are associated with a very high incidence of pain. The size and extension of the cavitary lesions, which are filled with fluid similar to the cerebrospinal fluid (CSF), vary immensely among patients. According to the most popular theory, hydromechanical forces are important for the development and expansion of these cavities. They start, therefore, in the center of the spinal cord, where the spinothalamic fibers cross the midline. Dissociated sensory loss (i.e., loss of pain and temperature sensation with preservation of touch) can occur. Indeed, this sensory abnormality was found in the vast majority of patients (14, 15). Boivie (5) reported that pain may be located in one of the upper extremities or the thorax, while few patients reported pain in the lower extremities. Burning, aching, and pressing were the most common qualities of pain. Boivie (5) stated that results of his own studies question the exclusive pain symptom production as a result of crossing spinothalamic tract fiber damage, since some patients may have strictly unilateral symptoms. It may be that the lesion in some affects the dorsal horns or the spinothalamic fibers before they decussate. In general the characteristics of pain in syringomyelia and syringobulbia are similar to those observed in traumatic spinal cord injuries (6). Unfortunately, pathological and magnetic resonance imaging (MRI) results are not available to correlate the extent of cavitary lesions with types, incidence, or severity of pain.

Pathophysiology of CP after Brain and Spinal Cord Lesions

Several theories have been put forward to explain CP. Some of the current concepts are as follows:

- The single most common anatomical lesion is an interruption of the spinothalamocortical nociceptive pathways.
- The lesion does not have to involve the dorsal column or medial lemniscal pathways (16). However, large fiber-dorsal column-medial lemniscus input may be involved in the generation of stimulus-evoked allodynia and dysesthesias (10).
- The lesion can be at any level of the neuraxis from the dorsal horn to the cerebral cortex.
- All kinds of diseases can cause CP, but the severity and incidence of CP may vary greatly among diseases.
- In SCI (a) loss of balance between different sensory channels, (b) loss of spinal inhibitory mechanisms, and (c) presence of pattern generators within the injured cord have been proposed as possible mechanisms of pain. Extensive discussion is beyond the scope of this chapter; see the extensive review by Yezierski (17) for details. Several studies in experimental models of SCI and in humans support the hypothesis that in spinal cord injury, alterations in the physiological properties of spinal neurons and the development of focal pattern generators are the result of anatomical and neurochemical changes collectively constituting a central injury cascade (17)

responsible for the development of the clinical symptoms. Furthermore, changes have been observed in supraspinal neurons. Lenz et al. (18) described changes in the thalamus of a patient with spinal cord injury. It is quite likely that more than one mechanism is involved in the appearance of CP, after either brain or spinal cord injury.

- While no single region has been considered crucial to the development of CP, Canavero (19) has further proposed that CP, irrespective of the location of the lesion, is generated by a "disturbance in the normal oscillatory mechanisms active between cortex and thalamus." Actually, both thalamic and cortical, parietal and/or frontal involvement in CP of both brain and spinal cord origin have been demonstrated via neurometabolic studies (20–25).

- Pain and hypersensitivity seem to be compatible with increased burst activity found in the ventroposterior thalamic nuclei in patients with spinal cord injury (26).

- Increased burst activity may be related to loss of afferent glutamate drive on NMDA (*N*-methyl-D-aspartate) receptors (26) or increased activity at NMDA receptor sites (27). The presence of glutamatergic hypertonus is suggested by the relief of CP by ketamine, (28) lamotrigine, (22) propofol (22), and barbiturates (2, 29). Canavero et al. (21) suggested that denervation (at whatever CNS level) induced a γ-aminobutyric acid (GABA) decrease that disinhibits the pain-coded thalamocortical loop and results in relative excitation. NMDA receptor-dependent neuronal hyperexcitability in the CNS is inhibited by GABA-A agonists (30), pointing to a functional relation between GABA and glutamate.

Treatment modalities for CP are multiple, and many of those are unproven. They include the following: (*a*) drugs (e.g., antidepressants, antiepileptics, antiarrhythmics, analgesics), (*b*) neuroaugmentative or stimulating procedures (e.g., transcutaneous nerve stimulation, spinal cord or brain stimulation), (*c*) ablative procedures (cordotomy, dorsal root entry zone lesions [DREZ], cordectomy, mesencephalic tractotomy, thalamotomy, and cortical and subcortical ablation), and (*d*) sympathetic blockade. The success is limited with any treatment, and multimodality therapies are generally used.

PAIN IN MULTIPLE SCLEROSIS

The reported prevalence of pain in multiple sclerosis (MS) varies from "uncommon" (31) to 82% (32). Four of the five most recent studies report prevalence figures of significant clinical pain in 54 to 65% of MS patients (33–37). Not all MS pain is of central origin. It is to be expected that patients with weakness, paralysis, spasticity, and movement disorders or incoordination can also develop nociceptive musculoskeletal pain, for example back pain. It is conceivable that neuropathic pain of peripheral origin can also occur. Accentuation of pain by superimposed depression must also be considered, but pain as part of a major psychiatric disorder appears to be rare (34). Pain syndromes in MS can be classified as follows:

1. **Acute pain syndromes** characterized by stereotypical paroxysmal attacks of pain are well-known but not common complications of MS. The incidence is probably less than 10% (38–40). The best-known acute pain syndrome is trigeminal neuralgia, which is indistinguishable from tic douloureux or idiopathic trigeminal neuralgia. It tends, however, to occur at an earlier age and may be bilateral. (41). Other paroxysmal pain syndromes include Lhermitte's sign (transient electrical sensation down the legs on neck flexion), very brief ticlike extremity pain or burning dysesthetic pain lasting less than a minute, and painful tonic seizures that may accompany paroxysmal dysesthetic pain or immediately follow it (42). These seizures may involve tetanic spasm of the hand, flexion of the elbow, and adduction of the shoulder and may even be contralateral to the sensory disturbance, a phenomenon called Brown-Séquard syndrome in reverse (40). Transaxonal ephaptic transmission may explain the spinal origin of these sensorimotor seizures (39). In terms of treatment, antiepileptic drugs, particularly carbamazepine, seem to be the drugs of choice for trigeminal neuralgia and other paroxysmal pains (42, 43). Baclofen is shown to be an effective alternative when carbamazepine fails or is not tolerated (44) and sometimes is given in combination with carbamazepine.

2. **Subacute pain syndromes** (39) last days to weeks. Optic neuritis may produce retro-orbital aching pain aggravated by eye movements. Good pain relief may be obtained with steroids. Painful compressive (ulnar and peroneal) neuropathies may occur in patients confined to wheelchairs, while immunosuppressive agents such as steroids or cyclophosphamide can produce osteoporosis and vertebral or other fractures or hemorrhagic cystitis, respectively.

3. **Chronic pain syndromes** are more common. The relation among pain, female gender, advancing age, and severity of the disease has been recognized. The most common chronic pain syndrome is dysesthetic extremity pain described as continuous burning discomfort, reported in 29% of 76 patients in one series (39), worse at night and with weather changes. All patients in one series had evidence of posterior column dysfunction, but fewer than two-thirds had signs of spinothalamic tract involvement (39). Antidepressants have been recommended for nonparoxysmal CP, but different studies have given conflicting results (33, 35). Also, these pains have been reported refractory to anticonvulsants (45) as well as spinal stimulation (46, 47). Back pain was reported in 14% of patients (39); it may be mechanical or myofascial, as a result of spastic weakness or poor posture. Many of these patients have scoliosis and significant degenerative disc changes (39). Painful leg spasms, which are quite serious in

patients with advanced disease, occur in 13% of patients with MS (39). Muscle relaxants (baclofen, diazepam, dantrolene sodium) help two thirds of the patients (39) but may produce undesirable weakness. Occasionally courses of high-dose steroids during relapses of MS have been advocated (48), and spinal opioids seem to have some value (49). Dorsal rhizotomy and intrathecal phenol can abolish spasticity but may inadvertently produce weakness or sphincter dysfunction (50). A minority of patients may suffer from visceral pain described as an aching, bloated periumbilical sensation and crampy abdominal pain as a result of constipation. Headaches can be quite frequent, with incidence as high as 27% compared with 12% in the general population (51).

PAIN AND EPILEPSY

Painful epileptic seizures were reported by Young and Blumme (51) in 24 (2.8%) of 858 epileptic patients. Of these patients 10 had pains in the face, arm, leg, or trunk unilaterally; in 11 pain was reported in the scalp or the calvarium; and 3 patients had painful abdominal seizures.

CLINICAL DISORDERS OF BASAL GANGLIA AND PAIN

Parkinson's disease is characterized by degeneration of striatonigral neurons followed by degeneration of dopaminergic nigrostriatal pathways. Approximately 40% of Parkinson's patients report sensory abnormalities (pain, headache, numbness, tingling, itching, coldness, burning, and cramping) summarized by Chudler and Willie (53). Pain particularly may occur in 10 to 29% of Parkinson's patients (54, 54a). Most describe pain as intermittent and poorly localized (55), but some patients report constant pain (56, 57). While headaches are quite common in this disorder, other pain sites include the face, neck, torso, and the extremities (summarized by Chudler and Willie, 53).

The painful symptoms have been classified as primary (originating from peripheral or central nervous system sites) and secondary (as the result of edema, dystonia, vascular problems, or muscle cramps) (58). Primary pain symptoms are not directly related to motor phenomena for the following reasons (53): (a) They may occur contralateral to the side with motor symptoms. (b) They can precede the diagnosis of Parkinson's by years. (c) The degree of rigidity, tremor, bradykinesia, and postural changes is not different between those with and those without pain or has no correlation with pain. (d) Anesthetic blocks that render painful parkinsonian limbs anesthetic do not alleviate pain. (e) Electrophysiological studies are usually normal in Parkinson's disease. (f) Antiparkinson medications may relieve both motor phenomena and pain in some patients, but in other cases they may only relieve motor phenomena or even increase the pain. Recent studies have demonstrated several abnormalities in

somatosensory function in patients with Parkinson's disease: abnormal spatial and temporal tactile discrimination thresholds (59, 60), abnormal blink and perioral reflexes (61), increases in pain threshold and pain tolerance measured by thermal and electrical stimuli (62, 63), but decreases in pain tolerance level measured by ischemic constriction of a painful limb (tourniquet test) (57). Changes in CSF monoamine metabolites (5-hydroxyindoleacetic acid) (57) and reduced levels of endorphins have been reported (64), as have enkephalins in both the CSF (65) and pallidal and striatal regions (66). Unfortunately, in these studies the relation between pain and opiate levels has not been examined. Some Parkinson's patients who have had adrenal medullary transplants into the caudate nucleus seem to have less pain and require less medication after abdominal (67, 68) or other surgeries (69, 70). In rats with experimental nerve injury (71, 72) or inflammatory arthritis (73) adrenal medullary transplants into the spinal subarachnoid space reduce pain behavior. Some of these effects are presumed to be mediated by release of opioids and catecholamines from the transplant, since naloxone or phentolamine pretreatment (an opioid and α-adrenergic antagonist, respectively) can block the antinociceptive effects of the adrenal medullary transplants (73).

In humans (74) and in mice, cats, and primates (60, 75–78), administration of 1-methyl-4-phenyl-1,2,3,6-tetrahydropyridine (MPTP) causes symptoms that mimic Parkinson's disease. Experiments in mice (46) have shown that MPTP treatment causing 62% reduction in striatal dopamine levels results in initial hyperalgesia in the tail flick test but produces analgesia in the hot plate test, with long-term hyperalgesia in both of these measures of pain. The results suggest that MPTP affects the responsiveness of somatosensory neostriatal, pallidal, or nigral neurons. It has been also hypothesized that some of the motor phenomena observed in Parkinson's patients is related to their inability to use tactile cues that may create delayed or abnormal signals preparing, initiating, or guiding movements (79, 80).

Case reports of other basal ganglia disorders with alteration in pain perception further indicate a role of the basal ganglia in pain: (a) Psychiatric patients on neuroleptics may develop extrapyramidal symptoms. In a recent study, patients with extrapyramidal symptoms had a much higher incidence of intermittent aches in the back and legs (81). These preliminary data may further suggest a role for central dopaminergic pathways in pain. (b) Few patients with Huntington's chorea, a neurodegenerative disorder with chorea and dementia associated with loss of cholinergic and GABAergic neurons in the striatum and cerebral cortex, have been described with severe intermittent pains (82). (c) Some patients with a hereditary sensorimotor neuropathy and delayed onset of parkinsonian symptoms develop pain (83). Levodopa treatment alleviated both pain and signs of Parkinson's disease. (d) Hemorrhage on the putamen or caudate nucleus has resulted in loss of pain withdrawal effects (84), while a lesion in the putamen and posterior limb of the internal capsule may alleviate phantom limb pain (85) and decrease sensation to light touch, pinprick, and temperature (86).

OTHER MOVEMENT-ASSOCIATED PAINFUL NEUROLOGICAL DISORDERS

Gilles de la Tourette's syndrome (GTS) is a disorder characterized by multiple motor and one or more vocal tics as defined by the fourth edition of *Diagnostic and Statistical Manual of Mental Disorders* (87). Self-injurious behavior has been reported in 25 to 50% of patients in some large series (88–90). These patients have normal intelligence but significant obsessive personality traits and psychopathology. Riley and Lang (91) reported that pain is associated in multiple ways with GTS and related tic disorders, caused by the tic, its suppression, or the resulting injury. They found that 15 to 20% of GTS patients volunteer some degree of pain associated with tics; however, direct questioning reveals a much higher incidence. Interestingly, Kurlan et al. (92) reported a high frequency of sensory tics (41%) and described three patients whose tics were a voluntary reaction to painful spontaneous sensations. The painful sensations responded very well to haloperidol in one patient and to clonidine in another, with considerable reduction of motor tics. Kurlan et al. (92) characterized the sensory tics as focal, localized, uncomfortable sensations for which patients attempt to obtain relief by producing movements in the uncomfortable body part.

The physiological basis of GTS has attracted significant attention. Decreased dynorphinlike immunoreactivity in striatal fibers projecting to globus pallidus was shown in a GTS patient (93) and was attributed to abnormalities in the synthesis, metabolism, or transport of the peptide. Animal data (94) implicate nigrostriatal dopamine denervation in self-injurious behavior. However, involvement of endogenous opioids in self-mutilation has also been considered. Herman et al. (95) treated three patients with self-injurious behavior, one of whom had GTS, with naltrexone, a long-lasting opioid antagonist, and produced a dose-dependent significant decrease of self-trauma in all patients. The authors concluded that their results supported the hypothesis of "enhanced brain opioid activity" in self-injurious behavior.

Sandyk and Bamford (96) studied luteinizing hormone (LH), follicle-stimulating hormone (FSH), and prolactin levels post naloxone challenge in a 13-year-old boy with GTS and self-injurious behavior. Based on abnormal responses compared to those of controls, they concluded that their findings supported deranged opioid-dopaminergic functions. In general the GTS literature has remarkably failed to elaborate on the potential relation of painful sensations and self-injurious behavior in a disorder whose biochemical abnormalities have received significant attention.

PHANTOM PAIN

Phantom sensations (persistent images of the missing body part) are quite common after limb amputation. Occasionally, severe pain develops in the phantom limb; this is phantom pain. Stump pain specifically refers to pain arising from the site of amputation. The frequency of limb pain after amputation ranges from 2 to 100% (97), but these figures include pains of variable origin in the missing limb. In particular, severe phantom pain is reported to occur in 0.5 to 5% of extremity amputees (98–100). The onset is within the first week of amputation in 50 to 75% of patients, but delays of months or years have also been reported (97). Phantom pain is mainly localized in the distal limb and described variably as burning, crushing, or squeezing (101, 102), associated at times with a distorted position of the missing limb (103). While it is generally assumed that phantom limb pain gradually diminishes, some authors report pain persisting many years after amputation (101, 103). The phantom limb experience undergoes important changes within the first 1 or 2 years after amputation, with telescoping (shrinking of the phantom, with the digits of the hand or foot gradually approaching the stump) or fading of the phantom limb pain or phantom shape (97). Spontaneous movements ranging from painful myoclonic jerks to clonic contractions of the stump, which may form part of the painful phantom, are rarely reported but may be quite frequent (104). Factors aggravating phantom sensations and pain include emotional distress, weather changes, stump touch or pressure, and so on, while relieving factors include rest, distraction, stump movements or massage, use of a prosthesis, and so on (97). Several studies have suggested that postamputation pain is more likely to occur in patients with preamputation pain and have features often resembling the preamputation experience (100, 105). Interestingly, lesions in the brain or spinal cord may dramatically alter the phantom sensations and pain. For example, both focal brain infarct (85) and partial seizures (106) have been reported to modify these experiences permanently and temporarily, respectively. Phantom sensations associated frequently with pain occur after amputation of other body parts, such as nose, eyeball, tongue, teeth, penis, rectum, and breast (97).

The literature rarely distinguishes phantom limb pain from stump pain. The incidence of the latter specifically is reported to vary from 13 to 27% in different studies summarized by Jensen and Rasmussen (97). Parkes (107) found that persistent stump pain may occur a year after stumps apparently have healed, with pains triggered by stump or scar stimulation lasting moments to days; the latter is called nerve storms by Sunderland (108). Local skin pathology, disturbances of the circulation, local infections of skin or underlying tissues, bone spurs, and neuromas (97) may account for stump pain.

Several mechanisms may be involved in the generation of phantom sensations and pain. These include peripheral mechanisms (i.e., in the stump or the central parts of the lesioned primary afferents), spinal cord changes (well known to occur after peripheral nerve section), and supraspinal mechanisms; case reports suggest that cortical and thalamic structures modulate phantom sensations and phantom pain (97).

Treatments for phantom pain are numerous, with generally limited results. Such treatments may be noninvasive or invasive. Noninvasive treatments include transcutaneous nerve stimulation (TENS), acupuncture, relaxation techniques, and hypnosis as well as local ultrasound, massage, manipulation, and stretching of the stump, which may be beneficial in some cases. Pharmaceutical treatments have some value. Intravenous calcitonin had some effect in phantom limb pain in a double-blind crossover study (109). Tricyclic antidepressants (110), carbamazepine (111, 112), and β-blockers (113) have been reported beneficial in case reports. Opioids can also be useful. Invasive techniques include stump revision with implantation of tender neuromas within deep tissue, DREZ, and spinal cord and brain stimulation. The latter two neuroaugmentative procedures are reported to provide good pain relief in more than half of amputees in some limited series (114, 115).

NEOPLASTIC AND PARANEOPLASTIC SYNDROMES AFFECTING THE NERVOUS SYSTEM

Neoplastic disorders may be accompanied by involvement of the nervous system by primary or metastatic tumors. Neurological symptoms then may arise from a multiplicity of tumor-related problems:

1. Primary tumors involving the brain, spinal cord, or peripheral nerves can cause symptoms by direct compression, infiltration, inflammation, and disturbance of the vascular supply.
2. Metastatic deposits commonly develop within the brain and rarely the spinal cord. Metastases may develop within the bony coverings with extension through the dura or compromise of the vascular supply. Diffuse metastatic involvement of the meninges may occur with leukemias and lymphomas.
3. Tumors can cause metabolic disorders (organ failures, endocrinopathies, nutritional problems, or tumor secretion of ectopic substances), which in turn may produce neurological symptoms.
4. Infections related primarily to immunosuppression (e.g., opportunistic infections with *Listeria, Cryptococcus,* or *Mycobacteria* involving the meninges) may produce neurological dysfunction.
5. Vascular disorders causing nervous system hemorrhages or infarctions (e.g., small vessel disease due to marked erythrocytosis or leukocytosis, intravascular clotting or bleeding diathesis associated with thrombocytopenia, clotting factor deficiencies, or the high serum viscosity state arising from macroglobulinemias) may be sequelae of different malignancies.
6. Treatment of primary or secondary malignancies with chemotherapy or radiation therapy may produce toxicity or fibrosis with resultant neurological manifestations. Fibrotic involvement of roots or the brachial plexus, for example after radiation therapy for breast or lung cancer, may be associated with intractable neuropathic pain.
7. Remote effects of malignancies (used interchangeably with the term paraneoplastic syndromes), specifically those *not* caused by infection, systemic metabolic disorders, vascular disease, or side effects of cancer therapy, can produce a host of physiological derangements relating to multiple systems and in particular can cause neurological symptoms.

Paraneoplastic neurological syndromes are either relatively common or quite rare, depending on how they are defined. Croft and Wilkinson (116) reported neurological symptoms in 6.6% of 1465 cancer patients, but many of the patients may have had subtle abnormalities of peripheral nerve or muscle function on either clinical or electrophysiological examination. Paraneoplastic syndromes may affect multiple neural structures as follows:

1. The brain and cranial nerves (e.g., paraneoplastic cerebellar degeneration, opsoclonus or myoclonus, limbic encephalitis, optic neuritis)
2. Spinal cord (necrotizing myelopathy, myelitis, subacute motor neuropathy, motor neuron disease)
3. Peripheral nerves and ganglia (subacute or chronic sensorimotor peripheral neuropathy, acute polyradiculopathy, Guillain-Barré syndrome, mononeuritis multiplex, brachial neuritis, sensory or autonomic neuronopathy)
4. Neuromuscular junction and muscle (e.g., Lambert-Eaton myasthenic syndrome, myasthenia gravis, dermatomyositis and polymyositis, acute necrotizing myopathy)
5. Encephalomyeloradiculitis (117)

Several hypotheses have been proposed (i.e., toxins secreted by tumor, competition for essential substrate, opportunistic infection, autoimmune processes) to explain these syndromes. Although individual paraneoplastic syndromes may have different etiologies and a given paraneoplastic syndrome (for example cerebellar degeneration) may have more than one etiology, an immune mechanism is now the most attractive hypothesis as a cause of most or perhaps all remote effects of cancer on the nervous system (118). The hypothesis posits that antigenic molecules or epitopes known as onconeural antigens are shared between certain tumors and cells of the central or peripheral nervous system (119). The immune system, recognizing the tumor antigen as foreign, directs a response to the tumor that is also misdirected against the shared epitopes in the nervous system. This immune response, while it may cause neurological dysfunction, also may retard tumor growth, which explains why so many tumors associated with paraneoplastic syndromes are small and very difficult to detect (118).

Certain paraneoplastic disorders affecting the nervous system may be associated with pain. Some examples (118) are as follows: Sensory neuronopathy (a rare syndrome associated with a variety of autoimmune conditions and malignancies, primarily small-cell carcinoma of the lung) usually presents with dysesthetic extremity pain and numbness (occasionally even beginning in the arms or face), with symptoms preceding the diagnosis of cancer in most cases. It progresses over days or weeks throughout the body, causing severe ataxia resembling cerebellar degeneration. Necrotizing myelopathy may be associated with lymphoma, leukemia, and lung or other cancers and may precede or follow the diagnosis of malignancy. Back pain or radicular pain may be the first manifestation, followed by rapidly ascending flaccid paraplegia. Subacute sensorimotor neuropathy can be induced by multiple mechanisms such as diabetes mellitus, nutritional deficiencies, alcoholism, vitamin B_{12} deficiency, toxin exposure, and cancer chemotherapeutic agents such as vincristine and cisplatin. When occasionally associated with cancer, most frequently of the lung and sometimes preceding the diagnosis by up to 5 years (120), it is predominantly a distal, symmetrical polyneuropathy with weakness and glove-and-stocking sensory impairment to all modalities as well as loss of deep tendon reflexes. The course is variable. In breast cancer there is a particular sensorimotor neuropathy with some additional features of myopathy or CNS dysfunction (121). It is frequently heralded by itching or muscle cramps, preceding identification of cancer. A very rare but clinically significant paraneoplastic disorder is acquired neuromyotonia (discussed later) characterized by progressive aching and stiffening of muscles associated with spasms or severe rigidity preventing muscle use (122). Electromyography (EMG) may indicate continuous muscle activity (123). Antibodies reacting with the cerebellum are found in both the paraneoplastic stiff-person syndrome associated with Hodgkin's disease (124) and breast cancer (125) and in the nonparaneoplastic entity (described later under acquired neuromyotonias). The syndrome has also been associated with lung cancer and thymoma (118). Pain is also associated with brachial neuritis and myelitis. Mailis recalls a woman presenting with impressive clinical manifestations of complex regional pain syndrome (CRPS) of the hand. Electrophysiological studies were consistent with C6-C7 root lesion, and MRI of the spine revealed a small spinal cord focal lesion at the level of C7 root. Chest radiographs disclosed a 1-cm nodule that proved to be an otherwise asymptomatic small-cell cancer. CRPS manifestations preceded the diagnosis of the malignancy by 2 years.

The major diagnostic challenge presented with paraneoplastic disorders occurs when the physician is confronted with a patient who has serious and often disabling symptoms for which no cause is apparent. Clues to the diagnosis are the subacute progression and then stabilization of the disorder, the severity of the symptoms, and occasionally neurological dysfunction in more than one part of the nervous system. Treatment is usually unsuccessful, and most paraneoplastic syndromes run a course independent of that of the tumor. Since extensive review of these entities is beyond the scope of this chapter, the reader is directed to other references (118, 126, 127).

ACQUIRED NEUROMYOTONIAS

The term neuromyotonia was introduced by Mertens in 1965 (128). It has been used to indicate that the delayed relaxation in Isaacs syndrome (discussed later) has its origin in the peripheral nerve axons throughout their length (associated with axolemmal ion channel disturbance) and not in muscle. Some authors caution that this term should not be applied to all forms of muscle stiffness and continuous muscle activity, as in the case of stiff-person syndrome, chondrodystrophic myotonia, anterior horn cell isolation, and so on, in which the abnormalities may involve either anterior horn cells or the postsynaptic neuromuscular junction (117). However, the term has received a much wider application in the literature, characterizing many disorders with continuous and painful muscle spasms (the paraneoplastic variety is discussed earlier). So continuous and painful muscle activity occurs predominantly in three clinical situations: Isaacs syndrome, stiff-person syndrome and jerking stiff-person syndrome.

Isaacs syndrome (129, 130), which was described in 1961, has subacute or chronic onset and is characterized by generalized stiffness with myokymia, fasciculations, and weakness; 50% of the patients present with autonomic dysregulation. The muscle stiffness and the continuous motor unit activity persist during sleep and spinal or general anesthesia. Drugs that reduce sodium channel conductance (phenytoin, carbamazepine, and tocainide) improve or abolish the abnormalities. Isaacs syndrome therefore is thought to be the result of an abnormality of axolemmal ion channels (131).

Stiff-person syndrome, which used to be called stiff-man syndrome, is a rare neurological disorder characterized by paroxysmal, fluctuating muscle spasms and rigidity predominantly affecting axial muscles (132–137). It has chronic onset with normal neurological examination, truncal stiffness, autonomic dysregulation, and continuous muscle activity at rest that disappears with sleep, general anesthesia, and nerve blocks. It seems to respond to benzodiazepines and valproic acid. Autoimmune origin has been suggested, since it seems to be associated with other autoantibodies as well as insulin-dependent diabetes mellitus. Antibodies against glutamic acid decarboxylase (GAD) have been found in the CSF of many patients, reducing the levels of available GABA at the CNS with decrease of the inhibitory input to anterior horn cells.

Jerking stiff-person syndrome, described in 1980, has subacute or acute onset with bulbar and cervical muscle rigidity, painful spasms and myoclonus, abnormal posturing, continuous muscle activity, and some response to phenytoin and benzodiazepines. Again, it is speculated to be anti-GAD antibody-mediated (138–140). The features of these disorders have been summarized by Jog et al. (141).

Neuromyotonia is clearly nonspecific and is encountered in many axonopathies and demyelinating neuropathies (hereditary motor sensory neuropathy type 2, paraneoplastic neuropathies discussed earlier, and so on).

PERIPHERAL NEUROPATHIES

Neuropathy Classification: Symptoms and Signs

The regions of involvement of the peripheral nervous system (PNS) are variable in neuropathies. Thus sensory and/or motor involvement can occur distally or proximally; may be symmetric, predominantly affecting the upper limbs; occasionally is complex; may be specific to cranial nerves; may be focal or multifocal; and may be predominantly motor or sensory. A simple classification scheme as per Table 7.1, adapted from Schaumburg et al. (142) and based on anatomy, leads to clinicopathological and electrodiagnostic correlation. Table 7.2 lists neuropathies in terms of pathogenesis. Table 7.3 classifies symptoms and signs seen in peripheral neuropathies (143). Table 7.4 lists the symptoms and signs of neuropathies. This chapter makes selective reference to neuropathies based on their association with pain.

Inflammatory and Demyelinating Neuropathies

Acute inflammatory demyelinating polyradiculoneuropathy (AIDP), otherwise known as Guillain-Barré syndrome or postinfectious polyneuropathy, is a rapidly evolving paralytic illness that may follow nonspecific viral infections and in some cases surgery, immunization, and infections with *Mycoplasma pneumoniae* or *Campylobacter jejuni* (144, 145). Endoneurial infiltration by mononuclear inflammatory cells, followed by widespread multifocal segmental demyelination with relative sparing of the axons is the hallmark of the disease (142). The findings are most pronounced in the ventral roots, limb girdle plexus, and proximal nerve trunks. It is generally believed that the disorder is immune-mediated. From the epidemiological point of view, AIDP is the most frequent cause of acute paralytic illness in young adults (1.2 cases per 100,000) in developed countries (146). The distribution is bimodal (young adults and those aged 45 to 64) (141). AIDP is a rapidly progressing, largely reversible motor neuropathy with progressive symmetrical ascending motor weakness combined with hyporeflexia. The final degree of paralysis is variable from the occasional individual who never has more than a mild foot drop to the patient with flaccid quadriplegia and breathing, swallowing, or speech difficulties. Facial weakness may be a striking feature of this neuropathy. Sensory symptoms, usually in the form of distal paresthesias, are present in most cases but rarely persist or progress. Marked sensory loss with pain or severe dysesthesias is unusual. When it does occur, the prognosis of the illness is worse than for the motor paralysis-only variant (147). However, it may occur in one third of cases with posterior root involvement, and the pain may be severe and lancinating. Autonomic dysfunction may lead to orthostatic hypotension and at times cardiac dysrhythmias. Several unusual regional patterns of involvement affect 15% of the patients (142). While most individuals have excellent functional recovery, the mortality rate is 5%, and more than 50% of patients have some degree of permanent PNS damage. Significant weakness persists in 16%, while another 5% remain severely disabled (142). Plasmapheresis is clearly the treatment of choice.

Chronic inflammatory demyelinating polyradiculoneuropathy (CIDP) may start with an illness similar to that in

Table 7.1.   Seldon's Nomenclature (1943) of Anatomical Lesions

Class 1
Neuropraxia
Transient
Delayed reversible
Conduction block due to ischemia
Demyelination
Class 2
Axonotmesis
Axonal interruption
Class 3
Neurotmesis
Axonal and endoneurial interruption
Class 4
Partial nerve section
Interruption of perineurium and epineurium, nerve continuity retained
Class 5
Complete nerve section
Complete transection

AIDP, but the course is either chronically relapsing or chronically progressive. While the pathogenesis of CIDP (as an autoimmune disorder of delayed supersensitivity) and the salient histological features are remarkably similar to those of AIDP, the nosological limits of CIDP remain poorly understood. Nevertheless, it may be a common neuromuscular disorder occurring throughout the world in all ages, with a peak incidence in the fifth and sixth decade. Men seem to be more often affected than women (148). Plasma exchange, corticosteroids, and human immunoglobulin therapy are the treatments of choice (142).

Infectious and Granulomatous Neuropathies

Herpes zoster results from infection of the nervous system with the varicella zoster virus. Inflammation and necrosis of the sensory ganglion neurons is the hallmark of this infection. It is associated with pain both during the acute stage and in the chronic form of postherpetic neuralgia. In the acute stage pain and paresthesias in the involved dermatomes often precede the appearance of vesicles. This common condition is described in Chapter 8 of this book.

Leprosy, the most common treatable neuropathy in the world, is the result of *Mycobacterium leprae* (Hansen's bacillus) infection. The lepromatous and tuberculoid forms are the polar extremes of the immunological response to *M. leprae,* with extensive, diffuse, symmetrical neuropathy in the former case (149) and focal or multifocal nerve lesions around the involved skin areas in the latter (150). Sensory loss with pain and temperature first affected and loss of sweat in involved areas are the early cardinal features. Dapsone (DDS) is the drug of choice.

Sarcoidosis produces a mixture of granulomatous infiltration and vascular compromise. Sarcoid-related neuropathies may be multifocal (affecting cranial or other nerves) or very rarely distal sensorimotor disorders that are indistinguishable from the symmetrical polyneuropathies of toxic or metabolic origin. Some cases respond to corticosteroids (151).

Table 7.2.   Anatomical Classification of Peripheral Neuropathies

Symmetrical Generalized Polyneuropathies

Distal axonopathies
    Toxic (drug or industrial chemical induced)
    Metabolic (uremia, diabetes, poryphria, endocrine, nutritional deficiency)
    Genetic (HMSN II)
    Malignancy associated (e.g., small cell lung carcinoma, multiple myeloma)
Myelinopathies
    Toxic (e.g., diphtheria, buckthorn)
    Immunological (AIDP, CIDP)
    Genetic (e.g., Refsum's disease, metachromatic leukodystrophy)
Neuronopathies
    Somatic motor
        Undetermined (amyotrophic lateral sclerosis)
        Genetic (hereditary motor neuronopathies)
    Somatic sensory
        Infectious (herpes zoster neuronitis)
        Malignancy associated
        Toxic (pyridoxine sensory neuronopathy)
        Undetermined (subacute sensory neuronopathy syndrome)
    Autonomic
        Genetic (hereditary dysautonomia)

Focal and Multifocal Neuropathies

Ischemic (polyarteritis, diabetes, rheumatoid arthritis)
Infiltration (leukemia, lymphoma, granuloma, schwannoma, amyloid)
Traumatic (severance, crush, compression, stretch, traction, entrapment)
Immunological

HMSN II, hereditary motor and sensory neuropathy type II; AIDP, acute inflammatory polyradiculoneuropathy; CIDP, chronic inflammatory demyelinating polyradiculoneuropathy; HSN IV, hereditary dysautonomia.

Table 7.3.   Etiopathological Classification of Peripheral Neuropathies

Inflammatory and demyelinating neuropathies
    Acute inflammatory demyelinating polyradiculoneuropathy
    (Guillain-Barré syndrome)
    Chronic inflammatory demyelinating polyradiculoneuropathy
Infectious and granulomatous neuropathy
    Herpes zoster
    Sarcoid neuropathy
    HIV-related peripheral neuropathy
    Lyme borreliosis
Diabetic neuropathies
    Symmetrical diabetic polyneuropathies
    Diabetic mononeuropathies
Endocrine neuropathies other than diabetes
    Hypothyroidism
    Acromegaly
Neuropathies associated with alcoholism, malnutrition, and malabsorption
    Alcohol-nutritional deficiency polyneuropathy syndrome
    Specific vitamin deficiency polyneuropathy syndromes
    Malabsorption neuropathies: postgastrectomy and sprue-related disorders
Ischemic neuropathies
    Neuropathy of peripheral vascular disease
    Necrotizing angiitis neuropathies
Neuropathy associated with paraproteinemias, dysproteinemias, and malignancy
    Paraproteinemic neuropathy (benign monoclonal gammopathy)
    Dysproteinemic neuropathies
    Malignancy-associated neuropathies
Neuropathy of systemic disease
    Amyloid neuropathy
    Uremic neuropathy
Inherited peripheral neuropathies
    Metabolic neuropathies (the porphyrias)
    Hereditary disorders of lipid metabolism
    Hereditary neuropathies without established metabolic basis (e.g., hereditary motor and sensory neuropathies, hereditary sensory and autonomic neuropathies)
Neuropathy associated with trauma and physical agents
    Acute nerve injury
    Compression and entrapment chronic neuropathies

Table 7.4.   Symptoms and Signs of Neuropathy

Negative motor symptoms
    Conduction block
    Interruption of motor axons
Positive motor symptoms
    Fasciculations, myokymia
    Muscle cramps
    Continuous motor unit activity
    Hemifacial spasm
    Painful legs, moving toes
    Restless leg syndrome
Tendon areflexia
Negative sensory symptoms
    Pain and temperature loss (small fiber loss)
    Joint position, vibration, touch-pressure loss (large fiber loss)
Positive sensory symptoms
    Spontaneous paresthesias
    Pain (spontaneous ongoing or paroxysmal, stimulus-evoked)
Autonomic involvement
    Ocular, cardiovascular, sweat gland, genitourinary, alimentary dysfunction
Skeletal deformities
Trophic changes
Nerve thickening

Peripheral neuropathy is a source of major morbidity in the *acquired immunodeficiency syndrome* (AIDS), and the incidence is estimated to be between 9 and 20% (142), but these figures are probably underestimates. Human immunodeficiency virus (HIV) neuropathies may signal HIV seroconversion, mark the transition from asymptomatic or less symptomatic stages to more severe ones, be treatable, or predispose to earlier and more severe onset of toxic neuropathies as the result of nucleoside antiviral agents (142). Clinical syndromes include acute and chronic inflammatory demyelinating neuropathy, distal symmetrical sensorimotor polyneuropathy, progressive polyradiculopathy, dorsal root ganglioneuritis, mononeuritis multiplex and cranial neuropathies, autonomic neuropathy, and finally iatrogenic neuropathies resulting from administration of various medications (isozianid, nitrofurantoin, DDS,, and antiviral agents such as ddC and ddI).

Lyme disease is a vector-borne disease caused by the spirochete *Borrelia burgdorferi* (152). Once it penetrates the skin, the spirochete uses hematogenous spread to reach the PNS and CNS. Lyme disease usually has three stages: stage 1 with a characteristic rash, erythema migrans, and a flulike illness; stage 2 with carditis, arthritis, and meningoradiculitis; and stage 3 with chronic skin, arthritic, and neurological manifestations (152).

The neurological manifestations consist of CNS disorders (meningitis and encephalomyelitis) and peripheral neuropathies involving the cranial nerves or multifocally affecting roots, plexus, and individual peripheral nerves. Radiculopathy is typically asymmetrical and painful, while the plexopathy pattern is usually brachial. Other forms include AIDP-like presentation and mononeuropathy multiplex; in the later stages a subtle generalized distal sensorimotor neuropathy may develop (142). Wide-spectrum antibiotics are the treatment of choice.

Diabetic Neuropathy

The prevalence of symptomatic diabetic neuropathy reportedly varies from 5 to 60% (summarized by Thomas and Tomlinson, 153). Diabetic neuropathy in general can be classified in two subtypes: (*a*) symmetrical polyneuropathy (distal sensorimotor, autonomic, symmetrical proximal lower limb) and (*b*) focal and multifocal neuropathy (cranial, trunk and limb, asymmetrical lower limb). Mixed forms also may exist. Patients with distal sensory or sensorimotor polyneuropathy may complain of tingling paresthesias, pain, and dysesthesias. The earliest sensory involvement affects the toes, since the neuropathy follows a typical length-related pattern (153).

Predominant *small-fiber neuropathy* is manifested with burning distal extremity pain, cutaneous hyperesthesia, autonomic dysfunction, loss of pain and temperature sensation, and preservation of deep tendon reflexes and large-fiber sensory modalities. *Acute painful neuropathy* (154) has been associated with precipitous and abrupt weight loss and severe unremitting burning distal leg pain, cutaneous hyperalgesia, and preservation of motor function. Establishment of adequate diabetic control usually leads to remission of symptoms. While autonomic neuropathy is painless, *lower limb asymmetrical motor neuropathy* (a term preferable to diabetic amyotrophy), manifested by asymmetrical muscle weakness and wasting in the proximal limb muscles, is often accompanied by pain in the thighs and occasionally the lumbar area or the perineum, more severe at night. The disturbance predominantly affects the lumbosacral plexus, but lesions have also been detected in peripheral nerves, roots, or spinal nerves. *Limb and trunk mononeuropathies,* primarily involving the ulnar, median, femoral, and lateral femoral cutaneous nerves of the thigh and peroneal nerves, may be insidious or abrupt in onset. When acute in onset, the pain maybe a prominent feature. Most often the lesions occur at the sites that are common for external pressure palsies. It seems that diabetic nerves are more susceptible to compression injury, although the reasons for this are not known (153). Cranial nerve palsies also occur more frequently in diabetic subjects, with the third nerve most commonly affected and the fourth, sixth, and seventh nerves less frequently affected. The onset is generally abrupt. In half the cases of third nerve palsy, pain may even precede the ophthalmoplegia by several days (155). The pain is usually retro-orbital and intense.

Management of pain in diabetic neuropathies is addressed first by strict diabetic control, second by symptomatic treatment of pain, and third by treatment of depression or through other supportive measures. Amitriptyline may be effective even in the absence of depression (156). Carbamazepine has a greater success rate than phenytoin but frequently is ineffective (157, 158). Mexiletine is sometimes beneficial (159). Simple analgesics are ineffective. TENS has been recommended with some success (160). Topical capsaicin has also been suggested (161). Many cases prove to be refractory.

Neuropathy Associated with Alcoholism, Malnutrition, and Malabsorption

Human studies have not been able to separate absolutely a direct toxic action of alcohol on the PNS from the effects of poor nutrition. Nevertheless, nutritional neuropathy in the Western world is almost synonymous with the multiple vitamin deficiency polyneuropathy associated with alcoholism (142). Selective vitamin B_{12} and B_6 (pyridoxine) deficiencies have become rare, while disorders such as beriberi and pellagra are now medical curiosities in Western medical practice. Symptoms of mild calf aching and discomfort are present in about half of patients with alcoholic polyneuropathy (162). In most severe cases a mixed sensorimotor neuropathy is the rule, with lower limb paresthesias, pain, and weakness in the distal extremities. About a quarter of the patients develop truly distressing symptoms in their feet. Burning feet syndrome develops gradually over weeks and months. The soles are initially affected with pricking, electric, stabbing, and at times intense burning pain associated with severe hyperesthesia to touch (163). Occasionally the syndrome is associated with some toxic and non-alcohol-related malnutrition state. Hand symptoms may also develop. In general, the alcoholic neuropathy may be only a part of the neurological manifestations of alcohol abuse associated with Wernicke's encephalopathy or Korsakoff 's syndrome. The treatment in general includes alcohol cessation and adequate balanced nutrition.

Ischemic Neuropathy in Peripheral Vascular Occlusive Disease and Vasculitis

Diseases producing nerve ischemia can be divided into those that affect (*a*) large arteries, (*b*) nerve microvessels, and (*c*) the rheological properties of the blood. *Acute arterial embolism and thrombosis* even after urgent restorative surgery may produce an ischemic monomelic neuropathy (164) with distal burning limb pain associated with glove-and-stocking sensory loss and distal muscle weakness persisting for months. *Iatrogenic acute arterial insufficiency* associated with painful neuropathies has been described in patients with transfemoral intra-aortic balloon pumps (165), brachial artery-antecubital vein fistulas for hemodialysis (166, 167), inadvertent intraarterial drug injections (168–170), and intentionally given intra-arterial injection of anticancer drugs (171). *Acute nerve ischemia* associated with extensive muscle necrosis occurs also in compartment syndromes, with most cases following trauma.

Neuropathy due to *chronic arterial insufficiency* severe enough to produce distal gangrene has been associated with mild abnormalities of nerve conduction studies and a variable degree of myelinated fiber loss expressed as multimodal sensory loss and absent ankle jerks. It is conceivable that in persons with intermittent claudication or even pain at rest without gangrene, nerve ischemia may contribute to pain, but good evidence to support or deny this concept is not available (172). There is a sizable literature about the syndrome of erythromelalgia (burning pain and erythema of distal feet) seen in conditions with *altered blood rheology* (polycythemia or essential thrombocythemia) (173, 174). Aspirin and indomethacin are reported to produce dramatic relief of this syndrome.

Vasculitic neuropathy is an important variant of hypoxic and ischemic neuropathy. In necrotizing vasculitis, inflammatory cell infiltration and necrosis of the walls of nutrient blood vessels cause segmental narrowing or occlusion, thrombosis or hemorrhage, with resultant tissue hypoxia and injury. Nerve ischemia produces axonal degeneration and segmental demyelination. Vasculitic neuropathy, a disease of adults, is seen in several distinctive syndromes: polyarteritis nodosa, vasculitis associated with connective tissue disease, Wegener's granulomatosis, hypersensitivity vasculitis, giant cell arteritis, Behçet's disease, and nonsystemic vasculitis of peripheral nerves (175). Vasculitic neuropathy usually presents as a syndrome of multiple mononeuropathies with abrupt onset of weakness, prickling paresthesias, or sensory loss often associated with local pain and occasionally involving several limbs in the same day. Limb and cranial neuropathies or brachial plexopathy can occur. Occasionally a distal symmetrical polyneuropathy may be seen.

Neuropathy of Systemic Disease: Amyloid and Uremic Neuropathy

Extracellular deposition of the fibrous protein amyloid is associated with nonhereditary (immunoglobulin derived) and hereditary (non-immunoglobulin derived) *amyloidosis.* In the former, sensory symptoms are prominent, with symmetrical numbness, dysesthesias, and spontaneous pain often predating systemic organ involvement (176). Autonomic manifestations may appear early, while distal motor weakness develops later. In the hereditary forms (with seven recognized forms of familial amyloid polyneuropathy) sensory and autonomic features may be significant. In some forms, attacks of stabbing pain with trophic changes and skin ulcerations can be prominent.

In *chronic renal insufficiency* and uremic states a distal symmetrical sensorimotor polyneuropathy appears. In hemodialysis centers it is shown to involve approximately half of all patients (142). Initially sensory symptoms may dominate the picture, and occasionally the burning feet syndrome develops, indistinguishable from that encountered in alcoholic and other nutritional deficiencies. Restless leg syndrome may accompany the sensory symptoms of early uremic neuropathy, and muscle cramps in distal extremities are common (177).

Inherited Peripheral Neuropathy with and without Associated Metabolic Defects

The *porphyrias* are a group of seven hereditary disorders characterized by disturbances in heme biosynthesis (178). Four of these disorders are associated with peripheral neuropathy. Porphyric neuropathy is a life-threatening illness occurring in acute episodes and often induced by drugs, hormones, or nutritional factors (179). Drugs such as barbiturates, sulfonamides, estrogens and oral contraceptives, ethanol, ergot compounds, rifampin, imipramine, and methyldopa, among others, have been reported to precipitate porphyric attacks. Acute intermittent porphyria (AIP) is usually manifested by acute attack of colicky abdominal pain with constipation, fever, and leukocytosis (possibly related to autonomic neuropathy). Mental disturbances may accompany or occasionally precede abdominal attacks. Peripheral neuropathy develops acutely or subacutely following the general manifestations of AIP, with limb weakness, proximal or distal, symmetrical or asymmetrical, and sensory symptoms that may be mild, or distressing with limb and facial or neck paresthesias that can be severe.

Other hereditary disorders related to metabolic problems are those of lipid metabolism. Among those worth noting is *Fabry's disease,* an X-linked recessive metabolic disorder associated with α-galactosidase A deficiency. It first appears in childhood and follows a steadily progressive course manifested by neurological, dermatological, ocular, cardiovascular, and renal disease complications. Fabry's disease should always be considered in the differential diagnosis when boys and young men present with intense burning sensations and pain in the distal extremities (180). The pains are often so severe that the patients cannot even walk moderate distances, and some may be bound to a wheelchair. Patients may obtain some relief from phenytoin (181), but the response has not been universal. Carbamazepine has been somewhat more effective but may exacerbate autonomic dysfunction (182).

Of the multiple hereditary nonmetabolic neuropathies that are either motor and sensory neuropathies (HMSN) or sensory and autonomic neuropathies (HSAN), HSAN type 1 (otherwise known as hereditary sensory neuropathy of Denny-Brown or maladie de Thévenard) is worth reporting because it is associated with episodes of lancinating extremity pain intermittently in about half of the cases, while burning feet pain may be bothersome in some patients (142).

Toxic Neuropathy

Drug toxicity may produce unacceptable side effects that may be either dose dependent or idiosyncratic. Peripheral neuropathy can be caused by drugs such as amiodarone, chloramphenicol, colchicine, DDS, nucleoside antiviral agents used in AIDS, ethambutol, ethionamide, gold, hydralazine, isoniazid, metronidazole, nitrofurantoin, phenytoin, pyridoxine, thalidomide, vincristine, and others. *Isoniazid,* introduced for the treatment of tuberculosis in 1952, is associated with painful peripheral neuropathy with initial symptoms consisting of acroparesthesias and numbness. While at this stage discontinuation of the drug reverses the symptoms rapidly, continuous treatment generates spreading burning pain. Distal weakness and tenderness in the muscles may ensue (183). *Misonidazole* (used to sensitize hypoxic neoplastic cells to the effects of radiation) may produce a dose-limiting peripheral neuropathy that is predominantly sensory; pain is a very troublesome feature (184). *Perhexiline maleate,* introduced in the early 1970s for the treatment of angina pectoris, was soon recognized to cause peripheral neuropathy (183). Susceptibility to this neuropathy is likely to be determined genetically. Distal acroparesthesias and pain are the first symptoms, followed by proximal and distal muscle weakness and autonomic disturbances. *Thalidomide* is an effective hypnotic that caused in 1960 and 1961 an epidemic of peripheral neuropathy in several European countries. In 1961 it was withdrawn from general use following recognition of its teratogenic effects. It is, however, still used in the treatment of leprosy and some other skin conditions, and early clinical trials suggest that it reverses cachexia. Mailis has actually successfully treated severe leg edema with thalidomide in a patient with chronic regional pain syndrome (CRPS). Thalidomide-induced neuropathy may be associated with paresthesias and numbness in the feet that spread upward. Leg cramps are common. Later on more proximal than distal limb weakness appears. The recovery from the peripheral neuropathy is fairly poor, and persistent painful paresthesias may be quite distressing and disabling (185).

Heavy metals can also cause neuropathies. *Arsenic* poisoning has the most typical history, starting with an acute gastrointestinal illness followed days later by burning, painful acroparesthesias and progressive distal muscle weakness (186). *Gold salts,* almost exclusively used in the treatment of rheumatoid arthritis, may produce a neuropathy with progressive symmetrical distal paresthesias followed by distal weakness and muscle atrophy. Burning facial discomfort has been described (186).

Neuropathy Associated with Trauma and Physical Agents

Table 7.1, adapted from Schaumburg et al. (142), shows different classifications of focal nerve injury. In acute traumatic nerve injuries certain rules apply: Nerve transection requires prompt surgical intervention. Lesions -in -continuity usually recover spontaneously, and most surgeons wait for 2 or 3 months before exploration. Chronic trauma to peripheral nerves is associated with (*a*) compression in tight spaces such as fibro-osseous tunnels (e.g., carpal, cubital, tarsal tunnels), (*b*) angulation and stretch (e.g., over anomalous fibrous bands or bony structures, under ligaments) or (*c*) recurrent external compression (occupational injuries to distal extremities). In nerve compression, as in carpal tunnel and similar syndromes,

the nerve appears constricted in the compressed site and enlarged above and below, with prominent demyelination at the compressed region (187, 188).

Pain is a frequent accompaniment of chronic nerve injuries. In the *upper extremities,* stretch or traction injuries of the brachial plexus over abnormal ribs or fibrous bands in certain types of thoracic outlet syndrome cause numbness, pain, and paresthesias (189). One of the most common entrapment neuropathies occurs at the carpal tunnel in the wrist, as the median nerve passes deep to the flexor retinaculum. Acroparesthesias, tingling, numbness, and burning sensations affect the first three fingers of the hand. Ulnar nerve entrapment is the second most common nerve entrapment in the arm, and it can occur in multiple sites. In the case of entrapment at the elbow sensory symptoms usually precede weakness, with numbness, paresthesias, and pain in the last two fingers of the hand. In the *chest wall,* damage of the intercostobrachial nerve can occur in mastectomies (190); postthoracotomy pain may arise from scar neuromas; and intercostal nerve damage is a very frequent accompaniment of aortocoronary bypass surgery with the use of internal mammary artery graft (191, 192). In the *abdominal and perineal wall,* entrapment of the genitofemoral nerve (originating from spinal roots L1-L2) as it passes through the psoas muscle and divides above the inguinal ligament and of the ilioinguinal nerve (originating from the L1 spinal root) as it passes around the abdominal wall to the inguinal canal may cause lower abdominal and inguinal pain. The pudendal nerve, the principal nerve of the perineum, which arises from S2-S4 spinal roots, when trapped or compressed, as in perineal operations or prolonged pressure such as bicycle riding, can produce perineal neuropathy with pain and penile numbness in men or perineal burning pain in women. In the *lower extremities,* obturator nerve entrapment after injury or occasionally during the third trimester of pregnancy produces groin and medial thigh pain. The lateral femoral cutaneous nerve of the thigh may be compressed under the inguinal ligament in cases of obesity, pregnancy, nerve injury during trauma, or application of external compression and may give rise to meralgia paresthetica with tingling or burning paresthesias and numbness at the lateral aspect of the thigh. The sciatic nerve can be damaged in any of several sites and circumstances (e.g., within the pelvis, the mass of the piriformis muscle, after hip surgery or trauma). Sensory and motor findings are extensive, and the distribution varies, affecting the total nerve, the tibial, or the common peroneal distribution. The tibial nerve can be compressed at the medial ankle (tarsal tunnel syndrome), with burning pain and tingling paresthesias in the sole of the foot, while pressure injury of the peroneal nerve at the head of the fibula may generate pain and paresthesias in the leg. The deep peroneal nerve or the superficial peroneal nerve branches can also be selectively involved. Multiple other sites of entrapment exist, as in the sural nerve at the back of the popliteal fossa, the plantar branches of the tibial nerve at or distal to the tarsal tunnel, and the digital branches of the plantar nerves (Morton's neuromas). Traumatic injuries to large nerves may give rise to causalgia (CPRS 2) in a minority of patients with severe spontaneous ongoing and paroxysmal as well as stimulus-evoked pains; hyperesthesia to multiple stimuli; sudomotor, vasomotor, and trophic changes.

Neuropathies of Unclear Etiology

Neuropathies of unknown or uncertain etiology are as follows: idiopathic facial paralysis (Bell's palsy), trigeminal sensory neuropathy, idiopathic cranial polyneuropathy (ICP), plexus neuropathies, critical illness polyneuropathy, idiopathic sensory neuronopathy syndrome, and acute pandysautonomic neuropathy. Pain is associated with trigeminal sensory neuropathy, with the sensory impairment preceded by or associated with unpleasant sensations (193). The pain differs from that of trigeminal neuralgia because it is spontaneous and ongoing, without a lancinating quality (142). ICP is heralded by subacute onset of aching, usually retro-orbital pain, while cranial nerve palsies develop soon after the onset of pain.

PLEXOPATHIES

Brachial Plexus Disorders

Brachial plexus disorders can be closed or open. Closed lesions can be due to any of several causes: traction, radiation, neoplasias, indirect postoperative complications, orthopaedic injuries, neuralgic amyotrophy (idiopathic brachial plexopathy), backpack palsy, burners syndrome, thoracic outlet syndrome, and so on. The degree of fiber injury varies from conduction block lesions (neuropraxia) to rupture and avulsion of anterior and/or posterior spinal roots. Although more common, upper plexus traction lesions are ruptures of the anterior primary rami or trunk levels (postganglionic and extraforaminal) and frequently can be repaired surgically. Severe lower plexus traction injuries are more likely to be preganglionic avulsion injuries and thus irreparable (for review see Wilbourn 194). In general, lesions of the brachial plexus are manifested by motor, sensory, and autonomic dysfunction of the shoulder and upper extremity with marked variability in extent, degree, and time course. Pain is a frequent symptom that can vary from mild to severe and from transient to permanent (195). Intense unremitting pain is common in brachial neuropathies caused by neoplastic infiltration (195a), avulsion of multiple roots (196), radiation injuries (197), and gunshot wounds (198). Pain is severe but temporary in idiopathic brachial plexopathy, an acute and painful illness characterized by brachial plexus dysfunction. It is also known as neuralgic amyotrophy, acute brachial radiculitis, and acute shoulder-girdle neuritis. The relation of this condition to serum or vaccine injections and toxic and hereditary brachial plexopathies is

uncertain, since the presentation is nearly identical (142). burners syndrome (burners, stingers) is almost limited to certain contact sports, particularly football in the United States. Sudden forceful depression of the shoulder creates abrupt, intense burning dysesthesias in the whole upper extremity associated with transient weakness. The symptoms resolve within minutes (199, 200). In contrast, pain is rarely a symptom of classic postanesthetic paralysis (201) or backpack palsy (202).

Pain from avulsion of brachial plexus roots merits specific mention. More than 80% of these patients develop pain, and half of those report the pain as severe. The incidence of severe pain is related to the number of roots avulsed. Avulsion pain is due to deafferentation. It often begins immediately, usually within the first 3 weeks (203, 204). It is characteristically described as spontaneous ongoing (crushing or burning, rarely varying in intensity) with superimposed brief paroxysmal pains of electrical shock-like quality, quite variable in frequency (203, 204). The duration of avulsion pain is variable. If it persists after 3 years, it is likely to last indefinitely (204). The treatment is exceedingly difficult. Stellate ganglion blocks, acupuncture, and faith healing are useless, while analgesics, carbamazepine, and antidepressants are seldom effective (194). Alcohol, hypnosis, and cannabis have been reported to be occasionally helpful (194). Multiple surgical procedures have been tried with poor results. The two most helpful procedures (at the opposite ends of the technological and medical spectrum) include distraction techniques (engaging the patient in distracting and enjoyable activities) (203, 205) and coagulation of the DREZ of the avulsed roots (206).

Lumbosacral Plexopathies

Although the lumbosacral plexus, which lies encased in the pelvic bony ring, is less susceptible to trauma than the brachial plexus, it is affected by a similar spectrum of disorders (for review see Donaghy, 207). Many plexus lesions are anatomically restricted in their initial stages, and they can be easily confused with lumbosacral root disease. The counterpart of idiopathic brachial plexitis is idiopathic lumbosacral plexitis. It is much less common than brachial neuritis, although the incidence is probably underestimated because of poor awareness of the condition. Nevertheless, muscle weakness is noted 5 to 10 days after the appearance of severe, usually unilateral anterior or posterior thigh pain. It may follow serum treatment, is occasionally bilateral, may follow intravenous injection of heroin, or may appear in individuals previously affected by brachial plexitis. Vasculitic plexopathy, usually in patients with other manifestations of systemic vasculitis, has been reported. Diabetic proximal neuropathy (known also as diabetic neuropathic cachexia, diabetic mononeuropathy multiplex, and so on) may appear with prominent anterior thigh pain followed by proximal muscle weakness. Herpes zoster infections can affect lumbosacral dermatomes with painful vesicular eruptions and segmental muscle weakness. Acute anorectal infection with herpes simplex may affect the lower part of the sacrococcygeal plexus with neuralgic pain, paresthesias, and dysesthesias of the perineum, buttocks, and posterior thighs followed by urinary retention, constipation, or erectile failure. Retroperitoneal hemorrhage can cause plexus compression within the psoas muscle or specific compression of the femoral nerve within the iliacus muscle. The latter can cause profound pain on forced hip extension. Fracture dislocations of the bony pelvic ring can cause lumbosacral plexus lesions with mostly the L5- and S1-innervated muscles affected. Inadvertent injections of vasotoxic or crystalline drugs into the inferior gluteal artery at the medial aspect of the buttock can produce ischemia or toxic vasospasm of the sciatic nerve (170). Obstetrical complications with compression of the plexus may cause postpartum foot drop, while laterally placed self-retaining retractor blades may compress the femoral nerve during pelvic operations such as abdominal hysterectomy or renal transplantation. Excessive stretch or angulation may be responsible for plexopathies and femoral or sciatic neuropathies following perineal surgeries. Tumors may variably infiltrate the plexus, while the late-onset radiation-induced lumbosacral plexopathy should be distinguished from postirradiation lower motor neuron syndrome and radiation-induced nerve sheath tumor (207).

NERVE ROOT DAMAGE AND ARACHNOIDITIS

Pain associated with root damage refers along the peripheral fiber distribution within the affected root or roots. Pain associated with cervical pathology (herniated disc or spondylosis with root compression) is constant, fluctuating, or intermittent, aggravated by activities, in particular neck movements, coughing, straining, and sneezing. Shooting pains may be superimposed on a background of constant pain. Similar characteristics may be seen in lumbosacral root pain due to disc protrusions. These pains very often are associated with paresthesias in the distribution of the affected root or roots and motor-sensory deficits. Lower sacral and coccygeal root pathology occasionally accounts for the burning pain of coccydynia. Multisegmental root involvement, as it occurs in spondylosis, may produce widespread motor and sensory abnormalities and reflex changes, not confined to single dermatomes. Neurogenic claudication, associated with a congenital or acquired narrow spinal canal, may produce painful leg paresthesias, particularly on walking, and must be differentiated from vascular claudication. Spinal arachnoiditis (particularly affecting the lumbosacral roots) is seen after repeated myelograms with oil-based contrast agents and other irritant chemicals, chronic lumbosacral root compression, spinal infections affecting the meninges, hemorrhage, and trauma, particularly after spinal surgeries, and it occasionally occurs congenitally. Inflammation of the pia of individual roots, followed by

fibroblast proliferation and adhesion of the roots to each other, may lead to atrophy of the roots and their encasement in collagen deposits (208). Pain, usually diffuse and frequently described as burning, may be ongoing or associated with paroxysmal lancinating pains. Sensory changes, if present, are not usually confined to a single dermatome except in the case of single-root fibrosis. While surgical decompression is useful in cervical or lumbar spondylosis or herniated discs after failure of conservative management, surgery is not beneficial in arachnoiditis. Epidural steroids are widely advocated, but there is limited literature to support their value. More commonly used is spinal cord stimulation, which has been reported to carry a 50% long-term improvement rate (209).

FACIAL PAIN AND TRIGEMINAL NEURALGIA

Trigeminal nerve lesions can be due to a multiplicity of causes (e.g., infectious and inflammatory, vascular hemorrhagic or ischemic, tumors primary or metastatic, aneurysms, demyelinating disorders, trauma, toxic, idiopathic). *Trigeminal neuralgia* is a characteristic syndrome consisting of brief paroxysmal facial pains in the territory of one or more divisions of the trigeminal nerve. The annual incidence is reported to be 4.3 per 100,000 (210). Women are more commonly affected than men, and the incidence increases with age. The pain is almost always unilateral, usually affecting the mandibular or maxillary territory. Triggers involve proprioceptive or tactile stimuli or movement during eating, talking, yawning, and so on (211). Trigger spots are most frequently found in the lips, nasolabial folds, upper eyelids, gums, or tongue. The paroxysms are brief, lasting seconds or 1 to 2 minutes, but they occur in clusters or episodes that may last for weeks (210). Between episodes patients are pain free. In idiopathic trigeminal neuralgia no sensory or motor deficit can be found on neurological examination, with the rare reports of transient slight increased or decreased sensitivity in the affected territory during and soon after bouts of pain. Occasionally trigeminal neuralgia is associated with ipsilateral hemifacial spasm, called tic convulsif by Cushing (212). The latter, which may occur on its own, has been shown to be usually due to compression of the facial and trigeminal nerve roots by arterial loops (213). Rare accompaniment of trigeminal neuralgia by glossopharyngeal neuralgia has been reported (214, 215). The association of trigeminal neuralgia and MS is well known. About 2% of patients with trigeminal neuralgia have MS, and 1% of MS patients have trigeminal neuralgia (41). Trigeminal neuralgia should be differentiated from glossopharyngeal neuralgia, temporomandibular joint disorders, and cluster headaches. Persistent sensory deficit indicates other conditions affecting the fifth nerve. Some authors have little doubt that trigeminal neuralgia is usually caused by compression of the trigeminal sensory roots by arterial loops (211), but certainly differences of opinion still exist (216). Carbamazepine is the basis of modern medical treatment, with success in about 70% of the patients (217). Phenytoin is less effective, while addition of a tricyclic antidepressant may help in some cases (211). A benzodiazepine, clonazepam, has been reported to have limited value (218), while baclofen has also been reported to have some effectiveness in resistant cases (219). Surgical treatments include ablative procedures most commonly addressed to the trigeminal ganglion (e.g., injections of phenol, alcohol, or glycerol; radiofrequency lesioning). Procedures causing sensory loss run the risk of anesthesia dolorosa. Microvascular decompression and percutaneous decompression of the trigeminal ganglion have been reported to have good success rates (211).

Rare but notable other facial neuralgias are as follows: (*a*) Glossopharyngeal neuralgia (idiopathic or secondary to structural lesion of cranial nerve XII) is characterized by paroxysmal pain at the base of the tongue referred to the external auditory meatus or the angle of the jaw and occasionally associated with trigeminal neuralgia. Coughing and swallowing are the main triggers. If paroxysms are frequent, syncope may occur (211). (*b*) Geniculate neuralgia of nerve VII probably originates from the nervus intermedius with paroxysmal pain felt around the ear.

Atypical facial pain is described as continuous pain with no pain-free intervals and without particular triggers. It is often bilateral or extends beyond the trigeminal nerve distribution. Unfortunately, the term is a wastebasket diagnosis (220) that may reflect several pain syndromes. Bilateral atypical facial pain occurs almost exclusively in middle-aged women who are agitated or depressed; there is no sensory loss; no evidence of pathology in teeth, gums, or sinuses is found; and treatment is generally ineffective (220). Unilateral facial pain may be due to injury to a branch of the trigeminal nerve (for example after facial lacerations), neoplasm, or infection at the base of the skull, at which time there occurs progressive trigeminal sensory loss, glossopharyngeal neuralgia, cluster headache, idiopathic benign trigeminal sensory neuropathy (193), myofascial trigger points, and local pathology of paranasal sinuses, jaws, teeth, or pharynx. It may also appear in patients with significant behavioral and psychological dysfunction preceding the onset of pain (221), in which case no pathology can be found. The latter again seems to be unresponsive to conventional treatments; hence aggressive interventions are not recommended.

COMPLEX REGIONAL PAIN SYNDROMES

CRPS has replaced the terms reflex sympathetic dystrophy and causalgia (now called CRPS type 1 and 2, respectively). CRPS 1 and 2 are described in *Classification of Chronic Pain* (1). They are purely phenomenological descriptors, without mechanistic connotations, of a variety of painful conditions that usually follow injury, occur regionally, have a

distal predominance of abnormal findings, exceed in both magnitude and duration the expected clinical course of inciting event, often result in impairment of the motor function, and show variable progression with time (222). They are described in detail in Chapter 12 of this book.

PRINCIPLES AND SUMMARY OF PHARMACOLOGICAL INTERVENTIONS IN NEUROPATHIC PAIN

There are several principles in the management of neuropathic pain (223):

- Removal of the cause when possible
- Promotion of healing or fiber regeneration
- Normalization of the nerve micromilieu and correction of metabolic parameters
- Normalization of sensory input and nerve transmission
- Modulation of central pathways
- Reduction of sympathetic overactivity
- Alteration of emotional and behavioral influences on pain interpretation

In regard to pharmacological interventions, the treating physician should do the following:

1. Have a basic understanding of the underlying pathophysiological mechanisms, the natural course of the disorder and the limiting medical conditions or contraindications. Understanding the pathophysiological mechanisms allows for *differential symptom* classification, each symptom possibly requiring specific management.
2. Use a *ladder approach,* starting from the least to the most invasive interventions considered appropriate for each disorder.
3. Follow a first-line approach that includes (*a*) mild analgesics and/or (*b*) specific neuropathic medications (e.g., tricyclics, anticonvulsants) and/or (*c*) physical modalities (e.g., exercises, application of TENS) depending on the disorder under treatment. Concomitant symptoms that are sequelae of chronic pain (e.g., anxiety, depression, insomnia) may be separate targets for management.
4. When it comes to neuropathic symptoms, start with *unimodality pharmacotherapy* based on differential symptom sensitivity. Be aware of contraindications to the use of each drug.
5. Observe desired *target effect* versus undesirable *adverse effect.*
6. When using multidrug pharmacotherapy, be aware of *drug-drug interactions* (224).
7. Institute multimodal drug treatment addressing neuropathic symptoms not simultaneously but *sequentially;* otherwise it is impossible to tell what works).

Table 7.5.   Differential Pain Symptom Sensitivity

Type of pain	Treatment
Burning, diffuse, poorly localized	Antidepressants (amitriptyline, imipramine); use trazodone in cardiac patients; for orthostatic hypotension, fluphenazine
Spontaneous (paroxysmal)	Anticonvulsants (carbamazepine, diphenylhydantoin, gabapentin) Membrane stabilizers (local anesthetics) Occasionally appropriate to add baclofen to anticonvulsants (i.e., resistant tic douloureux)
Touch-evoked	NMDA receptor blockers (e.g., dextromethorphan, memantine)
Deep tissue or muscle	NSAIDs Opioids
Vasoconstrictive symptoms	Calcium channel blockers (nifedipine)
Sympathetically maintained pain	α-Adrenergic blockers (e.g., phenoxybenzamine, prazosin, doxazosin) α_2-Adrenergic agonists (Clonidine)

Simultaneous analgesics may be required. First use simple analgesics, then combination of analgesics and opioids, finally opioids and substitutes. Do not hesitate to combine pharmacotherapy with physical modalities, exercises and/or supportive therapy at all times.

Table 7.6.   Concomitant Symptom Management

Symptom	Management
Depression	Tricyclics and nontricyclic antidepressants Selective serotonin reuptake inhibitors
Anxiety	Short-action benzodiazepines
Insomnia	Short-action benzodiazepines
Muscle spasm	Muscle relaxants (prn or short term); in spasticity-related pain, baclofen or dantrolene sodium

8. *Time is of the essence.* Use each drug in adequate dose and sufficient time to reach effect or side effect. If a drug is ineffective, do not hesitate to abandon it and institute another one. If the effect is partial, it may be desirable to add another drug. Examples are as follows: For (usually burning) ongoing pain amitriptyline should be initiated at 25 mg at bedtime and increased in 25-mg increments every 3 days or so. For elderly or fragile patients start with 10 mg. Analgesic effect if any will become apparent within 1 to 3 weeks, and usually doses up to 75 to 100 mg are adequate. For paroxysmal pains carbamazepine should be initiated at 200 mg daily for 2 to 3 days, and then the dose should escalate to 200 mg three or four times a day within a couple of weeks. Most neuropathic pain patients show an effect within 2 to 3 weeks. For gabapentin, the initial dose of 300 mg can be escalated daily by 300 mg to 1500 mg or more per day. A 2-week trial is adequate to demonstrate any analgesic effect.

9. *Monitor* treatment response frequently by documenting any change in the patient's basic condition (pain relief and alterations in function). Be aware that improvement may be the result of any of the following: (*a*) natural history of the disease with remissions due to regression to the mean; (*b*) placebo effect, or (*c*) actual physiological or pharmacological effect of the intervention. Be prepared to alter your treatment approach if necessary.

10. Be aware that patients tend to *prioritize* their pains. Elimination or reduction of the most prominent pain complaint may allow for previously covert or understated pain to surface. Therefore, *new complaints do not necessarily mean treatment failure.*

11. Neuropathic pain of peripheral and/or central origin often cannot be alleviated by opioids at doses that are free of side effects. While any of several mechanisms may be responsible for this—involvement of other than opioid-related pain systems, up-regulation of endogenous antiopioid substances such as the neuropeptide cholecystokinin (225), and so on—opioids are still valuable for selected patients. The physician prescribing opioids in neuropathic pain should be familiar with appropriate around-the-clock regimens of slow-release preparations; know equipotency values, modes of administration, and drug pharmacokinetics, types, and interactions; understand the differences among addiction, tolerance, and dependence; discriminate drug-seeking from pain relief-seeking behavior; and maintain good clinical practices (contract arrangement with the patient, detailed record keeping, documentation of pain and function alteration, and so on).

Pharmacotherapy suggestions based on differential pain symptom sensitivity and concomitant system management are listed in Tables 7.5 and 7.6, respectively.

References

1. Merskey H, Bogduk N, eds. Classification of chronic pain: descriptions of chronic pain and definitions of terms. 2nd ed. Seattle: IASP Press, 1994.

2. Tasker RR. Deafferentation pain syndromes: introduction. In: Nashold BS, Ovelmen-Levitt J, eds. Deafferentation pain syndromes: pathophysiology and treatment. Advances in Pain Research and Therapy, vol 19. New York: Raven Press, 1991;241.

3. Bonica JJ. Introduction: semantic, epidemiologic, and educational issues. In: Casey KL, ed. Pain and central nervous system disease: the central pain syndromes. New York: Raven Press, 1991;65.

4. Andersen G, Vestergaard K, Ingeman-Nielsen M, Jensen TS. The incidence of central post-stroke pain. Pain 1995;61:187.

5. Boivie J. Central pain. In: Wall PD, Melzack R, eds. Textbook of pain, 3rd ed. Edinburgh: Churchill Livingstone, 1994;871.

6. Tasker RR, de Carvalho G, Dostrovsky JO. The history of central pain syndromes, with observations concerning pathophysiology and treatment. In: Casey KL, ed. Pain and central nervous system disease: the central pain syndromes. New York: Raven, 1991;31.

7. Déjérine J, Roussy G. Le syndrome thalamique. Rev Neurol 1906;14:521.

8. Bonica JJ. Introduction. In Nashold BS, Ovelmen-Levitt J, eds. Advances in Pain Research and Therapy. Raven Press, New York, 1991, Vol. 19, pp. 1.

9. Jensen TS, Lenz FA. Central post-stroke pain: a challenge for the scientist and the clinician. Pain 1995;61:161.

10. Beric A. Central pain: "new" syndromes and their evaluation. Muscle Nerve 1993;16:1017.

11. Leijon G, Boivie J, Johansson I. Central post-stroke pain: neurological symptoms and pain characteristics. Pain 1989;36:13.

12. Donovan WH, Dimitrijevic MR, Dahm L, Dimitrijevic R. Neurophysiological approaches to chronic pain following spinal cord injury. Paraplegia 1982;20:135.

13. Beric A. Dimitrijevic MR, Wall PD. Modification of pain below the level of SCI. Pain 1990; Suppl 5:S279.

14. Foster JB, Hudgson P. Clinical features of syringomyelia. In: Barnett HJ, Foster JB, Hudgson P, eds. Syringomyelia. London: Saunders, 1973;1.

15. Schliep G. Syringomyelia and syringobulbia. In: Vinken G, Bruyn G, eds. Handbook of neurology. Amsterdam: North-Holland, 1978;255.

16. Boivie J. Hyperalgesia and allodynia in patients with CNS lesions. In: Willis WD Jr, ed. Hyperalgesia and allodynia. New York: Raven Press, 1992;363.

17. Yezierski RP. Pain following spinal cord injury: the clinical problem and experimental studies. Pain 1996;68:185.

18. Lenz FA, Tasker RR, Dostrovsky JO. Abnormal single unit activity recorded in the somatosensory thalamus of a quadriplegic patient with central pain. Pain 1987;31:225.

19. Canavero S. Dynamic reverberation: a unified mechanism for central and phantom pain. Med Hypotheses 1994;42:203.

20. Canavero S, Bonicalzi V. Cortical stimulation for central pain. J Neurosurg 1995;83:1117.

21. Canavero S, Bonicalzi V, Castellano G. Two in one: the genesis of central pain. Pain 1996;64:394.

22. Canavero S, Bonicalzi V, Pagni CA, et al. Propofol analgesia in central pain: preliminary clinical observations. J Neurol 1995;242:561.

23. Canavero S, Pagni CA, Castellano G, Bonicalzi V. SPECT, central pain. Pain 1994;57:129.

24. Canavero S, Pagni CA, Castellano G, et al. The role of cortex in central pain syndromes: preliminary results of a long-term technetium-99 hexamethylpropyleneamineoxime single photon emission computed tomographic study. Neurosurgery 1993;32:185.

25. Pagni CA, Canavero S. Functional thalamic depression in a case of reversible central pain due to a spinal intramedullary cyst: case report. J Neurosurg 1995;83:163.

26. Lenz FA, Kwan HC, Martin R, Tasker R, et al. Characteristics of somatotopic organization and spontaneous neuronal activity in the region of the thalamic principal sensory nucleus in patients with spinal cord transections. J Neurophysiol 1994;72:1570.

27. Koyama S, Katayama Y, Maejima S, et al. Thalamic neuronal hyperactivity following transection of the spinothalamic tract in the cat: involvement of N-methyl-D-aspartate receptor. Brain Res 1993;612:345.

28. Backonja M, Arndt G, Gombar KA, et al. Response of chronic neuropathic pain syndromes to ketamine: a preliminary study. Pain 1994;56:51.

29. Mailis A, Amani N, Umana M, et al. Effect of intravenous sodium amytal on cutaneous sensory abnormalities, spontaneous pain and algometric pain pressure thresholds in neuropathic pain patients: a placebo-controlled study. Pain 1997;70:69.

30. Goto T, Marota JJA, Crosby G. Pentobarbitone, but not propofol, produces preemptive analgesia in the rat formalin model. Br J Anesth 1994;72:662.

31. Tourtellotte WW, Baumhefner RW. Comprehensive management of multiple sclerosis. In: Hallpike JF, Adams CWM, Tourtellotte WW, eds. Multiple sclerosis. Baltimore: Williams & Wilkins, 1983;513.

32. Kassirer MR, Osterberg DH. Pain in chronic multiple sclerosis. J Pain Symptom Manag 1987;2:95.

33. Clifford DB, Trotter JL. Pain in multiple sclerosis. Arch Neurol 1984;41:1270.

34. Vermote R, Ketelaer P, Carton H. Pain in multiple sclerosis patients. Clin Neurol Neurosurg 1986;88:87.

35. Moulin DE, Foley KM, Ebers GC. Pain syndromes in multiple sclerosis. Neurology 1988;38:1830.

36. Osterberg A, Boivie J, Henriksson A, Holmgren H, Johansson I. Central pain in multiple sclerosis. Pain 1993;407.

37. Stenager E, Knudsen L, Jensen K. Acute and chronic pain syndromes in multiple sclerosis. Acta Neurol Scand 1991;84:197.

38. Espir MLE, Millac P. Treatment of paroxysmal disorders in multiple sclerosis with carbamazepine (Tegretol). J Neurol Neurosurg Psychiatry 1970;33:528.

39. Moulin DE. Pain in multiple sclerosis. In: Portenoy RK, ed. Pain mechanisms and syndromes. Neurol Clin 1989;7:321.

40. Osterman PO, Westerberg CE. Paroxysmal attacks in multiple sclerosis. Brain 1975;98:189.

41. Rushton JG, Olafson RA. Trigeminal neuralgia associated with multiple sclerosis: report of 35 cases. Arch Neurol 1965;13:383.

42. Shibasaki H, Kuroiwa Y. Painful tonic seizure in multiple sclerosis. Arch Neurol 1974;30:47.

43. Sweet WH. The treatment of trigeminal neuralgia (tic douloureux). N Engl J Med 1986;315:174.

44. Fromm GH, Terrence CF, Chattha AS. Baclofen in the treatment of trigeminal neuralgia: double-blind study and long-term follow-up. Ann Neurol 1984;15:240.

45. Swerdlow M. Anticonvulsant drugs and chronic pain. Clin Neuropharmacol 1984;7:51.

46. Rosen JA, Barsoum AH. Failure of chronic dorsal column stimulation in multiple sclerosis. Ann Neurol 1979;6:66.

47. Young RF, Goodman SJ. Dorsal spinal cord stimulation in the treatment of multiple sclerosis. Neurosurgery 1979;5:225.

48. Milligan NM, Newcombe R, Compston DAS. A double-blind control trial of high dose methylprednisolone in patients with multiple sclerosis: 1. Clinical effects. J Neurol Neurosurg Psychiatry 1987;50:511.

49. Erickson DL, Blacklock JB, Michaelson M, Sperling KB, Lo JN. Control of spasticity by implantable continuous flow morphine pump. Neurosurgery 1985;16:215.

50. Kasdon DL. Controversies in the surgical management of spasticity. Clin Neurosurgery 1986;33:523.

51. Watkins SM, Espir MLE. Migraine and multiple sclerosis. J Neurol Neurosurg Psychiatry 1969;32:35.

52. Reference deleted.

53. Chudler EH, Willie KD. The role of the basal ganglia in nociception and pain: review article. Pain 1995;60:3.

54. Sandyk R, Bamford CR, Iacono R. Pain and sensory symptoms in Parkinson's disease. Int J Neurosci 1988;39:15–25.

54a. Snider SR, Fahn S, Isgreen WP, Cote LJ. Primary sensory symptoms in parkinsonism. Neurology 1976;26:423.

55. Goetz CG, Tanner CM, Levy M, Wilson RS, Garron DC. Pain in Parkinson's disease. Mov Disord 1986;1:45.

56. Koller WC. Sensory symptoms in Parkinson's disease. Neurology 1984;34:957.

57. Urakami K, Takahashi K, Matsushima E, et al. The threshold of pain and neurotransmitter's change on pain in Parkinson's disease. Jpn J Psychiat Neurol 1990;44:589.

58. Snider SR, Sandyk R. Sensory dysfunction. In: Koller WC, ed. Handbook of Parkinson's disease. New York: Marcel Dekker, 1987;171.

59. Artieda J, Pastor MA, Lacruz F, Obeso JA. Temporal discrimination is abnormal in Parkinson's disease. Brain 1992;115:199.

60. Schneider JS, Diamond SG, Markham CH. Deficits in orofacial senso-rimotor function in Parkinson's disease. Ann Neurol 1986a;19:275.

61. Caligiuri MP, Abbs JH. Response properties of the perioral reflex in Parkinson's disease. Exp Neurol 1987;98:563.

62. Battista AF, Woolf BB. Levodopa and induced-pain response: a study of patients with parkinsonian and pain syndromes. Arch Intern Med 1973;132:70.

63. Guieu R, Pouget J, Serratrice G. Nociceptive threshold and Parkinson's disease. Rev Neurol (Paris) 1992;10:641.

64. Nappi G, Petraglia F, Martignoni E, et al. Beta-endorphin cerebrospinal fluid decrease in untreated parkinsonian patients. Neurology 1985;35:1371.

65. Baronti F, Conant KE, Giuffra M, et al. Opioid peptides in Parkinson's disease: effects of dopamine repletion. Brain Res 1991;560:92.

66. Taquet H, Javoy-Agid F, Hamon M, et al. Parkinson's disease affects differently Met5- and Leu5-enkephalin in the human brain. Brain Res 1983;280:379.

67. Tanner CM, Goetz CG, Gilley DW, et al. Behavioral aspects of intra-triatal adrenal medulla transplant surgery in Parkinson's disease. Neu-rology 1988;38(S):143.

68. Penn RD, Goetz CG, Tanner CM, et al. Adrenal medullary transplant operation for Parkinson's disease: clinical observations in five patients. Neurosurgery 1988;22:999.

69. Jankovic J, Grossman R, Goodman C, et al. Clinical, biochemical and neuropathologic findings following transplantation of adrenal medulla to the caudate nucleus for treatment of Parkinson's disease. Neurology 1989;38:1227.

70. Ostrosky-Solis F, Quintanar L, Madrazo I, et al. Neuropsychological effects of brain autograft of adrenal medullary tissue for the treatment of Parkinson's disease. Neurology 1988;38:1442.

71. Ginzburg R, Seltzer Z. Subarachnoid spinal cord transplantation of adrenal medulla suppresses chronic neuropathic pain behaviour in rats. Brain Res 1990;523:147.

72. Hama AT, Sagen J. Reduced pain-related behaviour by adrenal medullary transplant in rats with experimental peripheral neuropathy, Pain 1993;52:223–231.

73. Sagen J, Wang H, Pappas GD. Adrenal medullary implants in the rat spinal cord reduce nociception in a chronic pain model. Pain 1990;42:69.

74. Ballard PA, Tetrud JW, Langston JW. Permanent human parkinsonism due to 1-methyl-4-phenyl-1,2,3,6-tetrahydropyridine (MPTP): seven cases. Neurology 1985;35:949.

75. Burns RS, Chiueh CC, Markey SP, et al. A primate model of parkin-sonism: selective destruction of dopaminergic neurons in the pars com-pacta of the substantia nigra by N-methyl-4-phenyl-1,2,3,6-tetrahy-dropyridine. Proc Natl Acad Sci U S A 1983;80:4546.

76. Rosland JH, Hunskaar S, Broch OJ, Hole K. Acute and long term effects of 1-methyl-4-phenyl-tetrahydropyridine (MPTP) in tests of nociception in mice. Pharm Toxicol 1992;70:31.

77. Schneider JS, McLaughlin WW, Roeltgen DP. Motor and nonmotor behavioral deficits in monkeys made hemiparkinsonian by intracarotid MPTP infusion. Neurology 1992;42:1565.

78. Schneider JS. Responses of striatal neurons to peripheral sensory stim-ulation in symptomatic MPTP-exposed cats. Brain Res 1991;544:297.

79. Tatton WG, Eastman MJ, Bedingham W, et al. Defective utilization of sensory input as the basis for bradykinesia, rigidity and decreased movement repertoire in Parkinson's disease: a hypothesis. Can J Neurol Sci 1984;11:136.

80. Rothblat DS, Schneider JS. Response of caudate neurons to stimulation of intrinsic and peripheral afferents in normal, symptomatic, and recov-ered MPTP-treated cats. J Neurosci 1993;13:4372.

81. Decina P, Mukherjee S, Caracci G, Harrison K. Painful sensory symp-toms in neuroleptic-induced extrapyramidal syndromes. Am J Psychia-try 1992;149:1075.

82. Albin RL, Young AB. Somatosensory phenomena in Huntington's dis-ease. Mov Disord 1988;3:343.

83. Jaradeh S, Dyck PJ. Hereditary motor and sensory neuropathy with treatable extrapyramidal features. Arch Neurol 1992;49:175.

84. Lee JL, Wang AD. Post-traumatic basal ganglia hemorrhage: analysis of 52 patients with emphasis on the final outcome. J Trauma 1991;31:376.

85. Yarnitsky D, Barron SA, Bental E. Disappearance of phantom pain after focal brain infarction. Pain 1988;32:285.

86. Yang Y. Pure sensory stroke confirmed by CT scan. Chin Med J 1991;104:595.

87. American Psychiatric Association. Diagnostic and Statistical Manual of Mental Disorders. 4th ed. Washington: APA, 1994.

88. Comming DE, Comings BG. Tourette syndrome: clinical and psycho-logical aspects of 250 cases. Am J Hum Genet 1985;37:435.

89. Eldridge R, Sweet R, Lake CR, Shapiro AK. Gilles de la Tourette's syn-drome: Clinical, genetic, psychologic and biochemical aspects in 21 selected families. Neurology 1977;27:114.

90. Robertson MM, Trimble MR, Less AJ. Self-injurious behaviour and the Gilles de la Tourette syndrome: a clinical study and review of the liter-ature. Psychol Med 1989;19:611.

91. Riley DE, Lang AE. Pain in Gilles de la Tourette syndrome and related tic disorders. Can J Neurol Sci 1989;16:439.

92. Kurlan R, Lighter D, Hewitt BA. Sensory tics in Tourette's syndrome. Neurology 1989;39:731.

93. Haber SN, Kowall NW, Vonsattel JP, et al. Gilles de la Tourette's syn-drome: a postmortem neuropathological and immunohistochemical study. J Neurol Sci 1986;75:225.

94. Goldstein M, Kuga S, Kusano N, et al. Dopamine agonist induced self-mutilative biting behaviour in monkeys with unilateral ventromedial tegmental lesions of the brainstem: possible pharmacological model for Lesch-Nyhan syndrome. Brain Res 1986;367:114.

95. Herman BH, Hammock MK, Arthur-Smith A, et al. Naltrexone decreases self-injurious behavior. Ann Neurol 1987;22:550.

96. Sandyk R, Bamford CR. Deregulation of hypothalamic dopamine and opioid activity and the pathophysiology of self-mutilatory behaviour in Tourette's syndrome. J Clin Psychopharmacol 1987;7:367.

97. Jensen TS, Rasmussen P. Phantom pain and other phenomena after amputation. In: Wall PD, Melzack R, eds. Textbook of pain. 3rd ed. Edinburgh: Churchill Livingstone, 1994;651.

98. Ewalt JR, Randall GC, Morris H. The phantom limb. Psychosom Med 1947;9:118.

99. Melzack R, Loeser JD. Phantom body pains in paraplegics: evidence for a central "pattern generating mechanism" for pain. Pain 1978;4:195.

100. Jensen TS, Krebs B, Nielsen J, Rasmussen P. Immediate and long-term phantom limb pain in amputees: incidence, clinical characteristics and relationship to preamputation limb pain. Pain 1985;21:267.

101. Krebs B, Jensen TS, Kroner K, et al. Phantom limb phenomena in amputees 7 years after limb amputation. In: Fields HL, Dubner R. Cervero F, eds. Advances in pain research and therapy. vol 9. New York: Raven Press, 1985;425.

102. Brown WA. Postamputation phantom limb pain. Dis Nerv Syst 1968;29:301.

103. Sherman R, Sherman C, Parker L. Chronic phantom and stump pain among American veterans: results of a survey. Pain 1984;18:83.

104. Sliosberg A. Les algies des amputés. Paris: Masson, 1948.
105. Katz J, Melzack R. Pain "memories" in phantom limbs: review and clinical observations. Pain 1990;43:319.
106. Riddoch G. Phantom limbs and body shape. Brain 1941;64:197.
107. Parkes CM. Factors determining the persistence of phantom pain in the amputee. J Psychosom Res 1973;17:97.
108. Sunderland S. Nerves and nerve injuries. Baltimore: Williams & Wilkins, 1978.
109. Jaeger H, Maier C. Calcitonin in phantom limb pain: a double-blind study. Pain 1992;48:21.
110. Iacono RP, Sandyk R, Baumford CR, et al. Post-amputation phantom pain and autonomous stump movements responsive to doxepin. Funct Neurol 1987;2:343.
111. Elliott F, Little A, Milbrandt W. Carbamazepine for phantom limb phenomena. N Engl J Med 1976;295:678.
112. Patterson JF. Carbamazepine in the treatment of phantom limb pain. South Med J 1988;81:1100.
113. Marsland AR, Weekes JWN, Atkinson RL, Leong MG. Phantom limb pain: a case for beta blockers? Pain 1982;12:295.
114. Mundinger F, Neumüller H. Programmed transcutaneous (TNS) and central (DBS) stimulation for control of phantom limb pain and causalgia: a new method of treatment. In: Siegfried J, Zimmermann M, eds. Phantom and stump pain. Berlin: Springer Verlag, 1981;167.
115. Siegfried J, Cetinalp E. Neurosurgical treatment of phantom limb pain: a survey of methods. In: Siegfried J, Zimmermann M, eds. Phantom and stump pain. Berlin: Springer Verlag, 1981;148.
116. Croft PB, Wilkinson M. The incidence of carcinomatous neuromyopathy in patients with various types of carcinoma, Brain 1965;88:427.
117. Posner JB, Furneaux HM. Paraneoplastic syndromes. In: Waksman BH, ed. Immunologic mechanisms in neurologic and psychiatric disease. New York: Raven Press, 1990;187.
118. Posner JB. Paraneoplastic syndromes involving the nervous system. In: Aminoff MJ, ed. Neurology and general medicine. 2nd ed. Edinburgh: Churchill Livingstone, 1995;401.
119. Furneaux HM, Rosenblum MK, Dalmau J, et al. Selective expression of Purkinje-cell antigens in tumour tissue from patients with paraneoplastic cerebellar degeneration, N. Engl. J. Med. 1990;322:1844.
120. Croft PB, Urich H, Wilkinson M. Peripheral neuropathy of sensorimotor type associated with malignant disease. Brain 1967;90:31.
121. Peterson K, Forsyth PA, Posner JB. Paraneoplastic sensorimotor neuropathy associated with breast cancer. J Neurooncol 1994;21:159.
122. Halbach M, Homberg V, Freund HJ. Neuromuscular, autonomic and central cholinergic hyperactivity associated with thymoma and acetylcholine receptor-binding antibody. J Neurol 1987;234:433.
123. Garcia-Merino A, Cabello A, Mora JS, Lano H. Continuous muscle fiber activity, peripheral neuropathy and thymoma. Ann Neurol 1991;29:215.
124. Ferrari P, Federico M, Grimaldi LME, Silingardi V. Stiff-man syndrome in a patient with Hodgkin's disease: an unusual paraneoplastic syndrome. Haematologica 1990;75:570.
125. Folli F, Solimena M, Cofiell R, et al. Autoantibodies to a 128-kd synaptic protein in three women with the stiff-man syndrome and breast cancer. N Engl J Med 1993;328:546.
126. Owens AH, Baylin SB. Biology of human neoplasia. In: Harvey, Johns, McKusick, et al, eds. Principles of practice of medicine. 22nd ed. East Norwalk, CT: Appleton & Lange, 1988;368.
127. Posner JB. Paraneoplastic syndromes. In: Patchell RA, ed. Neurologic complications of systemic cancer. Neurol Clin 1991;9:919.
128. Mertens HG, Zschocke S. Neuromyotonie. Klin Wochenschr 1965;43:917.
129. Isaacs H. Syndrome of continuous muscle fiber activity. J Neurol Neurosurg Psychiatry 1961;24:319.
130. Sinha S, Newson-Davis J, Mills K, et al. Autoimmune etiology for acquired neuromyotonia (Isaac's syndrome). Lancet 1991;338:75.
131. Hahn AF, Parkes AW, Bolton CF, Stewart SA. Neuromyotonia in hereditary motor neuropathy. J Neurol Neurosurg Psychiatry 1991;54:230.

132. Blum P, Jankovic J. Stiff-person syndrome: an autoimmune disease. Mov Disord 1991;12.
133. Gordon EE, Januszko DM, Kaufman L. A critical survey of stiff-man syndrome. Am J Med 1967;42:582.
134. Howard FM Jr. A new and effective drug in the treatment of stiff-man syndrome: preliminary report. Proc Meet Mayo Clinic 1963;38:203.
135. Lorish TR, Thorsteinsson G, Howard FM. Stiff-man syndrome updated. Mayo Clinic Proc 1989;64:629.
136. Moersch FP, Woltman HW. Progressive fluctuating muscular rigidity and spasms ("stiff-man" syndrome): report of a case and some observations in thirteen other cases. Proc Staff Meet Mayo Clinic 1956;31:421.
137. Schmidt RT, Stahl SM, Spehlmann R. A pharmacologic study of the stiff-man syndrome: correlation of clinical symptoms with urinary 3-methoxy-4-hydroxy-phenyl glycol excretion. Neurology 1975;25:622.
138. Burn DJ, Ball J, Lees AJ. A case of progressive encephalomyelitis with rigidity and positive antiglutamic acid dehydrogenase antibodies. J Neurol Neurosurg Psychiatry 1991;54:449.
139. McCombe PA, Chalk JB, Searle JW. Progressive encephalomyelitis with rigidity: a case report with magnetic resonance imaging findings. J Neurol Neurosurg Psychiatry 1989;52:1429.
140. Weiner WJ, Lang AE. Movement disorders: a comprehensive survey. Mount Kisko, NY: Futura, 1989;506.
141. Jog MS, Lambert CD, Lang AE. Stiff-person syndrome. Can J Neurol Sci 1992;19:383.
142. Schaumburg HH, Berger AR, Thomas PK. Disorders of peripheral nerves. 2nd ed. Philadelphia: FA Davis, 1992.
143. Thomas PK, Ochoa J. Clinical features and differential diagnosis. In: Dyck PJ, Thomas PK, Griffin JW, et al., eds. Peripheral neuropathy. 3rd ed. Philadelphia: Saunders, 1993;749.
144. Arnason BG. Inflammatory polyradiculopathies. In: Dyck PJ, Thomas PK, Lambert EH, Bunge R, eds. Peripheral neuropathy, vol 2. 2nd ed. Philadelphia: Saunders, 1984;2050.
145. Ropper A. Campylobacter diarrhea and Guillain-Barré syndrome. Arch Neurol 1988;45:655.
146. Alter M. The epidemiology of the Guillain-Barré syndrome. Ann Neurol (Suppl) 1990;27:S7.
147. Dyck PJ, Low PA, Stevens JD. Diseases of peripheral nerves. In: Baker AB, Baker LH, eds. Clinical neurology. New York: Harper & Row, 1983.
148. McCombe PA, Pollard JD, McLeod JG. Chronic inflammatory demyelinating polyradiculoneuropathy. Brain 1987;110:1617.
149. Asbury AK, Johnson PC. Pathology of peripheral nerve. Philadelphia: Saunders, 1978.
150. Job CK. Pathology of peripheral nerve lesions in lepromatous leprosy: A light and electron microscopic study. Int J Lepr 1971;39:251.
151. Strickland GT, Moser KM. Sarcoidosis with a Landry-Guillain-Barré syndrome and clinical response to corticosteroids. Am J Med 1967;43:131.
152. Steere AC. Lyme disease. N Engl J Med 1989;321:586.
153. Thomas PK, Tomlinson DR. Diabetic and hypoglycemic neuropathy. In: Dyck PJ, Thomas PK, Griffin JW, et al., eds. Peripheral neuropathy. 3rd ed. Philadelphia: Saunders, 1993;1219.
154. Archer A, Watkins PJ, Thomas PK, et al. The natural history of acute painful neuropathy in diabetes mellitus. J Neurol Neurosurg Psychiatry 1983;46:491.
155. Zorilla E, Kozak GP. Ophthalmoplegia in diabetes mellitus. Ann Intern Med 1967;67:968.
156. Max MB, Culnane M, Schafer SC, et al. Amitriptyline relieves diabetic neuropathy pain in patients with normal or depressed mood. Neurology 1987;37:589.
157. Rull JA, Quibrera R, Gonzalez-Millan H, Lozano-Castaneda O. Symptomatic treatment of peripheral diabetic neuropathy with carbamazepine: double-blind cross-over study. Diabetologia 1969;5:215.
158. Wilton TD. Tegretol in the treatment of diabetic neuropathy. S Afr Med J 1974;48:869.

159. Dejgard A, Petersen P, Kastrup J. Mexiletine for treatment of chronic painful diabetic neuropathy. Lancet 1985;1:9.

160. Thorsteinsson G. Management of painful diabetic neuropathy. JAMA 1977;238:2697.

161. Ross DR, Varipapa RJ. Treatment of painful diabetic neuropathy with capsaicin. N Engl J Med 1989;321:474.

162. Lefebvre-D'Amour M, Shahani BT, Young RR, Bird KT. The importance of studying sural nerve conduction and late responses in the evaluation of alcoholic subjects. Neurology 1979;29:1600.

163. Bischoff A. Die alkoholische polyneuropathie: Klinische, ultrastucturelle und pathogenetische aspekte. Dtsch Med Wochenschr 1971;96:317.

164. Wilbourn AJ, Furlan AJ, Hulley W, Ruschhaupt W. Ischemic monomelic neuropathy. Neurology 1983;33:47.

165. Honet JC, Wajszczuk WJ, Rubenfire M, et al. Neurological abnormalities in the leg(s) after use of intra-aortic balloon pump: report of 6 cases. Arch Phys Med Rehabil 1975;56:346.

166. Bolton CF, Driedger AA, Lindsay RM. Ischemic neuropathy in uremic patients caused by bovine arteriovenous shunt. J Neurol Neurosurg Psychiatry 1979;42:810.

167. Wytrzes L, Markley HG, Fisher M, Alfred HJ. Brachial neuropathy after brachial artery-antecubital vein shunts for chronic hemodialysis. Neurology 1987;37:1398.

168. Cohen SM. Accidental intra-arterial injection of drugs. Lancet 1948;2:409.

169. Gammel JA. Arterial embolism: an unusual complication following the intramuscular administration of bismuth. JAMA 1927;88:998.

170. Stöhr M, Dicheans J, Dorstelmann D. Ischemic neuropathy of the lumbosacral plexus following intragluteal injection. J Neurol Neurosurg Psychiatry 1980;43:489.

171. Castellanos AM, Glass JP, Yung WKA. Regional nerve injury after intra-arterial chemotherapy. Neurology 1987;37:834.

172. Chalk CH, Dyck PJ. Ischemic neuropathy. In: Dyck PJ, Thomas PK, Griffin JW, et al., eds. Peripheral neuropathy. 3rd ed. Philadelphia: Saunders, 1993;980.

173. Michiels JJ, Abels J, Steketee J, et al. Erythromelalgia caused by platelet-mediated arteriolar inflammation and thrombosis in thrombocythemia. Ann Intern Med 1985;102:466.

174. Michiels JJ, van Joost T. Erythromelalgia and thrombocythemia: a causal relation. J Am Acad Dermatol 1990;22:107.

175. Chalk CH, Dyck PJ, Conn DL. Vasculitic neuropathy. In: Dyck PJ, Thomas PK, Griffin JW, et al., eds. Peripheral neuropathy. 3rd ed. Philadelphia: Saunders, 1993;142.

176. Glenner GG. Amyloid deposits and amyloidosis: The B-fibrillosis. N Engl J Med 1980;302:1283.

177. Tyler HR, Tyler KL. Neurologic complications. In: Eknoyan G, Knochel JP, eds. The systemic consequences of renal failure. Orlando: Grune & Stratton, 1984;302.

178. Keppes A, Saua S, Andersen KG. The porphyrias. In: Stanbury JB, Wyngaarden JB, Fredrickson DS, eds. The metabolic basis of inherited disease. 5th ed. New York: McGraw-Hill, 1983;1301.

179. Ridley A. The neuropathy of acute intermittent porphyrias. Q J Med 1969;38:307.

180. Brady RO. Fabry disease. In: Dyck PJ, Thomas PK, Griffin JW, et al., eds. Peripheral neuropathy. 3rd ed. Philadelphia: Saunders, 1993;1169.

181. Lockman LA, Krivit W, Desnick RJ. Relief of the painful crises of Fabry's disease by diphenylhydantoin. Neurology (Minn) 1971;21:423.

182. Filling-Katz MR, Merrick HF, Fink JK. Carbamazepine in Fabry's disease: effective analgesia with dose-dependent exacerbation of autonomic dysfunction. Neurology 1989;39:598.

183. Le Quesne PM. Neuropathy due to drugs. In: Dyck PJ, Thomas PK, Griffin JW, et al., eds. Peripheral neuropathy. 3rd ed. Philadelphia: Saunders, 1993;1571.

184. Dische S, Saunders MI, Lee ME, et al. Clinical testing of the radiosensitizer Ro 07-0582: experience with multiple doses. Br J Cancer 1977;35:567.

185. Fullerton PM, O'Sullivan DJ. Thalidomide neuropathy: a clinical, electrophysiological and histological follow-up. J Neurol Neurosurg Psychiatry 1968;31:543.

186. Windebank AJ. Metal neuropathy. In: Dyck PJ, Thomas PK, Griffin JW, et al., eds. Peripheral neuropathy. 3rd ed. Philadelphia: Saunders, 1993;1549.

187. Neary D, Eames RA. The pathology of ulnar compression in man. Neuropathol Appl Neurobiol 1975;1:69.

188. Neary D, Ochoa J, Gilliat RW. Sub-clinical entrapment neuropathy in man. J Neurol Sci 1975;24:283.

189. Schwartzman RJ. Brachial plexus traction injuries. Hand Clin 1991;7:547.

190. Assa J. The intercostobrachial nerve in radical mastectomy. J Surg Oncol 1974;6:123.

191. Boulias C, Mailis A. Intercostal nerve damage after aortocoronary bypass surgery utilizing internal mammary artery graft (IMA syndrome): prevalence and morbidity. Abstr VIII World Congress on Pain. Seattle: IASP Press, 1996;370.

192. Mailis A, Chan J, Basinski A, et al. Chest wall pain after aortocoronary bypass surgery using internal mammary artery graft: a new pain syndrome? Heart Lung 1989;18:553.

193. Leckey BRF, Hughes RAS, Murray NMF. Trigeminal sensory neuropathy: a study of 22 cases. Brain 1987;110:1463.

194. Wilbourn A. Brachial plexus disorders. In: Dyck PJ, Thomas PK, Griffin JW, et al., eds. Peripheral neuropathy. 3rd ed. Philadelphia: Saunders, 1993;911.

195. Tsairis P. Brachial plexus neuropathies. In: Dyck PJ, Thomas PK, Lambert EH, eds. Peripheral neuropathy. 1st ed. Philadelphia: Saunders, 1975;659.

195a.Thomas JE, Colby MY. Radiation-induced or metastatic brachial plexopathy. JAMA 1972;222:1392.

196. Wynn Parry CB, Thomas JE, Colby MY. Radiation-induced or metastatic brachial plexopathy. JAMA 1972;222:1392.

197. Terzis JK, Smith KL. The peripheral nerve: structure, function and reconstruction. New York: Raven Press, 1990.

198. Birch R. Lesions of the peripheral nerves: the present position. J Bone Joint Surg 1986;68B;1,20,21.

199. Hirshman EB. Brachial plexus injuries. Clin Sports Med 1990;9:311.

200. Robertson WC, Erchman PL, Clancy WG. Upper trunk brachial plexopathy in football players. JAMA 1979;241:1480.

201. Dawson DM, Krarup C. Perioperative nerve lesions. Arch Neurol 1989;46:1355.

202. Daube JR. Rucksack paralysis. JAMA 1969;208:2447.

203. Bruxelle J, Travers V, Thiebaut JB. Occurrence and treatment of pain after brachial plexus injury. Clin Orthop Rel Res 1988;23:87.

204. Wynn Parry CB. Pain in avulsion of the brachial plexus. Neurosurgery 1984;15:960.

205. Narakas AO. Traumatic brachial plexus lesions. In: Dyck PC, Thomas PK, Lambert PK, Bunge R, eds. Peripheral neuropathy. 2nd ed. Philadelphia: Saunders, 1984;1394.

206. Nashold BS, Friedman A, Bullitt E. The status of dorsal root entry zone lesions in 1987. Clin Neurosurg 1989;35:422.

207. Donaghy M. Lumbosacral plexus lesions. In: Dyck PJ, Thomas PK, Griffin JW, et al., eds. Peripheral neuropathy. 3rd ed. Philadelphia: Saunders, 1993;951.

208. Burton CV. Lumbosacral arachnoiditis. Spine 1978;3:24.

209. North RB, Eweend MG, Lawton MT, et al. Failed back surgery syndrome: 5-year followup after spinal cord stimulator implantation. Neurosurgery 1991;78:692.

210. Katusic S, Beard CM, Bergstralh E, Kurland LT. Incidence and clinical features of trigeminal neuralgia, Rochester, Minnesota. Ann Neurol 1990;27:89.

211. Hughes RAC. Diseases of the fifth cranial nerve. In: Dyck PJ, Thomas PK, Griffin JW, et al., eds. Peripheral neuropathy. 3rd ed. Philadelphia: Saunders, 1993;801.

212. Cushing HW. The major trigeminal neuralgias and their operations: varieties of facial neuralgia. Am J Med Sci 1920;160:157.

213. Fukushima T. Microvascular decompression for hemifacial spasm and trigeminal neuralgia: results in 4000 cases. J Neurol Neurosurg Psychiat 1990;53:811.

214. Brustowicz RJ. Combined trigeminal and glossopharyngeal neuralgia. Neurology 1955;5:1.

215. Henderson WR. Trigeminal neuralgia: the pain and its treatment. Br Med J 1967;1:7.

216. Adams CB. Microvascular compression: an alternative view and hypothesis. J Neurosurg 1989;70:1.

217. Heyck H. Drug therapy of trigeminal pain. In: Hassler R, Walker AE, eds. Trigeminal neuralgia: pathogenesis and pathophysiology. Philadelphia: Saunders, 1970;115.

218. Clarke RW. The trigeminal nuclei in pain. In: Holden AV, Winlow W, eds. The neurobiology of pain. Manchester, UK: Manchester University Press, 1984;70.

219. Fromm GH, Terrence CF, Chattha AS, Glass JD. Baclofen in trigeminal neuralgia: its effects on the spinal trigeminal nucleus: a pilot study. Arch Neurol 1980;37:768.

220. Loeser JD. Tic douloureux and atypical facial pain. In: PD Wall, R Melzack, eds. Textbook of pain. 3rd ed. Edinburgh: Churchill Livingstone, 1994;699.

221. Weddington WN, Blazer D. Atypical facial pain and trigeminal neuralgia: a comparison study. Psychosomatics 1979;20:348.

222. Boas RA. Complex regional pain syndromes: symptoms, signs and differential diagnosis. In: Janig W, Stanton-Hicks M, eds. Reflex sympathetic dystrophy: a reappraisal. Progress in Pain Research and Management, vol .6. Seattle: IASP Press, 1996;79.

223. Willner C, Low PA. Parmacologic approaches to neuropathic pain. In: Dyck PJ, Thomas PK, Griffin JW, et al., eds. Peripheral neuropathy. 3rd ed. Philadelphia: Saunders, 1993;1709.

224. Virani A, Mailis A, Shapiro L, Shear N. Drug interactions in neuropathic pain pharmacotherapy. Pain 1997;73:3.

225. Wiesenfeld-Hallin Z, Aldskogius H, Grant G, et al. Central inhibitory dysfunctions: mechanisms and clinical implications. Brain Behav Sci 1998 (in press).

CHAPTER 8

Zoster and Postherpetic Neuralgia: Pain Mechanisms and Current Management

Bradley S. Galer and Charles E. Argoff

INTRODUCTION

It has been well established that the varicella zoster virus (VZV) may be associated with a systemic infection, chickenpox, but that it may remain quiescent in the dorsal root ganglia long after the systemic VZV infection has cleared (1, 2). An outbreak of herpes zoster (HZ), also known as shingles or zona, results from the reactivation of VZV from these ganglia and its spread along corresponding sensory nerves (3). The initial complaint of dermatomal pain followed by the usual vesicular rash is typical of AHZ; however, the onset of pain may precede the rash by a variable amount of time (7 to 100 days) (4, 5). A minority of affected persons either have the pain when or after the rash appears, or rarely have the pain without the rash appearing at all (zoster sine herpete) (6). Two patients with VZV DNA in their cerebrospinal fluid have been reported with radicular pain and no rash (7). For many unfortunate persons the acute pain associated with the HZ outbreak persists well beyond the normal healing period and becomes associated with a different type of discomfort; this chronic pain syndrome is known as postherpetic neuralgia (PHN) (5).

EPIDEMIOLOGY OF ACUTE HERPES ZOSTER

The incidence of HZ infections is approximately 125/100,000 per year, and it is greatly influenced by age; those in their 80s have an incidence at least 20 times that of children (3, 8). There are no reported racial or seasonal differences; men and women are equally affected, and patients with various malignancies, especially lymphoproliferative disorders, are believed to have a higher than usual incidence (3, 8).

EPIDEMIOLOGY OF POSTHERPETIC NEURALGIA

There is little agreement as to when acute herpes zoster becomes PHN. Therefore, the incidence and prevalence of PHN have wide variability, depending on the definition used. Reports of PHN prevalence rates range from 9 to 34%, depending on the study's definition (8–11). Another complicating factor is that not all affected persons report continuous pain after the onset of AHZ. Reports of patients who have developed PHN despite having little or no AHZ-related pain, as well as reports of patients who have had painful periods followed by varying pain-free periods only to again experience pain makes it even more difficult to describe true prevalence rates (12).

DEFINING THE TRANSITION OF ACUTE HERPES ZOSTER TO POSTHERPETIC NEURALGIA

It is clear that the vast majority of patients who develop AHZ have a gradual resolution of their pain within a year, even without any treatment (3, 5, 8, 9). Dermatologic and painful manifestations included, the AHZ outbreak generally resolves within 3 weeks after onset; however, the variability of the clinical course is significant, complicating not only the nomenclature but also our ability to judge responses to therapeutic interventions (8). Even beyond 3 weeks, most patients with HZ-related pain report less pain over time; exactly when the pain associated with AHZ becomes PHN remains a matter of disagreement.

Some investigators define HZ-related pain lasting beyond a month after the outbreak as PHN; others suggest that PHN is pain that remains 3 months or more after an outbreak (9, 12–18). A recent attempt to create consensus definitions resulted in the establishment of three phases, acute, subacute, and chronic herpetic neuralgia. According to this classification, acute herpetic neuralgia is pain during the first 30 days after the rash outbreak. Subacute herpetic neuralgia is the pain that resolves within 3 months following the initial illness, and PHN, or chronic herpetic neuralgia, is the pain that persists 4 months or more beyond the outset. The proposed benefits of this newer classification scheme include the improved ability to use uniform standards for research as well as the use of criteria for differentiating between acute and chronic pain that are recognized by the International Association for the Study of Pain (19). To date, this classification scheme has not been widely accepted or implemented.

RISK FACTORS FOR THE DEVELOPMENT OF POSTHERPETIC NEURALGIA

The only definitive risk factor for developing PHN following AHZ is age; that is, the risk of developing persistent pain following AHZ increases significantly with the age of the person afflicted. While few patients under age 40 have pain a month beyond the rash healing period, 65% of affected individuals above age 60 report persistent pain for the same period, and the percentage of affected persons above age 70 increases to 75%. More than 50% of these latter two groups of patients continue in pain a year after the initial outbreak (8, 10).

Many other possible risk factors for the development of PHN have been described in the literature, although none has been conclusively proven. These other factors include greater severity of initial cutaneous manifestations, greater sensory dysfunction in the affected dermatome during AHZ, greater humoral and cell-mediated immune response during the AHZ outbreak, a painful prodrome prior to rash onset, and fever greater than 38° Celsius during AHZ (20). However, only age has been definitively shown to be a risk factor for the development of persistent pain following AHZ.

Risk factors for HZ and PHN may be different. Several studies conclude that there is no relation between age and the duration of HZ pain but that greater age is associated with greater duration of PHN (21, 22). In another study both acute pain severity and psychosocial stressors predicted the development of PHN, but only acute pain severity predicted pain extent 2 months after the onset of rash (23).

PATHOPHYSIOLOGY

The precise mechanisms of both AHZ-related pain and PHN remain to be defined and agreed upon. While some investigators have interpreted AHZ and PHN as a continuum, others have demonstrated evidence suggesting that these may be two clearly distinct disorders that should be viewed, studied, and treated as such.

An outbreak of HZ is most often associated with a vesicular skin rash. The virus spreads from the dorsal root ganglia along sensory nerve fibers into the skin and subcutaneous tissues. The anatomical distribution of the infection has been well described (5). In the elderly the thoracic region and the ophthalmic division of the trigeminal nerve are the most commonly affected areas (5). The facial nerve is the most commonly affected motor nerve, and sacral involvement, although uncommon, may result in bladder dysfunction. Rarely HZ results in encephalomyelitis, and a systemic response to AHZ, including

headache, nausea, meningismus, fever, and lymphadenopathy, is seen in approximately 5% of patients. Loss of vision can result from the severe conjunctivitis, keratitis, or iridocyclitis that may occur when the ophthalmic division of the trigeminal nerve is affected. Recurrent infection with HZ is uncommon; if this does occur, there is likely to be an underlying malignancy or other reason for immunosuppression. Pain or other abnormal sensation most often heralds the onset of the infection and continues to affect the individual after its outbreak (5).

Since 1861 inflammatory, hemorrhagic, and necrotic changes have been documented in the dorsal root ganglia, posterior nerve roots, spinal cord, and ascending spinal tracts (24). With the initial outbreak there is an extensive inflammatory response causing tissue damage, the most likely source of the pain (5). More-recent studies suggest that while morphologic changes persist in the dorsal horn of the spinal cord in persons with PHN, these do not occur in those without PHN who have had an HZ outbreak (25). It is common for the affected skin to demonstrate scarring and other visible changes even after resolution of the rash and even in the absence of pain (26).

Studies of pain quality reveal that sharp, stabbing pain is more commonly described by patients with AHZ pain and that burning pain appears to be more commonly described in patients with PHN. Allodynia has been described by both groups (27, 28). A recent study reported that the pain of PHN is similar to that of other neuropathic pain syndromes, such as diabetic neuropathy and reflex sympathetic dystrophy, but differs only in that PHN patients describe more itching, skin sensitivity, and sharp pains and less cold pain (29). The fact that the pain associated with AHZ is more responsive to steroids than is the pain associated with PHN may be an important distinction from a pathophysiological viewpoint (30, 31). In addition, PHN as a chronic pain disorder is more likely to raise health care utilization costs, disability, and psychological distress, further distinguishing it from AHZ-related pain (32). Some data regarding the proposed pathophysiologic mechanisms of both AHZ pain and PHN are summarized later in the chapter.

As in other cutaneous neural injuries, tissue inflammation and damage may sensitize and excite nociceptors, with resulting spontaneous discharge of these affected nociceptors, lowered nociceptor threshold for activation, and a greater than expected response to "normal" pain-producing stimuli. In addition, HZ is thought to produce pain by involvement of the nociceptors that surround the nervi nervorum (the sheaths covering the nerves and ganglia themselves) (33). Within the peripheral sensory nerves and their corresponding dorsal root ganglia, viral replication can directly cause a neurolytic injury to these structures, as well as damage from specific intraneural inflammation and hemorrhage as the result of the infection. The immediate net result of these events is that both the sensory nerve and the ganglia can become spontaneously active and demonstrate exaggerated responses to all of their inputs. A state of central hyperexcitability may also develop within the spinal cord, as has been demonstrated in normal human volunteers who received intradermal injections of capsaicin. In these subjects allodynia, hyperesthesia, and hyperpathia develop in a large area of skin beyond the injected site. These data may be interpreted as reflecting a spread of hyperexcitability to include cells within the central nervous system that were not initially activated directly by the neural injury. This nociceptor-evoked central hyperexcitability appears to be a normal consequence of tissue injury and is thought to be associated with the spread of pain in PHN. In the "normal" state the nociceptor sensitization and central hyperexcitability disappear with time and "normal" healing, regardless of the cause of the injury. This resolution is also true for the majority of those who have AHZ-related pain (34, 35).

Even in the absence of ongoing inflammation and injury, for example in a posttraumatic neuropathic pain state, there is evidence that acutely sensitized nociceptors may not normalize after healing, resulting in a state of continued inappropriate sensitization of C fiber nociceptors (36). This phenomenon, as seen in the ABC syndrome (angry backfiring C nociceptors) has not, however, been conclusively demonstrated in PHN patients. Data from animal experiments suggest that if C nociceptors travel through nerves that have survived damage to them, even though they are not in a constantly sensitized state, they are more than normally sensitive to circulating plasma norepinephrine. This phenomenon would result in more spontaneous and stimulus-evoked pain when these nociceptors were exposed to greater sympathetic efferent activity or greater amounts of circulating plasma catecholamines. In the attempt to find their peripheral targets, some regenerating axons may become misguided or trapped, and neuromas may form. Nociceptors and axonal sprouts in neuromas are known to be spontaneously active, more sensitive than normal to mechanical as well as to some forms of chemical stimulation, and more responsive than normal to thermal changes (35). A recent double-blind study revealed that subdermal injections of adrenaline directly into PHN skin increases pain and allodynia (36). Thus, these studies suggest that pain may in some cases be due to direct activation of C nociceptors in the skin and that allodynia may be centrally mediated and driven by abnormal C nociceptor input (36).

Although data to support these changes in PHN patients are more often based upon extrapolations of data from experiments done in animals with experimental nerve lesions, it has been demonstrated in PHN patients that large areas of skin that surround the infected nerve may have significant stimulus-evoked pain (38). These findings strongly suggest abnormalities of central nervous system function and sensory processing, because somatosensory neurons normally receive input from more than one nerve root. The death of some primary afferent neurons during an HZ outbreak has been associated with degeneration of their intraspinal connections, including a reduction in the number of intraspinal synapses. Whether this pathological change is in any way responsible for the development of PHN remains to be proved. Postmortem studies of

patients with PHN demonstrate notable atrophy of the spinal gray matter, most likely the consequence of damage occurring during a prior inflammatory response (37–41).

Nociceptor-related central hyperexcitability is known to involve spinal glutaminergic synapses through the N-methyl-D-aspartate (NMDA) receptor (34). NMDA receptor antagonists have been shown to prevent central hyperexcitability and suppress it once it is present (34). Thus, another postulated mechanism of PHN is damage or dysfunction of these dorsal horn neurons, which may contribute to a state of persistent sensory disinhibition (36).

Some investigators suggest that PHN is the result of anatomical injury to the primary afferent nerves and subsequent deafferentation of the dorsal horn neurons. However, it is clear that pain and allodynia do not directly correlate with loss of afferents and extent of sensory loss (17). Other investigators suggest that deafferentation may play only a minor role in PHN, noting that the patients with the most pronounced allodynia had minimal to undetectable sensory loss and that PHN pain was often the greatest in a zone of transition between areas of normal skin and the area of most significant sensory loss. Using quantitative sensory testing, these same investigators have shown that some patients with severe PHN and allodynia may demonstrate normal thermal sensory thresholds in the region of maximal pain (16). The conclusion is that for most PHN patients, pain severity is associated with preservation rather than loss of primary afferents. They did point out that a subgroup of patients, particularly those who had steady pain and little allodynia, were more likely to have pain in the region of maximal sensory loss, suggesting at least two mechanisms for PHN (16).

Therefore, both peripheral and central mechanisms for PHN have been postulated. Peripheral nervous system mechanisms include the development of spontaneous impulses from ectopic impulse generators from a neuroma, the axon, or the dorsal root ganglion itself. In addition, peripheral somatic nerve hypersensitivity to circulating catecholamines and the consequences of inflammation have been previously discussed. Central nervous system mechanisms include the loss of large nerve fiber (Aβ) afferent inhibition, deafferentation hyperactivity of central pain transmission neurons, aberrant central connections as a consequence of reorganization of the central nervous system, and central sensitization. Central sensitization can be demonstrated in normal human volunteers as summation, in which slowly repeated noxious stimuli become associated with an increase in pain. The neurophysiologic correlate to this may be the progressive increase in dorsal horn neuron response, also known as wind-up, that occurs when persistent similar noxious stimuli are steadily applied to the skin. Neuropeptides such as substance P and excitatory amino acids acting at the NMDA receptor have been shown to contribute to this response. Some large-diameter afferents, normally sensitive to light painless stimulation, may with central sensitization become capable of causing pain. Known as secondary hyperalgesia (primary hyperalgesia is the changes in primary afferents), this physiologic change may explain allodynia. This can also be observed without nerve damage and is considered a normal response to extensive nociceptive input (43–46).

In summary, many mechanisms most likely contribute to the pain associated with PHN. The fact that many pharmacological therapies with widely variant mechanisms of action may alleviate PHN pain also suggests the existence of multiple pathophysiological mechanisms, both peripheral and central, underlying the development and maintenance of PHN (34). Thus, current thought is that individual PHN patients differ with regard to pain mechanisms, hence also with regard to treatment effects.

TREATMENT OF HERPES ZOSTER

The treatment of pains associated with herpes zoster fall into two specific paradigms: (*a*) the pain of AHZ and (*b*) the pain of PHN. The pain of AHZ is an acute inflammatory, nociceptive, and neuropathic pain, whereas PHN is a chronic neuropathic pain. Thus, AHZ should be treated with an acute pain therapeutic paradigm, and PHN should be treated with a chronic neuropathic pain therapeutic paradigm.

However, these two "distinct" pains associated with HZ occur along a temporal continuum; that is, there is a defined evolution, the pain of PHN always evolving from AHZ. Yet the only factor that has well-documented supportive evidence of being a risk factor for this evolution is age of the patient; in fact, age is not a definitive factor either, since some patients with AHZ who are more than 80 years of age do not go on to develop PHN. Knowing that the acute pain of AHZ has the potential to transform into the chronic pain of PHN, clinicians have always looked for therapies that may be preventive, that is, treatments given during AHZ that may prevent PHN.

TREATMENT OF ACUTE HERPES ZOSTER

Corticosteroids

The largest controlled trial assessing the efficacy of corticosteroids given to patients with early AHZ (less than 72 hours after rash appearance) reported a significant decrease in the pain associated with AHZ and less analgesic use but failed to show an effect on the development of PHN (47). This study used 60 mg/day of prednisone with a 21-day taper.

Antiviral Drugs

Several antiviral agents are available for the treatment of AHZ, specifically acyclovir, valacyclovir, and famciclovir. The newer antiviral agents, valacyclovir and famciclovir, are more bioavailable when given orally than acyclovir and thus have a theoretical advantage over the older agent acyclovir. All three agents have been shown in large well-controlled studies to reduce the pain of AHZ similarly (48). Virology authorities do not consider any one of these agents clinically superior to another based on available clinical trial data (48).

Symptomatic Treatment

Pharmacotherapy

AHZ is an acute pain and should be treated with immediate symptomatic pain relief. Pharmacotherapy should be initiated immediately with around-the-clock dosing of opiate medication if necessary. NSAIDs may be useful adjuvants to moderate the pain of inflammation associated with the infection, although neither has been studied in a controlled fashion. Topical therapy using aspirin with diethyl ether has been described as helpful for AHZ (49, 50).

Nerve Blocks

Nerve blocks may provide immediate pain relief in AHZ. Many anecdotal reports and case series have described the efficacy of a variety of nerve blocks, including epidural, sympathetic, and peripheral blocks (51). However, no nerve block type has been studied in a controlled study, and so far no technique has been shown to be superior to another.

Are There Treatments That Prevent Postherpetic Neuralgia?

No, no therapies have been shown conclusively to prevent or reduce the incidence of PHN. However, several therapies are being promoted as reducing its incidence, mostly based on uncontrolled case series or statistical trends. *To tell a patient that a treatment will prevent PHN is setting up false expectations that cannot be guaranteed.* In addition, many PHN patients and their families have deep-seated anger toward themselves or physicians because of the belief that if the treatment (antiviral or nerve block) had been given earlier in the course of AHZ, PHN would not have developed. This anger can be an impediment to optimal treatment of PHN. The fact is that no therapy has been shown in well-controlled trials to significantly reduce the incidence of PHN.

Antiviral Therapy

Theoretically, antivirals if administered very early in the course of AHZ (during the gangliitis and before appearance of the rash) should minimize the damage to the nervous system and thus prevent PHN. Unfortunately, antivirals are most often prescribed too late in the course of the HZ to prevent nervous system injury. Most patients do not seek medical attention until after the rash has developed, and the patients who do seek medical attention prior to rash development are misdiagnosed with a cardiac or gastrointestinal disorder or cluster headache. Therefore, the antiviral drugs are prescribed *after* the zoster virus has extensively infiltrated neural structures, causing significant damage to them.

Studies indicate that antiviral therapy decreases the time of zoster-associated pain (52, 53). However, this end point of zoster-associated pain does not necessarily reflect the incidence of PHN. In fact, one of these studies did not show a reduction in PHN at 6 months (53), and the other study reported that 19% of subjects receiving valacyclovir continued to have pain at 6 months as compared with 26% who were given acyclovir (52). Thus, although all three antiviral agents are being promoted as reducing the time of zoster-associated pain or reducing the incidence of PHN, none has convincingly been demonstrated to reduce the incidence of PHN.

Nerve Blocks

Some anesthesiologists continue to promote the use of preemptive nerve blocks to prevent PHN (54). However, the data used to promote this procedure are uncontrolled (51). Since the natural history for most AHZ patients is a resolution of pain, no conclusion can be drawn from these uncontrolled case series. As pain anesthesiologist authority Fine has written, "[T]hese unsubstantiated claims must be regarded with healthy skepticism and held up to scientific scrutiny. These hopeful and tempting, but unproven, messages can not yet serve as standards for routine clinical practice" (51).

TREATMENT OF POSTHERPETIC NEURALGIA

Overview

Many patients continue to suffer needlessly with PHN. Unfortunately, patients are commonly told by their treating doctors, "There is nothing to do for your pain; you just have to live with it." The truth is that most patients with PHN can find some degree of pain relief.

Physicians are subject to the fallacy that PHN is a refractory condition because they have not been educated. The management of PHN is not taught in medical school and rarely in residency training; in fact, this sad fact holds for most chronic pain conditions. This lack of education results in most physicians not knowing *what* drugs to prescribe and *how* to prescribe the drugs properly.

In addition, quite often the PHN patient enters the doctor's office with preconceived ideas about treatment. Patients, especially the elderly, have unwarranted fears about taking pain medication. For them, pain medication means possible addiction. Another concern heard frequently is the misconception that taking an antidepressant means "the doctor thinks the pain is all in my head."

All of these issues that prevent proper management of PHN are easily rectifiable with proper education. The physician can easily learn about available therapies for PHN through many avenues, including books such as this one. Patients should learn about all therapies available for PHN at their doctor's office. Since the diagnosis of PHN is quite simple and the examination straightforward, the majority of time during the initial consultation should be devoted to educating the patient with PHN about the therapeutic options, allaying unwarranted fears and concerns, and providing optimism.

Table 8.1.   Medication Used to Treat PHN

Antidepressants
Tricyclic antidepressants
Venlafaxine
Antiepileptic drugs
Carbamazepine
Phenytoin
Gabapentin
Local anesthetic antiarrhythmic drugs
Intravenous lidocaine infusion
Mexiletine
Opioids
Topical drugs
Lidocaine
Capsaicin
Aspirin
Clonidine

Therapeutic Options

Several therapeutic approaches are available for the treatment of PHN. However, at present the gold standard of treatment is pharmacotherapy, that is, medication. Within the pharmacotherapeutic modality are many types of drugs that may relieve pain for any one PHN patient (Table 8.1). There are no means to predict which agent will work best for any patient. Therefore, each patient must be evaluated and treated empirically.

Even though many medications have been shown to alleviate the pain of PHN in some patients and have been shown to be safe, *no drug to date has an approved FDA indication for the treatment of PHN.* This lack of FDA approval should not be misinterpreted to mean that no drug alleviates PHN; rather, it reflects the lack of interest among the pharmaceutical industry to pursue an (expensive) indication.

Besides medication many other therapeutic modalities have been discussed in the medical literature, although none has been studied in a controlled protocol or recommended for PHN. These other therapeutic modalities include nerve blocks, central nervous system neuroaugmentation, neuroablative neurosurgery, and intrathecal drug delivery.

How to Prescribe Medication for Postherpetic Neuralgia

Pharmacotherapy remains the gold standard for PHN treatment. Within the past decade, many drugs have been studied in well-controlled protocols and shown to be efficacious for PHN. *However, no single drug or drug class has been shown to be effective in alleviating the pain in all PHN patients; there is significant individual variation.*

In clinical terms this principle means that some patients report significant pain relief and no side effects to drug X, while others (with the same symptoms) report no pain reduction and/or intolerable side effects to drug X. Moreover, some patients have a response (either positive or negative) at a certain drug dose and serum level, while others have a response at a dramatically different dose or serum level. Studies of many drugs have shown that there is *no correlation between drug dose, drug serum level, and the report of pain relief; again, there is significant individual variation.*

Thus, for the clinician this phenomenon translates into the necessity of sequential drug trials. Each drug must be titrated to assess its efficacy in any patient. To minimize confusion and potential side effects, only one drug should be titrated at any one time. The initial dose of each drug should be the lowest available dosage, and thereafter this dose should be increased every 2 to 7 days, depending on the drug being titrated, until the patient reports either significant pain reduction or intolerable side effects.

Another important element to proper pharmacotherapy is *assessment of the effect of each drug on the patient's different pain qualities.* Besides obtaining an overall rating of pain intensity, it is imperative that the treating physician obtain ratings of the different pain characteristics. Every PHN patient has several pains, such as burning, shooting, aching, itching and/or skin sensitivity (29). Although this factor is not thoroughly investigated to date, clinical experience has shown that a certain drug may significantly alleviate one type of pain yet have no effect on another. Therefore, a physician should ask how a drug has affected each pain quality when assessing a drug's efficacy. In addition, a physician should assess each drug's effect on allodynia and hyperpathia.

This phenomenon of individual variation with regard to a drug's efficacy may reflect the current hypothesis that PHN is not a single disease process but rather consists of a heterogeneous population with multiple different pain mechanisms within different PHN patients (29, 34).

DRUGS FOR POSTHERPETIC NEURALGIA

Antidepressants

Since the advent of the discovery that the tricyclic antidepressants can produce significant pain relief in PHN, every new antidepressant that becomes available is evaluated for efficacy in PHN. However, to date only the tricyclic antidepressants (TCAs) have several controlled trials that have reported significant benefit in some patients.

Tricyclic Antidepressants

Controlled Clinical Trials

The TCAs remain the best-studied class of drugs for the treatment of PHN. A review and meta-analysis of randomized trials in PHN concluded that only the TCAs offer "proven benefit" for PHN (55). Controlled studies have been reported with amitriptyline (11, 38, 56–58) and desipramine (59).

A randomized double-blind crossover study comparing amitriptyline, a mixed serotonin and norepinephrine reuptake inhibitor, with maprotiline, a tetracyclic with more-specific reuptake inhibition of norepinephrine, reported some interesting results (57). Although overall amitriptyline relieved more PHN patients' pain than maprotiline, four groups of patients were found: those with pain relief from both drugs, pain relief from only amitriptyline, pain relief from only maprotiline, and pain relief from neither drug. Thus, this study's results may be taken as evidence of individual variation with regard to response to different drugs and taken one step further, as evidence suggesting varying pain mechanisms among PHN sufferers.

Clinical Experience

Even though controlled trials have repeatedly shown that the TCAs are pain relievers in PHN, the clinical experience is not so good as the data suggest. A great many PHN patients either do not obtain significant pain relief or have intolerable side effects from TCAs.

Mechanism of Action

The mechanism of action of the TCAs is not known. Because these drugs are known to be reuptake inhibitors of the biogenic amines, until recently the only postulated pain mechanism has been that the TCAs act within the central nervous system's pain-modulating system, perhaps at the brainstem and dorsal horn (60). However, recently the TCAs have been shown to produce significant sodium channel blocking activity, which strongly correlates with the reduction in animal pain behavior in peripheral neuropathic pain models (61).

Recommendations

Recent controlled trials suggest that the TCAs must be recommended as the first-line choice for PHN. Yet the clinical experience of moderate efficacy and frequent intolerable side effects, especially in the elderly population, make the TCAs a tenuous gold standard.

Amitriptyline is the best-studied TCA, but many patients do not tolerate its side effects and may better tolerate an alternative TCA, such as desipramine or nortriptyline. The TCAs all differ significantly with regard to their serotonergic, noradrenergic, cholinergic, and histaminergic activity. Therefore, failure with one TCA, because of either poor pain relief or intolerable side effects, does not necessarily dictate failure with another TCA. Furthermore, because the TCAs produce sedation, a TCA may be used for the sole purpose of alleviating insomnia, even if the drug does not reduce the patient's pain. Insomnia is commonly seen among PHN patients and is another important symptom that should be treated.

Serotonin-Specific Reuptake Inhibitors

Controlled Clinical Trials

The only published controlled clinical trial of a specific serotonergic reuptake inhibitor (SSRI) for the treatment of PHN to date reported no effect with zimelidine (56). Recently a well-controlled parallel-design clinical trial compared the efficacy of fluoxetine, amitriptyline, and desipramine in patients with PHN (58). This study reported that all three antidepressants were statistically equally efficacious but that none produced a dramatic reduction in pain and all had significant side effects.

Clinical Experience

The clinical experience with the SSRIs for the treatment of PHN (and all other neuropathic pain conditions) is poor. Unfortunately, they do not appear to have a major role in the treatment of PHN.

Mechanism of Action

At present it is questionable whether the SSRIs actually relieve pain. Theoretically, like the TCAs, these drugs may act at the central nervous system pain-modulating sites. Fluoxetine has been shown to have some sodium channel blocking activity (61).

Recommendations

Based on current data the SSRIs cannot be recommended for treatment of PHN.

Venlafaxine

Controlled Clinical Trials

No controlled clinical trials assessing venlafaxine's efficacy in PHN have been published. Controlled clinical trials are under way.

Clinical Experience

A case series describing successful treatment of a variety of neuropathic pain conditions, including PHN, with venlafaxine has been presented (62). Physicians in pain clinics have used venlafaxine successfully in some patients who did not tolerate TCAs. However, even though venlafaxine does not cause the intolerable anticholinergic side effects of the TCAs, some patients are unable to tolerate venlafaxine because of nausea or agitation.

Mechanism of Action

Theoretically, venlafaxine's serotonergic and norepinephrine reuptake-inhibiting activity within the central nervous system may result in pain modulation. Venlafaxine also has local anesthetic properties.

Recommendations

Even though controlled clinical trials with venlafaxine have yet to be published, the clinical experience does suggest an emerging role for the treatment of PHN. Venlafaxine may be

prescribed for PHN patients after TCAs fail them. Dosing studies have yet to be published. The recommended starting dose is 25 mg per day and then thereafter titrated weekly to effect.

Antiepileptic Drugs

Phenytoin

Controlled Clinical Trials

No controlled trials assessing the efficacy of phenytoin in PHN have been published.

Clinical Experience

According to controlled clinical trials in other peripheral neuropathic pain conditions, especially painful diabetic neuropathy, clinicians have prescribed phenytoin for PHN for many years. However, phenytoin more often results in intolerable side effects than significant pain relief in the PHN patient.

Mechanism of Action

Phenytoin has strong sodium channel blocking activity.

Recommendations

Even though phenytoin has been prescribed for a variety of neuropathic pains, including PHN, its efficacy is low and its side effect profile in the elderly PHN patient is poor. Thus, phenytoin is a poor drug for PHN, especially with the emergence of newer drugs that appear to be more effective and better tolerated.

Carbamazepine

Controlled Clinical Trials

One small controlled trial reported that carbamazepine reduced the lancinating pains of PHN (63).

Clinical Experience

Although slightly better than phenytoin, carbamazepine also appears to have a poor efficacy-side effect ratio. Many more PHN patients report side effects than pain relief with carbamazepine.

Mechanism of Action

Carbamazepine has sodium channel blocking activity.

Recommendation

Based on the one small controlled study and vast clinical experience, carbamazepine should be prescribed for patients with PHN whom a TCA has failed in an adequate trial. But because of its modest efficacy and its proclivity to produce intolerable side effects, it is to be hoped that carbamazepine's role in PHN treatment will shrink in coming years.

Valproic Acid

Controlled Clinical Trials

No controlled clinical trial has reported utility of valproic acid for the treatment of PHN or any other neuropathic pain condition.

Clinical Experience

The clinical experience with valproic acid for the treatment of all neuropathic pains is poor. Moreover, valproic acid is often poorly tolerated by the elderly PHN patient.

Mechanism of Action

It appears that valproic acid does not possess any pain-relieving activity in neuropathic pain conditions.

Recommendation

It is recommended that valproic acid not be prescribed for the treatment of PHN.

Gabapentin

Controlled Clinical Trials

Controlled clinical trials of the use of gabapentin in treating PHN are under way.

Clinical Experience

The clinical experience among pain practitioners is that gabapentin appears to have significant efficacy for the treatment of PHN and other neuropathic pain. A published case report describes successful treatment of PHN with gabapentin (64). In addition, gabapentin appears to have a favorable side effect profile, with most patients able to tolerate clinically significant doses of the drug. Unlike other anticonvulsants, gabapentin does not have any hepatotoxicity, nor does it cause any blood dyscrasias. Gabapentin does not have any drug-drug interactions, making it safe for many elderly PHN patients on multiple other drugs.

Mechanism of Action

The mechanism of gabapentin's antiepileptic activity is not known. Glutamate antagonism has been proposed as a possibility.

Recommendation

Without results of a controlled clinical trial, gabapentin cannot be recommended as a first-line agent. However, the growing clinical experience, which demonstrates significant

efficacy and a laudable side effect profile, suggests that gabapentin should be prescribed for the PHN patient who does not respond to a TCA and carbamazepine. If the results of the controlled clinical trial mimic the apparent clinical experience, gabapentin may prove to be the drug of choice for PHN in the near future.

The dosage of gabapentin should be titrated until the patient reports significant pain relief or side effects. It is recommended that the uppermost dose be 3000 mg, although some clinicians have described patients who need up to 5000 mg (without side effects) before pain relief is reported.

Lamotrigine

Controlled Clinical Trials

No controlled trials on lamotrigine's efficacy in PHN or any other neuropathic pain condition have been reported.

Clinical Experience

A small uncontrolled study described pain reduction in patients with diabetic neuropathy following a trial of lamotrigine (65). To date, clinical experience has not suggested significant efficacy for PHN with lamotrigine, although the drug's side effect profile appears good.

Mechanism of Action

Lamotrigine has sodium channel blocking activity, suggesting a possible role in the treatment of peripheral neuropathic pain conditions, such as PHN.

Recommendation

Currently, lamotrigine should be reserved for the PHN patient whom conventional drugs have failed to treat.

Local Anesthetic Antiarrhythmics

Intravenous Lidocaine Infusion

Controlled Clinical Trials

A controlled study demonstrated that intravenous lidocaine infusion (5mg/kg body weight infused over 45 minutes) produced statistically more pain relief than placebo in PHN patients (66).

Clinical Experience

A large retrospective review of intravenous lidocaine infusions reported that most patients with peripheral neuropathic pains, including PHN, had a significant reduction in pain (67). However, even though an intravenous lidocaine infusion often produces a significant reduction in PHN, pain relief is transient, usually in the order of hours. Thus, this procedure cannot be used as maintenance therapy.

A prospective trial in peripheral neuropathic pain patients demonstrates that the response to an intravenous lidocaine infusion does predict subsequent response to a titrating trial of oral mexiletine (68). Thus, a patient who reports significant pain relief with a lidocaine infusion will most likely also respond to mexiletine, whereas a patient who does not report pain reduction with a lidocaine infusion will most likely not have clinically significant pain relief with mexiletine.

Mechanism of Action

Lidocaine is a strong sodium channel blocking agent.

Recommendation

An intravenous lidocaine infusion may be safely used in the PHN patient without a cardiac condition to predict whether a trial of mexiletine is warranted. The use of the intravenous infusion is one way to minimize the trial and error method of testing treatments.

Mexiletine

Controlled Clinical Trials

No published controlled trials have assessed the efficacy of mexiletine for PHN. However, controlled trials have demonstrated efficacy of mexiletine in the treatment of other neuropathic conditions, such as painful diabetic neuropathy (69).

Clinical Experience

No published clinical case series has described mexiletine for the treatment of PHN. Physicians in pain clinics have prescribed mexiletine for PHN with some beneficial results. Nausea is often a dose-limiting side effect.

Mechanism of Action

Mexiletine is a sodium channel antagonist.

Recommendation

Mexiletine should be reserved for the PHN patient without a cardiac history whom conventional therapies have failed. If possible, an intravenous lidocaine infusion should be performed before initiating a titrating trial of mexiletine.

Opiates

Controlled Clinical Trials

Recently, the first controlled trial that assessed an oral opiate for the treatment of PHN over several weeks was presented. This placebo-controlled study demonstrated statistical benefit from controlled-release oxycodone with minimal side effects (70). In addition, a prior placebo-controlled study

reported that an intravenous infusion of morphine produced significant pain relief in PHN (66).

Clinical Experience

A small open-label prospective study reported that PHN patients treated with a 2-month trial of controlled-release morphine, methadone, slow-release oxycodone, or hydromorphone had significant pain relief without intolerable side effects (71). The clinical experience among pain clinicians is that some PHN patients obtain the best balance of optimal pain relief and minimal side effects with time-contingent use of opiate medication.

Mechanism of Action

The opiates are active throughout the nervous system, with cortical, subcortical, spinal cord, and even peripheral nervous system sites of action.

Recommendation

Opiate use should be encouraged. Vast clinical anecdotal evidence suggests that some PHN patients obtain a significant amount of pain relief from time-contingent use of opiate medication without intolerable side effects and without developing tolerance. The clinician must demystify and debunk societal concerns of addiction by educating the patient. Opiates should be titrated like any other drug used to treat PHN, with the same end points, significant pain relief or intolerable side effects.

Topical Drugs

Topical drugs, (as opposed to transdermal drugs, which are applied on the skin but produce clinically significant drug levels in the blood) are those that are applied directly on the skin; have a mechanism of action locally in the skin, soft tissues, and peripheral nerves; and produce clinically insignificant serum drug levels. Thus, topical drugs have the theoretical advantage of producing pain relief without systemic side effects and drug-drug interactions.

Local Anesthetics

Controlled Clinical Trials

A new formulation of topical lidocaine, Lidoderm, has been shown in several single-session randomized double-blind, placebo-controlled trials to significantly reduce the pain of PHN when applied in both a gel and patch (15, 72).

The largest ever randomized parallel-design placebo-controlled study in PHN demonstrated efficacy with no side effects for Lidoderm patches following 4 weeks of treatment in 150 refractory PHN patients (73). The drug applied to the PHN skin via a topical patch appears to be particularly effective in reducing allodynia. Another formulation of topical local anesthetic, EMLA, composed of lidocaine and psilocaine, failed to demonstrate efficacy superior to that of placebo (74).

Clinical Experience

The two clinical sites, University of Washington and University of California at San Francisco, that have used lidocaine patches report that patients who use the drug for several years continue to obtain pain relief indefinitely, with some patients noticing a decrease in the size of the painful PHN region and others needing to apply the topical medication less and less frequently. No acute or chronic side effects have been reported.

Mechanism of Action

Lidocaine applied topically is thought to provide pain relief by reducing ectopic discharges in the superficial somatic nerves. In addition, the topical patch may protect the allodynic PHN skin from direct mechanical stimulation (72).

Recommendation

The only available topical local anesthetic drug, EMLA, does not appear to have significant efficacy for the treatment of PHN. If and when Lidoderm patches are approved by the FDA (at which point they will be the first drug to have an indication for the treatment of PHN), it is recommended that they be the first drug to be tried for several reasons: (a) good efficacy; (b) no need to titrate, a positive effect may begin within the first week of therapy; (c) no systemic side effects; (d) minimal overall side effects; (5) easy polypharmacy with oral agents if needed.

Capsaicin

Controlled Clinical Trials

All placebo-controlled trials of capsaicin are confounded by the fact that the drug causes burning upon application and therefore results in unblinding. The results of these controlled trials are mixed; two reported a benefit (75, 76) and one reported no benefit (77). The largest placebo-controlled study reported only a 15% reduction of pain from baseline with capsaicin (78).

Clinical Experience

The clinical experience among primary care physicians and pain specialists is poor. A review of capsaicin concluded that available formulations most often worsen the pain or provide no significant relief (79).

Mechanism of Action

Capsaicin selectively stimulates and then depletes substance P from nociceptive primary afferents, although this activity has not been proved to be the mechanism of action of capsaicin products. An alternative hypothesis is that capsaicin produces its effect on pain sensation by its counterirritant effect.

Recommendation

Available formulations of topical capsaicin are not recommended for the treatment of PHN because of its marginal efficacy and high prevalence of intolerable side effects.

Aspirin

Controlled Clinical Trials

A recently published double-blind, placebo-controlled crossover clinical trial with PHN subjects demonstrated statistically significant pain relief without any reported intolerable adverse reactions applying a topical aspirin-diethyl mixture (50). However, this study was only a single-session design, so long-term benefit and side effects were not assessed.

Clinical Experience

Several open-label studies and case series describe using topical mixtures of aspirin and chloroform or diethyl ether for the treatment of PHN (49, 80).

Mechanism of Action

Topically applied aspirin may desensitize the peripheral somatic nerve terminals that have been sensitized by an abnormal neurogenic inflammatory response (81).

Recommendation

Clinical experience is not very large, and the long-term efficacy of topical liquid aspirin is not yet known. However, the treatment does appear to have some efficacy and minimal side effects, and it is inexpensive.

Nonsteroidal Anti-Inflammatory Drugs

Controlled Clinical Trials

A single-session double-blind crossover study reported PHN efficacy for a topical diclofenac-diethyl ether mixture with no significant side effects (50). This same study reported that an indomethacin-diethyl ether topical mixture was not superior to placebo in a single-session protocol (50). Another single-session study observed significant pain reductions without complications with hydrous stupes (topical patches) containing indomethacin, ketoprofen, or flurbiprofen (82).

Clinical Experience

No long-term efficacy reports with topical anti-inflammatory drugs have been published.

Mechanism of Action

As with topical aspirin, topical NSAIDs theoretically may reduce primary afferent sensitization from an abnormal neurogenic inflammatory response (81).

Recommendation

Topical NSAIDs have not been well studied in a long-term controlled clinical trial for the treatment of PHN. However, available studies suggest that they may be a new type of therapeutic drugs that are effective, safe, and simple to use.

N-Methyl-D-Aspartate Antagonists

Controlled Clinical Trials

No published controlled clinical study has reported on use of NMDA antagonists for the long-term treatment of PHN. One published report assessed intravenous administration of ketamine 0.15 mg/kg in a double-blind crossover comparison with morphine and placebo (83). This single-session controlled study did report that ketamine produced significant pain relief and improvements in wind-up-like pain (i.e., pain evoked by repeatedly pricking the affected area) and mechanical allodynia. However, in this study all eight subjects reported either "bothersome" or "very bothersome" side effects with ketamine.

Clinical Experience

There is no large published clinical experience with the use of NMDA antagonists. Although several authorities hoped that dextromethorphan would be efficacious for PHN, a recent study failed to show efficacy, even though efficacy was reported for diabetic neuropathy (84).

Mechanism of Action

Animal models of peripheral neuropathic pain reveal that following a barrage of abnormal nociceptive input, a central hyperexcitability state develops and is maintained in the spinal cord; it involves activity at the spinal glutaminergic synapses of the NMDA type (34). NMDA antagonists both prevent the development of this hyperexcitability state and suppress its maintenance (34).

Recommendation

Today's NMDA antagonists cannot be recommended because there is no evidence suggesting efficacy, and ketamine carries a potential for significant side effects.

Phenothiazines

Controlled Clinical Trials

No published controlled studies have evaluated the efficacy of phenothiazines for PHN.

Clinical Experience

No large clinical experience with phenothiazines for the treatment of PHN has been published.

Mechanism of Action

Phenothiazines have not been shown to have analgesic qualities in neuropathic pain syndromes.

Recommendation

Phenothiazines should not be prescribed for the treatment of PHN because they lack efficacy and have short- and long-term adverse effects, especially in the elderly.

Sympatholytic Agents

Controlled Clinical Trials

No controlled clinical studies have assessed the efficacy of systemic sympatholytic drugs for the treatment of PHN. A single-dose placebo-controlled study demonstrated efficacy of oral clonidine in PHN subjects (85).

Clinical Experience

An open-label report observed pain reduction in PHN patients being treated with transdermal clonidine, with analgesic activity localized to the skin directly under the patch (86). An open-label study of intravenous phentolamine 35mg/kg over 30 minutes revealed significant pain relief and improvement of allodynia that lasted at least a week in 10 patients (87). Use of other sympatholytic agents has not been described.

Mechanism of Action

It has been postulated that in some patients with neuropathic pain syndromes, such as PHN, abnormal activity within the sympathetic nervous system may play a role in the maintenance of chronic pain. Postulated pathophysiologic mechanisms include abnormal activation of presynaptic (α_2-adrenoreceptors or ephaptic communication between the somatic and autonomic nerves (34).

Recommendation

These reports with use of clonidine in PHN and with transdermal clonidine's efficacy in a subpopulation of painful diabetic neuropathy patients as reported in a well-controlled trial (88) suggest that clonidine may be effective for some patients with PHN. Transdermal administration of clonidine may be preferable to the oral route, since it appears to be better tolerated and because a local peripheral effect from the topical application may be an independent mechanism of action.

Nerve Blocks

Controlled Clinical Trials

No placebo-controlled studies assessing the efficacy and safety of performing nerve blocks for the treatment of PHN have been performed.

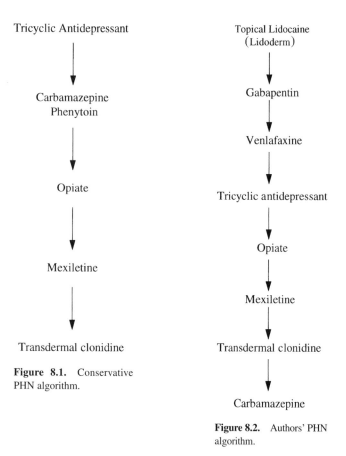

Figure 8.1. Conservative PHN algorithm.

Figure 8.2. Authors' PHN algorithm.

Clinical Experience

Although immediate pain reduction may or may not occur following somatic or sympathetic nerve block, long-term pain relief has not been shown to occur with single or series of such nerve blocks (51).

Recommendation

Nerve blocks are strongly advised against for established PHN. If pain relief does occur, it is short-lived, and repeated nerve blocks accrue the small but real potential complications of such invasive procedures.

Neuroaugmentation Therapies

Transcutaneous Nerve Stimulation

Controlled Clinical Trials

No well-controlled clinical trial has evaluated the use of transcutaneous nerve stimulation (TENS) for PHN.

Clinical Experience

Several small reports have described PHN pain reduction with TENS (89, 90). No large case series has been published. Today, the clinical experience of pain practitioners using TENS for PHN is not overwhelming. A small minority may report benefit, but the majority either have no significant pain relief or less commonly actually report a worsening of pain.

Recommendation

TENS should be given a 2-to 4-week trial in refractory PHN patients, since it is easy to use and it lacks serious side effects.

Spinal Cord Stimulation

Controlled Clinical Trials

No placebo-controlled trial has assessed the efficacy of spinal cord stimulation for PHN.

Clinical Experience

To date, there is no published large series of PHN patients treated with spinal cord stimulation. In a case series of 109 patients treated with spinal cord stimulation, 6 of 10 PHN patients were reported to have good pain relief (91).

Recommendation

At present spinal cord stimulation cannot be recommended for the treatment of PHN because of its lack of proven efficacy and its cost.

Surgery

Controlled Clinical Trials

No controlled study evaluating any surgical procedure for the treatment of PHN has been published.

Clinical Experience

Many ablative surgical procedures aimed at structures throughout the neuraxis have been described for the treatment of PHN, including undermining or excising skin, peripheral neurectomy, sympathectomy, myelotomy, cordotomy, thalamotomy, cingulotomy, and corticectomy, but none provides long-term pain relief (92). A recently published case series of dorsal root entry zone (DREZ) thermocoagulation in a variety of neuropathic pain conditions concluded that this surgery was not successful for PHN (93).

Recommendation

Pain neurosurgery authorities have cautioned against the use of surgery for PHN, especially neuroablative procedures (92).

PHN TREATMENT ALGORITHM

The treatment algorithm one chooses depends on one's practice style. A conservative physician practices medicine mostly according to proven therapies, that is, treatments that have undergone the rigors of placebo-controlled clinical trials, and thus are reluctant to use therapies based on anecdotal evidence. A less conservative physician may be willing to prescribe therapies with a certain degree of clinical experience but without published controlled trials. For this reason two separate algorithms are presented, one based on controlled clinical trials and medication available in 1997 (Fig. 8.1) and the other based on controlled studies, our clinical experience, and medication that will most likely be available in the coming years (Fig. 8.2).

References

1. Hope-Simpson RE. Studies on shingles: is the virus ordinary chicken pox virus? Lancet 1954;2:1299–1302.

2. Weller TH, Witton HM, Bell EJ. The etiologic agents of varicella and herpes zoster: isolation, propagation, and cultural characteristics in vitro. J Exp Med 1958;108:843–868.

3. Hope-Simpson RE. The nature of herpes zoster: a long-term study and a new hypothesis. Proc R Soc Med 1965;58:9–20.

4. Gilden DH, Dueland AN, Cohrs R, et al. Preherpetic neuralgia. Neurology 1991;41:1215–1218.

5. Loeser JD. Herpes zoster and postherpetic neuralgia. In: Bonica JJ, ed. The management of pain. 2nd ed. Philadelphia: Lea & Febiger, 1990;257–264.

6. Lewis GW. Zoster sine herpete. Br Med J 1958;2:418–421.

7. Gilden DH, Wright RR, Schneck SA, et al. Zoster sine herpete, a clinical variant. Ann Neurol 1994;35:530–533.

8. Ragozzino MW, Melton LJ III, Kurland LT, et al. Population-based study of herpes zoster and its sequelae. Medicine 1982;61:310–316.

9. Burgoon CF, Burgoon JS, Baldridge GD. The natural history of herpes zoster. JAMA 1957;164:265–269.

10. Hope-Simpson RE. Postherpetic neuralgia. J R Coll Gen Pract 975;25:571–575.

11. Brown GR. Herpes zoster: correlation of age, sex, distribution, neuralgia, and associated disorders. South Med J 1976;69:576–578.

12. Watson CPN, Watt VR, Chipman M, et al. The prognosis of postherpetic neuralgia. Pain 1991;46:195–199.

13. Rogers RS, Tindall JP. Geriatric herpes zoster. J Am Geriatr Soc 1971;30:359–365.

14. Max MB, Schafer SC, Culnane M, et al. Amitriptyline, but not lorazepam, relieves postherpetic neuralgia. Neurology 1988;38:1427–1432.

15. Harding SP, Lipton JR, Wells JCD. Natural history of herpes zoster ophthalmicus: predictors of postherpetic neuralgia and ocular involvement. Br J Ophthalmol 1987;71:353–358.

16. Rowbotham MC, Fields HL. Post-herpetic neuralgia: the relation of pain complaint, sensory disturbance, and skin temperature. Pain 1989;39:129–144.

17. Baron R, Saguer M. Postherpetic neuralgia: are C-nociceptors involved in signalling and maintenance of tactile allodynia? Brain 1993;116:1477–1496.

18. Rowbotham MC, Davies PS, Fields HS. Topical lidocaine gel relieves postherpetic neuralgia. Ann. Neurol. 1995;37:246–253.

19. Dworkin RH, Portenoy RK. Proposed classification of herpes zoster pain. Lancet 1994;343:1648.

20. Dworkin RH, Portenoy RK. Pain and its persistence in herpes zoster. Pain 1996;67;241–251.

21. Bean B, Deamant C, Aeppli D. Acute zoster: course, complication and treatment in the immunocompetent host. In: Watson CPN, ed. Herpes zoster and postherpetic neuralgia. Amsterdam: Elsevier, 1993;37–58.

22. Boon R. Efficacy and safety of famciclovir in the treatment of HZ. Paris: Second International Conference on the Varicella-Zoster Virus. 1994.

23. Dworkin RH, Hartstein G, Rosner HL, et al. A high-risk method for studying psychosocial antecedents of chronic pain: the prospective investigation of herpes zoster. J Abnorm Psychol 1992;101:200–205.

24. Head H, Campbell AW. The pathology of herpes zoster and its bearing on sensory localization. Brain 1900;23:353–523.

25. Bowsher D. Pathophysiology of postherpetic neuralgia: towards a rational treatment. Neurology 1995;45(Suppl 8): S56–S57.

26. Nurmikko T. Clinical features and pathophysiologic mechanisms of postherpetic neuralgia. Neurology 1995;45(Suppl 8): S54–S55.

27. Bhala BB, Ramamoorthy C, Bowsher D, Yelnoorker KN. Shingles and postherpetic neuralgia. Clin J Pain 1988;4:169–174.

28. Bowsher D. Sensory change in postherpetic neuralgia. In: Watson CPN, ed. Herpes zoster and postherpetic neuralgia. Amsterdam: Elsevier, 1993;97–108.

29. Galer BS, Jensen M. Development and preliminary validation of a pain measure specific to neuropathic pain: The Neuropathic Pain Scale. Neurology 1997;48:332–339.

30. Wood MJ, Johnson RW, McKendrick MW, et al. A randomized trial of acyclovir for 7 days or 21 days with and without prednisolone for treatment of acute herpes zoster. N Engl J Med 1994;330:896–900.

31. Portenoy RK, Duma C, Foley KM. Acute herpetic and postherpetic neuralgia: a clinical review and current management. Ann Neurol 1986;20:651–664.

32. Davies L, Cossins L, Bowsher D, Drummond M. The cost of treatment for postherpetic neuralgia in the UK. Pharmacoeconomics 1994;6:142–148.

33. Watson CPN, Deck JH, Morshead C, et al. Postherpetic neuralgia: further post-mortem studies of cases with and without pain. Pain 1991;44:105–117.

34. Fields HL, Rowbotham MC. Multiple mechanisms of neuropathic pain: a clinical perspective. In: Gebhart GF, Hammond DL, Jensen TS, eds. Proceedings of the VII World Congress on Pain, vol 2. Seattle: IASP Press, 1994.

35. Bennett GJ. Neuropathic pain. In: Wall PD, Melzack R, eds. Textbook of pain. 3rd ed. Edinburgh: Churchill Livingstone, 1994.

36. Choi B, Rowbotham MC. Effect of adrenergic receptor activation in post-herpetic neuralgia pain and sensory disturbances. Pain 1997;69:55–63.

37. Ochoa J. The newly recognized painful ABC syndrome: thermographic aspects. Thermology 1986;2:65–107.

38. Rowbotham MC, Fields HL. The relationship of pain, allodynia and thermal sensation in post-herpetic neuralgia. Brain 1996;119:437–454.

39. Zacks SI, Lagfitt TW, Elliot FA. Neurology 1964;14:744–750.

40. Watson CP, Evans RJ, Reed K. Neurology. Amitriptyline versus placebo in postherpetic neuralgia.1982;32:671–673.

41. Noordenbos W. Pain. Amsterdam: Elsevier, 1959.

42. Deleted.

43. Levine JD, Fields HL, Basbaum AL. Peptides and the primary afferent nociceptor. J Neurosci 1993;13:2273–2286.

44. Dickenson AH. NMDA receptor antagonists as analgesics. In: Fields HL, Liebeskind JC, eds. Progress in pain management and research, vol 1. Seattle: IASP Press, 1994;173–188.

45. Davies AM, Lodge LH. Evidence for involvement of N-methylaspartate receptors in "wind-up" of class 2 neurons in the dorsal horn of the rat. Brain Res 1987;424:402–406.

46. Price DD, Mao J, Frenk H, Mayer DJ. The N-methyl-D-aspartate receptor antagonist dextromethorphan selectively reduces temporal summation of second pain in man. Pain 1994;59:165–174.

47. Whitley RJ, Weiss H, Ghann J, et al. The efficacy of steroid and acyclovir therapy of herpes zoster in the elderly. J Invest Med 1995;43: (Suppl) 2:252A (abstract).

48. Kost RG, Straus SE. Postherpetic neuralgia: pathogenesis, treatment, and prevention. N Engl J Med 1996;335:32–42.

49. DeBenedittis G, Besana F, Lorenzetti A. A new topical treatment for acute herpetic neuralgia and post-herpetic neuralgia: the aspirin/diethyl ether mixture. An open label study plus double-blind controlled study. Pain 1992;48:383–390.

50. DeBenedittis G, Lorenzetti A. Topical aspirin/diethyl ether mixture versus indomethacin and diclofenac/diethyl ether mixtures for acute herpetic neuralgia and postherpetic neuralgia: a double-blind crossover placebo-controlled study. Pain 1996;65:45–61.

51. Fine PG. Nerve Blocks, herpes zoster, and postherpetic neuralgia. In: Watson CPN, ed. herpes zoster and postherpetic neuralgia. Amsterdam: Elsevier, 1993;173–185.

52. Beutner KR, Friedman DJ, Forszpaniak C, et al. Valacyclovir compared with acyclovir for improved therapy for herpes zoster in immunocompetent adults. Antimicrob Agents Chemother 1995;39:1546–1553.

53. deGreef H. Famciclovir, a new oral antiherpes drug: results of the first controlled clinical study demonstrating its efficacy and safety in the treatment of uncomplicated herpes zoster in immunocompetent patients. Int J Antimicrob Agents 1995;4:241–246.

54. Winnie AP, Hartwell PW. Relationship between time of treatment of acute herpes zoster with sympathetic blockade and prevention of postherpetic neuralgia: clinical support for a new theory of the mechanism by which sympathetic blockade provides therapeutic benefit. Reg Anesth 1993;18:277–282.

55. Volmink J, Lancaster T, Gray S, Silagy C. Treatments for postherpetic neuralgia: a systematic review of randomized controlled trials. Fam Pract 1996;13:84–91.

56. Watson CP, Evans RJ. A comparative trial of amitriptyline and zimelidine in postherpetic neuralgia. Pain 1985;23:387–394.

57. Watson CP, Chipman M, Reed K, et al. Amitriptyline versus maprotiline in postherpetic neuralgia: a randomised, double-blind, crossover trial. Pain 1992;48:29–36.

58. Davies P, Reisner-Keller L, Rowbotham MC. Randomized, double-blind comparison of fluoxetine, desipramine and amitriptyline in postherpetic neuralgia. International Association for the Study of Pain, 1996;193 (abstract).

59. Kishor-Kumar R, Max MB, Schafer SC, et al. Desipramine relieves postherpetic neuralgia. Clin Pharmacol 1990;47:305–312.

60. Basbaum AI, Field HL. Endogenous pain control mechanisms: review and hypothesis. Ann Neurol 1978;4:451–462.

61. Jacobson LO, Bley K, Hunter JC, Lee C. Anti-thermal hyperalgesic properties of antidepressants in a rat model of neuropathic pain. American Pain Society annual meeting, 1995;A-105 (abstract).

62. Taylor K, Rowbotham MC. Venlafaxine for chronic pain. American Pain Society annual meeting, 1995;A-105 (abstract).

63. Killian JM, Fromm GH. Carbamazepine with treatment of neuralgia. Arch Neurol 1968;19:129–136.

64. Segal AZ, Rordorf G. Gabapentin as a novel treatment for postherpetic neuralgia. Neurology 1996;46:1175–1176.

65. Eisenberg E, Alon N, Yarnitsky D, et al. Lamotrigine in the treatment of painful diabetic neuropathy. International Association for the Study of Pain, 1996;372 (abstract).

66. Rowbotham MC, Reisner-Keller LA, Fields HL. Both intravenous lidocaine and morphine reduce the pain of postherpetic neuralgia. Neurology 1991;41:1024–2028.

67. Galer BS, Miller KV, Rowbotham MC. Response to intravenous lidocaine differs based on clinical diagnosis and site of nervous system injury. Neurology 1993;43:1233–1235.

68. Galer BS, Harle J, Rowbotham MC. Response to intravenous lidocaine infusion predicts subsequent response to oral mexiletine: a prospective study. J Pain Symptom Manage 1996;12:161–167.

69. Dejgard A, Petersen P, Kastrup J. Mexiletine for treatment of chronic diabetic neuropathy. Lancet 1988;2:9–11.

70. Watson CPN, Babul N. Placebo-controlled evaluation of the efficacy and safety of controlled release oxycodone in postherpetic neuralgia. International Association for the Study of Pain, 1996;195 (abstract).

71. Pappagallo M, Raja SN, Campbell JN. Efficacy of opioids in the long-term management of postherpetic neuralgia. International Association for the Study of Pain, 1993;187 (abstract).

72. Rowbotham MC, Davies PJ, Verkempinck CM, Galer BS. Lidocaine patch: double-blind controlled study of a new treatment method for postherpetic neuralgia. Pain 1996;65:39–45.

73. Rowbotham MC, Davies PJ, Galer BS. Randomized, double-blind, placebo-controlled multicenter study assessing the efficacy of topical lidocaine patches in 126 patients with postherpetic neuralgia. International Association for the Study of Pain, 1996;184 (abstract).

74. Lycka BA, Watson CPN, Nevin K, Escobedo S. EMLA cream for treatment of pain caused by postherpetic neuralgia: a double-blind placebo controlled study. American Pain Society, 1996;A111 (abstract).

75. Bernstein JE, Korman NJ, Bickers DR, et al. Topical capsaicin treatment of chronic postherpetic neuralgia. J Am Acad Dermatol 1989;21:265–270.

76. Bruxelle J, Luu M, Kong-a-Siou D. Randomized double-blind study of topical capsaicin for treatment of postherpetic neuralgia. International Association for the Study of Pain, 1993;187 (abstract).

77. Drake HF, Harries AJ, Gamester RE, et al. Randomised double-blind study of topical capsaicin for treatment of postherpetic neuralgia. Pain 1990;(Suppl 5):S58 (abstract).

78. Watson CPN, Tyler KL, Bicker DR, et al. Randomized vehicle-controlled trial of topical capsaicin in the treatment of postherpetic neuralgia. Clin Ther 1993;15:10–26.

79. Watson CPN. Topical capsaicin as an adjuvant analgesic. J Pain Symptom Manage 1994;9:425–433.

80. King RB. Concerning the management of pain associated with herpes zoster and of postherpetic neuralgia. Pain 1988;33:73–78.

81. Rowbotham MC. Topical analgesic agents. In: Fields HL, Liebeskind JC, eds. Progress in pain research and management. Seattle: IASP Press. 1993.

82. Morimoto M, Inamori K, Hyodo M. The effect of indomethacin stupe for postherpetic neuralgia, particularly in comparison with chloroform-aspirin solution. Pain 1990(Suppl 5):S59 (abstract).

83. Eide PK, Jorum E, Stubhaug A, et al. Relief of post-herpetic neuralgia with N-methyl-D-aspartic acid receptor antagonist ketamine: a double-blind, cross-over comparison with morphine and placebo. Pain 1994;58:347–354.

84. Park KM, Nelson K, Robinovitz E, Max MB. High-dose oral dextromethorphan in diabetic neuropathy pain and post-herpetic neuralgia: a double-blind, placebo-controlled trial. American Pain Society annual meeting. 1995:A-115 (abstract).

85. Max MB, Schafer SC, Culnane M, et al. Association of pain relief with drug side effects in postherpetic neuralgia: a single-dose study of clonidine, codeine, ibuprofen, and placebo. Clin Pharmacol Ther 1988;43:363–371.

86. Kirkpatrick AF, Derasaria M, Piazza PA. Postherpetic neuralgia: a possible application for topical clonidine. Anesthesiology 1992;76:1065–1066.

87. Mekhail NA, Rodriguez RA, Hanna A. Role of systemic phentolamine in postherpetic neuralgia. Reg Anesth 1994;19(Suppl 2):84 (abstract).

88. Byas-Smith MG, Max MB, Muir J, Kingman A. Transdermal clonidine compared to placebo in painful diabetic neuropathy using a two-stage 'enriched enrollment design.' Pain 1995;60:267–274.

89. Nathan PW, Wall PD. Treatment of post-herpetic neuralgia by prolonged electrical stimulation. Br Med J 1974;1:645–647.

90. Loeser JD, Black RG, Christman A. Relief of pain by transcutaneous stimulation. J Neurosurg 1975;442:308–314.

91. Meglio M, Cioni B, Rossi GF. Spinal cord stimulation in management of chronic pain. J Neurosurg 1989;70:519–524.

92. Loeser JD. Surgery for postherpetic neuralgia. In: Watson CPN, ed. Herpes zoster and postherpetic neuralgia. Amsterdam: Elsevier Science, 1993;221–238.

93. Rath SA, Braun V, Soliman N, et al. Results of DREZ coagulations for pain related to plexus lesions, spinal cord injuries and postherpetic neuralgia. Acta Neurchir Wien 1996;138:364–369.

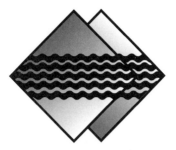

PART III

Regional Pain Disorders

CHAPTER 9

Spinal Cord Injury and Central Pain

Ronald R. Tasker

INTRODUCTION

The International Association for the Study of Pain (1) has defined central pain as "pain associated with lesions of the central nervous system," namely the spinal cord and brain. As such, it belongs to the group of neuropathic pain syndromes along with those caused by lesions of peripheral nerves and roots, with which it shares the unusual clinical features listed in Table 9.1 (2–5). It appears to be idiosyncratic; not every patient with a stroke or cord injury develops pain, even though the lesions involved may be identical. To support this notion, it is known that certain strains of rats and species of monkey are more prone to develop neuropathic pain than are others (6, 7). Central pain is caused by lesions of somatosensory pathways passing through the ventrocaudal nucleus (Vc) of thalamus, particularly the spinothalamic tract (8, 9). This is well demonstrated by its frequency after open mesencephalic tractotomy and by the fact that it never follows lesions of the kinesthetic pathways, such as those severed in thalamotomy for Parkinson's disease. It also never follows section of the nonspecific pain pathways passing through the medial thalamus that are divided during medial thalamotomy (10, 11). The pain is referred somatotopographically to the denervated area, and the causative lesion may be minimal, with no sensory loss or with total anesthesia. Sometimes only nonsomatosensory neurological signs and/or the circumstances of the case suggest subclinical damage to somatosensory pathways (5); or sensory loss may have been present when the causative lesion occurred, then faded with time. Pain onset may coincide with the occurrence of the lesion that caused the pain or may be delayed, increasing in severity and extent with time, suggesting a progressive central mechanism set in motion by the causative event. Central pain, like other types of neuropathic pain, commonly consists of several components. The most common of these are (*a*) steady, often causalgic and dysesthetic pain; (*b*) intermittent, neuralgic, and lancinating pain

Table 9.1. Features of Neuropathic Pain

It is idiosyncratic.
It is caused by lesions of primary somatosensory but not kinesthetic pathways, especially the spinothalamic tract.
Causative lesions may be minimal or massive.
Accompanying sensory loss ranges from none to complete anesthesia.
Pain onset is often delayed.
Pain has 3 common components, steady, neuralgic, and evoked (allodynia, hyperpathia).
Pain is in area of sensory change.
The steady element may be relieved temporarily by local anesthetic blockade but not by neural section at the same site.
The different components appear to have differing mechanisms and to respond differently to surgery.

and (*c*) evoked pain, such as allodynia and hyperpathia. Allodynia may be elicited by a single type of normally painless stimulus such as cold, particularly in brain central pain, (8, 9), or by several modalities, including kinesthetic stimuli. Of course, allodynia and hyperpathia can occur only in an area that is not completely denervated. However, evoked pain is not peculiar to neuropathic syndromes. Acute posttraumatic hyperesthesia is well known (12, 13), and physical compression of neuromas may cause a sensation like that of the neuralgic element of neuropathic pain. In my experience, unlike that of Riddoch (14), steady spontaneous pain is the most common feature of central pain syndromes, evoked and neuralgic pain being less frequent. Neuralgic pain is rare after stroke and most cord lesions except for those that affect the conus and cauda, where it is characteristic.

In an uncontrolled study (2) my colleagues and I found that the steady element of neuropathic pain was more responsive to the intravenous injection of sodium thiopental than of morphine sulfate, again suggesting a different mechanism from that of pain syndromes that are readily relieved with opiates. The steady element of neuropathic pain is usually temporarily relieved by proximal (2, 5) and distal (15) local anesthetic blockade but not by transection at the same site (2–5, 16–18), while the intermittent and evoked elements are relieved by both maneuvers. Thus, neuropathic pain consists of one or more components, each described consistently differently by the patients (19) and each of which appears to have a different pathophysiology requiring different strategies for therapy. For as discussed later, the evoked and neuralgic elements appear to be transmitted in pain pathways, but the steady element does not.

Many reviews of central pain (8, 9, 10, 11, 14, 20–21) are more or less in agreement with my experience as just briefly reviewed. I have never seen, however, an overreaction to pleasant stimuli such as described by Riddoch (14) and Foerster (22).

THE MECHANISM OF NEUROPATHIC PAIN

Table 9.2 lists some of the more popular proposals for the mechanism of neuropathic pain, including central pain (2, 3, 4, 10, 11, 23–26). Since I am unaware of any animal model for the chief element of central pain—that is, the steady, causalgic, or dysesthetic component—these proposals must depend on clinical observations. The main themes involve denervation neuronal hypersensitivity (27–40); somatotopographic reorganization (38–42), either through sprouting or more likely, opening up of inactive synapses; and mechanisms dependent on altered modulation within the central nervous system. Denervation neuronal hypersensitivity is often thought to be manifested by the appearance of bursting cells, which in turn in some way trigger the pain. Altered modulation may result from actual loss of inhibitory effects through damage to the pathway that mediates them by the causative injury, from imbalance between or among ascending pathways such as the neospinothalamic and spinoreticulothalamic, through selective damage to one of them (24), or by other means.

PAIN OF SPINAL CORD ORIGIN

Incidence

Various estimates of the incidence of pain following spinal cord lesions have been offered (Table 9.3). Since spinal cord lesions are usually the result of trauma, cord central pain affects males predominantly (76.4% of my series of 127 patients [54]). And the patients are usually young; 57.4% of my patients were under age 40. The median age in the series of Rose et al. (50) was the fourth decade.

Table 9.4 (54) lists the causation of cord central pain in my 127 patients, 65% of whom suffered from traumatic lesions. It is curious that a spinal cord lesion that results in no persistent clinically detectable neurological deficit (4% of our series) and one resulting in complete cord transection can both cause similar pain syndromes. There seemed little relation between the pain and its pattern and the level or completeness of a cord lesion; 42% of my patients suffered from cervical lesions—21%, T1 to T9 and 37%, T10 to L2; 32% had complete lesions; 64% had incomplete ones; and 4% had no sensory loss. Richards et al. (55) found cord central pain more common after gunshot wounds than other types of cord injury.

Table 9.2.   Possible Mechanisms of Central Pain

Denervation neuronal hypersensitivity usually correlated with the presence of bursting cells
Ephapses
Ectopic pulse generation
Somatotopic rearrangement with regeneration or with activation of quiescent synapses
Imbalance between excitatory and inhibitory pathways from damage by causative lesion
Disinhibition of pattern-generating systems
Selective destruction of neospinothalamic, sparing spinoreticulothalamic tract
Sympathetic influences
Hypothalamic disturbances

Table 9.3.   Published Estimates of Percent Incidence of Cord Central Pain after Spinal Cord Injury

Incidence (%)	Authors
6.4	Porter et al., 1966 (43)
7.5–10	White and Sweet, 1969 (44)
10–30	Casey, 1991 (42)
18–63	Mariano, 1992 (45)
25	Nepomuceno et al., 1979 (46)
26.8	Jefferson, 1983 (47)
27	Burke, 1973 (48)
33–94 (1/3 severe)	Yezierski, 1996 (49)
47–96	Yezierski, 1996 (49)
69.5 (49% severe)	Rose et al., 1988 (50)
77	Richards et al., 1980 (51)
80–94	Richardson et al., 1980 (52)
94	Botterell et al., 1954 (53)

Table 9.4.   Causation in 127 Cases of Cord Central Pain

Cause	Percent of Cases
Trauma	65
Iatrogenic causes	12
Inflammatory lesions	9
Neoplasm	6
Skeletal pathology	2
Vascular pathology	2
Congenital lesions	4

Delayed Onset

In a review of 72 cases (56) I found pain onset immediate in 17%, after less than 1 month in 13%, after 1 to 6 months in 19%, after 6 to 12 months in 8%, after 1 to 5 years in 13%, and after more than 5 years in 2%.

The Question of Syringomyelia

It is well known that spinal cord lesions of any type can lead to syringomyelia, which can progress and produce new neurological deficits to compound those caused by the original lesion. Unusually long latencies between the timing of the lesion responsible for cord damage and the onset of central pain raises concerns that the patient is developing a syrinx (seen in 16 of my 127 cases) (54). Some 37% of these patients with onset of pain delayed up to 1 year had a syrinx, as did 56% of those with delays of more than 1 year. Syringomyelia results in neuralgic pain related somatotopographically to the upper limit of the cyst, presumably caused by the cyst's impingement on certain cord structures as well as on steady causalgic dysesthetic pain over the area of the body in which the syrinx has introduced dissociated sensory loss. Milhorat et al. (57) have reviewed this subject very thoroughly.

The Phantom Phenomenon

Patients with complete spinal cord injury and amputees share the phenomenon of the phantom limb and sometimes phantom pain. Wall (58) and Carlen et al. (59) compared the two groups of patients, concluding that phantoms in paraplegics often did not appear immediately after the cord transection but rather after days to months, whereas they have immediate onset in amputees. Paraplegics' phantoms, which were not as vivid as those of amputees, tended not to telescope with time. Berger and Gerstenbrand (60) found that paraplegics lacked phantoms if they were comatose at the time of the cord injury; otherwise phantoms were usually present.

Quality of Cord Central Pain

Patterns of cord central pain are more complex than those in other neuropathic syndromes (49), the latter usually comprising only steady, neuralgic, and evoked components. White and Sweet (44) classified it as radicular (neuralgic), psychic, diffuse, sympathetic, and visceral. Pagni (11) listed visceral, radicular (most common in cauda equina lesions), and remote (causalgic and/or dysesthetic pain below the level of cord transection) pain. Other classifications include segmental, diffuse (burning or visceral), and lesional (projected or triggered) (61, 62). Rose et al. (50) recorded a 12.4% incidence of radicular and a 43% instance of constant pain in their patients. Berić et al. (63) found only a 13% incidence of what they called central dysesthesia syndrome, a spontaneous feeling of diffuse dysesthesia and causalgia. Davis and Martin (64) found that one third of their 471 cases had shocklike electric pain at or below the level of injury. Richards et al. (51) described musculoskeletal (in an innervated area), radicular (at the zone of injury and extending caudally), visceral, central (dysesthetic), psychogenic, lesional (at the zone of injury), reflex sympathetic dystrophy, and limb pain (from compression, mononeuropathy, especially in the upper limb). Nashold (65) described radicular, segmental, segmental with syrinx, phantom, and visceral pain; pain was a problem in 10% of his cases. Milhorat et al. (57) reported the pain patterns in the 71 patients of his series of 137 who had syringomyelia as "segmental dysesthetic in 51%, radicular in 36%, headache in 25%, suboccipital and cervical in 67%, in the back in 17%, in the face in 9%." The dysesthetic pain in their patients consisted of one or more of the following: burn-

Table 9.5.   Nature of Pain in 127 Cases of Cord Central Pain

Pain Quality	Percent of Cases
Burning	75
Numb, tingling	26
Shooting[a]	31
Evoked[b]	47
Musculoskeletal-like[c]	15
Visceral	3

[a]2% in isolation.
[b]4% in isolation.
[c]Below a complete level of sensory interruption.

ing, paresthetic, and a feeling of stretch or pressure, and they included trophic changes.

Table 9.5 lists the types of pain seen in my 127 patients. In contradistinction to the series quoted earlier, 96% suffered from steady, burning, or dysesthetic pain or both. In agreement with the observations of others, neuralgic shooting pain occurred most commonly with lesions of the conus and cauda between T10 and L2, and this type of pain occurred in 69% of patients with such lesions. On the other hand, 57% of patients with lesions at T10 to T12 in my series had such neuralgic pain.

Patients with cord central pain may suffer from two additional types of pain peculiar to cord lesions in addition to the usual steady, neuralgic, and evoked elements. Both of these are usually felt below a complete level of cord transection. Visceral pain resembles the pain of abdominal or pelvic disease and sometimes leads to extensive negative investigation and even surgery. The musculoskeletal pain resembles the pain of spinal instability or muscle tension, though it occurs in an area of anesthesia and is not associated with either of these features. I could find no particular correlation between pain quality and site or degree of cord lesion except for the association of visceral and musculoskeletal pain with complete lesions and of neuralgic pain with lesions of the conus and cauda; evoked pain can occur only in areas of incomplete sensory loss. More so than in other neuropathic syndromes, cord central pain may change or even lessen dramatically over time quite apart from the development of syringomyelia.

The Mechanism of Cord Central Pain

Yezierski (49) and Nashold (65) have reviewed cord central pain in detail, revealing the dearth of investigations into the understanding of its mechanism. Levitt and Levitt (6) studied the issue in monkeys. For pain to develop (as evidenced by autotomy), section of the anterolateral quadrant of the cord or hemisection preserving some sensation in ipsilateral nociceptive pathways seemed necessary. Pain never followed a posterior quadrant or funicular section, while simultaneous section of ipsilateral, lateral, or anterolateral cord quadrants, in addition to the ones whose section usually causes pain, prevented pain. Administration of morphine, subsequent transection of the cord rostral to the lesion, or subsequent rostral cord lesions identical to the ones that caused the pain failed to relieve it, and the researchers were unable to correlate the appearance of pain with any particular cord pathway.

Lenz (41) took advantage of thalamic exploration with microelectrodes for implantation of electrodes for deep brain stimulation (DBS) to study cord central pain. He found: (*a*) Receptive fields (RFs) were missing, as expected for the denervated part. (*b*) There was an increase in thalamic neurons without RFs. (*c*) There was takeover of part of the thalamic representation of the deafferented part by neurons with RFs in the border zone of the deafferentation resulting in an unusually large representation of these areas in the thalamic body map compared with what would be found in exploring, say, a patient with Parkinson's disease. (*d*) There was mismatch between the RFs and the projected fields (PFs) from stimulation at these sites. (*e*) In the area related to the deafferentation there were bursting cells whose spiking characteristics were typical of calcium spikes. These observations raised the question of a possible relationship between pain and the abnormal features described.

Pagni and Canavero (66) reported a patient with a spinal cord cyst at T9 associated with burning pain in the left leg, reduced temperature appreciation on the lateral aspects of both legs, and cold and deep pressure allodynia in the left leg. A single photon emission computed tomography (SPECT) scan showed diminished perfusion of the contralateral thalamus in this patient. Resection of the cyst both eliminated the pain and normalized the SPECT scan, an effect that they were also able to produce transiently by the intravenous administration of propofol. They related this observation to Hamby's account (67) of central pain relieved by removal of the causative lesion and to their own findings and those of Cesaro et al. (68) associating reduced thalamic activity in positron emission tomography (PET) or SPECT scans with contralateral stroke-induced peripheral neuropathic or cancer pain. In the latter, successful cordotomy normalized the thalamic scan. This suggested that whatever mechanism was responsible for the changes in the thalamic scan, it was not peculiar to neuropathic pain. It is particularly interesting that central pain can be reversible, suggesting that the responsible mechanism is not necessarily dependent on structural changes.

Surgical Treatment of Cord Central Pain

General Considerations

When central pain caused by cord lesions is sufficiently disabling and fails to respond to conservative measures, surgery is often considered. The choice among the options available depends not only on their efficacy, risk, and complexity but also on the nature of the pain from which the patient suffers. Though cord central pain can consist of five or more components, the two most frequently encountered in my experience are a steady, burning, dysesthetic element through-

out much or all of the body below the patient's level of cord interruption and intermittent shooting neuralgic pain, particularly running down the legs, characteristic of low thoracic and cauda lesions.

Table 9.6 (54) summarizes my experience, showing that evoked and neuralgic but not steady pain is relieved by destructive surgery (cordotomy, cordectomy, or dorsal root entry zone [DREZ] lesions) that interrupt pain paths, whereas the reverse is true for chronic stimulation techniques. The differences were statistically significant. Visceral and musculoskeletal pain are too rare for conclusions to be drawn. From these observations I have concluded that the steady pain does not depend upon transmission in pain pathways (2–4) but that neuralgic and evoked pain do. Neuralgic pain may arise from ephapses or from ectopic impulse generation at the site of injury, probably in the roots of the cauda equina (25, 26), with subsequent transmission in pain tracts. Evoked pain, especially allodynia, when caused by peripheral nerve or root lesions, is probably generated through perverted processing in the dorsal horn (69–71), whence transmission proceeds centrally in pain pathways. Such a mechanism may apply in lesions of the cauda equina and when such pain components occur in a radicular distribution associated with cord injury at higher levels. However, evoked pain also accompanies cord and brain lesions, in which case it is not related to roots when the mechanism must obviously be different. Even in the case of brain central pain, however, evoked pain can be relieved by chronic stimulation of the periventricular gray (PVG) so that it behaves as if transmitted in pain pathways (72); for PVG DBS is thought to depend upon blocking access of nociceptive stimuli into spinothalamic tract. When Nashold and colleagues (73–75) introduced the spinal DREZ procedure, they did not specify its mechanism of action. At about the same time, Sindou et al. (76) introduced the technique of making cuts with a scalpel in Lissauer's tract to relieve the pain of cancer at a lesion site very similar to that used by Nashold and Ostdahl (73). Although it has been popular to associate the Nashold DREZ procedure with the destruction of bursting cells whose presence is associated with deafferentation and neuropathic pain (27–41), Sindou's procedure clearly interrupted pain pathways. Thus, it does not seem unreasonable to me that the DREZ procedure, no matter how performed, should be particularly beneficial for the relief of the evoked and neuralgic elements of cord central pain because it interrupts pain pathways. The question of steady pain—its relation to bursting cells and its response to the DREZ operations—requires further study. My impression is that although the mechanism of steady burning dysesthetic pain is unknown, sometimes it can be reversed by chronic stimulation of nerve, spinal cord, or brain that produces paresthesias in the area of the pain. When neuralgic and steady pain occur together, the neuralgia is usually the more severe, so that procedures that relieve it may also appear to relieve the steady pain, because steady pain does not produce great disability after the neuralgic pain is gone. Nevertheless, not all patients conform to

Table 9.6.   Response of Common Components of Cord Central Pain to Surgery

| | | Percent of Patients with Good (>50%) and Fair (25–50%) Relief | | | | | |
| | | Steady | | Neuralgic | | Evoked | |
Procedure	No. of Patients	Good	Fair	Good	Fair	Good	Fair
Cordotomy	39	6	21	54	32	50	25
Cordectomy	12	0	30	60	40	80	20
DREZ	4	0	0	–		50	50
DCS	22[a]	27	14	0	0	0	25
DCS	11[b]	0	20	0	0	0	0
PPDBS	12	25	17	0	0	0	0

[a]Incomplete lesions
[b]Complete lesions

these guidelines, small numbers of our patients being relieved of steady pain by destructive lesions. White and Sweet (44) reported a patient relieved of burning leg pain by cordotomy.

As we review experience with surgical procedures to relieve cord central pain, we must keep in mind not only that its different components with their apparently differing mechanisms require differing therapeutic strategies but also that cord pain syndromes may consist of elements dependent both on cord and root damage.

Operations for Syrinx

It is my experience that decompression of a syrinx relieves any associated neuralgic pain but not the steady burning dysesthetic element. Milhorat et al. (57) addressed this subject in detail. They found that of 37 patients operated upon for syrinx who suffered from pain, 7 were totally and 15 partially relieved 6 weeks after the procedure; the rest were no better. After a year, 9 of the 37 patients were still better, but all complained of unpleasant symptoms. They concluded that syrinx surgery was disappointing with respect to pain relief, 41% of their patients showing either no change or aggravation of their pain postoperatively.

Destructive Surgery

Other surgical options in cord central pain can be divided into destructive and modulatory procedures.

Rhizotomy   Nashold (65) suggests that rhizotomy occasionally may be useful in "single root pain." In my experience it can be done, preferably percutaneously, to relieve allodynia in a single root distribution, for example at the upper end of a complete cord section. Of 72 of my patients with cord central pain, 5 had undergone rhizotomy and 1, intercostal neurectomy in other centers. In 2 of these patients a rhizotomy at C4 and T5–T12 respectively had relieved hyperpathia in the appropriate area.

Cordotomy   White (77) found cordotomy useful for relieving the radicular but not the steady element of cord central pain. White and Sweet (44) concluded that cordotomy "will relieve somatic pain following injury to the cauda equina, provided analgesia to the level of the xiphoid is achieved and maintained . . . pain, even when it follows injuries to the conus medullaris, can be relieved, at least in the majority. . . . With lesions situated in the thoracic portion of the spinal cord the operation is less likely to succeed." They wrote that 56% of their patients were relieved by high cordotomy. Bors (78) declared cordotomy useless for phantom pain in paraplegics (diffuse, dysesthetic pain below the injury level). Davis and Martin (64) did cordotomies on 18 of 126 paraplegics, relieving burning pain in only 1 but radicular pain in 50% of those who suffered from it. Botterell et al. (53) recognized the preferential effects of cordotomy on neuralgic over steady pain in 6 patients, the overall 67% success rate reflecting relief of neuralgic pain only. The experience of Porter et al. (43) was similar; 47% of their 34 patients enjoyed long-term relief.

However, patients with cord central pain survive a long time. Rosomoff et al. (79) reported that in their series of cordotomies, pain relief was achieved in 90% immediately after the procedure, 84% after 3 months, 61% after a year, 43% between 1 and 5 years, and 37% between 5 and 10 years. Of our patients, 25 with cord central pain underwent cordotomy, and pain is known to have recurred in 6 after 1, 1.1, 4, 5, 13 and 21 years, respectively, associated with fading of the analgesic level. Repetition of the cordotomy sometimes restored pain relief and the level of analgesia.

Cordectomy   The term cordectomy, referring to an operation long used in attempts to treat cord central pain, is applied to two procedures: actual removal of a segment of spinal cord and more often, cord transection above the level of the lesion causing the pain. Nashold (65) has reviewed the history of the procedure. Melzack and Loeser (80) failed to relieve 5 patients of cord central pain but achieved relief in another for 11.1 years before pain recurred. Other authors (81, 82) noted a preferential effect on the sharp but not the steady element of the pain. Pagni (11) failed to relieve pain in 6 patients with causalgic dysesthetic pain but was successful in 1 patient with intermittent sharp pain. Jefferson (47) studied cordectomy in more detail, noting that it was more successful with pain caused by lesions below T10, especially if the pain occurred in the anterior thighs and knees and especially if it was episodic. In 4 patients with cord lesions at or above T10 only 1 derived 25% pain relief. Of 15 patients with lower lesions (2 at T11, T12; 7 at T12, L1; 6 below L1), 7 enjoyed 100% pain relief, 7 more than 70% relief, and one, 50% relief; success occurred in what Jefferson called thighs, knees, or legs patterns. However he didn't think that such pain was necessarily radicular (Anthony Jefferson, personal communication, 1983). In 12 of my patients (Table 9.6) 100% were relieved of these elements and 30%, of steady pain. Druckman and Lende (81), however, report a seemingly suitable candidate for cordectomy with lancinating pain who failed to respond to previous cordectomy.

The Dorsal Root Entry Zone Procedure

Nashold and his group (65, 74, 75) reported the relief of cord central pain in 10 of 13 paraplegics, of whom 10 suffered from lesions of conus and cauda. In a subsequent report about half of 13 paraplegics were relieved. Richter and Seitz (83) reported partial relief in 2 of 10 paraplegics, and Sweet and Poletti (84), in 1 of 2.

Nashold and Bullitt (74) and Friedman and Bullitt (85) found the DREZ operation particularly effective for the "end zone" pain after spinal cord injury, reporting pain relief in 80% of 31 patients with pain starting at the level of the injury and extending distally and in 32% of 25 patients with diffuse sacral pain. Further reviews of the experience of this group with cord central pain have also been published (86, 87). Friedman et al. (88) divided cord central pain into two classes: Pain that extends into the dermatomes immediately caudal to the level of the injury is described as root pain, radicular pain, or end zone pain. Pain that extends into areas remote from the injury site is described as phantom, body, or diffuse burning pain. In such patients DREZ lesions were made beginning two spinal segments above and extending below the level of injury. Overall, 50% of 56 patients enjoyed good relief. However, 74% of the 31 patients who had pain starting at the injury level and extending caudally did well, but only 20% of the 25 patients with diffuse or predominantly sacral pain were relieved. Looked at another way, only 38% of 26 patients with a significant burning component did well. They quote Young's experience (89) with 57% of 14 patients gaining relief. Powers et al. (90) in a small series also described better results in patients with end zone than diffuse or sacral pain. Friedman et al. (88) conclude that DREZ procedures "are successful in relieving end zone pain following a spinal cord injury." In a literature review of 138 cases from 8 series, overall there was 54% good results. Selection of patients with end zone pain, which I interpret as including the neuralgic element, would doubtless enhance these results.

Destructive Stereotactic Lesions Published results after stereotactic lesions are difficult to analyze because the reported series tend to be small and to include patients with different types of chronic pain and because the lesions made are often at varied and/or multiple sites; often the pain syndromes from which the patient suffered are not stated. In a literature review (18), I found that 22 to 36% of 150 cases of central pain treated by thalamotomy at various sites resulted in good relief of pain, with 27% complications, compared with 60 to 70% success in cancer pain. After mesencephalic tractotomy Nashold (91) concluded from a literature review that 50% of patients with central pain benefited; Tasker (17), 27%; Cassinari and Pagni (10), Pagni (92), and Davis and Stokes (93), 50%. Pagni (92) reported 30% relief in his own experience. In published series of mesencephalic tractotomy the mortality ranged from 5 to 10%; the incidence of dysesthesia, from 15 to 20%; and that of oculomotor disturbances 15 to 20%. Gybels and Sweet (94) concluded from a literature review that mesencephalic tractotomy resulted in a 44% incidence of pain relief in neuropathic pain and 86% in cancer pain at the expense of 0 to 8% mortality.

Perhaps if stereotactic destructive procedures were reserved for patients with neuralgic pain, the results would be better.

Chronic Stimulation

Peripheral Nerve Stimulation Peripheral nerve stimulation usually has no role in the treatment of cord central pain (95).

Dorsal Column Stimulation The purpose of dorsal column stimulation (DCS) is to induce paresthesias in the patient's area of pain by inserting an electrode into the epidural space at the appropriate level (96, 97), although the mechanism of action is unclear. In cord central pain two technical matters often thwart success. First, prior spinal surgery may have made access to the extradural space at the appropriate level impossible for percutaneous insertion of an electrode and difficult or risky for those inserted by open laminectomy. In addition, cord lesions often damage the dorsal columns whose stimulation is necessary for the success of DCS. When the damage is severe, these structures "die back" to the dorsal column nuclei, preventing the induction of paresthesias by stimulation. Although seldom spelled out in the reports in the literature, these two issues probably account for the low success rate of DCS for cord central pain. For it is my experience that if appropriate paresthesias can be produced, pain relief may occur. Obviously a preliminary trial of DCS is important in these patients prior to internalization. Thus, in an earlier review (56), of 11 personal cases with complete cord lesions only 20% reported 25 to 50% (fair) relief of pain, and that in the narrow zone surrounding the patient's level of cord damage. Some 27% of patients with incomplete lesions had good results, and 14% had fair initial results. Neuralgic pain was never relieved, and 25% of those with allodynia and hyperpathia (3 patients) reported fair relief. In a longer-term review of 193 patients treated with DCS for various pain syndromes (98), 34 suffered from cord central pain. Of these 41% (14 patients) passed the test of trial stimulation, and 6% of the original 34, that is, 43% of those internalized, enjoyed significant long-term relief. All of these were patients with steady pain caused by lesions in the conus and cauda. Allodynia was also relieved in some of these patients, but actual numbers are not available.

Sweet and Wepsic (99) relieved postcordotomy dysesthesia in 2 of 7 patients with DCS, pain from cord lesions in multiple sclerosis in 1 of 3, pain from trauma in none of 4, and pain from various myelopathies in none of 5. Lazorthes et al. (100) relieved 2 of 9 cases of cord central pain during trial stimulation. Urban and Nashold (101) reported relief in 1 of 3 cases. Richardson et al. (52) stated that 5 of 10 of their paraplegic patients gained at least 50% pain relief during trial stimulation. Pagni (11) and Nashold (102) concluded that DCS was a poor operation for treating central pain.

Deep Brain Stimulation   In patients with steady pain in whom DCS is technically impossible, paresthesia-producing DBS (PPDBS) is worth considering, since no matter how complete the cord lesion, paresthesias (PFs) can still be produced below the patient's level by electrical stimulation of the medial lemniscus or thalamus. Unfortunately, cord central pain is often bilateral, requiring bilateral DBS.

Mention has already been made of the notion that the steady element of central pain appears not to be dependent on transmission in pain pathways and is therefore not relieved by cutting them but rather by inducing paresthesias in the area of pain; on the other hand, allodynia and neuralgic pain depend on transmission in pain pathways and are relieved by interrupting those pathways. If this is so, one would expect PPDBS to be useful in the treatment of steady but not of evoked or neuralgic pain and PVG DBS or DBS in periaqueductal gray (PAG) to be useful for the treatment of pain dependent on transmission in pain pathways, including evoked and neuralgic pain (103). Although there is not universal acceptance of this dichotomy, I implanted electrodes in both ventrocaudal nucleus (Vc) and PVG in 25 patients with steady neuropathic pain, inducing relief only by stimulating the Vc electrodes.

Mundinger and Salomao (104) reported one good, one fair, and one poor outcome with PPDBS in cord central pain. Adams (105) reported relief in 2 of 3 patients with postcordotomy dysesthesia and neither of 2 with spinal cord injury using PPDBS. Hosobuchi (106) relieved pain in 1 of 6 paraplegics with PPDBS. Richardson and Akil (107) relieved 2 of 5 paraplegics. Mundinger and Salomao (104) reported good pain relief with PVG DBS in 1 paraplegic. Turnbull (108) found cord central pain the least responsive neuropathic syndrome to PPDBS. In an early review (56) 6 patients with cord central pain underwent trials of PPDBS. Of these, 2 failed to respond, 2 lost their pain from the microthalamotomy effect of DBS electrode insertion, and 1 enjoyed ongoing relief

(109). Finally, 1 patient developed ventriculitis and died; he refused to allow removal of his electrode after developing a superficial infection because its stimulation relieved his pain. In a subsequent review (103) of PPDBS in 16 patients with cord central pain, 13 were test-stimulated and 6 internalized. In that trial 4 patients (31% of those undergoing trial stimulation, 67% of those internalized) derived long-term relief, but only of their steady element. Six published series reviewed by Tasker and Vilela (103) reported a 0 to 59% success rate. Our complications included 1.6% mortality from ventriculitis; 1.6% incidence of hematoma with permanent neurological deficit; 11.2% incidence of intracerebral hematomas, mostly detectable only on computed tomography (CT) or otherwise associated with transient symptoms; and 1.6% incidence of subdural hematoma requiring evacuation. There was 11% incidence of superficial infections and 44% incidence of technical problems with the hardware, such as lead migration and inadequate paresthesia production, many requiring surgical revision. All of these patients were implanted with monopolar electrodes anchored in various ways prior to our use of the much superior four-pole Medtronic 3387 electrode (Medtronic Corp., Minneapolis, Minnesota) with the bur hole ring and cap device provided to lock it in place. The use of this electrode, securely fixed to the skull, has dramatically reduced technical complications, and the use of prophylactic antibiotics has reduced the infection rate to 2%. Complications reported in the literature (103) included incidences of up to 1.6% mortality, 15% hematoma, 2.1% psychosis, 7.8% confusion, 8.5% mild hemiparesis, 5.2% deep infection, 15% superficial infection, 18% device failure, up to 30% equipment breakage and avulsion, and 27.5% lead migration. Levy et al. (110, 111) carried out PPDBS in 7 and PAG DBS in 7 of 11 patients with cord central pain. Of each group 2 patients were internalized, but none derived long-term relief. Of 5 patients with postcordotomy dysesthesia undergoing PPDBS, 2 were internalized and enjoyed long-term relief. Of 2 patients treated with PAG DBS, 1 was internalized but had no long-term relief. Complications included 0.7% mortality; 3.5% hematomas; 12.1% infections, including 0.7% meningitis; and 12.1% complications related to hardware.

BRAIN CENTRAL PAIN

Incidence

It has been estimated (42) that 1 to 2% of strokes give rise to pain. Andersen et al. (112) followed 207 stroke patients sequentially and found that 8% went on to develop central pain and 7% allodynia; pain was severe in 5%. Thus, like cord central pain, brain central pain is idiosyncratic.

Side of Responsible Lesion

Tasker and De Carvalho (113) reviewed 73 patients with brain central pain, of whom 43.9% had pain on the right side and 53.4% on the left side of the body. Of the 11 patients who had thalamic lesions either confined to thalamus (6) or extending to the cerebral cortex (5), 9 had left-sided pain and 2, right, confirming Kameyama's (114) finding of a preference for right thalamic lesions to cause pain.

The Role of Thalamus

Although Déjérine and Roussy's classical account (115) of brain central pain has led to the continued use of the term thalamic pain and to many attempts to correlate pain with a particular thalamic nucleus, the weight of published experience, even before the era of modern imaging, has gradually revealed that brain central pain does not depend on thalamic disease (56, 112). Although pain can follow brain lesions at any level from brainstem to cortex, cortical lesions are rarely associated with pain, pain rarely follows craniocerebral injuries or craniotomies, it is rare to induce pain by electrical stimulation of the brain (56), and epileptic seizures arising in somatosensory cortex rarely cause contralateral pain as part of the ictus (116). Marshall (117) found only 11 patients of 1000 with wounds confined to the cerebral cortex in whom appreciation of pain and/or temperature was altered; 2 had hyperpathia. When suprathalamic lesions cause pain, they tend to lie in the parietal area (56). I operated on a patient with a right parietal hemispheral meningioma who had contralateral central pain. This disappeared after total removal of the tumor, underlining the reversibility of central pain. It is suggested that the projection of spinothalamic tract to the second sensory cortex in the parietal lobe is involved in suprathalamic lesions causing pain.

Awareness of suprathalamic causes of brain central pain has increased with the use of CT and magnetic resonance imaging (MRI). Schmahmann and Leifer (118) studied 6 patients with brain central pain caused by parietal lesions. Of these lesions 4 were infarcts, 1 a stab wound, and 1 a hematoma that developed following resection of a meningioma. All caused dissociated hemibody sensory loss, preserving lemniscal function, and in each case the lesion involved the white matter deep to caudal ansa and the opercular region of the posterior postparietal cortex, sparing thalamus but including second somatosensory area.

Nevertheless, thalamic involvement in central pain is still important. Cesaro et al. (119) demonstrated thalamic hyperactivity in SPECT scans in 2 patients with stroke-induced pain who had an increased threshold to noxious stimulation on the side of the body contralateral to the stroke. Bogousslavsky et al. (120) studied 40 patients with thalamic infarcts, 3 of whom had central pain. The infarcts in all 3 involved the ventroposterior thalamic region. In fact, 17% of patients with such lesions had pain, whereas none with lesions elsewhere in thalamus did so. There is an interesting case report of a patient with a left hemispheric lacunar stroke inducing pain. The pain disappeared 7 years later, after the patient suffered a second left-sided stroke that affected the corona radiata, interrupting thalamoparietal interconnections (121).

In a review of 39 of my patients with stroke-induced pain in whom it was possible to localize the responsible lesion

(113), summarized in Table 9.7, 14 lesions were in the brainstem, 5 in the thalamus alone, 6 in thalamus with extension into suprathalamic structures, and 11 in suprathalamic structures, sparing thalamus. Of these patients 1 showed diffuse lesions and 2 no lesion at all on CT scanning, though the clinical picture suggested a supratentorial stroke. None of the patients with thalamic lesions had evoked pain. Degree of sensory loss predictably correlated with lesion size.

Clinical Features

Andersen et al. (112) found stroke-induced pain not related to the severity of the stroke. Onset was commonly delayed, pain occurring within a month of the stroke in 63%, between 1 and 6 months in 19%, and after 6 months in 19%. In a review of 50 of my cases (56), 52% of the patients were male and 83% were aged 41 to 70. Pain onset was immediate in 12% and delayed but within 6 months in 46%. Onset was between 6 and 12 months in 16% and over a year in 14%. Pain was left-sided in 44% and bilateral in 2%. Pain was always referred to a part of the body where sensation was abnormal or had been so at the time the stroke took place. In 45% it affected half of the body; in 12%, half of the face. In a later review of 73 cases (113), age at onset was between 51 and 80 in 67.2%, and onset of pain was immediate in 28.7% and delayed less than 6 months in 43.8%. Some 54.8% of the patients were men, and pain was right-sided in 43.9% and bilateral in 2.7%.

Causation

Any brain lesion that affects somatotopographically organized somatosensory pathways except the kinesthetic system can cause pain. For example, the lesion site in lateral thalamus for a stereotactic thalamotomy that involves the somatotopographically organized kinesthetic system to relieve movement disorder does not cause pain. Nor do lesions in the nonsomatotopographically organized sensory systems, such as those interrupted by medial thalamotomy. Cassinari and Pagni (10) found that pain occurred in 4 to 18% of reported patients undergoing thalamotomy in Vc for the relief of pain. Most of the responsible lesions are strokes, usually ischemic, as shown in Table 9.8 (113). In this series vascular events accounted for 91% of cases, 78% of them supratentorial; 74% of strokes were thrombotic, 16% hemorrhagic. Neoplasms are a rare cause (122). The causative lesion may be small or massive to the extent of producing virtual hemispherectomy (123), and the sensory loss may be severe, affecting all somatosensory modalities in half the body or none at all. In a literature review Boivie and Leijon (8) found that of 166 reported cases of brain central pain, 12.6% were caused by lower brainstem lesions, 22.9% of causative lesions included thalamus, 19.9% were supratentorial and extrathalamic, and 48% were supratentorial, involving both thalamus and suprathalamic structures. The delayed onset, location, and quality of pain found by them were similar to those in other series, including my own.

Table 9.7.   Lesion localization in 39 cases brain central pain

Location	Number of Cases
Infratentorial	14
Thalamic only	5
Thalamic and suprathalamic	6
Supratentorial extrathalamic	11
Diffuse	1
Not seen on CT (supratentorial stroke)	2

Table 9.8.   Causation in 73 Cases of Brain Central Pain

Cause	Overall Percentage[a]	Vascular[b]	Breakdown of Vascular Causes[b]
Vascular	90.6		
Supratentorial		78.1	
Thrombotic			67.1
Hematoma			11.0
Infratentorial		12.5	
Thrombotic			6.9
Hematoma			5.6
Infection	4.1		
Iatrogenic	1.4		
Syringobulbia	1.4		
Neoplasm	1.4		
Degenerative	1.4		

[a]Column does not add to 100% because of rounding error.
[b]Percent of overall causes.

Association with Dyskinesia

Some 8.2% of my patients (113) had accompanying dystonia as described by Déjérine and Roussy (115); 6.8% had accompanying tremor. Tremor occurred only in patients with both steady and evoked pain. The lesions responsible for tremor, which appeared to be in the brainstem, resulted in either no sensory loss or predominant loss of pain and temperature appreciation. Dystonia occurred in patients with or without evoked pain who had multimodality sensory loss associated with right- or left-sided lesions, all involving the thalamus.

Quality of Pain

In my series of 73 patients (113) steady pain occurred in 98.6%; intermittent neuralgic pain affected 16.4%, particularly patients with brainstem lesions; evoked pain affected 64.9%. Evoked pain might be stimulated by one or more than one sensory modality, and its presence did not correlate with degree or pattern of sensory loss except that it was uncommon in patients who had no clinically detectable sensory loss.

Leijon (124) correlated the presence of steady burning pain with an infratentorial brainstem lesion and with supratentorial lesions that did not involve thalamus, a distinction not evident in my patients. He found lancinating pain more common than I did and associated it with thalamic lesions, which was not the case in my patients.

Patterns of Sensory Loss

My 73 patients (113) showed the following:
46.5%, hemibody sensory loss affecting all modalities
20.5%, dissociated sensory loss affecting primarily pain and
    temperature appreciation
8.2%, multimodality sensory loss, preferentially affecting
    the spinothalamic system
6.8%, hyperpathia and/or allodynia without clinically
    detectable sensory loss
5.5%, loss of touch, position, and/or vibration sense but not
    of pain or temperature appreciation
5.5%, no clinically detectable sensory loss

In the 6.9% of our 73 patients with isolated facial pain, most showed facial dissociated sensory loss. The others showed this deficit plus various patterns of sensory loss on the opposite half of the body, usually dissociated sensory loss reflecting the effects of a medullary lesion. Pain distribution coincided with sensory loss, with no special predilection for any part of the body. The patterns of pain (steady, evoked, intermittent) did not correlate with patterns of sensory loss or with lesion location except that evoked pain was rare in the absence of sensory loss and intermittent pain was more prominent with medullary lesions and absent with thalamic ones.

Boivie and Leijon (8) concluded from a review of 63 patients studied with semiquantitative techniques that all stroke patients had sensory abnormalities, with impaired temperature and pain sensation being the key common factor. They do mention 1 patient outside their study who had no sensory loss. Many had normal thresholds for touch, vibration, and position sense. Allodynia affected 57% of the Swedish patients in their study and 23% of the British patients; hyperpathia occurred in 88% of the Swedish patients.

Andersen et al. (112) followed 207 patients with stroke who survived for at least 7 months, who were less than 81 years of age at the time of their stroke, and who could communicate; 16 developed central pain. The researchers concluded that the essential feature of the pain patients was interference with spinothalamic projection to cortex; appreciation of touch and vibration could be normal or impaired. Overall, 42% of their patients were recorded as having sensory abnormalities, and they could find no correlation between the presence of pain and degree of sensory loss, age, sex, side of lesion, site in brain, or general physical state. Some 15 of 16 of the patients who developed pain had allodynia or hyperpathia. The pain in their patients was usually lacerating or aching. They did find, however, that the patients with strokes who went on to develop pain had a more pronounced degree of abnormal sensitivity to cold and warmth than did those who did not develop pain. These abnormalities took the form of increased sensitivity to cold, decreased sensitivity to warmth, and allodynia or dysesthesia to touch or cold but not to warmth. 14 of the 16 pain patients showed cold allodynia or dysesthesia, but only 2 of 71 patients who did not go on to develop pain showed this abnormality. In general, lesions tended to be larger in the patients with pain.

Vestergaard et al. (125) studied sensory deficits in 11 stroke patients who suffered from pain. All demonstrated increased thresholds for pain appreciation in the affected area, and 10 of 11 showed increased cold thresholds. Cold pain and heat pain thresholds were always elevated but less strikingly. Of the 11, 4 showed enhanced threshold to touch using von Frey hairs and 3 to pain induced by an argon laser; 56% showed cold allodynia, 55%, touch allodynia. They concluded that damage to the spinothalamic pathway was the essential ingredient of stroke-induced pain.

Observations Based on Microelectrode Studies

In an unpublished study of 29 patients with brain central pain explored stereotactically, 22 with microelectrodes, brain mapping was correlated with CT findings, sensory loss, pain quality, and response to surgery in the hope of learning something more about the pathophysiology of stroke-induced pain. Spinothalamic sensory loss, usually associated with lemniscal loss, occurred in most patients, but a small number of patients had either no lemniscal loss or lemniscal loss without spinothalamic loss. Whether or not PFs and/or RFs could be found in the affected thalamus, whether the lesion was infratentorial or supratentorial, small or a virtual stroke hemispherectomy, pain was stereotyped (123). Even in these latter cases, however, with no PFs or Rfs in the thalamus on the side of the stroke, the pain must depend on somatotopographically organized pathways because of its discrete localization, raising the issue of ipsilateral mediation of residual sensation and pain after such severe strokes. Some of these patients with massive hemispheral destruction suffered from allodynia or hyperpathia, implicating ipsilateral pathways for evoked pain as well (126).

Various patterns of physiological findings occurred. RFs and PFs could both be intact, both be absent, or one or the other be present in isolation. The absence of RFs and preservation of PFs would therefore leave a relatively intact but deafferented thalamocortical set of circuits "in neutral" as potential generators of pain. I found that destructive lesions (Table 9.8) and Parrent et al. (72) found that PVG stimulation could relieve evoked pain, while PPDBS might relieve steady pain but not the reverse. These findings suggest that pain pathways are involved in the mediation of evoked pain caused by brain lesions but not of steady pain.

Thus, identical pain syndromes can be produced by lesions at any level and of any degree in the brain, sometimes depending on contralateral, at other times ipsilateral, presumably somatotopographically organized pathways.

The Issue of Bursting Cells

The question of bursting cells as markers of denervation neuronal hypersensitivity and as triggers of central pain has

been mentioned. In studies with microelectrodes in 29 patients with stroke-induced pain, I found bursting cells and somatotopographic reorganization in virtually every patient and no correlation between these factors and other features of the syndrome. I regard the presence of bursting cells as markers of deafferentation rather than of neuropathic pain because the same features commonly appear during stereotactic exploration of patients who have suffered from deafferentation but who do not have pain. Gorecki et al. (38) described similar observations. Bursting cells are found in patients with movement disorders who have had a previous thalamotomy and who are being reoperated on for recurrence of tremor but who do not suffer from pain. Both bursting cells and somatotopographic reorganization occur in patients with multiple sclerosis being operated on for the relief of tremor who do not have pain. The same applies in patients with secondary dystonia, including a patient with secondary dystonia after a stroke associated with hemibody sensory loss but who had never had pain: essentially a case of Déjérine-Roussy syndrome without pain (unpublished observations).

However, the issue has been raised that bursting cells with certain characteristics, such as those of calcium spikes (41, 127) or those occurring in Vc that fire regularly at regular intervals and that have RFs, may be related to pain (40) but that other bursting cells may not.

Rinaldi et al. (128) reported bursting cells in dorsomedian, central lateral, medial central, and parafascicular nuclei in 8 of 10 patients with deafferentation pain caused by various central and peripheral lesions, including 1 patient with stroke and 1 with spinal cord injury. Bursting cells occurred from the junction between lateral dorsomedian, central lateral, and central median nuclei to the inferior limit of central median nucleus. In the 2 patients without bursting cells some neurons in the intralaminar nuclei had RFs. Jeanmonod et al. (129) reported similar findings in 39 out of 45 patients with chronic pain; 29 of these had peripheral nerve or dorsal root lesions, 2 brachial plexus avulsion, 7 spinal cord, 2 brainstem, 2 thalamic, and 3 parietal lesions. Bursting cells were found clustered in and around central lateral nucleus, many with the characteristics of calcium spikes. Both Rinaldi's and Jeanmonod's groups appear to associate these bursting cells with the generation of neuropathic pain, Jeanmonod's group making destructive thalamotomy lesions among them with great success.

I have also frequently recorded bursting cells when directing a microelectrode parasagittally from anterodorsally into medial parafascicular nucleus 5 mm rostral to the posterior commissure and 2 mm lateral to the wall of third ventricle in the inferior portion of the dorsomedian nucleus at its junction with the parafascicular and have found this a useful physiological guide to that latter nucleus. However, I have assumed that the bursting cells represent normal activity of the dorsomedian nucleus rather than some pathological process. Clearly, this issue should be further explored.

Surgical Treatment of Brain Central Pain

There are few options for surgical treatment of brain central pain; data are sparse and outcome statistics usually only modestly impressive. The dichotomy between the steady component on the one hand and evoked and neuralgic components on the other, along with the differential response to destructive surgery and chronic stimulation, have been mentioned. In brain central pain my case numbers have been too few to produce convincing results, but they suggest a trend similar to that seen in cord central pain (Table 9.9), supporting this dichotomy.

In reading published surgical outcome data, it is difficult to find reports designating outcome after specific procedures in patients with brain central pain. Accounts usually include patients with varieties of pain syndromes undergoing a variety of surgical procedures.

Neurectomy

As expected, neurectomy failed to relieve pain in five of my patients except for relief of hyperpathia in one.

Stereotactic Destructive Lesions

Pagni (130) drew these conclusions from reviewing the literature: Peripheral procedures are ineffective in brain central pain. Sympathectomy may induce short term-relief. Cordotomy occasionally gives a few months' relief. Cordectomy fails. Cortical resections gave temporary relief. Finally, leukotomy may relieve pain at the expense of cognitive dysfunction.

Medial Thalamotomy

General overviews of outcome statistics in medial thalamotomy for neuropathic pain have been mentioned. After they made lesions in centromedian nucleus, Namba et al. (131) reported excellent relief in 4 and good but less significant relief in 4 more patients of 9 with brain central pain, but pain recurred within 2 years in all. Niizuma et al. (132) reported relief for up to 6 months in 17 similar patients. Pagni (130) reported that medial thalamotomy relieved 25% of patients with brain central pain. Jeanmonod et al. (129) reported relieving pain in 67% of 69 patients with brain central pain with stereotactic lesioning of centrolateral nucleus of thalamus (see section on bursting cells).

Mesencephalic Tractotomy

Pagni (130) states that Spiegel and Wycis failed to relieve brain central pain after mesencephalic tractotomy. He also reports that after Orthner extended the classical mesencephalic tractotomy lesion more medially from the neospinothalamic tract, more lasting relief of brain central pain was achieved. Amano et al. (133) reported relief of 64% of patients with brain central pain, and Shieff and Nashold

Table 9.9.   Response of Common Components of Brain Central Pain to Surgery

| | | Percent of Patients with >50% Relief | |
	No. of Patients	Steady	Evoked and neuralgic
Trigeminal stimulation	6	67	25
PPDBS	11	45[a]	13
Thalamotomy with or without mesencephalic tractotomy	11	30	67

[a]PPDBS was painful in three patients.

(134), of 62% by mesencephalic tractotomy extending medially toward the PAG. I carried out combined mesencephalic tractotomy and medial thalamotomy in 5 patients, mesencephalic tractotomy alone in 3, and medial thalamotomy alone in 3 patients with brain central pain (113). Of them 3 patients enjoyed ongoing pain relief, and review of the records shows that the 1 incidence of intermittent pain, 3 of the 5 incidences of evoked pain, and 3 of 7 incidences of steady pain were relieved (Table 9.9). Reported series (56) suggested early pain relief in 54% of cases of brain central pain after stereotactic destructive lesions. Levin et al. (135) reported relief of pain in 3 patients with stroke-induced pain after intrahypophyseal injection of alcohol. The complications of destructive procedures in brain central pain are similar to those reported with cord central pain.

Modulatory Treatment

Trigeminal Stimulation

Of the 34 patients in whom my colleagues and I (136) have used trigeminal stimulation, 7 had brain central pain, 3 lateral medullary syndrome, 1 an infarct in middle cerebral territory, 1 a massive infarct involving thalamus and internal capsule, 1 an infarct following ligation of the internal carotid artery, and 1 neuropathic pain following medullary tractotomy. Of the 7, 5 derived relief during test stimulation, went on to internalization, and enjoyed persistent relief of more than 50% of the pain. It was surprising to us that the group with central pain responded better to this treatment than did those with more peripheral lesions, though the numbers are small. Complications included an alarming 21% of superficial infections related to the hardware, a problem that has been greatly reduced by the use of prophylactic antibiotic therapy and by using different electrodes for trial and permanent stimulation, which is done a month after the trial in one sitting. In this series 29% suffered technical complications, particularly from lead migration, a problem that has been virtually eliminated by using a 4-pole Medtronic 3387 DBS electrode for the permanent implantation. However, 3 patients (9%) had increased facial sensory loss, presumably from trauma caused by the electrode insertion.

Dorsal Column Stimulation

Pagni (11) found DCS to have no benefit in brain central pain. I attempted DCS in 12 patients with brain central pain in a series of 193 patients treated with this modality. Of them 50% claimed significant pain relief during trial stimulation. After internalization, however, only 2 (17% of the original group) reported ongoing pain relief, 1 of these with pain caused by a thalamic glioma. Of these 12 patients, 8 suffered from evoked pain as part of their problem, and in 4 of the 8, dorsal column stimulation was painful, as Vc thalamic stimulation often is in such patients.

Deep Brain Stimulation

The dichotomy between PPDBS and PAG PVG DBS has been discussed. Mazars et al. (137) considered DBS ineffective for relieving brain central pain. Hosobuchi (106) and Hosobuchi et al. (138) reported relief in 4 of 5 cases of "thalamic syndrome" and 1 case of pain caused by a cortical lesion using DBS in medial lemniscus; 2 patients with lateral medullary syndrome were not helped. Adams (105) reported 8 of 10 cases of thalamic syndrome enjoying useful benefit, and Mundinger and Salamao (104) reported good relief in 2 of 5 patients with brain central pain, but a subsequent review (139) was less promising. Siegfried and Demierre (140) reported long-term relief in 7 of 9 cases of brain central pain with DBS through an electrode in Vc. Levy and Lamb (111) treated 25 stroke pain patients with DBS; 9 of 14 patients with electrodes placed in Vc, 1 of 6 of those with electrodes in internal capsule, and none of 3 with electrodes in PAG and/or PVG reported relief during trial stimulation and went on to internalization. Of the total, 6 (24%) reported long-term relief. There is anecdotal support for the notion that DBS in internal capsule is superior to that in other sites for controlling brain central pain (141), Hosobuchi (106) reporting 4 of 11 cases and Namba et al. (131) 3 of 7 cases so treated relieved of pain. PVG DBS has also been reported successful in the relief of brain central pain (105, 106).

Of our 62 patients treated with PP DBS (103), 17 suffered from brain central pain. Some 14 of these patients underwent trial stimulation and 8, internalization; 43% of those undergoing trial stimulation and 75% of those internalized derived useful ongoing relief. In 6 patients, all of whom suffered from marked allodynia and/or hyperpathia, PPDBS in ventrocaudal nucleus was painful, thwarting attempts to treat their pain, a problem that was uncommon in patients with neuropathic pain syndromes with allodynia and hyperpathia who did not have brain lesions (discussed later.). Parrent et al. (72) had 3 patients with stroke central pain who suffered from allodynia and/or hyperpathia and who reported reduction of their evoked pain with acute stimulation in PVG (72). They went on after internalization to long-term useful relief of this problem.

Painful Deep Brain Stimulation

Two features peculiar to brain central pain interfere with attempts to relieve it with DBS. The responsible brain lesion may so disrupt the anatomy that suitable targets cannot be found. Furthermore, patients who have allodynia and hyperpathia associated with brain central pain may find stimulation in ventrocaudal nucleus painful quite apart from the unpleasant effects that occur when stimulating PAG. It is normally difficult to induce pain by stimulating the central nervous system at threshold (142), and the induction of burning is also unusual. Even stimulating in the spinothalamic pathway usually induces warm or cold feelings. In our earlier experience with stereotactic mesencephalic tractotomy and medial thalamotomy to relieve intractable pain guided by macrostimulation, Tasker et al. (142) often induced burning or pain, the latter resembling the patient's own pain in many cases, while stimulating the midbrain medial to the neospinothalamic tract and the medial thalamic nuclei. Macrostimulation in these structures usually produces no conscious effect at all, for example in a patient with Parkinson's disease. Intrigued by this, we counted the number of sites where macrostimulation induced pain in 138 patients with movement disorders and in 22 with chronic pain, finding 26 pain points among the former 138 patients and 41 in the latter 22. Of the 22, 13 had cancer pain that appeared to be nociceptive in origin, and only 8 pain points were found in this group. However 33 pain points were located in the 9 patients with neuropathic pain, 5 of whom suffered from brain lesions, 2 from cord lesions, and 2 from peripheral neural lesions. Of the 9 patients with neuropathic pain, 6 (4 with brain lesions) reported pain on stimulation. In 7 of the 9 neuropathic pain patients stimulation produced burning in the same sites, either in isolation or in addition to pain. Thus, neuropathic pain, especially that caused by brain lesions, appeared to be related to the induction of pain by stimulation. Subsequent to this experience my colleagues and I began exploring ventrocaudal nucleus of thalamus, the tactile relay, to implant DBS electrodes, and we replaced macrostimulation by microelectrode recording and microstimulation for physiological guidance. Normally stimulation of Vc produces paresthesias even at four times threshold stimulation. In the posterior inferior rim of Vc, however, my colleagues and I (142) frequently encountered sites where macrostimulation induced feelings of warmth or cold attributed to stimulation in the parvocellular portion of Vc that is thought to be the spinothalamic relay. It would be natural to expect similar results to be obtained with microstimulation and nociceptive neurons to be recorded in this same region. However, as it turns out, it proved unusual to find neurons responsive to noxious or thermal stimulation anywhere in Vc, though those reported often turn up in the ventral posterior rim (143–145). Similarly, it was rare to induce a sensation of warmth, cold, or pain with microstimulation in the same region (146–150). Sometimes the effect induced was reported as burning, and sometimes the pain was referred to internal organs. Presumably these are normal responses reflecting the probe's entry into the spinothalamic relay.

However, in some patients, particularly those with brain central pain, stimulation throughout Vc may be painful, and the pain induced may resemble the patient's own pain, just as in the medial structures mentioned earlier (38, 127). There appears to be a higher incidence of stimulation-induced pain with microstimulation in Vc in poststroke patients than in others (146, 151). In a retrospective study of all our patients with stroke-induced pain explored stereotactically, the 18 patients in whom microstimulation in Vc was painful suffered from allodynia and/or hyperpathia, while only 5 of the 20 patients in whom such stimulation was not painful had allodynia and/or hyperpathia; burning was induced equally commonly in the 2 groups. The fact that stimulation of Vc in stroke patients may be painful reflected on success with PPDBS: 10 of 16 patients with brain central pain without an evoked element reported an initial success, while only 2 of 12 with allodynia and/or hyperpathia did so. These observations are in addition to those on 3 patients in whom PVG DBS relieved evoked pain.

Motor Cortex Stimulation

As a result of observations in laboratory studies, Tsubokawa et al. (152) treated 7 patients with brain central pain using chronic epidural motor cortex stimulation and reported excellent or good pain relief in all and no complications. In a subsequent report by the same group (153), in 12 patients with neuropathic pain, 10 caused by lesions in the brain, 90% of the cases of brain central pain reported ongoing relief after a year; 3 had required revision of electrode position. Hosobuchi (154) followed 6 patients with brain central pain for 9 to 30 months after inserting an extradural motor cortex stimulator. All reported initial relief, but in 3 the pain recurred after 2 to 3 months; the remaining 3 continuing to do well. A Resume (Medtronic Corp.) electrode is inserted through a bur hole under local anesthetic on the side of the lesion parallel with the central sulcus and overlying the motor cortex. For upper limb pain the electrode is inserted 3 to 4 cm; for lower limb pain, 1 cm lateral to the midline. The site can be identified with MRI, by using surface landmarks, or by evoked potential recording. In my experience, however, strokes often interfere with evoked potentials to the point that I find them not useful for localization. Stimulation is carried out below the threshold for a muscle twitch. Tsubokawa et al. (152, 153) used currents of less than 1.0 µA at 0.1 to 0.5 milliseconds pulsewidth at 50 to 120 Hz. The device can be internalized either to a radiofrequency-coupled Medtronic X-Trel or a totally programmable battery-powered Itrel device. More published experience must accumulate before this form of therapy can be assessed.

SUMMARY

Central pain is a distressing consequence of brain or spinal cord injury. It is difficult to understand how a person with a complete transection of the spinal cord can suffer from excruciating pain in his feet or how someone who has had a massive stroke rendering one whole cerebral hemisphere nonfunctional should have pain on the opposite side of the body. Our understanding of the mechanisms has progressed only modestly, and this is reflected in the outcome statistics from attempts to treat central pain either medically or surgically. Central pain commonly consists of three elements: steady, causalgic-dysesthetic; intermittent, often lancinating; and evoked (allodynia and hyperpathia). It is suggested that the mechanisms of each of these components is different, and therefore one would expect the surgical strategies used to treat them to be different as well. This seems to be borne out in the case of cord central pain, for which the amount of data is greater, and probably is also true in the case of brain central pain. It appears that therapy that interferes with transmission in pain pathways is beneficial for allodynia, hyperpathia, and neuralgic pain, whereas paresthesia-producing stimulation is preferable in the steady pain.

References

1. Merskey H. Classification of chronic pain: descriptions of chronic pain syndromes and definitions of pain terms. Pain 1986;3(Suppl):S1–S225.
2. Tasker RR. Deafferentation. In: Wall PD, Melzack R, eds. Textbook of pain. Edinburgh: Churchill Livingstone, 1984;119–132.
3. Tasker RR, Organ LW, Hawrylyshyn P. Deafferentation and causalgia. In: Bonica JJ, ed. Pain. New York: Raven Press, 1980;305–329.
4. Tasker RR, Tsuda T, Hawrylyshyn P. Clinical neurophysiological investigation of deafferentation pain. In: Bonica JJ, Lindblom U, Iggo A, eds. Advances in pain research and therapy. New York: Raven Press, 1983;713–738.
5. Livingston WK. Pain mechanisms: a physiologic interpretation of causalgia and its related states. 2nd ed. New York: Plenum, 1976.
6. Levitt M, Levitt JH. The deafferentation syndrome in monkeys: dysesthesias of spinal origin. Pain 1981;10:129–147.
7. Inbal R, Devor M, Tuchhendler O, Lieblich I. Autotomy following nerve injury: genetic factors in the development of chronic pain. Pain 1980;9:327–337.
8. Boivie J, Leijon G. Clinical findings in patients with central poststroke pain. In: Casey KL, ed. Pain and central nervous system disease. New York: Raven Press, 1991;65–75.
9. Boivie J, Leijon G, Johansson I. Central post-stroke pain: a study of the mechanisms through analyses of the sensory abnormalities. Pain 1985;37:173–185.
10. Cassinari V, Pagni CA. Central pain: a neurosurgical survey. Cambridge: Harvard University Press, 1969.
11. Pagni CA. Central pain due to spinal cord and brain stem damage. In: Wall PD, Melzack R, eds. Textbook of pain. Edinburgh: Churchill Livingstone, 1984;481–495.
12. La Motte RH, Thalhammer JC, Torebjörk HE, Robinson CJ. Peripheral neural mechanisms of cutaneous hyperalgesia following mild injury by heat. J Neurosci 1982;2:765–781.
13. Meyer RA, Campbell JN. Myelinated nociceptive afferents account for the hyperalgesia that follows a burn on the hand. Science 1981;213:1527–1529.

14. Riddoch G. The clinical features of central pain. Lancet 1938;1093, 1150, 1205.
15. Kibler RF, Nathan PW. Relief of pain in paraesthesia by nerve block distal to a lesion. J Neurol Neurosurg Psychiatry 1960;23:91–93.
16. Tasker RR, Organ LW, Hawrylyshyn P. Percutaneous cordotomy: the lateral high cervical technique. In: Schmidek HH, Sweet WH, eds. Operative neurosurgical techniques: indications, methods, and results. New York: Grune & Stratton, 1982:1137–1153.
17. Tasker RR. Stereotaxic surgery. In: Wall PD, Melzack R, eds. Textbook of pain. Edinburgh: Churchill Livingstone, 1984;639–655.
18. Tasker RR. Thalamic procedures. In: Schaltenbrand G, Walker AE, eds. Stereotaxy of the human brain: anatomical, physiological and clinical applications. New York: Thieme Verlag, 1982;484–497.
19. Boureau F, Doubrère JF, Luu M. Study of verbal description in neuropathic pain. Pain 1990;42:145–152.
20. Nashold BS Jr, Ovelmen-Levitt J, eds. Advances in pain research and therapy, vol 19. Deafferentation pain syndromes pathophysiology and treatment. New York: Raven Press, 1991.
21. Casey KL, ed. Pain and central nervous system disease: the central pain syndromes. New York: Raven Press 1991.
22. Foerster O. Die Leitungsbahnen des Schmerz-Zustände und die chirurgische Behandlung des Schmerzgefühls. Berlin: Urbani and Schwarzenberg, 1927.
23. Loeser JD. Definition, aetiology and neurological assessment of pain originating in the nervous system following deafferentation. Pain 1981;81(Suppl 1):981 (abstract).
24. Bowsher D. The problem of central pain. Verh Dtsch Ges Inn Med 1980;86:1525.
25. Raymond SA, Rocco AG. Ephaptic coupling of large fibres as a clue to mechanism in chronic neuropathic allodynia following damage to dorsal roots. Pain 1990(Suppl 5):S276.
26. Nordin M, Nystrom B, Wallin U, Hagbarth KE. Ectopic sensory discharges and paresthesiae in patients with disorders of peripheral nerves, dorsal roots and dorsal columns. Pain 1984;20:231–245.
27. Loeser JD, Ward AA Jr. Some effects of deafferentation on neurons of the cat spinal cord. Arch Neurol 1967;17:629–636.
28. Loeser JD, Ward AA, White LE. Chronic deafferentation of human spinal cord neurons. J Neurosurg 1968;29:48–50.
29. Anderson LS, Black RG, Abraham J, Ward AA. Neuronal hyperactivity in experimental trigeminal deafferentation. J Neurosurg 1971;35:444–452.
30. Apkarian AV, Hodge CJ, Martini S, Fraser A. Neuronal bursting activity in the dorsal horn resulting from dorsal rhizotomy. Pain 1984(Suppl 2):S442.
31. Black RG. Trigeminal pain. In: Crue BL, ed. Pain and suffering. Springfield, IL: Charles C. Thomas, 1970;119–137.
32. Black RG. A laboratory model for trigeminal neuralgia. Adv Neurol 1974;4:651–658.
33. Albe-Fessard D, Lombard MC. Animal models for pain due to central deafferentation: methods of protection against this syndrome. Pain 1981(Suppl 1):S80.
34. Albe-Fessard D, Lombard MC. Use of an animal model to evaluate the origin of and protection against deafferentation pain. In: Bonica JJ, Lindblom U, Iggo A, eds. Advances in pain research and therapy, vol 5. New York: Raven Press, 1983;691–700.
35. Albe-Fessard D, Nashold BS Jr, Lombard MC, et al. Rat after dorsal rhizotomy: a possible animal model for chronic pain. In: Bonica JJ, Liebeskind JC, Albe-Fessard DG, eds. Advances in pain research and therapy, vol 3. New York: Raven Press, 1979;761–766.
36. Lombard MC, Nashold BS Jr, Albe-Fessard D, et al. Deafferentation hypersensitivity in the rat after dorsal rhizotomy: a possible animal model of chronic pain. Pain 1979;6:163–174.
37. Lombard MC, Nashold BS Jr, Pelissier T. Thalamic recordings in rats with hyperalgesia. In: Bonica JJ, Liebeskind JC, Albe-Fessard DG, eds. Advances in pain research and therapy, vol 3. New York: Raven Press, 1979;767–772.
38. Gorecki J, Hirayama T, Dostrovsky JO, et al. Thalamic stimulation and recording in patients with deafferentation and central pain. Stereotact Funct Neurosurg 1987;52:219–226.
39. Lenz FA, Tasker RR, Dostrovsky JO, et al. Abnormal single-unit activity recorded in the somatosensory thalamus of a quadriplegic patient with central pain. Pain 1987;31:225–236.
40. Hirayama T, Dostrovsky JO, Gorecki J, et al. Recordings of abnormal activity in patients with deafferentation and central pain. Stereotact Funct Neurosurg 1987;52:120–126.
41. Lenz FA. The thalamus and central pain syndromes: human and animal studies. In: Casey KL, ed. Pain and central nervous system disease: the central pain syndromes. New York: Raven Press, 1991;171–182.
42. Casey KL. Pain and central nervous system disease: A summary and overview. In: Casey KL, ed. Pain and Central Nervous System Disease: The Central Pain Syndromes. New York: Raven Press, 1991;1–11.
43. Porter RW, Hohmann GW, Bors E, et al. Cordotomy for pain following cauda equina injury. Arch Surg 1966;92:765–770.
44. White JC, Sweet WH. Pain and the neurosurgeon: a forty-year experience. Springfield, IL: Charles C. Thomas, 1969;435–477.
45. Mariano AJ. Chronic pain and spinal cord injury. Clin J Pain 1992;8:87–92.
46. Nepomuceno C, Fine PR, Richards JS, et al. Pain in patients with spinal injury. Arch Phys Med Rehabil 1979;60:605–609.
47. Jefferson A. Cordectomy for intractable pain. In: Lipton S, Miles J, eds. Persistent pain, vol 4. New York: Grune & Stratton, 1983;115–132.
48. Burke DC. Pain in paraplegia. Paraplegia 1973;10:297–313.
49. Yezierski RP. Pain following spinal cord injury: the clinical problem and experimental studies. Pain 1996;68:185–194.
50. Rose M, Robinson JE, Ellis P, Cole JD. Pain following spinal cord injury: results from a postal survey. Pain 1988;34:101–102 (letter).
51. Richards JS, Meredith RL, Nepomuceno C, et al. Psychological aspects of chronic pain in spinal cord injury. Pain 1980;8:355–366.
52. Richardson RR, Meyer PR, Cerullo LJ. Neurostimulation in the modulation of intractable paraplegic and traumatic neuroma pains. Pain 1980;8:75–84.
53. Botterell EH, Callaghan JC, Jousse AT. Pain in paraplegia: clinical management and surgical treatment. Proc R Soc Med 1954;47:281–288.
54. Tasker RR, De Carvalho GTC, Dolan EJ. Intractable pain of spinal cord origin: clinical features and implications for surgery. J Neurosurg 1992;77:373–378.
55. Richards JS, Stover SL, Jaworski T. Effect of bullet removal on subsequent pain in persons with spinal cord injury secondary to gunshot wound. J Neurosurg 1990;73:401–404.
56. Tasker RR. Pain resulting from central nervous system pathology (central pain). In: Bonica JJ, ed. The management of pain. 2nd ed. Philadelphia: Lea & Febiger, 1990;264–280.
57. Milhorat TH, Kotzen RM, Mu HTM, et al. Dysesthetic pain in patients with syringomyelia. Neurosurg 1996;38:940–947.
58. Wall PD. On the origin of pain associated with amputation. In: Siegfried J, Zimmermann M, eds. Phantom and stump pain. Berlin: Springer-Verlag, 1981;2–14.
59. Carlen PL, Wall PD, Nodvorna H, Steinbach T. Phantom limbs and related phenomena in recent traumatic amputations. Neurology (Minneapolis) 1978;28:211–217.
60. Berger M, Gerstenbrand F. Phantom illusions in spinal cord injuries. In: Siegfried J, Zimmermann M, eds. Phantom and stump pain. Berlin: Springer-Verlag, 1981;66–73.
61. Pollock LJ, Brown M, Boshes B, et al. Pain below the level of injury of the spinal cord. Arch Neurol Psychiatry 1951;65:319–322.
62. Waisbrod H, Hansen D, Gerbershagen HU. Chronic pain in paraplegics. Neurosurgery 1984;15:933–934.
63. Berić A, Dimitrijevic MR, Lindblom J. Central dysesthesia syndrome in spinal cord injury. Pain 1988;34:109–116.
64. Davis L, Martin J. Studies upon spinal cord injuries: 2. Nature and treatment of pain. J Neurosurg 1947;4:483–491.

65. Nashold BS Jr. Paraplegia and pain. In: Nashold BS Jr, Ovelmen-Levitt J, eds. Deafferentation pain syndromes: pathophysiology and treatment. New York: Raven Press, 1991;301–319.

66. Pagni CA, Canavero S. Functional thalamic depression in a case of reversible central pain due to a spinal intramedullary cyst. J Neurosurg 1995;83:163–165.

67. Hamby WB. Reversible central pain. Arch Neurol 1961;5:528–532.

68. Cesaro P, Defer G, Moretti JL, Dagos JD. Central pain and thalamic activation. Pain 1990(Suppl 5):S433.

69. Lindblom U. Assessment of abnormal evoked pain in neurological pain patients and its relation to spontaneous pain: a descriptive and conceptual model with some analytical results. In: Fields HL, Dubner R, Cervero F, eds. Advances in pain research and therapy, vol 9. New York: Raven Press, 1985;409–423.

70. Woolf CJ. Evidence for a central component of post-injury pain hypersensitivity. Nature 1983;306:686–688.

71. Woolf CJ. Central mechanisms of acute pain. Pain 1990(Suppl 5):S218.

72. Parrent A, Lozano A, Tasker RR, Dostrovsky J. Periventricular gray stimulation suppresses allodynia and hyperpathia in man. Stereotact Funct Neurosurg 1992;59:82 (abstract).

73. Nashold BS Jr, Ostdahl RH. Dorsal root entry zone lesions for pain relief. J Neurosurg 1979;51:59–69.

74. Nashold BS Jr, Bullitt E. Dorsal root entry zone lesions to control central pain in paraplegics. J Neurosurg 1981;55:414–419.

75. Nashold BS Jr, Ostdahl RH, Bullitt E, et al. Dorsal root entry zone lesions: a new neurosurgical therapy for deafferentation pain. In: Bonica JJ, Lindblom U, Iggo A, eds. Advances in pain research and therapy, vol 5. New York: Raven Press, 1983;739–750.

76. Sindou M, Fischer G, Goutelle A, Mansuy L.. La radicellotomie postérieure sélective: premiers résultats dans la chirurgie de la douleur. Neurochirurgie 1974;20:397–408.

77. White JC. Anterolateral chordotomy: its effectiveness in relieving pain of non-malignant disease. Neurochirurgia (Stuttg) 1963;6:83–102.

78. Bors E. Phantom limbs of patients with spinal cord injury. AMA Arch Neurol Psychol 1951;66:610–631.

79. Rosomoff HL, Papo I, Loeser JD, et al. Neurosurgical operations on the spinal cord. In: Bonica JJ, ed. The management of pain. 2nd ed. Philadelphia: Lea & Febiger, 1990;2067–2081.

80. Melzack R, Loeser JD. Phantom body pain in paraplegics: evidence for a central "pattern-generating mechanism" for pain. Pain 1978;4:195–220.

81. Druckman R, Lende R. Central pain of spinal origin: pathogenesis and surgical relief in one patient. Neurology 1965;15:518–522.

82. Durward QJ, Rice GP, Ball MJ, et al. Selective spinal cordectomy: Clinico-pathological correlation. J Neurosurg 1982;56:359–367.

83. Richter HP, Seitz K. Dorsal root entry zone lesions for the control of deafferentation pain: experience in ten patients. Neurosurgery 1984;15:913–916.

84. Sweet WH, Poletti CE. Operations in the brain stem and spinal canal, with an appendix on open cordotomy. In: Wall PD, Melzack R, eds. Textbook of pain. Edinburgh: Churchill Livingstone, 1984;615–631.

85. Friedman AH, Bullitt E. Dorsal root entry zone lesions in the treatment of pain following brachial plexus avulsion, spinal cord injury and herpes zoster. Appl Neurophysiol 1988;51:164–169.

86. Friedman AH, Nashold BS Jr. DREZ lesions for relief of pain related to spinal cord injury. J Neurosurg 1986;65:465–469.

87. Friedman AH, Nashold BS Jr. Pain of spinal origin. In: Youmans JR, ed. Neurological surgery. Philadelphia: Saunders, 1990;3950–3959.

88. Friedman AH, Nashold JRB, Nashold BS Jr. DREZ lesions for treatment of pain. In: North RB, Levy RM, eds. Neurosurgical management of pain. New York: Springer-Verlag, 1997;176–190.

89. Young RF. Clinical experience with radiofrequency and laser DREZ lesions. J Neurosurg 1990;72:715–720.

90. Powers SK, Barbaro NM, Levy RM. Pain control with laser-produced dorsal root entry zone lesions. Appl Neurophysiol 1988;51:243–254.

91. Nashold BS Jr. Brain stem stereotaxic procedures. In: Schaltenbrand G, Walker AE, eds. Stereotaxy of the human brain: anatomical, physiological and clinical applications. Stuttgart: Thieme Verlag, 1982;475–483.

92. Pagni CA. Place of stereotactic technique in surgery for pain. In: Bonica JJ, ed. Advances in neurology, vol 4. New York: Raven Press, 1974;699–706.

93. Davis RA, Stokes JW. Neurosurgical attempts to relieve thalamic pain. Surg Gynecol Obstet 1966;123:371.

94. Gybels JM, Sweet WH. Neurosurgical treatment of persistent pain: physiological and pathological mechanisms of human pain. Basel: Karger, 1989.

95. Wall PD, Sweet WH. Temporary abolition of pain in man. Science 1967;155:108–109.

96. Shealy CN, Mortimer JT, Hagfors NR. Dorsal column electroanalgesia. J Neurosurg 1970;32:560–564.

97. North RB. Spinal cord stimulation. In: North RB, Levy RM, eds. Neurosurgical management of pain. New York: Springer, 1997;271–282.

98. Tasker RR, Parrent A. Outcomes of surgery for movement disorders and pain. In: Wilden JN, Swash M, eds. Outcomes of neurological and neurosurgical disorders. Cambridge, UK: Cambridge University Press, 1997; in press.

99. Sweet WH, Wepsic JG. Stimulation of the posterior columns of the spinal cord for pain control: indications, technique, and results. Clin Neurosurg 1974;21:278.

100. Lazorthes Y, Verdie JC, Arbus L. Stimulation analgésique médullaire antérieure et postérieure par technique d'implantation percutanée. Acta Neurochir (Wien) 1978;40:253–276.

101. Urban BJ, Nashold BS. Percutaneous epidural stimulation of the spinal cord for relief of pain. J Neurosurg 1978;48:323–328.

102. Nashold BS Jr. Central pain: its origins and treatment. Clin Neurosurg 1974;20:311–322.

103. Tasker RR, Vilela Filho O. Deep brain stimulation for the control of intractable pain. In: Youmans JR, ed. Neurological surgery. 3rd ed. 1996;3512–3527.

104. Mundinger F, Salomao JF. Deep brain stimulation in mesencephalic lemniscus medialis for chronic pain. Acta Neurochir Suppl (Wien) 1980;30:245–258.

105. Adams JE. Technique and technical problems associated with implantation of neuroaugmentative devices. Appl Neurophysiol 1977–1978;40:111–123.

106. Hosobuchi Y. The current status of analgesic brain stimulation. Acta Neurochir Suppl (Wien) 1980;30:219–221.

107. Richardson DE, Akil H. Long-term results of periventricular gray self-stimulation. Neurosurgery 1977;1:199–202.

108. Turnbull IM. Brain stimulation. In: Wall PD, Melzack R, eds. Textbook of pain. Edinburgh: Churchill Livingstone, 1984;706–714.

109. Tasker RR, Yoshida M, Sima AAF, Deck J. Stimulation mapping of the periventricular-periacqueductal gray (PVG-PAG) in man: an autopsy study. In: Samii J, ed. Surgery in and around the brain stem and the third ventricle. Berlin: Springer-Verlag, 1986;161–167.

110. Levy RM, Lamb S, Adams JE. Deep brain stimulation for chronic pain: long-term follow-up in 145 patients from 1972–1984. Pain 1984(Suppl 2):S115.

111. Levy RM, Lamb S, Adams JE. Treatment of chronic pain by deep brain stimulation: long-term follow-up and review of the literature. Neurosurgery 1987;21:885–893.

112. Andersen G, Vestergaard K, Ingeman-Nielsen, Jensen TS. Incidence of central post-stroke pain. Pain 1995;61:187–193.

113. Tasker RR, De Carvalho G. Pain in thalamic stroke. In: Proceedings of Stroke Rehabilitation: a conference and workshop on pain and ethical and social issues. Stroke Rehabilitation XIII Annual Scientific Meeting of the Inter-Urban Stroke Academic Association, Toronto, May 4–5, 1990.

114. Kameyama M. Vascular lesions of the thalamus on the dominant and nondominant side. Appl Neurophysiol 1976–1977;39:171–177.

115. Déjérine J, Roussy G. La syndrome thalamique. Rev Neurol (Paris) 1906;14:521–532.

116. Penfield W, Gage L. Cerebral localization of epileptic manifestations. Arch Neurol Psychiatry 1933;30:709–727.

117. Marshall J. Sensory disturbances in cortical wounds with special reference to pain. J Neurol Neurosurg Psychiatry 1951;14:187–204.

118. Schmahmann JD, Leifer D. Parietal pseudothalamic pain syndrome: clinical features and anatomic correlates. Arch Neurol 1992;1032–1037.

119. Cesaro P, Mann MW, Moretti JL, et al. Central pain and thalamic hyperactivity: a single photon emission computerized tomographic study. Pain 1991;47:329–336.

120. Bogousslavsky J, Regli F, Uske A. Thalamic infarcts: clinical syndromes, etiology and prognosis. Neurology 1988;38:837–848.

121. Soria ED, Fine EJ. Disappearance of thalamic pain after parietal subcortical stroke. Pain 1991;44:285–288.

122. Lozano AM, Parrent A, Dostrovsky JO, Tasker RR. Central pain from thalamic neoplasm. Stereotact Funct Neurosurg 1992;59:77 (abstract).

123. Parrent AG, Lozano AM, Dostrovsky JO, Tasker RR. Central pain in the absence of functional sensory thalamus. Stereotact Funct Neurosurg 1992;59:9–14.

124. Leijon G. Central post-stroke pain: clinical characteristics, mechanism and treatment. Linköping (Sweden) University Medical Dissertations No 281, 1988.

125. Vestergaard K, Nielsen J, Andersen G, et al. Sensory abnormalities in consecutive, unselected patients with central post-stroke pain. Pain 1995;61:177–186.

126. Parrent AG, Tasker RR. Can the ipsilateral hemisphere mediate pain in man? Acta Neurochir 1992;117:89 (abstract).

127. Lenz FA, Tasker RR, Dostrovsky JO, et al. Abnormal single-unit activity and responses to stimulation in the presumed ventrocaudal nucleus of patients with central pain. In: Dubner R, Gebhart GF, Bond MR, eds. Proceedings of the V World Congress on Pain. Amsterdam: Elsevier, 1988;158–164.

128. Rinaldi PC, Young RF, Albe-Fessard D, Chodakiewitz J. Spontaneous neuronal hyperactivity in the medial and intralaminar thalamic nuclei of patients with deafferentation pain. J Neurosurg 1991;74:415–521.

129. Jeanmonod D, Magnin M, Morel M. Thalamus and neurogenic pain: physiological, anatomical and clinical data. Neuroreport 1993;4:475–478.

130. Pagni CA. The treatment of central deafferentation pain syndrome. In: Nashold BS Jr, Ovelman-Levitt J, eds. Deafferentation pain syndromes. New York: Raven Press, 1991;275–283.

131. Namba S, Nakao Y, Matsumoto Y, et al. Electrical stimulation of the posterior limb of the internal capsule for the treatment of thalamic pain. Appl Neurophysiol 1984;47:137–148.

132. Niizuma H et al. Follow-up results of centromedian thalamotomy for central pain. Appl Neurophysiol 1982;45:324–325.

133. Amano K, Kawamura H, Tanikawa T, et al. Long term follow up study of rostral mesencephalic reticulotomy for pain relief: report of 34 cases. Appl Neurophysiol 1986;49:105–111.

134. Shieff C, Nashold BS. Stereotactic mesencephalic tractotomy for thalamic pain. Neurol Res 1987;0:101–104.

135. Levin AB, Remirez LF, Katz J. The use of stereotaxic chemical hypophysectomy in the treatment of thalamic pain syndrome. J Neurosurg 1983;59:1002–1006.

136. Taub E, Munz M, Tasker RR. Chronic electrical stimulation of the gasserian ganglion for the relief of pain in a series of 34 patients. J Neurosurg 1997;86:197–202.

137. Mazars G, Mérienne L, Cioloca C. Traitement de certains types de douleurs par les stimulateurs thalamiques implantables. Neurochirurgie 1974;20:117–124.

138. Hosobuchi Y, Adams JE, Rutkin B. Chronic thalamic and internal capsule stimulation for the control of central pain. Surg Neurol 1975; 4:91–92.

139. Mundinger F, Neumüller H. Programmed stimulation for control of chronic pain and motor diseases. Appl Neurophysiol 1982;45:102–111.

140. Siegfried J, Demierre B. Thalamic electrostimulation in the treatment of thalamic pain syndrome. Pain 1984;(Suppl 2):S116.

141. Hosobuchi Y, Adams JE, Fields HL. Chronic thalamic and internal capsular stimulation for the control of facial anesthesia dolorosa and the dysesthesia of thalamic syndrome. In: Bonica JJ, ed. Neurology, vol 4. New York: Raven Press, 1974;783–787.

142. Tasker RR, Organ LW, Hawrylyshyn PA. The thalamus and midbrain of man: a physiological atlas using electrical stimulation. Springfield, IL: Charles C. Thomas, 1982;154–172.

143. Lenz FA, Seike M, Lin YC, et al. Neurons in the area of human thalamic nucleus ventralis caudalis respond to painful heat stimuli. Brain Res 1993;623:235–240.

144. Lenz FA, Gracely RH, Rowland LH, Dougherty PM. A population of cells in human thalamic principal sensory nucleus respond to painful mechanical stimuli. Neurosci Lett 1994;180:46–50.

145. Dostrovsky JO, Davis KD, Kiss ZHT, et al. Evidence for a specific temperature relay site in human thalamus. Presented at IASP World Congress on Pain, Vancouver. Seattle IASP Press, 1996.

146. Davis KD, Kiss ZHT, Tasker RR, Dostrovsky JO. Thalamic stimulation-evoked sensations in chronic pain patients and in nonpain (movement disorder) patients. J Neurophysiol 1996;75:1026–1034.

147. Davis KD, Tasker RR, Kiss ZHT, et al. Visceral pain evoked by thalamic microstimulation in humans. Neuroreport 1995;6:369–374.

148. Dostrovsky JO, Wells FEB, Tasker RR. Pain sensations evoked by stimulation in human thalamus. In: Inoki R, Shigenaga Y, Yohyama M, eds. Processing and inhibition of nociceptive information. Amsterdam: Elsevier, 1992;115–120.

149. Lenz FA, Seike M, Richardson RT, et al. Thermal and pain sensation evoked by microstimulation in the area of human ventrocaudal nucleus. J Neurophysiol 1993;70:200–212.

150. Lenz FA, Gracely RH, Hope EJ, et al. The sensation of angina can be evoked by stimulation of the human thalamus. Pain 1994;59:119–125.

151. Davis KD, Dostrovsky JO, Tasker RR, et al. Increased incidence of pain evoked by thalamic stimulation in post-stroke pain patients. Soc Neurosci Abstr 1993;19:1572.

152. Tsubokawa T, Katayama Y, Yamamoto T, et al. Motor cortex stimulation for control of thalamic pain. Pain 1990;5(Suppl):491.

153. Tsubokawa T, Katayama Y, Yamamoto T, et al. Chronic motor cortex stimulation for the treatment of central pain. Acta Neurochir 1991;52 (Suppl):137–139.

154. Reference deleted.

CHAPTER 10

Headache

Dhirendra S. Bana

INTRODUCTION

Pain in the head has special significance to humans because the head is so primally associated with human happiness, self-image, and survival. Pain in a muscle or joint is annoying and interferes with normal activity. Pain from the heart forebodes death. Pain in the head, the seat of humans' unique and distinguishing intellect, is not only annoying and interfering but threatening; it brings with it despair, depression, and anxiety. It may occur not only when the head is traumatized or inflamed, but also when its complicated machinery strains to meet overwhelming mental and emotional stress.

Headache of migraine and tension type may stand for an alarm system of the body. The sensors for this alarm are probably set in more than one place, even though the "sound" of the alarm is the same. Thus migraine triggered by ingestion of specific food is similar to a headache brought on by stress. It is a good policy to pay heed to this alarm, identify triggering factors, and fix them while simultaneously shutting off the alarm. Stress, a precipitating factor for the alarm if ignored or shut up by a quick fix with medication, may lead to other bodily harms, even though the headache is under control.

The human with a headache needs relief and explanation. Both should be supplied by his or her physician. This requires time, patience, and a good therapeutic alliance between physician and patient.

QUESTIONS FOR THE PHYSICIAN

Faced in his or her office by a patient complaining of headache, a physician must consider the following questions:

1. Which structures in the head are potential sources of pain?
2. Where is pain from these structures felt?
3. Which sensory tracts carry the pain message?
4. What mechanisms can be responsible for the disturbance?
5. Which structures may be involved when pain is reported in a given location?

SOURCES OF PAIN IN THE HEAD

From personal experience, everyone recognizes that the eyes, teeth, ears, and their intricate mechanisms are sources of pain. The skin, sensory nerves, muscles of the face and head, and blood vessels overlying the skull are very sensitive to pain, as are the nasal turbinates and the ostia of the sinuses. The jaw joints and the periosteum of the skull are similarly sensitive.

The bones of the skull lack pain sensation, and the meninges lining the skull and covering the brain are sensitive only in certain areas, including the base of the skull and the areas immediately adjacent to the meningeal vessels. The great venous sinuses inside the head and the tributary veins carrying blood to them across the subarachnoid space are very sensitive to pain, as are the meningeal blood vessels.

The brain itself, the pial vessels, and the choroid and lining of the ventricles are insensitive. The great vessels bringing blood into the circle of Willis are very sensitive to pain; their extensions up into the brain from the circle of Willis remain pain sensitive for 1 or 2 inches above the circle and then lose their sensitivity as they become the pial vessels. The tentorium hurts when it is stretched up or down; sensory nerves and their ganglia within the cranium are very sensitive to pain.

With a few exceptions, pathological processes within the cranial cavity above the tentorium register their pain over the fifth cranial nerve and present it in the anterior half of the head. Disorders below the tentorium usually present pain via the upper cervical sensory roots in the posterior half of the head. Unfortunately for physicians, some painful events occurring below the tentorium are carried over the recurrent nerve of Arnold, a branch of the fifth cranial nerve that registers pain in the front of the head, although the process may be subtentorial.

Disturbances of the upper two posterior cervical sensory roots may cause pain in the ipsilateral temple. Other lesions, lower in the cervical spine, may bring about pain in the ipsilateral face and temple areas by muscle spasm, ligamentous strain, foraminal compression, or entrapment of sensory roots. Painful processes in the neck may be recorded in the brain via spread to the descending tract of the fifth cranial nerve and may be manifest by facial or temporal pain. Lesions in the neck that affect the sympathetic chain may lead to pain in the distribution of those nerves to the terrain of the carotid and vertebral artery systems as a result of inadequate constriction against noxious dilating substances. Pain from lesions in the middle fossa is carried over the ninth and tenth cranial nerves and felt in and around the ear and in the pharynx. Some sensory fibers associated with the facial nerve (the seventh cranial nerve) may be a source of pain in the ear canal.

Head pain may be a local phenomenon or referred from a distant or deep site. Pain from most superficial structures of the head is usually felt in the region of that structure. When the source is deeper, such as the sphenoid sinus ostium, the middle meningeal artery, or the tentorium, the pain may be referred to a superficial site. This usually is in close proximity to the source, but of necessity occasionally is somewhat remote. Before assuming that a deep structure is the source of referred pain from a remote spot, it is well to ensure that a pathological process is present in that structure. Thus, it is wise not to pull a tooth that is alleged to cause pain in the temple unless disease in the tooth can be demonstrated; similarly, it is appropriate not to operate on a turbinate or sinus for a remote pain unless definite local pathological conditions can be shown.

HEAD PAIN MECHANISMS

Eight mechanisms for head pain have been recognized for a long time. In addition, a central nervous system source of pain existing per se and affecting the threshold of pain from more peripheral afferent impulses has aroused great interest. This consists of disorders of the pain or nociceptive system itself, expressed by disturbed behavior of pain-related substances, such as endorphins, enkephalins, and their receptor systems. Disturbances of the brain itself or its blood vessels may initiate head pain through neurotransmitters, which carry news of damage or strain to be registered in consciousness via the sensory nociceptive system (1).

Conversion, or Hysterical, Headache

Conversion, or hysterical, headache is a head pain of psychogenic origin. Its mechanism is unknown in pathophysiological terms, but it is important to recognize that it is not imaginary. Such pain may arise in the unconscious workings of the brain and may be initiated in a thought or emotion that is converted to pain in the conscious state. Packard (2) provides an example of a young man who developed severe headache in situations reminiscent of troubles with his father.

Neuralgia

Neuralgia arises from disturbances in the physiological state of sensory nerve cells or ganglia or their communicating sensory tracts. The most common sources of cranial neuralgias are the fifth and ninth cranial nerves and the greater and lesser occipital nerves arising from upper cervical sensory roots. Rarely sensory fibers in the seventh cranial nerve also cause pain in the region of the ear canal. Damage by trauma, multiple sclerosis, inflammation, infection, circulatory disturbances, and disordered physiological states in the ganglion synapses may create this type of pain. Other mechanisms probably exist but are still unknown. The most common example of cranial neuralgia is tic douloureux, or trifacial neuralgia. This is usually a disease of patients more than 55 years of age, but occasionally it occurs in younger patients, in whom a local source of trouble such as multiple sclerosis, local tumor, or direct compression of the fifth ganglion by an entrapped artery may be demonstrable. A typical example is that of a 75-year-old woman who complains of a series of short, sharp bursts of electric shock-like pain limited to the second and third divisions of the fifth cranial nerve. Pain occurs in relation to any sensory stimulus in those areas. It is relieved by carbamazepine (Tegretol) or phenytoin (Dilantin) or by surgical interference with the fifth cranial nerve and its central connections.

Direct Pressure on Pain-Sensitive Structures

A posterior fossa tumor, cyst, or abscess directly pressing on the pain-sensitive tentorium or on the fifth cranial nerve itself is an example of pain from direct pressure.

Traction or Distortion

A space-occupying lesion that is insensitive to pain but that stretches, twists, or drags on pain-sensitive vessels, nerves, tributary veins, or vascular sinuses may result in pain. Thus, a brain tumor arising in the nonsensitive parietal brain substance may grow to a size that distorts the shape of the brain and drags on the pain-sensitive tributary veins anchoring it to the pain-sensitive sagittal sinus.

Excessive Generalized Dilation

Excessive generalized dilation of the pain-sensitive portions of intracranial vessels is an important feature of the headache arising from injection of histamine, injection or dermal application of nitroglycerine, or anoxia. The same process is involved in headache from fever, foreign-protein reactions, carbon dioxide intoxication, and toxic reactions to drugs and chemicals. Sudden rises in blood pressure, as happens in pheochromocytoma, and reactions to tyramine during monoamine oxidase inhibitor therapy are yet other examples of headache due to generalized vasodilation. Local vasoactive chemical factors are also implicated. The pial vessels are relatively insensitive to pain, but the main branches of the internal carotid artery, circle of Willis, and basilar artery and its branches are sensitive to pain.

Excessive Localized Vasodilation

Excessive localized vasodilation of branches of the external carotid artery, including the middle meningeal artery, which lies inside the cranium, can cause pain. Localized areas of the main branches of the internal carotid artery, the circle of Willis, and the proximal inch or two of the branches of the circle of Willis are also potential sources of localized pain. Other factors, such as the local accumulation of vasoactive substances that lower the pain threshold in the affected area and centrally, such as neurokinin and substance P, may be important contributors. This mechanism is largely responsible for headaches of the migraine type and many of the headaches associated with hypertension, other than those caused by sudden rises in pressure or hypertensive encephalopathy.

Prolonged Muscle Contraction

Prolonged contraction of face, head, or neck muscles is one of the mechanisms in creating tension and combined headaches. It may become a secondary contributor to the discomfort of any type of headache that calls for a response to keep the head and neck still to prevent worse pain. Headache that a secretary gets as the day grows more pressured and the boss becomes grouchy may well be based on this mechanism. The driver of a car who keeps his head and neck tense as he pushes home against traffic, lights, and rain is made miserable by this mechanism.

Inflammation

Inflammation of any pain-sensitive structure in the head caused by bacteria, viruses, immunological processes, cranial arteritis, lupus erythematosus, meningitis, or encephalitis from any agent creates generalized headache. Inflammation can occur intracranially as well as locally in sinusitis, lateral or cavernous sinus infection, iritis, dental and pharyngeal infections, and so forth. Headache in acquired immunodeficiency syndrome (AIDS) patients may be due to human immunodeficiency virus (HIV) encephalopathy or complication of this disorder by central nervous system involvement of cytomegalic virus, toxoplasmosis, *Candida,* or other fungal infection.

Headache rarely occurs in "pure culture." Combinations of several mechanisms are generally at work contemporaneously.

Structures Involved in Head Pain of a Given Location

Pain felt in a given region may have any of a variety of sources, both inside and outside the cranium. Thus, a pain

around the eye may arise from corneal ulceration; glaucoma; iritis; orbital tumor; cavernous sinus inflammation; temporal artery, middle meningeal, or carotid artery disease; or tumor in the pituitary fossa.

Similarly, pain in the occiput may indicate posterior fossa tumor, cyst, hemorrhage, infection, herpes zoster infection, cervical injury, arthritis, disk or congenital malformation, migraine, or incipient cluster headache. Differentiation of these possibilities is made possible by observation of the patient; a history of the headache attacks; a physical examination of the patient in the office and if possible during an attack; and selected laboratory, x-ray, and electroencephalograph (EEG) tests.

WORKUP OF THE HEADACHE PATIENT

Packard has pointed out that frequently the headache patient is searching as much for explanation and reassurance regarding the headache problem as for cure (3). At the outset of the patient's first visit, it may be wise to ask, "What do you want, and why now?" Patients often do not tell the physician what is worrying them about their symptoms. The physician may do well to identify any concern of a patient about his or her headache. Medical attention may be sought after a family member or a neighbor is diagnosed with brain tumor after a brief history of headaches, even though the patient has had headaches for years without any recent change. They want reassurance that they have not been living with brain tumor for all these years. If the secret worry is unearthed, appropriate reassurance can be provided.

The patient's headache history is by far the most important part of the workup. It is divided into two major parts, a profile of a given attack and a profile of the behavior of these attacks over the years in relation to life changes.

In addition, it is essential to accumulate facts about the patient's general medical background and emotional history. It is helpful to establish at the first interview whether the patient has more than one kind of headache. If so, attention should first be paid to the main headache, and the differences between it and others should be determined later.

The profile of an attack may be made in the physician's mind or better yet, on paper in the form of a diagram (Fig. 10.1). It should include the nature and timing of prodromal symptoms; the hour of onset; the time it takes for the pain to reach the peak level of intensity; and its duration in seconds, minutes, hours, or days. Factors that precipitate attacks should be noted as reported by the patient. Effect of sleep, emotion, fasting, foods, mood changes, light, sounds, smells, weather, exercise, sex, the Valsalva maneuver, and drugs is also recorded.

Presence of nausea, vomiting, prostration, confusion, visual symptoms, and neurological symptoms during headache aid in the diagnosis. Ask the patient what he or she does during a headache. Migraine patients prefer hibernation in a dark, quiet room with a cold cloth on the head; the cluster

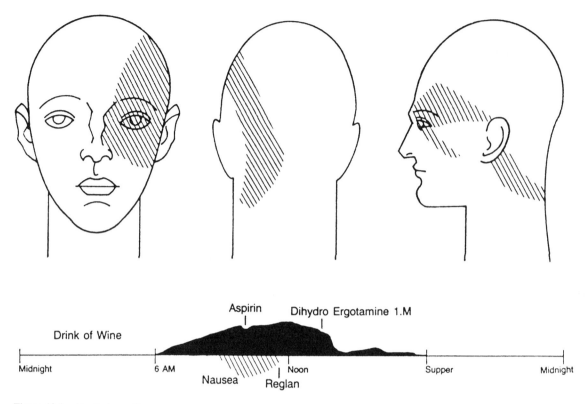

Figure 10.1. Headache profile.

headache sufferer is restless, paces the floor, jogs, or runs and may even become violent during an attack. A tension headache patient may not change his or her routine during a headache. Neurological disturbances may occur prior to the onset of headache and subside before the onset of headache. A note should be made if these symptoms persist or even outlast the headache phase.

Inquire about favorable or unfavorable responses to previous methods of treatment. Special attention should be paid to the effectiveness of ergotamine tartrate or sumatriptan. It is important to see that the ergotamine was properly taken. Ergotamine or sumatriptan effectiveness is a pointer in diagnosis and treatment because it rarely helps any headache other than migraine or cluster. The search for the precipitating factors of a given headache should be directed to the last few days before the headache and to the time the headache actually occurred.

Life profile of the headaches is also informative. It starts with a search into the family history for headache, especially of the migraine variety. Patients frequently report a family history of headaches as negative when they really mean, "negative as far as any headaches as bad as mine are concerned." A history of a father with "sinus headache" all his life may show on closer questioning a diagnosis of migraine, especially because chronic sinusitis rarely causes intermittent attacks of headache over many years. Early death of or separation from a parent also may hide a history of migraine. It is often useful to suggest to headache patients that they

inquire positively into the family history of headaches; this may reveal significant histories that have remained hidden because they were not considered important or for some other reason. About 70% of migraine headache patients have a family history of migraine; this is an important factor in making a diagnosis.

Age of the patient when headaches began is important. Frequently a patient fails to report minor headaches in early years because they were considered to be the "headaches like everyone has but nothing like the ones I have now." Forerunners of migraine should be looked for. Migraine frequently begins in early life with gastrointestinal upsets without headache. Colic in babyhood, carsickness, seasickness, and bilious attacks as a small child may herald migraine. The patient should be questioned about dyslexia and phobias, such as claustrophobia, because they are often missed despite the stress they create in the patient.

Valuable information about the nature of a headache problem is garnered by establishing relations between the onset, frequency, and severity of the attacks with major changes in life events. These include separations in the family, going to school and college, puberty, jobs, engagement, marriage, divorce, loss of important people and other supports, accidents, illnesses, pregnancy, toxemia of pregnancy, travel, vacations, illness, operations, menopause, depression, and retirement. When, where, and why the first headache appeared may be valuable guide to later events. The history may be greatly enriched by a detailed review of the patient's day or weekend, a picture of the people or pets in the house, and the family communication systems (e.g., telephone each other daily, twice daily, or not at all). The educational, religious, and employment background of parents often sheds light on the formation of habits in the patient when young, which may play a role in headache occurrence later on.

A review of medications and treatments that have been tried and succeeded, failed, or caused side effects is also very important to avoid useless or dangerous therapies.

The review of systems and medical and family history are, of course, important. In this connection it is best to ask how significant past events affected the life and emotional status of the patient. Physicians short on time who would like to know more about a patient with headache may gather a wealth of information by simply asking the patient to write about himself or herself and how headaches have changed plans in daily living. The diary can be reviewed on the next visit. Most patients are anxious to tell who they are and bring out pointers, which may aid in management of the headache.

Special Points in the Physical Examination of the Headache Patient

Physical and neurological examination of the headache patient should include evaluation of mood and behavior. Observe leonine facial features associated with cluster headache. Ipsilateral drooping of eyelid, tearing, nasal block, rhinorrhea, and meiosis may be seen during a cluster headache. Palpate and auscultate the head; look for signs of hypothyroidism, Cushing's disease, and acromegaly. Examine the skin for vascular nevi or lesions of neurofibromatosis. Search for dental occlusal defects. Examine the extremities for Raynaud's syndrome. Cardiac examination should include searching for murmurs, including signs of mitral valve prolapse. Palpate the scalp for engorgement or redness and tenderness of scalp blood vessels. Compression of the temporal artery may temporarily relieve migraine headache. Worsening of the pain by carotid artery palpation occurs in carotidynia. Head-neck traction applied by lifting the head off the neck helps to determine the role of neck as a cause of headache.

Warnings of Organic Disease from the Patient's History

Headache Accompanied by Unconsciousness

Although fainting is sometimes associated with migraine, episodes of blacking out during headache should prompt tests to rule out seizures, hemorrhages, posterior fossa lesions, and cervical spondylosis.

Headache with No History

A severe headache appearing suddenly for the first time may represent the beginning of a migraine history or the onset of cluster headache. However, it may indicate the first bleed from a vascular malformation, a sudden blood pressure rise from a pheochromocytoma, or an embolic event from a cardiac lesion or dissection of a carotid artery. Careful examination and testing are called for if a ready explanation cannot be determined.

Headache Accompanied by Neurological Abnormalities during and after the Head Pain

In migraine with aura (classic migraine) a short course of neurological symptoms precedes the onset of head pain. Occasionally they recur during the headache phase. In hemiplegic and ophthalmoplegic migraine, symptoms may begin during the headache and persist for hours, days, or weeks after the head pain. When neurological symptoms and signs occur *during* and *after* the head pain, a thorough investigation to rule out intracranial vascular lesion or tumor is necessary. Computed tomography (CT) with and without contrast and magnetic resonance imaging (MRI) with and without angiograms aid in the diagnosis. A radiology colleague often gives valuable advice as to which of these techniques is most appropriate (4). EEG abnormalities may suggest seizure activity.

Headache Associated with Fever or Stiff Neck

Fever associated with headache most often indicates underlying infection. It may be viral, bacterial, or parasitic. Fever may be associated with hemorrhage, vascular accidents such as emboli and stroke, malignant disease, central nervous system lues, or lupus. In older patients cranial arteritis should be suspected and immediately investigated with a blood test for sedimentation rates, antinuclear antibodies (ANA), and arterial biopsy.

Headache Developing after 50 Years of Age

Headache onset after 50 years of age is commonly associated with organic disease, such as cervical spondylosis or disc disease, onset of hypertension, menopause, hormonal change (especially thyroid deficiency), cranial arteritis, and tumor. Depression on retirement may also cause headaches for the first time at this age.

A Change in Character or Response to Treatment of Previous Headaches

When a headache suddenly changes in its location, quality of pain, or its response to a previously reliable treatment, a search for a new diagnosis is in order. If a migraine patient with unilateral headache begins to complain of bilateral pain that does not respond to previously effective ergotamine therapy suspect an organic cause. Suspicion of organic lesion is heightened if it is associated with numbness in the face that outlasts the headache or results in stiffness of the neck.

Headache Associated with Alteration in Personality and Habits

When a well-behaved, pleasant individual becomes unreasonable, uncleanly, forgetful, and disordered in daily work and habits, suspect organic lesions of the brain. Headache also may be a feature, and early on its location may point to the location of the organic disease. CT, MRI, a test for syphilis, a temperature chart, Doppler flow studies of cranial circulation, lumbar puncture for cells, India ink studies, and tests for abnormal pressures and proteins may be in order. Headache patients who are at risk for AIDS or AIDS-related complex (ARC) may need to be tested, with consent and counseling, for these disorders.

Headache Associated with Hypertension or Endocrine Disorders

Cushing's syndrome, parathyroid tumors, hypothyroidism from radioactive thyroid therapy or other causes, and hypertensive episodes from pheochromocytoma may first present clinically as headache. The development of essential hypertension in the middle years of life is not uncommon in migraine (5). When this happens, single, infrequent episodes of migraine may change into the daily wake-up headache of the hypertensive patient. Treatment of the hypertension usually helps the headache problem.

Headache Initiated by the Valsalva Maneuver

When a headache is precipitated by the Valsalva maneuver, such as coughing, sneezing, bending, straining, coitus, or lifting, a search must be made for organic disease, although the Valsalva maneuver can accentuate a preexisting headache of vascular origin, such as a migraine or the flu. When this maneuver *brings on* headache, a search for an organic lesion such as vascular malformation, posterior fossa tumor pressing on the brainstem, a cyst obstructing spinal fluid flow, and serious neck lesions compromising the lumen of the cervical spinal canal is essential.

Headache Due to Other Causes

If headaches do not fit the well-recognized functional classification and occur with physical changes such as straining, turning, and lying on one side, suspect organic cause. Organic headaches last a short time, only to come back unexpectedly. Nausea or vomiting and disturbances of vision, gait, or cognitive functions are common. Their very failure to follow the rules of well-established functional headache patterns may be the clue to serious organic disease demanding further investigation.

Tests Useful in the Diagnosis of Organic versus Functional Causes of Headache

1. Temperature chart reveals infection, systemic disease, cranial arteritis or abscess, autoimmune disorders.

2. Minnesota Multiphasic Personality Inventory (MMPI), Zung scale, or other personality evaluation tests reveal hidden emotional factors or depression conversion symptoms.

3. Cognitive testing discovers organic cerebral dysfunction.

4. Skull radiographic films show fractures, pituitary size, metastases, acoustic neuroma, tumors, bone destruction, Paget's disease, calcified arteriovenous malformation (AVM), shift of midline, parathyroid disease, multiple myeloma, platybasia, erosion of bone, sickle cell disease, and others.

5. Neck radiographic films show fractures old and new; disc disease; arthritis (especially abnormality of odontoid ligament in rheumatoid arthritis); congenital malformations; cervical spondylosis; tumors; dislocation.

6. Noninvasive Doppler studies discover blood flow in major cranial arteries; vascular spasms; obstructions; reverse flow phenomena.

7. Technetium scans show inflammation (abscess); secondary syphilis and other granulomatous disorders; blood flow studies; tumors; AVM related to abnormal presence and flow of blood.

8. EEG reveals seizure disorders; sleep disorder; space-occupying lesions; metabolic and hyperkinetic disorders; brain damage and deterioration.
   A. Sleep EEG sometimes shows abnormalities not shown in regular EEG.
   B. Brain electrical activity map (BEAM) EEG may disclose small foci of seizure activity, posttraumatic damage, or dyslexia.

9. Magnetoencephalogram (MEG) discloses changes in brain during migraine attack and in between attacks (6).

10. Visual evoked potential discovers differentiating migraine from other neurological or ocular condition (7).

11. Transcranial Doppler evaluation shows pathophysiology of migraine (8).

12. CT of head and neck reveals intracranial bleeding; space-occupying lesions; atrophy; nose and throat disease; orbital lesions; abscess; AVM; coronal section of sinuses for sinusitis; special body scan tests for cervical lesions, such as discs and syringomyelia; tumor and vascular malformations in brain and cervical spine. CT may miss small aneurysms and other small lesions, especially in the posterior fossa. Noninvasive CT, despite its cost, may be both economically and medically preferable to a whole series of other less effective tests, which taken together cost as much or more.

13. MRI with gadolinium-diethylenetriaminepentaacetic acid-dimeglumine (Gd-DTPA) is probably the most specific test to rule out intracranial space-occupying lesions. Combined with angiography of cervical and intracerebral vessels, it is a sensitive test to rule out carotid or vertebral artery dissections and aneurysms.

14. Lumbar puncture shows infection, protein abnormalities, pressure abnormalities, disc disease, tumor cells in cerebrospinal fluid. Care should be exerted in performing lumbar puncture in the presence of suspected posterior fossa space-occupying lesions or abnormalities near the foramen magnum for fear of creating brainstem coning. Patients usually avoid post-lumbar puncture headache when they maintain a prone position with the buttocks raised or the foot of the bed raised slightly for 6 to 8 hours after the procedure.

15. Overnight continuous oxygen saturation study by finger oxymetry for sleep apnea syndrome may show a typical sawtooth pattern of saturation and desaturation during sleep. If positive, it should be followed by a full sleep study to differentiate between central neurological and upper airway obstruction for sleep apnea. History of snoring and morning headache is an indication to rule out sleep apnea syndrome.

Reassuring the patient, a necessary therapeutic maneuver, may require special testing to document that no serious organic disease is present.

CLASSIFICATION OF HEADACHE

In 1988 the International Headache Society (IHS) published a classification of headache (9). Prior to this Ad Hoc Committee classification was in vogue (10). An abbreviated version of IHS classification is listed under Table 10.1

The Migraines

Migraine with Aura (Classic Migraine)

Migraine with aura is characterized by succinct neurological prodrome, sometimes occurring without headache, usually lasting 20 to 45 minutes and followed by a headache. The headache is most often unilateral, lasts several hours, and often is associated with nausea and vomiting.

Migraine without Aura (Common Migraine)

Common migraine is characterized by familial unilateral or bilateral periodic attacks of headache, occasionally preceded over some hours by vague mood changes and autonomic symptoms. It may be accompanied by nausea, vomiting, diuresis, and prostration over 12 to 72 hours.

Ophthalmoplegic and Hemiplegic Migraine

Periodic attacks of severe headache associated with paralysis of the third nerve (ophthalmoplegic) or motor paralysis of one side of the body (hemiplegic) that outlasts the headache but eventually clears in several weeks or days characterize ophthalmoplegic and hemiplegic migraines. In some patients there is family incidence of similar disorders. Hemiplegic migraine may have a genetic predisposition.

Retinal Migraine

In retinal migraine young patients develop repeated episodes of transient dimness or complete loss of vision in one or both eyes without a preceding visual fortification spectrum. Visual symptoms, which can be triggered by bright light, vary in severity and frequency. Impaired vision lasts about 10 minutes, but on rare occasions it may be prolonged to an hour. Sometimes it leaves a permanent visual deficit. Headache never occurs during or soon after the visual phenomenon, but migraine headache may be present at other times, or the patient may not give any history of migraine at all. There may be a history of bilious vomiting in childhood (a migraine equivalent). The cause of retinal migraine is probably reversible narrowing of the ophthalmic artery. These symptoms in older age groups must be distinguished from amaurosis fugax, an embolic phenomenon from atheromatous plaque in the ipsilateral internal carotid artery near the bifurcation of the common carotid artery. Treatment is the same as for migraine headache (11).

Cluster Headache

A cluster headache, almost always an excruciating unilateral headache, occurs mostly in men and usually in short attacks lasting 10 to 120 minutes once or several times a day or night. Prominent autonomic symptoms and signs, such as ipsilateral partial Horner's syndrome, tearing, conjunctival redness, ptosis, meiosis, nasal block and rhinorrhea, unilateral or bilateral sweating, and frantic pacing accompany it. Clusters of daily headaches last for a few weeks or months, followed by weeks, months, or years of remission. When cluster headaches continue daily for more than a year, they are termed chronic cluster headaches. Primary chronic cluster headache occurs if there is no break in the headache from the outset. Secondary chronic cluster headache is preceded by several cycles of episodic clusters. The laterality of the pain and autonomic symptoms may change in some patients over the years, during one attack, or in different clusters. Rare instances of bilateral attacks have been observed.

A subset of cluster headache is chronic paroxysmal hemicrania. This is much more common in women than in men, is shorter in duration (15 to 30 minutes) than cluster headache, and occurs many (5 to 30) times per day. It is remarkable for prompt response (in a few hours), specifically to indomethacin. These attacks may occur in periodic or chronic patterns.

Lower-Half Headache, or Atypical Facial Neuralgia (10)

Lower-half headache is possibly related to migraine. The symptoms are unilateral facial pain occurring at first in episodes similar to common migraine, then more and more frequently until the patient is in constant pain. Psychoses may lie (not too deeply buried) beneath this disabling symptom.

Table 10.1.   IHS Headache Classification

1. Migraine
   With or without aura; familial hemiplegic; basilar, ophthalmoplegic, retinal
	8. Substances or their withdrawal
	   Birth control pills or estrogens

2. Tension
   Episodic; chronic
	9. Noncephalic infection
	   Bacterial or viral infections, septicemia

3. Cluster, chronic paroxysmal hemicrania	10. Metabolic disorder

4. Miscellaneous, not associated with structural lesion
   Idiopathic stabbing; external compression headache; cold stimulus
   headache; benign cough, benign exertional; associated with sexual activity
	Hypoxia
	   High altitude
	   Sleep apnea
	   Hypercapnia
	   Hypoglycemia
	   Dialysis

5. Head trauma
   Acute; chronic
	11. Headache or facial pain or disorder of facial or cranial structures
	   Cranial bone, neck, eyes, ears, nose and sinuses
	   Acute sinus headache, teeth, jaws, and related structures
	   Temporomandibular joint disease

6. Vascular disorder
   Acute ischemic cerebrovascular disease
   Transient ischemic attack
   Thromboembolic stroke
   Intracranial, intracerebral subdural and epidural hematomas
   Subarachnoid hemorrhage
   Arteriovenous malformation
   Saccular aneurysm
   Giant cell arteritis
   Other systemic arteriolitis
   Carotid or vertebral artery dissection
   Carotidynia (idiopathic)
   Postendartectomy headache
   Venous thrombosis
   Arterial hypertension
   Acute pressor response to exogenous agent
   Pheochromocytoma
	12. Cranial neuralgias, nerve trunk pain, and deafferentation pain
	   Persistent (in contrast to ticlike) pain of cranial nerve origin
	   Compression or distortion of cranial nerves and second or third cervical roots
	   Demyelination of cranial nerves
	   Optic neuritis (retrobulbar neuritis)
	   Infarction of cranial nerves
	   Diabetic neuritis
	   Inflammation of cranial nerves
	   Herpes zoster
	   Chronic postherpetic neuralgia
	   Tolosa-Hunt syndrome
	   Neck-tongue syndrome
	   Trigeminal neuralgia
	   Glossopharyngeal neuralgia
	   Idiopathic glossopharyngeal neuralgia
	   Symptomatic glossopharyngeal neuralgia
	   Nervus intermedius neuralgia
	   Superior laryngeal neuralgia
	   Occipital neuralgia
	   Anesthesia dolorosa
	   Thalamic pain

6. Malignant (accelerated) hypertension Preeclampsia and eclampsia	13. Headache not classifiable

7. Nonvascular intracranial disorder
   High or low cerebrospinal fluid pressure
   Post–lumbar puncture
   Cerebrospinal fluid fistula
   Intracranial infection
   Intracranial sarcoidosis and other noninfectious inflammatory diseases
   Related to intrathecal injections
   Intracranial neoplasm	

Tension-Type Headache (9)

Commonly known as tension headache, tension-type headache is usually an overall head and neck discomfort occurring during periods of anxiety and stress. Demonstrable increase in head and neck muscle contraction is present in many cases but not in others with similar symptoms. Often periodic headaches gradually become constant.

Combined Headache (10)

In combined headache, factors of both migraine and muscle contraction headache are prominently and contemporaneously active, producing an overall head and neck discomfort and pain; it is often called mixed headache.

Headache of Nasal Vasomotor Reaction (10)

Headache of nasal vasomotor reaction is associated with a constant sense of fullness, pressure, and pain in the region of the eyes, nose, and anterior upper face that is not related to allergy but is often associated with deep-seated emotional problems.

Headache of Delusional, Conversion, or Hypochondriacal State (10)

Headache of delusional, conversion, or hypochondriacal state is a manifestation of an illness in which the prevailing clinical disorder is a delusional or conversion reaction and a peripheral pain mechanism is nonexistent or minimal. These headaches are related to subconscious emotions or to mood changes, such as depression.

Nonmigrainous Vascular Headaches

Head pain may result from many sources of dilation of cranial arteries, such as fever; anoxia; foreign protein, toxic, or allergic reactions; hypercapnia; or vasodilating drugs, such as nitrites and histamine.

Traction Headache (10)

Traction headache results from traction on pain-sensitive intracranial structures by space-occupying lesions or distortion of brain structures by changes in intracranial pressure.

Headache Caused by Overt Cranial Inflammation (10)

Some headaches are due to readily recognized inflammation of cranial structures by hemorrhagic, allergic, chemical, or infectious causes that produce meningitis, arteritis, or phlebitis.

Headache from Noxious Stimulation (10)

Headaches may result from noxious stimulation of ocular, aural, nasal, dental, or other local structures of the head by any of various agents, such as trauma, spasm, new growth, inflammation, or allergic reaction.

Cranial Neuritides (10)

Cranial neuritides are due to direct injury to nerves by new growths, trauma, or inflammation.

Cranial Neuralgia

The cranial neuralgias include trigeminal, glossopharyngeal, and greater and lesser occipital nerve neuralgias producing lancinating, jabbing pain in rapid succession for several minutes or longer in an area limited to the distribution of the affected nerve.

Chronic Posttraumatic Headache

Chronic posttraumatic headache may arise from any one or all of several mechanisms, including muscle contraction; vascular dilation; direct nerve, vessel, scalp, or neck injury; or conversion or hypochondriacal reactions. This chapter discusses the mechanism and management of these headaches but does not attempt to cover the details of headaches caused by specific organic disease processes, the alleviation of which is based on treatment of the underlying disorder.

MIGRAINE WITH AURA (CLASSIC MIGRAINE)

Description (9)

Migraine with aura is an idiopathic, recurring disorder manifesting with attacks of neurological symptoms unequivocally localizable to cerebral cortex or brainstem, usually gradually developed over 5 to 20 minutes and usually lasting less than 60 minutes. Headache, nausea, photophobia, or a combination of these usually follows neurological aura symptoms directly or after a free interval of less than an hour. The headache usually lasts 4 to 72 hours but may be completely absent.

Diagnostic Criteria (9)

Migraine with aura is characterized by at least two attacks with any three of the following four characteristics:

1. One or more fully reversible aura symptoms indicating focal cerebral cortical or brainstem dysfunction occurs.
2. At least one aura symptom develops gradually over more than 4 minutes or two or more symptoms occur in succession.
3. No aura symptom lasts more than 60 minutes. If more than one aura symptom is present, accepted duration is proportionally increased.
4. Headache following aura with a free interval of less than 60 minutes (may also begin before or simultaneously with the aura); history, physical, neurological examinations required to rule out any organic disorder; laboratory investigation if indicated to rule out organic cause

The attack profile of migraine with aura (Fig. 10.2) includes a prodrome that may take the form of succinct neurological disturbance, such as visual scotoma; hemianesthesia; aphasia; flashing lights; confusion; micropsia; heightened sensitivity to light, noise, and smells; and other neurological symptoms. These phenomena usually last 20 to 30 minutes, but as they move from one area to another, they may last longer; rarely, they recur during the headache phase of the attack.

As the sharply defined neurological fireworks clear, the headache usually but not always follows. It takes about 30 to 60 minutes to reach its peak, is often unilateral, and most commonly is on the side of the head opposite from the symptoms of the prodrome. The pain is steady, often throbbing with the pulse, lasts 1 to 6 hours, and often is accompanied by nausea and vomiting. It may always occur on the same side of the head but commonly changes sides from attack to attack. Change in location is a reassuring feature, because it argues strongly against a fixed organic cause.

During the prodromal phase of the attack, changes in the blood circulation of the brain have been recorded. Recent studies suggest that these start with a sudden short increase in cerebral blood flow followed by a decreased blood flow. These disturbances may be generalized but are especially pronounced in the area of cerebral dysfunction. Increasing blood flow by breathing carbon dioxide or very small amounts of amyl nitrite (12) may alleviate the condition and help to abort the prodrome and at times the whole attack. Pathophysiology of migraine with aura is not yet established. Factors studied include vasomotor spasm (13), generalized or local (14); hyperviscosity of blood of a transient nature related to aggregation of platelets (15), increased protein or lipoprotein (16), or free fatty acid content of serum (17); opening of arteriovenous shunts (18); and disturbed metabolic or electrical events in brain cells leading to circulatory reactions, as in the spreading depression (19). Substance P is probably the agent for transmitting this noxious condition into the brain, where it is registered as pain.

Treatment of the prodrome phase of the attack is often not successful. Treatments include the following:

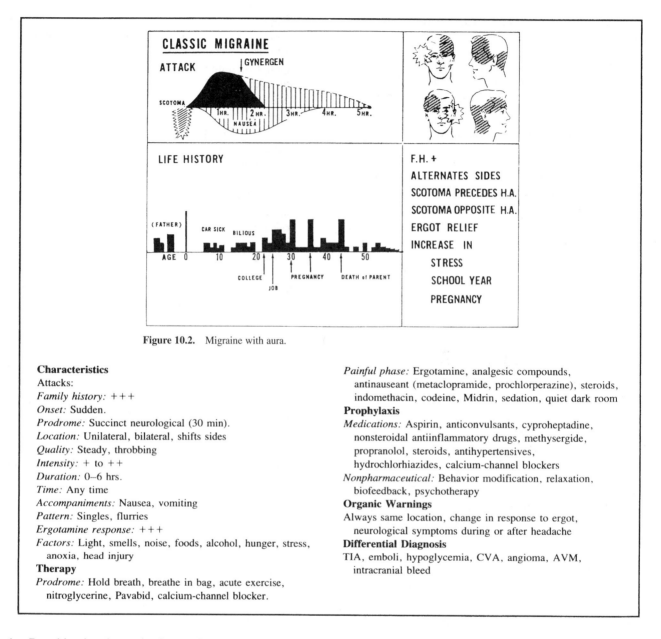

Figure 10.2. Migraine with aura.

Characteristics
Attacks:
Family history: +++
Onset: Sudden.
Prodrome: Succinct neurological (30 min).
Location: Unilateral, bilateral, shifts sides
Quality: Steady, throbbing
Intensity: + to ++
Duration: 0–6 hrs.
Time: Any time
Accompaniments: Nausea, vomiting
Pattern: Singles, flurries
Ergotamine response: +++
Factors: Light, smells, noise, foods, alcohol, hunger, stress,
   anoxia, head injury
Therapy
Prodrome: Hold breath, breathe in bag, acute exercise,
   nitroglycerine, Pavabid, calcium-channel blocker.

Painful phase: Ergotamine, analgesic compounds,
   antinauseant (metaclopramide, prochlorperazine), steroids,
   indomethacin, codeine, Midrin, sedation, quiet dark room
Prophylaxis
Medications: Aspirin, anticonvulsants, cyproheptadine,
   nonsteroidal antiinflammatory drugs, methysergide,
   propranolol, steroids, antihypertensives,
   hydrochlorhiazides, calcium-channel blockers
Nonpharmaceutical: Behavior modification, relaxation,
   biofeedback, psychotherapy
Organic Warnings
Always same location, change in response to ergot,
   neurological symptoms during or after headache
Differential Diagnosis
TIA, emboli, hypoglycemia, CVA, angioma, AVM,
   intracranial bleed

1. Breathing in a large-sized paper bag (may be carried folded), which is put over the head to rest lightly on the shoulders for 10 to 15 minutes
2. Holding the breath as long as possible, alternating with short periods of breathing
3. Breathing a whiff of amyl nitrite or putting 0.3 mg nitroglycerine under the tongue.

When the prodrome has cleared and the head pain begins, there is a "luxury suffusion" of blood in the brain, especially in the affected area, and an increased amplitude of pulsation of the branches of the ipsilateral external carotid artery, which become the seat of most of the pain. Chapman et al. (20) described the presence of a bradykinin-like substance that lowers the pain threshold. Others suggest that the pain is determined by changes in the biochemistry of the central nociceptive nervous system, perhaps in the limbic system. Whichever of

these theories is correct, it is clear that physical or pharmaceutical measures that result in contraction of dilated vessels and possibly in closure of abnormally open shunts are related to the alleviation of pain. Treatment of the painful phase of migraine is described further in the section on common migraine.

The life profile of migraine with aura includes the following important points: a positive family history of the migraines and forerunners of migraine in childhood, such as biliary colic, carsickness, or cyclic vomiting attacks.

Headaches occur either as single separate attacks or as intermittent flurries of several attacks in a week separated by periods of freedom from headache. These attacks tend to occur at times of major physiological or psychological change and bodily adjustment, such as beginning school, puberty, a job, marriage, pregnancy, menopause, or onset of hypertension.

Oddly enough, classic migraine attacks tend to occur or recur during pregnancy and cause alarm to the patient and the obstetrician. They also may appear after years of absence in middle and old age, perhaps as a complication of arterial changes, brain cell dysfunction, changed vasomotor tone, or disease associated with increased blood viscosity. In rare instances, permanent neurological lesions may persist after prolonged or severe attacks (complicated migraine).

Treatment of complicated migraine with anticoagulants is indicated. Drugs commonly used include aspirin 325 mg daily; dipyridamole (Persantine) 50 mg three times a day. If the patient continues to have complicated migraine while on aspirin or dipyridamole, warfarin sodium (Coumadin) should be tried. The dose of warfarin is adjusted to keep prothrombin time in the therapeutic range (international normalized ratio [INR] between 2 and 3). Calcium channel blockers may also be effective. The use of ergotamine, however, should be avoided because it may cause vascular occlusion.

MIGRAINE WITHOUT AURA (COMMON MIGRAINE)

Description

Common migraine is an idiopathic, recurring headache disorder manifesting in attacks lasting 4 to 72 hours. Typical characteristics of this headache are its unilateral location, pulsating quality, moderate or severe intensity, aggravation by routine physical activity, and association with nausea, photophobia, and phonophobia (9).

Diagnostic Criteria (9)

Common migraine consists of at least five attacks lasting 4 to 72 hours (untreated or unsuccessfully treated) and having at least two of these characteristics:

1. Unilateral location
2. Pulsating quality
3. Moderate or severe intensity (inhibits or prohibits daily activities)
4. Aggravation by walking stairs or similar routine physical activity

During the headache at least one of the following is present:

1. Nausea, vomiting, or both
2. Photophobia and phonophobia

An organic cause for these symptoms should be ruled out by history, physical and neurological examinations, and laboratory tests, if indicated. Common migraine (Fig. 10.3), the old-fashioned sick headache, is the source of more disability from headache than any other type. It occurs about three times as often in women as in men. In some patients (possibly about 25%), there is a vague, prolonged prodrome that precedes the painful phase by several hours rather than by several minutes. These symptoms are mood disturbances, such as euphoria, depression, or irritability, or bouts of excessive yawning, sneezing, or hunger occurring the night before the attack.

The patient awakes with a headache that is usually but not always unilateral, slowly mounts in severity, and unless stopped by rest, sleep, or appropriate medication, usually lasts until the patient goes to bed. In severe cases the headache may last several days. Nausea, vomiting, polyuria, chills, and cold hands and feet are common. Sensitivity to sound, light, and smell is frequent. Patients prefer to hibernate in a dark room, begging for quiet and freedom from people and problems.

Migraine sufferers who come to physicians for help usually have already tried the ordinary analgesics. There are two excellent medications, ergotamine and triptans, for treatment of headache attack. These work for both classic and common migraine.

The backbone of therapy for the painful phase of the attack is the proper use of ergotamine tartrate (Table 10.2). Ergotamine tartrate controls the attack by its special predilection for constricting branches of the external carotid artery, by possibly closing shunts, and by some central nociceptive actions. The sooner it is used, the better it works. Convenience of administration is important in the effectiveness of the product. Because nausea is frequently a feature of the migraine attack or the result of drugs used for its relief, an antiemetic is the first step in treatment. Metoclopramide (Reglan) 10 or 20 mg orally is used for nausea. Rectal suppositories of chlorpromazine (Thorazine) 25 mg, prochlorperazine (Compazine) 25 mg, or trimethobenzamide hydrochloride (Tigan) 100 mg may be beneficial, followed 20 to 30 minutes later by a selected dose of ergotamine. When ergotamine is used for the first time, try only half of the dose listed in Table 10.2. Response to ergot is variable, and a bad first reaction to this valuable drug may steer the patient away from it forever.

The route and content of ergot use must be tailored to the individual and his or her activities, bearing in mind that early use is desirable. Ergotamine efficacy is least by oral route, better by nasal (21) or rectal route, and best as an intramuscular injection. Intravenous dihydroergotamine has been used for the treatment of acute migraine attacks and refractory headaches (22–24). After three doses of oral ergot-containing drug, it is usually not helpful to take more for any given attack. Ergotamine should not be used more than 3 or 4 days in a given week. Daily use can lead to the development of ergotamine dependency (i.e., the ergot cycle, which can lead to daily rebound headaches).

Contraindications to the use of ergotamine tartrate are pregnancy, cardiovascular disease, severe hypertension, significant renal or liver disease, fibroses resulting from previous use of methysergide (Sansert) therapy, Raynaud's disease, and valvular heart disease. The steady simultaneous use of ergotamine and β-blockers or methysergide requires careful monitoring to avoid compromise of the peripheral circulation. Avoid ergot use for the first time in patients more than 60 years of age or in poor health. The exception is the older patient who has used ergot drugs without any harmful effects for many years and who has no heart condition; such persons may be allowed to use it under careful watch.

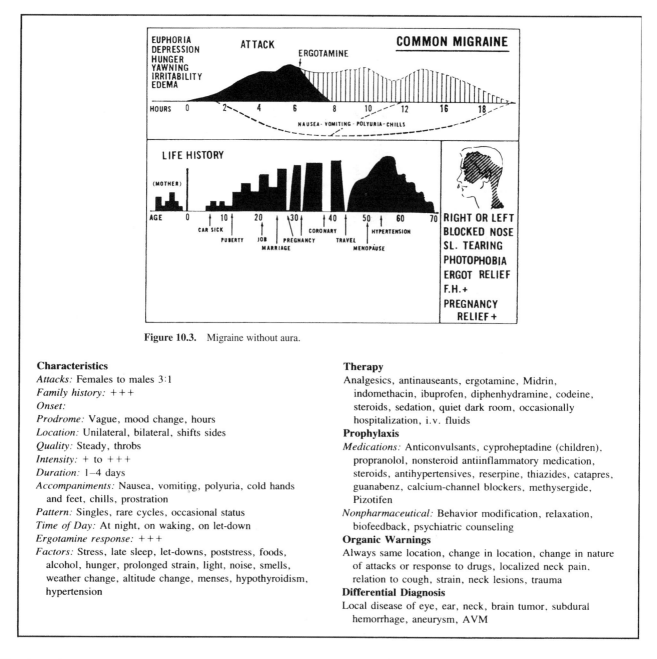

Figure 10.3.   Migraine without aura.

Characteristics

Attacks: Females to males 3:1
Family history: +++
Onset:
Prodrome: Vague, mood change, hours
Location: Unilateral, bilateral, shifts sides
Quality: Steady, throbs
Intensity: + to +++
Duration: 1–4 days
Accompaniments: Nausea, vomiting, polyuria, cold hands
    and feet, chills, prostration
Pattern: Singles, rare cycles, occasional status
Time of Day: At night, on waking, on let-down
Ergotamine response: +++
Factors: Stress, late sleep, let-downs, poststress, foods,
    alcohol, hunger, prolonged strain, light, noise, smells,
    weather change, altitude change, menses, hypothyroidism,
    hypertension

Therapy

Analgesics, antinauseants, ergotamine, Midrin,
    indomethacin, ibuprofen, diphenhydramine, codeine,
    steroids, sedation, quiet dark room, occasionally
    hospitalization, i.v. fluids

Prophylaxis

Medications: Anticonvulsants, cyproheptadine (children),
    propranolol, nonsteroid antiinflammatory medication,
    steroids, antihypertensives, reserpine, thiazides, catapres,
    guanabenz, calcium-channel blockers, methysergide,
    Pizotifen
Nonpharmaceutical: Behavior modification, relaxation,
    biofeedback, psychiatric counseling

Organic Warnings

Always same location, change in location, change in nature
    of attacks or response to drugs, localized neck pain,
    relation to cough, strain, neck lesions, trauma

Differential Diagnosis

Local disease of eye, ear, neck, brain tumor, subdural
    hemorrhage, aneurysm, AVM

Treatment

Intravenous Dihydroergotamine Protocol

Dihydroergotamine (DHE) is an α-adrenergic blocking agent and an antiserotonin compound. It causes vasospasm of peripheral and cranial blood vessels. It is not an analgesic.

Indications

Intravenous DHE is used for continuous intractable daily headaches of vascular type or vascular headaches complicated by analgesic abuse.

Method

Place an intravenous heparin lock. Give metoclopramide 10 mg intravenous diluted in 50 mL of normal saline or dex-

trose 5% in water. Run it in 30 minutes (100 mL/hour). After the metoclopramide drip is finished, give 0.5 mL (1 mg/mL) DHE 45 directly through the heparin lock. Administer it slowly over 3 minutes.

Observe the response to this dose. Whether to repeat the dose of DHE depends on response to the first dose. If after the first injection there was improvement in headache and no side effects were reported, repeat 0.5 mL of undiluted DHE every 8 hours for a total dose of 3 mL (3 mg). If the patient continues to complain of headache but no side effect is reported from the first dose of DHE, give another dose of 0.5 mL intravenously an hour after the first dose. Repeat DHE 1 mL intravenously slowly every 8 hours for a total of 6 doses. The dose of DHE can be titrated down if side effects were noted with 0.5 mL of DHE (23). Side effects of DHE include nausea, vomiting, numbness or tingling in the fingers or toes, muscle

Table 10.2.   Ergotamine Products for Migraine Attacks

Product	Route	Ergotamine	Caffeine	Initial dose	Repeat dose	Maximum dose
Ergotamine tartrate (Ergomar)	Sublingual	2 mg	None	2 mg	2 mg at 30-min interval	Not more than 6 mg in 24 hr and not more than 10 mg in a wk
Dihydroergotamine mesylate (Migranal)	Nasal spray	2 mg (0.5 mg/spray)	10 mg	1 spray in each nostril	1 spray in each nostril 15 min later	Not more than 3 mg in 24 hr and not more than 4 mg in a wk
Ergotamine tartrate (Cafergot, Ercaf, Ergo-Caff, Gotamine, Generic)	Tablet	1 mg	100 mg	1–2 tablets	1 tablet q 30 min; max 6 tablets/attack	Not more than 10 tablets in a wk
Ergotamine tartrate and caffeine (Wigraine)	Tablet	1 mg	100 mg	2 tablets	1 tablet q 30 min; max 6 tablets/attack	Not more than 10 tablets in a wk
Ergotamine tartrate and caffeine (Cafergot, Cafertine, Cafetrate, Migergot, Wigraine, Generic)	Rectal	2 mg	100 mg	1/4 (50 mg) to 1 supp (2 mg)	1/4 to 1 supp in 30 min	2 suppositories for each attack, not more than twice a week, preferably 5 days apart
Dihydroergotamine mesylate	IM	1 mg	None	1 mL (1 mg)	1 mL	Not more than 3 mL in 24 hr and not more than 6 mL in a wk
Dihydroergotamine mesylate	IV	1 mg	None	0.5 mL (0.5 mg)	1 mL	See details in text

pain or weakness in arms or legs, chest discomfort, palpitations, and swelling or itching.

A continuous infusion of DHE by IV pump has been found safe and effective in patients with intractable headaches. Mix 3 mg DHE in 1 L normal saline and administer at 42 mL/hour. Give metoclopramide 10 mg every 8 hours intravenously. Common side effects of continuous intravenous DHE are nausea, diarrhea, vomiting, and leg cramps (25).

Contraindications to Intravenous Ergot Use

Avoid DHE in patients with peripheral arterial disease, coronary artery disease, sepsis, shock, vascular surgery, uncontrolled hypertension, or severely impaired hepatic or renal function. It is also contraindicated during pregnancy.

Metoclopramide may be repeated if nausea persists. A word of caution about metoclopramide: although rare, extrapyramidal signs (involuntary limb movements, grimacing, torticollis, oculogyric crisis, rhythmic protrusion of tongue, or laryngospasm) can be caused by this drug. Diphenhydramine hydrochloride (Benadryl) 50 mg intramuscularly is an effective antidote.

Sumatriptan

Sumatriptan is a serotonin agonist at the vascular $5HT_{1D}$ receptor site. $5HT_{1D}$ receptor consists of two subtypes, alpha and beta. β-$5HT_{1D}$ receptors aid in constriction of large vessels of the head that gives relief in headaches. Sumatriptan does not penetrate the blood-brain barrier. It does however, contract the internal carotid artery.

Dosage

A 6-mg subcutaneous injection produces significant improvement in headache intensity within 15 minutes. There is improvement in the nausea and vomiting that commonly accompany migraine. The maximum recommended dose in a 24-hour period is two 6-mg injections (12 mg) separated at least by 1 hour.

A physician's supervision is recommended when this drug is used for the first time. It can cause transient chest pressure, heaviness of arms, and shortness of breath. Most often these symptoms disappear spontaneously within a few minutes. If symptoms last longer, the patient needs evaluation of cardiac status.

Oral sumatriptan (Imitrex) is available in 25- and 50-mg tablets. An initial dose of 25 mg should be tried at the onset of headache, although it is also affective if taken when the headache has been present for some time. If the first dose is ineffective, a repeat dose up to a maximum of 100 mg may be tried in 2 hours. Maximum daily dose tried has been 300 mg.

Side Effects

A flushed feeling in chest and neck is transient but may be disabling. There may also be transient heaviness of the arms, chest pressures, shortness of breath, and palpitations. Sumatriptan may induce anginal symptoms, acute myocardial infarction, and cardiac arrhythmia. However, the cause of these symptoms in patients with no underlying heart disease is unclear.

Contraindications

Avoid sumatriptan in patients with coronary artery disease and hypertension. Patients who may be at risk for having a heart condition (history of smoking, high cholesterol, family history of heart disease, diabetes mellitus) should have their cardiac status evaluated before sumatriptan is used. Do not use an ergot preparation with sumatriptan, as vasoconstriction caused by both drugs can be cumulative. Avoid concomitant use of sumatriptan and methysergide for migraine prophylaxis.

In spite of some serious side effects, sumatriptan is a major breakthrough in treatment of migraine. Most patients with no underlying heart condition tolerate this drug well. In some cases this is the only drug that helped them to salvage the day previously lost to headache. Some patients have described it as the best thing to come along since sliced bread.

Other Drugs Useful in Migraine

Isometheptene mucate 65 mg with dichloralphenazone 100 mg and acetaminophen 325 mg (Midrin) is useful chiefly because of its octin content, which produces mild vasoconstriction. The usual dose is 2 capsules at the onset of headache followed by 1 capsule every hour until relieved, up to 5 capsules within a 12-hour period.

Indomethacin (Indocin) 25, 50, or 75 mg may be useful in stopping an attack or in lessening intensity of headache. Indomethacin rectal suppository is the preferred route because nausea is a prominent symptom.

Prednisone 30 to 40 mg may be taken on the first day, tapered to 20 mg the next day and 10 mg on the day following. Lidocaine intravenous in a standard dose of 100 mg (25 mg/minute) can temporarily relieve the pain of common migraine (26). Occasionally breathing 100% oxygen by face mask for 20 minutes helps.

A select group of patients get relief from their headaches only by butalbital 50 mg, aspirin 325 mg, and caffeine 40 mg (Fiorinal) one or two capsules every 4 hours. Total daily dose should not exceed 6 tablets or capsules. Butalbital can be habit forming, and daily use should be discouraged.

Use of narcotics for migraine is to be discouraged but not necessarily forbidden. Their use must be monitored by one physician and except in very rare situations, never put in the hands of another member of the patient's family.

Prevention is the key word in managing migraine. The physician must become acquainted with the factors that set off a migraine attack in susceptible patients and must have the patience and take the time to teach the patients how their attacks may be modified. Building blocks for migraine attacks may be assembled from the external, the physiological, and the psychological environments; if they are stacked high, attack results. Common precipitating factors include external, physiological, and psychological environment.

External Environment

Attacks may be precipitated by hot, muggy weather or extreme changes in weather, barometric pressure, or altitude, such as during air flights from the seashore to the Rockies. Close, smoke-filled rooms; carbon monoxide in cars, garages, and houses; and toxic fumes can start a migraine. Strong smells, perfumes, bright flickering lights, and loud noise are yet other environmental trigger factors for migraine attack.

For some patients, foods containing tyramine (cheddar cheese, pickled herring, liver, pods or broad beans, yeast, coffee, ianti wine and beer), phenylethylamine (chocolate), nitrites and nitrates (smoked fishes, bologna, salami, pepperoni, bacon, frankfurters, corned beef, canned ham, and sausages) are triggers. Nitrites and nitrates used create a pink color and give cured flavor interact with blood to form methemoglobin. Nitrite-induced headache is caused by vasodilation. Food containing monosodium glutamate (Chinese food, canned soups, some potato chip products, gourmet seasonings, some dry-roasted nuts, certain processed meats, instant gravies, and TV dinners) can cause a headache by neurotoxic property of glutamate.

Medications can also induce migraine headaches. Atenolol has been observed to cause visual prodromes in classic migraine patients (27). Other agents known to cause headaches include dapsone (4,4′diaminodiphenyl sulfone) (28); the antiviral agent acyclovir (29); the calcium channel blocker nitrendipine (30); the cholesterol-lowering medication gemfibrozil (31); the nasal vasoconstrictor phenylpropanolamine (32); and barium enema (33). Antacids, such as famotidine and ranitidine but not cimetidine (34), can cause headaches. Also, nonsteroidal anti-inflammatory drugs, although used commonly in the treatment of migraine, in rare instances can induce an attack (35). Cardiac drugs containing coronary vasodilators may bring back migraines that had long since disappeared.

Physiological Environment

Attacks may be precipitated by sleeping late and by missing or postponing meals. Menstrual migraine occurs at the onset or end of menstrual periods or in midcycle, at the time of ovulation. Ingestion of oral contraceptives in a migraine patient is a cause of frequent migraine attacks. Prolonged mental strain, excessive physical exercise, and extreme changes in the pace of living are well known headache predictors to a migraine sufferer.

Psychological Environment

Anger (especially when suppressed), anxiety, fear, guilt, depression, or a combination of these may precipitate a headache in the migraine patient. The physician must examine these factors with the patient in hopes of changing the patient's lifestyle in some respects. The help of a psychiatric social worker, a psychologist, or a psychiatrist may be required for some patients. However, modifying behavior within the medical model is suitable and helpful for the majority of patients if the physician has the time and interest for it. A simple and efficient way for physicians to learn more about the lifestyle of a headache patient is to ask him or her to write an autobiography (36). Most patients are pleased to be asked to do this, and many reward the physician with many illuminating facts that help to manage their problem.

Biofeedback, behavioral therapy, meditation, relaxation techniques, and hypnosis may also be useful in treatment of migraine patients. Young people are especially good at these techniques. In all of these regimens involving modification of behavior, a well-cultivated relationship between the patient and the therapist is essential.

Medicines for Migraine Prevention

Despite all efforts to modify migraine by nonpharmaceutical means, there is a hard core of headache sufferers who do not benefit from behavioral techniques but who can be helped by medications for prevention of a headache. Some of these medications are listed next.

Anticonvulsants are especially useful for patients with borderline EEGs with asymmetry and spike-wave features. Phenytoin sodium, the anticonvulsant primidone (Mysoline), and carbamazepine may be used with benefit in patients with these findings.

Divalproex sodium (Depakote), a delayed release antiepileptic medication, is effective for migraine prophylaxis (37). Standard dose is 250 mg twice a day. Start 125 mg twice a day and gradually increase the dose according to the response. Maximum dose is 1000 mg daily. Monitor dosage by measuring blood level for divalproex sodium. The aim is to keep the trough level between 3 and 13 µg/mL. Monitor liver function tests before starting treatment and monthly for the first 6 months.

Drug Interactions with Divalproex Sodium

Simultaneous administration of aspirin decreases protein binding and inhibition of metabolism of valproic acid, resulting in a fourfold increase in valproate free fraction. Concurrent use of valproic acid and clonazepam may induce absence seizures in patients with history of absence seizures. Diazepam's free fraction is increased by 90% when used with valproic acid. Valproic acid inhibits phenobarbital metabolism. Phenytoin sodium becomes more effective because of decreased hepatic metabolism and increased availability of the free fraction of phenytoin. Divalproex sodium is secreted in breast milk.

Side Effects

In addition to abnormal liver function tests, alopecia, thrombocytopenia, acute pancreatitis, hyponatremia, serum inappropriate antidiuretic hormone (SIADH) secretion, hyperammonemia, hearing loss, and reversible cerebral atrophy are some of the side effects to caution the patient and to monitor divalproex sodium levels on return visits.

Monoamine oxidase inhibitors, such as phenelzine sulfate tablets (Nardil 15 mg three times a day) or isocarboxazid (Marplan 10 mg three times a day), are useful. The patient should avoid cheese and tyramine-containing foods and drinks.

Amitriptyline is useful in some patients; start with small doses, 12.5 mg at bedtime and gradually increase to 150 to 200 mg/day if side effects (dry mouth, weight gain, postural hypotension) are tolerable.

Antihistamines, such as diphenhydramine hydrochloride 50 mg at bedtime or if tolerated, three or four times a day, are occasionally effective. In children cyproheptadine (Periactin) 4 to 16 mg daily is useful.

β-Blockers, such as propranolol (Inderal) 80 to 320 mg daily, metoprolol (Lopressor) 100 to 450 mg daily, atenolol (Tenormin) 50 to 100 mg daily, nadolol (Corgard) 40 to 80 mg daily, and timolol (Blocadren) 20 to 60 mg daily can reduce the frequency and severity of migraine attacks. Start with a small dose and gradually increase it. Monitor heart rate and blood pressure. β-Blockers are especially useful if the patient also has mild hypertension. Addition of small doses of hydrochlorothiazide to this regimen is useful.

Nonsteroidal anti-inflammatory agents help some patients. Ibuprofen (Motrin) 400 mg three times a day or naproxen (Naprosyn) 250 mg tablets, three tablets at the onset of headache and total of 1250 mg in 24 hours was shown to have marginal improvement in migraine. Fenoprofen calcium (Nalfon) 200 mg three times a day, indomethacin 150 to 250 mg in three divided doses, and mefenamic acid (Ponstel) 500 mg three times a day have also been shown effective in migraine prophylaxis. Old standby aspirin 650 mg twice a day may occasionally achieve migraine prophylaxis. Gastrointestinal disturbance and kidney and hematopoietic complications should be carefully monitored.

Methysergide, a potent antiserotonin compound, is effective in migraine prophylaxis. It should be considered in migraine patients who are refractory to other medications. The starting dose is 2 mg two or three times a day. Maximum dose is 8 mg daily. If the headache has not improved after 3 weeks, it is unlikely to be effective. If methysergide is used for long duration, a 3- to 4-week medication-free period every 6 months is mandatory. Cardiac and pulmonary fibrosis has been reported with continuous use of methysergide. These complications do not occur if there is a 3- to 4-week interruption in methysergide administration every 6 months. Other side effects include gastrointestinal and vascular disturbances, edema, and weight gain. It is contraindicated in hypertension, coronary artery disease, collagen vascular disease, peripheral vascular disease, and renal or hepatic disease. Careful instruction and close follow-up of the patient are necessary.

Calcium channel blockers, such as verapamil (Isoptin or Calan) 80 to 120 mg three times a day, diltiazem (Cardizem) 180 to 240 mg daily, and nifedipine (Procardia) 10 to 40 mg three times a day, are beneficial in migraine prophylaxis and may be used when vascular or cardiac complications preclude the use of ergotamine. Nimodipine, a class II calcium channel blocker, is a specific inhibitor of cerebral vasospasm in subarachnoid hemorrhage; however, as yet there are conflicting reports about its effectiveness in the prophylaxis of migraine headache.

Newer Drugs

Although sumatriptan, a very potent drug, works within 15 to 20 minutes, the effect wears off within few hours. Quite often migraine headache resurfaces. Newer drugs are in various stages of trial. Some have lesser side effects than sumatriptan; others work as fast orally as subcutaneous sumatriptan; and yet others have longer duration of action, so the headache breakthrough is less likely.

Zolmitriptan (Zomig)

Like Sumatriptan, zolmitriptan is a serotonin $5HT_{1D}$ receptor agonist. It is specific for beta subtype. It does penetrate the blood-brain barrier and acts on the trigeminal nerve nucleus to inhibit nociceptive stimulus and acts peripherally as a vasoconstrictor. It is given orally; a 2.5- or 5-mg tablet relieves migraine within 2 hours. It is 2 to 3 times as potent as sumatriptan, but headache breakthrough is common. Almost half of migraine patients require a second tablet (38).

Naratriptan

Naratriptan (Amerge) is also a selective $5-HT_{1D}$ receptor agonist with a long half-life. Indicated for long-duration migraine headache, it is available in 1- and 2.5-mg tablets. Precautions for its use are the same as with sumatriptan.

Alniditan

Alniditan, a benzpyrene derivative, is a serotonin $5-HT_{1D}$-receptor agonist. It is given as a subcutaneous 1.4-mg dose and is as effective as sumatriptan. The effect of alniditan lasts longer than sumatriptan. The half-life of alniditan is 7 to 12 hours; the half-life of sumatriptan is only 2 hours (39). Other antimigraine drugs acting as serotonin receptor agonists under study are rizatriptan, avitriptan, and IS-159.

CLUSTER HEADACHE

Description (9)

Cluster headaches are attacks of severe strictly unilateral pain orbitally, supraorbitally, temporally, or a combination of these, lasting 15 to 180 minutes and occurring every other day to eight times a day. They are associated with one or more of the following: conjunctival injection, lacrimation, nasal congestion, rhinorrhea, forehead and facial sweating, meiosis, ptosis, and eyelid edema. Attacks occur in series lasting for weeks or months (so-called cluster periods) separated by remission periods that usually last months or years.

Diagnostic Criteria

Cluster headaches are characterized by at least five attacks of severe unilateral orbital, supraorbital, and/or temporal pain, lasting 15 to 180 minutes when untreated, and associated with at least one of the following signs, which must be present on the pain side:

- Conjunctival injection
- Lacrimation
- Nasal congestion
- Rhinorrhea
- Forehead and facial sweating
- Meiosis
- Ptosis
- Eyelid edema

The underlying organic lesion must be ruled out by history, physical and neurological examination, and investigations if indicated. Cluster headache (Fig. 10.4) is chiefly a man's disease, as opposed to common migraine, which is more prevalent in women. It presents in closely packed groups or clusters consisting of short attacks of unilateral pain of excruciating severity accompanied by marked autonomic symptoms of tearing, meiosis, salivation, nasal blocking and rhinorrhea, drooping of the eyelid, and occasionally slowing of the pulse. During the cluster period alcohol, nitroglycerine, and histamine can produce an attack. A seasonal pattern with attacks in the fall and spring is common. Frequently attacks occur during periods of relaxation after stressful mental or physical activity and thus ruin vacations and spoil the rewards of hard work and stress.

Headaches occur with clocklike regularity. The usual time is during rapid eye movement (REM) sleep. The hallmark of cluster headache pain is abrupt onset, reaching peak intensity within minutes and rapid descent to complete pain relief within minutes after the start of decline in pain intensity. In contrast to migraine, the cluster headache patient feels relatively well after the attack. If the attack occurs during the day, the patient can resume work after the attack. Pain is felt in and around the eye and sometimes at the back of the neck; the maxillary area is also involved. Pain is described as sharp, knifelike, as if someone is piercing a hot poker through the eye. Vision is not affected. Headaches last 20 to 40 minutes. Although headaches last only a short time, patients describe it as sheer hell, the worst pain that can ever be imagined. On a scale of 0 to 10 cluster headache patients rate their pain as 11. Their worst fear is that the pain may never end. Attacks occur on the same side during one cluster period. The headache may switch sides during next attack. Each cluster period may last 4 to 6 weeks.

Unlike common migraine sufferers, who withdraw or "hibernate" during attacks, cluster headache patients tend to pace the floor, bite a pillow, bang on the wall, cry for help, resist physical assistance, lock themselves away from the family, or even go into a trancelike state.

Approximately 80% of cluster headache patients are male. Female patients often show a number of masculine physical features. Many men with cluster headache are tall, square-jawed, and leonine in their facial appearance. Thick, pitted facial skin, which is well furrowed and creased, and facial cutaneous telangiectasia are common. Hazel eyes are common in cluster patients.

Psychologically, cluster headache patients are ambitious, with a strong sense of upward social mobility. They strive hard to live up to their husky masculine appearance, yet they often present an inner side that has strong dependency needs. They may show powerful feelings of guilt, anger, and inadequacy, leading to a tendency to brief hysterical behavior under pressure and periods of underlying depression. Bizarre behavior, such as striking those who try to help them, violence, yelling, pleading, trancelike states, amnesia, pacing, running, pounding walls, breaking furniture, and in rare instances criminal behavior, make problems for the patient, family, friends, and at times the police.

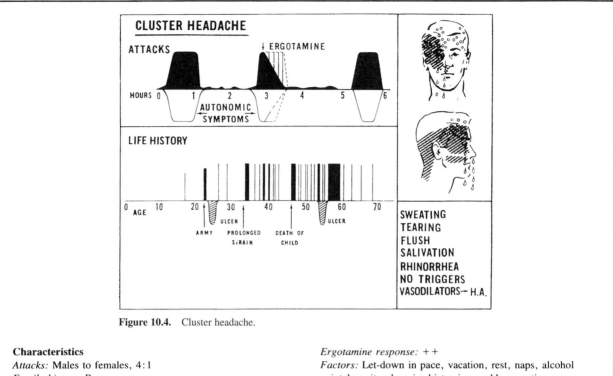

Figure 10.4. Cluster headache.

Characteristics

Attacks: Males to females, 4:1
Family history: Rare
Onset: Sudden
Prodrome: None or short "burning" (5 min)
Location: Unilateral, rarely shifts sides, some pain in neck
Quality: Steady, twisting, pulling, burning
Intensity: + + + +
Duration: 10–90 min, rarely, longer
Time of onset: After stress, after work, after nap, during sleep, night or day
Accompaniments: Ipsilateral tearing, sweating (bilateral or ipsilateral), nasal block, rhinorrhea, flush or pallor, meiosis, partial Horner's syndrome, slow pulse, gastric acid increase, pacing, crying out, banging hand or head on wall
Pattern: 1–6 attacks per 24 hr in clusters lasting weeks, months, and rarely, years, with freedom for weeks or months or years in between

Ergotamine response: + +
Factors: Let-down in pace, vacation, rest, naps, alcohol intake, nitroglycerin, histamine, sudden emotion, depression, injury to head or neck

Therapy

Breathe O$_2$, violent exercise (5 min), ergotamine, analgesics, codeine, occasionally meperidine, Decadron IM, Nembutal or diazepam IV in hospital, methysergide, steroids, lithium, calcium-channel block, estrogen, progesterone, cyproheptadine, indomethacin, behavior modification, neurosurgery

Differential Diagnosis

Tic douloureux, acute sinusitis, scratched cornea, chronic paroxysmal hemicrania, aneurysms, AVM, Raeder's syndrome, Tolosa-Hunt syndrome

Frequently these leonine men are led into the physician's office by a petite but powerful spouse. Peptic ulcer was present at one time or another in about 25% of cluster headache patients (40).

Treatment

Acute Attack

1. The immediate use of very hot or very cold applications to the painful area
2. 5 to 10 minutes of exercise
3. Breathing of 100% oxygen (8 to 10 L/minute for 10 to 15 minutes)
4. Prompt use of sumatriptan 6 mg subcutaneous is remarkably effective and well tolerated for cluster attack (41). For details about sumatriptan use, see under migraine treatment.
5. Ergotamine in a readily accessible form, such as two whiffs from an inhaler or an oral, sublingual, rectal, or injectable dose, whichever the patient finds most effective.

A substantial dose of analgesic medication taken when the ergotamine is given may help to bring the attacks under control. In a hospital setting the intravenous use of 30 mg pentobarbital (Nembutal), or 15 mg diazepam (Valium) may be justifiable in extreme cases. Repeated and frequent resort to narcotic medication is to be avoided as much as possible.

Prophylaxis

Younger patients and those with no contraindication to ergotamine use may try ergotamine (Cafergot, Wigraine) two, three, or four times a day during a cluster period to prevent headaches. Methysergide 2 mg two or three times a day can be very effective. Gradual tapering of the dose is required as the condition improves.

Prednisone 40 to 60 mg/day in divided doses may be very useful in shortening cluster headaches and preventing the individual attacks. It should be tapered by 5 mg every 2 to 4 days. It should not be continued for more than a month because of potential for serious side effects. Consider concurrent use of H$_2$ blockers (cimetidine 300 mg three times a day, nizatidine 150 mg twice a day) to prevent gastric erosion, since cluster headache patients are prone to peptic ulcer disease. Cyproheptadine 4 mg three to four times daily may be effective. In women with cluster headache, oral contraceptives may be beneficial when taken for several months. In postmenopausal women, moderate doses of estrogen are worth a trial. In both men and women, progesterone gives relief to some patients who cannot use or have not improved with other medications. Progesterone has been used in menstrual migraine (42).

Lithium (Eskalith) 300 mg three or four times a day to achieve blood levels of 0.5 to 1.2 mEq/L is very effective in cluster headache. It can be used for months. Long-term use of lithium causes a defect in the renal concentrating mechanism and hypothyroidism. If there is suspicion of diabetes insipidus, monitor renal function, including blood urea nitrogen (BUN), serum creatinine, urine specific gravity, 24-hour urine volume, and renal concentration tests under supervision. The combination of a neuroleptic drug and lithium can result in an encephalopathic syndrome (weakness, fever, tremor, confusion, extrapyramidal symptoms, leukocytosis, and elevation in blood sugar and BUN). Concurrent use of indomethacin, piroxicam, enalapril, or captopril increases plasma lithium level. Use of calcium channel blockers and lithium may increase the risk of neurotoxicity (ataxia, tremors, nausea, vomiting, diarrhea, and tinnitus).

Methysergide 2 mg three or four times a day can stop cluster attack. It can be given for 2 to 3 months. Long-term use can cause cardiac and pulmonary fibrosis. It should be avoided in patients with underlying heart disease, hypertension, or peripheral vascular insufficiency.

Experience with the calcium channel blockers—nimodipine (Nimotop) 30 mg four times a day, verapamil 240 mg daily, nifedipine 10 mg four times a day—shows they are all effective. The dosage is increased gradually, and results may not appear for 2 to 4 weeks. These medications are particularly useful in patients who cannot take ergotamine or methysergide. Monitor cardiac status and blood pressure closely as the dosage is gradually increased.

Melatonin 10 mg daily for 14 days may be effective in some patients. It can be tried in patients who cannot tolerate other drugs.

Transdermal clonidine patch (Catapres-TTS .2) releases 0.2 mg of clonidine daily. The patch is changed every 7 days. It can reduce frequency, severity, and duration of cluster headaches (43). Clonidine acts in the central nervous system at the hypothalamus and locus ceruleus as an agonist of presynaptic adrenoreceptor.

The response of chronic paroxysmal hemicrania (described later) pain to indomethacin suggests that a 2-day trial of 50 to 75 mg daily in cluster headache can sometimes be extremely effective. β-Blockers, such as propranolol 40 mg three or four times a day, may be suitable in cluster headache.

Biofeedback and behavioral therapy have little role in cluster headache treatment. When medical treatment has failed or threatens to cause serious side effects, including addiction, surgical means of relief may be sought. In refractory chronic cluster headache surgical treatment may offer the only hope of relief. Various surgical procedures claim to offer relief. Resection of the greater superficial petrosal nerve, section of the nervus intermedius, sphenopalatine ganglionectomy, cryosurgery of the facial arteries, trigeminal root section, percutaneous rhizotomy of the trigeminal ganglion, and radiofrequency lesions of the trigeminal nerve have all been tried. These procedures have limited success. Discussion of surgical procedures is beyond the scope of this chapter. However, these should be considered and carried out, if at all, only by neurosurgeons well acquainted with chronic cluster headache.

An interesting subgroup of cluster headache that is more common in women than in men is called chronic paroxysmal hemicrania (CPH) (44). It is characterized by 15- to 20-minute attacks of pain in the temple, eye, cheek, and occasionally the suboccipital area and is associated with ipsilateral nasal blocking and tearing. It occurs in attacks both day and night 5 to 15 times a day. CPH patients do not respond to the usual cluster headache remedies but improve dramatically within a few hours after taking indomethacin. The usual dose is 50 to 75 mg in three divided doses daily. The dosage should be increased up to 150 to 200 mg per day to before it is declared ineffective. Gastric upset is frequent side effect. Use of an H$_2$ blocker is recommended with indomethacin.

Migraine without aura may occur in clusters every day for weeks and then disappear for weeks or months. It is aptly described as *cyclical migraine*. Headaches respond favorably to lithium for prophylaxis. Indomethacin may also prove useful. A continuous daily unilateral headache associated with ipsilateral visual blurring has been described. It responds specifically to the administration of indomethacin. Other headaches responsive to indomethacin include cervical lesion-related headaches, characterized by short sharp episodes of pain (jabs and jolts).

OPHTHALMOPLEGIC MIGRAINE

This rare condition often begins in childhood. Headache attacks are recurrent and episodic. Third nerve paralysis causes dilated pupils and diplopia. The neurological abnormalities may outlast the headache by several days or occasionally weeks and then may clear. As attacks recur repeatedly over the years, the third nerve paralysis may be permanent.

Frequently there is a history of migraine or ophthalmoplegic migraine. Despite a family history of migraine or even of ophthalmoplegic migraine, it is important to carry out tests to rule out organic causes of headaches. Aneurysms in the vicinity of the third cranial nerve produce a similar picture following repeated small intracerebral bleeds. MRI with angiography is useful to rule out berry aneurysms in the circle of Willis or the anterior or posterior communicating arteries. These studies should be done within a few days after an attack. Arteriography may be necessary if suspicion of aneurysm is high. Lumbar puncture helps to rule out small bleeding if aneurysm is not seen by other studies.

After fixed organic lesions have been ruled out and the migrainous nature of the disorder has been established, it may be treated as for common migraine, both during the attack and prophylactically. Ergotamine can be very helpful, and if the paralysis is long lasting, steroids may be useful. Tapering down from 40 mg/day over the course of 3 or 4 days discontinues the use of prednisone.

HEMIPLEGIC AND BASILAR ARTERY MIGRAINE

These rare forms of migraine occur mostly in female patients below age 30 years who have a family history of classic or common migraine. Vasospasm of cerebral vessels is most likely to be the underlying cause of diverse symptoms. Dysarthria, aphasia, ataxia, tinnitus, vertigo, visual loss, transient global amnesia, and unconsciousness accompany headache. Motor and sensory disturbances are part of the syndrome. Such attacks are prone to occur around menstrual periods. Smoking and stress also precipitate hemiplegic headache. A genetic predisposition is suggested in familial hemiplegic migraine (45).

Treatment

Attendance by a friend during these frightening and dangerous experiences is essential. The following treatments may also be beneficial.

1. Patient should lie flat.
2. Propranolol 20 mg orally daily should be administered.
3. A small dose of amyl nitrite should be inhaled.
4. Calcium-channel blockers can be effective.
5. Papaverine hydrochloride (Pavabid) 150-mg capsule twice a day provokes vasodilation without nociceptor stimulation.
6. Ingestion of 15 mg of prednisone orally immediately and again after 4 hours may be effective.
7. Naloxone 0.4 mg intravenously may be beneficial (46).

If attacks are frequent, prophylaxis may include one or more of the following:

1. Aspirin 150 mg and/or dipyridamole 50 mg daily for prevention of platelet hyperaggregability may prevent frequent attacks.
2. Propranolol 20 mg daily is recommended.
3. Use of calcium-channel blocker such as flunarizine 10 mg daily was effective in children with alternating hemiplegic migraine.
4. Avoid smoking.
5. Avoid oral contraceptives.
6. Avoid ergot preparations in the presence of severe ischemia in the vertebrobasilar system.

Closely connected to such episodes are global amnesia and the locked-in syndrome (LIS), in which a conscious patient can move only the eyes because the rest of the body is paralyzed. Although LIS is apt to indicate an organic lesion in the pons that may be fatal, an episode with spontaneous recovery in a migraine patient has been reported. The lateral medullary syndrome has been reported in a patient with basilar artery migraine, and neurologic deficits may be permanent (47).

LOWER-HALF HEADACHE AND ATYPICAL FACIAL NEURALGIA

Lower-half headache (10) is distinguished by its lack of associated symptoms and its constant chronic dull facial and neck pain that lasts for months or years. Fortunately, lower-half headache, or atypical facial neuralgia, is rare. Although its relation to migraine is questionable, this headache often grows out of intermittent headache attacks that resemble common migraine and increase in frequency until pain becomes constant.

In the early stages lower-half headache often responds to migraine therapy; in the late stages, it loses this response. Antidepressant agents and supportive psychotherapy are the mainstays of management. Attempts to cure this condition with medical treatment may induce psychotic behavior. Narcotic addiction is a real danger. Patients suffering with this disorder frequently end up having several surgical procedures with a hope for cure. Any surgical relief should be sought only after psychiatric evaluation. Transcutaneous electric stimulation may be beneficial in some patients.

MUSCLE CONTRACTION OR TENSION-TYPE HEADACHE

Description

Muscle contraction or tension-type headache consists of recurrent episodes of headache lasting minutes to days. The pain is typically pressing or tightening in quality, mild or moderate in intensity, and bilateral, and it does not worsen with routine physical activity. Nausea is absent, but photophobia or phonophobia may be present (9).

Diagnostic Criteria proposed by the International Headache Society (9)

According to IHS, these headaches last 30 minutes to 7 days. At least two of the following pain characteristics must be present:

1. Pressing or tightening (nonpulsating) quality
2. Mild or moderate intensity (may inhibit but does not prohibit activities)
3. Bilateral location
4. No aggravation by walking stairs or similar routine physical activity

At least 10 previous headache episodes with the following must have occurred:

1. No nausea or vomiting (anorexia may occur)
2. Photophobia or phonophobia but not both may be present

Frequency must be fewer than 15 days with headache per month (fewer than 180 days per year). Frank or occult lesions of the head and neck can mimic tension-type headaches. History and physical examination are mandatory to rule out organic lesion.

Sometimes the frequency of migraine or tension-type headache increases to almost daily. When seen for the first time with daily headache, it may be difficult to determine whether the origin was tension type or migraine. It is episodic tension-type headache that most frequently transforms into chronic daily headache. Overuse of analgesic drugs frequently becomes counterproductive and may contribute to daily headache. Discontinuation of daily analgesic intake often helps.

Muscle contraction or tension-type headache (Fig. 10.5) is sometimes not even a headache when examined closely, but rather is a discomfort more accurately described as a tight band, pressure, viselike compression, or cap applied tightly to the head and neck. When this pressure is severe, it does become pain. The IHS recommends separation of tension-type headache into those with and those without muscle involvement (9). Muscles of the face, head, and neck may be involved. In some instances this finding is not present, and other physiological factors, as yet unidentified, must be postulated.

Unlike migraine, which *follows* stress, tension headache occurs *during* stress. Whereas the migraine patient is apt to suppress anger and frustration, the tension headache patient is likely to complain about the circumstances leading to the symptoms and to stop the activity or retreat from the emotional disturbance that may have precipitated the attack.

Tension headache may be a consequence of maintenance of a fixed position of the head or neck. Typing, knitting, reading, and driving against traffic are commonly associated with tightening of head and neck muscles. Rain, change in barometric pressure, and bright lights can reflexly cause tightening of muscles. Muscle contraction is probably the most important causative factor in headache related to disorders of the bite and temporomandibular joint disorder.

Analgesic over-the-counter drugs are effective in the beginning. Regular use of analgesic agents, especially those containing phenacetin and acetaminophen, may lead to analgesic abuse, which may perpetuate the headache. Excessive caffeine intake for headache relief sets the patient up for a caffeine withdrawal headache later in the day or night. Tranquilizers are useful for brief periods, but these should be avoided for long-term relief. Some patients with chronic daily headaches need admission to the hospital or pain center to withdraw from analgesics under supervision.

Treatment

The nonpharmaceutical approach is the first line of treatment. Behavior modification therapy, relaxation techniques, biofeedback, and hypnosis have all proved effective. Young patients are very good subjects and enjoy relief from headache. In selected patients, formal psychotherapy (48) or counseling by a psychiatric social worker may prove rewarding. An interested nonpsychiatric physician willing to devote time to listen to the patient's concerns and offer common-sense suggestions regarding his or her problems can make a huge difference in the patient's well-being.

Drug treatment of tension type of headache includes a combination of aspirin, butalbital, and caffeine or substitution of acetaminophen for aspirin (Fioricet). These combinations are very effective and without any problem if used in moderation. Some patients who use these combinations find that they must gradually increase the dosage to get relief in headaches. Dependence on these drugs or other analgesics can be real. Other drugs useful in tension type of headaches include ibuprofen 400 mg three times a day or naproxen sodium (Anaprox) 275 mg three times a day. Transcutaneous electrical nerve stimulation (TENS) is sometimes useful. Tricyclic antidepressant drugs, such as amitriptyline (Elavil) (49) in full amounts of 150 mg/day given in one dose at bedtime may strikingly relieve constant daily headache even when no overt depression is present.

COMBINED (MIXED) HEADACHE (10)

Combined headache is a throbbing and pounding pain in conjunction with the viselike pressure of tension headache. It may be associated with nausea and vomiting in severe attacks, similar to migraine. It may wake the patient from sleep, but unlike migraine, its pain is bilateral or all over. It is accentuated at the time of menstruation. These features suggest a vascular component operating simultaneously with muscle contraction as the source of discomfort. Drugs effective in treating migraine symptomatically and prophylactically may be useful in combined headache. Propranolol is especially beneficial. Modification of lifestyle and habits and solution of family and work problems may offer a hope for cure in the long run. Such patients have a tendency to become drug dependent and may require admission to a pain center to withdraw from excessive use of medication.

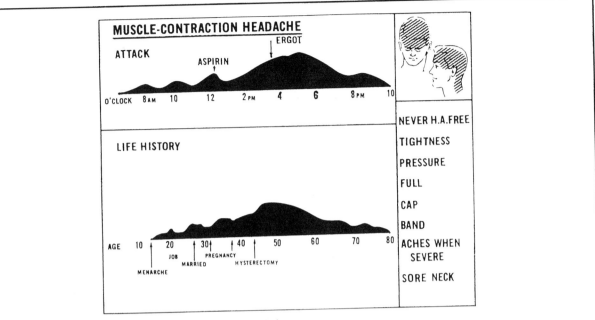

Figure 10.5.   Muscle contraction headache.

Characteristics

Family history: Occasionally +

Male:female ratio: In clinics, females 2:1

Attacks: Prodromes − 0

Location: All over head and in neck, occasionally localized

Quality: Tightness, pressure, vise, cap, band, sore, occasionally throbs

Duration: Hours, all day, continuous

Accompaniments: Anxiety, irritability, depression, overt anger

Pattern: Increases as day goes on, singles, constant for several days during stress; daily for weeks, months, or years

Ergotamine response: None or worsens, alcohol helps

Factors: Deadlines; obsessiveness; difficult boss, relative, or situation; anxiety about personal performance, pressure of work, ideas, children

Therapy

Limited analgesics, temporary tranquilizers, tricyclics, antidepressants, supportive therapy by physician, help from counselor, social service, stress management, behavioral modification with relaxation training and biofeedback, psychotherapy, travel vacation, change of job

Differential Diagnosis

Migraine, conversion headache, scleroderma, caffeine withdrawal, medication dependency, brain tumor, psychosis

Organic Warnings

Psychotic behavior, cognitive deficiencies, memory or performance change; check for chronic viral infections including AIDS and ARC

HEADACHE OF NASAL VASOMOTOR REACTION (VASOMOTOR RHINITIS) (10)

Constant pain at the bridge of the nose, cheeks, lower forehead, and near the eye is a frequent complaint. Pain is usually mild to moderate in intensity but very annoying because of its constancy. Nose and sinus examination is normal. This headache seems to be a bodily response to deep-seated psychogenic factors, often at an unconscious or subconscious level. Surgical approaches, such as corrections of septal deviations and turbinectomies and operations on the sinuses to obliterate cysts, do not relieve headaches. Psychotherapy may be helpful for patients who can discuss their inner feelings with the therapist. More often this approach is unprofitable; a patient, supportive medical therapy may be more acceptable.

In such instances the physician's role is to listen, reassure, and prevent unnecessary or even harmful surgery. Antidepressant medication, such as amitriptyline or phenelzine, may be cut down the effects of emotional troubles and life pressures on the patient. The physician may do a great service by keeping such patients away from addiction, polysurgery, and drug reactions. Occasionally joint counseling of family or husband and wife may be useful. Behavior modification, hypnosis, and relaxation training may be useful.

HEADACHES OF DELUSIONAL, CONVERSION, OR HYPOCHONDRIACAL STATES (PSYCHOGENIC HEADACHE) (10)

Patients with psychogenic headache complain of pressure, exploding sensation, or fullness or extra weight on their head or neck. Headache is on their mind every waking hour. Vision may be blurry and show concentric narrowing of the visual fields. Light-headedness, faintness, and inability to concentrate are frequent accompaniments. The symptoms interfere with almost all activities. It has been recommended to limit use of the term psychogenic headache to patients with psychiatric illness whose primary complaint is headache (50). Symptoms are based on the unconscious, and their causes are hard to determine except by psychotherapy, hypnotism, or sodium amytal interview. When symptoms occur in a young person, early referral to a psychiatrist may be very successful.

Patients with conversion headache can relate their pain of long duration to events that they were unable to talk about for years. Others may experience severe headache in episodes that mimic many features of migraine when guilt or anger feelings residing in the unconscious break through in somatic form to their consciousness.

In recent years depression has replaced syphilis as the great impostor. One of its favorite roles is headache, often expressed in forms resembling muscle contraction headache or vascular (combined) headache. Psychotherapy with or without antidepressant drugs, such as the tricyclic compound doxepin (51) and amitriptyline (49), is effective. Ventilating feelings is one of the greatest forms of relief for the patient, and the physician must recognize that he or she treats the patient by simply listening. Supportive encouragement, suggestions, and recommendations about vacation exercise, activities, and a trial of new attitudes are well within the training and capabilities of most physicians. Deeper problems may need psychotherapy. Specific questions about suicide thought must be asked by the physician, and the patient, who may have been suffering in silence, often welcomes such queries.

NONMIGRAINOUS VASCULAR HEADACHE (10)

Nonmigrainous vascular headaches are related to a long list of causes that lead to throbbing generalized or localized headache resulting from excessive amplitude of intracranial blood vessel pulsation. The disorders are numerous, and treatment of pain is usually correction of the underlying disturbance. Systemic infections; hypoxia and hypercapnia; nitrites, histamine, alcohol; and other vasodilating substances are well-known causes of headache. Caffeine withdrawal, steroid withdrawal syndromes, intracranial circulatory insufficiency, and hypoglycemia can present as headache. Abrupt elevations or decreases of blood pressure, essential hypertension, renal disease, drainage or leaking of spinal fluid, postconvulsive states, and renal dialysis are some of the other known causes of nonmigrainous vascular headaches. Only a few special situations are mentioned here.

Steroid Withdrawal

Sudden withdrawal of steroids may precipitate vascular headaches similar to migraine or cluster headache. The hypoadrenal may temporarily unearth a previously hidden diathesis for migraine or cluster headaches. Headaches improve after reinstitution of steroid therapy (52). A gradual reduction of the steroids after increasing the dose is recommended.

Hypertension

Hypertensive headaches resemble migraine. Mild to moderate hypertension usually does not cause a headache. A migraine sufferer, on the other hand, may have a recurrence of migraine when blood pressure is mild or moderately elevated. Malignant hypertension and hypertensive encephalopathy are invariably accompanied by headache. Hypertensive headaches commonly occur upon awakening. Frequently headaches occur as blood pressure falls from a very high to a normal or low level. Treatment consists of control of the blood pressure with single-agent or combined drugs such as β-blocking agents, centrally acting drugs such as clonidine or guanabenz, hydrochlorothiazide, and calcium channel blockers. A low-salt diet may improve the headache.

Renal Disease

Headache may be an early indication of renal insufficiency. These headaches are throbbing, unilateral, and similar to migraine in the absence of migraine history. Headaches may occur even with normal blood pressure. Headache-prone renal failure patients have frequent headaches if they go on chronic renal dialysis.

Renal Dialysis

For some weeks or months when a patient first starts the dialysis program, headache occurs on dialysis, especially if the patient has previously been subject to headache. Big swings in serum sodium osmolality during dialysis are likely to cause the headache. Raising the sodium content of the dialysate so that the washout of sodium and change in osmolality of blood plasma is reduced can control headache. Nephrectomy of the diseased kidney and successful transplant are frequently associated with relief of headache. Return of headaches after a successful transplant may be the first symptom of transplant rejection (53).

Carotid Artery Dissection

Dissection of the carotid artery may cause headache, neck pain, and carotid artery tenderness. Dissection can occur spontaneously or follow trauma, exercise, strain, anger, or vomiting (54). The pain is felt in the ipsilateral frontal, orbital, and adjacent regions. Rarely pain in the neck may be the only manifestation. The head or neck pain may be present for several days or even weeks before the diagnosis is made. Patients have visual disturbances on the side of the lesion and can hear a sound in their head. Horner's syndrome may be a tip-off to this diagnosis. Stroke is a feared complication. The diagnosis can be made by noninvasively by MRI with angiography. Anticoagulation is employed to prevent transient ischemic attacks or strokes.

Mitral Valve Prolapse

Mitral valve prolapse has an increased incidence in a migraine patient (55), although cardiac arrhythmia in a migraine patient is more frequent than in the nonmigraine population. Atrial and ventricular arrhythmia is even more prevalent if the patient also has mitral valve prolapse. β-Blocker therapy such as propranolol is the treatment of choice for both migraine and arrhythmia. Calcium channel blockers are also useful.

RHEUMATOID SPONDYLITIS

Rheumatoid spondylitis may lead to degeneration and weakening of the odontoid ligament and painful instability of the ligaments and joint capsules at C1 and C2. Headache is felt in the temporal area. Diagnosis is made by radiographic study of the mobility between the odontoid and the body of C1 during flexion and extension.

VITAMIN A MEGADOSES

Acne may lead young people to take excessive amounts of vitamin A (200,000 to 300,000 USP units daily or more). The U.S. recommended daily allowance of vitamin A is 5,000 units. Pseudotumor cerebri and headache have been associated with vitamin A megadoses. Vitamin A remains in body fat for weeks or months after ingestion. Additional dietary intake of carotene and vitamin A-containing yellow fruits and vegetables and beef liver may prolong or accentuate body content of vitamin A.

RAYNAUD'S DISEASE

Cold hands and feet are common among migraine sufferers with Raynaud's disease, especially during attacks. Some migraine patients have these symptoms to such a degree that color changes and pain in the hands and feet as well as the head are prominent features of headache. Calcium channel blockers, especially nifedipine, are effective therapy for Raynaud's attacks and sometimes for migraines. Collagen vascular disorders such as systemic lupus erythematosus, scleroderma, and mixed collagen disorders can cause Raynaud's syndrome. Serum ANA and immunoelectrophoresis are good screening diagnostic aids. Blood tests should also include sedimentation rate, lupus anticoagulant, and anticardiolipin antibodies. Patients with positive ANA need further screening tests to establish a diagnosis. Propranolol, sumatriptan, and ergotamine preparations should be avoided to prevent iatrogenic peripheral vasoconstriction.

TRACTION HEADACHE

Space-occupying lesions in the head cause headache by traction on pain-sensitive structures in the brain. Brain tumors, cysts, abscesses, hematomas, and hygromas can dis-tort and drag on such pain-sensitive structures. Although brain substance is insensitive to pain, intracerebral large veins; venous sinuses; meningeal vessels; pain-sensitive portions of the carotid, vertebrobasilar, cerebellar, and cerebral arteries; and tentorium are pain sensitive.

Headache is caused by change (increase or decrease) in intracranial volume. Headache may be generalized or localized and may shift sides during the same attack. Onset of headache may be acute or subacute. Obstruction in the venous sinus drainage of the head from venous sinus thrombosis or intermittent obstruction to free flow of spinal fluid such as in colloid cyst of the third ventricle (56) can cause headaches. Headache from intermittent obstruction of third ventricle may be episodic or continuous and often accentuated or precipitated by change in position or by coughing. Swelling of the brain itself, whether local or generalized, may lead to obstruction and distortions of pain-sensitive structures, such as in herniation of the temporal lobe through the tentorium or herniation of cerebellar tonsils into the foramen magnum.

A headache of sudden comings and goings, with abrupt onset of nausea, vertigo, or other neurological symptoms, should alert the physician to search for an organic cause. Favorable response to antimigraine or tension headache therapy does not rule out a possibly serious underlying cause. A detailed description of the headache and its accompaniments is most useful in diagnosing traction headache, since often there are no objective findings on examination. A change in familiar headache pattern of migraine or tension headache is a tip-off of serious underlying cause. Investigation with CT scan with contrast or MRI is indicated when there is change in the usual headache pattern. Traction headaches may also originate from abnormalities in the upper cervical region, such as congenital malformations of the first and second cervical vertebrae, platybasia, Arnold-Chiari malformation, and metastatic tumor in the high cervical region.

A decrease in cerebrospinal fluid volume from severe dehydration or leakage following lumbar puncture or a tear in the dural sleeves of spinal nerves after a blunt trauma can produce traction headache. Headaches caused by low cerebrospinal fluid pressure are position dependent. Headache is felt in upright position and improves on lying down. There may be a history of sudden discharge of clear fluid from the nose on bending or coughing. Glucose in this fluid suggests spinal fluid leakage. Diagnosis is made by inability to obtain spinal fluid under low pressure with a well-placed spinal needle.

The site of headache may have localizing value in the early stages of traction. With widespread disruption of intracranial structures, the headache loses its localizing significance. For instance, posterior fossa lesions cause pain in the back of the head at first but become more general later.

The excessive use of vitamin A (200,000 to 300,000 U per day), tetracycline ingestion, and use of amitriptyline, indomethacin, or penicillin in infants are known causes of pseudotumor cerebri (benign intracranial hypertension).

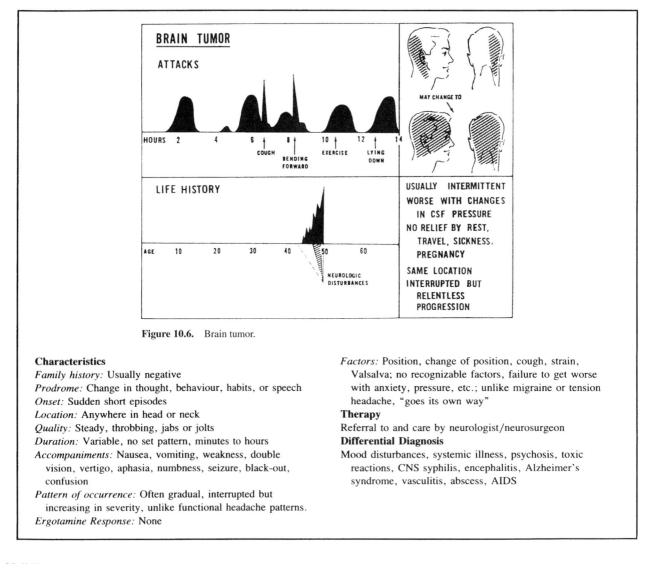

Figure 10.6. Brain tumor.

Characteristics

Family history: Usually negative

Prodrome: Change in thought, behaviour, habits, or speech

Onset: Sudden short episodes

Location: Anywhere in head or neck

Quality: Steady, throbbing, jabs or jolts

Duration: Variable, no set pattern, minutes to hours

Accompaniments: Nausea, vomiting, weakness, double vision, vertigo, aphasia, numbness, seizure, black-out, confusion

Pattern of occurrence: Often gradual, interrupted but increasing in severity, unlike functional headache patterns.

Ergotamine Response: None

Factors: Position, change of position, cough, strain, Valsalva; no recognizable factors, failure to get worse with anxiety, pressure, etc.; unlike migraine or tension headache, "goes its own way"

Therapy

Referral to and care by neurologist/neurosurgeon

Differential Diagnosis

Mood disturbances, systemic illness, psychosis, toxic reactions, CNS syphilis, encephalitis, Alzheimer's syndrome, vasculitis, abscess, AIDS

Nalidixic acid, sulfonamides, and nitrofurantoin have been associated with the syndrome. Pseudotumor cerebri has also been reported in ingestion of phenothiazines and oral contraceptives and in corticosteroid treatment and withdrawal. Hypoparathyroidism, Addison's disease, Conn's syndrome, hyperthyroidism, obesity, and menstrual irregularities are yet other causes of this syndrome. Exposure to metals, including lead, nickel, zinc, and tin have been implicated in this condition. Other causes include intracranial venous thrombosis, iron deficiency anemia and hyperalimentation therapy, and organochlorine insecticide chlordecone (Kepone). Increased CSF pressure, headache papilledema, and sixth nerve palsy are common. There may be permanent impairment of visual acuity and complete external or even bilateral total (internal and external) ophthalmoplegia with unilateral seventh nerve palsy.

Treatment

Treatment includes repeated lumbar punctures, corticosteroids, acetazolamide, lumboperitoneal shunts, and optic nerve fenestration. Visual loss may be slow but progressive. Visual field testing, fundus examination for papilledema, and visual evoked potentials should be performed in follow up-examination. Visual loss is higher in patients with a history of systemic hypertension. The prognosis is good after offending agents are removed.

Brain Tumor

Brain tumor (Fig. 10.6) is the most feared and least likely cause of a severe headache. In children a space-occupying lesion is suspected when headaches are less than 6 months in duration, there is no family history of headaches, headaches are sleep related, and there is vomiting, confusion, abnormal neurological findings, and absence of visual symptoms. CT or MRI is indicated under these conditions (57). In adults, headache is a common finding in brain tumor. It is a short-lasting, steady, intermittent pain of mild to moderate intensity. Headache onset after age 40 should raise suspicion of brain tumor (58, 59). Change in the usual headache pattern or failure to respond to previously successful forms of headache

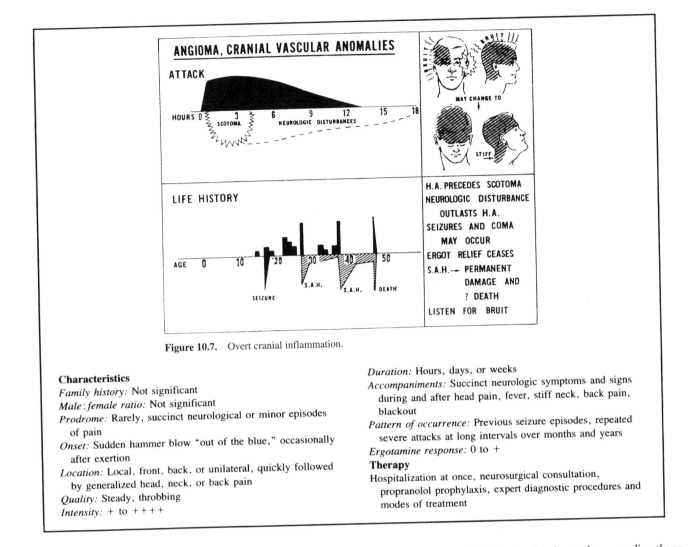

Figure 10.7.   Overt cranial inflammation.

Characteristics

Family history: Not significant

Male:female ratio: Not significant

Prodrome: Rarely, succinct neurological or minor episodes of pain

Onset: Sudden hammer blow "out of the blue," occasionally after exertion

Location: Local, front, back, or unilateral, quickly followed by generalized head, neck, or back pain

Quality: Steady, throbbing

Intensity: + to + + + +

Duration: Hours, days, or weeks

Accompaniments: Succinct neurologic symptoms and signs during and after head pain, fever, stiff neck, back pain, blackout

Pattern of occurrence: Previous seizure episodes, repeated severe attacks at long intervals over months and years

Ergotamine response: 0 to +

Therapy

Hospitalization at once, neurosurgical consultation, propranolol prophylaxis, expert diagnostic procedures and modes of treatment

---

therapy is a clue to organic cause. Nausea and vomiting are more common in brain tumor than they are in migraine. MRI is the best test to search for brain tumor.

HEADACHE CAUSED BY OVERT CRANIAL INFLAMMATION

Cranial inflammation (Fig. 10.7) is a frequent source of headache, usually of a nonrecurrent type. Its recognition is a part of general medicine. The source of inflammation may be infectious or sterile. It may result from leakage of blood, reaction to chemicals, or autoimmune processes. Treatment is directed toward the underlying condition.

Although headache is often a prominent symptom of such illnesses, it is usually not the presenting symptom. In some instances, however, the symptoms of a generalized systemic disease are not prominent, and the patient seeks relief for the most troublesome symptom of headache.

In subarachnoid hemorrhage arising from rupture of an intracranial aneurysm or leakage of blood from an AVM, headache is a primary complaint. Nonbleeding cerebral aneurysm or AVM usually does not cause headache. Exceptions

to this occur when the lesion is enlarging and presses directly on or distorts a pain-sensitive structure in the head. In AVM recurrent attacks of generalized or focal seizures may precede a major bleed. Vascular malformations on the skin, especially of the face, head, and neck, may warn of similar intracranial lesions. A steady headache concentrated in one particular area of the head is common. More common, however, is generalized headache, fever, and stiff neck as a result of bleeding into the subarachnoid space with meningeal irritation and inflammation.

A hallmark of subarachnoid hemorrhage is the sudden onset of severe headache arising out of the blue or sometimes in relation to a physical or emotional strain. Stiff neck and focal neurologic signs, depending on the location of the lesion and the amount of brain damage, follow. The first episode of headache and stiff neck may be short lasting and without focal neurologic signs. Prompt investigation with noncontrast CT and a lumbar puncture for presence of blood or xanthochromia is mandatory even if the episode is short. Magnetic resonance angiography frequently gives details of intracranial and extracranial blood vessels and identifies the source of aneurysmal rupture or localizes vascular malformations. A combination of β-blockers and anticonvulsant therapy and surgical evaluation is recommended.

Cranial arteritis is an important form of overt cranial inflammation in patients over 55 years of age. It may be a part of a generalized collagen vascular disease such as polyarteritis nodosa or polymyalgia rheumatica. Temporal arteritis is probably an autoimmune process against arterial internal elastic lamina. Proliferation of mononuclear cells and giant cells may lead to occlusion of ophthalmic or retinal arteries. Monocular or even binocular blindness is the most feared complication.

In cranial arteritis the patient usually feels ill all over, has a poor appetite, often runs a low-grade fever, and has a nagging, moderately severe headache that moves slowly over days or weeks to one area of the head after another. The temporal area of the head is the most common site, and the disease may manifest as swollen, tender, reddened temporal vessels in which the pulse has disappeared; neighboring tissues also participate in the inflammation. (Temporal arteries during the migraine or cluster headache attack also are swollen and tender but have increased amplitude of pulsation and regress to normal size after the attack).

The early symptoms of cranial arteritis often involve "angina" of the tongue during eating or of the jaw muscles during chewing. Pain from inflammation of the mandibular artery may lead to extraction of healthy teeth. Depression is a prominent symptom at times and may be erroneously considered the cause of the headache in an older or retired patient.

Joint and muscle pains of polymyalgia rheumatica may point to the headache diagnosis as being one component of a generalized vasculitis. The sedimentation rate is almost always significantly elevated, although there are very rare exceptions. White blood cell counts are frequently elevated, and titers of antinuclear antibodies in the blood are often elevated. The diagnosis is confirmed by longitudinal biopsy of the sorest and most swollen stretch of cranial artery available, because the disease is disseminated in a spotty fashion in the cranial vascular tree. It is important to obtain a biopsy as soon as possible to establish the diagnosis definitely for reassurance during the long months of steroid treatment that lie ahead.

Prednisone 40 mg daily should be started without waiting for the final tissue diagnosis, which is positive in genuine cases, even after few days of steroid therapy. Delay in the onset of therapy can result in sudden blindness. The dose of steroids may be tapered or manipulated in accordance with the improvement in symptoms, the course of fever, and sedimentation rate. Final recovery may take months or years, during which time attention must be directed to the prevention and detection of complications of prolonged steroid therapy. Other generalized systemic inflammatory processes in the cranium that may cause headache include polyarteritis nodosa, Takayasu's vasculitis, Wegener's granulomatosis, and cerebral venous thrombosis of pregnancy and lupus erythematosus.

Intermittent, recurrent headache can be caused by attacks of meningitis related to infection via spinal fluid leaks. Secondary syphilis, tuberculous meningitis, fungal meningitis, and undulant fever are yet other examples of infections causing headaches. In recurrent polyserositis, allergic reaction to intraspinal anesthetic or contrast agent headache may be a conspicuous symptom. Physicians should be alert to factitious fever, in which mentally disturbed patients induce fever and headache by ingestion or injection of abnormal substances, such as lighter fluid, typhoid vaccine, or dishwater.

AIDS

Patients with AIDS or ARC may have headache as the only manifestation of central nervous system involvement in this disease. Other common complaints in AIDS include seizure, confusion, and hallucination. Common causes of headache in AIDS include acute aseptic meningitis; chronic headache and persistent pleocytosis; cryptococcal, syphilitic, tuberculous, or lymphomatous meningitis; toxoplasmosis; cryptococcoma, *Candida* abscess, primary central nervous system lymphoma, progressive multifocal leukoencephalopathy, herpes simplex virus encephalitis, and drug-induced headache from zidovudine use. In addition to these specific conditions, AIDS patient can also have migraine, tension, or sinus-related headaches, as in the non-AIDS population.

Recommended work includes evaluation for depression or drug abuse and a review of all medications. Obtain CD counts and serum antibody titers for *Toxoplasma gondii, Treponema pallidum,* and *Cryptococcus neoformans.*

In early disease (CD4 count greater than 500 cells/mm^3) if exposure to syphilis is documented, even if treated in the past, obtain a brain MRI and a lumbar puncture. For patients with a new-onset headache or worsening of a preexisting headache disorder and a CD4 count below 500 cells/mm^3, perform a brain MRI and a lumbar puncture. In addition to routine studies, cerebrospinal fluid studies include culture and stains for bacteria, *Myobacteria,* viruses, fungi, cryptococcal antigen titer, and a cerebrospinal fluid Venereal Disease Research Laboratory (VDRL) titer and cytologic analysis (60).

Treatment of AIDS is rapidly changing, with hope of containment of disease. Triple therapy is the norm, and polydrug cocktail also offers promise of improvement. Headache treatment should be based on the underlying cause and current recommendations of AIDS therapy by infectious disease experts.

HEADACHE CAUSED BY DISEASES OF CRANIAL OR NECK STRUCTURES

Only a few of the disorders of these structures that cause head pain are mentioned here because their symptoms are usually called to the attention of specialists in the respective fields and their cure depends on correction of the specific underlying disorder.

Eyes

Glaucoma and corneal ulceration frequently cause headaches and photophobia. Retinitis pigmentosa may manifest initially as headache rather than night blindness or loss of visual fields (61).

Sinuses

Headache is common in acute sinusitis. Many patients with recurrent headaches readily agree to ill-advised surgery for chronic sinusitis and retention cysts, looking for cure of their headaches. Headaches rarely improve after these procedures. Flexible rhinolaryngoscopy is an indispensable tool in visualizing active infection in a headache patient (62, 63).

Ears

In herpes zoster of the eardrum and external canal, vesicles on the drum can be visualized. Malignancies in the pharynx and fossa of Rosenmüller can cause constant ear pain. CT helps to detect malignancies in nasal, sinus, and aural regions. Purulent drainage, headache, and fever are early symptoms of neurological complications of otitis media (64). Complications of chronic mastoiditis may include headache (65).

Teeth

Avoid extraction of a healthy tooth even though pain is focused in the suspected tooth. Radiographic or other definite evidence of disease or cracks in teeth should be obtained before extraction for painful conditions. Often a new pain condition follows extraction of a healthy tooth, particularly if extraction was technically difficult or only a partial extraction was possible. Often extraction of a normal tooth leads to chronic atypical facial neuralgia, a condition that may be impossible to treat.

Oromandibular Dysfunction (9)

Oromandibular dysfunction used to be called myofascial pain dysfunction syndrome, temporomandibular joint pain dysfunction syndrome, Costen's syndrome, or craniomandibular dysfunction.

Diagnostic Criteria for Oromandibular Dysfunction

Three or more of the following are necessary for the diagnosis: temporomandibular joint noise on jaw movements, limited or jerky jaw movements, pain on jaw function, locking of jaw on opening, clenching of teeth, gnashing of teeth (bruxism), other oral parafunction (tongue, lips, or cheek biting or pressing).

Pain in the region of the temporomandibular joint, mouth, temples, cheek, and at times neck frequently emanates from disease of the temporomandibular joint or its cartilage and from significant degrees of malocclusion. Major factors in these conditions are tension and anxiety in the patient, leading to bruxism and habits of tensing muscles of the face and scalp in response to adverse life situations. Improvement in facial pain is likely to be successful if a psychologist, physical therapist, and dentist with temporomandibular joint expertise evaluate the patient in a multidisciplinary approach.

Neck

Disorders of the neck play an important role in the generation of headache in the back of the head, neck, and remotely in the eye and temporal regions. The source of the pain can be blood vessels, sensory and autonomic nerves, plexuses, facets, bones and joints, ligaments, discs, muscles and foramina, and lymph nodes. Pain may result from injury, inflammation, entrapment, spasm, autonomic disturbance, tumor, or congenital abnormalities of these structures.

Injury, inflammation, or physical displacement of structures in one part of the neck may evoke protective painful spasm in the other parts of the neck and head. Impairment of autonomic function in the sympathetic nerves emanating from cervical outlets to the blood vessels may alter their capacity to respond properly to vasodilating and vasoconstricting demands.

Intermittent compression of sensory cervical roots may cause sudden zap pains radiating to the occipital and eye regions, and injury and irritation to these nerves may produce causalgia, neuralgia, and pain of vascular origin. Cervical rib disorders, scalenus anticus syndrome, disc degeneration, and foramen impingement by cervical osteoarthritis may cause pain in the head directly or by the reactive spasm of protective muscle groups.

Obstruction to the free exchange of cerebrospinal fluid flow and pressure between head and neck may give rise to cough and exertional or coital headache. Entrapment of the sensory root of C1 with the occipital artery in the trapezius canal may cause painful unilateral headache resembling common migraine.

When the head is significantly injured, some cervical injury is also very common. Manual traction on the head (lifting it off the shoulders) may relieve head pain and point to a cervical origin for pain. Sudden pressure on the head may exacerbate head pain and indicate a cervical component. At times indomethacin has a specific effect on headaches of cervical origin. Prolonged use of a cervical collar may lead to weakening of cervical supporting muscles and is to be avoided. During sleep the use of a plastic collar that is individually fitted to the patient to keep the head in a neutral to slightly flexed position may prevent wake-up headache caused by excessive cervical motion during sleep. Look for areas of increased tenderness on pressure in the neck in fixed unilateral headache problems, especially in the region of the occipital nerve and artery in the trapezius canal. Surgical relief of entrapment of these structures may be beneficial.

CT and MRI may show soft-tissue injury in the neck commonly missed by ordinary x-ray techniques. Techniques for nerve blocks and surgical intervention in localized pain arising in the neck are proving useful. Consultation with a conservative neurosurgeon or anesthetist is suggested. Early referral for physical therapy, ultrasound treatments, transcutaneous nerve stimulation, anti-inflammatory medication, and graduated exercise is prudent in neck injuries leading to head pain problems.

CRANIAL NEURITIDES CAUSED BY TRAUMA, NEW GROWTH, OR INFLAMMATION (10)

Direct trauma to sensory nerves may cause injury and impaired function leading to causalgic pain of a steady or jabbing nature. Such trauma may occur during orbital or jaw fractures that damage or cause entrapment or neuroma formation of sensory nerves. Direct injury to sensory and sympathetic nerves in blood vessel walls in head injury of the temple or occiput may create causalgic pain.

Infection and inflammation, such as lymphadenitis, in the immediate vicinity of cranial sensory nerves may lead to ticlike jabs of pain. Lymph node enlargement at the base of the scalp and in the vicinity of the cervical plexus may be the culprit. Inflammation of the ear may cause pain as well as facial paralysis as in Bell's palsy and may respond to corticosteroid therapy.

Postherpetic neuralgia (shingles) following herpes zoster involving the fifth cranial nerve poses a serious problem. During the acute phase, acute inflammation similar to burn causes tissue damage and pain. Nociceptor fibers are excited. Spontaneous discharge, lowered activation threshold and exaggerated response to normal painful stimuli contribute to pain that appears out of proportion to the visible damage. Postherpetic neuralgia is most likely due to failure of nociceptors to return to normal after the acute phase (66). Treatment includes acyclovir, analgesics, local anesthetics, and opioids in the acute phase and chronically in postherpetic neuralgia. Mechanisms and management of this disorder are discussed in detail in Chapter 8.

CRANIAL NEURALGIA

Tic douloureux, or trifacial neuralgia (Fig. 10.8), is the most common and most severe of the true neuralgias affecting the head. It usually occurs in patients over 55 to 60 years of age. When it develops in younger patients, a search must be made for multiple sclerosis or a tumor causing local disturbances to the branches, ganglion, or central tracts of the fifth cranial nerve. Repeated bursts of electric shock-like pains limited to the distribution of the branches of the fifth cranial nerve, usually V2 or V3 and less frequently V1 is characteristic. Each shock lasts 1 or 2 seconds and is repeated every few seconds for minutes or hours. The jabs of pain are frequently set off by sensory trigger mechanisms, such as hot soup, cool air, touching or moving the face, chewing, or swallowing. Drug treatment includes phenytoin, carbamazepine, chlorphenesin carbamate, gabapentin or combinations of these. When medications are not effective or cause side effects, surgical relief may be sought.

Surgical techniques include local peripheral nerve blocks with lidocaine or alcohol, radiofrequency lesions of the nerve rootlets, injection of glycerol into Meckel's cave, surgical section of the sensory rootlets, posterior fossa microvascular decompression, and bulbar tractotomy of sensory pain tracts. The results of surgery are usually rewarding.

The profiles of headache depicting trigeminal neuralgia should be compared with those of cluster headache, with which it is sometimes confused (Figs. 9.5 and 9.9), since treatment of these two conditions differs.

Glossopharyngeal neuralgia is probably more correctly described as glossopharyngeal and vagal neuralgia, since the distribution of pain is in the territory of both nerves. It occurs between ages 40 and 70 years. Chewing, swallowing, or yawning precipitates pain. Sudden onset of pain of increasing intensity, which radiates from the throat to the ipsilateral ear, is typical. The pain lasts 20 to 30 seconds and is often followed by a burning sensation lasting 2 to 3 minutes in these same areas (67).

Identifiable causes include elongation of the styloid process, atheromatous plaques of the vertebral artery, compression of the ninth and tenth cranial nerves by arachnoiditis, and an arterial loop of the posterior inferior cerebellar artery. Tuberculous laryngitis, ossification of the stylohyoid ligament, posttonsillectomy tumors, and nasopharyngeal and intracranial tumors are also known causes of glossopharyngeal neuralgia, although in the vast majority of cases it is idiopathic. Patients with glossopharyngeal neuralgia are at risk for cardiac arrhythmia, asystole, and cardiac arrest. Arterial hypotension, syncope, and convulsions have also been reported in association with glossopharyngeal neuralgia.

Carbamazepine, baclofen, lithium, or intravenous phenytoin is usually effective. Surgeries include intracranial section of the glossopharyngeal nerve and upper two rootlets of the vagus nerve and microvascular decompression of the posterior inferior cerebellar artery.

CHRONIC POSTTRAUMATIC HEADACHE SYNDROME

Acute injury to the head and neck can cause severe headache and neck pain by hemorrhage and direct injury to many pain sensitive structures. Usually pain improves in a few weeks. In some patients it lingers on for weeks, months, or even years, causing increasing discomfort, depression, and disability.

Transformation to chronic posttraumatic headache is considerably increased by the circumstances in which the trauma took place and the personality and lifestyle of the patient. Accidents leading to head and neck injury at home are less likely to lead to a chronic pain than those that occur on the job. When accidents are one's own fault, there is less anxiety and tension than when someone else is liable for the injury.

Anger at one's assailant, anxiety about courts, lawyers, family, and the whole system of remuneration, and a long-drawn-out court process introduce a sense of frustration and poor attitude. Prompt resolution of the case and early rehabilitation therapy offer hope for speedy recovery and gainful employment. But in real life posttraumatic headache victims find that it is not easy to fight the system.

Posttraumatic pain syndrome may result from chronic subdural hematoma, seizures, accentuation of previous vascular headache, injury to sensory nerves, or neuromas. Onset of cluster or muscle contraction headache sometimes is linked to head injury. Following head trauma the patient may have bad

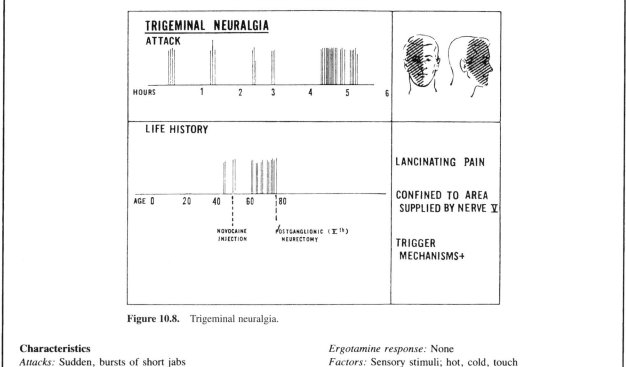

Figure 10.8. Trigeminal neuralgia.

Characteristics

Attacks: Sudden, bursts of short jabs

Family history: Not significant

Age: Elderly

Location: Limited to domain of CN V, usually V2, V3.

Quality: Lancinating

Intensity: + to +++

Duration: Repeated 2- to 3-seconds jabs or jolts in repeated bursts of 10 to 15 min all day

Accompaniments: Wincing, salivation, occasionally flushing, avoidance of stimuli

Pattern: As above, in groups, lasting weeks, months, or years

Ergotamine response: None

Factors: Sensory stimuli; hot, cold, touch

Therapy

Medications: Phenytoin, carbamazepine, chlorphenesin, antidepressants, thioridazine (Mellaril)

Surgical: Novocaine, alcohol blocks, radiofrequency lesion, surgical or glycerol destruction of CN V rootlets, Janetta procedure, tractotomy, implants in central gray matter

Differential Diagnosis

Multiple sclerosis in patients under 55 to 60 years of age, tumor near Gasserian ganglion, dental lesions, sinusitis, cluster headache

dreams, phobias, and fears of repeat injury. Inability to concentrate, poor sleep, and irritable personality are frequently part of chronic pain syndrome. Dependency on tranquilizing and analgesic drugs also becomes a major problem in effective management of headaches.

Early and active rehabilitation, the open discussion of bad dreams and sources of tension and anger, the use of antidepressant drugs rather than analgesic and tranquilizing medications, the avoidance of narcotics, early settlement of legal issues, and return to work should be advocated. Surgical relief of definite demonstrable lesions is indicated. However, polysurgery should be avoided.

Chronic posttraumatic pain may be caused by injury to muscle, bone, joint, nerve, emotion, teeth, jaw, or brain. Pain of multifactorial origin needs a team approach of corresponding specialties. Positive outcome is likely in a multidisciplinary setting. Patience, genuine interest in the victim's life situation, and perseverance in pursuit of pain management goals on the part of health care providers are important to successful outcome.

References

1. Moskowitz MA, Buzzi MG. Neuroeffector functions of sensory fibers: implications for headache mechanisms and drug actions. J Neurol 1991;238(suppl 1):S18–22.
2. Packard RC. Conversion headache. Headache 1980;20:266–268.
3. Packard RC. What does the headache patient want? Headache 1979;19:370–374.
4. Kuhn MJ. A comparative study of magnetic resonance imaging and computed tomography in the evaluation of migraine. Comput Med Imaging Graph 1990;14:149–152.
5. Leviton A, Malvea B, Graham, JR. Vascular disease, mortality, and migraine in the parents of migraine patients. Neurology 1974;24:669–672.
6. Barkley GL, Tepley N, Nagel-Leiby S, et al. Magnetoencephalographic studies in migraine. Headache 1990;30:428–434.
7. Mortimer MJ, Good PA, Marsters JB. The VEP in acephalgic migraine. Headache 1990;30:285–288.
8. Thie A, Fuhlendorf A, Spitzer K, Kunze K. Transcranial Doppler evaluation of common migraine and classic migraine: 2. Ultrasonic features during attacks. Headache 1990;30:209–215.
9. Headache classification committee of the International Headache Society. Classification and diagnostic criteria for headache disorders, cranial neuralgias, and facial pain. Cephalalgia 1988;8(Supp 7):1–96.

10. Ad Hoc Committee Classification of headache. JAMA 1062;179:717–718.
11. Carroll D. Retinal migraine. Headache 1970;10:8–12.
12. Wolff, HG. Headache and other head pain. ed 4. Dalessio DJ, ed. New York: Oxford University Press, 1980;71–73.
13. Skyhoj OT, Friberg L, Lassen NA. Ischemia may be the primary cause of the neurological deficits in classic migraine. Arch Neurol 1987;44:156–161.
14. O'Brien MD. Cerebral blood changes in migraine. Headache 1971;10:139–143.
15. Deshmukh SV, Meyer JS. Cyclic changes in platelet dynamics and the pathogenesis and prophylaxis of migraine. Headache 1977;17:101–108.
16. Leviton A. Migraine associated with hyper-pre-beta lipoproteinemia. Neurology 1969;19:963–965.
17. Anthony M. Role of individual free fatty acids in migraine. Res Clin Stud Headache 1978;6:110–116.
18. Saxena PR. Arteriovenous shunting and migraine. Res Clin Stud Headache 1978;6:89–102.
19. Tepley N, Barkley GL, Moran JE, et al. Observation of cortical spreading depression in migraine patients. In: Williamson S, Kaufman L, et al., eds. Biomagnetism. New York: Plenum Press, 1990;327–330.
20. Chapman LF, Ramos AO, Goodell H, et al. A humoral agent implicated in vascular headache of the migraine type. Arch Neurol 1960;3:223–229.
21. The Dihydroergotamine Nasal Spray Multicenter Investigators. Efficacy, safety, and tolerability of dihydroergotamine nasal spray as monotherapy in the treatment of acute migraine. Headache 1995;35:177–184.
22. Callaham M, Raskin N. A controlled study of dihydroergotamine in the treatment of acute migraine headache. Headache 1986;26:168–71.
23. Raskin NH. Repetitive intravenous dihydroergotamine as therapy for intractable migraine. Neurology 1986;36:995–997.
24. Silberstein SD, Schulman EA, Hopkins MM. Repetitive intravenous DHE in the treatment of refractory headache. Headache 1990;30:334–339.
25. Ford, RG, Ford KT. Continuous intravenous dihydroergotamine in the treatment of intractable headache. Headache 1997;37:129–136.
26. Maciewicz R, Chung RY, Strassman A, et al. Relief of vascular headache with intravenous lidocaine: clinical observations and a proposed mechanism. Clin J Pain 1988;4:11–16.
27. Kumar KL, Cooney TG. Visual symptoms after atenolol therapy for migraine. Ann Intern Med 1990;112:712–713 (letter).
28. Willie RC, Morrow JD. Case report: dapsone hypersensitivity syndrome associated with treatment of the bite of a brown recluse spider. Am J Med Sci 1988;296:270–271.
29. Arndt KA. Adverse reactions to acyclovir: topical, oral, and intravenous. J Am Acad Dermatol 1988;18:188–190.
30. Vanov SK, Pun EF, Taylor RJ. The safety of nitrendipine in the treatment of essential hypertension: a review of 61 clinical studies. Angiology 1988;39:113–122.
31. Alvarez-Sabin J, Codina A, Rodriguez C, Laporte JR. Gemfibrozil-induced headache. Lancet 1988;2(8622):1246 (letter).
32. LeCoz P, Woimant F, Rougemont D, et al. Benign cerebral angiopathies and phenylpropanolamine. Rev Neurol (Paris) 1988;144:295–300.
33. Kutt E, Hall MJ, Booth A, Virjee J. Barium enemas are a headache. Clin Radiol 1988;39:9–10.
34. Hirsch E. Famotidine and ranitidine, but not cimetidine, cause severe, disabling headache. Am J Gastroenterol 1989;84:202–203 (letter).
35. Sylvia LM, Forlenza SW, Brocavich JM. Aseptic meningitis associated with naproxen. Drug Intell Clin Pharm 1988;22:399–401.
36. Bana DS, Graham JR, Spierings ELH. Headache patients as they see themselves. Headache 1988;28:403–408.
37. Mathew NT, Saper JL, Silberstein SD, et al. Migraine prophylaxis with divalproex. Arch Neurol 1995;52:281–286.
38. Fletcher PE, Lowy MT. Evaluation of long-term safety and efficacy of Zolmitriptan 311C90 in the treatment of migraine. In Olesen J, Tfelt-Hansen P, eds. Headache treatment trial methodology and new drugs. Philadelphia: Lippincott-Raven 1997:273–278.
39. Goldstein J, Schellens R, Diener HC, et al. Alniditan, a novel nonindole 5-HT$_{1D}$ Receptor agonist: a subcutaneous dose finding trial in acute migraine. In: Olesen J, Tfelt-Hansen P, eds. Headache treatment trial methodology and new drugs. Philadelphia: Lippincott-Raven 1997:279–285.
40. Graham JR. Cluster headache. Headache 1972;11:175–185.
41. Sumatriptan Cluster Headache Study Group. Treatment of acute cluster headache with sumatriptan. N Engl J Med 1991;325:322–326.
42. Dalton K. Progesterone suppositories and pessaries in the treatment of menstrual migraine. Headache 1973;12:150–158.
43. D'Andrea G, Perini F, Granella F, et al. Efficacy of transdermal clonidine in the treatment of cluster headache. In: Olesen J, Tfelt-Hansen P, eds. Headache treatment trial methodology and new drugs. Philadelphia: Lippincott-Raven 1997:335–340.
44. Sjaastad O, Dale I. Evidence for a new treatable headache entity. Headache 1974;14:105–108.
45. Joutel A, Bousser M, Biouses V, et al. A gene for familial hemiplegic migraine maps to chromosome 19. Nat Genet 1993;5:40–45.
46. Centonze V, Brucoli C, Macinagrossa G, et al. Non-familial hemiplegic migraine responsive to naloxone. Cephalalgia 1983;3:125–127.
47. Solomon GD, Spaccavento LJ. Lateral medullary syndrome after basilar migraine. Headache 1982;22:171–172.
48. Martin MJ. Tension headache: a psychiatric study. Headache 1966;6:46–53.
49. Diamond SS, Baltes BJ. Chronic tension headache treated with amitriptyline: a double-blind study. Headache 1971;11:109–115.
50. Weatherhead AD. Psychogenic headache. Headache 1980;20:47–54.
51. Morland TJ, Storli OV, Mogstad TE. Doxepin in the prophylactic treatment of mixed vascular and tension headache. Headache 1979;19:382–383.
52. Graham JR. A "cluster" of complications and correlations. Headache 1976;16:46–51.
53. Graham JR, Bana DS, Yap AV. Headache, hypertension and renal disease. Res Clin Stud Headache 1978;6:147–154.
54. Fisher CM. The headache and pain of spontaneous carotid dissection. Headache 1982;22:60–65.
55. Litman GI, Friedman HM. Migraine and the mitral valve prolapse syndrome. Am Heart J 1978;96:610–614.
56. Young WB, Silberstein SD. Paroxysmal headache caused by colloid cyst of the third ventricle: case report and review of the literature. Headache 1997;37:15–20.
57. Medina LS, Pinter JD, Zurakowski D, et al. Children with headache: clinical predictors of surgical space-occupying lesions and the role of neuroimaging. Radiology 1997;202:819–824.
58. Rushton JG, Rooke ED. Brain tumor headache. Headache 1962;3:146–151.
59. Forsyth PA, Posner JB. Headaches in patients with brain tumors: a study of 111 patients. Neurology 1993;43:1678–1683.
60. Holloway RG, Kieburtz KD. Headache and the human immunodeficiency virus type i infection. Headache 1995;35:245–255.
61. Heckenlively JR, Yoser SL, Friedman LH, Oversier J. Clinical findings and common symptoms in retinitis pigmentosa. Am J Ophthalmol 1988;105:504–511.
62. Castellanos J, Axelrod D. Flexible fiberoptic rhinoscopy in the diagnosis of sinusitis. J Allergy Clin Immunol 1989;83:91–94.
63. Stammberger H, Wolf G. Headaches and sinus disease: the endoscopic approach. Ann Otol Rhinol Laryngol 1988;134(Suppl):3–23.
64. Ryan RE Jr, Eugene B, Kern EB. Rhinologic causes of facial pain and headache. Headache 1978;18:44–50.
65. Schwaber MK, Pensak ML, Bartels LJ. The early signs and symptoms of neurotologic complications of chronic suppurative otitis media. Laryngoscope 1989;99:373–375.
66. Bennett GJ. Hypothesis on the pathogenesis of herpes zoster associated pain. Ann Neurol 1994;35(Suppl):38–41.
67. Bruyn GW. Glossopharyngeal neuralgia. Cephalalgia 1983;3:143–157.

CHAPTER 11

Facial Pain and Craniomandibular Disorders

Donald F. Booth and Michael J. Hunter

In this chapter we outline the basic and most widely accepted methods of treatment of facial pain syndrome, craniomandibular disorders (CMD), and temporomandibular joint (TMJ) pain. It is not our intention to downgrade the success of other modalities but rather to instill in the reader a high level of suspicion when referring pain patients to other specialists who claim high success rates for their treatments.

CMD includes a host of disease entities with various symptoms and causes. CMDs are characterized by tenderness in the muscles of the jaw, head, neck, and back; painful TMJs; limited mandibular movements; joint noises; double vision and blurred vision; loss of balance; and facial deformities. Headaches, earaches, neck aches, and toothaches are frequently listed as complaints.

The facial pain patient presents a clinical challenge to the health care provider. In determining the causative factors of facial pain, the challenge arises because of the overlapping of the somatic and psychological components of pain, the similarities between diagnoses, and the influence of anatomical structures. In approaching the facial pain patient, the somatic and psychological components of the pain must be considered. One must assess the patient's behavior resulting from pain, consider contributing factors, examine reasons for pain reinforcement, and identify physiological and anatomical processes involved. Facial pain characteristics influenced by anatomical structures are often overlooked. Local disease conditions can produce pain by causing pressure on a nerve. Facial pain may also be limited to the distribution of a particular nerve. The total evaluation of the facial pain patient should be the synthesis of a detailed history, a physical examination, appropriate studies, and consultations.

PATIENT'S HISTORY AND INFORMATION

During the history taking, the information in (Table 11.1) should be obtained as accurately as possible (1).

CLINICAL EXAMINATION

We recommend that the practitioner make a thorough examination of the areas described in Table 11.2. Notes on clinical findings should be descriptive and complete.

EVALUATED MOUNTED DIAGNOSTIC CASTS

The integration of all facets of an evaluation of a facial pain patient is indeed a complex problem, and all aspects of the case should be considered. The causative factors of facial pain may range from a "simple" toothache to a complex central entity such as trigeminal neuralgia. Table 11.3 is a general classification of facial pain (2).

CAUSATION

The causative factors of CMDs are multiple. They include genetic, developmental, physiological, traumatic, pathological, environmental, mental, and behavioral factors. There are various theories of causation. De Boever (3) organizes these concepts into the following five basic theories.

Mechanical Displacement Theory

The mechanical displacement theory includes the TMJ theories of Costen (4) and others (5, 6), who thought that the distal displacement of the condyles after loss of posterior teeth caused impingement on various structures in the region with resultant symptoms. Sicher (7) and others later showed that the anatomical basis of Costen's syndrome was invalid. However, mandibular overclosure (reduced vertical relation of occlusion) as a causative factor has remained prevalent in many current concepts.

The position of the condyle is dictated by the occlusion. When occlusal problems result from missing teeth, prematurities (deflective occlusal contacts), or insufficient eruption of the posterior teeth causing a deviation of the condyles from

Table 11.1.   Patient's History

I. Personal information	(4) Tension or fatigue
A. Name	2. Limit in function
B. Age	3. Clicking
D. Date of birth	B. Duration
E. Telephone numbers (work and home)	C. Changes with time
F. Height	D. Initiating or precipitating traumatic factors
G. Weight	1. Whiplash
H. Referring doctor	2. Sports injury
I. Medical insurance	3. Facial trauma
J. Dental Insurance	4. Intubation (hyperextension)
II. Medical history	5. Cervical trauma
A. Hospitalizations (with dates and reasons)	6. Hyperextension of joint
B. Allergies	7. Extraction (difficult)
1. Medications	8. Prolonged opening of mouth
2. Foods	E. Exacerbating factors
3. Other	F. Ameliorating factors
C. Medications taken in the past year	G. What does this complaint stop the patient from doing?
D. Heart condition	H. Previous treatment for this complaint
1. Valve disorder	1. Medical
2. Rheumatic fever	2. Dental
E. Psychiatric and psychological therapy (with dates and diagnosis)	I. Patient's evaluation of results of previous treatment
F. Contributory family history	J. Examiner's evaluation of results of previous treatment
III. Chief complaint	1. Orthodontics
A. Description: determine quality, frequency, location, and type	2. Restorative dentistry
1. Pain	3. Equilibration
a. Quality	4. Other
(1) Mild	K. Patient's narrative report of the complaint
(2) Severe	IV. Current health information
(3) Spontaneous	A. Other illnesses or disabilities
(4) Paroxysmal	B. Amount of exercise
(5) Dull	C. Nutrition
(6) Burning	1. General dietary habits
(7) Aching	2. Food and drink
b. Duration	a. Alcohol
(1) Continuous	b. Sugar
(2) Recurrent	c. Caffeine
(3) Intermittent	3. Smoking habits
(4) Momentary	D. Harmful oral habits
c. Location	1. Bruxism (clenching or grinding)
(1) Local	2. Chewing gum
(2) Diffuse	3. Chewing ice
(3) Radiating	4. Chewing fingernails, pencil, pipe, or other objects
d. Affected by	5. Occupational (e.g., work, posture, use of telephone)
(1) Jaw movement	6. Tongue thrusting
(2) Tongue movement	E. Habitual chewing pattern
(3) Head or body position	F. Sleeping posture

their normal centric position, the muscles become involved, creating dysfunction and pain. The mechanical displacement group relies heavily on the use of radiographic examinations and diagnostic casts for diagnosis and the determination of proper mandibular position.

Muscle Theory

Muscle tension increases and results in pain and spasm as a manifestation of Selye's general adaptation syndrome when the stresses of everyday life do not have an adequate outlet or release. Muscles are primarily involved as part of a general rather than local reaction.

Psychological Theory

The psychological theory includes several diverse thoughts with published studies by various authors producing conflicting results. However, it is generally agreed that emotional and behavioral factors play some role in TMJ disorders, either as modifying or initiating factors.

Some authors, such as Moulton (8) and Lupton (9), believe that psychological factors are capable of initiating TMJ pain and dysfunction. The patient is psychologically predisposed or pain prone, with occlusal changes or trauma merely serving as trigger factors. Others, such as Mozak (10), believe the psychological factors found in patients with TMJ

Table 11.2.   Physical Examination of the Patient

I. Joint and muscle palpation	D. Protrusion
A. Joint	E. Deviation of sagittal
1. Lateral	1. Opening
2. Dorsal (through the external auditory meatus)	2. Closing
B. Muscle	F. Deviation of protrusion
1. Extraoral	G. Pattern and quality
a. Deep masseter	1. Bradykinesia
b. Superficial masseter	2. Dyskinesia
c. Anterior (through the posterior temporalis)	III. TMJ sounds (auscultation may be performed by stethoscope, Doppler, and so on)
d. Vertex	A. Type
e. Posterior cervicals	1. Popping, clicking
f. Trapezius	2. Crackling, crepitus
g. Spine	B. Consistency
h. Sternocleidomastoid	C. Loudness
I. Posterior digastric	D. Frequency
j. Angle mandible	E. Mandibular position coincident with sound
k. Anterior digastric	F. Can click be eliminated by repositioning the mandible?
l. Suprahyoid	G. Is sound associated with pain?
m. Infrahyoid	IV. Tooth contact relationship
2. Intraoral	A. Mandibular reference positions
a. Temporal tendon	1. Muscular position
b. Lateral pterygoid	2. Maximum intercuspation
c. Medial pterygoid	3. Centric relation occlusion
II. Mandibular range of motion	B. Mandibular excursive movements
A. Sagittal range of motion	1. Lateral movements
B. Right lateral excursion	2. Protrusive movements
C. Left lateral excursion	

Table 11.3.   General Classifications of Facial Pain

1. Extracranial
2. Intracranial
3. Vascular
4. Myofacial
5. Rheumatic, temporomandibular joint
6. Neuralgic
7. Causalgic
8. Psychogenic

disorders are a result of the patients' living with long-term, constant pain resulting from occlusal disharmonies, jaw imbalances, or both. Treatment depends on whether the clinician subscribes to the concept of eliminating the psychological factors first or initially treating the occlusion.

Neuromuscular Theory

The proponents of the neuromuscular theory consider occlusion as the major influence on the functional remodeling and development of arthrosis in the joint. Occlusion is responsible for causing parafunctional habits such as grinding or clenching, provided that a background of psychic tension, stress, or anxiety is present. Laskin (11) believes that the reverse is true. He suggests that the emotional disturbances trigger the parafunctional habits, which then lead to emotional interferences. In either instance emotional factors figure prominently in causation.

Psychophysiological Theory

In the psychophysiological theory masticatory muscle spasm is considered the main factor causing pain and dysfunction. Overextension, overcontraction, or muscle fatigue may initiate the spasm and result in occlusal disharmonies and pathological joint changes. This group stresses that occlusal changes occur in response to or as a result of muscle spasm. The American Academy of Craniomandibular Disorders, whose membership lists the major academicians, clinicians, researchers, lecturers, and authors of texts on the subject, have divided the causative factors into three categories, as follows:

Predisposing factors include structural (size and/or shape) discrepancies with any of the tissues of the masticatory system. In addition, physiological disorders such as neurological, vascular, nutritional, or metabolic disorders can predispose the patient to craniomandibular problems. Pathological factors include systemic disease and infections, neoplasias, and orthopedic imbalances. Behavioral factors relate to the personality profile of the patient and how the patient responds to stress. They can be expressed as noxious habits such as bruxism and tooth clenching. Precipitating (initiating) factors include trauma not only to the masticatory system itself but to the entire head and neck of the patient, an adverse stress response, iatrogenic problems, infection, and idiopathic factors. Perpetuating (sustaining) factors are manifested primarily by the myospasm-pain-spasm cycle. They can be related to any one or a combination of the above predisposing or precipitating factors.

TRIGEMINAL NEURALGIA

According to some estimates, trigeminal neuralgia, or tic douloureux, afflicts 15,000 new patients per year in the United States (12). It is characterized by brief paroxysmal episodes of severe pain that are usually unilateral and occur within the distribution of the trigeminal nerve (Fig. 11.1). There is no sensory loss involved with the attacks; this differentiates trigeminal neuralgia from the trigeminal neuropathies (Fig. 11.2). The pain may, however, be bilateral and have cyclical features in which attacks are most frequent during the day. The attacks are brief, lasting a few seconds to a minute, and may occur in clusters, with the pain spreading to involve adjacent facial areas. The pain rarely extends below the mandible or posterior auricular area. The third branch of the trigeminal nerve (V_3) is more commonly affected than the second branch (V_2). V_1, or the first branch, is rarely involved. The right side is more commonly involved than the left. Women are affected more frequently than men, with the average age of onset of around the fifth decade of life. Frequently trigger zones are associated with initiating an attack, and patients avoid touching these areas. Common trigger zones include the lips, the alar base or nasolabial fold area, and the gingiva. Trigger points may be distant from the site of pain. A brief refractory period, during which time a new attack cannot be initiated, follows an attack. Attacks vary in frequency and may last several months or years. Spontaneous remissions may occur.

The causative factors of trigeminal neuralgia is not well understood. Various proposed theories include trigeminal root compression by blood vessels and elevation of the petrous portion of the temporal bone, resulting in improper angulation of the trigeminal nerve; demyelinating plaque caused by multiple sclerosis or tumor; segmental demyelination; and microneuroma formation (12–14). A recent study found vascular contact and/or compression of the trigeminal nerve at the root entry zone to the brainstem in 14 of 18 patients undergoing intracranial rhizotomy (15). Multiple sclerosis is found in fewer than 5% of patients with trigeminal neuralgia. The onset of trigeminal neuralgia associated with multiple sclerosis occurs in the fourth decade of life. However, multiple sclerosis trigeminal neuralgia may involve more than one trigeminal branch and may also occur bilaterally. Tumors of the middle cranial fossa and cerebellopontine angle may also present as trigeminal neuralgia. Recently bone cavities in the jaws with connecting passages to trigeminal nerve branches have been cited in trigeminal neuralgia (16). It is believed that these cavities develop after extraction of an abscessed tooth.

Treatment of trigeminal neuralgia involves medical or surgical measures. Carbamazepine (Tegretol), often the drug of choice, results in effective management in a number of patients. If results are not achieved in 1 week on a maximum dose regimen, increased effectiveness is not likely. See Table 11.4 for one reported dose regimen (13). Phenytoin (Dilantin) may be used concurrently with carbamazepine to increase effectiveness. Baclofen has also been used to treat trigeminal

Table 11.4.   Drug Treatment of Trigeminal Neuralgia

1. Start with 100 mg BID and increase by 100 mg daily in divided doses TID until
   A. Relief is obtained
   B. Toxicity occurs (dizziness, nausea, ataxia, diplopia)
      1. Decrease dose and wait 2 to 3 days
      2. Add phenytoin (100 mg TID)
2. If relief is obtained, taper by 100 mg every 3 days to the lowest maintenance dose possible
3. Continue maintenance dose for 2 to 3 mo, then taper 100 mg/wk, hoping for remission
   A. If no symptoms occur without medication, observe until next attack
   B. If pain recurs, restart maintenance dose
4. Obtain complete blood count initially and after 2 wk, 1 mo, then monthly; also obtain baseline liver function tests
   A. If white blood cell count is mildly decreased (3000 to 4000) at 2 wk, observe with weekly counts; most return to baseline by 1 mo
   B. If white blood cell count is markedly decreased (<3000 or mildly but persistently decreased after reducing the dosage of the drug, discontinue it
5. If initially ineffective or benefit unsustained, add phenytoin 100 mg TID (allow 1 wk to assess results)
   A. If the combination is effective, maintain for 2 to 3 mo; taper one drug at a time, hoping for remission
   B. If ineffective, consider other medical or surgical therapy

neuralgia secondary to multiple sclerosis. Before prescribing any agent, the health care provider should review the pharmacological properties, side effects, and interactions of the agents.

Surgical management of trigeminal neuralgia has taken many approaches. Alcohol and phenol injections are used with varying success. Anesthesia dolorosa, a painful zone of paresthesia in denervated tissues, is a possible complication of injection. Trigeminal pain has a tendency to recur following injection (15). Thermal differential rhizotomy is being used with greater success and can be repeated if symptoms recur. An occipital craniotomy to reposition tortuous branches of the cerebellar arteries that compress the trigeminal nerve is a more aggressive approach that has met with good results. Curettage of bone cavities has proved effective in the management of trigeminal neuralgia in which jaw bone concavities are found.

ATYPICAL TRIGEMINAL NEURALGIA

Often no specific entity or cause of facial pain is found. Many of these patients are diagnosed as having atypical trigeminal neuralgia, a catchall diagnosis. The differentiation between atypical trigeminal neuralgia and other entities, including trigeminal neuralgia, is difficult. The clinical criteria that distinguish atypical trigeminal neuralgia from trigeminal neuralgia are specific. The patient with atypical trigeminal neuralgia describes a steady, continuous aching pain that is long lasting and is neither initiated nor relieved by specific actions (17). This steady pain, which has been described as aching or burning, may extend to the neck or posterior scalp. Superimposed on this steady pain are sharp, paroxysmal pains that last a short time. These pains are provokable by stimulation and may be associated with symptoms of autonomic activity such as lacrimation, facial flushing, and edema. In addition, sensory

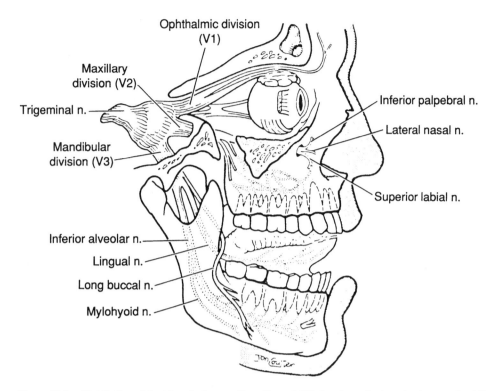

Figure 11.1.   Distribution of the trigeminal nerve. From Bennett CR. Local anesthesia and pain control. ed 7. St Louis: Mosby, 1984.

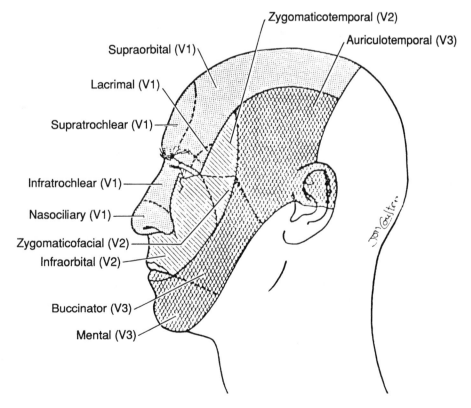

Figure 11.2.   Superficial sensory nerves of head and neck regions (after original drawing of TW Brand). From Bennett CR. Local anesthesia and pain control. ed 7. St Louis: Mosby, 1984.

abnormalities occur within the distribution of the trigeminal nerve. As is true of trigeminal neuralgia, atypical trigeminal neuralgia may be associated with other pathological conditions, such as multiple sclerosis, vascular lesions, or tumors. Mass lesions, such as cerebellopontine angle tumors, affecting the fifth cranial nerve proximal to the gasserian ganglion are frequently associated with atypical trigeminal neuralgia. The mechanisms involved with these associations are not understood. Medical treatment of atypical trigeminal neuralgia and trigeminal neuralgia is similar, and results of treatment are comparable. Surgical intervention, if the cause is a tumor, depends on the condition involved.

GLOSSOPHARYNGEAL NEURALGIA

Glossopharyngeal neuralgia, which occurs less frequently than trigeminal neuralgia, involves the sensory, motor, and autonomic components of the glossopharyngeal and vagus nerves. The pain ranges from a sharp, shooting pain that may last up to a minute to a dull, burning pain that may last several hours (18). The pain may occur in the tonsillar pillars, base of the tongue, soft palate, and external auditory canal. Many patients complain of an altered sensation, such as a foreign body in the throat, before the onset of pain. Trigger zones are poorly delineated, but trigger mechanisms such as swallowing or coughing are common. Patients may report a spread of pain to contiguous areas not within the area of the glossopharyngeal and vagus nerves (trigeminal). Some patients with this entity have syncopal attacks, convulsions, lacrimation, salivation, and vertigo associated with the pain attacks. The onset of pain is usually in the fourth decade of life. There is no clear predilection for either sex, and the pain is usually unilateral. Some patients have both glossopharyngeal and trigeminal neuralgia, and the identification of each entity is made on the anatomical distribution of the pain.

The causative factors of glossopharyngeal neuralgia include demyelination of the nerve with possible vascular compression including aneurysm. This pain entity has been associated with paratonsillar infections and an ossified and elongated stylohyoid ligament.

Both nonsurgical and surgical treatments are being used. Carbamazepine and phenytoin alone or in combination, as in the management of trigeminal neuralgia, are used effectively. Surgery entails extracranial avulsion of the glossopharyngeal nerve or if classic symptoms exist, intracranial sectioning of the glossopharyngeal nerve and upper rootlets of the vagus nerve. Pain in the inner ear has been managed by sectioning the nervus intermedius of the facial nerve in addition to the glossopharyngeal nerve.

NERVUS INTERMEDIUS NEURALGIA

Nervus intermedius neuralgia presents as pain in the external auditory canal and auricular area (19). Somatic afferent fibers of the seventh cranial nerve are the origin of the pain. The pain, which has been described as similar to trigeminal neuralgia, may be intermittent or continuous, superficial or deep, provokable or nonprovokable. No discernible trigger mechanism has been identified, but the external ear has been cited as a probable trigger zone. It may be difficult to differentiate this entity from atypical facial pain. Females are affected more often than males, and the average time of onset is young adulthood. Surgical sectioning of the nervus intermedius is the treatment of choice.

SPHENOPALATINE NEURALGIA

Patients with this neuralgia have paroxysmal pain over the middle third of the face. The unilateral pain follows the distribution of the sphenopalatine ganglion, and as a result pain is referred to the eye, teeth, nose, palate, and pharynx. Pain has even been reported to radiate to the shoulder and arm. Autonomic stimulation may result in lacrimation, rhinorrhea, salivation, and sneezing. No discrete trigger zone can be identified. The cause is an irritation of the sphenopalatine ganglion, and treatment consists of local anesthetic injection, alcohol injection, or resection of the ganglion.

PARATRIGEMINAL NEURALGIA

Also known as Raeder's syndrome, paratrigeminal neuralgia is characterized by ocular and periocular pain, along with an incomplete Horner's syndrome in which miosis and ptosis are present. A dual presentation may occur with this entity. In the first presentation recurring migraine headaches are caused by an irritation. The second type displays a sudden onset with no history of events, and the cause is often a carotid aneurysm, basilar skull trauma, or a tumor. Management is directed toward the underlying cause.

VIDIAN NEURALGIA

Vidian neuralgia is closely related to sphenopalatine neuralgia, because the vidian nerve passes into the sphenopalatine ganglion. The paroxysmal attacks involve not only the face and contiguous structures but also the neck and shoulder. Women are more frequently affected than men, and attacks may have a cyclical feature, occurring at night. The cause is an inflammation of the vidian nerve and hence the sphenopalatine ganglion. Treatment is chemical cauterization by alcohol injection or surgical resection. Many other less common neuralgias exist; a neurology text should be consulted for the appropriate information.

TRIGEMINAL NEUROPATHY AND NEURITIS

Trigeminal neuropathy is facial numbness that may or may not be accompanied by a steady, dull pain, with or without superimposition of sharp attacks of pain in the distribution of the trigeminal nerve. The presentation may be unilateral or bilateral. Trigeminal neuritis is a form of neuropathy caused by inflammation. Its distinguishing feature is that a neurological examination reveals sensory as well as motor loss (20–22). There are many causes of trigeminal neuropathy, but it is most commonly caused by a tumor (Table 11.5) (13).

Table 11.5.   Potential Causes of Trigeminal Neuropathy

Tumors, 50%	Syringobulbia
Nasopharyngeal carcinoma	Pseudotumor cerebri
Neurinoma	Paget's disease, acromegaly
Metastatic tumors	Postherpetic
Cerebellopontine angle tumors	Basilar artery or cavernous sinus carotid aneurysm
Pontine glioma	Vascular compression
Idiopathic	Amyloidosis
Multiple sclerosis, 10%	Toxins; hydroxy stilbamidine, trichloroethylene
Sarcoidosis	Syphilis
Connective tissue disease	Déjérine-Sottas neuropathy
Posttraumatic or postsurgical	Arnold-Chiari malformation

Sensory loss in the trigeminal nerve distribution may be the presenting symptom in a connective tissue disease such as scleroderma. Sensory loss most commonly involves the second and third branches of the trigeminal nerve. Some reports indicate that women are affected more often than men, and the average age of onset is the fourth and fifth decades of life. Benign trigeminal neuropathy caused by vascular compression of the nerve has been treated by craniotomy to relieve the compression.

ATYPICAL FACIAL PAIN

Atypical facial pain is characterized by pain outside of the trigeminal nerve distribution. The pain is unilateral or bilateral and is more frequently constant than intermittent. The patient has difficulty in precisely describing the pain and precipitating and alleviating factors. Many patients with atypical facial pain have psychological problems that are believed to contribute to or cause the symptoms. The examination of the patient may reveal a slight sensory loss in an unexplainable location. Pathological causes of atypical facial pain include dental problems, trigeminal neuritis, tumors, TMJ problems, and otolaryngologic problems. Surgical or pharmacological treatment meets with varying success depending on the causative factors. Mood elevators and psychiatric counseling may help the patient with pain of a psychological basis.

SINUS DISEASE

Sinus disease is an often-overlooked origin of facial pain. In particular, maxillary sinus disease can produce symptoms ranging from a dull, aching sensation to a more acute pain. An expanding mass in the maxillary sinus tends to cause a dull, aching sensation initially over the cheek area. The pain may increase as the mass expands or becomes infected. Because of the proximity of other structures, pain may be referred to the eye or teeth. Conversely, pain may also be referred to the sinus from the teeth. Acute sinusitis may have an odontogenic cause or be the result of dental manipulation. Acute sinusitis causes pain overlying the area; it may intensify with positional change. At times, the patient may even be aware of fluid shifting within the sinus. Frontal sinusitis produces the same

type of pain over its area. Treatment is aimed at determining the causative factors and eliminating the source of the problem. Surgical or pharmacological intervention is commonly used in the management of sinus disease.

CAROTIDYNIA

Carotidynia (23) is a facial pain syndrome of vascular origin. The pain is usually confined to one side and tends to throb over the carotid area. Carotid tenderness, muscle stiffness, and referred pain to the muscles of the head and neck are also present. The patient has difficulty extending the head away from the affected side. The pain is episodic and occurs over a long period. Women are more commonly affected than men, and the average onset is around the fourth decade of life. The pain syndrome may be related to migraine headaches.

Treatment is very similar to the treatment of migraine headaches. Agents commonly administered include ergotamine, propranolol, and prednisone. Stress reduction techniques such as hypnosis and biofeedback may prove beneficial in the management of this disorder.

FIBROMYALGIA

Fibromyalgia is a painful syndrome in which there has been at least 3 months of diffuse pain, and the pain is evident by digital palpation in at least 11 of 18 tender points distributed throughout the cervical spine, anterior chest, thoracic spine, and/or low back (24). This long-standing pain at defined spots is felt deep within muscles, ligaments, or tendons and is defined as deep aching, radiating, gnawing, shooting, or burning.

The relation between fibromyalgia syndrome (FMS) and CMD is a matter of interest and investigation. Both include chronic pain primarily affecting women, although CMD is reported in a younger population of women (20 to 40 years old) and appears to decrease in prevalence with age, whereas the prevalence of FMS (mean age, 40 years) increases with age. It has been reported that a small proportion of patients with CMD (18.4%) also has FMS but that most individuals with FMS (75%) also have myofascial CMD. CMD is often considered to be a local or focal disease or disorder, whereas FMS is essentially a generalized syndrome with clinical signs and symptoms of pain in multiple craniofacial and skeletal regions. Treatments for FMS are in many instances palliative and often include patient education, physical therapy, and counseling (24).

EAGLE'S SYNDROME

Eagle's syndrome (25), or elongated styloid process syndrome, may be divided into two categories. The classical syndrome develops after a tonsillectomy and is characterized by referred ear pain, pain on swallowing, and the feeling of a sore throat. The other category is the carotid artery syndrome, which is typified by carotidynia. Pain may radiate to the face and neck along the distribution of the carotid arteries. The pain is produced by impingement of the styloid process on the external or internal carotid artery. Diagnosis is made by noting an elongated styloid process on a radiograph and production of the pain by palpation over the styloid process. Treatment requires the surgical reduction of the styloid process or processes (Table 11.6) (26).

TEMPOROMANDIBULAR JOINT DISEASE

When evaluating the origins of pain in the head and face region, consideration should be given to the TMJ apparatus. This unique and highly specialized joint can be the cause of pain in the face, temple, posterior auricular area, and neck and jaw. This joint is involved in the entire masticatory system, which includes the muscles of mastication, the dental occlusion, the trigeminal nerve, and the internal apparatus of the joint itself. The TMJ is a freely movable (diarthrodial) joint that differs from other joints in the body in several respects:

1. Its position is determined by the occlusion of the teeth.
2. It is a bilateral joint, with each side working symmetrically with its counterpart.
3. Its articular surface is covered by a combination of fibrous tissue and cartilage (fibrocartilage).
4. It provides both hinge movement and gliding movement.

The position of the condyle in the fossa of the temporal bone is critical to the normal painless functioning of the TMJ. This position is determined by the dental occlusion. Changes in the normal dental occlusion, through wear, dental restoration, orthodontic movement of teeth, or missing teeth, alter the position of the condyle and thus alter the normal relation between the muscles of mastication and the TMJ. Once the normal position of the masticatory muscles has been altered, muscle hyperactivity and muscle spasm lead to pain in the region innervated by the trigeminal nerve.

The hallmarks of a disturbance in the masticatory system are pain and abnormal mandibular function. The two most common disturbances of TMJ function are myofascial pain dysfunction (MPD) syndrome and internal joint derangement. Other joint disturbances, such as ankylosis, degenerative joint disease, rheumatoid involvement, trauma, and neoplasia, are less common and are not covered in this section.

MYOFASCIAL PAIN DYSFUNCTION SYNDROME

MPD syndrome is characterized by pain, muscle tenderness, and disturbance of mandibular movement. Equally important to the diagnosis are two negative findings, lack of joint sounds (clicking or grinding) and lack of specific joint pain. The pain of MPD can exhibit itself as facial pain in the region of the masseter muscle or preauricular area; as headache in the temple region, retro-orbital region, or occipital area; or as pain in the neck region. The pain often has a time relationship. Patients who have pain in the morning may have such nighttime habits as bruxism, which puts added stress on the TMJ. Patients with pain in the early evening may be the victims of job stress. A good history may elicit some previous trauma to the area or recent dental treatment. Recent dental therapy may lead to dysfunction caused by dislocation or stretching of the joint during a long dental appointment or to a change in dental occlusion. Placement of new restorations or orthodontic treatment to move teeth into new positions can change the relation between the patient's bite and the TMJ.

When the TMJ is working normally and without pain, there is a harmonious relationship between the internal joint structures consisting of the condylar head, fossa, and meniscus; the muscles of mastication; and the dental occlusion. Minor disturbances in any of these three components of the TMJ apparatus lead to MPD syndrome.

OCCLUSAL PROBLEMS

The position of maxillary and mandibular teeth determines the position of the closed mandible. Inclinations of the cusp of the teeth guide the mandible into occlusion with the maxilla. The normal closed position of the dental occlusion, when all muscles are in a normal position and the condyle is seated normally in the fossa, is called centric relation (CR). When teeth are repositioned, either through orthodontic movement, drifting as a result of loss of teeth, or recontouring of the dental anatomy by restorative procedures, the mandible assumes a new position called centric occlusion (CO). It is this discrepancy between CR and CO that causes muscular strain and hyperactivity, leading to pain and muscle tenderness.

MUSCULAR PROBLEMS

Hyperactivity of the muscles of mastication caused by oral habits such as bruxism or excessive use in stressful situations can lead to muscular pain and TMJ tenderness.

TEMPOROMANDIBULAR JOINT CHANGES

Bony changes in the normal articular surface of the condyle can lead to pain in the joint itself. Degenerative arthritis occurs most commonly in older patients with a history of long-standing TMJ problems or acute traumatic injuries affecting the joints. Degenerative arthritis is not the most common cause of TMJ pain and should not be placed high on the list when looking for the cause of MPD syndrome.

PSYCHIC STRESS

Psychological problems play a significant role in some cases of MPD syndrome. Whether acting as an initiating factor or playing a supporting role, psychic stress places excessive strain on the masticatory muscles, causing muscular pain and spasm. Psychological counseling may be necessary to determine to what degree psychological problems are contributing to the overall pain pattern.

Table 11.6.   Summary Chart

	Trigeminal neuralgia	Atypical neuralgia	Trigeminal neuropathy	Facial pain	Glossopharyngeal neuralgia	Intermedius neuralgia	Sphenopalatine neuralgia	Carotidynia	Eagle's syndrome
Average age of onset	5th decade	Adult	4th–5th decade	3rd–4th decade	4th decade	2nd decade	None	4th decade	None
Sex distribution	F	No	F	F	No	F	No	F	No
Trigger zone	Yes	?	No	No	Yes	Possible	No	No	Yes
Cyclical	Yes	No	No	No	Yes	No	No	No	No
Sensory change	No	Yes	Yes	Vague	Yes	No	No	Variable	Yes
Unilateral/ bilateral	U/B	?	U/B	U/B	U	?	U	U	U/B
Pain type	Sharp paroxysmal	Aching paroxysmal	Steady dull	Vague	Sharp/dull	Variable	Variable	Throbbing	Dull/sharp
Pain duration	Brief	Long	Variable	Variable	Variable	Variable	Variable	Variable	Variable
Area of distribution	CN V	CN V	CN V	Variable	CN IX, X	Auricular	Sphenopalatine	Carotid	Carotid
Autonomic signs	No	Possible	Possible	Possible	Possible	No	Possible	No	No
Possible underlying disease	Yes	Yes	Yes	Yes	Yes	Yes	Yes	?	Yes
Psychological component	Variable	Yes	Variable	Strong	Variable	Variable	Variable	Yes	Variable

CN, cranial nerve.

Clinicians have long recognized the association between depression and chronic pain syndromes, including facial pain (27). This relation has been interpreted in several ways. Blumer and Heilbronn (28) suggested that patients with chronic pain have an underlying depression that is masked and represented only by somatic symptoms that are not accompanied by the usual mood and neurovegetative symptoms. Others have conceptualized depression as a secondary maladaptive response to chronic pain (29). However, in light of present knowledge, it is much more likely that chronic pain and depression share a common pathophysiological basis and that the division of symptoms into psychological and physical is an artificial one (27).

The problems just enumerated do not act alone in causing MPD, but rather work in a circular or interlocking pattern. Stress increases muscular activity, which, compounded by a malocclusion, causes pain and spasm, leading to more stress. It is necessary when dealing with the treatment of MPD to carefully judge all aspects of the problem so that a successful solution can be reached.

EXAMINATION

In examining the patient for muscle tenderness, the clinician should carefully outline the areas of pain. Bimanual palpation of the muscles elicits areas of pinpoint tenderness and muscle spasm. It is not unusual for pain from the muscles of mastication to be referred to surrounding areas.

RESTRICTION OF MANDIBULAR MOVEMENT

Whenever there is muscle pain and spasm, it is possible to have restricted mandibular movement. The most common problems are trismus, the inability to open the jaw to a normal degree (approximately 30 mm, or two fingerbreadths), and deviation of the mandible to the side of the muscle involvement on opening. Any opening of less than 30 mm should be considered a dysfunction of the TMJ apparatus. If the mouth opening can be stretched to 30 mm, the source of restriction is most likely a muscle problem. If the mouth opening cannot be stretched to a normal 30 mm, there may be internal disc problems preventing full rotation of the mandibular condyle. To test for mandibular movement, the patient should be asked to protrude the mandible and to move it in left and right lateral excursions. If there is muscle trismus, the mandible will deviate to the side of involvement on a protrusive movement.

TREATMENT OF MYOFASCIAL PAIN DYSFUNCTION

The first step in the treatment of MPD syndrome is the recognition of a pattern of facial pain that involves the muscles of mastication and the TMJ. Thorough examination and evaluation of the dental occlusion, palpation of the masticatory muscles, and observation of the movements of the mandible are necessary to arrive at a proper diagnosis. Although there are various forms of treatment for TMJ pain, it is a well-accepted practice to institute the most conservative and most reversible therapy first to prevent further damage to the TMJ apparatus. An occlusal splint disengages the occlusion and allows the jaws to assume a more natural position. Use of the splint for 24 to 48 consecutive hours helps to eliminate some if not all of the pain if the dental occlusion plays a major causative role. The splint is constructed to fit over the upper teeth and provide a flat plane of plastic, which the lower teeth can contact. Eliminating the interlocking aspects of the tooth anatomy allows the lower jaw to assume a passive position and therefore rest the muscles that are in spasm and producing pain. Splinting is diagnostic and not meant to be therapeutic. If the pain is relieved by the splint, treatment must be aimed at reestablishing the dental occlusion in a proper relationship to the TMJ. This may include restorative dental treatment, major prosthetic rehabilitation, including full-mouth overlays or crowns, or orthodontic treatment to move the teeth into a more normal position.

Rarely is it necessary to take an immediate surgical approach to the correction of TMJ pain. It is generally agreed that only 5% of patients with TMJ pain require surgery. One must keep in mind that surgical intervention in the area of the TMJ changes the normal anatomy of the joint area and thus adds to the asymmetrical function between the two joints. It is not uncommon to see patients who have had a surgical procedure on one joint return with new pain in the opposite joint. Surgery must be limited to cases in which there are demonstrated anatomical interferences within the joint or on the condylar surface.

INTERNAL JOINT DERANGEMENT

A second cause of TMJ pain is derangement of the internal architecture of the TMJ. The joint includes the head of the condyle, which articulates in the glenoid fossa of the temporal bone. Interposed between the condylar head and the articulating surface of the fossa is an avascular fibrous disc, the meniscus. This disc is biconcave, with a thick posterior band, a thinner intermediate zone, and a somewhat thick anterior band. When the mouth is closed, the disc is situated in the glenoid fossa so that the articulating surface of the condyle rests just below the thickened posterior band of the disc. The disc is attached anteriorly to the condyle and the external pterygoid muscle. Posteriorly, it is attached to the TMJ capsule and the condyle by a band of tissue called the bilaminar zone. This tissue consists of muscle and elastic tissue interspersed with blood vessels and nerve fibers.

As the mandible opens, the first movement is a rotation of the condyle on the posterior band of the disc. As further opening occurs, the mandible slides forward and articulates on the intermediate zone of the disc. As full opening occurs, the disc moves forward in conjunction with the forward movement of the condylar head. As the jaw closes, the disc moves back, maintaining its position interposed between the condylar head and the glenoid fossa. It is not known specifically what causes

the forward and backward movements of the disc. However, it is speculated that the external pterygoid helps to bring the disc forward during opening and that the bilaminar zone helps to pull the disc backward on closing.

It is possible—as a result of either macrotrauma, such as direct forceful blows to the facial skeleton, or microtrauma, such as a change of dental occlusion—to dislocate the disc into an anterior position. In this situation the disc is forward of the condyle during closure, and the condyle rests on the bilaminar zone. Because of the vessels and nerves in the bilaminar zone, pain can be associated with this situation. As the jaw opens, the condyle comes in contact with the posterior band of the dislocated meniscus (disc). As further opening occurs, the condyle rides over the posterior band, causing a noise known as an opening click. As the jaw closes, the reciprocal closing click is heard. Clicking of the TMJ in conjunction with pain in the joint area that can be palpated through the external auditory canal (endaurally) is characteristic of internal joint derangement and disc displacement. As this condition continues, a second condition may arise. At some point the patient may be unable to open the jaw fully because of impingement of the condyle on the posterior portion of the disc. At this point there is no clicking, as the condyle does not ride over the disc, but the opening is limited because the disc blocks the full excursion of the condyle in the fossa. This condition, known as closed lock, should be considered whenever a patient cannot fully open the jaw.

Unfortunately, the exact role of disc displacement has only questionable importance in TMJ dysfunction. In cases of TMJ pain, reduction of the disc does not eliminate pain in every case, and significant improvement can be gained without returning the disc to a normal position. Although disc displacement is present in many cases of osteoarthrosis of the joint, no evidence has been found to suggest that it is a cause of osteoarthrosis. The relation of disc displacement to mandibular growth disturbance is also unsubstantiated. Not all growing patients with disc displacement grow abnormally, and not all patients with growth deficiencies have disc displacement. At present the precise relation between disc displacement and TMJ disease is questionable, as many patients exhibit disc displacement and have completely normal function without pain (30).

Internal joint derangement can be associated with the three MPD syndrome symptoms: pain, muscle tenderness, and disturbance of mandibular movement. The distinguishing factors between the two conditions are the addition of endaural pain and joint sounds in patients with internal derangement.

Long-term anterior dislocation may lead to perforation of the bilaminar zone. This allows contact between the condylar head and the glenoid fossa, resulting in degenerative arthritic changes in the articulating surface of the condyle. When the disc is perforated, it is quite common to hear a grinding noise in the TMJ area.

Treatment of internal joint derangement consists of correction of the initiating cause of the disc displacement. If the patient has an opening and reciprocal click, conservative methods are used. The construction of splints is used to try to recapture the disc. Recapturing consists of placing the occlusion in an anterior position so that the condyle rests on the anteriorly displaced disc. If recapturing the disc in this fashion eliminates the clicking and pain associated with the internal derangement, the mandible can be repositioned into this forward position by either orthodontic treatment or prosthetic reconstruction of the occlusion. Sometimes, however, it is not possible to recapture the disc in this manner, and consideration must be given to surgically repositioning the disc in its normal position. Surgery should be contemplated only if the anteriorly displaced disc is causing pain to the patient. Numerous studies have indicated that patients with internal derangement who are treated conservatively can have good long-term results (31, 32). A mere click is not justification for surgery.

DOCUMENTATION OF DISC POSITION

Before surgery on a displaced disc, it is necessary to document its position. This can be done by the use of three modalities: arthrograms, computed tomography (CT), and magnetic resonance imaging (MRI).

In TMJ arthrogram, dye is injected into the inferior joint space and the movement of the condyle and disc is observed under fluoroscopy. Spot films or tomograms can then be taken of the jaw in the closed, preclick, and postclick positions. The advantages of the arthrogram are that it gives the surgeon a dynamic record of the movement of the joint in relation to the position of the disc and shows any disc perforations as well as displacements. The disadvantage is that it is an invasive procedure that can cause pain in an inflamed joint.

CT of the TMJ gives a static record of the position of the disc in relation to the condyle. The advantage of CT is its noninvasive nature. However, CT does not reveal any perforation, nor does it give the surgeon a dynamic view of the situation.

Most surgeons document the position of the TMJ disc with MRI. This procedure uses a magnetic field to produce a picture similar to radiograph. Its advantage over CT is that it delineates soft tissue and thus can show the position of the disc more clearly than CT. Patients who are claustrophobic may require oral sedation because it frequently requires an hour in a very confined environment.

With so many modalities available to visualize the TMJ apparatus, it is common for radiographs of the TMJ to be ordered early in the diagnostic phase of treatment. Patients with MPD syndrome usually do not have a bony disturbance in the TMJ; therefore radiograph shows only a lack of movement of the condyle. Radiographs should not be ordered for patients with MPD until such time as conservative therapy has failed to resolve the pain problem. When radiographs are made of a patient with MPD, maximum diagnostic benefit can be achieved from tomographic studies of the TMJ. It is important that the tomograms be corrected for the axial angulation of the condyle to the lateral plane of the head so

that a clear view of the entire extent of the condyle is obtained. It is possible on tomographic studies to document areas of erosion, hyperplasia, osteophytic formation, and deformities. CT also gives a clear view of the bony architecture of the TMJ. When anterior disc displacement is suspected, MRI is most helpful for documenting it. Radiographs, CT, MRI, or a combination of these should be secondary procedures and should not be ordered routinely on all patients with TMJ problems.

SURGICAL TREATMENT OF INTERNAL JOINT DERANGEMENT

It is generally accepted that the least invasive procedure possible should be used in the management of TMJ dysfunction. In the past several years many surgeons have had great success with a minimally invasive technique known as arthrocentesis (33). An 18-gauge needle is placed in the superior joint space and approximately 100 mL of sterile saline or lactated Ringer's solution is flushed through the joint, with a second needle acting as a means of egress. It is thought that "pumping" the solution into the joint with pressure prior to the placement of the second needle may help to break up adhesions that are holding the disc in its anterior position. It is also thought that arthrocentesis helps to equilibrate the "negative pressure" that has been found within a joint suffering from a closed lock (34). At the same time, lubrication of the articular surfaces is achieved and inflammatory factors are flushed out. Obviously, the disc position itself is not changed by arthrocentesis, but it is thought that the disc is able to glide more freely within the superior joint space. This procedure can easily be performed in the office setting with local anesthesia only, or with intravenous sedation, and is associated with minimal morbidity. Good long-term results have been achieved in the treatment of acute closed lock, but its efficacy in the management of other types of TMJ disorders has not yet been demonstrated (35, 36).

Another modality used in the treatment of internal derangement is arthroscopy of the TMJ. Arthroscopy of the TMJ is very similar to arthroscopy of other joints. The procedure is performed with the patient under general anesthesia on an ambulatory basis. A small arthroscope is placed in the involved joint, and the image is portrayed on a television monitor. At present, treatment with arthroscopy is usually limited to exploration of the superior joint compartment and the release of fibrous bands, but some surgeons have been able to reposition the disc through the arthroscope. These more advanced procedures are performed by only a few surgeons, and there seems to be a rather steep learning curve. Good results from arthroscopic surgery have been reported in approximately 80% of cases, with decreases in pain and increases in mobility being common. Recent studies, however, have shown no statistical difference in outcome between arthroscopic lysis and lavage and the much less expensive procedure of arthrocentesis (37).

The purpose of the surgical approach to the treatment of an anteriorly displaced disc is to replace the disc into its normal anatomical position. This is accomplished through the standard preauricular or postauricular approach to the condyle. After surgical exposure of the superior and inferior joint spaces, it is possible to see the anterior dislocation of the disc. At this point a wedge is removed from the bilaminar zone, the disc is replaced in its normal position, and the bilaminar zone is plicated with a nonresorbable suture. The success of this surgical procedure depends on the correction of the original cause of the displacement. If the disc displacement was due to microtrauma caused by a posteriorly positioned occlusion, failure to correct the occlusion will lead to redislocation of the disc. Surgery should be undertaken only after due consideration of the conservative approach to internal derangement. One should recognize that open surgery on the TMJ will materially change the anatomy of that joint. This usually has some long-term effect on the contralateral joint.

Occasionally the disc is so badly damaged that it cannot be repositioned or repaired, necessitating its removal. Most surgeons advocate replacing the disc with an autogenous graft, and good results have been reported with dermis, temporalis muscle or fascia, and auricular cartilage. Discectomy without replacing the disc has demonstrated excellent long-term results in several studies (38, 39).

A discussion about the surgical management of internal derangement of the TMJ would not be complete without some mention of the use of alloplastic materials. In the early 1980s many patients underwent discectomy, with a Proplast-Teflon interpositional implant being placed. Subsequently microfragmentation and inflammatory giant cell reactions have caused a great deal of pain and joint destruction, with some patients even incurring an erosion into the middle cranial fossa. These patients are difficult to treat, and several treatment protocols have been proposed (40, 41). These patients seem to do best with complete debridement of all Proplast-Teflon and inflammatory particles, followed by an alloplastic total-joint prosthesis (40), although some clinicians advocate a temporalis muscle and fascia graft (41). The problems with the Proplast-Teflon implant led to a total ban on all TMJ alloplastic materials by the FDA, but several well-tested total joint prostheses are being introduced to the marketplace.

Experience with surgery for internal derangement of the TMJ has shown that the vast majority of patients have an improvement of their condition with conservative treatment only (31, 32) and that the likelihood of success decreases with each subsequent surgical procedure (42, 43).

References

1. Lunn RH. Report of the committee on principles, concepts and practices of the management of craniomandibular diseases. Comp Am Equilib Soc 1987;20:186–189.
2. Fricton J, Kroening R. Practical differential diagnosis of chronic craniofacial pain. Oral Surg Oral Med Oral Pathol 1982;54:628–634.
3. De Boever JA. Functional disturbances of the temporomandibular joint. In: Zarb GA, Carlsson GE, eds. Temporomandibular joint function and dysfunction. St. Louis: Mosby, 1979;78–91.
4. Costen JB. Syndrome of ear and sinus symptoms dependent upon distributed function of the temporomandibular joint. Ann Otol Rhinol Laryngol 1934;43:1.
5. Monson GG. Occlusion as applied to crown and bridge work. Natl Dent Assoc J 1921;7:399.
6. Prentiss HJ. Preliminary report upon the temporomandibular joint in the human. Dent Cosmos 1918;60:505.
7. Sicher H. Temporomandibular articulation in mandibular overclosure. J Am Dent Assoc 1948;36:131.
8. Moulton RE. Psychiatric considerations in maxillofacial pain. J Am Dent Assoc 1955;51:408.
9. Lupton EE. Psychological aspects of the temporomandibular joint dysfunction, J Am Dent Assoc 1969;79:131.
10. Mozak H. Does a "TMJ personality" exist? In: Gelb H, ed. Clinical management of head, neck and TMJ pain and dysfunction. Philadelphia: Saunders, 1977;198.
11. Laskin DM. Etiology of the pain-dysfunction syndrome, J Am Dent Assoc 1969;79:147.
12. Sweeny PJ. Tic douloureux. Am Fam Physician 1981;23:153.
13. Hart R, Easton JD. Trigeminal neuralgia and other facial pains. Mo Med 1981;78:11.
14. Mahan PE, Alling CC. Facial pain. Philadelphia: Lea & Febiger, 1991.
15. Turgut M, Benli K, Ozgen T, et al. Twenty-five years experience in the treatment of trigeminal neuralgia: comparison of three different operative procedures in forty-nine patients. J Craniomaxillofac Surg 1996;24:40–45.
16. Roberts A, Person P. Etiology and treatment of idiopathic trigeminal and atypical facial neuralgias. Oral Surg Oral Med Oral Pathol 1979;48:298–308.
17. Cusick J. Atypical trigeminal neuralgia. JAMA 1981;245:2328–2329.
18. Rushton J, Stevens JC, Miller RH, et al. Glossopharyngeal neuralgia. Arch Neurol 1981;38:201.
19. Kruger G, ed. Textbook of oral and maxillofacial surgery. St. Louis: Mosby, 1979.
20. Blau JN, Harris M, Kennett S. Trigeminal sensory neuropathy. N Engl J Med 1969;281:873–876.
21. Eggleston DJ, Haskill R. Idiopathic trigeminal sensory neuropathy. Practitioner 1972;208:649–655.
22. Goldstein NP, Gibilislo JA, Rushton JG. Trigeminal neuropathy and neuritis: a study of etiology with emphasis on dental causes. JAMA 1963;184:458–462.
23. Scheitler L, Balciunas BA. Carotidynia. J Oral Maxillofac Surg 1982;40:121–122.
24. Slavkin HC. Chronic disabling diseases and disorders: the challenges of fibromyalgia. J Am Dent Assoc 1997;128:1583–1589.
25. Lawrence FR, Cornielson E. Eagles syndrome. J Oral Maxillofac Surg 1982;40:307–309.
26. Chase DC, Zarmen A, Bigelow WC, McCay JM. Eagle's syndrome: a comparison of intraoral and extraoral surgical approaches. Oral Surg Oral Med Oral Pathol 1986;62:625–629.
27. Korszun A, Ship JA. Diagnosing depression in patients with chronic facial pain. J Am Dent Assoc 1997;128:1680–1686.
28. Blumer D, Heilbronn M. Chronic pain as a variant of depressive disease: the pain-prone disorders. J Nerv Ment Dis 1982;170:381–406.
29. Dworkin SF. Illness Behavior and dysfunction: review of concepts and application to chronic pain. Can J Physiol Pharmacol 1991;69:662–671.
30. Dolwick MF. Intra-articular disc displacement: 1. Its questionable role in temporomandibular joint pathology. J Oral Maxillofac Surg 1995;53:1069–1072.
31. Sato S, Kawamura H, Nagasaka M, et al. The natural course of anterior disc displacement without reduction in the temporomandibular joint: follow-up at 6, 12, and 18 months. J Oral Maxillofac Surg 1997;55:234–238.

32. De Leeuw R, Boering G, Stegenga B, deBont LGM. TMJ articular disc position and configuration 30 years after initial diagnosis of internal derangement. J Oral Maxillofac Surg 1995;53:234–241.

33. Nitzan DW, Dolwick MF, Martinez GA, et al. Temporomandibular joint arthrocentesis: a simplified treatment for severe, limited mouth opening. J Oral Maxillofac Surg 1991;49:1163–1167.

34. Nitzan DW, Mahler Y, Simkin A, et al. Intra-articular pressure measurements in patients with suddenly developing, severe limited mouth opening. J Oral Maxillofac Surg 1992; 50:1038–1042.

35. Nitzan DW, Samson B, Better M, et al. Long-term outcome of arthrocentesis for sudden onset, persistent, severe closed lock of the temporomandibular joint. J Oral Maxillofac Surg 1997;55:151–157.

36. Dimitroulis G, Dolwick MF, Martinez A, et al. Temporomandibular joint arthrocentesis and lavage for the treatment of closed lock: a follow-up study. Br J Oral Maxillofac Surg 1995;33:23–27.

37. Fridrich KL, Wise JM, Zeitter D, et al. Prospective comparison of arthroscopy and arthrocentesis for temporomandibular joint disorders. J Oral Maxillofac Surg 1996;54:816–820.

38. Trumpy IG, Lyberg T. Surgical treatment of internal derangement of the temporomandibular joint: long-term evaluation of three techniques. J Oral Maxillofac Surg 1995;53:740–746.

39. Takau S, Toyoda T. Long-term evaluation of discectomy of the temporomandibular joint. J Oral Maxillofac Surg 1994;52:722–726.

40. Henry CH, Wolford LM. Treatment outcomes for temporomandibular joint reconstruction after Proplast-Teflon implant failure. J Oral Maxillofac Surg 1993;51:352–358.

41. Kearns GJ, Perrott DH, Kaban LB, et al. A protocol for the management of failed alloplastic temporomandibular joint disc implants. J Oral Maxillofac Surg 1995;53:1240–1247.

42. Wolford LM, Cottrell DA, Henry CH, et al. Temporomandibular joint reconstruction of the complex patient with the techmedica custom-made total joint prosthesis. J Oral Maxillofac Surg 1994;52:2–10.

43. Henry CH, Wolford LM. Reconstruction of the temporomandibular joint using a temporalis graft with or without simultaneous orthognathic surgery. J Oral Maxillofac Surg 1995;53:1250–1256.

Suggested Reading

1. Greene M, Van Sickels J. Survey of TMJ arthroscopy in oral and maxillofacial surgery residency programs. J Oral Maxillofac Surg 1989;47:574.

2. Katzberg RW, Bessette RW, Tallents RM, et al. Magnetic resonance surface coil images of the normal and abnormal TMJ. Radiology 1986;158:183.

3. Moses J, Sartoris D, Glass R, et al. The effect of arthroscopic surgical lysis and lavage of the superior joint space on TMJ disc position and mobility. J Oral Maxillofac Surg 1989;47:674.

4. Murakami K, Matsuke M, Iizulea T. Diagnostic arthroscopy of the TMJ: Differential diagnosis in patients with limited jaw opening. J Craniomand Pract 1986;4:118.

5. Ohnishi M. Clinical application of arthroscopy in temporomandibular joint diseases. Bull Tokyo Med Dent Univ 1980;27:141.

6. Sanders B. Arthroscopic surgery of the temporomandibular joint: treatment of internal derangement with persistent closed lock. Oral Surg Oral Med Oral Pathol 1986;62:361.

7. Sanders B, Buoncristiani R. Diagnostic and surgical arthroscopy of the temporomandibular joint: clinical experience with 137 procedures over a 2-year period. J Craniomand Dis 1987;1:202.

8. Greene C, Laskin D. Long term evaluation of treatment for myofascial pain-dysfunction syndrome: a comparative analysis. JAMA 1983;107:235.

9. Peterson LJ, Ellis E, Mupp Jr, et al. Contemporary Oral and Maxillofacial Surgery. 2nd ed. St. Louis: Mosby, 1993.

CHAPTER 12

Complex Regional Pain Syndrome: A New Name for Reflex Sympathetic Dystrophy

Michael D. Hicks

PROLOGUE

It is clear that the sympathetic nervous system is involved in preserving the *milieu interne* (1), or homeostasis, of the organism and its responses to noxious challenges (stress) (2, 3). A complex, diverse, and functionally specific number of preganglionic and postganglionic sympathetic neurons are pathways to numerous target organs containing enteric neurons, smooth muscle, syncytial muscle, and striated muscle. It is also evident that the sympathetic nervous system is associated with pain, demonstrating both a general and a specific local reaction to supratentorial components including confrontational aspects that are represented in the dorsolateral periaqueductal gray and associated with nonopioid analgesia. Rest and quiescence are represented in the ventrolateral periaqueductal gray and in contradistinction are associated with endogenous opioid analgesia (4, 5).

Hypothalamomesencephalic and spinal levels of integration are associated with the adrenocortical and hypothalamohypophyseal axis to protect the organism under normal biological conditions. A secondary reaction of the sympathetic nervous system that may occur with or without any obvious nerve lesion is associated with a diffuse burning dysesthesia and hyperalgesia; is correlated with changes in blood flow (vasomotor), sudomotor, and muscle activity (dystonia, tremor); and may be associated with trophic changes of the integument. Such pain syndromes have been described during the past 100 years by Sudeck (6), Mitchell et al. (7), Bonica (8, 9), and Evans (10).

The manner in which the sympathetic nervous system is involved with pain following trauma, in particular injuries of the extremities, has given rise to considerable confusion as to the underlying mechanism and its diagnosis. In fact, a parallel may be seen in some other pain states, such as irritable bowel syndrome, interstitial cystitis, angina pectoris, and nonulcer dyspepsia, in which the sympathetic nervous system may be causally involved (11).

HISTORY

In 1864 Mitchell et al. (7) drew attention to the exaggerated response and pain that occurred in soldiers in the Civil War who had received a penetrating wound near a major nerve. A French surgeon, Leriche (12), described the relief of pain that could be achieved in wounded soldiers during World War II by stripping the sympathetic plexus from large arteries in the lower extremities. In a series of articles Sudeck (6) provided detailed descriptions of the osteopathic abnormalities that occurred in many patients with autonomic dysfunction. What has in German-speaking countries come to be known as Morbus Sudeck is known as reflex sympathetic dystrophy in most other countries (10). However, the many pseudonyms used to describe these conditions include posttraumatic sympathetic dystrophy, shoulder-hand syndrome, chronic traumatic edema, posttraumatic spreading neuralgia, posttraumatic osteoporosis, reflex neuromuscular dystrophy, neurovascular dystrophy, and sympathalgia, to name but a few. Evans (10) was obviously influenced by the research and writings of his contemporary, Livingston (13), who proposed the concept of *a vicious circle* involving the spinal cord at the level of sensory interneurons that are maintained in a state of abnormal repetitive firing from the periphery. The words *reflex, sympathetic, and dystrophy,* by implying a mechanism, also invite treatment based on an unsubstantiated mechanism. At about the same time, Lewis (14) suggested that nocifensor nerves became irritated in causalgic states, potentiating the condition. Lewis, who was interested in humoral processes and physiology, suggested that a disturbance in secretory function might be responsible for the dystrophic changes and atrophy of the integumentary structures, although he did not attribute these clinical features to a disturbance of autonomic function.

Walker and Nulsen (15), who were interested in autonomic physiology, investigated patients who had undergone thoracic sympathectomy for causalgia and were able to elicit burning and tingling paresthesias by continuous electrical stimulation of the sympathetic trunk. These observations were also confirmed by White and Sweet (16). These and other results have collectively supported the contention that a sympathetically dependent mechanism is responsible for the disturbance seen in patients with causalgia and reflex sympathetic dystrophy. However, even Bernard (1) demonstrated that interruption of the sympathetic nervous system is succeeded by an altered stimulus response sensitivity in the dependent region.

Observations supporting a sympathetic role in pain are the relief by local anesthetics that are applied to paravertebral ganglia (8, 9, 17) and by other sympathetic procedures such as intravenous regional guanethidine, bretylium, or systemic intravenous phentolamine (18–21). Even placebo-controlled, double-blind studies of intravenous regional sympathetic blocks in patients with a diagnosis of reflex sympathetic dystrophy have been shown to produce significant analgesia (21). Stanton-Hicks et al. (22), Jänig and Schmidt (23), Blumberg and Jänig (24), Jänig (25, 26), and Häbler et al. (27) have described clinical observations that argue strongly in favor of a role for the sympathetic nervous system in the generation of pain in such patients. Also, pain may be rekindled when β-adrenoceptor agonists are applied to a previously affected extremity by iontophoresis or injection in spite of the fact that the patients may have been in remission for a period exceeding 15 years (28–31). Furthermore, the injection of epinephrine into a chronic neuroma elicits or aggravates pain in humans (32).

Roberts (33) introduced the hypothesis in which he suggested that sympathetically maintained pain occurring in reflex sympathetic dystrophy develops at some point in its natural history from tonic activity in myelinated low-threshold mechanoreceptors (LTM), types I and II, Aβ-fibers (Fig. 12.1). He suggests that the activity is induced by postganglionic sympathetic action on sensory afferents, which in turn elicits tonic firing in previously sensitized wide dynamic range (WDR) multireceptive neurons, maintaining the status quo, and symptoms. In part, this hypothesis is supported by animal experiments demonstrating an activation of mechanoreceptors by sympathetic postganglionic sympathetic efferents.

Interestingly, there is neither a lowering of nociceptor mechanical threshold nor relief of pain by C fiber blockade. The data are supported in part by observations of Torebjörk and Hallin (34), who demonstrated analgesia by differential ischemic (tourniquet) block in patients who were hyperalgesic after a nerve injury (the hyperalgesia was mediated by large myelinated primary efferents). Campbell et al. (35) and Raja et al. (20) claim that the cause of sympathetically maintained pain resides in the periphery and suggest that an expression of α_1-adrenoceptors on primary afferent nociceptors in turn are stimulated by sympathetic activity, which may in fact be normal but because of their increased number induce pain.

INTERLUDE

Because of the considerable confusion regarding what constitutes reflex sympathetic dystrophy and the seemingly heterogeneous approaches to its treatment, members of the Special Interest Group (SIG), Pain and the Sympathetic Nervous System of the International Association for the Study of Pain (IASP) met in 1990 at the Sixth World Congress on Pain in Adelaide, Australia, to develop a consensus statement. The intent of this statement was to stimulate clinical and basic research and provide at least an initial operational definition of reflex sympathetic dystrophy. In fact, the statement is a contraction of an earlier definition that resulted from a meeting held in Germany in 1988 (Schloss Rettershof), Stanton-Hicks et al. (1989) (36).

CONSENSUS STATEMENT

Reflex Sympathetic Dystrophy is a descriptive term meaning a complex disorder or group of disorders that may develop as a consequence of trauma affecting the limbs, with or without an obvious nerve lesion. RSD may also develop after visceral disease, central nervous system lesions, or rarely without an obvious antecedent event. RSD consists of pain and sensory abnormalities, abnormal blood flow, decreased or increased sweating, abnormalities of the motor system, and changes in the structure of both superficial and deep tissues (trophic changes). It is not necessary that all components be present. The name "Reflex Sympathetic Dystrophy" is used in a descriptive sense and does not imply specific underlying mechanisms.[1]

The foregoing consensus statement by Jänig et al (37a) and the many articles on reflex sympathetic dystrophy in the scientific literature in the past 10 years, while attempting to redefine and characterize certain aspects of the conditions reflex sympathetic dystrophy, causalgia, sympathetically maintained pain, and sympathetically independent pain (SIP), have tended more to increase the level of misunderstanding simply because of the plethora of new terms and hypotheses. If there is to be a new classification of these clinical syndromes, certainly the terms most commonly recognized, namely, reflex sympathetic dystrophy and causalgia, should be retained in parentheses to facilitate their recognition and communication.

To this end, a closed workshop was convened in conjunction with the annual scientific meeting of the American Pain Society in Orlando during November 1993 (37). This workshop developed clinical descriptions characterizing the features of these medical entities, provided criteria for their differential

---

[1]Reprinted from Jänig W Blumberg H, Boas RA, Campbell JA. The reflex sympathetic dystrophy syndrome: consensus statement and general recommendations for diagnosis and clinical research. In: Bond MR, Charlton JE, Wool CS, eds. Proceedings of the V World Congress on Pain, Pain Research and Clinical Management, vol 4, 1991; 372–375, with kind permission from Elsevier Science NL, Sara Burgerhartstraat 25, 1055 KV Amsterdam, The Netherlands.

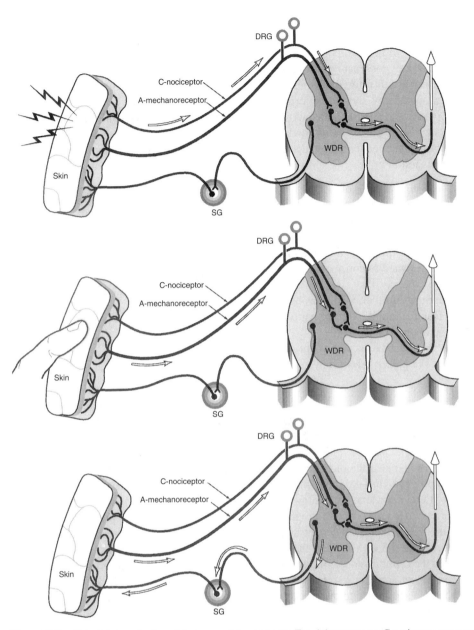

Figure 12.1.   Roberts's hypothesis and its temporal development. **Top,** injury causes a C-nociceptor response with propagation to the WDR neurons and central transmission. **Middle,** WDR neurons remain sensitized and become reactive to activity in large-diameter A-mechanoreceptors that are stimulated by light touch. This response represents allodynia. **Bottom,** The WDR neurons respond to A-mechanoreceptor activity, which is now elicited by sympathetic efferent action at the sensory receptor. No cutaneous stimulation is necessary for this effect. This last phase represents sympathetically maintained pain. DRG, dorsal root ganglion; SG, sympathetic ganglion. (Reprinted with permission from Roberts WJ. A hypothesis on the physiological basis for causalgia. Pain 1986;24:297–311.)

diagnosis, and developed a new classification. In conjunction with the contemporary revision of the IASP classification of chronic pain syndromes, this new classification not only spelled out the definitions of these medical entities but clearly defined what is meant by the term *sympathetically maintained pain.* It was also agreed that any such change in the taxonomy must be open to continued modification as better understanding of the pathophysiological processes is derived from future scientific investigations (38).

REQUIREMENTS FOR A NEW TAXONOMY

Fundamental to a diagnosis of reflex sympathetic dystrophy is pain that is abnormal in intensity and spontaneous; that is, occurring without external cause. Evoked pain, such as allodynia or hyperalgesia, is disproportionate to both nonnoxious and noxious stimuli. Although in some rare cases pain may be absent, it is the crux of a diagnosis of reflex sympathetic dystrophy. Other features essential to a diagnosis are vasomotor disturbances. Though tremor, dystonia, and muscle weakness are frequently found, they are considered to be motor impairment and are not necessary for a diagnosis of reflex sympathetic dystrophy. Furthermore, while osteoporosis is seen in many cases, because of its lack of consistency, it was not considered to be a cardinal feature of this disease complex. Also, as stated earlier, any new taxonomy should conform to the convention already adopted by the IASP Subcommittee on Taxonomy (39) and as such should have as its fundamental purpose the facilitation of communication and understanding of the medical condition, as follows:

1. The taxonomy should suggest lines of basic science research and the development of animal models that clarify how the sympathetic nervous system is involved.
2. The taxonomy should pose questions that will promote clinical investigation designed to corroborate its elements.
3. The differential diagnosis of other conditions having similar but not all features found in reflex sympathetic dystrophy should be improved.
4. Any taxonomy should suggest tests that might support a diagnosis of reflex sympathetic dystrophy.

NEW TAXONOMY

In conformity with the linguistic convention adopted by the Subcommittee on Taxonomy for inclusion in the classification of chronic pain, the term *complex regional pain syndrome* (CRPS) was chosen to replace the older terminology, reflex sympathetic dystrophy and causalgia. Not only is this new term an umbrella for these disorders, but it allows for the later inclusion of a variety of painful conditions that may occur after injury; that are manifested regionally, mostly in an extremity, predominantly distal; and with findings that exceed in magnitude and duration the expected course following such an inciting event. However, in some cases these disorders occur on the trunk or the face and spread to other body areas. Not infrequently there is impairment of motor function, evident as tremor, dystonia, or muscle weakness. Because a temporal sequence is not always followed, the terms *complex* and *regional* were necessary to distinguish the syndrome. While the clinical features tend to commence in the distal part of an extremity, the symptoms tend to extend proximally and involve the musculature of the shoulder or pelvic girdles, depending on which extremity is affected.

Because the most common disorder is reflex sympathetic dystrophy, the term CRPS type I was adopted for it, and causalgia is called CRPS type II. This is a reversal of the original IASP classification (38), which in deference to the historical description of causalgia by Mitchell was cited first. In fact, the description of CRPS type II has been well described by Richards (40) and Bonica (8, 9, 17).

While the terminology for CRPS types I and II makes allowance for spontaneous pain or touch-evoked pain such as allodynia or hyperalgesia, these symptoms may be concurrent in affected areas. Pain of either class is considered to be the cardinal symptom in these medical disorders, notwithstanding that in rare cases pain is absent but all other clinical features satisfy the diagnosis.

Since some patients do not fulfill the criteria for a diagnosis of CRPS type I or II, allowance was made in the taxonomy for a third type of CRPS, not otherwise specified (NOS). In this manner the taxonomy encourages the clinician to identify specific types or subgroups of CRPS types I and II. As an example, one patient group may have met all of the specific criteria for CRPS type I but uniformly have in addition another specific symptom or clinical finding. Should the response of this group be different from that of the main type I group, or the temporal course of their disease process follow a uniformly different course, the classification could be allowed to include this as a specific subgroup within the main CRPS type I group. While Bonica thought staging was important to the description of these diseases, its utility for diagnosis or course of treatment was not considered important to the taxonomy. Of course, experience with the new taxonomy may suggest a reappraisal and its inclusion in the future.

Although the epidemiology of CRPS has not been described, both anecdotal and recent evidence suggests that certain patients have a predisposition to the development of CRPS types I and II. In fact, the clinical report by Mailis and Wade (44) of genetically similar profiles in white women with CRPS type I and the genetically selected predisposition for neuropathic pain in laboratory animals by Devor and Raber (45) and Bhatia et al. (46) lend some credence to this concept. Motor symptoms and signs are a frequent finding in patients with CRPS types I and II. These are often discounted as being a consequence of pain rather than a specific movement disorder (41–43). Because there is virtually no research into their causation, it was thought that they should not be included as standard criteria, but they are mentioned in the draft criteria of the taxonomy. Similarly, the role of sympathetic blocks is removed from the taxonomy of CRPS types I and II and is discussed separately as sympathetically maintained pain and other neuralgias.

To prevent the inclusion of clinical entities and syndromes in which the findings are consistent with a particular injury, it was necessary to introduce specific exclusion criteria to the definitions of CRPS types I and II. One such example might be a patient whose criteria meet those for causalgia but in whom the signs and symptoms lie outside of the territory of the injured nerve. Obviously, should the clinical findings occur within the regional territory of a nerve, they could still satisfy inclusion criteria under this definition. Another exception to the rule may be a patient whose clinical findings are localized, on the trunk or face for example, and are not associated with a particular injured nerve. These could be classified as a subset within the main definition. However, such an entity, like the primary classification, must have signs and symptoms that are completely disproportionate in nature and severity to the injury.

The classification makes clear that at the time of examination, signs of vasomotor instability may not be present.

Therefore, the historical reporting by a patient of swelling, color and temperature changes or sweating abnormalities would be sufficient to satisfy diagnostic criteria for CRPS.

DIFFERENTIAL DIAGNOSIS

A large number of medical entities may have characteristics that in part are similar to the clinical features of CRPS. While these conditions are most frequently found in the distal part of an extremity, they must be distinguished from other neuropathic pain conditions. Complicating the issue is their positive response to sympatholysis, at least during their early presentation. Pain relief after sympatholysis is specific for neither reflex sympathetic dystrophy nor causalgia but is merely a reflection of a functioning sympathetic nervous system. The manner in which the sympathetic nervous system is responsible for this component of pain (sympathetically maintained pain), which is found in association with many neuropathic pain states, such as postherpetic neuralgia and diabetic neuropathy and possibly some nociceptive pain conditions, is yet to be determined. Another factor complicating the diagnosis of CRPS is the temporal variation in sensitivity and the exacerbations of dysfunction that may satisfy some but not all of the criteria for diagnosis.

Many patients with myofascial pain syndrome, a frequent accompaniment of CRPS, may be considered to have another type of CRPS. Such cases may demonstrate regional temperature differences and even mechanical hyperalgesia yet still have inadequate features to substantiate a diagnosis of reflex sympathetic dystrophy. Perhaps the most difficult group of clinical entities that have assumed the broad terminology of pain dysfunction syndromes are those with clinical signs and symptoms that *almost* satisfy the requirements for a diagnosis of CRPS but that are not in sufficient proportion to merit such a diagnosis. These medical entities, which include overuse syndrome (47), repetitive strain injury (48), cumulative trauma disorder (49, 50), tennis elbow, and nerve entrapments (51, 52) will be discussed in more detail later. A number of conditions that may partially satisfy a diagnosis of CRPS are listed:

Fracture, sprain
Pain dysfunction syndromes (cumulative trauma disorder, repetitive strain injury, overuse syndrome)
Thoracic outlet syndrome
Peripheral nerve entrapment
Fibromyalgia
Myofascial pain syndrome
Inflammatory disorders
Biologic toxins
Insect bite
Disuse
Posttraumatic vasospasm
Raynaud's phenomenon
Thrombophlebitis
Neurogenic inflammation
Rheumatological conditions
Factitious disease

As discussed earlier, while motor dysfunction is not among the inclusion criteria for CRPS, its frequent finding is mentioned in the classification (41, 46, 53, 54). Weakness, dystonia, and limitation of movement should be carefully distinguished from a lack of voluntary effort, pain-limited movement, or a joint frozen from disuse.

While accepting the requirement under the taxonomy that pain is out of proportion to what one would expect from a particular injury, the differential diagnosis of causalgia can be distinguished from a nerve injury in which the neurogenic inflammation is also associated with pain. The distinction for a qualifying diagnosis of causalgia requires that edema, skin temperature, color changes, and sudomotor changes are all found in association with the painful nerve injury. While one or more of these signs and symptoms may dominate, all should be found at some time. Put another way, pain, including allodynia or hyperalgesia without vasomotor changes, by itself does not satisfy the criteria for CRPS. Rarely, patients with all or most of the clinical features of CRPS have no pain. The temporal course and response to treatment modalities is identical to that of CRPS. At present the taxonomy requires that such patients must remain outside of the CRPS umbrella.

Although some patients with CRPS types I and II may have premorbid psychological or psychiatric disturbances, their occurrence is not a basis for excluding a diagnosis of CRPS (55, 56). Furthermore, malingering and factitious disease are well-recognized clinical entities and as such are also excluded from the diagnosis of CRPS but must be included in the differential diagnosis (57–59). Similarly, conversion disorders and somatization, while well recognized in association with chronic pain, have their own specific criteria and may occur separately or in association with CRPS types I and II. However, sometimes the diagnosis is difficult, and its interpretation is often possible only after medical treatment has been instituted (60, 61). The sine qua non of CRPS is pain. This is primarily a neuropathic pain and as such is a symptom of many other medical conditions. One form of neuropathic pain, so-called sympathetically maintained pain, which is associated with many conditions (e.g., postherpetic neuralgia, diabetic neuropathy) can be demonstrated in most cases of CRPS types I and II, particularly early in their course (33, 62) (Fig. 12.2).

SYMPATHETICALLY MAINTAINED PAIN

Sympathetically maintained pain is defined as *pain that is maintained by sympathetic efferent innervation or by circulating catecholamines* (33, 62). Historically, a positive response to sympatholysis (sympathetic blocks) was axiomatic to a diagnosis of CRPS (8, 9, 17). How the sympathetic nervous system is involved in the pathophysiology of these conditions is open to conjecture (63–65). Clinical practice has perpetuated a convention that only after a positive response to sympathetic blockade can a diagnosis of CRPS be supported. This of course has led to persistent measures of sympathetic blocking whether or not pain of CRPS type I and II was independent of

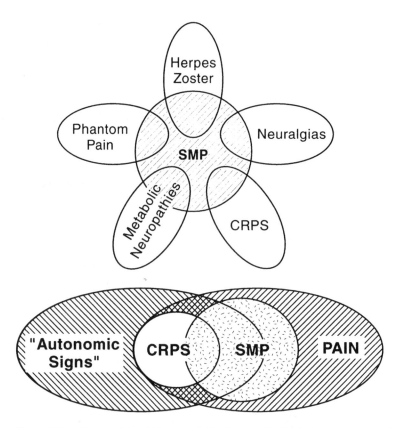

Figure 12.2. A concept in which sympathetically maintained pain is a component of selected painful conditions. It does not indicate the magnitude or proportion of pain that is sympathetically maintained pain. Also, sympathetically maintained pain may exist without an associated medical condition. (Reprinted with permission from Stanton-Hicks M. Reflex sympathetic dystrophy: changing concepts and taxonomy. Pain 1995;63:127–133.)

sympathetic activity, that is, SIP. Figure 12.3 illustrates a situation in which a symbolic patient may be seen at one time when the pain is mostly sympathetically maintained but during the course of the disease, it becomes more and more sympathetically independent. On the other hand, these may be two separate patients who at the time of their physical examination exhibit pain that is either sympathetically maintained, sympathetically independent, or some proportion of each. While the link between pain and the sympathetic nervous system appears established and is undergoing promising and extensive investigation in various countries, the manner in which it is related to these medical entities is incomplete (66–68).

However, sympathetic blocking can contribute to the other clinical signs and symptoms that make up diagnostic criteria (8, 9, 17, 69). Numerous tests, including temperature measurements, sudomotor function, skin blood flow, and skin resistance, have been developed to assess sympathetic activity (9, 22, 70–73). A mechanism for sympathetically maintained pain was proposed by Roberts (33) as a tonic activity in myelinated mechanoreceptor types I and II that occurs as a consequence of sensitization of the WDR neurons in lamina V of the dorsal horn. This response occurs in individuals who are predisposed to develop CRPS and as suggested by the hypothesis, become sensitized to the initial C-polymodal

nociceptor input from the traumatized area. The hypothesis, supported by animal experiments, proposes an increased tonic activity in postganglionic sympathetic efferents which in turn stimulate mechanoreceptor neurons to maintain WDR activity. This concept is demonstrated in Figure 12.3.

The conclusion is that while sympathetically maintained pain is invariably present at some point in the course of CRPS, it cannot be included other than as a contributory phenomenon or symptom and therefore is not a defining characteristic of this disease (62).

PAIN DYSFUNCTION SYNDROME AND OTHER PAIN PROBLEMS

In a manner similar to that in which the International Classification of Diseases (ICD-10) defines medical entities that do not satisfy specific diagnostic criteria for a certain condition and are therefore described as NOS codes, the diagnostic criteria for CRPS types I and II use a similar device (39). An example, pain in a limb without the other characteristics of CRPS would be defined as limb pain, NOS type III. The IASP classification of chronic limb pain conditions provides a code for such instances: XI.19 pain in the limbs, NOS: Upper limb (S) 2XX.XXZ, and lower limb (S) 6XX.XXZ.

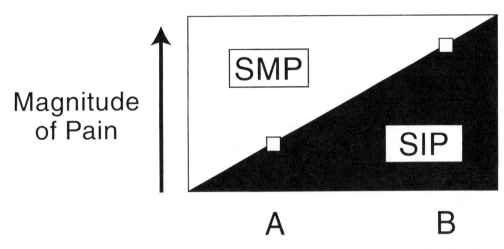

Figure 12.3.   The relative contribution of sympathetically maintained pain to overall pain at any given time. An individual whose pain is sympathetically maintained is represented by point A, therefore highly responsive to sympatholysis. Point B represents pain that has little sympathetic component. Points A and B may represent different patients or the same patient at different times. (Reprinted with permission from Stanton-Hicks M. Reflex sympathetic dystrophy: changing concepts and taxonomy. Pain 1995;63:127–133.)

Pain in the hand that does not meet the criteria for CRPS might be diagnosed as pain dysfunction syndrome, mentioned earlier under differential diagnosis (50). While this is not a standard classification of a medical disease, it belongs to contemporary terminology used to describe a number of medical conditions, including cumulative trauma disorder (49), repetitive strain injury (48), overuse syndrome (47), and tennis elbow (51, 74). These conditions all fall under the general term musculoskeletal conditions, which include a large number of diseases and syndromes, such as carpal tunnel syndrome (75, 76). Obviously, some of these conditions that are associated with pain, mechanical hyperalgesia, and temperature change may be CRPS type III or a myofascial pain syndrome. The differential diagnosis of a condition in which tenderness and hyperalgesia are found specifically over particular muscle groups and epicondylar regions may easily favor that of occupational overuse, bursitis, a nerve entrapment, or tennis elbow, for example. Though there is generally a long antecedent history, patients with fibromyalgia demonstrate hyperresponsiveness with associated headache, fatigue, sleeplessness, depression, and other subjective symptoms, all or some of which may also be present in CRPS. Finally, the particular specialty of the physician making the diagnosis may influence the primary or secondary diagnosis when its differential, namely a diagnosis of CRPS, may not be satisfied by sufficiently stringent criteria.

SUMMARY

The new classification using the umbrella term CRPS is an attempt to remove any preconceived ideas suggesting mechanistic connotations, particularly those that might set the course for treatment failure. The classification is based on historical practice and clinical symptoms and signs that underscore the salient features of reflex sympathetic dystrophy and causalgia while allowing for anomalies and a third type of subgroup that awaits future definition. Disorders that were attributed a sympathetic basis are now confined to conditions having neuropathic pain that responds positively to sympathetic block, namely, sympathetically maintained pain. This characteristic may or may not be present when a diagnosis of CRPS is made. Patients with sympathetically maintained pain may support a diagnosis of many painful conditions, including CRPS. Therefore, CRPS may have both sympathetically maintained and sympathetically independent pain either at the same or at different times (Fig. 12.3). The clinical presentation of these disorders is dynamic, varying within patients and throughout the temporal course of the disease. The pain is both spontaneous and touch-evoked (allodynia or hyperalgesia) and by definition must be associated with vasomotor disturbances, sweating abnormalities, edema, temperature changes, and not infrequently, sensory and/or motor disturbances. Trophic changes may occur. The pain and skin signs may respond favorably to sympatholysis. These features generally occur in the distal part of an extremity, spread beyond the original initiating noxious influence, are disproportionate to the inciting event, and may occur on other parts of the body including trunk and face. Because the diagnosis of CRPS type I (reflex sympathetic dystrophy) is a diagnosis of exclusion, tests of the clinical features that contribute to and are reproducible for such conditions should remain a part of any standard diagnostic protocol. Therefore, sympatholysis, whether pharmacological or by conduction block, is one such test (22). It is the intent that introduction of the new nomenclature for reflex sympathetic dystrophy and causalgia should stimulate a more pragmatic approach to their diagnosis and as a corollary, improved clinical management.

References

1. Bernard CL. Influence du grand sympathique sur la sensibilité et sur la calorification. CR Soc Biol (Paris) 1851;3:163–164.
2. Cannon WB. Organization for physiological homeostasis. Physiol Rev 1929;9:399–431.
3. Cannon WB. The wisdom of the body. New York: Norton, 1939.
4. Bandler R, Shipley MT. Columnar organization in the mid-brain peri-aqueductal gray: modules for emotional expression? Trends Neurosci 1994;17:379–388.
5. Jänig W. Vegetatives Nervensystem. In: Schmitt RF, Thewes G, eds. Physiologie des Menschen. 26th ed. Berlin: Springer-Verlag, 1995;340–369.
6. Sudeck P. Über die akute (trophoneurotische) Knochenatrophie nach Entzündungen und Traumen der Extremitäten. Deutsch Med Wschr 1902;28:336–342.
7. Mitchell SW, Morehouse GR, Keene WW. Gunshot wounds and other injuries of nerves. Philadelphia: Lippincott, 1864.
8. Bonica JJ. The management of pain. Philadelphia: Lea & Febiger, 1953.
9. Bonica JJ. Causalgia and other reflex sympathetic dystrophies. In: JJ Bonica, ed. The management of pain. 2nd ed. Philadelphia: Lea & Febiger, 1990:220–243.
10. Evans JA. Reflex sympathetic dystrophy. Surg Clin North Am 1946;26:780–790.
11. Jänig W, Häbler HJ. Visceral-autonomic integration. In: GF Gebhart, ed. Visceral pain: progress in pain research and management, vol 5. Seattle: IASP Press, 1995;311–348.
12. Leriche R. La Chirurgie del la Douleur. Paris: Masson, 1939.
13. Livingston WK. Pain mechanisms: a physiologic interpretation of causalgia and its related states. New York: Macmillan, 1943.
14. Lewis T. Pain. London: Macmillan, 1942.
15. Walker AE, Nulsen F. Electrical stimulation of the upper thoracic portion of the sympathetic chain in man. Arch Neurol Psychiatry 1948;59:550–560.
16. White JC, Sweet WH. Pain and the neurosurgeon, Springfield, IL: Charles C. Thomas, 1969.
17. Bonica JJ. Causalgia and other reflex sympathetic dystrophies. In: JJ Bonica, JC Lieberskind, DG Alb-Fessard, eds. Advances in pain research and therapy, New York: Raven Press 1979:141–166.
18. Hannington-Kiff JG. Pain relief. Philadelphia: Lippincott, 1974.
19. Arnér S. Intravenous phentolamine test: diagnostic and prognostic use in reflex sympathetic dystrophy. Pain 1991;46:17–22.
20. Raja SN, Treede RD, David KD, Campbell JN, Systemic alpha-adrenergic blockade with phentolamine: a diagnostic test for sympathetically maintained pain. Anesthesiology 1991;74:691–698.
21. Hord H, Rooks MD, Stephens BO, et al. Intravenous regional bretylium and lidocaine for treatment of reflex sympathetic dystrophy: a randomized, double-blind study. Anesth Analg 1992;74:818–821.
22. Stanton-Hicks M, Raj PP, Racz GB. Use of regional anesthetics for diagnosis of reflex sympathetic dystrophy and sympathetically maintained pain: a critical evaluation. In: Jänig W, Stanton-Hicks M, eds. Reflex sympathetic dystrophy: a reappraisal. Progress in pain research and management, vol. 6. Seattle: IASP Press, 1996;217–237.
23. Jänig W, Schmidt FR, eds. Reflex sympathetic dystrophy: pathophysiological mechanisms and clinical implications. Weinheim: BCH Verlagsgesellschaft, 1992.
24. Blumberg H, Jänig W. Clinical manifestations of reflex sympathetic dystrophy and sympathetically maintained pain. In: Wall PD, Melzack R, eds. Textbook of pain. 3rd ed. Edinburgh: Churchill Livingstone, 1994;685–697.
25. Jänig W. The sympathetic nervous system in pain: physiology and pathophysiology. In: Stanton-Hicks M, ed. Pain and the sympathetic nervous system. Boston: Kluwer, 1990;17–89.
26. Jänig W. Pain and the sympathetic nervous system: pathophysiological mechanisms. In: Bannister R, Mathias CJ, eds. Autonomic failure. 3rd ed. Oxford, UK: Oxford University Press, 1992;231–251.
27. Häbler HJ, Jänig W, Koltzenburg M. Activation of unmyelinated afferents in chronically lesioned nerves by adrenalin and excitation of sympathetic efferents in the cat. Neurosci Lett 1987;82:35–40.
28. Wallin G, Torebjörk HE, Hallin RG. Preliminary observations on the pathophysiology of hyperalgesia in the causalgic pain syndrome. In: Zottermann Y, ed. Sensory Functions of the skin in primates. Oxford, UK: Pergamon, 1976;489–499.
29. Torebjörk HE. Clinical and neurophysiological observations related to psychophysiological mechanisms in reflex sympathetic dystrophy. In: Stanton-Hicks M, Jänig W, Boas RA, eds. Reflex sympathetic dystrophy. Boston: Kluwer, 1990;71–80.
30. Davis KD, Treede RD, Raja SN, et al. Topical application of clonidine relieves hyperalgesia in patients with sympathetically maintained pain. Pain 1991;47:309–317.
31. Torebjörk HE, Wahren LK, Wallin G, et al. Noradrenalin-evoked pain in neuralgia. Pain 1995;63:11–20.
32. Chabal C, Jacobson K, Russell LC, Burchiel KJ. Pain response to perineuronal injection of normal saline, epinephrine, and lidocaine in humans. Pain 1992;49;12.
33. Roberts J. A hypothesis on the physiological basis for causalgia and related pains. Pain 1986;24:297–311.
34. Torebjörk HE, Hallin RG. Perceptual changes accompanying controlled preferential blocking of A and C-fiber responses in intact human skin nerves. Ext Brain Res 1973;16:321–332.
35. Campbell JN, Meyer RA, Raja SN. Is nociceptor activation by alpha-1 adrenoceptors the culprit in sympathetically maintained pain? Am Pain Soc J 1992;1:3–11.
36. Stanton-Hicks M, Abram SE, Blumberg H, et al. Definition of reflex sympathetic dystrophy (RSD). In: Stanton-Hicks M, Jänig W, Boas RA, eds. Reflex sympathetic dystrophy. Boston: Kluwer, 1990;209–210.
37. Jänig W, Stanton-Hicks M. Reflex sympathetic dystrophy: a reappraisal. In: Jänig W, Stanton-Hicks M, eds. Progress in pain research and management, vol 6. Seattle: IASP Press, 1996;ix–x.
37a. Jänig W, Blumberg H, Boas RA, Campbell JA. The reflex sympathetic dystrophy syndrome: consensus statement and general recommendations for diagnosis and clinical research. In: Bond MR, Charlton JE, Wool CS, eds. Proceedings of the V World Congress on Pain, Pain Research and Clinical Management, vol 4. Amsterdam: Elsevier, 1991;372–375.
38. Merskey H, Bogduk N, eds. Classification of chronic pain: descriptions of chronic pain syndromes and definition of pain terms. 2nd ed. Seattle: IASP Press, 1994.
39. IASP Subcommittee on Taxonomy. Pain terms: a list with definitions and notes on usage. Pain 1979;6:249–252.
40. Richards RL. Causalgia: a centennial review. Arch Neurol 1967;16:339–350.
41. Schwartzman RJ, Kerrigan J. The movement disorder of reflex sympathetic dystrophy. Neurology 1990;40:57–61.
42. Veldman PHJM, Reyner HM, Arntz IE, Goris RJA. Signs and symptoms of reflex sympathetic dystrophy: a prospective study of 829 patients. Lancet 1993;342:1012–1016.
43. Hunker CJ, Backonja M. The progression of movement disorders in patients with RSD. Soc Neurosci Abstr 1992;18:1593.
44. Mailis A, Wade J. Profile of Caucasian women with possible genetic predisposition to reflex sympathetic dystrophy: a pilot study. Clin J Pain 1994;10:210–217.
45. Devor M, Raber P. Heritability of symptoms in an animal model of neuropathic pain. Pain 1990;42:51–67.
46. Bhatia KP, Bhatt MH, Marsden CD. The causalgia-dystonia syndrome. Brain, 1993;116:843–851.

47. Fry HJH. Overuse syndrome in musicians: prevention and management. Lancet 1986;11:728–731.

48. Browne CD, Nolan BM, Faithfull DK. Occupational repetitive strain injuries: Guideline for diagnosis and management. Med J Aust 1984;140:329–332.

49. Viikari-Juntura E. The role of physical stressors in the development of hand/wrist, and elbow disorders. In: Gordon SL, Blair SJ, Armstrong, et al., eds. Pathophysiology and clinical factors in upper extremity repetitive motion syndromes. Bethesda: American Academy of Orthopaedic Surgeons, 1995.

50. Schottland JR, Kirschberg GJ, Fillingim R, et al. Median nerve latencies in poultry process workers: an approach to resolving the role of industrial "cumulative trauma" in the development of carpal tunnel syndrome. J Occup Med 1991;33:627–631.

51. Webster BS, Snook SH. The cost of compensable upper extremity cumulative trauma disorders. J Occup Med 1994;36:713–727.

52. Silverstein BA, Fine IJ, Armstrong TJ. Hand and wrist cumulative trauma disorders in industry. Br J Ind Med 1986;43:779–784.

53. Jancovic J, van der Linden C. Dystonia and tremor induced by peripheral trauma: predisposing factors. J Neurol Neurosurg Psychiatry 1988;51:1512–1519.

54. Deuschl G, Blumberg H, Lücking CH. Tremor in reflex sympathetic dystrophy. Arch Neurol 1991;481247–1252.

55. Haddox JD, Abram SE, Hopwood MH. Comparison of psychometric data in RSD and radiculopathy. Reg Anesth 1988;13:27.

56. Haddox JD. Psychological aspects of reflex sympathetic dystrophy. In: Stanton-Hicks M, ed. Pain and the sympathetic nervous system, Boston: Kluwer, 1990.

57. Carlson MJ, Linscheid RL, Lucas AR: Recognition of factitial hand injuries. Clin Orthop 1977;122:222–227.

58. Weintraub MI. Chronic pain in litigation: what is the relationship? Neurol Clin 1995;13:341–349.

59. Jarventausta TH, Telaranta TK. Factitious pain and swelling of the upper arm: case report. Acta Chir Scand 1987;153:71–72.

60. Weintraub MI. Regional pain is usually hysterical. Arch Neurol 1988;45:914–915.

61. Merskey H. Regional pain is rarely hysterical. Arch Neurol 1988;45:915–918.

62. Stanton-Hicks M, Jänig W, Hassenbusch S, et al. Reflex sympathetic dystrophy: changing concepts and taxonomy. Pain 1995;63:127–133.

63. Price DD, Bennett JG, Raffii A. Psychophysical observations on patients with neuropathic pain relieved by a sympathetic block. Pain 1989;36:273–288.

64. Price DD, Long S, Hewitt C. Sensory testing of pathophysiological mechanisms of pain in patients with reflex sympathetic dystrophy. Pain 1992;49:163–173.

65. Bennett JG. Neuropathic pain. In: Wall PD, Melzack R, eds. Textbook of pain. 3rd ed. Edinburgh: Churchill-Livingstone, 1994;201–224.

66. McLachlan EM, Jänig W, Devor M, Michaelis M. Peripheral nerve injury triggers non-adrenergic sprouting within dorsal root ganglia. Nature 1993;363:543–545.

67. Levine JD, Taiwo YO, Collins SD, Tam JK. Noradrenalin hyperalgesia is mediated through interaction with sympathetic postganglionic neuron terminals rather than activation of primary afferent nociceptors. Nature 1986;323:158–160.

68. Devor M, Jänig W, Michaelis M. Modulation of activity in dorsal root ganglion (DRG) neurons by sympathetic activation in nerve-injured rats. J Neurol Physiol 1994;71:38–47.

69. Stanton-Hicks M. Blocks of the sympathetic nervous system. In: Stanton-Hicks M, ed. Pain and the sympathetic nervous system. Boston: Kluwer, 1990:125–164.

70. Cousins MJ, Bridenbaugh PO. Neural blockade. 2nd ed. Philadelphia: Lippincott, 1988.

71. Kurvers AJ, Jacobs MJ, Buck RJ, et al. Reflex sympathetic dystrophy: result of autonomic denervation. Clin Sci 1994;87:663–669.

72. Low PA, Caskey PE, Tuck RR, et al. Quantitative pseudomotor axon reflex test in normal and neuropathic subjects. Ann Neurol 1983;14:573–580.

73. Low PA, Amadio PC, Wilson PR, et al. Laboratory findings in reflex sympathetic dystrophy: a preliminary report. Clin J Pain 1994;10:235–239.

74. Dimberg L. The prevalence and causation of tennis elbow (lateral humeral epicondylitis) in a population of workers in an engineering industry. Ergonomics 1987;30:573–580.

75. Hales TR, Habes D, Fine L, et al. John Morell and Coe. NIOSH HETA Report 88–180-1958. Cincinnati: National Institute for Occupational Safety and Health, 1989.

76. Moore JS. Carpal tunnel syndrome. In: Moore JS, Garg A, eds. Occupational medicine, state-of-the-art reviews: ergonomics: low back pain, carpal tunnel syndrome and upper extremity disorders in the workplace. Philadelphia: Hanley and Belfus, 1992;741–763.

CHAPTER 13

Joint Pains and Associated Disorders

William N. Pachas

INTRODUCTION

Joint pains are common complaints in the general population. Since joint pain is likely to affect the person's ability to function, there is a need to alleviate the discomfort as early as possible. In response to that need there is a whole industrial complex devoted to providing short-term solutions to painful ailments. Indeed, in many instances, musculoskeletal aches and pains can be mitigated without medical intervention, for instance if they are due to self-limited processes such as the aches and pains that may accompany a viral illness. In other examples, however, an identifiable rheumatic disorder is the cause of the joint pains, and medical intervention becomes necessary. This chapter presents an overview of common rheumatological disorders with emphasis on their clinical manifestations and their pathogenesis and offers some useful clues for diagnosis and treatment.

EVALUATION OF THE PATIENT WITH JOINT PAIN

In the initial evaluation of a rheumatological disorder, the physician should try to obtain a detailed history of the painful event and its characteristics, including the number of joints involved and any other symptoms that accompany the onset and course of the disease. Sometimes one is faced with diagnostic difficulties because multiple conditions affect the same region of the body. The most common example is the back pain that occurs in an elderly person in whom degenerative joint disease coexists with osteoporosis and spinal stenosis or disc disease. The physical examination becomes critical; it may disclose significant anatomical changes in bones and joints. This, together with careful functional assessments, should provide information regarding not only possible diagnosis but also the degree of impairment or disability due to bone and joint damage. Diagnostic clues obtained from the history and physical examination should be complemented by radiographic studies and appropriate laboratory tests that may help the physician to formulate a diagnostic workup and possible treatments. Valuable assistance may be obtained from computed tomography (CT) or magnetic resonance imaging (MRI). One must be careful, however, to ascertain the pertinence of these studies, and consultations with appropriate professionals are advisable to maximize the efficiency of these new technologies.

TYPES OF JOINT PAINS

Synovial Pain

Synovial pain is usually associated with inflammation. It may be monoarticular or affect more than one joint. In addition to pain, there is swelling, warmth, and a variable degree of deformity of the joint, depending on the intensity and duration of the inflammatory process. Passive and active motion of the joints with direct pressure over the swollen area can either provoke or aggravate a preexisting pain. Joint stiffness sometimes precedes the onset of inflammatory synovitis in rheumatoid arthritis, and morning stiffness is characteristic of the disease. Chronic synovitis can result in joint destruction and deformity. When the articular cartilage is lost, the apposition of bone upon bone during motion creates a grinding sensation known as joint crepitus. Muscle atrophy may follow as a consequence of joint immobility and deconditioning. Nerve entrapment syndromes and corresponding neuropathy fairly commonly result from compression of nerves by hypertrophic synovium. Synovitis is then a complex joint disorder that affects the joint itself, as well as the neighboring structures.

Bone Pain

The pain of bone disease is usually deep and often localized in the shaft of the long bones such as the tibia, femur, and humerus. Disorders such as hypertrophic idiopathic osteoarthropathy and Paget's disease of bone are likely to cause bone pain. In the first example, the pain is due to hypervascular changes occurring in the thickened, multilayered periosteum. The bone pain of Paget's disease, often more severe at night, is due to the hypermetabolic state of accelerated bone remodeling. Sometimes the pain of Paget's disease occurs near joints and suggests arthritis. Degenerative joint disease is fairly common near pagetic bone. Bone infarcts are also painful, and they may occur near the joints, such as in sickle cell anemia crisis. Other causes of bone pain include osteomyelitis and metastatic disease. These processes should be suspected in accordance with the overall clinical situation.

Tendinous and Ligamentous Pain

Pain originating from an inflammatory process or traumatic tears in tendons and ligaments may be elicited with certain specific movements of the joints. For instance, with tendinitis of the rotator cuff in the shoulder joint, the pain appears when the shoulder is brought into abduction between 60 and 100°. The rotator cuff is compressed at the acromion within this range of motion of the shoulder. When the supraspinatus tendon is affected, one should immobilize the scapula and position the shoulder in abduction and external rotation; the pain can usually be increased by resisted abduction. In subscapularis tendinitis, pain usually increases with resistance to external rotation. Full-thickness tears of the rotator cuff are identified when the shoulder is passively brought into 90° of abduction and the shoulder drops when the assistance to the movement is withdrawn. Tendinitis of the bicipital tendon can be identified by direct external pressure on the tendon groove during rotation of the arm. Another maneuver for bicipital tendinitis is Speed's test, in which pain is induced in the anterior aspect of the shoulder by resisted arm elevation while the elbow is fully extended. Another typical tendon pain is tennis elbow, or epicondylitis. In both the medial and the lateral epicondyles of the humerus, the epicondylitis is easily identified by obtaining a painful response to pressure directly on the medial or lateral epicondyle. In the ankle, pain in the Achilles' tendon is most commonly due to sprain; and the pain occurs on weight-bearing and plantar flexion of the foot. When a full-thickness tear of the Achilles' tendon occurs, likely after a traumatic event, there is severe pain at the tear site and inability to flex the foot down.

Ligamentous strain is best illustrated in the knee. The pain is often due to a traumatic injury affecting the cruciate ligaments. The physical examination may reveal an abnormal displacement of the tibia on the femur with the knee in flexion at 90°. Anterior displacement and pain identify an anterior cruciate ligament rupture. With posterior ligament rupture, the pain occurs with the posterior displacement of the tibia with the knee flexed at 90°. The medial and lateral collateral ligaments are commonly subject to strain; on forceful varus or valgus, strain may produce pain on the medial or lateral aspect of the knee, respectively.

Bursal Pain

Bursal pain is most commonly noted in the shoulder in the subacromial or subdeltoid bursa. In the hip the site of pain is noted over the greater trochanter area. In the elbow it manifests in the olecranon bursa, and in the knee, in the prepatellar bursa. Acute inflammatory processes affecting the superficial bursal structures such as the prepatellar and olecranon bursae are easily identified by the swelling, erythema, warmth, and pain that increase with range of motion and with direct external pressure, which causes further distension of the bursa. Subdeltoid bursitis is suspected when the patient reports pain when leaning on the affected shoulder, such as when trying to sleep on that side. During examination the pain greatly increases when the shoulder is placed in abduction and external pressure is applied laterally about an inch below the acromial prominence. Involvement of the subacromial bursa is suspected when the shoulder is brought into abduction and pain occurs at the top of the shoulder because of impingement of the bursa.

Capsular Pain

Capsular pain, or capsulitis, is an acute and chronic inflammatory and rapidly fibrotic process that causes marked restriction of motion in the affected joint, most commonly the shoulder, where the term frozen shoulder truly reflects chronic adhesive capsulitis. This rather serious disease entity appears to have a totally independent course; it responds to anti-inflammatory drugs, physical therapy maneuvers, and surgery. This process may resolve spontaneously in 2 to 3 years. Adhesive capsulitis has been associated with some acute illnesses, including stroke, myocardial infarction, and pulmonary disease. It is clear, however, that the most frequent association of adhesive capsulitis is with diabetes mellitus. The reason for this association is unclear. It does not appear to correlate with the state of diabetic control. The hip is another site for adhesive capsulitis, and when it occurs it can cause severe pain and restriction of motion. Surgical treatment of the hip may be more effective than in the shoulder.

Periosteal Pain

Periosteal pain is characteristically seen in idiopathic hypertrophic pulmonary osteoarthropathy, in which the pain is most severe in the para-articular areas and along the diaphysis of bone. Direct external pressure over the bone surface causes exquisite pain. This condition seen in association with malignancies of the lung is also seen in other pulmonary and nonpulmonary conditions. The radiological changes are characteristic of the thickened periosteum in the affected areas. Reactive periosteitis may also be seen in a patient with renal osteodystrophy and primary hyperparathyroidism. The characteristic radiological changes include subperiosteal bone resorption with tunneling of cortical bone.

RHEUMATOID ARTHRITIS: CAUSATION AND PATHOGENESIS

Rheumatoid arthritis is a chronic inflammatory disease of the joints unique to the human race. It can affect persons at any time during the course of their lives; therefore, children, adults, and the elderly share the risk for developing this disease. Its prevalence in the general population is about 1 to 3%. Peak incidence of rheumatoid arthritis occurs between ages 30 and 40. It is seen worldwide and affects women more frequently than men. Certain ethnic groups also appear to be particularly susceptible to it. The role of genetic and environmental factors has been the subject of intensive investigation. The cause of rheumatoid arthritis is unknown, but whatever the cause, the basic process is these unknown factors leading to the inflammatory reaction in the joints. The inflammatory process in many ways is similar to the inflammatory reactions induced by infectious agents. As such, viruses and bacteria have been intensely investigated as possible causative factors, but, to date none has been found. If infectious agents are involved in some way in the cause of rheumatoid arthritis or in its pathogenesis, it probably requires a special host in whom the needed interaction between the agent and the immune system can take place. In this regard some facts are of interest. For instance, women appear to be at higher risk for developing rheumatoid arthritis. This suggests a possible role for hormones, such as estrogen, by unknown mechanisms increasing women's susceptibility to it. Moreover, the role of hormones may be further highlighted during pregnancy. It appears that pregnancy affords a protective effect against rheumatoid arthritis. Although it does not shed light on the causation or pathogenesis of rheumatoid arthritis, other important information suggests precipitating or activating factors. For instance, psychological stress may be a determining factor to the beginning of joint symptoms or exacerbations in otherwise stable disease state.

The inflammation of the joints in rheumatoid arthritis and their subsequent destruction requires the participation of an activated immune system that responds to an antigenic stimulation (antigen unknown) followed by a biotransformation of the synovial membrane. The result is synovial hypertrophy and a hypersecretory state that clinically manifests by swelling, pain, and stiffness; and progressive joint destruction and deformity. The activation of the inflammatory process requires the participation of the cells of the immune system, such as the macrophage and T and B cells, which are activated by lymphokines: interleukin-1, tumor necrosis factor, and other cytokines and growth factors that appear to play a fundamental role in maintaining both the inflammatory state and the pannus formation once the disease becomes well established. As noted earlier, it appears that certain genetic elements may increase the risk for developing rheumatoid arthritis. It is now well established that those with the DR-4 gene are at higher risk for it. Along with contribution of other genes, DR-1 appears to determine the ultimate course of the disease. The gene expressions of DR-1 and DR-4 on the surface of the appropriate T cells contain a five-amino acid sequence motif that is shared by these antigens; it is called the shared epitope HLADRB-1. It is intriguing that this same epitope is present in the dnaJ class of heat shock proteins of gram-negative bacteria and the capsid protein of the Epstein-Barr virus. The pathogenetic significance of these findings, if any, remains to be established. Some recent work on the mechanism of pannus formation appears to point out a failure in the mechanism of synovial cell apoptosis (programed cell death) as an important source of synovial hypertrophy. The research into the nature of cell interactions and humoral factors leading to inflammation has continued at a very intense pace, and much will be learned about the pathogenesis of this very important human disease in the not too distant future. The antigen that drives the immune response, however, remains elusive.

Clinical Manifestations

Rheumatoid arthritis is a systemic disease that usually begins in the joints. The joint involvement at the outset may be single or multiple, and when polyarticular, it often follows a symmetrical distribution. The affected person has joint stiffness that is more marked in the mornings, as well as joint pains. The joint stiffness usually clears after some hours but returns during the course of the day when the patient is idle. The subsequent course of the disease is unpredictable. Sometimes the arthritis has a chronic course without remission; most commonly partial remissions and sometimes complete remissions occur. Because of the insidious nature of the disease, many times the diagnosis cannot be established with certainty before all of the criteria required by the American College of Rheumatology (ACR) are satisfied. These diagnostic difficulties are well recognized, and the ACR in its diagnostic criteria still accepts the categories of possible, probable, and definitive rheumatoid arthritis.

The hallmark of the disease is synovitis, which is clinically defined as thickening of the synovial tissue, but to the hand of the examiner there is a sensation of bogginess. The hypertrophy of synovial tissue can extend into adjacent areas, including the tendon sheath. Since the synovium is in a hypersecretory state, the examiner is likely to find joint effusions of variable size. The effusions may be quite large, especially in the knees and shoulders. During the joint examination, pain may be elicited by motion and by direct pressure over the inflamed tissue. Maneuvers such as squeezing of the metacarpophalangeal (MCP) and metatarsophalangeal (MTP) joints can elicit severe pain. Along with the inflammatory and hypertrophic synovial changes, joint deformation sometimes adopts typical shapes having a swan neck or boutonniere appearance. Ulnar deviation and subluxation can be found in chronic advanced cases. Fibrous ankylosis of the fingers, either in flexion or extension, severely restrict the joint function. In the feet, the subluxation of the MTP joints may be the source of major complications, as is reviewed later in this chapter. It is important to examine the patient not only at the bedside but also in functional activities such as sitting, standing, and walking or during the performance of activities of daily living, such as dressing, grooming, writing, and food preparation, to obtain an overall picture of the degree of disability resulting from the joint deformities. But one must not forget that rheumatoid arthritis is a systemic disease, and consequently internal organs such as lungs and the serous membranes can be affected. The radiological abnormalities and the laboratory tests provide further insight to the severity and degree of activity of the disease. The sedimentation rate has been used for many years to measure disease activity.

Important Clinical Clues in the Evaluation of Joints

The discussion in the previous paragraph encompasses the generalities of the joint examination in rheumatoid arthritis. This section presents more specific discussion of the anatomical changes by regions.

Neck

Begin the evaluation by noticing the position and movement of the cervical spine. All motions of the neck should be explored, and this includes flexion, extension, rotation, and tilting of the neck. One should appreciate any pain or limitation of motion with any of these movements. Sometimes by the time the patient comes for the first examination, the neck is already in an abnormal position, most commonly in flexion. Underlying pathology may include apophyseal joint disease or subluxation of the intervertebral joints with displacement in the anterior or posterior planes. Careful flexion of the neck is always warranted in patients with chronic rheumatoid arthritis because of the frequent cervical involvement, the potential for atlantoaxial subluxation, causing neurological symptoms due to spinal cord compression during flexion of the neck. The neck motion is often decreased and painful, especially toward the end of the movement. Tilting of the head may be quite painful and should be avoided. Crepitus may be elicited with any neck motion. Radiographs of the cervical spine and occasionally MRI may be necessary to complete the assessment of the cervical spine in rheumatoid arthritis. MRI is most helpful in assessing joint instability, especially at the C1-C2 level, and in the lower part of the cervical spine, where stepladder deformity commonly causes significant narrowing of the spinal canal. Both of these abnormalities create significant risk of injury to the spinal cord.

Shoulder

Again, all movements should be tested, including true abduction, which is normally 90° with the scapula fixed. Other shoulder movements include anterior and posterior flexion, external and internal rotations, and elevation of the arms above the shoulder level anteriorly and laterally. Frequent abnormal findings are decreased abduction, subluxation of the humeral head, which is commonly associated with damage to the rotator cuff and associated tendons, and painful crepitus during movement. Once there is total loss of the rotator cuff, the head of the humerus migrates up and becomes anchored in the glenoid, and the humerus moves together with the scapula when the scapula swings. When the shoulder joint reaches this state of damage, the functional disability is severe and the patient cannot perform certain activities of daily living, such as dressing, toileting, and grooming, and therefore needs continued assistance. Patients having this kind of functional limitation may not be able to live independently and may require institutionalization if the needed family support is not available.

Elbow

The normal elbow is capable of flexion and extension as well as pronation and supination. Rheumatoid arthritis often affects this joint, and pain, warmth, and swelling are present, usually on the sides of the olecranon. Pronation and supination may be limited by pain, fibrous ankylosis, and subluxation. Olecranon bursitis is common and usually painless, and rheumatoid nodules may also be noted in this area. Because of the natural tendency for the elbow to be flexed during significant parts of the day, this joint is at high risk for becoming fixed in flexion. Once fibrous ankylosis develops, the elbow motion lacks significant extension and flexion, also resulting in serious functional disability.

Wrists

There are many changes to be noted in wrist joints. Most common is the synovial swelling, both at the volar aspect of the joint and over the dorsum. Sometimes the inflammatory process affects the tendon sheath, posing a risk of tendon rupture when the synovitis is uncontrolled. Subluxations of the wrists are common. The characteristic drift is toward the ulnar side in conjunction with resorption of the ulnar styloid. Sometimes the wrists show extensive resorption of the carpal bones, giving the impression that the metacarpals are sitting directly on the radius. Carpal tunnel syndrome may arise from compression of the median nerve by the hypertrophied synovium. A wrist drop may be due to radial nerve compression or rupture of the extensor tendons eroded by the synovitis. This type of joint damage is also extremely incapacitating; fusion procedures or stabilizing devices sometimes dramatically improve the function of the hand.

Metacarpophalangeal and Proximal Interphalangeal Joints

The metacarpophalangeal (MCP) and proximal interphalangeal (PIP) joints are frequently affected in rheumatoid arthritis. In the initial stages one sees swelling and sometimes redness and increased warmth. It is possible to see that the MCP and PIP joints that are most involved with function tend to develop more inflammatory changes and deformities in the long term. Characteristic subluxation of the MCPs are ulnar deviations and subluxations of the proximal phalanx and of the metacarpal heads. Contractures and bone resorption with shortening of the metacarpals and phalanges may be prominent. When the PIP joints are subluxed in hyperextension, they cause a deformity called swan neck. If the PIPs develop flexion deformity accompanied by hyperextension of the corresponding distal interphalangeal (DIP), the resultant deformity is a boutonniere finger. These two types of deformities often coexist in the same patient. The DIP joints are rarely affected in rheumatoid arthritis.

Hips

Pain and limitation of hip motion are characteristics of late disease, and radiography may reveal total loss of the cartilage space. Erosion of the articular surfaces may cause crepitus with motion. In advanced cases, protrusio, the hip deformity due to thinning of the roof of the acetabulum, gives way to the mechanical forces bearing down on the femoral head and transmitted into the acetabulum, drive the acetabulum into the pelvic cavity. Protrusion often shortens the affected limb and causes compensatory lumbar scoliosis.

Knees

The most prominent finding in the knees is swelling due to synovial hypertrophy with increased production of synovial fluid. The swelling may be noted on each side of the patella and in the suprapatellar compartment. Sometimes the swelling occurs in the popliteal fossa, producing a fluctuant tender mass or Baker's cyst. The Baker's cyst is better appreciated when the patient is standing. These popliteal cysts may reach very large dimensions and sometimes dissect down toward the calf. When the pressure inside the cyst is too great, it may rupture and extravasate into the surrounding tissue, resulting in diffuse swelling and pain, sometimes confused with thrombophlebitis.

Apart from the changes due to the synovitis, the knee may undergo significant loosening of ligaments and erosion of cartilage and bone, resulting in joint instability in either varus or valgus positions. The straining caused by these deformities on the ligaments of the knee further weakens these structures in addition to causing considerable pain. The progressive shortening of the hamstring tendons causes stiffening of the knee in flexion and significant gait disorder, forcing a compensatory flexion of the hip and stooping.

Ankles

In the ankles the synovial swelling may be prominent above the malleoli and over the anterior compartment. Chronic syn-

ovitis can induce joint instability through collapse of the ligamentous structures that maintain the ankle in alignment with the foot. Collapse of the foot arch often accompanies the ankle deformity. At this stage of joint damage, the mechanics of walking are completely distorted, and any weight bearing may be intolerable because of the severe pain. Sometimes stabilizing devices help temporarily; joint arthrodesis may be the most effective way to restore stability, but it requires prolonged periods of not bearing weight to allow full healing.

Toes

The most common deformity of the toes in rheumatoid arthritis is the hyperextension of the MTP joints and combined flexion of the DIP joints. Called the cocked-up deformity, it is often the source of significant morbidity. The progressive subluxation of the MTP joint causes upward displacement of the first phalanx, leaving the metatarsal heads bearing down on the soft tissues of the sole of the foot. This sharp pressure of the metatarsal heads leads to the formation of painful calluses that tend to break down, become infected, and ulcerate, causing major management problems requiring complex surgical debridements and intravenous antibiotic treatments if there is osteomyelitis. Sometimes these types of subluxation of the toes require the resection of the metatarsal heads and realignment with the first phalanx. The cocked-up deformities are also predisposed to develop ulcers at pressure sites on top of the toes. These ulcers are painful and difficult to heal. Rheumatoid nodules can also appear in pressure areas of the feet and are prone to breakdown, with increased risk for infection and nonhealing ulcers.

There is no doubt that the loss of function in one joint, such as the shoulder, may be terribly frustrating for someone whose income-earning ability depends on the intact function of that joint, such as a musician and some athletes. This situation can be magnified to the degree of losing the capability of self-care and performance of normal daily activities. Given the way rheumatoid arthritis can affect the joints, it is not inconceivable that some patients with major joint involvement and increments of dysfunction of the high-function joints such as those in the hands may be irreversibly totally disabled. Having said that, one should emphasize that the situation is not without hope. The disease can certainly be arrested, although not cured. Appropriate orthopaedic surgery may restore the ability to walk and sit, and rehabilitation medicine may offer modalities to reduce pain and discomfort and optimize functional capabilities with joint supports and functional tools that can return at least some functional independence.

Treatment of Rheumatoid Arthritis

Nowadays, the rationale for treatment of many diseases is based on the knowledge that the disease has a known cause and a specific treatment. The best example of this type is seen in the field of infectious diseases; specific treatments can be given according to the organism causing the disease. In other instances, when the cause is not known, some strategies for treatment can be designed if one knows some important elements of the pathogenesis of the disease. Rheumatoid arthritis falls into this second category; the physician attempts to control a complex condition whose cause or causes remain unknown. Not so long ago, the treatment of rheumatoid arthritis was bed rest and aspirin. With the advent of new technologies there is a better understanding of the pathogenesis of the inflammatory process and the tissue destruction in rheumatoid arthritis. New efforts to influence the course of the disease by blocking certain crucial steps of the inflammatory reaction are being made. From the therapeutic point of view, there have been significant advances in the development of new anti-inflammatory drugs, which are easier to administer and hence improve compliance.

However, the anti-inflammatory drugs address only one of the mechanisms of the disease process. They do not treat the autoimmunity and immune complex disease or the synovial hypertrophy with destructive pannus, which destroys cartilage and bone. It is clear then that no single drug can address all of the mechanisms involved in the inflammation and tissue destruction. For this reason, drug treatment of rheumatoid arthritis has been staged according to the degree of activity of the disease process. In the early stages, drugs that suppress the inflammatory activity or nonsteroidal anti-inflammatory drugs (NSAIDs) may suffice. Unfortunately, the disease has a progressive course, and disease-modifying antirheumatic drugs (DMARD) must be used. These drugs probably work at the cellular line of the immune system, including the macrophage and the activated T-cell lymphocytes. On the horizon are a series of new drugs that have been developed for specific targeting of factors with a fundamental role in the inflammatory process, such as tumor necrosis factor-α, interferon-γ, and blocking agents of the tumor necrosis factor receptor. Cyclosporine is proved to be effective in some patients with rheumatoid arthritis by a mechanism of inhibition of interleukin-1 production. Of the drugs available for the treatment of rheumatoid arthritis, methotrexate has been used successfully in the treatment of this disease, inducing significant remission for as long as the patient remains on the drug. Minocycline 100 mg twice a day and sulfasalazine (Azulfidine) 1 to 3 g/day are effective in the management of moderately active disease. Long-term studies are desirable to establish their place in the therapeutic armamentarium against rheumatoid arthritis.

Steroids are very important drugs in the overall management of rheumatoid arthritis, especially during periods of disease exacerbation or resistance to other drugs. In these situations, steroids are used in relatively high doses, usually greater than 30 mg a day. Steroids have also been used for the treatment of chronic rheumatoid arthritis in low doses, 5 to 10 mg a day, in conjunction with NSAIDs or disease-modifying drugs. In spite of the advances in understanding the pathogenesis of rheumatoid arthritis and the advent of more powerful and target-specific drugs, the treatment of rheumatoid arthritis remains more art than science. No two patients respond the same to a given drug or drug combination. It is clear that each disease course has its own pattern, which may be predictable in regard to overall disease severity but is much less clear in terms of response to drugs.

The Role of Rehabilitation Medicine and Reconstructive Surgery in Rheumatoid Arthritis

So far this discussion addresses the treatment of rheumatoid arthritis only from the point of view of drug use to control inflammation, pain, and disease activity. In all stages of the disease—acute, chronic, and flaring up—other disciplines become equally important, because joint and bone damage may occur in spite of adequate drug treatment. A patient with rheumatoid arthritis may become functionally impaired and ultimately disabled by the severe damage in the joints. The early changes characterized by joint swelling, pain, and stiffness may progress to joint deformities due to subluxations and fixed fibrous and bony ankylosis, tendon ruptures, and general debilitation and deconditioning. Rehabilitation medicine faces a formidable challenge as it addresses these problems. The main goal is to restore function and decrease the pain and discomfort to the joints. An appropriate rehabilitation program requires the participation of physical and occupational therapy specialists along with experts in pain control with proper modalities. Rehabilitation also necessitates stabilization of unstable joints by the use of suitable devices, patient education about strategies of joint protection, and a host of devices that allow the patient to perform activities of daily living even in a handicapped condition. Significant recovery of joint function can be accomplished with exercises and careful strengthening of affected body segments. Pain control modalities in general soothe the patient but may also be used to prepare the patient for physical therapy activities. Heat and cold are commonly used to treat painful joints, but it has not been clearly established whether one modality is superior to the other. The patient decides which modality is best for reducing joint discomfort and pain. Theoretically, cold may be preferable to heat, because heat may favor the activation of proteolytic enzymes within the joint, increasing the risk of cartilage degradation. Finally, the role of exercise cannot be stressed too strongly, especially in view of new information clearly showing the beneficial effects of exercise in reducing pain and fatigue without exacerbating the symptoms of rheumatoid arthritis.

The management of rheumatoid arthritis cannot be complete without pain management. The pain may limit the ability to move the joints and therefore the ability of the person to participate in activities of daily living; because of these disadvantages the patient may be at risk for losing his or her social independence. It is in this context that the treatment of pain should be addressed. It is clear that some of the NSAIDs also have an analgesic effect, though sometimes they do not suffice to control the rheumatoid pain. When these agents do not provide adequate analgesia, one must resort to other drugs, such as acetaminophen and propoxyphene. These drugs are most effective in mild to moderate cases of rheumatoid arthritis. They are not effective in very severe cases or during acute exacerbations of the disease. Short-term use of opioids in appropriate doses is therefore a very effective way to control severe pain that cannot be controlled by NSAIDs or regular analgesics. Finally, local steroid injections can be very helpful in reducing inflammation and pain unresponsive to systemic treatment. When joint deformities are beyond the reach of the medical management, depending on the problem, one should obtain the advice of a qualified orthopaedic surgeon familiar with joint reconstruction. There is no doubt that with the present advances in prosthetic joint design and other technical improvements, one can look forward to successful joint reconstructions that will both eliminate pain and more important, restore lost function for long periods.

OSTEOARTHRITIS

Osteoarthritis is a progressive degenerative disease of articular cartilage. Its cause is unknown, but probably multiple factors contribute to cartilage degeneration. From the clinical point of view, the patient affected by osteoarthritis may develop pain in the affected joints at any time during the course of the disease or no pain at all in spite of severe loss of cartilage. In the classical situation, as the joint cartilage degenerates, joint deformities begin to appear, most significantly, hypertrophy of bone in the form of osteophytes. As the stress forces operating in the joints further overload the areas undergoing cartilage degeneration, straining of the ligaments and tendons aggravates the symptoms. In the end stages the joint pain and the joint deformity become more severe, resulting in limitation or loss of motion and disability. For some unclear reasons, osteoarthritis affects individuals in their late middle years of life and frequently sets in after 65 years of age. There is no sex preference, but in certain forms of osteoarthritis genetic predisposition may be significant, such as in osteoarthritis affecting the distal interphalangeal joints, which is more frequent in women by a ratio of 10:1. Some factors, such as trauma, may influence the biology of the cartilage in a way that causes degeneration. These may be seen in those who practice certain stressful sports in which they are exposed to repetitive injury, such as soccer players and weight lifters. Some overweight persons also develop degenerative arthritis, but one must be careful in ascribing to the overweight the direct responsibility for the cartilage loss because in other overweight individuals the cartilage is intact even after many years of excessive weight. Also, osteoarthritis can occur in persons who are actually underweight. At any rate, the degenerative process of the cartilage seems to be slow and progressive, but the initiating cause of the cartilage damage is unknown.

Pathogenesis

In the early stages, there is swelling of the involved cartilage and increased production of collagen. Subsequently there is an increase in the number of chondrocytes and increased collagen production. It is also apparent that the synovial membrane becomes hyperactive, with increased production of synovial fluid. In a more advanced stage of cartilage degeneration there is an increase in the water content of the cartilage, and microfissures begin to appear together with cloning of the chondrocytes in scattered islandlike arrays. This process precedes their disappearance and final loss of cartilage, leaving the rough surface of bone against bone and the crepitus sign during joint motion. Recent data show that the synovium in osteoarthritis is an important source of interleukin-1 and tumor necrosis factor-α. The role of these factors in cartilage degeneration is not yet clear, but it is thought that they may stimulate the production of collagenase and stromelysin, two powerful collagen degrading enzymes. It is likely that in the not too distant future the present concept about cartilage degeneration may be advanced by further clarification of the role of the synovium in osteoarthritis.

Clinical Manifestations

The dominant symptom of osteoarthritis is articular pain. However, as noted before, joints may degenerate and for some unclear reason not be symptomatic at all. Hips and knees are the most frequently affected weight-bearing joints. Osteoarthritis also frequently occurs in non-weight-bearing joints such as the shoulders, elbows, the interphalangeal joints. The pain of osteoarthritis is usually aggravated by activity. It becomes more severe as the cartilage loss becomes more evident. In the final stages the pain may be spontaneous, occurring at rest and very much aggravated by motion and weight bearing. Nocturnal pain in the knees and hips can be extremely disturbing and often prompts the patient to seek orthopaedic advice, especially when in addition to pain there is severe limitation of motion and functional incapacity. It is clear, however, that the process of cartilage degeneration has quite a various clinical behavior, according to the part of the body in which it occurs. In the cervical and lumbar spine, in addition to pain the patient may have neurological problems arising from nerve compression syndromes, whereas in the distal interphalangeal joints of the hands, for instance, after a certain period of painful activity, the osteoarthritic symptoms often disappear in spite of the cartilage loss. Although it seems logical to think that when a joint becomes denuded of cartilage, leaving bone on bone, it is enough to explain the pain of osteoarthritis, it is clear that this is not always true. The clinical examples mentioned pose intriguing questions to the mechanisms that may turn pain on and off in the osteoarthritic joint.

Laboratory and Radiological Findings

In osteoarthritis there are no systemic manifestations. Therefore, laboratory studies such as a sedimentation rate and a hematocrit are normal unless altered by some other disease or dysfunction. The synovial fluid has good viscosity, the white blood cell count is made up mainly of mononuclear cells, and it rarely exceeds 1000 cells per cubic millimeter.

Radiologically, osteoarthritis has characteristic findings that include narrowing of the articular space, subchondral cyst formation, and bony sclerosis usually noted at the margin of the articulating surfaces. Osteophytes may occur in the lateral margins of the joints. In the knee, for instance, they can be seen in the lateral aspect of the femoral condyles, as well as posteriorly and in the superior and inferior poles of the patella. In very advanced cases there is total loss of the articular space, and some bone resorption may be seen. In the hip and other joints pathological fractures and avascular necrosis are rarely seen as complications of osteoarthritis, and actually the reverse may be true. Cartilage calcification can be seen in the knee joints, in the intervertebral space, and in the shoulders and wrists.

Treatment

Until recently the treatment of osteoarthritis was limited to pain control by the use of analgesics and NSAIDs. On occasions the intra-articular steroid injection was given with some beneficial effects, although they were never long lasting. When there was significant deformity and it was believed that the instability was the cause of the pain by overstretching the periarticular structures, the realignment of the joint by appropriate bracing provided temporary help. In this regard, the point should be made that unless the brace was well fitting and comfortable, there was a high likelihood that the patient would not wear it. It appears that under certain conditions of training, the pain of osteoarthritis of the knee may be alleviated. The benefit of exercise in preventing and improving the pain of osteoarthritis has been demonstrated in several recent studies. It is clear then, that management of osteoarthritis encompasses the judicious administrations of NSAIDs and pain control regimens, the use of stabilizing devices when appropriate, steroid injections, and especially exercise that may have a fundamental beneficial effect on the biology of the degenerative cartilage.

Finally, very recently two new approaches in the management of osteoarthritis are the subject of intensive clinical evaluation. First, intra-articular injections containing cross-linked hyaluronan have been shown to diminish the pain of osteoarthritis; however, experience with this product, is still too limited. The second approach, the implantation of cartilage grafts, thus far used only for osteoarthritis of the knee, has produced some encouraging early results. For the time being and until new therapies become established, joint replacement surgery is one of the mainstays for the restoration of function in end-stage osteoarthritis.

CRYSTALLINE ARTHROPATHIES: GOUT AND PSEUDOGOUT

Gout

Gout, an acute and sometimes chronic rheumatological disorder, is caused by the generation of sodium urate crystals in the joints and periarticular tissues, followed by an acute inflammatory reaction resulting from the activation of multiple inflammatory factors released in the affected joints after phagocytosis of the sodium urate crystals by polymorphonuclear leukocytes. There is a clear relation between the serum concentration of uric acid and the development of gouty arthritis, men being at higher risk than women; rates are 13.6 per 1000 men and 6.4 per 1000 women. Blacks may be at higher risk for developing gouty arthritis. A high uric acid level indicates a higher risk for developing gout but is not necessarily the determining factor for gouty arthritis. It is well known that persons with normal or even low uric acid levels may also develop gout. Therefore, factors other than hyperuricemia may be at play in the development of gouty arthritis. Peak incidence of the disease in men is in the fifth decade of life, and after menopause the incidence of gout in women is probably as high as in men. The development of gouty arthritis is unrelated to socioeconomic class and to excesses in eating or drinking alcoholic beverages. Alcohol consumption, on the other hand, may be a precipitating factor in a predisposed person, because of its interference with the renal elimination of uric acid and resulting hyperuricemia. Diet as the cause of hyperuricemia has only secondary significance. Genetic factors affecting uric acid metabolism such as familial gout, overproduction of uric acid, and diseases due to the enzyme phosphoribosyl transferase (HGPRT) or severe deficiency of it can cause hyperuricemia and gout. Certain drugs such as diuretics may cause hyperuricemia gout. In the elderly diuretics are possibly the most common cause of hyperuricemia and gout. Diseases characterized by high uric acid turnover, such as in patients with myeloproliferative disorders, are risk factors for gout and renal failure due to uric acid overload of the kidney.

Pathogenesis

Uric acid is a poor solute. Saturation occurs at a concentration of 7 mg/100 mL. It is remarkable that supersaturated solutions of uric acid in the tissues can maintain the stability of the uric acid without precipitating. This appears to be due to local factors such as serum proteins and the chemical constitution of the interstitial tissue. The mechanism by which uric acid nucleates to form crystals is unknown. As the crystal is formed, a sequence of metabolic changes releases inflammatory factors, and the whole sequence of inflammation-activating compounds cooperate to produce the acute inflammatory arthritis. The sequence of events may be as follows: First neutrophils adhere to the endothelial cells under the influence of interleukin-1 and tumor necrosis factor-α. Then chemotactic factors are secreted as interleukin-8 and the complement component c5A and crystal-induced chemotactic factor enhances the entrance of polymorphonuclear leukocytes into the tissues. To become activated, polymorphonuclear leukocytes initiate phagocytosis of uric acid crystals, which then release proteolytic enzymes lowering the tissue pH, in turn causing precipitation of new uric acid crystals. Prostaglandins and other vasodilating factors are released, resulting in increased vasodilation and edema production. The outcome is a self-perpetuating inflammatory reaction clinically represented by the intense joint pain, swelling, and heat so characteristic of the disease.

Clinical Manifestations

Gout is perhaps one of the most dramatic painful disorders in medical practice. In the early stages of the disease, clinical gout is monoarticular and occasionally pauciarticular and is frequently self-limited. The reason for the self-limitation of the gouty attacks is unclear. If the disease remains untreated and enters into a more chronic advanced stage, the attacks of gout become more frequent and often systemic manifestations such as general malaise and fever may be present. Both the sedimentation rate and the white blood cell count may be moderately elevated. Chronic polyarticular gout may be extremely debilitating and difficult to treat. In this state, uric acid may accumulate in the tissues as large deposits of sodium urate called tophi. Sometimes these deposits are superficial enough that they easily erode the overlying skin and drain a white toothpastelike or chalky material. Because of poor circulation in the area of the tophus, healing is impaired and skin ulcerations may form. Tophaceous deposits may also occur in the kidneys and other tissues, and uric acid crystals deposited in the renal parenchyma may cause renal failure. For instance, an abrupt increase in the load of uric acid to the kidney during treatment of a myeloproliferative disorder may cause uric acid precipitation in the renal tubes and lead to acute tubular necrosis. Fortunately, this complication is rare. More commonly uric acid stones may in individuals who are overproducers of uric acid.

Acute Attack

The acute attack of gout occurs suddenly and without a prodromal state. There is no joint stiffness or achiness preceding the attack. The person with gout may awaken in the middle of the night with a painful joint, often the great toe, and by the morning the attack is fully established with excruciating joint pain. The attack of gout may last for hours or a few days or longer, but eventually it may resolve spontaneously.

The attacks may occur many years apart or more frequently and eventually involve more joints. In the chronic tophaceous stage, the attacks of gout may be so severe that the patient is totally incapacitated, and fever and other toxic symptoms may be present. Because patients are quite ill, they may require hospitalization because of decompensation in other organs and systems and because septic arthritis may accompany gout. With proper treatment, the attack of gout can be brought under control, the patient may gradually resume usual activities, and joint function may be restored to baseline. When the diagnosis of gout is made, the patient should be told the nature of the condition and the value of the prophylactic treatment of the gout. During the early stages of the disease, it may not be necessary to treat the hyperuricemia as a prophylactic measure because the levels of uric acid are subject to spontaneous fluctuations, and unless a precipitating factor exists, the hyperuricemia may not constitute the only risk factor for gout. The patient with frequent attacks of gout or chronic tophaceous gout requires both treatment of the attack and the prophylactic treatment.

Laboratory and Radiological Findings

The diagnosis of gout is established by the identification of uric acid crystals in the joint fluid. Under polarized light microscopy, the uric acid crystals are negatively birefringent and may be seen within polymorphonuclear leukocytes with their typical needlelike shape. Often these leukocytes contain more than one crystal. The leukocyte count in the fluid is usually more than 5,000 and commonly between 15,000 and 30,000. The fluid obtained from joint aspiration has a yellow-green hue and some turbidity due to the presence of cells. It is always a good idea to send the fluid for culture because of the possibility of a concomitant septic process. This is especially important in the elderly.

Radiological Abnormalities

In the absence of tophi, the most characteristic finding is periarticular swelling and perhaps some osteopenia of the affected joint. In chronic tophaceous gout, the tophi may cause erosion of bone preferentially in para-articular areas, sometimes with speckles of calcifications within the tophus. Material available from aspiration of a tophus or from spontaneous drainage should be examined under polarized light microscopy for proper identification of sodium urate crystals.

Treatment

The pain of acute gout can be excruciating. Therefore, pain measures with appropriate medications such as narcotics are desirable. After the diagnosis is made, treatment with colchicine, NSAIDs, steroids, or adrenocorticotropic hormone (ACTH) may be given. If only one or a few joints are involved, the treatment of choice is colchicine 0.5 to 0.6 mg every hour until the acute attack is controlled or the patient develops gastrointestinal toxicity or a maximum dose of 6 to 8 tablets is reached. As a general rule, no more than 10 to 12 tablets should be given to treat the attack. Colchicine may be contraindicated in patients with preexisting gastrointestinal disease, liver disease, and chronic renal failure. When the intravenous route is preferred, it may be given at 2 mg in a proper diluent, usually normal saline, and the dose can be repeated in 12 hours. After this treatment no further colchicine should be given for at least 5 to 7 days because of the potential for bone marrow toxicity. Bone marrow function should be carefully monitored, especially in patients with borderline renal disease. In patients with polyarticular gout, colchicine may not be effective. NSAIDs can be effective, especially indomethacin 25 to 50 mg four times a day until the attack subsides. Maintenance treatment may be adequate with twice or thrice daily dosing. Other NSAIDs in high doses may also be effective; however, they may cause significant gastrointestinal and renal side effects.

Patients with chronic tophaceous gout are always at risk for new attacks of gout when the prophylactic regimen is discontinued, especially if it is allopurinol, whose effect of decreasing uric acid synthesis may create a gradient from the saturated tissues to the blood and in the process allow noninflammatory sodium uric acid crystals to dissolve and recrystallize in the monohydrate form, which is highly inflammatory. ACTH and prednisone are useful agents in the treatment of acute gouty arthritis. They are especially recommended in patients who have risk factors for the use of colchicine or NSAIDs. ACTH gel 40 units may be given once or twice daily for several days until the attack is controlled. Patient may receive colchicine for long-term prophylaxis along with the hypouricemic agent allopurinol. If the patient is allergic to allopurinol, the hyperuricemia may be treated with probenecid or sulfinpyrazone. But neither probenecid nor sulfinpyrazone should be used in patients who are overproducers of uric acid because of the risk of uric acid stone formation. The standard initial dose of probenecid is 500 mg/day, which is gradually increased to a maximum dose of 2 g. Sulfinpyrazone is given at 200 to 400 mg/day, with a maximum of 800 mg in two divided doses. Allopurinol is given to reduce uric acid synthesis; the usual dose is 300 mg/day but smaller doses of 100 or 200 mg/day may be sufficient to bring the uric acid back within normal range. Allopurinol has special indications in uric acid stone formers because it reduces their overproduction of uric acid. In spite of the progress in the understanding of the pathogenesis and treatment of gouty arthritis, many important issues remain to be solved. These include crystal nucleation and the role of tissue factors that are important in maintaining the stability of the uric acid in its solute state.

Pseudogout

The arthritis of pseudogout is due to the release of calcium pyrophosphate crystals into the joint space, resulting in acute or chronic inflammatory reaction. Calcium pyrophosphate crystals are preferentially seen in the cartilage of joints such as the knees, shoulders, wrists, and hips and in the intervertebral disk space. In spite of the recognized inflammatory property of the calcium pyrophosphate crystals, the disease does not occur in every patient with demonstrated calcium pyrophosphate deposition in joint cartilage. Both chondrocalcinosis and pseudogout are commonly associated with degenerative joint disease, although a clear pathogenetic relation between these conditions has not been established. Chondrocalcinosis is also frequently associated with diabetes, hypoparathyroidism, hemochromatosis, aging, and occasionally rheumatoid arthritis and other unrelated disorders.

Causation and Pathogenesis

There are two clinical forms of the disease, hereditary and sporadic. The hereditary form has been described in pedigrees in Czechoslovakia and Chile; the sporadic form can be associated with degenerative joint disease and the metabolic disorders described earlier in the chapter. Aging is an important factor for the development of chondrocalcinosis. Careful studies have shown an incidence of 6% in people over 70 years of age, and the incidence increases to 20 to 25% by the ninth decade of life. The factors leading to the deposition of calcium pyrophosphate crystals in the cartilage joints are unknown. Some persons with chondrocalcinosis shed crystals from the cartilage into the joint space, giving rise to an inflammatory reaction, most commonly in the knee joints and thereafter in order of frequency in the wrists, hips, carpals, elbows, shoulders, and the metacarpophalangeal joints. The inflammatory reaction is probably elicited by phagocytosis of the calcium pyrophosphate crystals by polymorphonuclear leukocytes. The synovial cells then undergo cell division, probably induced by the high intracellular calcium levels derived from the digestion of the calcium pyrophosphate crystals. The end result is the development of hypertrophic synovium and the secretion of the enzymes collagenase, stromelysin, and gelatinase, all having the property of destroying cartilage. The generation of calcium pyrophosphate crystals is complex and requires the presence of the chondrocytes, adenosine triphosphate (ATP), and nucleoside 5′-triphosphatase (NTPase), as demonstrated in experiments in vitro.

Clinical Manifestations

The general manifestations in pseudogout are pleomorphic, and a variety of clinical syndromes have been described. Most commonly, a patient has acute attacks of arthritis affecting one or a few joints, sometimes after physical activity and sometimes after surgery, especially surgery for hyperparathyroidism. The attack may last for hours, a few days, many days, or sometimes weeks. Once the attack resolves, the patient may remain asymptomatic until the next attack. In some cases, at the beginning the symptoms may occur sporadically, but later the attacks present more frequently and become chronic and polyarticular, sometimes with a rheumatoidlike course of evolution. The joint deformities that may occur are usually osteoarthritic. The definitive diagnosis is made by the identification of the positively birefringent calcium pyrophosphate crystals in the joint fluid with the polarizing microscope. Radiological findings of chondrocalcinosis alone may not be sufficient for diagnosis of pseudogout, because pseudogout without chondrocalcinosis has been described. Neurological symptoms due to calcium pyrophosphate crystal deposition in the spine with a picture of pseudomeningitis and cervical myelopathy from synovial hypertrophy have been reported.

Radiological Changes

The radiological findings in chondrocalcinosis are characteristic and most frequently found in the knee joints. The calcium deposits may be seen as a linear calcification in the meniscal cartilage or as a punctate deposit in the hyaline cartilage. Similar deposits may be found in the hips, wrists, symphysis pubis, and the intervertebral discs in the annulus fibrosus. In addition to the calcific deposits, the radiological changes in pseudogout, which are similar to those of degenerative joint disease, may also include subchondral cysts and involvement of the patellofemoral joints. On occasion, destructive joint disease with neuropathic appearance is seen. On the other hand, true Charcot arthropathy may be accompanied by calcium pyrophosphate deposition disease.

Treatment

In mild to moderate cases of pseudogout, joint aspiration alone may be sufficient to control the joint inflammation. In the more acute and severe cases NSAIDs such as indomethacin (Indocin) may be necessary. Colchicine orally or intravenously may also be helpful, and appropriate rest of the affected joint is part of the treatment of the acute attack. In the chronic polyarticular pseudogout indomethacin may be given for long periods, frequent joint aspirations are necessary to eliminate the crystals, and occasionally intra-articular steroid therapy has been helpful. Patients with the pseudorheumatoid form of the disease, after successful treatment with an NSAID, may show complete regression of the synovial hypertrophy, recovery of range of motion, and disappearance of the periarticular osteoporosis. These observations may be helpful in distinguishing chronic polyarticular pseudogout from true rheumatoid arthritis, in which these favorable changes are not likely to occur with NSAID treatment alone.

Arthritis Caused by Apatite Crystals

Several syndromes of acute arthritis and periarthritis have been described in association with hydroxyapatite crystals in and around joint tissues. Because the crystals are not birefringent, they cannot be seen with the polarizing microscope. The apatite crystals and other basic calcium phosphate crystals are quite small, varying in length from 50 to 500 nm. They tend to form conglomerates that can be visualized when stained with the alizarin red S stain. The individual crystals can be seen only with the electron microscope. The joint manifestations may be acute, with severe inflammatory changes and moderate to high white blood cell counts in the joint fluid. The joints most frequently affected are the shoulders, hips, elbows, wrists, and fingers; the attacks of arthritis or periarthritis may respond to NSAIDs, ACTH injections, and colchicine. It is appropriate to try joint lavage in persistent cases.

RHEUMATOID VARIANTS, PSORIATIC ARTHRITIS, ANKYLOSING SPONDYLITIS, AND REITER'S SYNDROME

Psoriatic arthritis is a very aberrant disease in terms of its clinical presentation and response to treatment. The disease can affect the peripheral joints as well as the axial skeleton. It is equally distributed between men and women, with the men presenting spondylitis more frequently and the women, the symmetric polyarthritis. The disease occurs most frequently in whites, and it appears to be associated with certain genes, including HLA Cw6, and HLA B27 may be associated when there is ankylosing spondylitis. The prevalence of the disease is about 0.1% in this country. Approximately 30% of the patients are positive for HLA B27. At the beginning, the disease has a tendency to affect the joints in a nonsymmetrical fashion, but later it becomes symmetrical. Joint involvement is progressive and sometimes severe, with destruction of the articular cartilage, and bone resorption may be quite dramatic. The pathogenesis of the disease is complex, requiring genetic, environmental, and immunological factors that determine disease propensity and the clinical features. The fact that the psoriasis usually precedes the onset of joint disease has led to some speculation regarding the role of gram-positive cocci commonly associated with the psoriatic plaque in the pathogenesis of psoriatic arthritis, with the possible release of superantigens resulting in a reaction in both the skin and joints.

Clinical Manifestations

Disease may be monoarticular or pauciarticular, affecting mainly the large joints. In about 30 to 50% of the cases it is fairly symmetrical and similar to rheumatoid arthritis and less frequently involves the axial skeleton. The sacroiliac joint may be involved in asymmetrical fashion, and ankylosing spondylitis may be distributed along the spine in an irregular fashion. The sacroiliac and spine involvement may be the source of severe pain, which can be difficult to treat. Involvement of the DIP joints is characteristic of this disease, and erosive changes are typical. Pitting of the fingernails and hyperkeratosis may be present. Sometimes the psoriasis and the arthritis have a parallel course, but many times they are totally independent of each other. Arthritis mutilans is a form of psoriatic arthritis of the fingers characterized by extensive bone resorption and destruction that causes typical telescoping of the joints. Bony ankylosis, especially of the distal and proximal interphalangeal joints, is fairly common. Enthesopathy characteristic of psoriatic arthritis is clinically manifested by severe pain due to inflammation at the attachment site of tendons and ligaments, the heel being the most commonly affected.

Radiological Changes

The radiological manifestations include erosion of the articular surfaces, sometimes with significant periosteal reaction and frequently affecting the distal interphalangeal joints, which is rare in rheumatoid arthritis. The ankylosing spondylitis is asymmetrical, and syndesmophytes appear to be of the nonmarginal type, arising from the midportion of the vertebral body and extending to the midportion of the vertebral body above or below. Sacroiliitis with irregular and asymmetric involvement is common. Other typical joint changes include pen-and-cup deformity and fluffy periosteitis.

Treatment

NSAIDs should be the first line of treatment but in disease that is progressive and unresponsive to them, methotrexate 15 to 20 mg weekly may help to control both the psoriasis and the arthritis. Sulfasalazine 2 to 3 g/day may be helpful for the arthritis but not for the psoriasis. Other antirheumatic drugs, such as antimalarials, gold, azathioprine (Imuran), and others, usually in combination therapy, have been used with some success.

Reiter's syndrome is a form of reactive arthritis that affects usually young males, who may carry the HLA B27 gene. The syndrome is characterized by a clinical triad of conjunctivitis, nongonococcal urethritis, and arthritis. Sexual exposure often precedes it, but sometimes it follows a diarrheic disease caused by enteric pathogens such as *Shigella, Salmonella,* and *Campylobacter,* whereas *Chlamydia trachomatis* is associated with sexually transmitted disease arthritis. The disease may affect the peripheral joints as well as the axial skeleton. Nonarthritic clinical manifestations include lesions in the skin and oral mucosa. Keratoderma blennorrhagicum commonly affects the soles or the palms, appearing in the form of papular lesions that later evolve into hyperkeratotic lesions resembling psoriasis. Fingernails and toenails adopt a thickened structure without pitting. Circinate balanitis characteristically affects the glans or shaft of the penis. The lesions have a serpiginous appearance and are often located around the meatus. Mucosal ulcers are also frequent. This disease may be self-limited, but it may also be chronic and develop a chronic polyarthritis and ankylosing spondylitis. Other systemic involvement includes cardiac and aortic disease, neurological manifestations, and peripheral neuropathy. In immunosuppressed persons, such as those with acquired immunodeficiency syndrome (AIDS), the disease may be particularly severe and resistant to treatment.

Urethritis is characterized by clear urethral secretion and absence of gonorrhea. In the dysenteric form the diarrhea follows infection with enteric pathogens, but some patients also develop nongonococcal urethritis. Conjunctivitis is common, and acute anterior uveitis of an intermittent or chronic course is seen in about 20% of patients. The conjunctivitis is moderately intense and resolves spontaneously in a few days. The arthritis of Reiter's syndrome is typically pauciarticular, affecting mainly the large joints of the lower extremities, such as the knees and ankles, also the small joints of the feet and the fingers. The arthritis is exquisitely painful, and when it affects the digits, the entire finger may be swollen, giving the finger a sausagelike appearance. Sacroiliitis is noted in about 17% of the patients and spondylitis in 7%. Pericarditis, sometimes complicated with aortic valve regurgitation and heart block, is rare but may require intervention with valve replacement and pacemaker implant, respectively.

Patients with the chronic form of the disease develop anemia. Leukocytosis is common, usually low grade, and the sedimentation rate is elevated. These patients tend to develop immunoglobulin (Ig) A antibodies to the organism thought to trigger it, such as *Chlamydia.* Some 60 to 70% of patients with reactive arthritis are HLA B27 positive. The joint fluid may reveal moderate to high white blood cell count with predominance of polymorphonuclear leukocytes and mononuclear cells displaying nucleophagocytosis. The complement level may be normal or elevated in the joint fluid and in the serum. Arthritis of Reiter's syndrome is often self-limited, but while it is active, treatment with NSAIDs may be helpful. In severe cases short periods of bed rest, nutritional care, and a regimen of exercise to restore muscle mass and fitness are useful complements to the anti-inflammatory drug regimen. Analgesics may be used for pain control. Patients with AIDS present a tremendous challenge because often these patients develop a more severe and accelerated course of the disease.

ARTHROPATHY ASSOCIATED WITH CHRONIC INFLAMMATORY BOWEL DISEASE

Ulcerative colitis and Crohn's disease may be complicated by peripheral joint disease and ankylosing spondylitis. The peripheral joint disease affects large joints and is often monoarticular and rarely polyarticular. In ulcerative colitis, the arthritis follows very closely the course of the bowel symptoms, whereas in Crohn's disease this correlation is less likely. The joint symptoms are self-limited and the joint fluid is inflammatory, containing mainly polymorphonuclear leukocytes. Rheumatoid factor is negative. The ankylosing spondylitis of inflammatory bowel disease is clinically similar to the idiopathic type and radiologically shows the typical bamboo spine appearance. Treatment of the arthropathy is symptomatic, with NSAIDs. The laboratory tests often show anemia, elevated erythrocyte sedimentation rate, and antineutrophil cytoplasmic antibodies specifically directed against lactoferrin or pANCA. This antibody is formed in about 60% of patients with ulcerative colitis and rarely in patients with Crohn's disease.

Ankylosing Spondylitis

Ankylosing spondylitis is a disease of the axial skeleton affecting the sacroiliac joints, often the entire spine, and occasionally the large para-axial joints such as the hip and shoulder joints. The disease appears to be systemic because of involvement of the eye (with iritis), aorta, and lungs and development of amyloidosis, which may complicate the course of the disease. Ankylosing spondylosis affects young men more frequently than women by 3:1 to 4:1 ratio. The disease may have a chronic indolent course compatible with a fully productive life, but it can also be incapacitating and deforming. Its cause is unknown. Genetic factors appear to be important in view of the fact that HLA B27 antigen is present in over 90% of the patients. The most common symptom is low-back pain accompanied by progressive decrease of motion in the lower spine due to early involvement of the sacroiliac joints and the lumbar spine. The diagnosis may not be obvious initially because of the subtle nature of the discomfort and the intermittent nature of the back pain. The peripheral joint involvement occurs in about 20% of cases. The natural course of the disease is chronic, progressively fusing the spine, often uniformly from the top of the spine to the lumbosacral junction. Characteristically there is progressive immobilization of the lumbar, thoracic, and cervical spines due to fusion of the apophyseal joints. The fusion of the costovertebral joints causes restrictive chest expansion and puts the patient at risk for respiratory problems due to restrictive lung disease. Fusion of the cervical spine may cause important distortions in the alignment of the neck, and the patient may end up with a fixed flexion of the neck or even flexion of the entire thoracic spine. Patients with this type of spinal and neck deformities are unable to look forward and often adapt by flexing their knees in order to have a limited forward visual field. Many lose their spine mobility without being aware that the spinal fusion is taking place because the fusion is painless. Although the diagnosis of ankylosing spondylitis is mainly clinical and radiological, testing for HLA B27 may help in establishing the diagnosis in early cases, when the symptoms are not very clear-cut. In patients with well-established disease, the HLA B27 test is not necessary.

Radiological Changes

Radiographs of the spine may show the early changes in the sacroiliac joints, with erosions of the iliac side of the sacroiliac joint and subcortical osteitis. Later, the sacroiliac joint fuses, and as the disease progresses, one may see a squaring of the vertebral bodies, fusion of the apophyseal joints, calcification of the anterior and posterior spinal ligaments, calcification of the annulus fibrosus, and the production of marginal syndesmophytes. When the entire spine is affected by these changes, it acquires the typical appearance of bamboo spine. The joints most commonly affected and at risk for sustaining significant cartilage loss are primarily the hip joints. The shoulders may be symptomatic, but usually there is no appreciable joint destruction. Patients with end-stage hip disease may require joint arthroplasties; however, postoperatively these procedures may complicate with myositis ossificans and bony bridging that may cause severe immobility to the operated joint. To minimize this complication, patients are usually given low-dose radiation to inhibit ectopic bone formation. Enthesitis, or inflammation and pain, at the site of attachment of tendons and ligaments on bone is common. In ankylosing spondylitis, enthesitis occurs especially in

the heel at the site of insertion of the Achilles tendon in the os calcis. Ankylosing spondylitis may present a number of extraskeletal conditions including acute anterior uveitis, which is characterized by photophobia, blurred vision and increased tearing, thus the pupils may become irregular if posterior adhesions form. Aortitis of the ascending aorta produces aortic regurgitation and the patient may require aortic valve replacement. The lungs may show apical fibrosis on chest radiographs.

Treatment

The appropriate use of NSAIDs in ankylosing spondylitis is reserved for the time during which the spine is symptomatic. But when patients fuse the spine without pain, no treatment is necessary. An important point is to make sure that the patient understands the nature of the disease and the actual progression toward fusion of the spine. It is important to establish prophylactic measures to prevent skeletal deformities that may cause significant disability and be a risk factor for other complications, such as falls. Falls are particularly dangerous in patients with ankylosing spondylitis because of the markedly decreased flexibility of the spine and the inability to cushion a mechanical impact on the spine due to the bony ankylosis and immobility. The fractures tend to be through fractures. If serious displacement occurs, the patient may be at risk for spinal cord damage. In general, a program of exercise to maintain fitness and good diaphragmatic function as well as good posture may help prevent serious complications over the long term. Steroids are usually not effective in the treatment of ankylosing spondylitis. There has been some success in the use of sulfasalazine, especially in patients whose inflammatory bowel disease is associated with ankylosing spondylitis. The prognosis of the illness is generally good, especially if serious skeletal deformities can be prevented or minimized. If this can be accomplished by allowing fusion of the spine to occur as physiologically as possible and by the judicious use of NSAIDs, complemented by appropriate exercise programs and hygienic measures to prevent deformities, these patients may achieve fully productive lives.

BACTERIAL AND VIRAL ARTHRITIS

Septic arthritis is usually secondary to a blood-bone infection. Only rarely it is due to direct infection such as complicated prosthetic joint surgery or penetrating injuries. The important predisposing elements in the pathogenesis of septic arthritis are preexisting joint damage due to bone trauma or degenerative joint disease, chronic inflammation, aging, malnutrition, drug abuse, diabetes, steroid treatment, and an immunosuppressed state. Septic arthritis should be suspected in an individual with persistent joint pain and inflammation occurring in the course of an illness of unclear nature or in the course of a well-documented infection, such as pneumococcal pneumonia, staphylococcal sepsis, or urosepsis. Often one joint is involved, but sometimes two or more are. The intensity of the local symptoms range from minimal to extremely severe, with rapid incapacitation due to joint destruction. Aspiration of joint fluid must be done as soon as possible to identify organisms with the Gram stain, and appropriate cultures must be processed at once. The white blood cell count in the joint fluid may vary from 5,000 cells to more than 100,000, with 90% of the cells being polymorphonuclear leukocytes. The appearance of the fluid may vary from cloudy to purulent. Occasionally septic arthritis coexists with either gout or pseudogout. Close attention should be paid to patients who are immunosuppressed or markedly debilitated and to those on steroid therapy, because of their blunted fever mechanism and decreased inflammatory response. Antibiotic treatment should have good coverage with broad-spectrum antibiotics until the specific infectious agent is isolated and a more specific treatment can be given. Frequent joint aspirations are recommended to eliminate the pus and prevent development of fibrous adhesions, which can greatly limit the range of motion of the affected joint. The postinfectious inflammation may last for many weeks. Bacterial products are eliminated slowly and are probably the source of a biochemically induced inflammatory reaction. The role of bacterial products in the pathogenesis of reactive arthritis has been demonstrated in patients with *Yersinia* infections. Infections in prosthetic joints may present acutely or in a low-grade smoldering fashion. If an infection is suspected in a prosthetic joint, the workup should include a sedimentation rate and direct joint aspirations. The treatment of an infected prosthesis includes the removal of the hardware and intravenous antibiotic treatment for 6 to 8 weeks. Reimplantation of a new prosthesis may be possible if after the antibiotic treatment, the joint aspiration proves sterile.

Viral Arthritis

Viral infections may be complicated with arthralgias and arthritis. In hepatitis B joint symptoms appear during the prodromal state prior to the clinical onset of jaundice. A low-grade fever is common, as are pleomorphic skin rashes and lymphadenopathy. The fingers, knees, shoulders, and ankles are involved, usually symmetrically, and the wrists and elbows are affected less frequently. The joints may appear red and swollen and quite painful with movement, or they may be only mildly inflamed. The articular symptoms disappear spontaneously after a few days or weeks, but sometimes NSAIDs are necessary to control joint pain. Rubella can cause polyarthritis of symmetrical distribution when the rash is still present. This complication occurs mainly in women and tends to be self-limited. Salicylates are effective treatment, but other NSAIDs are equally satisfactory. A second type of rubella arthritis is seen in children who have received vaccination. The joint symptoms last 2 to 4 weeks, and their course is benign. The treatment is bed rest and aspirin. Varicella, mumps, and other viral illnesses rarely cause joint symptoms. Parvovirus B19 infection, or fifth disease, causes a symmetrical polyarthritis in children and in adults. The joint involve-

ment suggests rheumatoid arthritis; in some cases the disease may last longer, but characteristically it is a nonerosive articular disease.

POLYMYALGIA RHEUMATICA AND TEMPORAL ARTERITIS

Polymyalgia rheumatica usually affects people over 50 years of age and may be associated with temporal arteritis. Whites and women are at highest risk for it. The symptoms may be initially subtle, with generalized stiffness and pain, and as the disease progresses, the stiffness and pain become more severe. Synovitis may not be clinically detectable, but it may show up on synovial biopsy specimens, especially those taken from the shoulder. The sedimentation rate is usually accelerated, over 60 mm per hour.

When temporal arteritis is associated with polymyalgia, the patient may have temporal headache, claudication of the jaw, diplopia, and motor and sensory symptoms involving the cranial nerves and the upper extremities. The most serious complication is visual loss, which is irreversible. The temporal artery may be prominent and painful to touch and the temporal artery pulse absent. Biopsy of the temporal artery reveals giant-cell arteritis. The treatment of polymyalgia rheumatica requires 10 to 15 mg of prednisone a day. This is usually sufficient to induce a remission. Treatment of temporal arteritis requires high steroid dosage, 40 to 60 mg of prednisone a day. The duration of the treatment in either situation is guided by the clinical manifestations and the sedimentation rate but is generally long term. After a year of treatment, nearly half of the patients have a relapse and require additional steroid treatment, sometimes for several years. When steroid tapering is difficult, cyclophosphamide in doses of 50 to 100 mg daily may facilitate steroid reduction, decreasing the risk of complications deriving from long-term steroid treatment.

Rheumatological Disorders in Patients Infected with HIV

It has been recognized for some time that patients with human immunodeficiency virus (HIV) infection may present peculiar rheumatological complaints and diseases. Diffuse body aches and pains without arthritis are fairly common among HIV patients. For some unclear reasons, these symptoms tend to worsen with the progression of the viral infection. The neuropathic disorder of HIV may cause severe to excruciating pain and is extremely difficult to treat. A painful form of arthritis whose causation and pathogenesis are unclear has been associated with HIV. Preexisting rheumatological disorders may present an accelerated and unusually severe course, such as is seen with Reiter's syndrome and psoriatic arthritis. These diseases may also appear after the onset of HIV infection and may have a clinical course very similar to the primary disease. A form of ankylosing spondylitis has also been described. Painful inflammation of muscle with CD8 lymphocytes typical of HIV may be the source of severe disability and discomfort. The muscle enzymes may be normal or elevated and the electromyograph pattern is characteristic of polymyositis. Because of the immunosuppressed state, these patients are likely to develop numerous infectious complications. Muscle infection with bacterial pathogens is a serious complication and must be recognized early. An autoimmune disorder with lupuslike features has also been described. A more benign course of rheumatoid arthritis has been observed in HIV-infected persons. This is thought to be due to the decrease of CD4 lymphocytes. Perhaps an important clue in the differential diagnosis of these rheumatological syndromes in HIV patients with a primary rheumatic disease is the low frequency with which autoimmune antibodies are found. The treatment of these disorders in HIV patients should be carried out with caution, but there is no contraindication to the use of NSAIDs, low-dose steroids, and even methotrexate.

CONCLUSION

In the past 10 years, there has been an explosion of new information regarding the nature of rheumatological disorders, some of which are discussed in this chapter. It is clear that in the years to come, further understanding of the basic disease mechanisms, pathogenesis, and causes will be brought forward. It is to be hoped that the new knowledge will serve as the basis for new treatments that in turn will help to decrease the pain and discomfort that these diseases cause and to decrease or prevent disability. I also suspect that as we enter the new millennium, there may be real cures for some of these rheumatological disorders.

References

1. Murphey MD, Quale JL, Martin NL, et al. Computed radiography in musculoskeletal imaging: state of the art. AJR Am J Roentgenol 1992; 158:19–27.
2. Statsny P. Association of the B-cell alloantigen Drw4 with rheumatoid arthritis. N Engl J Med 1978;298:869–871.
3. Gregersen PK, Silver J, Winchester RJ. The shared epitope hypothesis: an approach to understanding the molecular genetics of susceptibility to rheumatoid arthritis. Arthritis Rheum 1987;30:1205–1213.
4. Wilkins RF, Nepom GT, Marks CR, et al. Association of HLA-Dw16 with rheumatoid arthritis in Yakima Indians. Arthritis Rheum 1991;34:207–214.
5. Elliott MJ, Maini RN, Feldmann M, et al. Randomised double-blind comparison of chimeric monoclonal antibody to tumor necrosis factor alpha (cA2) versus placebo in rheumatoid arthritis. Lancet 1994; 344:1105–1110.
6. Weyand CM, Hicok KC, Conn DI, Goronzy JJ. The inflammation of HLA-DRB1 genes on disease severity in rheumatoid arthritis. Ann Intern Med 1992;117:801–806.
7. Albani S, Carson DA, Roudier J. Genetic and environmental factors in the immunopathogenesis of rheumatoid arthritis. Rheum Dis Clin North Am 1992;18:729–740.
8. Albani S, Keystone EC, Ollier WER, et al. Positive selection in autoimmunity: abnormal immune responses to a bacterial dnaJ antigen determinant in patients with early rheumatoid arthritis. Nat Med 1995;1:488–452.
9. Carson DA, Tan EM. Apoptosis in rheumatic diseases. Bull Rheum Dis 1995;44:1–3.
10. Mountz JD, Wu J, Cheng J, Zhou T. Autoimmune disease: a problem of defective apoptosis. Arthritis Rheum 1994;37:1415–1420.
11. Arnett FC, Edworthy SM, Bloch DA, et al. The American Rheumatism Association 1987 revised criteria for the classification of rheumatoid arthritis. Arthritis Rheum 1988;31:315–324.
12. Krane SM. Mechanisms of tissue destruction in rheumatoid arthritis. In: McCarthy DJ, Koopman WJ, eds. Arthritis and allied conditions. 12th ed. Malvern, PA: Lea & Febiger, 1993;763–779.
13. Weinblatt ME, Kaplan H, Germain BF, et al. Methotrexate in rheumatoid arthritis: a five-year prospective multicenter study. Arthritis Rheum 1994;37:1492–1498.
14. O'Dell JR, Haire CE, Palmer W, et al. Treatment of early rheumatoid arthritis with minocycline or placebo: results of a randomized, double-blind, placebo-controlled trial. Arthritis Rheum 1997;40:842–848.
15. Kirwan JR. The effect of glucocorticoids on joint destruction in rheumatoid with regard to early and aggressive treatment of people with RA: The Arthritis and Rheumatism Council Low-dose Glucocorticoid Study Group. N Engl J Med 1995;333:142–146.
16. Ettinger WH, Burns R, Messier SP, et al. A randomized trial comparing aerobic exercise and resistance exercise with a health education program in older adults with knee osteoarthritis: the fitness arthritis and seniors trial (FAST). JAMA 1997;277:25–31.
17. Fries JF, Gurkirpal S, Morfeld D, et al. Relationship of running to musculoskeletal pain with age: a six-year longitudinal study. Arthritis Rheum 1996;39:64–72.
18. Terkeltaub R. Pathogenesis and treatment of crystal-induced inflammation. In: McCarthy DJ, Koopman WJ, eds. Arthritis and allied conditions. 13th ed. Baltimore: Williams & Wilkins, 1996;2085–2102.
19. Paul H, Reginato AJ, Schumacher HR. Alizarin red S staining as a screening test to detect calcium compounds in synovial fluid. Arthritis Rheum 1983;26:191–200.
20. Tomfohrde J, Silverman A, Barnes R, et al. Gene for familial psoriasis susceptibility mapped to the distal end of human chromosome 17q. Science 1994;264:1141–1145.
21. Hammer RE, Maika SD, Richardson JA, et al. Spontaneous inflammatory disease in transgenic rats expressing HLA-B27 and human B2m: an animal model of HLA-B27-associated human disorders. Cell 1990;63:1099–1112.
22. Nickoloff BJ, Turka LA. Immunological functions of nonprofessional antigen-presenting cells: new insights from studies of T-cell interactions with keratinocytes. Immunol Today 1994;15:464–469.
23. Panayi GS. Immunology of psoriasis and psoriatic arthritis. Bailliere's Clin Rheumatol 1994;8:419–427.
24. Duerr RH, Targan SR, Landers CJ, et al. Neutrophil cytoplasmic antibodies: a link between primary sclerosing cholangitis and ulcerative colitis. Gastroenterol 1991;100:1385–1391.
25. Inman RD. Rheumatic manifestations of hepatitis B virus infection. Semin Arthritis Rheum 1982;11:406–420.
26. Smith CA, Petty RE, Tingle AJ. Rubella virus and arthritis. Rheum Dis Clin North Am 1987;13:265–274.
27. Howson CP, Howe CJ, Fineberg HV, eds. Adverse effects of pertussis and rubella vaccines: a report of the committee to review the adverse consequences of pertussis and rubella vaccines. Washington: National Academy Press, 1991;187–205.
28. White DG, Woolf AD, Mortimer PP, et al. Human parvovirus arthropathy. Lancet 1985;1:419–421.
29. Naides SJ, Scharosch LL, Foto F, et al. Rheumatologic manifestations of human parvovirus B19 infection in adults: initial two-year clinical experience. Arthritis Rheum 1990;33:1297–1309.
30. Calabrese LH. Human immunodeficiency virus infection and arthritis. Rheum Dis Clin North Am 1991;19:477–488.
31. Workowski K, Agudelo CA. Musculoskeletal infections in patients with human immunodeficiency virus infection. Medicine (Balt) 1997; 76:284–294.

CHAPTER 14

Controversies in Fibromyalgia and Myofascial Pain Syndromes

Don L. Goldenberg

DEFINITIONS AND HISTORICAL PERSPECTIVES

The concept of fibrositis and fibromyalgia syndromes dates back to the early 1800s. Balfour and Valleix, as well as Gowers, provided very accurate descriptions of the shooting pains reported by patients and the painful soft-tissue points found with palpation (1). However, the term fibrositis was used loosely and applied to many musculoskeletal disorders, some of which eventually proved to have specific pathophysiological explanations, such as polymyositis or brachial neuritis. Furthermore, the initial report of inflammatory hyperplasia of the connective tissue in muscle was never confirmed. Thus fibrositis fell out of favor in academic circles for most of this century. Many considered it to be a nonentity. Others equated fibrositis with psychogenic rheumatism because no objective abnormalities could be found.

CURRENT DEFINITION OF FIBROMYALGIA

Smythe and Moldofsky (2) in the mid-1970s reported that certain anatomical locations, termed tender points, were useful to distinguish patients with fibromyalgia from normal subjects. They also reported that patients with fibromyalgia had a stage 4 sleep disturbance and that experimental selective stage 4 disturbance produced the symptoms and muscle tenderness consistent with fibromyalgia.

The term fibromyalgia was substituted for fibrositis in the 1980s. Diagnostic criteria for fibromyalgia were suggested, each based on the exclusion of rheumatic and systemic diseases and the presence of certain symptoms and tender points. The location of these tender points were often identical to soft-tissue areas most tender in regional pain conditions such as tennis elbow, costochondritis, and cervical strain syndromes. The American College of Rheumatology 1990 criteria for the classification of fibromyalgia have been widely adopted for clinical and research studies (Table 14.1) (3). In that study 293 patients with fibromyalgia and 265 control patients were interviewed and examined by trained, blinded assessors. Controls were matched for age and sex, and controls had a rheumatic disorder that could be easily confused with fibromyalgia, such as "possible" rheumatoid arthritis or neck and back pain syndromes.

The combination of widespread pain, defined as above and below the waist in both extremities and axial, and at least 11 of 18 specified tender points yielded a sensitivity of 88.4% and a specificity of 81.1%. There were no significant differences in patients considered to have primary or concomitant versus secondary fibromyalgia, and for classification purposes, such distinctions were to be discarded. No exclusions were made for laboratory or radiographic findings.

CURRENT DEFINITION OF MYOFASCIAL PAIN SYNDROMES

Myofascial pain, historically and currently, has been thought to be a regional pain syndrome (4, 5). Myofascial pain has been defined by the presence of trigger points, a localized area of deep muscle tenderness in a taut band of muscle (Table 14.2). Pressure on the trigger point refers pain to well-defined areas distal to the actual trigger point. Some authors also insist on the presence of a local twitch response, a visible or palpable contraction of the muscle produced by a rapid snap of the examining finger of the taut band of muscle. Trigger points may be latent, that is, not associated with pain until they are activated by pressure or trauma.

The most important difference between fibromyalgia and myofascial pain is the presence of trigger points and the notion that myofascial pain is a localized or regional pain disorder, whereas fibromyalgia causes generalized pain (Table 14.3). Furthermore, the pain of myofascial syndrome is said to be immediately and often permanently relieved by local treatment methods, such as application of a cold spray and passive stretch of the involved muscle (4). Such treatment has not been

Table 14.1.　The American College of Rheumatology 1990 Criteria for the Classification of Fibromyalgia

1. History of widespread pain
   Definition. Pain is considered widespread when all of the following are present: pain in the left side of the body; pain in the right side of the body; pain above the waist; and pain below the waist. In addition, axial skeletal pain (cervical spine, anterior chest, thoracic spine, or low back) must be present. In this definition, shoulder and buttock pain is considered as pain for each involved side. "Low-back" pain is considered lower segment pain.
2. Pain in 11 of 18 tender point sites on digital palpation.
   Definition. Pain, on digital palpation, must be present in at least 11 of the following 18 tender point sites:
     Occiput: bilateral, at the suboccipital muscle insertions
     Low cervical: bilateral, at the anterior aspects of the intertransverse spaces at C5–C7
     Trapezius: bilateral, at the midpoint of the upper border
     Supraspinatus: bilateral, at origins, above the scapula spine near the medial border
     Second rib: bilateral, at the second costochondral junctions, just lateral to the junctions on upper surfaces
     Lateral epicondyle: bilateral, 2-cm distal to the epicondyles
     Gluteal: bilateral, in upper outer quadrants of buttocks in anterior fold of muscle
     Greater trochanter: bilateral, posterior to the trochanteric prominence
     Knee: bilateral, at the medial fat pad proximal to the joint line
   Digital palpation should be performed with an approximate force of 4 kg. For a tender point to be considered "positive," the subject must state that the palpation was painful. "Tender" is not to be considered "painful."

For classification purposes, patients are said to have fibromyalgia if both criteria are satisfied. Widespread pain must have been present for at least 3 months. The presence of a second clinical disorder does not exclude the diagnosis of fibromyalgia. From Wolfe F, et al. The American College of Rheumatology 1990 criteria for the classification of fibromyalgia: report of the multicentre criteria committee. Arthritis Rheum 1990;33:160–172.

Table 14.2.　Definition of Myofascial Pain (Trigger Points)

- Found in muscle belly, tender on palpation when "active"
- Located within a taut band of muscle
- Snapping across the trigger point elicits a local twitch response
- When "active," trigger points refer pain in specific zone

successful in fibromyalgia, which is usually a chronic pain disorder. Most important, trigger points are classically associated with regional pain, whereas the pain of fibromyalgia is generalized and not necessarily related to tender points.

The term repetitive strain syndrome has often been used when the myofascial pain followed activities involving repetitious movement or postural changes (6). In the mid-1980s an epidemic of such syndromes was reported in Australia (6). By the early 1990s the condition had again receded to a low endemic rate similar to that observed a decade earlier. These changes were related to medicolegal and societal issues rather than specific workplace modification.

Unfortunately, the literature on myofascial pain has been largely uncontrolled, and until recently there have been no studies of comparable groups of patients with fibromyalgia and myofascial pain. Therefore, the concept that myofascial pain is limited to a single anatomical region, improved or cured with local treatment, and not associated with fatigue and sleep disturbances may be a result of anecdotal studies and failure to assess chronicity and systemic symptoms. Particularly important has been the absence of longitudinal studies of myofascial pain to determine whether a subset of patients do indeed have chronic pain and whether such pain evolves into a more characteristic fibromyalgia syndrome.

My colleagues and I examined fibromyalgia and myofascial pain patients, as well as normal controls, for tender points and trigger points (7). The myofascial pain patients reported less painful sites. Systemic complaints, such as fatigue, were most frequent in the fibromyalgia patients but were also common in myofascial pain. With direct pressure, tender points referred pain less often than trigger points. Muscle tenderness was present in more than 75% of muscle examined in both patient groups. Most important, tender points were present in more than half the sites evaluated in myofascial pain patients, yet trigger points were found in fewer than 20% of both myofascial pain and fibromyalgia patients. Furthermore, latent trigger points, taut muscle bands, and muscle twitch were found equally in both patient groups and normal controls. However, there was significant variation among raters in finding trigger points.

Table 14.3.　Distinguishing Fibromyalgia from Myofascial Pain Syndromes

Characteristic	Fibromyalgia syndrome	Myofascial pain syndrome
Prevalence	4%–6% of general medical patients	30%–60% of patients in chronic pain clinics
Sex	10:1 female	Equal
Onset	50% idiopathic; 20% physical trauma; 20% viral; 10% emotional	Trauma or strain
Sleep disorder, fatigue	Always	Often
Pain	Diffuse	Localized
Pain referral (trigger point)	?	Specific patterns
Tenderness (tender point)	Multiple spots at tendon insertion, in muscle belly, or over bone	Few spots in muscle belly only
Palpable taut band with twitch response of muscle	?	Present
Treatment	Medications, exercise	Local myofascial "release"
Outcome	Usually chronic	Usually self-limited

The definition of a trigger point, central to the concept of myofascial pain, is controversial and varies from one author to another (7). There is significant variation among raters and in individual raters in performing an examination for trigger points. In contrast, the tender point examination is very simple and has been found to have good validity and reliability (8). Many investigators consider that myofascial pain is simply localized fibromyalgia, more often affecting the upper body.

Because neither condition has any known pathological explanation, such disorders cannot be convincingly demonstrated to be based on hard scientific facts. The absence of objective physical signs, laboratory tests, and radiologic features makes the diagnosis suspect. However, during the past decade diagnostic criteria—largely employing patients' symptoms—have been applied to large groups of patients with fibromyalgia. This has allowed investigators to promote the notion that fibromyalgia is a definable syndrome. With application of such clinical criteria to ambulatory general medical patients, fibromyalgia has been found in 4 to 6% of the population (9). Fibromyalgia syndrome is one of the second or third most common diagnoses made by rheumatologists in practice, and 4 million to 6 million Americans may have fibromyalgia. Thus far, rigid diagnostic criteria for myofascial pain syndrome have not been applied to general medical patients, and therefore there are no good estimates of comparable frequency.

DIAGNOSIS AND DIFFERENTIAL DIAGNOSIS

The two cardinal features of fibromyalgia are generalized chronic pain and diffuse tenderness at discrete anatomic locations, termed tender points (3) (Table 14.1). The majority of patients also complain of fatigue, sleep disturbances, headaches, irritable bowel syndrome, paresthesias, Raynaud-like symptoms, depression, and anxiety. The fatigue is often as debilitating as the pain. About 80 to 90% of patients are women, and the peak age of onset is 30 to 50 years. However, fibromyalgia is common in children and the elderly. The point prevalence of fibromyalgia is 2% of the population and up to 7% in women between ages 60 and 70.

On examination, patients usually appear well, with no obvious systemic illness or articular abnormalities. Many patients describe some joint or soft-tissue swelling, but no obvious synovitis is present. Fibromyalgia may be present concurrently with systemic arthritis, so the presence of osteoarthritis or rheumatoid arthritis does not exclude coexistent fibromyalgia. Patients invariably complain of muscle weakness; however, formal muscle testing does not reveal significant weakness provided the pain does not prevent the patient from achieving maximal effort. Numbness and tingling, especially in the extremities, are present in more than 75% of patients, yet a neurologic examination does not demonstrate any significant abnormalities.

Thus the only reliable finding on examination is multiple tender points. The examiner must gain experience with the

Table 14.4.   Performing a Tender Point Examination

Select 4 to 9 sites as suspected tender points, and check these same sites bilaterally in all suspected fibromyalgia patients.
Similarly, select 2 to 3 sites for control (i.e., nontender points).
Palpate over site gently and feel for spasm; examine skin for tenderness or redness
Apply increasing pressure with your thumb or one finger until the patient (a) tells you to stop because of pain, (b) withdraws, or (c) grimaces.
Compare tenderness in suspected and control points, and compare with your experience in other patients and in normal controls (or on yourself). Inspect site examined for erythema "flare."

technique and the location of these sites (Table 14.4). The patient should be seated comfortably on the examination table and queried as to the presence of pain following the palpation of each bilateral anatomical site. Palpation should be done with the thumb or forefinger, applying pressure approximately equal to a force of 4 kg (8). Excessive force may elicit pain in anyone. A systematic palpation of each of the proposed nine tender point pairs should be followed. Control anatomical sites, such as over the thumbnail, mid-forearm, and forehead, should also be palpated. These sites are not as painful on pressure as the selected anatomical sites, although most patients with fibromyalgia are more tender to palpation than normal controls in many muscle and soft-tissue sites.

The diagnostic utility of a tender point evaluation has been objectively documented with the use of a dolorimeter or algometer, pressure-loaded gauges that accurately measure force per area, as well as by manual palpation (3, 8). Such instruments are useful in controlled studies, but in the clinic digital palpation is usually adequate. Other common findings on examination include muscle spasm, or taut bands of muscle, sometimes referred to by patients as nodules; skin sensitivity in the form of dermatographism; or purplish mottling of the skin, especially of the legs following exposure to cold.

As noted earlier, the definition of myofascial pain is more subjective and varies with the technique of the trigger point examination. Generally, patients describe regional pain, often in the head and neck, and trigger or tender points are localized to that region. Many patients do report the same degree of fatigue, sleep disturbances, and mood disturbances as patients with fibromyalgia.

Laboratory and radiological investigations in fibromyalgia or myofascial pain are largely unrevealing and primarily useful for excluding other conditions. At an initial evaluation baseline blood tests should include a complete blood count, erythrocyte sedimentation rate, standard blood chemistry, and thyroid function studies. These all are usually normal in fibromyalgia. Unless there is evidence of an associated arthritis or possible cervical or lumbar radiculopathy, plain radiographs, CT, nuclear scans, and MRI are not generally necessary. Unless there is a clinical suspicion of a systemic connective tissue disease or Lyme disease, routine ordering of serologic tests such as rheumatoid factor, antinuclear antibodies, or Lyme antibody assays is not recommended. Such assays are often false positive.

The somewhat vague and nebulous symptoms of chronic, generalized pain and fatigue are present in many rheumatic and nonrheumatic diseases. Nevertheless, the characteristic synovitis and systemic features of the connective tissue disorders are not features of fibromyalgia. Certain nonrheumatic systemic illnesses, particularly hypothyroidism, may initially mimic fibromyalgia. In fact, there are some reports of fibromyalgia as a presenting manifestation of hypothyroidism (10). Peripheral neuropathies, entrapment syndromes such as carpal tunnel syndrome, and neurologic disorders, such as multiple sclerosis and myasthenia gravis, are sometimes considered in the differential diagnosis. However, the standard neurological examination, as well as electromyography (EMG) and nerve conduction velocity (NCV), are normal in fibromyalgia.

Chronic fatigue syndrome (CFS) overlaps with fibromyalgia and may be considered part of the fibromyalgia spectrum (11, 12). One of the major differences has been the notion that CFS has an infectious cause. During the mid 1980s, the concept of chronic Epstein-Barr viral (EBV) infection as a cause of what is now termed CFS became popular. However, despite elevated antibody titers to EBV antigens in many patients, there is no evidence that EBV or any other single infection is causally associated with the vast majority of patients with CFS (13).

The cardinal symptom of CFS is chronic, debilitating fatigue, initially characterized as not resolving with bed rest and severe enough to reduce average daily activity by at least 50% (11, 14). Neurocognitive and musculoskeletal symptoms have been present in 75 to 95% of patients with CFS (13–15). Demographic, immunological, and psychiatric studies, as well as investigations of muscle fatigue, have also demonstrated similarities with fibromyalgia (12). We also reported that the manual and dolorimeter mean tender point scores of CFS patients with myalgias were nearly identical to those of fibromyalgia patients (12). Thus the majority of CFS patients met historical and tender point diagnostic criteria for fibromyalgia.

ARE THESE PSYCHIATRIC DISORDERS?

It is not surprising that many authors have concluded that fibromyalgia is a psychiatric illness or a manifestation of psychophysiological abnormalities. Patients look well, and the physical examination, laboratory, and radiological findings do not account for the chronic symptoms. Many of the symptoms of depression, such as fatigue, lack of energy, and sleep disturbances are identical to those in fibromyalgia, and some authors have proposed that fibromyalgia is a manifestation of depression. Furthermore, many patients do report depression, anxiety, and high levels of stress. Thus, fibromyalgia is often considered to be a form of masked depression or a somatization disorder, termed psychogenic rheumatism.

Depression is more common in fibromyalgia than in normal controls or in rheumatoid arthritis (RA) (16–18) (Table 14.5). Approximately 25 to 35% of fibromyalgia patients have current major depression, and 50 to 70% have a lifetime history of major depression. Somatization disorder has been noted in 5 to 20% of fibromyalgia patients. However,

Table 14.5.   Conclusions of Studies Evaluating the Psychiatric Aspects of Fibromyalgia

1. Previously used psychologic and psychiatric instruments do not control for pain, falsely elevating scores for neurosis and depression in fibromyalgia.
2. There is a greater prevalence of depression in patients with fibromyalgia than in controls—and possibly than in patients with RA. However, symptoms of depression usually antedate those of fibromyalgia, and the two diagnoses are often discordant temporarily.
3. The majority of patients with fibromyalgia do not meet DSM-IV criteria for an active psychiatric disorder.

75% of fibromyalgia patients do not have a current psychiatric illness. Irritable bowel syndrome and migraine, which have been noted in more than 50% of patients, generally develop concurrently with fibromyalgia (18, 19). These disorders have also been linked to psychiatric or psychosomatic illness. Hudson et al. (18) have used the term affective spectrum disorder to account for the association of fibromyalgia, chronic fatigue syndrome, migraine, irritable bowel syndrome, and depression.

The frequency of psychiatric disorders may not be intrinsically related to fibromyalgia but may be more related to the decision of patients to seek medical care. For example, the frequency of lifetime psychiatric disorders was compared in 64 fibromyalgia patients, 28 fibromyalgia nonpatients, and 23 healthy controls (20). The fibromyalgia nonpatients met diagnostic criteria for fibromyalgia but had not sought medical care for their symptoms. The fibromyalgia patients had significantly more psychiatric diagnoses than did the nonpatients and the controls. Nonpatients did not differ from healthy controls in psychiatric diagnoses but did have greater levels of psychological distress than healthy controls.

DO DIAGNOSTIC LABELS HELP OR HURT?

The diagnosis of fibromyalgia and myofascial pain have been criticized because of the lack of objective criteria or pathological findings. We have acknowledged that all diagnostic criteria are based on circular reasoning when there is no diagnostic tissue or laboratory gold standard (21). However, the absence of a tissue gold standard does not preclude the diagnosis of an illness. Performing a simple tender point examination in people with widespread pain provides excellent specificity and sensitivity in differentiating fibromyalgia from other chronic rheumatic pain disorders (3). A recent study validated the fibromyalgia criteria as applied to the general population (9). Every specialty of medicine has assigned diagnostic labels to chronic illness where causation and pathophysiology are not understood. Examples of such labels include migraine, causalgia, irritable bowel syndrome, and major depression.

Certain authors have suggested that these diagnostic labels promote sickness behavior (Table 14.6). For example, Bohr wrote that fibromyalgia patients exaggerate their disability and pain, "in contradistinction to patients with genuine rheumatologic disease, such as rheumatoid arthritis" (22).

Table 14.6.   Negative Physician Comments about Fibromyalgia and Myofascial Pain Syndromes

Hadler: Fibromyalgia patients are "out of sorts."

Bohr: Fibromyalgia patients exaggerate their disability and pain "in contradistinction to patients with genuine rheumatologic disease, such as rheumatoid arthritis."

Bohr: The label of fibromyalgia has promoted physician–attorney collusion for financial self-interest.

Table 14.7.   The Spectrum of Illness

X	X	X
Normotensive	Labile hypertension	Chronic hypertension

X	X	X
No pain	Mild, intermittent pain	Chronic, severe pain

Hadler, a rheumatologist, equated fibromyalgia with being "out of sorts" (23). He asserted that we all have bad days characterized by stiffness and achiness, easy fatigue, loss of well-being, and awareness of our bowels. Hadler claimed that the diagnosis of fibromyalgia "teaches people to be sick." Another author suggested that the terms fibromyalgia, myofascial pain, and soft-tissue injury promote abnormal illness behavior that is reinforced by society, which provides advantages for the sick role (24).

Although muscle pain, fatigue, headaches, and depression are common in the general population, persistent and debilitating symptoms are much less common. However, the syndrome label of fibromyalgia describes a degree of suffering that is well out of the norm. Such symptoms define a syndrome of poor health. Hypertension is an apt analogy (Table 14.7). Chronic pain, chronic fatigue, depression, and headaches are similarly best viewed on a continuum of normal to abnormal in the population. People suffering with such chronic symptoms are a homogeneous and well-defined group. Appropriate diagnostic criteria have been established for migraine, depression, and chronic fatigue syndrome, as well as fibromyalgia. Therefore, physicians can accurately diagnose people with the syndrome of fibromyalgia, just as they can diagnose migraine or depression.

A diagnostic label alleviates uncertainty and fear for the fibromyalgia patient. A label of fibromyalgia is also cost effective, since patients generally stop doctor shopping and undergoing costly and invasive diagnostic studies. Most patients with fibromyalgia have 5 to 7 years of symptoms before the diagnosis is made (3, 25). Once the diagnosis is made, hospitalizations and health care utilization drop dramatically (26).

CAN A DISORDER BE DEMONSTRATED?

The cause of fibromyalgia and myofascial pain is unknown. Trauma is often linked to these conditions, but often patients do not remember a specific factor that triggered their symptoms. The most common factors that patients do identify are a flulike or viral illness; minor or substantial physical trauma, such as a fall or a motor vehicle accident; emotional trauma; or changes in medication, especially withdrawing corticosteroids (25, 27).

Fibromyalgia has been noted to follow various viral diseases, including human immunodeficiency virus (HIV) infection and Lyme disease (28–30). About 25 to 40% of patients with documented Lyme disease who were treated appropriately with antibiotics developed persistent pain and fatigue, consistent with fibromyalgia or chronic fatigue syndrome. In these reports there is no evidence of persistent microbial infection. The infection may act similarly to other stressors and initiate both neurohormone and psychosocial dysfunction (28).

Fibromyalgia and myofascial pain have traditionally been considered to be caused by muscle disease. However, the search for possible abnormalities in muscle structure and function have been largely unrewarding (31). With recent studies using phosphorus magnetic resonance spectroscopy, no differences in the levels of phosphocreatine, inorganic phosphate, and intracellular pH after exercise were found in women with fibromyalgia compared with sedentary control women (32).

The first laboratory or objective abnormality found in fibromyalgia was the report that patients had an abnormal slow wave sleep pattern, termed alpha-delta sleep (2). Those researchers also experimentally induced the same nonrestorative sleep in normal controls, and the controls developed symptoms of fibromyalgia as well as tender points in their muscles. Unfortunately, the significance of these findings has been debated because of the absence of large, well-controlled studies. Although a number of laboratories have confirmed the finding by electroencephalography of an alpha sleep anomaly in fibromyalgia, such sleep patterns are common in RA and CFS and can be seen in healthy people. Furthermore, many fibromyalgia patients do not have the alpha-delta sleep abnormality (33), and other sleep disturbances, such as nocturnal myoclonus and obstructive sleep apnea, have been reported in fibromyalgia (34).

Most recent investigations focused on the role of the central and peripheral nervous system in causing altered pain perception in fibromyalgia and myofascial pain syndromes. For example, the level of substance P in the cerebrospinal fluid was three times as high in fibromyalgia patients as in normal controls (35). Fibromyalgia patients have reduced pain tolerance to pressure, heat, and electrical pulse, both at classic tender points and control points (36, 37). The regional cerebral blood flow, as detected by single photon emission computed tomography, was lower in the left and right hemithalami and the right heads of the caudate nuclei in fibromyalgia than in controls (38). These areas of the brain are important in pain perception.

Two studies have demonstrated reduced levels of growth hormone in some patients with fibromyalgia (39, 40). Growth hormone, which is important in muscle homeostasis, is excreted primarily during stage 4 sleep. Fibromyalgia patients were noted to have low urinary free cortisol and a decreased cortisol response to corticotropin-releasing hormone (41, 42). Plasma neuropeptide Y levels were also low in fibromyalgia.

DOES POSTTRAUMATIC FIBROMYALGIA EXIST?

Approximately 25% of patients with fibromyalgia attribute the onset of their pain to an injury or physical trauma. However, there is no evidence that any single factor causes fibromyalgia. The American College of Rheumatology does not recognize the term secondary fibromyalgia (3). A recent consensus document specifically recommends that the term posttraumatic fibromyalgia not be used (Table 14.8) (43). Rheumatologists have also consistently argued against the concept that myofascial pain is caused by repetitive strain (6, 44). This does not preclude a physician from declaring that a patient may be disabled from the symptoms of pain, fatigue, mood, and sleep disturbances. A Canadian court decision denied a fibromyalgia patient's claim, since the symptoms were "largely psychogenic in origin." Such court decisions are not in keeping with current concepts of pain and mind-body interactions.

CAN IT BE TREATED?

During the past 10 years there have been a number of controlled therapeutic trials in patients with fibromyalgia. These have included medications and nonmedicinal therapies. The choice of specific therapeutic approaches has in some situations been largely empirical. However, possible pathophysiological abnormalities such as peripheral and central hyperalgesia, sleep disturbances, mood disturbances, and altered blood supply to muscle and superficial tissues form a basis for certain therapeutic modalities.

Medications

Despite the fact that there is no evidence of tissue inflammation in fibromyalgia, anti-inflammatory medications are often used and have been studied in controlled trials. "Therapeutic" doses of naproxen and ibuprofen and 20 mg daily of prednisone were not significantly better than placebo in clinical trials (45). Nonsteroidal anti-inflammatory drugs may have a synergistic effect when combined with central nervous system (CNS) active medications (46) but may be no more effective than simple analgesics.

In contrast, certain CNS active medications, most notably the tricyclic antidepressants amitriptyline and cyclobenzaprine, have performed better than placebo in controlled trials (45, 47, 48). The doses of amitriptyline studied have been 25 to 50 mg, usually given as a single dose at bedtime. Cyclobenzaprine 10 to 40 mg in divided doses also improved pain, fatigue, sleep, and tender point count (48). However, clinically meaningful improvement with the tricyclic medications occurred in only 25 to 45% of patients in these studies (45). Furthermore, the efficacy of these medications may decrease over time (45).

Table 14.8.   Recommendations from report of fibromyalgia and disability*

1.) *Causality:*

Since the cause of FM is not known, any relationship to a precipitating factor must be reviewed by the physician on a case by case basis. Precipitating events may include physical trauma, emotional trauma, infection, surgery, and stress. The terms "reactive" and "post-traumatic fibromyalgia" should be eliminated.

2.) *Assessing work capacity:*

The assessment of symptom severity and work capacity should include pain levels, functional ability, and psychosocial distress, using appropriate assessment tools. Validated work assessment tools need to be developed.

3.) *Prognosis:*

The majority of patients with FM have chronic symptoms that wax and wane in severity. Most are capable of working, although job modifications and flexibility are often useful.

4.) *Therapy:*

A comprehensive treatment approach is important. Duration of treatment should be specified with the goal of therapy to make the patient independent. Testing methods to aid patients in their rehabilitation are needed and should be supported by the insurance industry.

*Modified from Wolfe FM. The fibromyalgia syndrome: A consensus report on fibromyalgia and disability. J Rheumatol 1996:23(3):534–539

My colleagues and I (49) found that 20 mg of fluoxetine improved the pain and global well being of patients with fibromyalgia. There was comparable efficacy of the fluoxetine with that of 25 mg of amitriptyline given at bedtime. Both were better than placebo, and the combination of fluoxetine and amitriptyline was better than either alone. Other tricyclics and different classes of CNS-active medications, including alprazolam, temazepam, and clonazepam, as well as 5-hydroxytryptophan and an analgesic containing carisoprodol and paracetamol, have been found to be somewhat effective in preliminary studies.

Nonmedication treatments that have been helpful in controlled studies include cardiovascular fitness training (50), EMG biofeedback (51) and hypnotherapy (51). It is important to instruct patients in the principles and methods of gradual incremental cardiovascular fitness programs. Low-impact aerobic activities, such as fast walking, biking, swimming, and water aerobics, are most successful. However, the type and intensity of the program should be individualized, and physical therapists or exercise physiologists can provide helpful instruction. Other uncontrolled reports have evaluated transcutaneous nerve stimulation (TENS), acupuncture, laser treatment, and tender point injections in fibromyalgia patients. Uncontrolled studies have found that cognitive behavioral treatment (52), mindfulness meditation programs (53) and multidisciplinary treatment with physical medicine and mental health professionals (54) have helped patients with fibromyalgia. A team employing nurse-educators, psychiatrists or other mental health workers, physiatrists, and physical therapists is especially useful in difficult cases.

CAN IT BE DISABLING?

The few longitudinal studies in fibromyalgia have demonstrated persistent pain and significant interference with function (55). Factors associated with improved outcome include a younger age and lower global and pain scores at the time of the initial survey. Fibromyalgia symptoms are also remarkably stable over time in a single patient, although they vary greatly between patients. Pain is the most important determinant of severity, but psychological status and functional disability contribute independently to severity (27).

With regard to function in fibromyalgia, studies have reported varying disability rates from 9 to 44% (56–58). Using a computer-assisted work simulator, fibromyalgia patients and RA patients had comparable ability to perform standardized work tasks, and both were only 60% of that done by normal controls (57). The Stanford Health Assessment Questionnaire was the best predictor of work ability in both groups of patients. Patients in tertiary referral practices with a special interest in fibromyalgia may represent the tip of the iceberg in terms of severity and functional disability. Community-based fibromyalgia patients have fared much better in outcome (59). Nearly half of community fibromyalgia patients no longer met criteria for the diagnosis 2 years after conservative treatment was begun (59).

Fibromyalgia has become an important medicolegal condition. Fibromyalgia was responsible for disability payments in 9% of cases at a major Canadian life insurance company, which translates to $200 million (Canadian) per year paid out in Canada in long-term disability claims for fibromyalgia (45). Rheumatologists have in general recommended guidelines that promote staying in the workplace and avoiding litigation (43, 60). The relation of the injury to fibromyalgia is best approached by using the term precipitating factor or temporal relationship of the injury to the onset of symptoms. We certainly do not know the cause of fibromyalgia, and it would be inappropriate to tackle issues of causation.

The prognosis is impossible to predict in any chronic condition. However, it should be stressed that the majority of patients are working full time. Reports do describe significant work loss, work modifications, and work disability. What is such disability related to, since there are no objective measures of physical impairment? Pain is more prominent than in many disabling conditions, such as RA. Fatigue may also cause disability. However, according to some countries' social security guidelines, pain without objective physical or laboratory abnormalities is not a sufficient factor in disability determinations. Tender points may be used as an objective measure of pain and dysfunction. Public education, standardized diagnostic criteria, and emphasis on rehabilitation, not compensation, are necessary to interrupt the expanding area of disability in fibromyalgia (Table 14.8).

The variable severity of fibromyalgia must be considered in any discussion of prognosis and outcome. The somewhat bleak outcome reported from tertiary referral clinics with a specialty interest in fibromyalgia may not be representative of the general community. Less problematic patients may often do well with simple reassurance, education, and attention to physical fitness and ergonomic issues. Many patients respond well to very low doses of tricyclics or other CNS medications, and particularly as their sleep improves, they cope well and find fibromyalgia to be a no worse than a nuisance.

In conclusion, fibromyalgia is a common condition that despite being well described 150 years ago is just beginning to be accepted as a discrete syndrome. Controversy regarding the presence of inflammation and confusion regarding terminology and overlap with other pain syndromes has resulted in a healthy skepticism about its existence. Many physicians still believe that it is a wastebasket term for any nonspecific ailment. However, recent epidemiologic studies conclude that fibromyalgia is a discrete syndrome with a uniform set of symptoms and signs that can be readily distinguished from other causes of chronic musculoskeletal pain. This recognition will undoubtedly lead to a better understanding of the complicated pathophysiologic mechanisms involved and ultimately to a better treatment for this perplexing syndrome.

References

1. Gowers WR. Lumbago: its lessons and analogues. Br Med J 1904;1:117–121.
2. Smythe HA, Moldofsky H. Two contributions to understanding the "fibrositis syndrome." Bull Rheum Dis 1978;26:928–931.
3. Wolfe F, Smythe HA, Yunus MB, et al. The American College of Rheumatology 1990 criteria for the classification of fibromyalgia: report of the Multicenter Criteria Committee. Arthritis Rheum 1990;33:160–172.
4. Travell JG, Simons DG. Myofascial pain and dysfunction: the trigger point manual. Baltimore: Williams & Wilkins, 1983.
5. Simons DG. Referred phenomena of myofascial trigger points. In: Vecchiet L, Albe-Fessard D, Lindblom U, eds. New trends in referred pain and hyperalgesia. Amsterdam: Elsevier, 1993;341.
6. Littlejohn GO. Fibrositis/fibromyalgia syndrome in the workplace. Rheum Dis Clin North Am 1989;15:45–60.
7. Wolfe F, Simons DG, Fricton J, et al. The fibromyalgia and myofascial pain syndromes: a preliminary study of tender points and trigger points in persons with fibromyalgia, myofascial pain syndrome and no disease. J Rheumatol 1992;19:944–951.
8. Tunks E, McCain GA, Hart LE, et al. The reliability of examination for tenderness in patients with myofascial pain, chronic fibromyalgia and controls. J Rheumatol 1995;22:944–952.
9. Wolfe F, Ross K, Anderson J, et al. The prevalence and characteristics of fibromyalgia in the general population. Arthritis Rheum 1995;38:19–28.
10. Wilke WS, Sheeler LR, Makarowski WS. Hypothyroidism with presenting symptoms of fibrositis. J Rheumatol 1981;8:626–631.
11. Komaroff AL, Goldenberg D. The chronic fatigue syndrome: definition, current studies and lessons for fibromyalgia research. J Rheumatol Suppl 1989;19:23–27.

12. Goldenberg DL, Simms RW, Geiger A, Komaroff AL. High frequency of fibromyalgia in patients with chronic fatigue seen in a primary care practice. Arthritis Rheum 1990;33:381–387.

13. Schluederberg A, Straus SE, Peterson P, et al. Chronic fatigue syndrome research: definition and medical outcome assessment. Ann Intern Med 1992;117:325–331.

14. Fukuda K, Straus SE, Hickie I, et al. The chronic fatigue syndrome: a comprehensive approach to its definition and study. Ann Intern Med 1994;121:953–959.

15. Komaroff AL, Fagioli LR, Geiger AM, et al. An examination of the working case definition of chronic fatigue syndrome. Am J Med 1996;100:56–64.

16. Hudson JI, Hudson MS, Pliner LF, et al. Fibromyalgia and major affective disorder: a controlled phenomenology and family history study. Am J Psychiatry 1985;142:441–446.

17. Goldenberg DL. Psychiatric and psychologic aspects of fibromyalgia syndrome. Rheum Dis Clin N Am 1989;15:105–114.

18. Hudson JI, Goldenberg DL, Pope HG Jr, et al. Comorbidity of fibromyalgia with medical and psychiatric disorders. Am J Med 1992;92:363–367.

19. Triadafilopoulos G, Simms RW, Goldenberg DL. Bowel dysfunction in fibromyalgia syndrome. Dig Dis Sci 1991;36:59–64.

20. Aaron LA, Bradley LA, Alarcon GS, et al. Psychiatric diagnoses in patients with fibromyalgia are related to health care-seeking behavior rather than to illness. Arthritis Rheum 1996;39:436–445.

21. Goldenberg DL. Fibromyalgia: why such controversy? Ann Rheum Dis 1995;54:3–5.

22. Bohr T. Problems with myofascial pain syndrome and fibromyalgia syndrome. Neurology 1996;46:593–597.

23. Hadler NM. Is fibromyalgia a useful diagnostic label? Cleve Clin J Med 1996;63:85–87.

24. Awerbuch M. Different concepts of chronic musculoskeletal pain. Ann Rheum Dis 1995;54:331–332.

25. Goldenberg DL. Fibromyalgia syndrome: an emerging but controversial condition. JAMA 1987;257:2782–2787.

26. Cathey MA, Wolfe F, Kleinheksel SM, Hawley DJ. Socioeconomic impact of fibrositis: a study of 81 patients with primary fibrositis. Am J Med 1986;81:78–84.

27. Goldenberg DL, Mossey CJ, Schmid CH. A model to assess severity and impact of fibromyalgia. J Rheumatol 1995;22:2313–18.

28. Goldenberg DL. Do infections trigger fibromyalgia? Arthritis Rheum 1993;36:1489–1492.

29. Steere AC, Taylor E, McHugh GL, Logigian EL. The overdiagnosis of Lyme disease. JAMA 1993;269:1812–1816.

30. Hsu VM, Patella SJ, Sigal LH. "Chronic Lyme disease" as the incorrect diagnosis in patients with fibromyalgia. Arthritis Rheum 1993;36:1493–1500.

31. Jacobsen S. Chronic widespread musculoskeletal pain: the fibromyalgia syndrome. Dan Med Bull 1994;41:541–564.

32. Simms RW, Roy SH, Hrovat M, et al. Lack of association between fibromyalgia syndrome and abnormalities in muscle energy metabolism. Arthritis Rheum 1994;37:794–800.

33. Carette S, Oakson G, Guimont C, Steriade M. Sleep electroencephalography and the clinical response to amitriptyline in patients with fibromyalgia. Arthritis Rheum 1995;38:1211–1217.

34. May KP, West SG, Baker MR, Everett DW. Sleep apnea in male patients with the fibromyalgia syndrome. Am J Med 1993;94:505–508.

35. Russell IJ, Orr MD, Littman B, et al. Elevated cerebrospinal fluid levels of substance P in patients with the fibromyalgia syndrome. Arthritis Rheum 1994;37:1593–1601.

36. Gibson SJ, Littlejohn GO, Gorman MM, et al. Altered heat pain thresholds and cerebral event-related potentials following painful CO2 laser stimulation in subjects with fibromyalgia syndrome. Pain 1994;58:185–193.

37. Lautenbacher S, Rollman GB, McCain GA. Multimethod assessment of experimental and clinical pain in patients with fibromyalgia. Pain 1994;59:45–53.

38. Mountz JM, Bradley LA, Modell JG, et al. Fibromyalgia in women: abnormalities of regional cerebral blood flow in the thalamus and the caudate nucleus are associated with low pain threshold levels. Arthritis Rheum 1995;38:926–938.

39. Bennett RM, Clark SR, Campbell SM, Burckhardt CS. Low levels of somatomedin-C in patients with the fibromyalgia syndrome: a possible link between sleep and muscle pain. Arthritis Rheum 1992;35:1113–1116.

40. Griep EN, Boersma JW, de Kloet ER. Pituitary release of growth hormone and prolactin in primary FS. J Rheumatol 1994;21:2125–2130.

41. Crofford LJ, Pillemer SR, Kalogeras KT, et al. Hypothalamic-pituitary-adrenal axis perturbations in patients with fibromyalgia. Arthritis Rheum 1994;37:1583–1592.

42. Griep EN, Boersma JW, de Kloet ER. Evidence for neuroendocrine disturbance following physical exercise in primary fibromyalgia syndrome. J Musculoskeletal Pain 1993;1:217–222.

43. Wolfe F, Aarflot T, Bruusgaard D, et al. Fibromyalgia and disability: report of the Moss International Working Group on medico-legal aspects of chronic widespread musculoskeletal pain complaints and fibromyalgia. Scand J Rheumatol 1995;24:112–118.

44. Littlejohn G. Medicolegal aspects of fibrositis syndrome. J Rheumatol 1989;16(Suppl 19):169–173.

45. Goldenberg DL. Treatment of fibromyalgia syndrome. Rheum Dis Clin North Am 1989;15:61–71.

46. Hench PK. Evaluation and differential diagnosis of fibromyalgia: approach to diagnosis and management. Rheum Dis Clin North Am 1989;15:19–29.

47. Goldenberg DL, Felson DT, Dinerman H. A randomized, controlled trial of amitriptyline and naproxen in the treatment of patients with fibromyalgia. Arthritis Rheum 1986;29:1371–1377.

48. Bennett RM, Gatter RA, Campbell SM, et al. A comparison of cyclobenzaprine and placebo in the management of fibrositis: a double-blind controlled study. Arthritis Rheum 1988;31:1535–1542.

49. Goldenberg DL, Mayskiy M, Mossey CJ, et al. A randomized, double-blind crossover trial of fluoxetine and amitriptyline in the treatment of fibromyalgia. Arthritis Rheum 1996;39:1852–59.

50. McCain GA, Bell DA, Mai FM, Halliday PD. A controlled study of the effects of a supervised cardiovascular fitness training program on the manifestations of primary fibromyalgia. Arthritis Rheum 1988;31:1135–1141.

51. Goldenberg DL. Management of fibromyalgia syndrome. Rheum Dis Clin N Am 1989;15:499–512.

52. Nielson WR, Walker C, McCain GA. Cognitive behavioral treatment of fibromyalgia syndrome: preliminary findings. J Rheumatol 1992;19:98–103.

53. Kaplan KH, Goldenberg DL, Galvin-Nadeau M. The impact of a meditation-based stress reduction program on fibromyalgia. Gen Hosp Psychiatry 1993;15:284–289.

54. Bennett RM, Burckhardt CS, Clark SR, et al. Group treatment of fibromyalgia: a 6 month outpatient program. J Rheumatol 1996;23:521–528.

55. Felson DT, Goldenberg DL. The natural history of fibromyalgia. Arthritis Rheum 1986;29:1522–1526.

56. Hawley DJ, Wolfe F, Cathey MA. Pain, functional disability, and psychological status: a 12-month study of severity in fibromyalgia. J Rheumatol 1988;15:1551–1556.

57. Cathey MA, Wolfe F, Kleinheksel SM. Functional ability and work status in patients with fibromyalgia. Arthritis Care Res 1988;1:85–98.

58. Kennedy MJ, Goldenberg DL, Felson DT. A prospective long-term study of fibromyalgia. Arthritis Rheum 1994;37(Suppl):S213 (abstract).

59. Granges G, Zilko P, Littlejohn GO. Fibromyalgia syndrome: assessment of the severity of the condition 2 years after diagnosis. J Rheumatol 1994;21:523–529.

60. Wolfe F, Vancouver Fibromyalgia Consensus Group. The fibromyalgia syndrome: a consensus report on fibromyalgia and disability. J Rheumatol 1996;23:534–539.

CHAPTER 15

Differential Diagnosis and Management Strategies of Low Back Pain

Paul A. Glazer and Liane M. Clamen

INTRODUCTION

Low back pain has a tremendous cost to society. Its damage is felt not only in the morbidity of afflicted individuals, but also through lost productivity and increased health care costs. Low back pain is the second leading cause of work absenteeism in this country, and it leads to more productivity loss than any other medical condition (1).

In 1990 alone, the number of people in the United States who sought professional health care for back pain was 24 million (9.4% of the population), according to population surveys. Every year in the United States, more than $33 billion is spent on health care for low back pain. When additional costs such as disability and lost productivity are included, total costs for low back pain in this country are more than $100 billion per year (2).

Approximately 80% of adults in this country at some point during their lives have low back pain that affects their activities of daily living; 1 to 2% of these require surgery (3). The first episode of low back pain typically occurs in the third decade of life. The incidence of low back pain peaks between ages 55 and 64 and then decreases. The severity of pain at onset increases with age of presentation. About 10 to 12% of patients with low back pain have concomitant sciatica.

One way to improve health care treatment of low back pain is to increase the frequency with which the various causes of back pain are properly diagnosed. We hope this chapter will prove useful to health care providers as they attempt to differentiate and treat different types of low back pain.

RISK FACTORS FOR LOW BACK PAIN

It is difficult to define risk factors for low back pain because associations between low back pain and specific variables do not necessarily imply a causal link. This fact may help explain the often conflicting results from various studies on risk factors for low back pain. The literature emphasizes two categories of risk factors associated with back pain: extrinsic and intrinsic. Extrinsic risks include heavy physical labor, frequent bending and twisting, lifting and forceful movements, repetitive work, vibration, sedentary office work, and smoking. Truck drivers (4–6), athletes (7), and nurses (8) are more likely than others to suffer from back pain. Intrinsic risk factors for disc degeneration include anthropometrics, spinal abnormalities, and genetic predispositions.

Heavy Physical Labor and Lifting

Heavy physical labor is often associated with low back pain. One study found that people whose jobs required reaching and twisting to lift more than 25 pounds at least 25 times a day were at more than three times as much risk of developing low back pain as were controls (9). In a recent 5-year prospective study, people who reported heavy physical labor were almost twice as likely to report low back pain as those who described their work as sedentary (10). One study compared nonoccupational lifting in patients with confirmed herniated discs and in matched controls; the researchers found that frequent lifting of 25 pounds or more, with knees straight and back bent, conferred a relative risk of 3.95 for lumbar disc prolapse (11).

Sedentary Labor

There is no consensus on the contribution of sedentary labor to low back pain. Although some investigators (11–14) noted a positive relation between sedentary occupations and low back pain, others (15–17) demonstrated no significant relation. Researchers attribute the positive associations to increased intradiscal pressures while sitting versus those while standing, fluid exudation from the nucleus leading to harmful load transfer to the anulus, and a decrease in normal nutrient delivery due to intermittent disc compression (18, 19). The lack of consensus on this topic may be because most studies on sedentary labor do not account for confounding factors such as variations in work history and nonoccupational activities.

Driving and Vibration

There is a strong association between disc prolapse and vehicle driving. The risk ratio of disc herniation for truck drivers is as high as 3:1 in the United States (20) and 4.6:1 in Finland (16). This increased risk of back disorders in drivers has been attributed to both posture and vibration (11, 12, 17, 20). Whole-body vibration has harmful effects on the spine, especially at 4.5 to 6 Hz; this vibration frequency is both the natural frequency of the human spine and a major component of motor vehicle vibration (21, 22). Vibration reportedly causes damage to the back via a reduction of strength and stiffness of ligaments, disc fluid loss, and disc hardening (23, 24).

Athletics

Studies have shown a correlation between low back pain and participation in sports such as golf, gymnastics, rowing, and bowling (25, 26). In a survey of 142 athletes who did soccer, tennis, wrestling, and gymnastics, 50 to 85% reported low back pain and 36 to 55% had radiological spinal abnormalities. These radiological findings included reduced disc height, Schmorl's nodes, and abnormalities of vertebral body configuration (27, 28). On the other hand, insufficient exercise has also been linked to an increased risk of disc herniation (11). In general, good muscle strength and overall fitness are suggested for reducing the risk of low back pain and disc herniation (29–32).

Smoking

A number of retrospective (17, 33–35) and prospective (29, 36) studies report a positive association between smoking and back pain. One hypothesis to explain the connection is that repetitive increases in intradiscal pressure, as occurs with frequent coughing, may cause discogenic back pain (6, 33, 37). This theory is supported by the observation that coughing and chronic bronchitis among nonsmokers have also been associated with back pain (13).

In addition to the biomechanical risk factor of increased intradiscal pressure with coughing, smoking has been shown to reduce vertebral blood flow (35) and to inhibit diffusion to the intervertebral disc (37). An MRI study of smoking and nonsmoking identical twins found that those who smoked had an increased frequency of disc degeneration throughout the entire lumbar spine. This supports the hypothesis that smoking interferes with systemic nutrient delivery and that this decrease in nutrients may facilitate disc degeneration (36).

Anthropometrics

Height, weight, and body build have been correlated with disc prolapse (7, 13, 16, 38, 39). A study of the association between height and disc herniation found that men taller than 180 cm (5′ 11″) had a relative risk of disc prolapse of 2.3, and women taller than 170 cm (5′ 7″) had a relative risk of 3.7 (16). The average increase in risk relative to height was 5% per centimeter for men and 4% per centimeter for women. In general, men's discs have been shown to degenerate earlier than women's discs, but this may be due to differences in work history (40).

In a study of 1128 patients undergoing surgery for disc herniations, there were strong associations between the likelihood of developing a prolapse requiring surgery and both tallness and large body mass (38). Obesity independent of height has been positively associated with both disc degeneration, as diagnosed by radiographic abnormalities, (41) and low back pain (33, 42).

Although tall and large people probably place greater loads on their intervertebral discs, they also typically have correspondingly large discs (43). Therefore, people of different statures should not have significant differences in disc stress related to a given task. Rather, the increased disc disease in individuals of large stature may be explained by factors such as problems with nutrient diffusion (44) or the fact that large persons are likely to work in awkward postures (18).

Genetic Predisposition

Postacchini et al. (45) suggested that there may be a genetic predisposition for disc herniation. In a review of 63 patients under age 21 who had lumbar disc herniations, 32% had a family history of that same lesion; in the control group only 7% had a family history (46). Although no genetic markers have been proposed, certain congenital spinal abnormalities such as asymmetrical facet orientation (47) and a small vertebral canal (48–50) hypothetically predispose certain individuals to symptomatic disc herniations (51).

Genetic deficiencies leading to inadequate healing responses or inordinate sensitivity to mechanical stress may make an individual susceptible to a disc prolapse. A review of 101 surgical cases of herniated lumbar discs in patients under 20 years of age reported that the most significant causative factors for disc prolapse were congenital lumbosacral malformations, early onset of disc degeneration, and repetitive trauma (52).

EVALUATION OF LOW BACK PAIN

History

A careful history is one of the most important components of the evaluation of a patient with low back pain. A good history can help the health care provider formulate a differential diagnosis for each patient's specific type of low back pain. When speaking with the patient, have him or her clearly describe the nature of the pain, including the presence or absence of associated leg pain. Ask whether there were any precipitating events or the onset of the pain was more insidious in nature. Find out whether the patient's low back pain is a recurrent or a progressive problem. Ask when the pain occurs and whether it is exacerbated or alleviated when the patient lies down. Mechanical low back pain is an ache; it is typically worse toward the end of the day and better with rest. Discogenic pain is often burning and aching, and it may be constant. Radicular pain radiates below the knee, may be coupled with numbness and/or paresthesias, and often improves with rest. Spinal tumors are frequently associated with boring pain that is worse at night and unrelieved by bed rest.

Ask the patient whether there are any aggravating or alleviating factors. Flexion of the spine often causes an increase in pain related to discogenic disease, whereas extension worsens facet pain. Determine any history of systemic disease that may be affecting the spine. Find out about any family history of back problems or psychiatric illness. It is important to know the medications and alternative treatments (e.g., spinal manipulations) being used by the patient and how long they have been used. Also ask the patient what medications and treatments he or she has tried in the past and why those modalities were abandoned. Note the occupation and social circumstances of the patient and whether or not there is any litigation involved with the illness (53).

A careful neurological history is essential. In the elderly one often has to distinguish between neurogenic and vascular claudication. For example, neurogenic claudication is often alleviated by walking uphill or by leaning forward in a chair and exacerbated by walking downhill. Vascular claudication, however, is exacerbated by any exercise and alleviated with rest.

Question the patient about paresthesias and weakness. If paresthesias are present, determine their exact location. Pain drawings are often helpful in demonstrating the dermatomal distribution of the patient's radicular pain. These pain drawings in conjunction with Waddell signs (described later) help in distinguishing nonorganic pain patterns. Patients with weakness of the lower extremities, incontinence, or constipation of either bowel or bladder require an immediate neurological evaluation.

Physical Examination

The physical examination of a patient with low back pain should begin with observation of gait, mobility, and posture. Many clues to the diagnosis can be acquired through observation. For example, the patient with acute pain and spasm avoids bending and twisting motions.

To perform a thorough physical examination, it is essential to have the patient completely disrobe. Inspect the skin over the lower back; hairy patches, lipomas, or neurofibromas may indicate spinal dysraphism. Check for asymmetry or scoliosis. Determine whether there is a normal lumbar lordosis. The loss of lordosis may be secondary to a loss of disc height

or anterior compression fractures. Conversely, an exaggerated lumbar lordosis is characteristic of obese patients and those with a high grade spondylolisthesis.

Palpate all tender areas. Sciatic notch tenderness may indicate a radicular disorder. Low back spasm, which can be appreciated by manual palpation, may be associated with a scoliosis or loss of lordosis. An accurate measurement of range of motion of the spine is difficult. Furthermore, there is a wide variance in normal range of motion in the general population. But one can easily test flexion motion quantitatively by assessing how far the patient can bend forward as if to touch the toes with the knees straight. If the patient cannot touch the floor, measure the distance from the fingertips to the floor with a tape. Similarly, one can determine whether the range in lateral bending and hyperextension is decreased or whether it causes an increase in pain. Spondylolisthesis, spondylolysis, and spinal stenosis cause increased back pain with extension (53).

The Neurological Examination

The neurological examination of the lower extremities, as it relates to the lumbar spine, consists of a careful evaluation of motor strength, sensation, vibratory sense, reflexes, and evidence of nerve tension signs. True muscle weakness is the most reliable indicator of persistent nerve compression. Muscle strength should be assessed on a scale of 0 to 5 points. One should carefully document the strength of hip flexion, extension, abduction, and adduction; knee flexion and extension; ankle dorsiflexion and plantar flexion; extensor and flexor hallucis and digitorum communis; and peroneal and posterior tibialis muscles. Fatigue testing, as with repetitive isolated calf raises, is often beneficial. It is good to note sensory changes but important to remember that they are subjective.

Much can be learned by testing knee and ankle reflexes. Hyperreflexia may indicate an upper motor neuron lesion. Upper motor neuron dysfunction may also be indicated by the absence of the superficial abdominal reflex, the superficial cremasteric reflex, and the superficial anal reflex. A positive Babinski sign may be elicited in the presence of an upper motor neuron lesion.

Vibratory sensation is lost in peripheral neuropathy, spinal stenosis, and in the elderly. One should accurately record the proximal level of intact vibration sense. Proprioceptive function, indicative of posterior column disease, should also be assessed. Lower motor neuron problems, as seen in degenerative lumbar spinal stenosis, can cause pain, dysesthesias, motor weakness, and diminished reflexes.

With the straight-leg-raise test, one can assess the extent of nerve root tension by noting the angle made between the table and the extended leg when pain is produced. The test is considered positive only if the pain extends below the knee. The straight-leg-raise test should be performed on both legs. Radicular pain in the affected leg during straight leg raising of the unaffected leg is a positive contralateral test. A variation of this test can be performed sitting. Have the patient sit on the examination table and extend the patient's knee while the patient grips the side of the examination table. The test is positive if the patient leans backward and complains of radicular pain as the leg is lifted.

As one performs the physical examination, it is important to remember extraspinal sources of low back pain. Abdominal aortic aneurysms and renal disease secondary to nephrolithiasis can also cause low back pain. Rectal and pelvic examinations should be performed to evaluate for prostatic or rectal, cancer since they may present as low back pain.

To evaluate whether a patient has nonorganic disease such as malingering, Waddell developed a series of five tests. Three of five positive Waddell signs implies a high probability of nonorganic disease. The first sign is tenderness in a nonanatomical distribution. The second is use of axial pressure on the skull or rotation of the pelvis and shoulders in the same plane to reproduce low back pain. The third sign is symptoms that disappear when the patient is distracted. The fourth sign is a giving way or voluntary release during testing of muscle strength or a nondermatomal distribution of sensation loss. The fifth sign is overreaction to stimuli (54).

Diagnostic Studies

Plain radiographs in the anteroposterior and lateral planes of all patients with persistent lower back pain should be taken with the patient standing to assess the effect of gravity on any deformity. The diagnosis of spondylolisthesis may be missed if plain films are taken with the patient supine, as 30% of spondylolistheses reduce in this position. Carefully document any decompensation in the frontal and lateral planes in patients with severe kyphosis or scoliosis.

Magnetic resonance imaging (MRI) is the gold standard for evaluating patients who may have disc problems, infections, or stenosis. Computed tomography (CT) is the study of choice in trauma because of its ability to assess the spine's bony architecture. Myelography in conjunction with CT is the imaging modality of choice in patients with deformity. Radionuclide imaging or bone scans allow evaluation of any process that disturbs the normal balance of bone production and resorption. Discography, which involves the injection of saline into the disc to determine a concordant pain response, remains a controversial technique (55).

Laboratory Tests

In patients who have suspected malignancies, infections, or metabolic abnormalities, a complete blood count with differential is helpful. The erythrocyte sedimentation rate (ESR) is nonspecific but is often a useful indicator of disease severity. Calcium and alkaline phosphatase activity may demonstrate an increased osteoblast activity secondary to malignancy or to metabolic diseases such as Paget's disease of bone. Protein electrophoresis of urine and serum are helpful in demonstrating the presence of multiple myeloma. HLA-B27 antigen testing provides evidence for ankylosing spondylitis and Reiter's syndrome.

GENERAL MANAGEMENT STRATEGIES

Treatment of low back pain should be directed to the patient's specific diagnosis. Remember that the differential diagnosis includes the following extraspinal diseases, which may produce symptoms similar to those caused by degenerative spinal disorders: hip osteoarthritis, diffuse idiopathic skeletal hyperostosis, cervical spinal stenosis, central neurological syndromes, psychological disorders, tumors, renal disease, abdominal aortic aneurysms, and peripheral vascular disease. Surgery for spinal disorders is the conservative approach in some cases. Nonsurgical treatment for low back pain may include short-term (1 to 3 days) bed rest and the use of nonsteroidal anti-inflammatories.

No specific exercise or physical therapy regimens have been demonstrated to be better than any other in the prevention of back pain. However, patients may benefit from physical therapy regimens, as these modalities encourage them to take a more active role in their recovery process (56). Braces offer little biomechanical support but can provide a proprioceptive function and may subjectively reduce back pain (57).

Epidural steroid injections are commonly used to treat low back pain. They have also been shown to provide temporary relief in patients with sciatica. However, epidural steroid injections have inherent risks as well. These include the systemic effects of the steroids, persistent cerebrospinal fluid leak, and meningitis (58, 59). Furthermore, they have been found to have a decreased efficacy in patients with previous surgery, those with symptoms greater than a year in duration, and in smokers. I advocate steroid injections only for temporary relief of symptoms and only for patients who have either spinal stenosis or disc herniations with sciatica and who are not candidates for surgery.

In the United States approximately 40% of patients with back pain seek chiropractic care (2). Many studies have attempted to demonstrate the benefit of spinal manipulation for patients with low back pain (60–62). However, recent reviews indicate that the efficacy of spinal manipulation has not been demonstrated by sound randomized clinical trials (63, 64).

DIFFERENTIAL DIAGNOSIS AND SPECIFIC MANAGEMENT STRATEGIES

Muscle Strain

Acute muscle strain is a common cause of low back pain (Table 15.1). When a patient has a history of pain after exertion without evidence of neurological deficits or structural abnormalities, the most likely diagnosis is acute muscle strain. The majority of muscle strains improve with rest and with soft-tissue modalities such as ultrasound, ice, heat, and massage. Prolonged bed rest should be avoided, as muscle atrophy and stiffness may result. In addition, bed rest longer than 2 to 3 days

Table 15.1.   Differential Diagnosis of Low Back Pain

Musculoskeletal
Spinal degenerative diseases
   Disc degeneration
   Disc herniation
   Spinal stenosis/osteoarthritis/facet degeneration
   Degenerative spondylolisthesis/osteoarthritis
   Facet degeneration
   Spinal instability (normal loads producing abnormal motion)
Spinal deformities
   Scoliosis
   Spondylolisthesis
   Kyphosis
   Hyperlordosis
   Spina bifida
Trauma
   Spondylolysis
   Spondylolisthesis
Systemic problems
   Metabolic: Paget's disease, osteoporosis
   Infections: discitis, osteomyelitis
   Neoplasia
   Inflammatory: rheumatoid, Reiter's syndrome, ankylosing, spondylitis
   Back pain during pregnancy
Iatrogenic
   Flat back
   Instability

may induce a dependency role. Nonsteroidal anti-inflammatory drugs and flexibility and strengthening exercises are often beneficial. Patients whose symptoms persist longer than 3 weeks after initiation of treatments should be further evaluated for other structural or systemic abnormalities. Disorders such as fibromyalgia must be considered in the differential diagnosis when patients have prolonged pain in multiple muscle groups.

Spinal Degenerative Diseases

Disc Degeneration and Herniation

Intervertebral disc disease is a common cause of low back pain (65). Disc disorders encompass many conditions, from subtle disc degeneration to dramatic disc herniation. Annually, an estimated 4.1 million people in the United States report a prolapsed disc. From 1985 to 1988 intervertebral disc disorders were the cause of an average of 334,000 hospitalizations annually, or 2.3 million annual hospital days (1). After chronic ischemic heart disease and osteoarthritis, intervertebral disc herniation is the third most frequent condition for which worker disability is granted (51).

As common and troubling as intervertebral disc disorders are, there is little agreement regarding their causation. While some researchers (66) believe that disc disruption is primarily an acute or traumatic injury, others (67, 68) argue that it generally results from a chronic or degenerative process. Researchers agree, however, with the observation that disc degeneration tends to occur in people who exercise either too much or too little. To understand intervertebral disc disorders, it is useful to review the anatomy of the disc.

Anatomy of the Intervertebral Disc

A complex structure, the fibrocartilaginous intervertebral disc supports the weight of the upper body while permitting a significant range of motion. Because it is viscoelastic, the disc damps the impulses applied to the body. The disc is able to withstand forces of compression, bending, shear, and torsion because of the unique combination of materials that form the disc. The disc is composed of three histologically different yet functionally and physically interdependent elements: the nucleus pulposus, the anulus fibrosus, and the cartilaginous endplates.

A viscid mucoprotein gel, the nucleus pulposus lies in the center of the disc. The nucleus has a high water content, high fixed charge density, and random orientation of collagen fibrils. The composition of the nucleus allows it to function under hydrostatic pressure to distribute loads from the spine onto the superior and inferior vertebral body endplates as well as onto the inner lamina of the anulus fibrosus (51).

Positioned on the periphery of the nucleus, the anulus fibrosus forms the outer lateral boundary of the disc. The anulus fibrosus consists of a series of 15 to 25 lamellae that create a network between the adjacent vertebral bodies (69). The lamellae are composed of coarse collagen fibers that run parallel within each lamella and obliquely at approximately a 60° angle to the fibers in adjacent lamellae (70). Occasional areas of asymmetry interrupt this tidy arrangement of collagen fiber bundles. In particular, the posterolateral portions of the anulus have the majority of incomplete laminae and asymmetrical collagen fiber bundle organization. Like the arrangement of plies in a modern automobile tire, the organization of collagen fibers and laminae in the anulus fibrosus allows the anulus to contain hydrostatic pressure loads. The anulus is also able to provide resistance to minor displacements of the adjacent vertebral bodies because of the variation in fiber orientation.

The endplate provides the cranial and caudal surfaces of the intervertebral disc while serving as the interface between the nucleus pulposus and the neighboring intervertebral bodies. Although it is composed of a thin layer of hyaline cartilage, the endplate lacks the zones of fibrillar and cellular organization that characterize articular hyaline cartilage. The endplate's collagen fibers are oriented horizontally and parallel to the vertebral body surface. With its collagen fibers in this orientation, the endplate can best withstand the tension generated in the inner anulus. Another level of support is derived from the continuity between these collagen fibers of the endplate and the fibers of the inner third of anular lamellae (71). At the juncture between the anulus and the vertebral epiphysis, elastin fibers contribute to the disc's flexibility and durability (72).

The avascular nucleus receives most of its nutrients via diffusion through the endplate. Solutes are transported between the well-vascularized vertebral body and the disc nucleus via capillaries as well as areas of the vertebral bone marrow that have direct contact with the hyaline cartilage of the central endplate (42, 73–76).

Epidemiology of Degenerative Disc Disease

While many patients with low back pain have disc degeneration, a significant number of patients with degeneration are completely asymptomatic. Consequently, disc degeneration is not a precise indicator of back pain. As a corollary, in a patient with both back pain and disc degeneration, the degeneration does not always account for the pain.

Approximately 95% of herniated intervertebral discs occur at the L4 and L5 levels in people between ages 25 and 55 years (77, 78). The high prevalence of disease at L4 and L5 can be explained by several factors unique to the lower lumbar spine. First, the posterior longitudinal ligament is narrow and thus provides less support to the posterior anulus. Second, this site undergoes a great deal of flexion, bending, and torsion, placing great structural demands on the connective tissue. Finally, lumbar lordosis causes the vertebrae at L4 and L5 to bear more force in shear (79). Although the disc between L5 and S1 is usually the smallest of the lower three lumbar discs, it bears the heaviest loads. Thus, L5–S1 disc stresses are much greater than those found in the other lumbar discs (37) (Fig. 15.1). While disc degeneration typically begins in the lower lumbar spine, it progresses to successively higher levels as the affected discs become stiffer and an increased demand is placed on the superiorly adjacent discs (80, 81). The pathophysiology of disc degeneration helps one to understand why disc degeneration is more likely to occur in people who exert themselves either too much or too little.

Treatment for Disc Herniation

Surgical intervention is indicated for patients who have pain refractory to 6 to 8 weeks of nonoperative therapy. Any patient with a neurological deficit secondary to disc herniation should initially be considered a candidate for surgery. Surgical interventions for isolated herniated discs include microdiscectomy, routine laminotomy, and modern endoscopic approaches (82–84). Because these procedures are minimally invasive, length of hospital stay and overall cost for these procedures have been dramatically reduced.

Spinal Stenosis, Osteoarthritis, and Facet Degeneration

Degenerative lumbar spinal stenosis results from chronic disc degeneration, facet arthropathy secondary to osteoarthritis, spinal instability, and the body's attempt to compensate for these changes. The disease spectrum ranges from minimal symptoms of mechanical low back pain caused by early facet degeneration to severe spinal stenosis. Stenosis can lead to compression of the cauda equina or exiting nerve roots and to significant pain and functional disability (85). Symptoms may include isolated nerve root irritation, back pain, and frank neurogenic claudication (86).

Primarily a diagnosis of the elderly, lumbar spinal stenosis is the most common diagnosis among Medicare patients undergoing lumbar spine surgery (87). Each year more than 30,000 surgeries are performed for degenerative spinal stenosis (88). The direct medical cost of these procedures is approximately $1 billion (85).

Treatment

Spinal stenosis is caused by a combination of hypertrophy of the facet joints and degeneration of the ligamentum flavum. Therefore, surgical intervention for spinal stenosis consists of decompression of the neural elements. This is accomplished with laminectomies, partial facetectomies, bilateral foraminotomies, and removal of the hypertrophic soft tissue. Decompression should provide adequate space for the passage of the nerve roots through the foramen.

Preoperative assessment of the structural integrity of the spine should be performed to assess whether fusion should also be performed. The indications for fusion include degenerative spondylolisthesis, scoliosis and/or kyphosis, or recurrent spinal stenosis. Intraoperative structural alterations that require fusion include excessive facet joint removal (greater than 50% bilaterally) and radical disc excision. In patients who are not candidates for surgery, temporary relief of symptoms may be achieved through the use of epidural steroid injections.

Degenerative Spondylolisthesis

Degenerative spondylolisthesis is a form of spinal stenosis caused by chronic disc degeneration and consequent motion segment instability (Fig. 15.2). Patients with a sagittal orientation of their facet joints are predisposed to this form of spinal stenosis. Conservative treatment is similar to that for spinal stenosis.

Treatment

Surgery for degenerative spondylolisthesis is indicated when symptoms become functionally incapacitating despite 2 to 3 months of nonoperative treatment. About 10 to 15% of patients have surgery as a result of failure of conservative treatment. Operative treatment is decompression with stabilization and/or fusion. Pedicle screws have been found efficacious in the treatment of multisegmental instability of the lumbar spine, such as degenerative spondylolisthesis (89–91). Pedicle screws allow fixation of the strongest portion of osteopenic vertebra, maintain lordosis, and achieve torsional stability.

Spinal Deformities

Scoliosis

When viewed from behind, a normal spine appears straight. A scoliotic spine has a lateral curvature. Patients with scoliosis have the appearance of leaning to one side. This should not be confused with poor posture. Many patients with thoracic and lumbar scoliosis have one shoulder higher and one scapula more prominent than the other. With the arms at

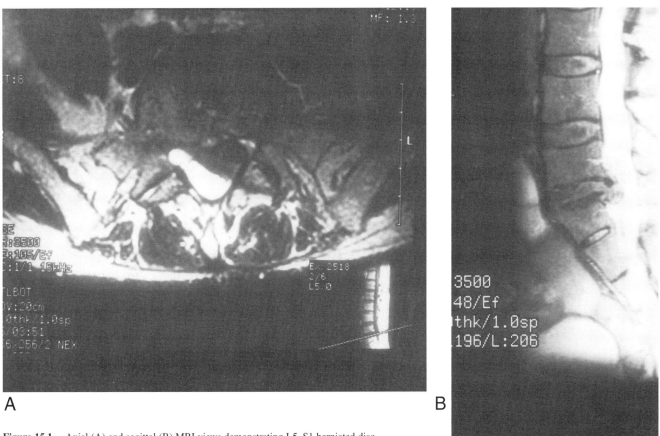

Figure 15.1.   Axial (A) and sagittal (B) MRI views demonstrating L5–S1 herniated disc.

the side, more space is seen between the arm and body on one side than on the other, and one hip appears higher. Often the head is not centered over the pelvis.

The majority of scoliosis (85%) is idiopathic, having no known cause. It commonly affects adolescents during the growth spurt. It has been found to run in families, showing some genetic or hereditary influences. Congenital scoliosis is due to defects of the spinal vertebrae present at birth. Neuromuscular scoliosis is due to chromosomal abnormalities or to disorders of the central nervous system, muscle, and connective tissue. Representative examples of neuromuscular scoliosis include cerebral palsy, arthrogryposis, Marfan's syndrome, and Down's syndrome.

More than 500,000 adults in the United States have scoliosis greater than 30°. Scoliosis greater than 50° may progress after skeletal maturation. Furthermore, untreated spinal deformity of childhood can lead to severe back pain, cardiopulmonary dysfunction, and neurological compromise.

Many adults lack documentation of the progression of their scoliosis. Patients notice an increasing deformity with loss of overall height. There is a high incidence of pain in adult patients with thoracolumbar or lumbar curves greater than 45°. Standing anteroposterior and lateral plain radiographs of the lumbar spine demonstrate an apical vertebral rotation and coronal imbalance. Neurological dysfunction is uncommon. Rather, patients have radiculopathy and signs and

symptoms of spinal stenosis. Paraplegia secondary to scoliosis has not been reported.

Radiographic studies should include standing anteroposterior, lateral, and bending radiographs. Pulmonary function testing should be considered in those with significant thoracic scoliosis and pulmonary compromise. MRI and CT myelograms should be used to evaluate the neural axis. In the older adult population with scoliosis, it is often beneficial to perform a thorough medical evaluation. These patients may have cardiorespiratory problems, nutritional deficiency, poor body conditioning, and osteopenia.

Treatment

Nonoperative treatment for scoliosis includes soft-tissue modalities, analgesics, and NSAIDs. Exercises demonstrated by a competent therapist with a sports medicine approach can restore many patients to a higher degree of overall function. Bracing does not permanently change the curvature of an adult. However, braces may provide pain relief for older patients.

The indications for surgical intervention include progression of deformity, pain, deterioration of pulmonary function, and cosmesis. The surgical goals are to improve and arrest deformity. Surgery involves the fusion of the spine at the optimum degree of safe correction of the deformity. Correction in adults in general does not equal that of adolescents, who have

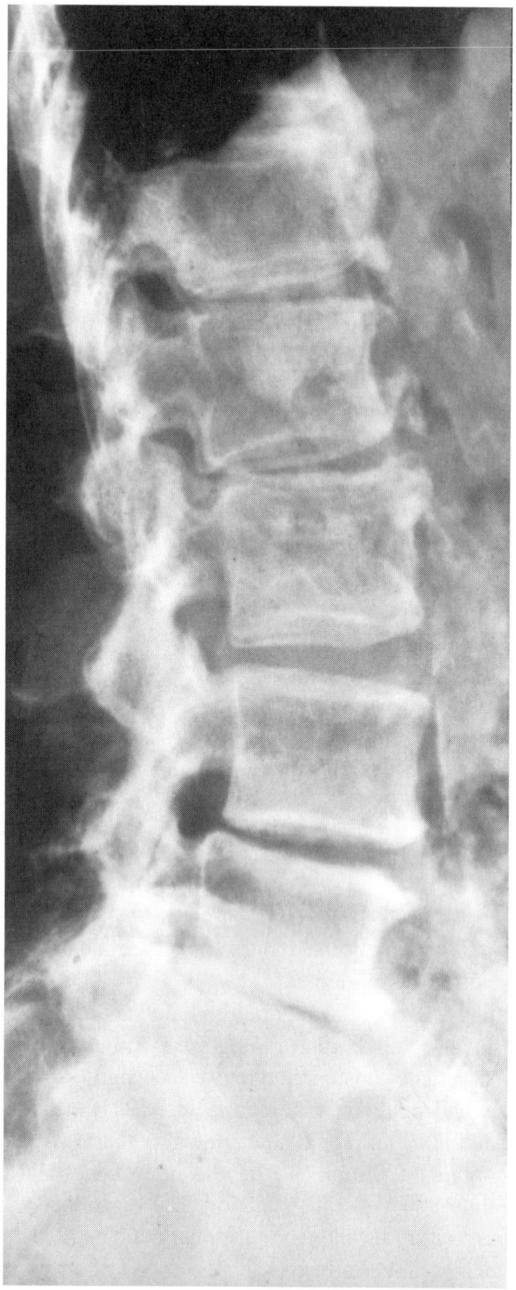

Figure 15.2. Lateral radiograph demonstrating severe spondylosis and degenerative spondylolisthesis.

more flexible curves. The surgical complications include pseudarthrosis (0 to 25%), residual pain (5 to 15%), neurological problems (1 to 5%), and infection (0.5 to 5%).

Spinal fusion instruments include metallic rods, hooks, and screws that hold the spine in the corrected position while the fusion heals. The instruments are rarely removed. Modern scoliosis surgical techniques provide maximum stability with early postoperative mobilization of patients. Combined anterior and posterior procedures allow greater correction of the curves and obtain higher fusion rates. Comprehensive preoperative conferences involve discussion of the risks versus benefits of surgical intervention.

Kyphosis, Hyperlordosis, and Spina Bifida

The lumbar spine has a natural swayback, or lordosis. The thoracic spine has a normal kyphosis. Patients who have an excessive thoracic curvature (kyphosis) often compensate to maintain sagittal plane balance by increasing their lumbar lordosis. This commonly causes pain in the lumbar region secondary to the hyperextension stress on the facet joints. Treatment should be directed to correct the thoracic deformity.

Hyperlordosis can be a congenital deformity but most commonly is secondary to obesity with weakness of the anterior wall musculature. Treatment should include an appropriate nutritional regimen and exercise program.

Spina bifida is a congenital absence of a portion of the bony elements of the posterior spine. There is a wide spectrum of the defect. Most people are not aware that they have this abnormality (thus the term spina bifida occulta). Typically no treatment is necessary for patients who have no neurological deficit. However, there is an increased incidence of spina bifida in patients with lumbar spondylolysis or defects in the pars interarticularis.

Trauma

Adolescents

Low back injuries from trauma often happen to adolescents. Adolescents have a high susceptibility to back injury because of the young spine's immature bony and ligamentous structures. Sports such as football and gymnastics can cause low back pain secondary to the hyperlordotic postures required by these sports. Conservative treatment of this type of low back pain caused by muscle strain consists of rest, abstinence from sports, and flexibility exercises for the hamstrings as well as strengthening exercises for the abdominal muscles (92).

If the back pain persists despite conservative treatment, further evaluation should be performed to determine whether the patient has spondylolysis, fracture in the pars interarticularis. This type of fracture may lead to a spondylolisthesis, or slippage, of one vertebra on another. On physical examination these patients often have pain exacerbated when they assume a hyperlordotic stance. This diagnosis can be confirmed with the use of plain films and CT. If no disease is seen with these studies, it is often useful to use bone scans and single-photon emission computed tomography (SPECT). Nonoperative treatment includes the use of a brace and NSAIDs. If the pain persists despite these interventions, operative treatment involves either a direct repair of the pars interarticularis fracture or a fusion in situ (93–95).

Adults

Evaluation of a patient after a serious traumatic insult requires a thorough history and physical evaluation including a neurological examination. Plain radiographs, including flexion-extension views, provide information regarding lumbar spine stability. CT and MRI are also beneficial in assessing bony and soft-tissue injuries. The principles of treatment of fractures in the spine are similar to those for the management of long bone fractures. It is essential to obtain immediate stability so that early mobilization of the patient can occur. One fuses the involved spinal segments only, attempting to maximize the remaining number of levels for motion.

Systemic Problems

Metabolic Diseases

Paget's Disease of Bone

Paget's disease of bone is a common disorder in adults over 40, affecting up to 10% of the general population of octogenarians. It is an idiopathic disorder of skeletal remodeling. The primary dysfunction involves an increase in osteoclastic resorption of bone, with the production of structurally weak and immature woven bone, which leads to deformities and fractures. Paget's disease is usually asymptomatic. However, aching bone pain may be present in severe cases. The progressive enlargement of vertebral bodies involved with Paget's may cause a secondary spinal stenosis. Patients with extensive disease may have high-output congestive heart failure. One must be aware of the possibility of the development of a secondary sarcoma in pagetoid bone.

Pain may be associated with an increase in metabolic activity. The major therapeutic agents used to relieve clinical symptoms are bisphosphonates and calcitonin. Surgical interventions are indicated for nerve compression, fractures, and end-stage arthritis.

Osteoporosis

Osteoporosis affects 20 million individuals in the United States (96). It is characterized by decreased bone mass and increased susceptibility to fracture. Given the increasing longevity of the general population, the number of people who sustain osteoporotic compression fractures grows each year. Although osteoporosis is the most common cause of vertebral compression fractures in the elderly, such fractures may also be secondary to other metabolic bone diseases that affect the spine, such as osteomalacia. Therefore, any elderly patient with a compression fracture requires a thorough medical workup to assess the true cause of the patient's osteopenia. Osteoporosis is now a subject of major interdisciplinary research efforts, and treatment should be focused on prevention.

Infections

The goal of treatment of spinal infections includes early diagnosis with eradication of infection and prevention of neurological deficit. This requires an aggressive approach to prevent osteomyelitis and secondary deformities. The incidence of postoperative infections has been greatly reduced with the use of antibiotic regimens. However, there has been a resurgence of diseases such as tuberculosis of the spine in patients with compromised immune systems. In this population of immunocompromised patients, any suspicion of spinal infections should be promptly investigated.

Most epidural abscesses are associated with vertebral osteomyelitis, discitis, or postoperative infections. These abscesses occur commonly in the lumbar region. The imaging modality of choice for the diagnosis of epidural abscesses is MRI. Treatment with surgical decompression and antibiotics must be performed immediately, because the prognosis is directly related to the timing of the intervention.

Tumors

Although primary malignancies of the spine are rare, many types of cancers metastasize to the spine. The most common tumors that metastasize to the vertebral column include breast, prostate, lung, kidney, and thyroid.

Tumors may cause progressive low back pain that is not relieved with rest. Many patients report severe night pain. Suspicion of metastatic involvement can be evaluated with the use of plain radiography and bone scans. Treatment goals include the maintenance of spinal stability and oncologic treatment of the primary cancer.

Inflammatory Diseases

Low back pain may be secondary to inflammatory diseases such as rheumatoid arthritis, ankylosing spondylitis, and Reiter's syndrome. Severe spinal deformities and pain may occur in patients with these diseases. Surgical intervention should be considered in coordination with rheumatological consultation. In certain conditions, such as ankylosing spondylitis, the surgical correction of spinal deformities may provide patients with a dramatic improvement in overall outlook and quality of life.

Back Pain during Pregnancy

In a recent prospective study of 200 pregnant women, 76% reported back pain at some time during pregnancy, with 61% having new onset of their back pain during the present pregnancy. The prevalence of pain in the latter group declined to 9.4% after delivery. Some 30% of the pregnant women with back pain reported significant difficulty with activities of daily living and significant time lost from work (97).

Iatrogenic Spinal Deformities

One of the most common and preventable forms of iatrogenic lumbar spine deformities is the flat back syndrome, which consists of a loss of lordosis in the lumbar spine. It is most commonly created by the use of distraction instruments. Historically, use of Harrington instruments was the primary reason for this severe iatrogenic deformity. Patients lose sagittal plane imbalance and have a flexed hip and knee posture. Surgical correction of this deformity involves anterior and posterior spinal reconstruction with osteotomy of the spine.

CONCLUSION

Low back pain, a common ailment in our society, may be due to any of a variety of conditions. To provide appropriate care and minimize disability, it is essential to obtain the appropriate diagnosis and institute the proper treatment.

References

1. Praemer A, Furner S, Rice DP. Musculoskeletal conditions in the United States. Park Ridge, IL: American Academy of Orthopaedic Surgeons, 1992.
2. Waddell G. Low back pain: a twentieth century health care enigma. Spine 1996;21:2820–2825.
3. Kelsey JL, White AA. Epidemiology of low back pain. Spine 1980;6:133–142.
4. Fishbein W, Salter L. The relationship between truck and tractor driving and disorders of the spine and supporting structures. Ind Med Surg 1950;19:444–445.
5. Heliovaara M. Body height, obesity, and risk of herniated lumbar intervertebral disc. Spine 1987;12:469–472.
6. Kelsey J. An epidemiological study of the relationship between occupations and acute herniated lumbar intervertebral disc. Int J Epidemiol 1975;4:197–205.
7. Hrubec Z, Nashold B. Epidemiology of lumbar disc lesions in the military in World War II. Am J Epidemiol 1975:366–376.
8. Chaffin DB, Park KS. A longitudinal study of low-back pain as associated with occupational weight lifting factors. Am Ind Hyg Assoc J 1973;34:513–525.
9. Harber P, Billet E, Gutowski M, et al. Occupational low-back pain in hospital nurses. J Occup Med 1985;27:518–524.
10. Leboeuf-Yde C, Lauritsen JM, Lauritzen T. Why has the search for causes of low back pain largely been nonconclusive? Spine 1997;22:877–881.
11. Kelsey J, Ostfeld A. Demographic characteristics of persons with acute herniated lumbar intervertebral disc. J Chron Dis 1975;28:37–50.
12. Andersson G. Epidemiologic aspects on low-back pain in industry. Spine 1981;6:53–60.
13. Gyntelberg F. One year incidence of low back pain among male residents of Copenhagen aged 40–59. Dan Med Bull 1974;21:30–36.
14. Magora A. Investigation of the relation between low back pain and occupation. Ind Med 1970;39:504–510.
15. Frymoyer EA. Epidemiological studies of low-back pain. Spine 1980;5:419–423.
16. Heliovaara M. Occupation and risk of herniated lumbar intervertebral disc or sciatica leading to hospitalization. J Chron Dis 1987;40:259–264.
17. Kelsey J, Golden A, Mundt D. Low back pain/prolapsed lumbar intervertebral disc. Rheum Dis Clin North Am 1990;16:699–716.
18. Nachemson A. The effect of forward leaning on lumbar intradiscal pressure. Acta Orthop Scand 1965;35:314–328.
19. Frymoyer J, Cats-Baril W. Predictors of low back pain disability. Clin Orthop 1987;221:89–98.
20. Kelsey J, Hardy R. Driving of motor vehicles as a risk factor for acute herniated lumbar intervertebral disc. Am J Epidemiol 1975;102:63–73.
21. Panjabi MM, Takata K, Goel UK. Kinematics of lumbar intervertebral foramen. Spine 1983;8:348–357.
22. Weinstein J, Pope M, Schmidt R, Seroussi R. Neuropharmacological effects of vibration on the dorsal root ganglion: an animal model. Spine 1988;13:521–525.
23. Pope MH. Vibration of the spine and low back pain. Clin Orthop 1992;279:49–59.
24. Pope MH, Rosen JC, Wilder DG, Frymoyer JW. The relation between biomechanical and psychological factors in patients with low-back pain. Spine 1980;5:173–178.
25. Keene JS, Alber MJ, Springer SL, et al. Back injuries in college athletes. J Spinal Disord 1989;2:190–195.
26. Mann DC, Keene JS, Drummond DS. Unusual causes of back pain in athletes. J Spinal Disord 1992;4:337–343.
27. Farfan H, Huberdeau R, Dubow H. Lumbar intervertebral disc degeneration. J Bone Joint Surg Br 1972;69B:699–703.
28. Sward L, Hellstrom M, Jacobsson B, et al. Back pain and radiologic changes in the thoraco-lumbar spine of athletes. Spine 1990;15:124–129.
29. Biering-Sorenson R, Thomsen D. Medical, social and occupational history as risk indicators for low back trouble in a general population. Spine 1986;11:720–725.
30. Chaffin D, Herrin G, Keyserling W. Preemployment strength testing. J Occup Med 1978;20:403–408.
31. Nutter P. Aerobic exercise in the treatment and prevention of low back pain. Occup Med 1988;3:137–145.
32. Troup JD. Causes, prediction and prevention of back pain at work. Scand J Work Environ Health 1984;10:419–428.
33. Deyo R, Bass E. Lifestyle and low-back pain: the influence of smoking and obesity. Spine 1989;14:501–506.
34. Frymoyer EA. Risk factors in low-back pain: an epidemiological survey. J Bone Joint Surg Am 1983;A65:213–218.
35. Svensson H, Andersson G, Johansson S, et al. A retrospective study of low-back pain in 38- to 64-year old women. Spine 1988;13:548–552.
36. Battie M, Videman T, Gill K, et al. Smoking and lumbar intervertebral disc degeneration: an MRI study of identical twins. Spine 1991;16:1015–1021.
37. Holm S, Nachemson A. Nutrition of the intervertebral disc: acute effects of cigarette smoking: an experimental animal study. Ups J Med Sci 1988;93:91–99.
38. Bostman OM. Body mass index and height in patients requiring surgery for lumbar intervertebral disc herniation. Spine 1993;18:851–854.
39. Lloyd M, Gauld S, Soutar C. Epidemiological study of back pain in miners and office workers. Spine 1986;11:136–140.
40. Miller J, Schmatz S, Schultz A. Lumbar disc degeneration: correlation with age, sex, and spine level in 600 autopsy specimens. Spine 1988;13:173–178.
41. Kellgren J, Lawrence J. Osteo-arthritis and disk degeneration in an urban population. Ann Rheum Dis 1958;17:388–397.
42. Brown M, Tsaltas T. Studies of the permeability of the intervertebral disc during skeletal maturation. Spine 1976;1:240–244.
43. Colombini D, Occhipinti E, Grieco A, Faccini M. Estimation of lumbar disc areas by means anthropometric parameters. Spine 1989;14:51–55.
44. Stairmand JW, Holm S, Urban JPG. Factors influencing oxygen concentration gradients in the intervertebral disc. Spine 1991;16:444–449.
45. Postacchini F, Lami R, Pugliese O. Familial predisposition to discogenic low-back pain. Spine 1988;13:1403–1406.
46. Varlotta G, Brown M, Kelsey J, et al. Familial predisposition for herniation of a lumbar disc in patients who are less than twenty-one years old. J Bone Joint Surg Am 1991;73A:124–128.
47. Farfan H, Sullivan J. The relation of facet orientation to intervertebral disc failure. Can J Surg 1967;10:179–185.
48. Heliovaara M, Vanharanta H, Korpi J, et al. Herniated lumbar disc syndrome and vertebral canals. Spine 1986;11:433–435.
49. Ramani PS. Variations in size of the bony lumbar canal in patients with prolapse of lumbar intervertebral discs. Clin Radiol 1976; 27:301–307.
50. Verbiest H. Further experiences on the pathological influence of a developmental narrowness of the bony vertebral canal. J Bone Joint Surg Br 1955;37B:576–583.
51. Lotz J, Donlon BS, Glazer PA, et al. Intervertebral disc herniation: a review (in press).
52. Savini R, Martucci E, Nardi S, et al. The herniated lumbar intervertebral disc in children and adolescents: long-term follow-up of 101 cases treated by surgery. Ital J Orthop Traumatol 1991;17:505–511.

53. Gates SJ. Musculoskeletal primary care. In: Gates SJ, Mooar PA, eds. Primary care for nurse practitioners: management of musculoskeletal problems. Philadelphia: Lippincott-Raven, 1997 (in press).

54. Waddell G, McCulloch JA, Kummel E, Venner RM. Nonorganic physical signs in low-back pain. Spine 1980;5:117–125.

55. Guyer RD, Ohnmeiss DD. Contemporary concepts in spine care: lumbar discography. Spine 1995;20:2048–2059.

56. Wheeler AH, Hanley EN Jr. Nonoperative treatment for low back pain: rest to restoration. Spine 1995;20:375–378.

57. Nachemson AL, Schultz A, Andersson G. Mechanical effectiveness studies of lumbar spine orthoses. Scand J Rehabil Med 1983;15:139–149.

58. Mamourian AC, Dickman CA, Drayer BP, Sonntag VK. Spinal epidural abscess: three cases following spinal epidural injection demonstrated with MRI. Anesthesiology 1993;78:204–207.

59. Shantha TR, Bisese J. Subdural blood patch for spinal headache. N Engl J Med 1991;325:1252–1254.

60. Twomey L, Taylor J. Exercise and spinal manipulation in the treatment of low back pain. Spine 1995;20:615–619.

61. Postachini F, Facchini M, Palieri P. Efficacy of various forms of conservative treatment in low-back pain: a comparative study. Neuroorthop 1988;6:28–35.

62. Meade TW, Dyer S, Browne W, Frank AO. Randomised comparison of chiropractic and hospital outpatient management for low back pain: results from extended follow up. Br Med J 1995;311:349–351.

63. Assendelft WJJ, Koes BW, Knipschild PG, Bouter LM. The relationship between methodological quality and conclusions in reviews of spinal manipulation. JAMA 1995;274:1942–1948.

64. Koes BW, Assendelft WJJ, Van der Heijden GJMG, Bouter LM. Spinal manipulation for low back pain: an updated systematic review of randomized clinical trials. Spine 1996;21:2860–2873.

65. Vanharanta H, Guyer RD, Ohnmeiss DD, et al. Disc deterioration in low-back syndromes: a prospective, multi-center CT/discography study. Spine 1988;13:1349–1351.

66. Adams MA, Hutton WC. Prolapsed intervertebral disc: a hyperflexion injury. Spine 1982;7:184–191.

67. Lipson SJ. Metaplastic proliferative fibrocartilage as an alternative concept to herniated intervertebral disc. Spine 1988;13:1055–1060.

68. Saunders JB, Inman VT. Pathology of the intervertebral disk. Arch Surg 1940;40:389–416.

69. Marchand F, Ahmed AM. Investigation of the laminate structure of lumbar disc anulus fibrosus. Spine 1990;15:402–410.

70. Horton W. Further observations on the elastic mechanism of the intervertebral disc. J Bone Joint Surg Br 1958;40B:552–557.

71. Inoue H. Three-dimensional architecture of lumbar intervertebral discs. Spine 1981;6:139–146.

72. Johnstone B, Urban JPG, Roberts S, Menage J. The fluid content of the human intervertebral disc. Spine 1992;17:412–416.

73. Crock H, Yoshizawa H. The blood supply of the lumbar vertebral column. Clin Orthop 1976;115:6–21.

74. Maroudas A. Biophysical chemistry of cartilaginous tissues with special reference to solute and fluid transport. Biorheology 1975;12:233–245.

75. Nachemson A. Towards a better understanding of back pain: a review of the mechanics of the lumbar disc. Rheumatol Rehabil 1975;14:129.

76. Ogata K, Whiteside L. Nutritional pathways of the intervertebral disc. Spine 1981;6:211–216.

77. Friberg S, Hirsch C. Anatomical and clinical studies on lumbar disc degeneration. Acta Orthop Scand 1949;19:222–242.

78. Schultz A, Andersson G, Ortengren R, et al. Loads on the lumbar spine. J Bone Joint Surg 1982;64A:713–720.

79. Hickey DS, Hukins DWL. Relation between the structure of the annulus fibrosus and the function and failure of the intervertebral disc. Spine 1980;5:106–116.

80. Hsu K, Zucherman J, Shea W, et al. High lumbar disc degeneration: incidence and etiology. Spine 1990;15:679–682.

81. Powell M, Wilson M, Szypryt P, et al. Prevalence of lumbar disc degeneration observed by magnetic resonance in symptomless women. Lancet 1986;13:1366–1367.

82. Kambin P, Zhou L. History and current status of percutaneous arthroscopic disc surgery. Spine 1996; 21:57S–61S.

83. Andersson GBJ, Brown MD, Dvorak J, et al. Consensus summary on the diagnosis and treatment of lumbar disc herniation. Spine 1996;21:75S–78S.

84. McCulloch JA. Focus issue on lumbar disc herniation: macro- and microdiscectomy. Spine 1996;21:45S-56S.

85. Katz JN, Lipson SL, Chang LC, et al. Seven- to 10-year outcome of decompressive surgery for degenerative lumbar spinal stenosis. Spine 1996;21:92–98.

86. Frymoyer JW, ed. Orthopaedic knowledge update 4. Rosemont, IL: American Academy of Orthopaedic Surgeons, 1993:491–501.

87. Deyo RA, Ciol MA, Cherkin DC, et al. Lumbar spinal fusion: a cohort study of complications, reoperations, and resource use in the Medicare population. Spine 1993;18:1463–1470.

88. Taylor VM, Deyo RA, Cherkin DC, Kreter W. Low back pain hospitalization: recent United States trends and regional variations. Spine 1994;19:1207–1213.

89. Zdeblick TA. A prospective, randomized study of lumbar fusion: preliminary results. Spine 1993;18:983–991.

90. Bridwell KH, Sedgewick TA, O'Brien MF, et al. The role of fusion and instrumentation in the treatment of degenerative spondylolisthesis with spinal stenosis. J Spinal Disord 1993;6:461–472.

91. Mardjetko SM, Connolly PJ, Schott S. Degenerative lumbar spondylolisthesis. A meta-analysis of literature, 1970–1993. Spine 1994;19:2256S–2265S.

92. Micheli LJ. Low back pain in the adolescent: differential diagnosis. Am J Sports Med 1979;7:362–364.

93. Micheli LJ, Wood R. Back pain in young athletes. Arch Pediatr Adolesc Med 1995;149:15–18.

94. Saraste H, Brostrom LA, Aparisi T. Prognostic radiographic aspects of spondylolisthesis. Acta Radiol 1984;25:427–432.

95. Scaglietti O, Frontino G, Bartolozzi P. Technique of anatomical reduction of lumbar spondylolisthesis and its surgical stabilization. Clin Orthop 1976;117:165–175.

96. Sandhu HS, Lane JM. Osteoporosis of the spine. In: Garfin SR, Vaccaro AR, eds. Orthopaedic knowledge update: Spine. Rosemont, IL: American Academy of Orthopaedic Surgeons, 1997:227–234.

97. Kristiansson P, Svardsudd K, Von Schoultz B. Back pain during pregnancy. Spine 1996; 21:702–709.

CHAPTER 16

Facts and Fallacies of Spinal Disorders: A Neurosurgeon's Viewpoint

Charles A. Fager

Remarkably, most pain in neck, head, and back gradually disappears. The natural history of degenerative and arthritic change, at times punctuated by protrusion or rupture of a disc, is one of slow, gradual progression over the years. The bouts of lumbago and even sciatica in most persons tend to occur in erratic cycles, often with complete freedom of pain for years at a time. With advancing age the radiographic appearance of the spine worsens, but the patient is little worse, perhaps losing some height and mobility. Some of the lumbar and cervical spines that radiographically show the most degeneration are not troublesome at all.

The back that goes out, often called the acute back syndrome and far more common than the acute neck, has usually been attributed to paravertebral muscle spasm. The pain, often intense, may be attended by severe immobility and sometimes scoliotic listing. This is probably the least understood of all back pains. Spinal radiography initially may show no abnormality. Commonly, as years go by, evidence of degenerative disc space narrowing or facet arthropathy begins to appear. Change in position, often with turning from side to side in bed, is difficult. Pain, however, is prominent in the lumbosacral and sacroiliac areas, often on the same side in repeat attacks, and infrequently extends to the posterior hip, groin, or anterolateral thigh. Occasionally sciatic pain is referred below the knee. Despite the severity of the attack, it does not pose a serious problem; pain and spasm usually subside in 3 to 10 days, and the patient returns to full activity. The greatest concern is usually anticipation of the next episode, which may not occur for months or years.

After consultation with physicians, chiropractors, osteopaths, and acupuncturists, the patient with recurring back pain comes to the orthopaedic or neurological surgeon. He or she frequently has had diverse opinions regarding the cause and is anxious and fearful that some type of surgery will be necessary. Reassurance that surgery is not necessary is an important first step in palliation. A logical explanation of the cause is not always so easy, especially when the physician finds it difficult to explain the mechanics of the pain. Patients seem to accept the belief that an inherent weakness renders the human spine vulnerable to mechanical disorders. The lower lumbar spine bears the burden of enormous stresses, holds a person upright, and returns the body (even without a load) to the vertical position from sitting, lying, or especially from a bent-over position. Characteristically, degenerative change, ruptured disc, and facet arthritis develop at the lowest two lumbar segments (that is, L4-L5 and L5-S1) where the greatest weight, torsion, and shearing stresses occur. At times, however, these changes extend up to L3-L4. Degenerative changes in the cervical spine also develop, most often at the lowest two cervical disc spaces (that is, C5-C6 and C6-C7), the levels of greatest wear and tear from movement of the head and neck.

These lumbar and cervical changes sometimes develop at an early age, even in the 20s; this is beyond our understanding. It suggests some underlying problem that is not the result of excessive repetitive movement or injury. It has been said that there is a chemical basis for metabolic abnormality in the disc tissue, but this theory remains a mystery. At times there appears to be a familial tendency toward early degenerative change. Disc space narrowing, because it alters the relation of the vertebral bodies to each other, may lead to secondary and more typically, arthritic changes involving facet joints.

Some patients prefer heat for relief of pain and others use cold, with no common ground for choice. Although muscle-relaxing agents help a number of patients, equal relief has been obtained from taking simple analgesics. The many other drugs often used for acute back pain are overkill and are frequently ineffective. Rest in a bed or a recliner may be mandatory for several days during times when virtually all motion is impossible. The concept of manipulative therapy has intrigued physicians as well as chiropractors. Many persons with painful acute back spasm have reported dramatic relief, jumping down from the chiropractor's table after a single "adjustment." I can only speculate that some minor subluxation of a facet induced the spasm and may be rearranged by these maneuvers. Other patients with more chronic forms of back pain seem to improve more slowly after this type of therapy, probably despite the treatment rather than because of it. I have found that chiropractic treatment may be hazardous rather than beneficial. A number of patients have developed serious neurological signs when chiropractic was used in the presence of rupture of a disc. Cervical manipulation has at times been responsible for dissecting aneurysm of the vertebral artery and brainstem stroke.

In many patients who have low-back pain, the underlying cause is poor muscle tone, especially among those who lead sedentary lives. The most important definitive treatment is a disciplined exercise routine after the acute event subsides, with a long-term commitment to strengthening abdominal, gluteal, quadriceps, and other supportive muscles. Few persons are willing to make the commitment. Those who have been faithful to an exercise routine for many years have done exceptionally well in reducing the severity and number of attacks.

Many patients accept the fact that common back problems are not serious and that acute flare-ups come and go and will interfere only briefly with their usual physical activities. They respond to encouragement and are no worse off for pushing ahead with tennis, golf, skiing, or sailing. Others, however, shop around, accepting injections, stimulators, mechanical devices, and rolfing, none of which can possibly have any curative effect.

NEURAL ENTITIES AND SURGERY

Some patients with a history of recurring back pain eventually rupture a disc, suggesting that from the onset the problem may have been intervertebral disc degeneration, dissolution of normal cartilage structure, and disruption of surrounding fibrous tissue in so-called anulus fibrosis and longitudinal ligament. Early changes may not be detectable by radiography, and impairment of resiliency of the disc may lead to instability. Others, after years of recurring episodes, are found to have narrowing of the disc space indicative of chronic degenerative change, but protrusion or rupture of the disc, the most common causes of sciatica, never develops. The degenerative loss of disc substance, however, often is associated with abnormalities of the facet posteriorly, referred to as facet arthritis or arthropathy. As the facets thicken, enlarge, and expand in the lumbar region, they also crowd nerve roots or cauda equina, at times leading to serious irreversible entrapment and the symptoms of neurogenic claudication in the lower extremities. In the lower cervical region most of the degenerative changes arise from the intervertebral disc areas, although facets do become involved at times. Serious encroachment on the spinal cord leads to myelopathy in addition to the well-known pinched nerve or radiculopathy,

resulting in pain in the arm or femoral or sciatic pain in the lower limbs. Some of this comes about because spinal canals differ in size (1–4), with the smaller ones providing less room for their enclosed neural elements and rendering them more susceptible to compression, whether acute or chronic.

Time and experience have shattered many misconceptions about herniations of the intervertebral disc. The cartilaginous nucleus, as it degenerates, may protrude through its surrounding fibrous anulus in response to compressive spinal forces (Fig. 16.1) or it may rupture through the anulus and through the overlying tough posterior longitudinal ligament (Fig. 16.2), which extends throughout the anterior wall of the spinal canal. The common path for extrusion of fragments of ruptured lumbar disc is posterolateral, so that they present immediately anterior or anterolateral to the nerve root coursing over the disc space. Larger fragments extruding more laterally and superiorly may also compress the root above, at its neural foramen. This escape route develops more often because of midline tenacity and thickness of the longitudinal ligament. Attenuation of this ligament, however, permits some fragments to extrude in a median or paramedian position and to extend above or below the disc space when in the open spinal canal (Fig. 16.2). This may result in varying forms of cauda equina compression, which is far more serious than involvement of one or two nerve roots alone.

One of the most important elements in the biomechanics of a disc rupture or extrusion is that a large fragment of disc material is often displaced through a relatively small opening or tear in anulus and ligament. This retropulsion, which is probably the result of forces applied within the intervertebral space against a degenerative portion of disc that has lost its continuity, frequently results in the incarceration of the ruptured fragment at its stem, the mushroomlike expansion trapped beneath neural elements (Fig. 16.1). Some disc fragments become totally free and lodge in a nest as a sequestrum, at times actually hollowing out a saucer in the posterior portion of vertebral body.

Only a small number of patients have this type of rupture or extrusion on presentation. Although some patients with disc or spondylotic disorders require surgery, most patients with disc protrusion producing nerve root pain in the arm or leg, either cervical or lumbar, get better. Spontaneous recovery from protrusion or even small rupture of a disc comes about because the initial compression or pinch of the nerve responsible for sciatica or pain in the arm produces nerve root swelling. As the swelling subsides, if the nerve finds enough room, whether in the spinal canal or at its foramen, the pain subsides and disappears, usually in 4 to 6 weeks but sometimes in 2 to 4 months. With lessening of pain, slight or moderate neurological symptoms also clear. The cartilaginous fragment, which has protruded or even ruptured, undergoes some resorption, with decrease in its size; at times later thickening and often calcific or osteophytic changes occur, much the same as in the degenerative process. Without disc rupture, the soft, fragmented cartilage seems gradually to melt away completely or in time is replaced by hardened tissue.

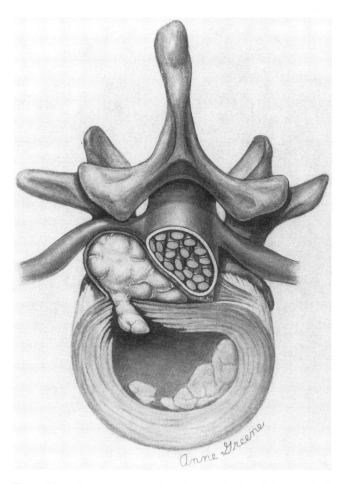

Figure 16.1.   Herniation of disc through the anulus fibrosis but contained within the posterior longitudinal ligament. Note compression of nerve root posterolaterally and indentation of cauda equina. (Courtesy of Lahey Clinic, Burlington, Massachusetts.

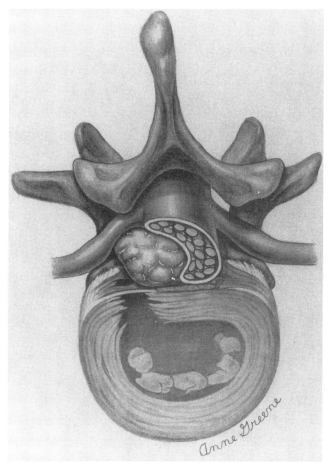

Figure 16.2.   Complete extrusion of paramedian disc fragment compressing cauda equina and nerve root. (Courtesy of Lahey Clinic, Burlington, Massachusetts.

It seems to make little difference, except from the standpoint of comfort, whether the patient with nerve root compression stays at rest, uses a cervical collar or lumbar support, or applies traction, which is a device I have never recommended other than for spinal fracture because the mechanical logic of its use has never been clear. In general, however, patients are advised to avoid exercise and of course, excessive physical activity. Many times they have already found a position of comfort; this, of course, implies less pressure on nerve root and may be salutary. The primary role of surgical treatment is relief of unremitting neural compression (5–7). When radicular pain associated with neurological symptoms or signs persists, which is evidence that a sizable fragment of disc has extruded, surgery provides dramatic relief of pain and return to full activities, although it obviously does nothing for the underlying disorder.

The large disc ruptures compressing the cauda equina and the more chronic forms of spondylotic change closing in on spinal cord or nerve roots require more extensive, more difficult, and more serious surgical procedures (Fig. 16.3 and 16.4). Spinal fusion is seldom necessary.

Contrary to most belief, trauma is only rarely the cause of disc rupture. Rupture of a disc after weight lifting or after injury probably occurs because of some degenerative change that was not evident or symptomatic before. Most of the injury responsible for acute and chronic forms of back pain is clearly the result of muscular strain and ligamentous sprain. As with similar injury elsewhere in the body, these are best treated by early return to full activity and an aggressive approach to exercise, but it may be difficult to persuade a squeamish or histrionic patient whose back hurts to follow these instructions. Unfortunately, many patients with this type of injury after an industrial or vehicular accident have undergone surgery for removal of a disc, which only adds to their problems and prolongs disability, sometimes permanently.

Although it is now well documented that the colloquial failed back is the result of faulty selection of patients not suitable for surgery initially, instances of residual pain and deficit ranging from foot drop to cauda equina damage result from inappropriate surgery (8). In cervical injury also, many patients have undergone anterior cervical discectomy and cervical spine fusion after whiplash injury without any evidence of a ruptured disc.

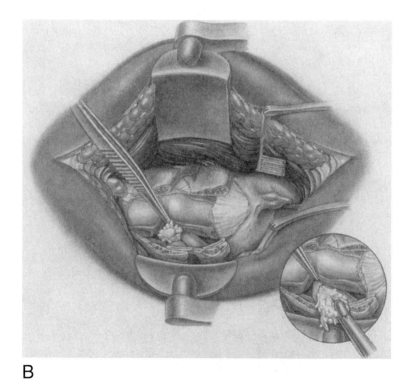

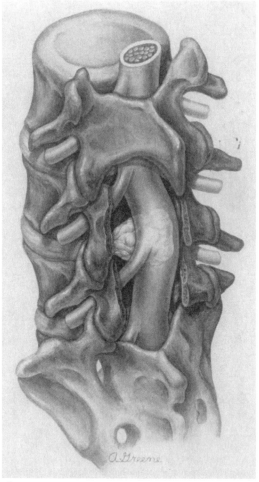

Figure 16.3. **A.** Conceptual drawing of median or paramedian disc rupture displacing neural structures, showing posterior neural arch removed as with laminectomy. **B.** Surgical view from left posterolateral approach showing liberation and extraction of disc fragment extruded beneath nerve root and cauda equina. (Courtesy of Lahey Clinic, Burlington, Massachusetts.)

A

Several factors add to the disarray in spinal surgery. The spurious belief that prominence of the disc or midline bulging seen in the past in lateral myelographic films and more recently by computed tomography (CT) or magnetic resonance imaging (MRI) may require surgery has resulted in ill-advised excision or injection of an enzyme (9), often at more than one level. Spondylotic constriction, or waistlike myelographic deformities, have often been misinterpreted as midline disc protrusions, leading to removal of the disc through small, frequently bilateral, surgical exposures. This type of surgery, rather than relieving nerve root or cauda equina compression, intensifies constriction because of contusion, early nerve root edema in a confined canal, later epidural fibrosis, and cohesion of nerve roots so often called adhesive arachnoiditis.

As welcome as CT and MRI have been to the diagnostic inventory, these procedures have compounded the problem of unnecessary and irrelevant studies. Each day of my consulting practice, one or more patients are seen carrying spinal MRI films reported to show disc problems, often questioning the need for surgery. Many of these imaging procedures have been ordered by their physicians or chiropractors at considerable expense, primarily for back pain with nothing in the clinical presentation to suggest a ruptured disc or radiculopathy.

Regrettably, all too frequently radiologists who do not understand the pathogenesis or biomechanical factors in disc disorders and spondylosis report "disc herniation" when the image clearly shows degenerative disc space narrowing with a typical hypertrophic change associated with prominence of the anulus so commonly seen in the ventral spinal canal (Fig. 16.5). Similar reports of "mild posterior protrusion" or "bulging" are frequently given when findings represent nothing more than normal prominence of a disc, especially at the L4-L5 level. The prevalence of abnormal findings on MRI of the lumbar spine in persons without back pain or other symptoms is well known. In one study (10), only 36% of 98 asymptomatic subjects had normal discs at all levels, confirming the irrelevance of so-called disc bulges or protrusions.

Nevertheless, imaging procedures are without question the most practical method of confirming the diagnosis of nerve root, cauda equina, or spinal cord compression by disc herniation or spondylotic change. They usually provide the surgeon with adequate information as to the location of the offending lesion, so that when surgery is necessary, it can be undertaken with accuracy directed at the specific area of involvement (Figs. 16.6 and 16.7). In the lumbar region, when the clinical diagnosis of disc herniation at either of the lower

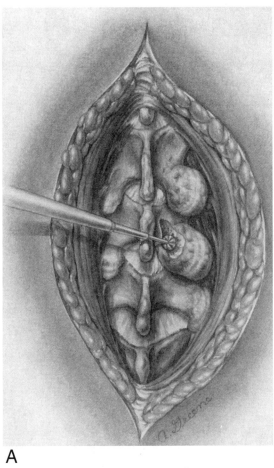

A

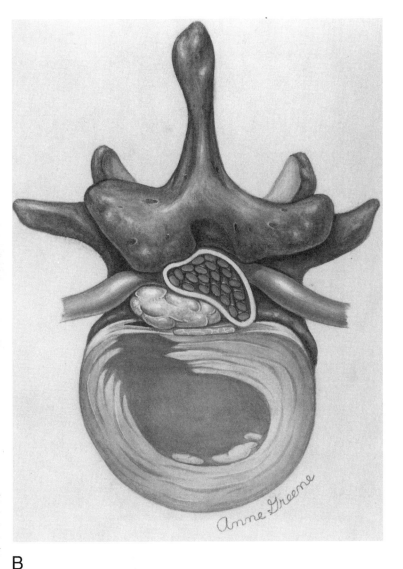

B

Figure 16.4.   A. Marked expansion of facets on right side of lumbar spine. Bone drilled down and thinned out before laminectomy and foraminotomy. **B.** Extruded disc associated with lumbar spondylosis. Note compression of cauda equina and nerve roots by arthropathic enlarged facets and by fragment of disc. (Courtesy of Lahey Clinic, Burlington, Massachusetts.)

three disc spaces is neurologically apparent, CT is usually adequate to confirm the diagnosis and localize the herniation. Should there be suspicion of a tumor or other lesion at a higher level, MRI that displays the lower spinal cord and cauda equina may be necessary. In lumbar spinal stenosis, the facet arthropathy and expansion are usually better detailed by CT. In the cervical region, however, MRI is more likely to disclose cervical disc herniation, although disc herniation is even more commonly confused with osteophyte formation in the cervical spine than in the lumbar spine. In any event and at any level, myelography combined with CT remains the ideal procedure for outlining neural elements and observing the degree of compression.

FALLACIES AND FADS

The procedure known as discography, long since laid to rest, has undergone a rebirth. Proponents of its use in the treatment of so-called discogenic pain believe that this type of pain may result from "internal disruption syndrome," anular tear, or even the chemical irritation said to result from leakage of an enzyme produced by disc material through such a tear (11). Discographers, some of whom are skillful and experienced, believe that pain coming from such a disc that is not herniated or protruded can be reproduced by direct injection, and this may be associated with leakage of the contrast material that is injected as well. This belief, supposedly reproducing the patient's pain, has resulted in surgery, at times more extensive than anyone can believe, discectomy at multiple levels, and multiple level lumbar spinal fusion that has at times been less than helpful and has added to disability. Most spinal disorders requiring surgery are readily diagnosed by history, physical examination, and imaging studies. Searching for a cause of elusive pain in patients with a poorly explained back syndrome has in general not proved rewarding. I have never found it necessary to use electromyography or nerve conduction studies to diagnose disc disorders. Although this is performed routinely in many centers, it adds nothing to the

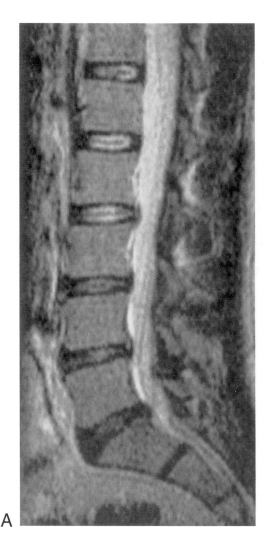

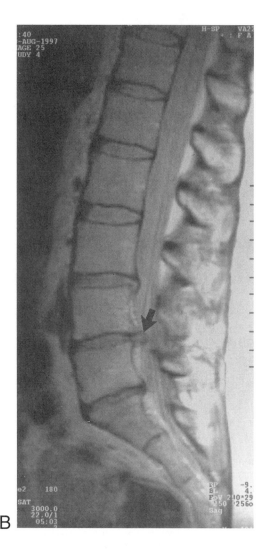

Figure 16.5.   **A.** Sagittal MRI shows degenerative changes at three lowest disc spaces as shown by desiccation, narrowing, and dark appearance in T2 image. Note the prominence of anulus seen with degeneration at all three levels—not disc herniation. **B.** Sagittal MRI of another patient with a similar degenerative change at lowest three levels with typical prominence at L3-L4 and L5-S1 levels that are not symptomatic and herniated disc at L4-L5 (arrow) with sciatica and L5 nerve root compression.

clinical diagnosis, although it may, of course, confirm the involvement of one particular nerve root or another. Electrodiagnostic studies may be more helpful when other possible causes—peripheral neuropathy, motor system disease, nerve entrapment syndromes—may explain the neurological syndrome that may not be caused by neural compression.

Other fallacies concern the neurosurgeon. Many patients have had surgery for removal of two and sometimes three discs at once. Many others have undergone intradiscal procedures, either by chemonucleolysis or automated nucleotome or laser at more than one level (12–14). After caring for thousands of patients who require surgery, I have yet to see the first with simultaneous symptomatic rupture of multiple intervertebral discs from more than one space. This must be extremely rare. Multilevel discectomy intended to relieve pain has at times only made the condition worse, and much of the disability of patients with chronic back pain remains iatrogenic at present. Multilevel discectomy should not, of course,

be confused with multilevel laminectomy for spinal stenosis, usually an effective palliative procedure.

The annals of medicine are filled with drugs and procedures that did not withstand the test of time or were not always proclaimed a boon to humanity. Oliver Wendell Holmes (15), in 1860, is quoted as saying, "If the whole materia medica, as now used, could be sunk to the bottom of the sea, it would be all the better for mankind—and all the worse for the fishes." His exception was wine, which he ranked with opium, quinine, anesthetics, and mercury among the boons to humanity. Except for quantitative population and inflationary change, the same problems exist in the 20th century. Lister (16), in 1975, recalled an Irish woman who said to him, "You know, if only you doctors could find a cure for these wretched antibiotics, you would be doing us all a good turn, and anyway all of my family in Ireland died, whether of TB or DT's, and they were a damned sight happier than us lot being kept alive with your lousy drugs."

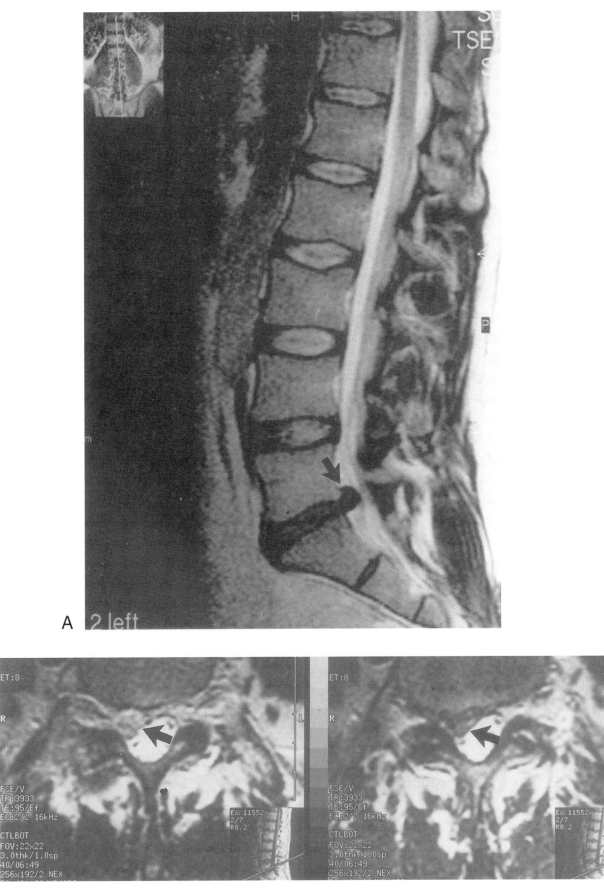

Figure 16.6.   Sagittal (**A**) and axial (**B**) MR images of patient with disc herniation (arrows) at L5-S1 requiring surgery.

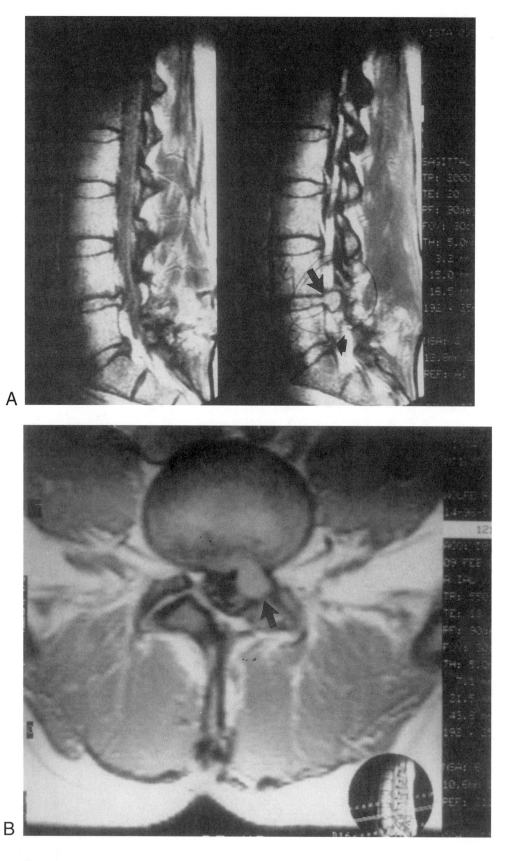

Figure 16.7.   Sagittal **(A)** and axial **(B)** MRI of patient with disc herniation at L4-L5 (arrows) requiring surgery.

In recent years the technological explosion has brought an abundance of instruments, techniques, drugs, and procedures, some of which have proved useful. Many of the numerous nonsteroidal anti-inflammatory agents are being employed immediately at the onset of spinal or extremity pain when conventional analgesics may be just as effective. With the increasing interest in so-called pain management, the proliferation of pain treatment centers, and the reluctance of orthopaedic and neurological surgeons to deal with chronic pain problems, patients are now being channeled into these areas where they are willing to accept repeated trigger point injections, facet blocks, and the ultimate epidural steroid injections. These are given usually with bupivacaine (Marcaine), initially three times at 2-week intervals.

I have talked with some patients in whom these epidural steroid injections have inexplicably brought dramatic relief. However, there have also been many patients in whom the logic for such a procedure is far from understandable. One would expect that the concept of bathing the epidural space, whether cervical or lumbar, with the intent of providing anti-inflammatory response to the exiting nerve roots would be undertaken in the assumption that the nerve roots were involved in some inflammatory process; this is highly speculative in the vast majority of patients who have been subjected to this procedure. It is being done on a wide range of patients with back pain who have no radicular symptoms or signs at all.

Furthermore, some disasters have occurred. On a number of occasions the dura has actually been penetrated, resulting in local reaction as with a spinal anesthesia, and at times persistent and severe spinal headache has occurred. I observed one case in which the needle penetrated the spinal cord at the C6 level, resulting in a serious spinal cord lesion, with complete paralysis of the right hand. It seems likely that many of the good results in patients with disc herniation, similar to the so-called good results after chiropractic manipulation, acupuncture, and myotherapy, occur despite these procedures and not because of them. A double-blind study of epidural corticosteroid injections for sciatica caused by herniated disc concluded that although there may be short-term improvement in sciatica from disc herniation, this treatment offers no significant functional benefit, nor does it reduce the need for surgery (17). Because most patients with sciatica resulting from a herniated disc can expect spontaneous recovery in an average of 6 weeks, it is easy to be misled into believing that one procedure or another has been effective. At any rate, the placebo effect cannot be disregarded.

Modifications of surgical intervention developed over the years have produced better approaches, less-invasive procedures, and far better recovery with greatly reduced hospital stays. In fact, in a number of institutions surgery for herniated cervical or lumbar disc is now being performed on an outpatient ambulatory basis. In most centers hospitalization is rarely more than 24 hours. The operating microscope has added tremendously to limited dissection and less discomfort, albeit the operative approach must still conform to the surgical principles of providing adequate exposure and decompression of neural element (18). There has been reported a unique percutaneous procedure that in my opinion establishes an approach to the epidural space for removal of disc fragments that have ruptured (19). Percutaneous procedures that previously were entirely limited to the disc space itself could not possibly address discs that have ruptured beyond the discal compartment, especially when the biomechanics shown in Figures 16.1 and 16.2 prevailed. The theory once proposed that reducing intradiscal contents decreased the pressure on herniated fragments, allowing regression, has never had scientific confirmation. In fact, it is abundantly clear that there is resorption of disc tissue so that it actually shrinks within the epidural space in patients who make a spontaneous recovery without any treatment (20).

For patients who require spinal fusion because of instability from spondylolisthesis, postlaminectomy subluxation, fracture dislocation, and bony tumors, it seems evident that the use of internal fixation with pedicle screws and plates and at times the more extensive use of rods and other internal fixation devices has provided an element of stability that clearly allows for a higher percentage of satisfactory fusion among patients who may require it.

References

1. Alexander E Jr. Significance of the small lumbar spinal canal: Cauda equina compression syndromes due to spondylosis: 5. Achondroplasia. J Neurosurg 1969;31:513–519.
2. Clark K. Significance of the small lumbar spinal canal: cauda equina compression syndromes due to spondylosis: 2. Clinical and surgical significance. J Neurosurg 1969;31:495–498.
3. Enhi G. Significance of the small lumbar spinal canal: cauda equina compression syndromes due to spondylosis: 1. Introduction. J Neurosurg 1969;31:490–494.
3a. Enhi G. Significance of the small lumbar spinal canal: cauda equina compression syndromes due to spondylosis: 4. Acute compression artificially induced during operation. J Neurosurg 1969;31:507–512.
4. Wilson CB. Significance of the small lumbar spinal canal: cauda equina compression syndromes due to spondylosis: 3. Intermittent claudication. J Neurosurg 1969; 31:499–506.
5. Fager CA. Surgical approaches to lumbar disc lesions and spondylosis. Surg Clin North Am 1980;60:649–663.
6. Fager CA. Lumbar disc disease: surgical treatment. In: Hardy RW Jr, ed. Lumbar disc disease. New York: Raven Press, 1993;105–122.
7. Scoville WB, Corkill G. Lumbar disc surgery: technique of radical removal and early mobilization. J Neurosurg 1973;39:265–269.
8. Fager CA, Freidberg SR. Analysis of failures and poor results of lumbar spine surgery. Spine 1980;5:87–94.
9. Fager CA. Commentary: chymopapain. In: Schmidek HM, Sweet WH, eds. Operative neurosurgical techniques. 2nd ed. New York: Grune & Sratton, 1988;1443–1448.
10. Jensen MC, Brant-Zawadzki MN, Obuchowski N, et al. Magnetic resonance imaging of the lumbar spine in people without back pain. N Engl J Med 1994;331:69–73.
11. Fager CA. The argument against discography. Neurosurg Q 1996;6:154.

12. Freidman WA. Percutaneous discectomy: an alternative to chemonucle-olysis? Neurosurgery 1983;13:542–547.

13. Kambin P, Schaffer JL. Percutaneous lumbar discectomy: prospective review of 100 patients. Clin Orthop 1989;238:24–34.

14. Maroon JC, Onik G. Percutaneous automated discectomy: a new method for lumbar disc removal. J Neurosurg 1987;66:143–146.

15. Holmes OW. Currents and countercurrents in medical science. In: Medical Essays: 1842–1882. Boston: Houghton Mifflin, 1883;173–208.

16. Lister J. By the London Post: Christmas Books. N Engl J Med 1975; 292:467–469.

17. Carette S, LeClaire R, Marcoux S, et al. Epidural corticosteroid injections for sciatica due to herniated nucleus pulposus. N Engl J Med 1997;336:1634–1640.

18. Fager CA. Microsurgical intervention for lumbar disk disease: A critique. In: Williams RW, McCulloch JA, Young PH, eds. Microsurgery of the lumbar spine. Rockville, MD: Aspen, 1990;249–262.

19. Ditsworth DA. Endoscopic transforaminal lumbar diskectomy and reconfiguration: A posterolateral approach into the spinal canal. Surgical Neurology, in press.

20. Fager CA. Observations on spontaneous recovery from intervertebral disc herniation. Surg Neurol 1994;42:282–286.

CHAPTER 17

Evaluation and Management of Back Pain: Preventing Disability[1]

Gerald M. Aronoff and David N. Dupuy

INTRODUCTION

Ongoing musculoskeletal pain has become a major public health problem which in addition to the pain and suffering involved, is also associated with huge economic loss to individuals and to society. Second only to the complaint of headaches in frequency, musculoskeletal pain is the most common pain complaint brought to health care providers, with back pain the most common musculoskeletal complaint. Because there are so many myths and misconceptions regarding its treatment, the topic will be covered in this paper to review those aspects of evaluation and management, which we believe, have adequate documentation for us to recommend them as useful as opposed to others where the data is less compelling. We want to acknowledge that two recent excellent reviews of the topic of back pain have contributed to what will follow in this paper, as we have incorporated many of the principles and treatment recommendations into our practices. These reviews are *Acute Low Back Problems in Adults* (1), published in 1994 by the Agency for Health Care Policy and Research to offer clinical practice guidelines, and *Back Pain in the Workplace* (2), published by the International Association of the Study of Pain, Task Force on Pain in the Workplace.

DEFINITION OF PAIN AND BACK INJURY

Pain is a complex, personal, unpleasant, subjective sensory and perceptual experience which may or may not be related to bodily injury or tissue damage. Psychosocial, ethnocultural, motivational, biological, chemical, and other factors (3) influence it. In managing a patient with intractable chronic pain and the inevitable accompanying suffering that

often leads to chronic debilitation, it is important to recognize the associated dysfunctional pain behaviors which are maladaptive and help define what is often referred to as a chronic pain syndrome (CPS). Pain is a symptom and not a disease. CPS is a symptom complex. All pain is real to the sufferer (with the possible exception of malingering) and those of us involved in its evaluation must attempt to understand its persistence even if we are unable to define its etiology. Not to do so will undermine our ability to form a therapeutic relationship with the patient.

Loeser's paradigm (4) in conceptualizing chronic pain syndromes (Fig. 17.1) is clinically useful.

It is suggested that the initial noxious stimulus leading to nociception appears less important in the management of CPS than the suffering, which is an emotional experience, and the pain behaviors, which the patient exhibits. This implies that while nociception may have initiated the pain process, in CPS, central more than peripheral factors may be prolonging the suffering and disability. Nociception, if still present, may not be directly treatable by conventional techniques, such as peripherally acting analgesics, nerve blocks, or surgery. Indeed, clinical experience caring for patients with chronic musculoskeletal pain suggests that often-environmental reinforcers, life stressors, depression, and cognitive distortions are more likely to prolong resolution of chronic pain and disability than are structural spinal factors. That is, they may serve as perpetuating factors, especially in many of the myofascial pain syndromes.

MAGNITUDE OF THE PROBLEM

Epidemiology

Recent estimates suggest that 2% of the U.S. work force suffer from chronic back pain, costing the U.S. economy $50 billion annually. It is estimated that the annual incidence rate

[1.] This chapter is reprinted with permission from Aronoff GM, Dupuy DN. Evaluation and management of back pain: preventing disability. J Back Musculoskeletal Rehab 1997;9:109–124.

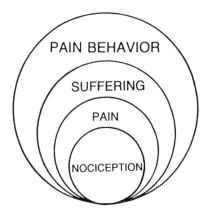

Figure 17.1. Pain in the framework of sequential input. Suggested by Loeser (4).

of low-back pain in the U.S. is 2 to 5% of the adult population (5). There is a wide incidence range from 0.2% to greater than 10% dependent on the type of work performed. In general, there is a higher incidence of back injuries found in those doing heavy work than in sedentary work (6). The lifetime incidence or risk ranges from 60 to 90% (7, 8). There is a yearly prevalence of 15 to 20% (9). Impairments of the low back are the most frequent cause of activity limitations among those under age 64 (10) and are the common cause of a decrease in work capacity in persons aged 25 to 44 (9). About 1% of the U.S. population is temporarily disabled from back problems (at any given time) and the same percentage is chronically disabled (9). Although costs involved with direct medical care are more easily calculated, costs related to work-days lost, workers' compensation, decreased efficiency and work productivity are also staggering. When one combines these with direct medical costs, estimates are between $26.8 billion and $56 billion (Clark WL. Occupational low back pain (unpublished manuscript). The frequency and impact of chronic back pain are expected to increase over the next decade as the average age of the work force increases (12).

CAUSATION

Most cases of low-back pain are idiopathic, and more often than not, the exact etiology of low-back pain is obscure (13–15). Dillane et al. (16) found that the cause was unknown for 79% of first episodes of low-back pain in men and 89% of first episodes in women. They divided lumbar spinal pain into three categories: (*a*) degenerative and traumatic, the most common, (*b*) structural abnormalities, and (*c*) musculoligamentous dysfunction. The degenerative process represents the general wear and tear which results from aging. Therefore, it should not be considered a disease process. The traumatic process can arise either from an isolated injury or repeated and cumulative trauma contributing to degeneration (e.g., repeated trauma incurred by professional football linemen). Structural abnormalities such as spondylolisthesis (a pars interarticularis defect), or leg length discrepancy are fairly rare (fewer than

5%). Among the latter group overuse syndromes are the most common and myofascial pain is increasingly being recognized as a significant cause of chronic back pain.

As an industrial or personal injury, back pain often results from an unwitnessed event. The patient presents with a subjective complaint and gives a history, which may or may not be based in fact. It is essential that we make every attempt to clarify and when possible verify the history, especially if the initial physical examination either reveals no objective findings or the findings are inconsistent with the history and subjective complaints. We should avoid using the term acute back strain in the absence of findings suggestive of an acute soft-tissue process. Use of that term without objective findings legitimizes ongoing symptoms (without signs) and the subsequent diagnosis of chronic back strain, giving credibility to a disease process which may have never existed. This becomes especially important in a medical-legal context where one is often asked to comment on causality. Often the more appropriate initial diagnosis is that of nonspecific low-back pain or back pain of undetermined etiology not suggestive of spinal disease. The IASP Task Force on Pain in the Workplace (2) describes known causes for specific back pain as follows:

- Disk herniation
- Spondylolisthesis, usually in the young
- Spinal stenosis, usually in the elderly
- Vertebral fractures, tumors, infections, and inflammatory diseases
- Definite instability exceeding 4 to 5 mm on flexion–extension radiographs

They note that fewer than 15% of persons with back pain can be assigned to one of these categories (17) and suggest the diagnostic label of nonspecific low-back pain (NSLBP) for many of the others with back pain. They describe NSLBP as a disorder of activity intolerance and work incapacity and have developed algorithms to interrupt the process at various stages (Fig 17.2).

DIAGNOSTIC EVALUATION

Guidelines from the Agency for Health Care Policy and Research (AHCPR) and "Back Pain in the Workplace" suggest that in the absence of red flags, trauma, or evidence to suggest underlying spinal disease minimal diagnostic testing should be performed the first month following the onset of back pain (1). A summary of AHCPR (18) findings regarding commonly used diagnostic studies will be presented.

Pain studies and discography were found to be of questionable use and generally not indicated for NSLBP (19). The AHCPR Task Force concluded that there was "limited" evidence that discography could help select patients who would benefit from spinal fusion and "no" evidence that it was helpful in patients with acute low-back pain. Also, the use of discography or CT discography to diagnose herniated discs was felt to offer no significant advantage over other imaging techniques with less potential morbidity (MRI, CT). How-

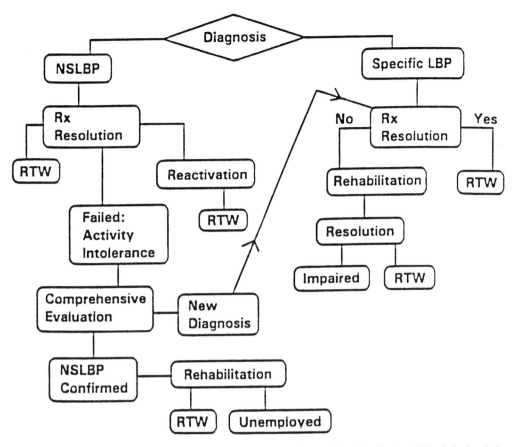

Figure 17.2.   Algorithm of management of low back (Reprinted with permission from Fordyce WE, ed. Back pain in the workplace. Seattle: IASP Press, 1995.)

ever, infrequently in orthopaedic practice Dupuy notes anecdotally that discography may be useful as an adjunct to support or refute the diagnosis.

Electrodiagnostic testing (EMG) and H-reflex tests to clarify the etiology of radiating lower extremity pain lasting longer than 3 to 4 weeks appear to be useful to (*a*) document the presence or absence of radiculopathy or neuropathy (*b*) to clarify presence of specific nerve root compromise, and (*c*) to help distinguish between acute and chronic nerve root dysfunction.

Sensory evoked potentials (SEPs) were found to be helpful in diagnosing spinal stenosis and spinal cord myelopathy. F-wave tests and surface EMGs were not considered effective for assessing acute low back problems.

Bone scan was found to be a "moderately" sensitive test for detecting suspected tumor, infection or occult vertebral fractures in patients with low-back pain but not for specifying the diagnosis. Positive bone scan will generally require confirmation by other diagnostic tests or procedures. Bone scanning can assist in detecting spinal metastases in patients with prior cancer and was found to be effective in detecting tumor, fracture, or infection in patients where these are clinically suspected. Studies have also failed to document efficacy for *thermography* for diagnosing low back disorders (20), and it is felt that thermography is nonspecific, adding no useful information in most spinal diseases (21).

Plain lumbar x-rays were found to be useful in detecting spinal fractures but not in diagnosing lumbar nerve root impingement from a herniated disc, spinal stenosis or in ruling out cancer or infection. Use of lumbar x-rays was not felt to be effective to screen for spinal degenerative changes, congenital anomalies, spondylolysis, spondylolisthesis, or scoliosis. It was specifically concluded that x-rays done to screen for the presence of spondylolisthesis are unnecessary in adults during the first 3 months of symptoms.

Computed tomography (CT), magnetic resonance imaging (MRI), myelography, and CT myelography were only recommended during the first month of symptoms in the presence of red flags suggesting serious conditions such as cauda equina syndrome or progressive neurological deficits. When clinical findings strongly suggest tumor, infection, fracture, or other spinal space-occupying lesions, spinal imaging and/or specialty consultation is suggested. In patients who have had prior back surgery, MRI with contrast is the recommended study to distinguish disc herniation from scarring associated with prior surgery. CT myelography and myelography are invasive and because of associated morbidity are indicated only when required for preoperative planning.

Wiesel (22) suggests cautious interpretation of radiographic studies. He notes that many spinal radiographic abnormalities are unrelated to pain syndromes. Table 17.1 lists

Table 17.1.   Cautious Use and Interpretation of Radiographic Studies: Many spinal Radiographic Abnormalities Are Unrelated to Pain Syndromes (22, 54)

Spina bifida occulta
Spondylosis
Most facet joint problems
Lumbarization of sacral vertebra
Sacralization of lumbar vertebra
Hyperlordosis
Schmorl's notes

some of these. In his review of lumbar CT scans, he noted that 20% of normal subjects (without a history of back symptoms) under age 40 demonstrated a herniated nucleus pulposis and 50% over age 40 showed abnormalities including disc herniation, facet degeneration, and stenosis. Furthermore, he emphasizes that findings which are not clinically correlated may lead to unnecessary diagnostic studies and surgery.

TREATMENT CONSIDERATIONS

Most episodes of acute low-back pain do not cause significant incapacity and are self-limited. We may move incorrectly, exercise excessively without proper conditioning, be under excessive stress, or fall. Generally health care personnel are not consulted, and within days to weeks the problem resolves either with no treatment or with a variety of over-the-counter nonprescription remedies. Indeed, studies have shown that in uncomplicated back injuries resolution of symptoms can be expected in most within 1 to 2 weeks and 80 to 90% within 4 to 8 weeks regardless of treatment (1, 2). As such, back pain generally is a benign, self-limited condition more than 90% of the time. However, the remaining 5 to 10% have prolonged incapacity and unfortunately have a disproportionately high utilization of resources. A study at the Boeing plant in Washington state found that 10% of the back injury claims accounted for 79% of the cost (23). This is consistent with other studies from Liberty Mutual (24), which found that 25% of their cases accounted for 93% of costs and 10% of the cases accounted for 78% of costs. The high-cost cases had more frequent hospitalization, surgery, litigation, and psychological impairment. Hadler (25) has noted that in NSLBP (which he refers to as regional low-back pain without radiculopathy) often the prognosis worsens as individuals move from being a person in pain with a predicament (a self-limited process) to a patient in pain undergoing diagnostic evaluation, treatments, pharmacologic trials, blocks, surgery, and so on who now has a diagnostic label, "an illness," to a claimant with pain (resolution now complicated by health care and legal systems). Aronoff (26) has noted that some back pain patients with prolonged disability do not necessarily have more significant impairment than the group that returned to work but do have significant differences in terms of negative attitude, marginal motivation, poor support systems, and often a chronic disability conviction based more on cognitive distortions than on objective impairment.

In 1985 Snook (27) found that the average cost per back pain claim was nearly $6000 and significantly affected company profits to the extent that it was concluded that industry needed to find better ways to control back pain costs. Ergonomic considerations were recommended.

Social Security statistics also note an alarming trend. From 1957 to 1976 while the population of the U.S. approximately doubled and the SSDI awards for all medical conditions rose about 350%, the awards for low-back pain rose by nearly 2700% (28). This is despite the fact that there was no significant change in the incidence or prevalence of back pain. More recent statistics suggest that disability from back pain continues to rise at more than 14 times the population growth (1) and that $110 billion is spent annually on Social Security disability for chronic pain. These statistics are suggestive of a disturbing change in societal values, especially in work ethic, job dissatisfaction, and litigation trends. Disability is now often seen as a socially acceptable alternative to work. This trend not only threatens societal health and well being and those of societal funded programs for health care and disability, but also threatens the health of the injured worker, as has been discussed by Aronoff in prior publications on chronic pain and the disability "epidemic" (29–32). Injured patients with ongoing musculoskeletal pain are often overly evaluated and treated and are susceptible to develop iatrogenic complications and iatrogenic disability.

OCCUPATIONAL CONSIDERATIONS

Exposure to Risk Factors

The risk of injury is innate to certain occupations and activities. This is clear in the case of some professional sports and daredevil stunts; however, it is also too often unrecognized in certain industries. Simultaneous bending and twisting as well as exposure to excessive vibration carry a statistically significant increased risk for the development of low-back pain. Material handling and occupations with heavy physical demands generally impact the musculoskeletal system, especially when workers cannot modify body mechanics to prevent injury. Cumulative-trauma disorders result from sustained exposure to repetitive forces such as vibration or abnormally sustained postures including prolonged sitting such as in those whose livelihood involves prolonged driving or sitting (33).

Individual Risk Factors

Cigarette smoking has been shown to increase the risk of back pain by diminishing oxygenation and diffusion of nutrients to the disks as well as via problems associated with excessive coughing (34). Aging brings with it multiple degenerative and metabolic changes which may adversely affect one's ability to perform certain occupations and may increase the risk of injury (35).

Studies on gender differences suggest that back pain generally is as frequent in males as females but in occupational settings males have their highest incidence around age 40 without substantial subsequent increase with further aging. In part, this was attributed to men placing less physical demands on their back in later years, whereas women had an increased incidence from 40 to 55, this being attributed to increasing osteoporosis (36). Postural deformities and leg length discrepancy generally have not been found to predispose to low-back pain (37, 38). There has been extensive study on the effects of physical conditioning, job training, and body mechanics as risk factors. Nachemson (39) believes that there is no direct correlation between trunk muscle weakness and low-back pain. However, studies are discrepant, and some suggest that physical conditioning minimizes the risk of injury. Battie (40) in her literature review stated that she is "aware of no studies demonstrating that strength, flexibility, or aerobic capacity play a significant role in back pain reporting in occupations of light or moderate physical demands." There is evidence that the at-risk population includes workers with premorbid psychosocial problems including substance abuse, depression, and anxiety disorders (41). Certainly these issues may adversely impact on concentration and attentiveness, which often contribute to injuries through no fault of the employer or the workplace. Other nonoccupational risk factors include those who are poorly educated, in low paying, boring, repetitive jobs without significant chance for advancement. Table 17.2 lists individual factors felt to increase risk for involvement in a disabling injury.

Multiple studies have supported the view that nonmusculoskeletal and indeed nonphysical factors are often the crucial variables in workers prone to chronic disability following a work-related injury (4–43). Among these are difficulty dealing with stress, the perception of one's job as stressful, non–work related personal and home problems, feeling devalued by one's employer, and strain in relationships with coworkers or supervisors. It has also been shown that risk of a claim for compensable injury is more frequent early in employment, especially the first several years (44). Much has been written about the pain-prone personality in individuals who have a striking developmental history prominent for unmet dependency needs, physical and/or sexual abuse, hyperresponsibility at an early age, and family members who themselves were chronically ill or disabled (45). Aronoff has often found in evaluation of these individuals that after even a minor injury they fail to recover as would be expected, and it is as if their injury was their way of saying, "Now it's my turn to be taken care of."

Certain industries have a high prevalence of work injuries. Materials handlers, truck drivers, nursing assistants, and helicopter pilots (vibration) are at increased risk for back injury (46). Occupational risk factors are listed in Table 17.3. One of the highest risk factors for repeat back injury is a history of prior back injury. Under the Americans with Disabilities Act (ADA) an employer is not permitted to inquire about a history of prior back injuries (47).

Table 17.2.   Individual Risk Factors

Aging and gender: men have higher incidence of back pain until early 40s, but women have a substantial increase after age 40 to about 55
History of back pain
Physical deconditioning
Pregnancy
Smoking
Psychosocial stressors
Premorbid psychopathology
Morbid obesity
Job dissatisfaction

Table 17.3.   Occupational Risk Factors for Back Pain

Heavy manual labor
Vibration
Prolonged sitting or driving
Confined spaces with difficulty using proper body mechanics
Heavy lifting
Twisting
Bending
Years of employment: first few years higher risk

Socioeconomic Factors

The American workplace has evolved, and although some of the changes benefit workers, others have merely been designed to increase efficiency and productivity without concern about the impact on the worker. No longer can workers be assured of job stability until retirement. Corporate downsizing, a changing economy, reinventing jobs, and the evolving multiethnic and cross-cultural character of our modern work force has influenced the morale of American workers. Such psychosocioeconomic influences may lead to prolonged illness and disability following a work-related injury and act as barriers to recovery. For many, the job site has changed from a source of emotional and financial security to a major life stressor. Unable to cope, some may view the injury as a socially acceptable way out of a stressful situation.

PATHOPHYSIOLOGY OF WORKPLACE MUSCULOSKELETAL BACK INJURIES

Certain work injuries have well-defined management and recovery time. When the pathophysiology can be clearly identified and the subjective complaints are consistent with the clinical and other diagnostic findings, the course of recovery is generally predictable. Expectations of the physician and patient in these treatment situations are positive, even with compensated illness and work injury. More unpredictable, however, is the treatment of musculoskeletal injuries, which are poorly defined and defy a clear diagnosis. When back pain is vague and diffuse and there are disincentives to work return, recovery time often is prolonged. In these cases, early recognition of treatment failure and operant influences is imperative.

Injuries from prolonged exposure to high repetition and high-force jobs are theorized to result from microtears, inflammation, and degeneration of tendons, ligaments, and possibly synovial tissue and muscle (48). How myofascial pain syndromes and fibromyalgia relate to this particular topic is unclear; some physicians advocate these as defined disorders (49–51), and others do not (52, 53). However, in both the pathophysiology is unclear, frequently complicated by coexisting anxiety, depression, or other psychopathology which are likely to contribute to poor outcome. Furthermore, a strictly anatomical or mechanical explanation for the cause of nonspecific low back and leg pain is inadequate. Though pathology affecting the disc has been attributed as a popular cause of low back and leg pain, cases of asymptomatic disc herniation are commonly identified on CT and MRI of the lumbar spine. A study of asymptomatic individuals revealed abnormalities of lumbar spine MRI in 64%. (54). Additionally, the extent of disc protrusion to create clinical symptoms often does not correlate. Degenerative change and injury to spinal structures reportedly produces low back and leg pain in various combinations which are similar in that activities such as prolonged sitting and standing are aggravating and changing positions or reclining are alleviating. Mechanical conditions of the spine, including disc disease, spondylosis, spinal stenosis, and fractures account for up to 15% of cases of low-back pain (55), with the remainder comprising the category of NSLBP.

GENERAL MANAGEMENT OF MUSCULOSKELETAL BACK PAIN

Acute and Subacute Injuries

Initial evaluation (history and physical examination) of all musculoskeletal injuries is similar. The physician evaluation determines the degree of structural or tissue disruption and the tissues involved—that is, bone, joint, or soft tissues such as ligaments, tendon, and muscle—and the integrity of neurovascular structures. If fracture or joint subluxation is possible due to the magnitude or character of trauma, then initial plain x-ray films are appropriate. Unless red flags are present, x-rays are usually not indicated and generally should not be performed simply to alleviate the concern of the patient, his or her family, or the plaintiff's attorney. If ligamentous disruption and joint instability are suspected, then motion radiographs may be necessary. In cases with neurovascular compromise, CT scan to assess bony structures and identify acute hemorrhage or lumbar disc herniations are considered. MRI is useful to assess spinal canal, soft tissues, and neural structures and may be preferred to CT for herniated discs. Minor or incidental injuries causing marked or severe pain and disability may warrant medical, neurological, orthopaedic, psychiatric, or other subspecialty investigation.

Rest is a time-honored treatment for musculoskeletal injury; however, the amount prescribed for acute back pain (in the absence of neuropathology) is generally grossly excessive. Studies have shown that when indicated at all, bed rest should be limited to 2 to 4 days, after which there should be progressive return to normal activity. Further bed rest contributes to progressive deconditioning, illness behavior, and functional disability (56). Some studies have found modalities of equivocal benefit, and the summary report from the AHCPR indicates that the use of physical agents and modalities in the treatment of acute low-back pain is of insufficiently proven benefit to justify their cost (1). Anecdotal reports from patients, however, document efficacy in individual situations. Our findings are consistent with those of the AHCPR panel suggesting that training patients in the self-application of heat or cold should be considered as a treatment option. Modalities such as ice are advocated early. A study at the Boston Pain Center with a heterogeneous group of patients with chronic low-back pain found that ice massage was a more effective modality for analgesia than either cold or hot packs (57) (Fig. 17.3). Some industrial settings allow such modalities to be applied by the worker at his or her workplace and therefore establish a psychological continuum that reinforces return-to-work goals.

Trigger point injections with corticosteroids are generally not recommended for back pain (1); however, in many clinical settings successful outcomes have been noted. Epidural or selective nerve root injections are advocated by many both therapeutically and diagnostically in the acute stages of acute low-back pain without radiculopathy or neural compromise, but the AHCPR found no evidence to support this practice. However, they found that epidural steroid injections are an option for short-term relief of radicular pain in patients refractory to conservative treatment who are attempting to avoid surgery. Chiropractic spinal manipulation has been suggested as being effective especially in older individuals with primarily back pain in the first 2 weeks following injury, although these studies may be flawed (58). McKenzie exercises, dynamic lumbar stabilization exercises, and back school, when effectively administered, are likely cost effective and beneficial. Active exercise has been clearly demonstrated as an effective intervention in maintaining activity level and preventing (or reversing) debilitation, as has back care education; however, whether these interventions are preventive is unclear (59). Treatments found by the AHCPR Task Force to be ineffective in the management of acute low-back pain include transcutaneous electrical nerve stimulation (TENS), shoe lifts when leg length discrepancy is less than 2 cm, lumbar corsets or support belts, spinal traction, biofeedback, trigger point and ligamentous injections, facet joint injections, and acupuncture.

Acute injuries, when minor, are best managed by activity restriction, but not necessarily away from the workplace. Positive personal interaction between the injured worker and employer–supervisor during the acute period has been shown to reduce injury-related disability, specifically back pain. Modified work and light duty may also favorably impact work injury disability and reduce the cost of lost productivity. This should be the goal of treatment within 2 to 4 weeks in most routine back injuries (nonspecific back pain, lumbar strain, and myofascial pain). With more moderate levels of injury,

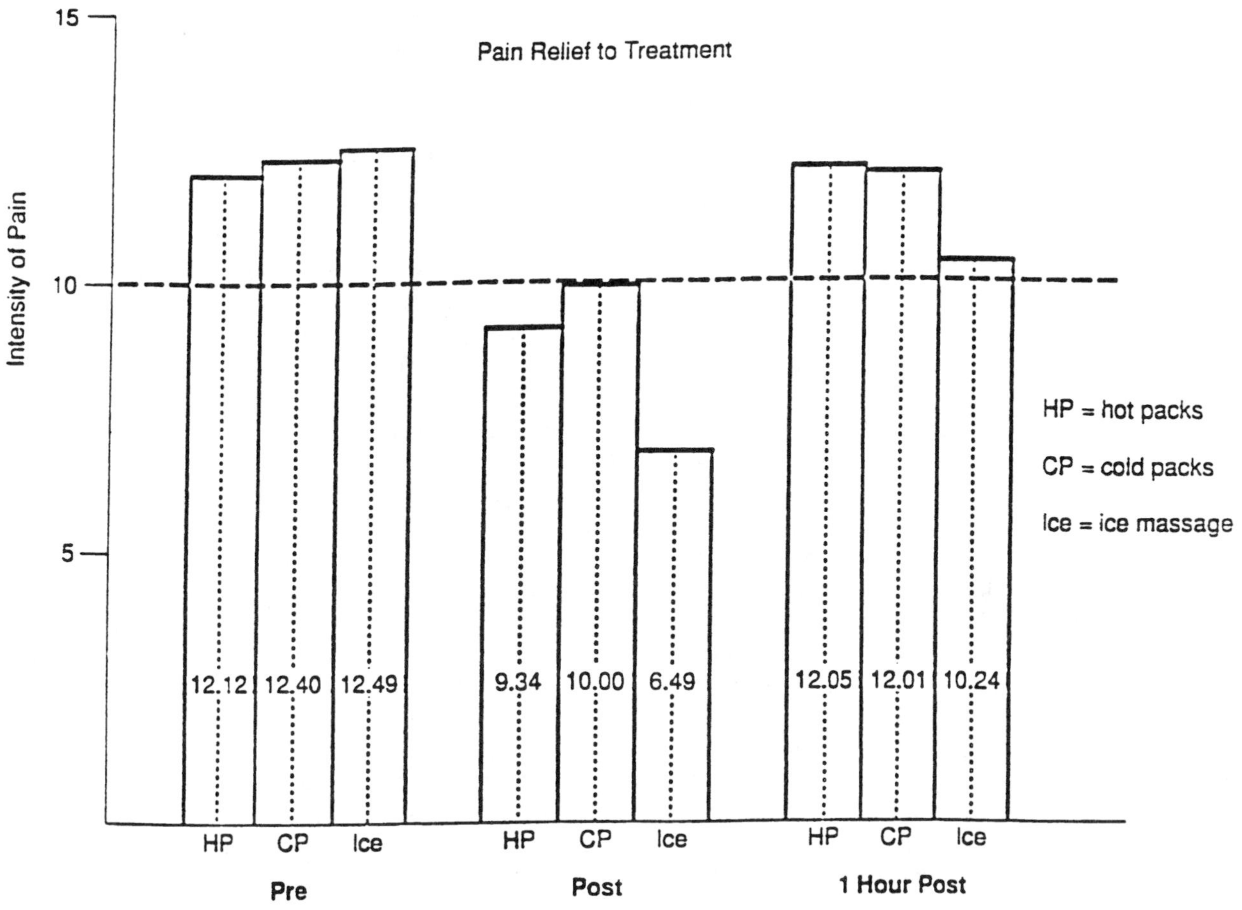

Pain Relief to Treatment

HP = hot packs

CP = cold packs

Ice = ice massage

Figure 17.3. Ice massage as a therapeutic modality for back pain compared with heat and cold packs. (Reprinted with permission from Roberts DJ, Walls CM, Carlile JA, et al. Relief of chronic low-back pain: heat versus cold. In: Aronoff GM, ed. Evaluation and treatment of chronic pain. 2nd ed. Baltimore: Williams & Wilkins, 1992;299–301.)

the patient should be involved in a supervised physical therapy program by the second week to include progressive increasing functional activities, exercise with strength and flexibility training, and aerobic activities. In certain cases such conditioning should be followed by supervised work simulation to address body mechanics. Health club programs which overlap return to work are beneficial and may promote general overall health benefits and wellness behaviors.

Subacute and Chronic Work-Related Injuries

When musculoskeletal injuries cause pain and disability lasting longer than 6 to 12 weeks, they are classified as subacute or chronic, respectively. Working patients return to physical demands, which are approved by the treating physician. Restrictions and limitations should be predictably removed in a logical, physiological, goal-oriented way, designed by medical provider and endorsed by the patient. At the work site, wellness behaviors need continued reinforcement. On-site physical therapy consultation may provide important feedback for physician, patient, and supervisory personnel. Industrial medical personnel and the employee's supervisor can

often supervise well-planned modification of activities back to a normal level. When medical care is incorporated into the workplace routine and recognized as a job responsibility by both employee and supervisor, work injury and disability can be prevented. Furthermore, such programs, including on-site management of the injury, show the injured worker that he or she is valued by the company and also satisfies the employee's sense of entitlement among working peers who are in observance. Prevention and awareness are also heightened in these cases.

The nonworking patient with subacute or chronic injury should be referred for appropriate multidisciplinary evaluation if the signs and symptoms suggest development of a chronic pain syndrome (CPS) which interferes with return to function. CPS is not a diagnostic term but rather descriptive of a process in which, in addition to the pain, there are dysfunctional pain behaviors, impaired coping, diminished functional activities of daily living (generally self-imposed), excessive reliance on the health care system, and global life disruption. With medical clearance, these patients are often best managed in chronic pain programs which are geared toward physical reconditioning, functional restoration, and aggressive physical and emotional rehabilitation as opposed to programs in which despite interventions (blocks and medication) patients are maintained on disability.

Pharmacological Management

Oliver Wendell Holmes stated, "If the whole materia medica, as now used, could be sunk to the bottom of the sea, it would be all the better for mankind—and all the worse for the fishes." Although certainly an oversimplification of a very complex issue, long term use of analgesic medication for back pain is a double-edged sword. While occasionally of assistance in providing analgesia, diminishing suffering, and improving function and the quality of life, the converse is also frequently seen. Physicians' prescriptions may in the patient's mind validate the belief that he or she has a significant underlying pathological process in need of treatment, when in the case of nonspecific low-back pain, the problem often is more one of activity intolerance, deconditioning, conditioned pain behaviors, and a disability conviction based on cognitive distortions.

Medications are often useful acutely and short term. When analgesics are indicated for mild to moderate pain, it is reasonable to begin with acetaminophen, aspirin, or an NSAID, taking into account potential side effects. For most patients with chronic back pain it is difficult to justify long-term use of NSAIDs. Although some may work well in specific individuals, there are no clear data that support the use of costly NSAIDs as more beneficial. When an NSAID is desired but benefit is lacking, switching to a drug within another chemical family through sequential trials may eventually assist identifying a therapeutic NSAID when such benefit is felt absolutely necessary.

Muscle relaxants and spasmolytics are frequently utilized in the management of back pain despite a paucity of studies demonstrating their clinical efficacy, although some did in the acute pain phase. Indeed, our clinical experience is consistent with studies suggesting that most commonly used muscle relaxants may have a sedative action and are therefore somewhat anxiolytic but appear ineffective for true muscle spasm associated with chronic pain. Some have a potential for physical dependency. There appears to be no significant benefit noted combining a muscle relaxant and NSAID over using an NSAID alone (1). Oral steroids, such as methylprednisolone (Medrol Dosepack), may be effective when used within the first several weeks of back pain onset but are rarely effective when treatment is delayed.

Although opioids are often clinically indicated for severe acute pain, their use in chronic nonspecific back pain is generally not recommended, and even in chronic back pain with underlying spinal disease they should be used cautiously. Many patients will respond to a combination of physical reconditioning in combination with acetaminophen, aspirin, or an NSAID and perhaps use of an adjuvant analgesic. However, there is a subgroup of patients who can be appropriately maintained for prolonged periods on opioids (62) (Chapter 32). Generally use of a long-acting opioid is preferable to one with a shorter action. Guidelines for chronic opioid therapy are suggested in Table 17.4.

Role of Physical Therapy

There is much anecdotal support for physical therapy interventions in acute and persistent back pain but few controlled outcome studies. Studies suggest that higher levels of physical fitness are associated with a decrease in the incidence and severity of low-back pain disability (63). Aerobic exercise is generally associated with improved endurance and strength and less fatigue. This may be important, as fatigue often leads to diminished use of proper body mechanics and increased risk of injury. Involvement in aerobic exercise should be coupled with good nutrition, better sleep, and no smoking. Aerobic conditioning exercises should be an integral part of all back pain rehabilitation programs. Weakness of the back and abdominal muscles has been associated with increased incidence of low-back pain and related disability costs (63, 64). However this too is controversial, and Battie (40) stated, "The investigator is aware of no studies demonstrating that strength, flexibility, or aerobic capacity play a significant role in back pain reporting in occupations of light or moderate physical demands." We believe that early mobilization to prevent physical and mental deconditioning also serves the purpose of interrupting the process of learned, conditioned dysfunctional pain behaviors from emerging. Cognitive distortions often develop after prolonged inactivity, as do inadvertent reinforcement of pain behaviors either from health care providers or significant others. Aronoff et al. (65) have indicated that to promote rehabilitation and prevent iatrogenic disability physical therapists must evaluate whether a patient's statements about inability to perform essential activities of daily living are based on objective impairment or are self-imposed due to gradually conditioned dysfunctional pain behaviors.

Surgical Intervention

Immediate surgical decompression is indicated when the patient has intractable pain associated with progressive neurological dysfunction or a cauda equina syndrome. If after 4 weeks, sciatica is worsening and imaging (CT, MRI) confirms abnormalities on the same level and side of symptoms, surgery may be considered. Decompressive laminectomy and microdiscectomy are generally preferred over chemonucleolysis or percutaneous discectomy (66). The key to successful surgical intervention is for the correct surgeon to select the correct patient for the correct procedure at the correct time. A problem in any of these factors may be an explanation for a poor surgical result. It is estimated that less than 1% of patients with acute back and leg pain will have a treatment course ultimately requiring surgery. Furthermore, it is often the case that the decision to perform surgery is more a func-

Table 17.4.   Guidelines for Maintenance Opioid Use in Chronic Nonmalignant Pain

1. Document that a medical condition is the initiating and sustaining cause of pain.
2. Document that prior systemic therapeutic trials of alternative pain control regimens (analgesics, adjuvants, psychosocial interventions, appropriate medical treatments, and behavioral approaches) have been unsuccessful.
3. Document that nonopioid treatments have resulted in (a) inadequate analgesia impairing functional activities of daily living and (b) continued suffering.
4. Prior to initiating opioid maintenance, obtain consultation with a specialist in pain medicine and consider consulting a specialist in the management of the specific problem being treated. These consultation reports should document concurrence with the need for maintenance opioid treatment.
5. Document detailed discussion of short- and long-term effects and risks. Patients should sign an informed consent with a detailed behavioral contract.
6. Identify one physician as responsible for writing prescriptions, which should be on a time-contingent rather than pain-contingent basis, and for monitoring clinical progress. To titrate doses to stable levels, we recommend that the initial frequency of appointments should be at least monthly. Also, clinical progress should be monitored for the need for continuing opioids.
7. Identify one pharmacy for all prescriptions.
8. Document that maintenance opioids improve pain control and functional activities of daily living and diminish suffering.
9. Use the lowest clinically effective opioid dose. Peripherally acting nonnarcotics and adjuvants used concurrently and nonpharmacological pain control (e.g., ice, TENS, relaxation, stretching) may allow less opioid usage.
10. A history of substance dependence or abuse is a precaution.
11. Any evidence of drug-seeking behavior, obtaining opioids from multiple sources, or frequent requests for dose escalation without documentation of significant worsening of the clinical condition should be a cause for careful review and reconsideration of maintenance opioid use.
12. Concurrent treatment by a clinician or service experienced in substance abuse may be a condition of continued treatment.

tion of a compressive radiculopathy causing extremity pain than because of axial pain alone. The decision should never be based solely on the basis of a demanding patient with persistent pain just because he or she has failed conservative treatment. To do so is to participate in the making of a low-back loser. It is important to recall that prior to 1934, when Mixter and Barr discovered the technical surgical procedure for "the herniated disc," patients recovered from these herniations without surgery. To be sure, some had permanent neurological residua; however, most fully recovered. Table 17.5 lists Aronoff's recommendations for mandated second opinions for elective back surgery (67). In a recent review, Millander (68) set forth four situations in which surgery should proceed with caution:

1. The clinical features are not clear.
2. Pain is the predominant complaint.
3. There are major psychosocial issues.
4. The surgery is unlikely to restore the patient to his or her job.

PREVENTION OF DISABILITY

Physicians cannot prove or disprove the existence of pain clinically. A person complaining of pain may or may not have nociception, suffering, pain behavior, impairment, or disabil-

Table 17.5.   Second Opinions Prior to Elective Surgery

Two or more pain-related surgeries without beneficial results
One or more pain-related surgeries with negative findings
Attorney-referred patients involved in pain-related litigation
Known or highly suspected major psychopathology
History of unjustified excessive use of the health care system

ity. When diagnostic evaluation has ruled out treatable nociception and when impairment has been addressed, targets for intervention include the suffering component (emotional distress), pain behaviors, and disability issues.

Since pain behaviors are often conditioned, learned, and goal-directed, they are amenable to behavioral intervention. In recent years it has been established that with CPS, patients develop cognitive distortions regarding themselves, their future, and their environment. A goal of treatment is to extinguish or modify these maladaptive behaviors and cognitive distortions and replace them with more adaptive coping skills.

This is most likely to occur in a specially structured therapeutic milieu using a cognitive-behavior–based rehabilitation model directed toward helping patients understand the nature and implications of their physical symptoms and involving them in a physical reactivation/functional restoration program to reverse the effects of deconditioning from inactivity. Concurrently psychosocial, pharmacological, and disability issues are addressed and in the latter part of the treatment program work simulation activities can be assessed.

Chronic pain often leads to a chronic disability syndrome (69), in which even in the absence of significant documented physical impairment, the patient has a conviction of being disabled and unable to return to work. Findings from the Boston Pain Center (Aronoff), the Mid-Atlantic Center for Pain Medicine (Aronoff), and clinical orthopaedic practice (Dupuy) have shown that injured workers maintained on workers compensation may be at increased risk for developing CPS unresponsive to conventional treatments and iatrogenic disability. These individuals may have significant financial, psychosocial, and environmental reinforcement for maintenance of their disability and little incentive to return to work. Often there is no direct correlation between objective impairment and an individual's request for disability status. For patients who have had prior back surgery, unless there are significant objective deficits, we do not recommend arbitrarily restricting a patient's activity on or off the job simply because he or she had prior surgery, solely based on a subjective complaint. More important than the absolute weight limit of lifting is the person's conditioning, use of proper body mechanics, and favorable ergonomics at the workplace.

Aronoff has found that in patients with work-related chronic back pain unresponsive to conventional treatment approaches, whether the problem is nonspecific low-back pain or whether there is underlying structural pathology not amenable to or appropriate for a curative procedure, the treatment of choice is use of a directive return-to-work approach in the context of a pain rehabilitation program designed to emphasize functional restoration. This was shown to be effective in earlier studies by Catchlove and Cohen (70), who found that when patients entering a rehabilitation-oriented treatment program are told from the outset that they are expected to return to work after completion of treatment (in spite of residual pain), they are more likely to do so than when the decision is left to the patient. In addition, when followed over time they demonstrated the ability to remain at work and used fewer health care resources than the second group. Patients will either live up to our expectations that they can get on with their life in spite of pain or they will become disabled unnecessarily (iatrogenic) through a process of learned helplessness. The belief system of clinicians treating chronic pain may be a determining factor in whether patients are rehabilitated or remain disabled.

The Task Force for Pain in the Workplace has offered an alternative to the current management protocol for individuals with NSLBP by suggesting that disability benefits be time limited followed by a change in status to unemployment. Our experience from the Boston Pain Center (Aronoff) Mid-Atlantic Center for Pain Medicine (Aronoff), and office practice of orthopaedic surgery (Dupuy) is consistent with the findings of the task force that "a significant subset of injured workers, who are suffering and are burdened with difficulties in coping with life and work demands, have problems that have been misidentified as stemming from injury to the low back" (2). The task force makes a cogent argument for the demedicalization of suffering. Their document is an attempt to improve the quality of care for a patient population currently often receiving suboptimal care by practitioners who often benefit far more than their patients; a population which has contributed to a public health problem that if not corrected threatens to bankrupt medical insurance and disability reimbursement systems. Hadler (52) states, "If you have acquired the illness of work incapacity in the context of a backache, worker's compensation is the most appealing recourse generally available in our society."

As disability-evaluating physicians, we applaud their efforts to contain runaway disability costs. As treating physicians, however, we are concerned about the consequences of having deserving patients with NSLBP who have been compliant with treatment recommendations and algorithms, have not been found to have significant spinal disease, yet continue to suffer with back pain severe enough to prevent their return to work through no fault of their own but who lose their health care and disability benefits. Do they become sacrificial lambs for the benefit of society as a result of years of system abuse by a relatively small segment of the injured worker population? For some, their suffering may constitute a psychiatric impairment, in which case, despite a minimal physical impairment, they would qualify for temporary (and for a small group, permanent) psychiatric disability. However, most would not qualify. An alternative proposal would be to improve our ability to distinguish which of the NSLBP group would benefit from more pro-

longed medical/disability services from those less likely, in which case the benefits would be terminated as proposed.

CONCLUSION

As advocates for patients, and in the best interest of society, we should encourage rehabilitation, not disability. Certification of disability because of chronic pain sometimes occurs as a direct result of collusion between health care providers and patients. We must address invalidism and learned helplessness. The individual who has chronic pain suffers less when his or her life has purpose and meaning. Gainful employment frequently serves as a distraction from pain. Individuals with legitimate painful injuries should be appropriately compensated for pain and suffering. But we need an alternative to the current reimbursement system, which often rewards people more for remaining in a body jacket than for wearing a sports jacket (26). In discussions of "the disability epidemic" Aronoff has noted that if this epidemic is to be reversed, the compensation and disability systems must be changed so that they encourage early intervention, prevention of chronicity with incentives toward rehabilitation, and early return to work (26, 32).

References

1. U.S. Department of Health and Human Services. Acute Low Back Problems in Adults. AHCPR Pub 95–0642, Washington, December 1994.
2. Fordyce WE, ed. Back pain in the workplace. Seattle: IASP Press, 1995.
3. Aronoff GM. Evaluation and treatment of chronic pain. 2nd ed. Baltimore: Williams & Wilkins, 1992.
4. Loeser J. Schematization of Pain. In: Stanton-Hicks M, Boas R, eds. Chronic low back pain. New York: Raven Press, 1982;145–148.
5. Frymoyer JW, Cats-Baril W. An Overview of the incidences and costs of low back pain. Orthop Clin North Am 1991;22:263–271.
6. Snook SH, Webster BS. The cost of disability. Clin Orthop 1987; 221:77–84.
7. Spengler D, Bigos S, Martin NA, et al. Back injuries in industry: a retrospective study: 1. Overview and cost analysis. Spine 1986;11:241–245.
8. Von Korff M, Dworkin S. An epidemiological comparison of pain complaints. Pain 1989;32:173–183.
9. Anderson GBJ. The epidemiology of spinal disorders. In: Frymoyer JW, ed. The adult spine: principles and practice. New York: Raven Press 1991;107–146.
10. Cunningham LS, Kelsey JL. Epidemiology of musculoskeletal impairments and associated disability. Am J Public Health 1984;74:574–579.
11. Deleted.
12. Schwartz GE, Watson SD, Galvin DE, Lipoff E. The disability management sourcebook, vol 6. Washington Business Group on Health/Institute for Rehabilitation and Disability Management 1989.
13. Nachemson AL. Advances in low-back pain. Clin Orthop 1985; 200:266–278.
14. Nachemson AL. Newest knowledge of low back pain: a critical look, Clin Orthop 1992;279:8–20.
15. Deyo R, Tsui-Wu Y. Descriptive epidemiology of low back pain and its related medical care in the United States. Spine 1987;12:264.
16. Dillane JB, Fre J, Kalton G. Acute back syndrome: a study from general practice. Br Med J 1966;2:82.
17. Spitzer W, LeBlanc F, et al. Scientific approach to the assessment and management of activity-related spinal disorders: report of the Quebec Task Force on Spinal Disorders. Spine Eur Ed 1987;12:7S(Suppl 1):S1–S59.

18. U.S. Department of Health and Human Services. Acute low back problems in adults. AHCPR Pub 95–0642. Washington: 1994;79–81.

19. U.S. Department of Health and Human Services. Acute low back problems in adults. AHCPR Pub 95–0642, Washington: 1994;65–67.

20. Frymoyer JW, Haugh LD. Thermography: a call for scientific studies to establish its diagnostic efficacy. Orthopaedics 1986;9:699.

21. Mahoney L, McCulloch J, Csima A. Thermography in back pain: 1.Thermography as a diagnostic aid in sciatica. Thermology 1985;1:43.

22. Wiesel SW, Tsourmas N, Feffer HL, et al. A study of computer-assisted tomography: the incidence of positive CAT scans in an asymptomatic group of patients (1984 Volvo Award in Clinical Sciences). Spine 1984;9:549–551.

23. Svensson HO, Anderson GBJ. Low back pain in 40 to 47 year old men: work history and work environment. Spine 1983;8:272.

24. Snook S, Webster B. The cost of disability. Clin Orthop 1987;221:27.

25. Hadler NM. Occupational musculo-skeletal disorders. New York: Raven Press, 1993.

26. Aronoff GM. Chronic pain and the disability epidemic. Clin J Pain 1991;7:330–338.

27. Snook SH. The costs of back pain in industry. Spine State Art Rev 1987;2:1.

28. Social Security Disability Supplement, 1977–1979. 1979;129.

29. Aronoff GM. Chronic pain and the disability epidemic. Clin J Pain 1991;7:361.

30. Aronoff GM. Psychiatric aspects of chronic pain and disability. J Disabil 1993;3:63–79.

31. Aronoff GM. Psychiatric aspects of chronic pain and disability. Curr Rev Pain 1997;1:2:93–98.

32. Aronoff GM. The disability epidemic. Clin J Pain 1989;5:203–204 (editorial).

33. Pope MH, Andersson, GBJ, Chaffin DB. The workplace. In: Pope MH, Andersson GBJ, Frymoyer JW, Chaffin DB, eds. Occupational low back pain. Chicago: Mosby–Year Book, 1991;117–131.

34. Frymoyer JW, Pope MH, Clements JH, et al. Risk factors and low back pain: an epidemiological survey. J Bone Joint Surg 1983;65:213.

35. Andersson GBJ, Pope MH. The patient. In: Pope MH, Andersson GBJ, Frymoyer JW, Chaffin DB, eds. Occupational low back pain. Chicago: Mosby–Year Book, 1991;132–145.

36. Biering-Sorensen F, Thomsen C. Medical, social, and occupational history as risk indicator for low back trouble in a general population. Spine 1986;11:720–725.

37. Magora A. Investigation of the relation of low back pain and occupation. Scand J Rehabil Med 1975;7:146.

38. Pope MH, Bevins T, Wilder DG, et al. The relationship between anthropometric, postural, muscular, and mobility characteristics of males age 18–55. Spine 1986;11:720–725.

39. Nachemson AL. Newest knowledge of low back pain: a critical look. Clin Orthop 1992;279: 8–20.

40. Battie MC. Minimizing the impact of back pain: workplace strategies. Semin Spine Surg 1992;41:20–28.

41. Weinstein MR. The concept of the disability process. Psychosomatics 1978;19:94–97.

42. Ellard J. Psychological reactions to compensable injury. Med J Aust, 1970:8:349–355.

43. Aronoff GM. Pain treatment programs: do they return workers to the workplace? Spine State Art Rev 1987;2:123–136.

44. Bigos SJ, Spengler DM, Martin NA, et al. Back injuries in industry: a retrospective study: 3. Employee related factors. Spine 1986; 11:252.

45. Blumer D, Heilbrun M. Chronic pain as a variant of depressive disease. J Nerv Ment Dis 1982;170:381–406.

46. Mandell P, Lipton MH, Bernstein J, et al. Low back pain: an historical and contemporary overview of the occupational, medical, and psychosocial issues of chronic back pain. Thorofare, NJ. Slack, 1989;1–35.

47. American Medical Association. Americas with Disabilities guidelines: guide to the evaluation of permanent impairment. 4th ed. Chicago: AMA, 1993;304.

48. Myers ML, Withers PC, Johnson JA. Program of the National Institute of National Safety and Health. U.S. Dept of Health & Human Services Pub. 84–107, 1984.

49. Wolfe F, Smyth HA, Yunus MB, et al. American College of Rheumatology 1990 criteria for the classification of fibromyalgia: report of the multicentre criteria committee. Arthritis Rheum 1990;33:60–172.

50. Yunus MB. Diagnosis, etiology, and management of fibromyalgia syndrome: an update. Compr Ther 1988;14:8–20.

51. Goldenberg DL. Controversies in fibromyalgia and myofascial pain syndrome. In: Aronoff M, ed. Evaluation and treatment of chronic pain. 2nd ed. Baltimore: Williams &Wilkins, 1992;165–175.

52. Hadler NM. The dangers of the diagnostic process: iatrogenic labeling as in the fibrositis paralogism. In: Hadler NM. Occupational musculoskeletal disorders. New York: Raven Press, 1993;16–36.

53. Bohr TW. Fibromyalgia syndrome and myofascial pain syndrome: do they exist? Neurol Clin 1995;13:365–384.

54. Boden SD, Davis DO, Dina TS, et al. Abnormal magnetic-resonance scans of the lumbar spine in asymtomatic subjects. J Bone Joint Dis 1990;72A:403–408.

55. Deyo RA. Back pain revisited: newer thinking of diagnosis and therapy. Consultant 1993;33:88–100.

56. Deyo R, Diehl A, Rosenthal M. How many days of bed rest for acute low back pain? A randomized clinical trial. N Engl J Med 1986;315:1064–1070.

57. Roberts DJ, Walls CM, Carlile JA, et al. Relief of chronic low-back pain: heat versus cold. In: Aronoff GM, ed. Evaluation and treatment of chronic pain. 2nd ed. Baltimore: Williams & Wilkins, 1992;299–301.

58. U.S. Department of Health and Human Services. Acute low back problems in adults. AHCPR Pub. 95–0642. 1994;41.

59. Battle MC, Bigos SJ, Fisher LD, et al. Isometric lifting strength of a predictor of industrial back pain reports. Spine 1989;14:851–856 .

60. Holmes OW. Currents and countercurrents in medical science. In: Medical essays: 1842–1882. Boston: Houghton Mifflin, 1883;173–208.

61. Deleted.

63. Cady LD, Thomas PC, Karwasky RJ. Program for increasing health and physical fitness of firefighters. J Occup Med 1985;27:110.

64. Valbonna C. Bodily responses to immobilization. In: Stillwell, Lehman, eds. Kottke, Krusen's handbook of physical medicine and rehabilitation. Philadelphia: Saunders, 1982.

65. Aronoff GM, Layden M, Green E, Goodall R. Assessment and prevention of disability. In: Wittink H, Michel TH, eds. Chronic pain management for physical therapists. Butterworth-Heinemann, 1997;239–246.

66. U.S. Department of Health and Human Services. Acute low back problems in adults. AHCPR Pub. 95–0642. 1994;88.

67. Aronoff GM, McAlary PW. Pain centers: treatment for intractable suffering and disability resulting from chronic pain. In: Aronoff GM, ed. Evaluation and treatment of chronic pain. 2nd ed. Baltimore: Williams & Wilkins, 1992;416–429.

68. Millender LH, Conlon M. An approach to work-related disorders of the upper extremity. J Am Acad Orthop Surgeons 1996;4:134–142.

69. Strang JP. Chronic low back pain and disability. In: Aronoff GM, ed. Evaluation and treatment of chronic pain. 2nd ed. Baltimore: Williams & Wilkins, 1992;484–498.

70. Catchlove R, Cohen K. Effects of a directive return to work approach in the treatment of workers' compensation patients with chronic pain. Pain 1982;14:181–191.

CHAPTER 18

Interstitial Cystitis: A Complex, Progressive Visceral Pain Syndrome

Grannum R. Sant, Andrew W. Sukiennik, and Richard M. Kream

Interstitial cystitis (IC) is a debilitating inflammatory condition of the urinary bladder characterized by excessive urinary frequency, urgency, and pain (1, 2). The inflammation in IC is initiated by various stimuli, and IC tends to have its onset among young to middle-aged persons, 90% of whom are women (2–4). Urinary frequency and nocturia are the quintessential symptoms of IC. However, many IC patients have pain (1, 3), ranging from a mild burning or discomfort to excruciating pain in the bladder, lower abdomen, perineum, and vagina, as well as the low back and thighs (5). Although pain in IC is most often associated with filling of the bladder and alleviated by urination, it sometimes lacks any relation to voiding (1, 2, 4).

Hunner's ulcers, accompanied by marked inflammation and a reduced bladder capacity, occur in about 10% of cases of IC (4, 5). A less severe but much more common form of IC is characterized by petechial bladder mucosal hemorrhages (glomerulations) in the absence of ulceration (6). Pain, urinary urgency, and frequency are not specific to IC; they can accompany other conditions, such as bacterial, chemical, and radiation-induced cystitis and bladder carcinoma (2). However, these symptoms suggest IC, and together with the cystoscopic findings of Hunner's ulcers or glomerulations provide for reliable diagnosis (6, 7).

The natural history of IC involves periods of symptomatic flares and remissions, and the condition tends to be chronic (2, 4). At the time of definitive diagnosis, the typical IC patient has had symptoms for 3 or 4 years (2). The symptoms usually plateau within 5 years of onset and do not progress (5). Menstruation tends to aggravate the symptoms of IC in some patients, and 75% of affected women claim that sexual intercourse exacerbates their symptoms (5). There is no evidence that the nonulcerative form of IC progresses to the ulcerative form, although progressive fibrosis and shrinkage of the bladder can occur (2).

The symptoms of IC create substantial psychological, social, and hygienic problems (5, 8, 9), and chronic pain and sleep loss from nocturia contribute to depression in patients with IC. Patients typically consult several physicians before their condition is diagnosed (9). Because of the similarity of IC symptoms to those of acute bacterial urinary tract infections, many patients are mistakenly treated with multiple courses of antibiotics (10)

EPIDEMIOLOGY

The underreporting of IC and the similarity of its symptoms to those of other urological diseases make its true incidence difficult to determine, particularly in the less severe, nonulcerative form of the condition (6, 9). The true prevalence (number of patients per 100,000 population) of IC is unknown, and published studies have used various diagnostic criteria and methodologies. Prevalence estimates range from 10 cases per 100,000 in Finland based on hospital record review (11) to 30 cases per 100,000 in the United States according to a postal survey of urologists (9) to as high as 510 cases per 100,000 using participant's self-reports from the 1989 U.S. National Health Interview Survey (12). The prevalence in women is higher, ranging from 18 to 865 cases per 100,000 (12). None of these studies employed the National Institutes of Health and National Institute of Digestive Diseases and the Kidney (NIH-NIDDK) criteria for diagnosis.

The nonulcerative form of IC, which occurs in approximately 90% of cases in the United States, is typically seen in patients who are an average of 10 years younger than those with the ulcerative form (2, 6). In the United States IC appears to be more common among whites (5) but occurs in all racial and ethnic groups (13). Although it has been described in children (14), research criteria established by the NIDDK exclude its diagnosis for research purposes in persons under 18 years of age (3, 15). Questionnaire surveys suggest that IC occurs commonly in patients with allergies, irritable bowel syndrome, inflammatory bowel disease, systemic lupus erythematosus, and fibromyalgia (16).

PATHOPHYSIOLOGY

The causes of IC remain unknown (1, 2, 17). Autoimmune, allergic, and infectious causes have all been suggested, as have neurological, vascular, and circulatory abnormalities, mechanical injury to the bladder, infiltration of the bladder wall by excessive numbers of mast cells, and damage to the mucosal lining of the bladder permitting the entry of allergenic or toxic substances into underlying tissues (4, 17).

Although the diagnostic criteria for IC include sterile urine, infection has been postulated because of scanning electron microscopic findings and the culture of microorganisms embedded in the bladder wall of patients with IC (18). Further evidence of an infectious cause includes bacterial ribosomal 16S r RNA in bladder biopsy tissue from patients with IC (19). However, the consensus, which is based on conventional and molecular biological techniques, speaks against an infectious (bacteria, viruses) cause (18).

Another hypothesis is reflex sympathetic dystrophy (1, 20). Injury to peripheral nerves from prior infection, hysterectomy, or childbirth may interrupt the sympathetic innervation of the bladder, prompting a compensatory increase in sympathetic α-adrenoceptors (21), with increased transmission of pain-producing impulses from the bladder and reduced circulatory perfusion facilitating infiltration by inflammatory cells and bladder ulceration, fibrosis, and atrophy (20). Findings supporting reflex sympathetic dystrophy include the ability of pharmacological blockade of spinal sympathetic tracts and transcutaneous electrical nerve stimulation (TENS) to alleviate pain in patients with IC (2, 20).

Evidence for an immunological basis of IC is inconsistent (17, 21). Evidence favoring autoimmunity includes the detection of antinuclear antibodies (ANAs), increased urinary excretion of eosinophilic cationic protein (ECP) (9), and the tendency of IC, like systemic lupus erythematosus, to affect women and periodically flare up and remit (1, 2, 16). Further supporting a role for autoimmunity in IC are the findings of immunoglobulin (Ig) M in the urothelium, immune deposits in vessel walls, and aggregates of T- and B-cell nodules, including germinal centers containing suppressor cytotoxic cells (22). However, the symptoms of IC do not consistently respond to anti-inflammatory or immunosuppressive drugs. Delayed hypersensitivity in the skin of IC patients exposed to their urine may be a direct toxic response (8).

A primary role for mast cells in the causation of IC is a matter of controversy (2, 17). Mast cell degranulation releases histamine, prostaglandins, leukotrienes, and other vasoactive substances, as well as inflammatory mediators, all with proven effects on smooth muscle and nerve terminals in the bladder wall (23). A third to half of patients with IC have increased numbers of mast cells in the bladder wall (23), and both light microscope and electron microscope studies have documented mast cell activation and degranulation (24). Other findings supporting the role of mast cells in IC include the increased numbers of peptidergic nerve fibers in close proximity to mast cells in the bladders of patients with IC (25) and the presence of estrogen receptors on mast cells (26). Mast cell degranulation may promote the symptoms of IC by stimulating sensory nerves in the bladder wall (23). The exacerbation of pain, urgency, and frequency reported by many IC patients during menstruation may be due to mast cell degranulation triggered by altered female sex hormone levels (26).

The concept of IC as originating from a defect in the mucin coating of the bladder urothelium maintains that alterations (qualitative and quantitative) in the glycosaminoglycans (GAGs) that constitute this coating permit solutes and other substances in urine to penetrate the bladder wall (27). This results in tissue irritation and injury, mast cell degranulation, inflammation, sensory nerve depolarization, and development of the symptoms of IC (28). Support for the GAG hypothesis in IC includes reduced urinary levels of GAGs, the suburothelial presence of Tamm-Horsfall proteins, and the symptomatic benefit that accompanies the use of sulfated polysaccharides, such as pentosan polysulfate sodium (PPS; Elmiron) in treating IC (1, 17, 29).

DIAGNOSIS

The diagnosis of IC requires a complete history and cystoscopy under anesthesia with bladder hydrodistention (2, 3). Bladder biopsy is useful but not essential for the diagnosis (2, 30). The differential diagnosis includes carcinoma in situ, infectious cystitis, tuberculosis of the bladder, chemical- and radiation-induced cystitis, urinary tract degeneration from estrogen deficiency, malakoplakia, neuropathic bladder dysfunction, invasive tumors of the bladder and uterus, prostatitis, vaginitis, urethritis, and bladder stones (3, 30).

Gynecological examination should be done to rule out vaginitis, vulvar lesions, and urethral diverticula, and urine microscopy, culture, and cytology are important to exclude bacterial cystitis and transitional cell carcinoma of the bladder. Diseases that mimic the symptoms and cystoscopic appearance of IC can be ruled out on the basis of laboratory, histological, and cytological findings (2, 30). IC must also be distinguished from detrusor irritability caused by involuntary contraction of the detrusor muscle (1). Eosinophilic cystitis may also be confused with IC because of the similarity of symptoms, but eosinophilic cystitis is rarer and is characterized by an inflammatory response that involves the detrusor muscle and often the perivesical fat of the bladder, neither of which occurs in IC (8).

Although pain, urgency, and urinary frequency are essential to the diagnosis of IC, their intermittent nature and dependence on individual patient perception complicate their quantification (9, 30). A symptom scoring index for IC has recently been developed and validated, and this may help clarify the natural history of IC and the efficacy of various treatments (31).

In severe IC, cystometry may reveal hypersensitivity and a reduced bladder capacity (15). In advanced IC, intravenous pyelography may reveal a diminished bladder capacity and moderate dilation of the upper urinary tract (2). Cystoscopy for IC is typically done under general or regional anesthesia (3, 30), with hydrodistention and visual examination of the bladder (2, 30). The bladder is filled with water under passive gravity infusion at a pressure of 60 to 80 cm H_2O for about 2 to 3 minutes. IC is confirmed by the cystoscopic findings of Hunner's ulcers and/or submucosal hemorrhage and glomerulations (6) (Table 18.1). Hunner's ulcers are discrete hemorrhagic lesions with an erythematous, velvety appearance closely resembling that of carcinoma in situ (4, 10). Cystoscopy in cases of advanced ulcerative IC may disclose a fibrous and contracted bladder with a pale mucosa.

The more common nonulcerative form of IC is characterized by the cystoscopic finding of petechial hemorrhages or glomerulations (2, 6). These strawberry-red spots may number from only 1 or 2 to as many as 50 per cystoscopic field of view, and upon hydrodistention often coalesce into areas of hemorrhage. They are generally most prominent on the dome, posterior wall, and side walls of the bladder and are rare on the trigone.

Bladder biopsy (usually a small cold-cup biopsy) not only is useful in excluding specific bladder diseases such as dysplasia and carcinoma in situ but is also helpful in documenting the degree and type of bladder inflammation. Specific mast cell stains (Giemsa, toluidine blue) identifies a subset of patients with bladder mastocytosis that respond to treatment with oral hydroxyzine (23).

TREATMENT

Drugs

Because of the chronicity and indefinite causation of IC, treatment is largely directed at alleviating symptoms (2, 32). To reduce the patient's discontent and permit the institution of other treatment as needed, the absence of a specific cure and the rationale for use of a specific treatment should be explained to the patient before treatment is begun (2) (Table 18.2).

First-line treatment of IC is usually with oral drugs such as antihistamines, tricyclic antidepressants, or PPS. Hydroxyzine, an antihistamine, is used on the hypothesis that histamine released by mast cell degranulation may be responsible for the symptoms of IC (23). Nifedipine, a calcium channel blocker that inhibits smooth muscle, has been reported in an uncontrolled study to alleviate symptoms in some patients with IC (1, 15).

Although their efficacy in treating IC has not been established in randomized controlled studies, amitriptyline and other tricyclic drugs have found application in treating IC on the basis of their analgesic, antihistaminic, anticholinergic, and sedative properties, as well as their antidepressant effect (1, 3, 15).

Table 18.1.   Cystoscopic Findings in Interstitial Cystitis

Use of general or spinal anesthesia
Glomerulations
Bloody cystoscopic effluent
  Post hydrodistention
Ulcers
  Rare
  Mucosal crack
  True Hunner's ulcers
Nonulcer IC
  Most common
  Bladder capacity >400 mL
  No ulcers
Classic IC
  Rare
  Bladder capacity <400 mL
  Ulcers
Bladder biopsy
  Optional
  Excludes specific diseases
  Confirms mastocytosis

Table 18.2.   Treatment of Interstitial Cystitis

First-line oral drugs
  Tricyclic antidepressants
  Antihistamines
  Sodium pentosanpolysulfate
Intravesical therapy
  DMSO
  DMSO plus
    Steroids
    Heparin
    Bicarbonate
    Lidocaine
Rescue intravesical therapy
  Oxychlorosene sodium
  Hyaluronic acid
  BCG
  Interferon

PPS, a highly sulfated semisynthetic GAG with chemical and structural similarities to the naturally occurring GAGs in the bladder mucin layer (33), is the only oral agent approved by the U.S. Food and Drug Administration (FDA) for the treatment of IC, and apart from dimethyl sulfoxide (DMSO), the only drug approved for IC. Its use is based on the hypothesis that IC originates from abnormalities in the mucin GAG component (27, 33). PPS eases pain, urinary frequency, and other symptoms of IC in a substantial proportion of patients (29). In a physicians compassionate use study begun in 1986 and involving more than 3000 patients with IC in whom other treatments had failed to provide relief, PPS at a total daily dose of 300 mg produced significant relief of pelvic pain in 42% of patients treated for up to 6 months and 60% of those treated for 2 years. It also reduced urinary frequency in 44% of patients and decreased the frequency of nocturia in 55% of patients treated for more than 6 months. In two multicenter studies PPS produced overall improvement in 28% and 32% of treated patients, respectively, as opposed to 13% and 16% improvement in groups receiving placebo (29, 33). Neither study found significant clinical side effects or complications of PPS, and it appears to be safe and well tolerated, with a high therapeutic index. Several months of treatment, usually at least 3, are typically needed before PPS begins to produce symptomatic relief.

Passive hydrodistention of the bladder at the time of diagnostic cystoscopy provides temporary symptomatic relief in many patients with IC (2), and it may be repeated as an elective therapeutic procedure (1, 15). Hydrodistention with the Helmstein balloon, which produces greater distention than passive hydrodistention, is especially useful in patients with bladder capacities of less than 300 to 400 mL (2, 32). Symptomatic benefit from both direct and balloon hydrodistention typically lasts for several months, after which further hydrodistention is required.

Intravesical DMSO was the first drug approved by the FDA for the treatment of IC. In uncontrolled studies DMSO has been reported to induce symptomatic remission in up to 70% of patients with classic ulcerative IC and 90% of those with the nonulcerative form of the disease for periods up to 24 months (15, 32). Intravesical therapy with DMSO requires anesthetization of the urethra and bladder with 2% lidocaine jelly, followed by urethral catheterization and the sterile instillation of 50 mL of a DMSO solution (RIMSO-50) through a size 8 to 10 Fr urethral catheter, with the patient instructed to retain the solution in the bladder for at least 15 minutes before voiding. Four to eight such treatments are given at 1- to 2-week intervals, after which the treatment intervals are increased until symptomatic relief or treatment failure occurs (1, 2, 32).

After DSMO therapy a small number of patients have exacerbated symptoms that are eased by oral anticholinergic agents or belladonna and opium suppositories. For patients who do not respond to an initial course of DMSO, hydrocortisone can be added (32). Sodium bicarbonate may be added to the DMSO-hydrocortisone combination for its enhancing effect on steroid activity (4).

Heparin, both alone and in conjunction with DMSO, can also be used intravesically (32). Heparin may help compensate for the GAG defect postulated in the cause of IC. Significant symptomatic relief has been reported in about 50% of patients treated with intravesical heparin (33). DMSO with heparin reduces the relapse rate among patients who respond to DMSO (33). DMSO can be self-administered by patients who are taught sterile self-catheterization. Patients who fail to respond to DMSO or heparin and those with more severe symptoms of IC can be treated intravesically with silver nitrate or oxychlorosene sodium, both of which are proved to be safe but neither of which has been evaluated in controlled clinical studies (32).

Intravesical silver nitrate concentrations range from 1:5000 to as high as 2%, with intravesical dwell times rang-ing from 2 to 10 minutes. The treatment, which is given at intervals averaging 6 to 8 weeks, requires anesthesia. Intravesical oxychlorosene sodium (Clorpactin) is generally reserved for patients who fail to benefit from DMSO alone or in combination with hydrocortisone, heparin, and so on (32). The painful effects of oxychlorosene sodium require either regional or general anesthesia. Because severe urinary urgency, frequency, and dysuria (6) often persist for 24 to 48 hours after treatment with oxychlorosene sodium, an indwelling Foley catheter may be needed during this period, in addition to narcotic analgesics and anticholinergics (2). This technique produces long-term remission in only about a third of patients, necessitating repeated courses of therapy (6). However, repeated courses of treatment and the repeated use of general anesthesia that accompanies each treatment pose the risks of damage to the bladder mucosa and anesthesia-related morbidity (32).

Agents for which pilot studies have shown recent promise in IC are intravesical bacillus Calmette-Guérin (BCG), hyaluronic acid (Cystistat), and PPS (15, 32). The common treatment options for IC are summarized in Table 18.2.

Surgery

In addition to the medical therapies used for IC, endoscopically guided transurethral resection, fulguration, or laser irradiation can be used to eliminate Hunner's ulcers from the bladder (34). About 5% of patients who have incapacitating IC and who do not respond to more conservative treatment modalities require surgery (1, 2, 15). For patients with a diminished bladder capacity, supratrigonal cystectomy and substitution cystoplasty may be done to enlarge the bladder, or a neobladder may be created from a segment of bowel anastomosed to the urethra (35). As a procedure of last resort for patients in whom medical therapy and more conservative surgery have failed, total cystectomy may be performed, with the diversion of urine into an ileal reservoir or continent pouch (2, 34).

The results of bladder surgery for IC are variable (34). Many patients develop a neurogenic bladder with a return of pain and urinary frequency or require permanent catheterization. IC has been reported to recur in the anastomosed bowel segment following substitution cystoplasty, and many patients who undergo cystectomy continue to report persistent suprapubic and pelvic pain even after such surgery (36, 37).

NEUROGENICALLY MEDIATED PAIN

Afferent nerve fibers in the gut and bladder shift their response characteristics from distention insensitive (silent, or sleeping) to distention sensitive in the presence of inflammation, and this may explain the visceral hyperalgesia in nonulcer dyspepsia, noncardiac chest pain, irritable bowel syndrome, and the inflammatory bowel syndromes (38, 39).

There is functional evidence linking activated substance P (SP) expressing sensory systems to the pain and hyperalgesia associated with peripheral inflammatory states. Furthermore, summated second pain following sustained C fiber afferent stimulation is partly driven by SP receptors in conjunction with activated spinal cord N-methyl-D-aspartate (NMDA) receptors. The end result is a form of central sensitization (perceived as allodynia and hyperpathia) to peripheral nociceptive stimuli manifested by enlargement of primary receptive fields, automaticity, and alterations in stimulus-response relations.

A putative involvement of SP-expressing neural systems in the pathophysiology of IC has been suggested. A significant population of bladder unmyelinated C fiber and lightly myelinated delta-A fiber afferents contains SP (40). Furthermore, in a rat model of chemical cystitis, altered peripheral nociceptive fields are functionally linked to activated dorsal horn neurons expressing neurokinin 1 receptors, thereby indicating plasticity of SP-expressing afferent systems as positive effectors of increased bladder pain (41).

Increased NK1 receptor density has been observed in Crohn's disease, a painful inflammatory bowel syndrome (42). Our Interstitial Cystitis Research Group has recently demonstrated increased numbers of immunoreactive SP-positive nerve fibers in the suburothelial bladder layer (25) and increased expression of NK1 receptor-encoding messenger RNA (mRNA) overlying vascular endothelial cells in IC patients (43).

The NK1 receptor is a G_q-coupled integral membrane protein. Upon activation, the NK1 receptor promotes increased phospholipase C (PLC) activity with resultant increases in intracellular levels of inositol 1, 4,5-triphosphate (IP3) and diacylglycerol (DAG). Increased formation of IP3 effectively raises levels of intracellular Ca^{2+}, which synergizes with DAG in the activation of isoforms of protein kinase C (PKC). PKC activation results in translocation of isoforms from the cytosolic compartment to the perinuclear region, consistent with functionally linked changes in phosphorylation of key cellular metabolic enzymes, signaling proteins, and cytoskeletal components. PKC activation appears to be involved in the central sensitization and persistent pain following tissue injury (44) and may be involved in peripheral mechanisms of nociceptor activation and sensitization.

Bladder distention may engender pain via mechanical stimulation of normally silent nociceptive bladder afferents (45). Antidromic propagation of these signals to collateral terminals on vascular elements via local axon reflex may effectively result in SP release at perivascular sites. Although the bladder equivalent of the local axon reflex is speculative, similar neurogenic mechanisms mediating reflex vasodilation have been demonstrated in the esophagus (46). Perivascular release of SP may promote a number of inflammatory responses with NK1 receptor-mediated activation of bladder endothelial cells initiating and potentiating IC-associated vasodilation and inflammation (47).

Immunohistochemical analysis using a highly specific antibody for the carboxy-terminal domain of SP (48) demonstrated the presence of immunoreactive SP-positive fibers in IC (25). The fibers were typically varicose in nature and distributed in the suburothelial zone, perivascularly in the submucosa, and in the detrusor lamina. Image analysis confirmed a statistically significant (p < .05) increase of immunoreactive substance P positive fibers in the submucosa.

We have employed immunohistochemical techniques to quantitate the density of immunoreactive SP- and CGRP-positive fibers and the frequency of their colocalization in IC. There was a significant increase in the percent of immunoreactive calcitonin gene-related peptide (CGRP) positive fibers containing immunoreactive SP in IC biopsies, suggesting that SP expression is induced in CGRP expressing fibers previously devoid of SP. There is also considerable evidence for the expression of NK1 receptors in the rat and guinea pig bladder (49). The distribution of NK1 receptor-encoding mRNAs in human bladder biopsies from IC patients has been studied (43). Computer-assisted image analysis of the autoradiographic data revealed the NK1 receptor-encoding mRNA signal overlying blood vessels was considerably higher in biopsy material from IC versus non-IC patient controls: 58.8 plus or minus 7.37 fCi/mm^2 (mean plus or minus SEM) versus 27.7 plus or minus 4.52 fCi/mm^2, respectively.

Immunoreactive SP has been measured in 50 mL aliquots of acidified urine from IC and age- and sex-matched non-IC controls. Samples were extracted according to our published procedures using SEPAK cartridges and increasing concentrations of acetonitrile (50). Extracts were dried and reconstituted and levels of immunoreactive SP-like immunoreactivity were quantified using a highly sensitive and specific radioimmunoassay. Values of immunoreactive SP were 1.31 plus or minus 0.26 fmol/mL (mean plus or minus the standard deviation [SD]) vs. 0.58 plus or minus .07 fmol/mL for IC and non-IC patients, respectively (p < .001), indicating significant increases in levels of immunoreactive SP in the urine of IC patients (Sant GR, Kream RJ, Marchard J, unpublished data).

In sum, our studies have demonstrated a significant increase in the density of immunoreactive SP-positive fibers in the bladders of IC patients, no change in the density of immunoreactive CGRP-positive fibers, and a significant increase in the frequency of colocalization of immunoreactive SP-positive with immunoreactive CGRP-positive nerve fibers. The final item strongly suggests that the increase in immunoreactive SP-positive fiber density is not due to sprouting of new immunoreactive SP-positive fibers but the result of new expression of immunoreactive SP in afferent fibers previously devoid of this peptide. These data support the hypotheses that selective expression of immunoreactive SP by newly activated nociceptive afferent fibers corresponds to the conversion of silent to active nociceptors and that peripheral and central release of SP may mediate the positive peripheral feedback in IC and the central signaling of pain in the spinal cord.

PAIN MANAGEMENT

Pain management in patients with IC is a significant challenge. Similar to other chronic pain patients, many IC patients are depressed and exhibit dysfunctional behaviors that are detrimental to a functional lifestyle. The pain in IC is unique because it is visceral and not easily examined or measured. Prior to diagnosis most patients have seen several physicians who failed to diagnose or appropriately treat this chronic condition (2). Some patients are labeled as suffering from a psychosomatic disorder. This further intensifies their frustration and illness behaviors. In addition patients may seek solace in support groups that include members who complain of their symptoms and lack of compassion from the medical community. This disease can, if not managed properly, affect the patient's ability to work, especially when urinary frequency and urgency predominate. Last, this disease interferes with sexual relations and marital life. The overall quality of life of IC patients is dismal—reportedly worse than that of chronic renal failure patients (2, 9).

The Multidisciplinary Pain Clinic at the New England Medical Center has developed significant expertise and experience in the management of IC pain. There are multiple causes to account for the symptoms of IC, and the rule *primum non nocere* (first do no harm) must always be adhered to, especially in IC, which has no clear-cut cause. The pain complaints of IC patients at the pain clinic are remarkably similar. The intensity of pain varies within and among individuals (5, 9). A burning, cramping, at times sharp and stabbing pain is felt in the pelvis and lower abdomen. It may radiate to the back, genitalia, and upper thighs. In addition, the majority of patients have urgency and frequency of urination and suprapubic and/or pelvic discomfort. The two major approaches used to treat the pain associated with IC are pharmacotherapy and neural blockade (Table 18.3).

Pharmacotherapy

The use of intravesical pharmacotherapy to control the symptoms of IC was discussed earlier. Several systemic medications control IC pain unresponsive to standard urological treatments. In our practice we initially use nonopioid medications to control pain and add medications as required. Opioids are used only after a thorough psychological screening to identify any contraindications to their use. Since many of the IC patients referred to the pain clinic are depressed, it is necessary to rule out the risk of suicide. Diagnosis of a mood disorder and its type guides the practitioner to appropriate pharmacological management. Incorrectly prescribing antidepressants to a patient with a bipolar disorder who is mistaken to suffer only from reactive depression can precipitate a manic episode. Psychological examination further aids in the diagnosis of patients who are oversomatizing or who have poor impulse control, deranged illogical thought processes (psychotic), or a history of medication abuse.

Table 18.3.   Pain Management in Interstitial Cystitis

Pharmacotherapy
  Intravesical
  Systemic
    Opioids
    Tricyclics
    Calcium channel blockers
    Antihistamines
Neural blockade
  Hypogastric plexus
  Continuous epidurals
  Spinal opioid infusions
  Spinal column stimulation

Substance abuse is almost always an absolute contraindication to opioid use unless one can tightly control the patient's use of the medication by dispensing small quantities, performing random drug screens, and demanding compliance. A drug contract should be incorporated into the treatment plans of all IC patients.

There is ample information on the use of opioids in the treatment of chronic pain (51, 52). In general, one should establish the opioid dose required to give the patient adequate pain control (visual analog scale [VAS] score below 5). This can be done by intravenous titration of an opioid to establish an analgesic dose without side effects. This dose is then prescribed, according to the pharmacokinetics of the drug, for a 24-hour period. For instance if methadone 20 mg intravenously is required to achieve analgesia, 10 mg may be given every 12 hours. This is based on the fact that methadone has up to a 36-hour elimination half-life and a bioavailability of 80%. The patient needs to take this medication around the clock. Breakthrough pain medication must be provided, since patients may have exacerbation of pain beyond their baseline levels. If the patient consistently requires breakthrough pain medication, his or her basal opioid dose should be raised. In our opinion no opioid on the market offers an overwhelming advantage over other opioids, but patients may have unacceptable responses to certain opioids. The selection of the opioid should be based on the patient's analgesic response and side effects profile. Cost enters into the equation if a patient is uninsured or if the medical insurance plan does not include these drugs on their formulary. Methadone offers a cost-effective alternative to many of the recently introduced opioids.

In our clinic opioids have been used with some success in IC, but they are not a panacea in the battle against IC pain. Opioids exert most of their analgesic effects via central nervous system actions. At times IC pain is so severe that alternative routes of administration are selected. Subarachnoid administration of opioids is discussed later.

Tricyclic antidepressants have been used to treat a variety of painful conditions, including IC (2, 15, 53). Their proposed mechanism is amine pump inhibition and an increase in serotonin and norepinephrine, which are responsible in modulating pain. Amitriptyline is the most efficacious tricyclic for pain management. However, its anticholinergic side effects may make it difficult to tolerate. We usually start the patient on a 10-mg dose and escalate by 10 mg every 3 days to 50 to 100 mg. The tricyclic antidepressants are frequently used to commit suicide. Thus it behooves the physician to evaluate and seek help, when necessary, in diagnosing suicidal ideation and depression.

Calcium channel blockers such as nifedipine have been reported to afford relief from the cramplike pain associated with IC (15, 54). It is recommended that the patient take the medication consistently for up to 3 months before relief can be expected. Side effects such as headache and orthostasis can be problematic but are fortunately rare. We have seen good relief in a small subset of patients using 30 mg of a long-acting nifedipine.

Much has been written about the role of histamine in promoting mucosal inflammation in IC (55, 56). Antihistamines have been used with good results in several patients. The patient usually notes a decrease in frequency after about a month of therapy. Some patients use it as the sole agent to decrease their IC symptoms. Further placebo-controlled studies are needed to corroborate these findings.

The pain symptoms of IC may be promulgated at different levels of the nervous system: from the primary nociceptive afferents, spinal nerve roots, posterior horns of the spinal cord, and the brain. Research indicates a link between the central nervous system and peripheral inflammation (57). Several studies indicate that IC pain is also linked to neurogenic inflammation (25, 55). Nitric oxide is implicated in mucosal inflammation in *Clostridium difficile* diarrhea (58). Blocking the production of nitric oxide actually may promote mast cell and neutrophil activity. Nitric oxide may also affect smooth muscle function in IC patients and may be responsible for the cramplike sensations and the voiding disturbances seen with this disease (59). Thus nitric oxide appears to have a multitude of effects in neural transmission and certain chronic pain states. Research at our institution is examining the effects of several neuropeptides on the inflammatory state of IC.

Neural Blockade

It is theorized that inflammation can be brought under control by blocking either the immune response or reducing contribution of the neural component of IC pain. The reductions of primary afferent signals from the bladder to the posterior horns of the spinal cord, therefore, should reduce antidromic release of neuropeptides from the dorsal root ganglia and posterior horns and thus reduce inflammation. Lumbar epidural blockade using a local anesthetic has been used to reduce IC pain. Pain relief was obtained for days beyond the local anesthetic effect. Urinary frequency issues were not affected by this technique (60). After neuroconductive studies and cystoscopy to identify IC, vesicoureteric plexus ablation was conducted to reduce pain. Some 45 of the 175 women in the study, who were followed for 2 years, had complete relief

(61). We have conducted several placebo-controlled individual trials of hypogastric plexus blocks, using 0.5% bupivacaine to treat IC pain. Many patients have a marked reduction in their symptoms except urinary frequency. Most have a reduction in pain that lasts for weeks. Some patients who have inadequate control of their pain have been hospitalized for continuous epidural infusion of a local anesthetic, especially when opioid management is problematic and ineffective. We avoid epidural opioids to prevent bladder catheterization. The epidural catheter is placed at a T 11–12 interspace and a 0.05% solution of bupivacaine instilled so as to avoid difficulty with walking. We have been encouraged by the results, with some patients getting months of relief from their symptoms and reducing their opioid use. More work should be done to evaluate these initial findings.

Light lumbar nerve root decompression has been used in some IC cases to control pain. Magnetic resonance imaging of the lumbar spine showed compression of the fifth lumbar nerve root in 10 patients. When the lateral foramen was decompressed in these patients, 9 of them were pain free for 6 months (62). Perhaps these studies and anecdotal experiences indicate that persistent stimulation of the posterior horn second-order neurons, namely the wide dynamic range ones, are partially responsible for the symptoms that result from mucosal inflammation and in severe cases, the bladder wall in its entirety.

Spinal opioids are used successfully in controlling visceral pain (63). We reserve this intervention for when more conservative methods fail and use it only after a thorough psychological evaluation. We admit the patient to hospital and conduct a trial of spinal morphine, monitoring for pain relief, somnolence, urinary retention, and respiratory depression. We indicate to the patient that little is known about the long-term effects of opioids on the spinal cord.

Electrical stimulation of the spinal nerve roots and cord is used to treat a variety of neuropathic conditions. Percutaneous placement of epidural leads stimulates the posterior horns and releases antinociceptive substances to reduce pain. We try a dual lead system to achieve pain control in a patient who cannot tolerate the side effects of opioids. The procedure is reversible and has minimal morbidity.

IC patients with chronic pain symptoms unresponsive to urological treatment need management in a multidisciplinary pain clinic. Many of these patients are physically deconditioned, with a decrease in physical capacity that predisposes to increased morbidity. They often have marked pain behaviors that isolate them from a functional lifestyle and promote disability. A multidisciplinary approach to pain control in IC patients is recommended. Some patients benefit from a functional restoration program to help them cope with the pain. With early intervention, within the year of the onset of IC, we have been successful in returning patients to work, even when urological treatments failed. It is not our experience to see a reduction in pain followed up by a return to work unless behavioral and physical conditions are addressed concomitantly. This is accomplished by a behavior modification program and an intensive aerobic and strength-training program. This reflects our experience with other chronic pain patients. A single modality approach in any chronic pain patient, including IC, is less than successful. Patients must be treated in a holistic fashion and be optimistic about their future. With each passing year new discoveries and treatments bring us closer to understanding this disease which afflicts an increasing number of patients worldwide.

CONCLUSION

Despite its chronicity and the mysterious nature of its causation, IC can be treated with a number of modalities that are safe and have the capacity to alleviate symptoms. Chief among these are hydrodistention and intravesical therapy with DMSO, either singly or in combination with other drugs. PPS, the first orally available agent to be approved for treating IC, has shown substantial promise in controlled studies for alleviating its symptoms without the risks of intravesical therapy. Surgery for IC has had varying results and should be reserved for the small minority of patients in whom all other treatment modalities fail.

References

1. Thompson AC, Christmas TJ. Interstitial cystitis: an update. Br J Urol 1996;78:813–820.
2. Sant GR. Inflammatory diseases of the bladder. In: Gillenwater JY, Grayhack JT, Howards SS, Duckett JW, eds. Adult and pediatric urology. St. Louis: Mosby, 1996;1327–1354.
3. Hanno P, Levin RM, Monson FC, et al. Diagnosis of interstitial cystitis. J Urol 1990;143:278–281.
4. Sant GR, Meares EM Jr. Interstitial cystitis: pathogenesis, diagnosis, and treatment. Infect Urol Jan/Feb 1990;3:24–30.
5. Koziol JA. Epidemiology of interstitial cystitis. Urol Clin North Am 1994;21:7–20.
6. Messing EM, Stamey TA. Interstitial cystitis. Urology 1978;12:381–392.
7. Ruggieri MR, Chelsky MJ, Rosen SI, et al. Current findings and future research avenues in the study of interstitial cystitis. Urol Clin North Am 1994;21:163–176.
8. Jensen H, Nielsen K, Frimodt-Moller C. Interstitial cystitis: a review of the literature. Urol Int 1989;44:189–193.
9. Held PJ, Hanno PM, Wein AJ, et al. Epidemiology of interstitial cystitis. In: Hanno PM, Staskin DR, Krane RJ, Wein AJ, eds. Interstitial cystitis. Berlin: Springer-Verlag, 1990;29–48.
10. Parivar F, Bradbrook RA. Interstitial cystitis. Br J Urol 1986;58:239–244.
11. Oravisto, KJ. Epidemiology of interstitial cystitis. Ann Chir Gynaecol 1975;64:75–77.
12. Jones C, Nyberg L. Epidemiology of interstitial cystitis. Urology 1997;49(Suppl 5A):2–9.
13. Sant GR. Interstitial cystitis in minority women. J Assoc Acad Minor Phys 1993;4:89–92.
14. Close CE, Carr MC, Burns MW, et al. Interstitial cystitis in children. J Urol 1996;156:860–862.
15. Wein AJ, Broderick GA. Interstitial cystitis: current and future approaches to diagnosis and treatment. Urol Clin North Am 1994;21:153–161.
16. Alagiri M, Chottiner S, Ratner V, et al. Interstitial cystitis: unexplained associations with other chronic disease and pain syndromes. Urology 1997;49(Suppl 5A):52–57.

17. Ratliff TL, Klutke CG, McDougall EM. The etiology of interstitial cystitis. Urol Clin North Am 1994;21:21–30.
18. Duncan JL, Schaeffer AJ. Do infectious agents cause interstitial cystitis? Urology 1997;49(Suppl 5A): 48–51.
19. Domingue G, Choniem G, Bost K, et al. Dormant microbes in interstitial cystitis. J Urol 1995;153: 1321–1326.
20. Irwin PP, James S, Watts L, et al. Abnormal pedal thermoregulation in interstitial cystitis. Neurourol Urodynam 1993;12:139–144.
21. Erickson DR, Simon LJ, Belchis DA. Relationships between bladder inflammation and other clinical features in interstitial cystitis. Urology 1994;44:655–659.
22. Johansson SL, Fall M. Pathology of interstitial cystitis. Urol Clin North Am 1994;21:55–62.
23. Sant GR, Theoharides TC. The role of the mast cell in interstitial cystitis. Urol Clin North Am 1994;21:41–51.
24. Theoharides TC, Sant GR, El-Mansoury M, et al. Activation of bladder mast cells in interstitial cystitis: a light and electron microscopic study. J Urol 1995;153:629–636.
25. Pang X, Marchand J, Sant GR, et al. Increased number of substance P positive nerve fibers associated with bladder mast cells in interstitial cystitis. Br. J Urol 1995;75:744–750.
26. Pang X, Cotreau-Bibbo MM, Sant GR, Theoharides TC. Bladder mast cell expression of high-affinity oestrogen receptors in patients with interstitial cystitis. Br. J Urol 1995;75:154–161.
27. Parsons CL, Lilly JD, Stein P. Epithelial dysfunction in nonbacterial cystitis (interstitial cystitis). J Urol 1991;145:732–735.
28. Nickel JC, Emerson L, Cornish J. The bladder mucus (glycosaminoglycan) layer in interstitial cystitis. J Urol 1993;149:716–718.
29. Mulholland SG, Hanno P, Parsons CL, et al. Pentosan polysulfate sodium for therapy of interstitial cystitis: a double-blind placebo-controlled clinical study. Urology 1990;35:552–558.
30. Hanno PM. Diagnosis of interstitial cystitis. Urol Clin North Am 1994;21:63–66.
31. O'Leary MP, Sant GR, Fowler FJ, et al. The interstitial cystitis symptom index and problem index. Urology 1997;49(Suppl 5A):58–63.
32. Sant GR, LaRock DR. Standard intravesical therapies for interstitial cystitis. Urol Clin North Am 1994;21:73–83.
33. Parsons CL. The therapeutic role of sulfated polysaccharides in the urinary bladder. Urol Clin North Am 1994;21:93–100.
34. Irwin PP, Galloway NTM. Surgical management of interstitial cystitis. Urol Clin North Am 1994;21:145–151.
35. Hughes ODM, Kynaston HG, Jenkins BJ, et al. Substitution cystoplasty for intractable interstitial cystitis. Br. J Urol 1995;76:172–174.
36. Nurse DE, Parry JRW, Mundy AR. Problems in the surgical treatment of interstitial cystitis. Br J Urol 1991;68:153–154.
37. Baskin LS, Tanagho EA. Pelvic pain without pelvic organs. J Urol 1992;147:683–686.
38. Sengupta JN, Gebhart GF. Mechanosensitive afferent fibers in the gastrointestinal and lower urinary tracts. In: Visceral pain. Gebhart GF, ed. Seattle: International Association for the Study of Pain, 1995;75.
39. Mayer EA, Munakata J, Mertz H, et al. Visceral hyperalgesia and irritable bowel syndrome. In: Visceral pain. Gebhart GF, ed. Seattle: International Association for the Study of Pain, 1995;429.
40. Shankey KA, Williams RG, Schultzberg M, Dockray GJ. Sensory substance P-innervation of the urinary bladder: possible site of action of capsaicin in causing urine retention in rats. Neurosci 1983;10:861–868.
41. Lu Y, Jin S, Xu T, et al. Expression of c-fos protein in substance P receptor-like immunoreactive neurons in response to noxious stimuli of the urinary bladder: an observation in the lumbosacral cord segments of the rat. Neurosci Lett 1995;198:139–144.
42. Mantyh CR, Gates TS, Zimmerman RP, et al. Receptor binding sites for substance P, but not substance K or neuromedin K, are expressed in high concentrations by arterioles, venules, and lymph nodules in surgical specimens obtained from patients with ulcerative colitis and Crohn's disease. Proc Natl Acad Sci U S A 1988;85:3235–3239.

43. Marchand JE, Sant GR, Kream RM. Increased expression of substance P receptor-encoding mRNA in bladder biopsies from patients with interstitial cystitis. Br J Urol 1998;81:224–228.

44. Coderre TJ. Contribution of protein kinase C to central sensitization and persistent pain following tissue injury. Neurosci Lett 1992;140:181–184.

45. Maggi CA, Meli A. The role of neuropeptides in the regulation of the micturition reflex. J Auton Pharmacol 1986;6:133–162.

46. Bass BL, Trad KS, Harmon JW, Hakki FZ. Capsaicin-sensitive nerves mediate esophageal mucosal protection. Surgery 1991; 110:419–425.

47. Brider MA. Endothelium and inflammation. JAMA 1992;203:300–302.

48. Kream RM, Schoenfeld TM, Mancusco AN, et al. Precursor forms of substance P in nervous tissue: detection with antisera to SP, SP-gly and SP-gly-lys. Proc Natl Acad Sci U S A 1985;82: 4832–4836.

49. Nimmo AJ, Morrison JFB, Whitaker EM. A comparison of the distribution of substance P and calcitonin gene-related peptide receptors in the rat bladder. Q J Exper Physiol 1988;73:789–792.

50. Shimonaka H, Marchand JE, Connelly CS, Kream RM. Development of an antiserum to the midportion of substance P: applications for biochemical and anatomical studies of substance P-related peptide species in CNS tissues. J Neurochem 1992;59:81–92.

51. Dickenson A. Where and how do opioids act? In: Gebhart GR, Hammond DL, Jensen TS, eds. Proceedings of the VII World Congress on Pain, Progress in Pain Research and Management, vol. 2. Seattle: IASP Press, 1994;525–552.

52. Portenoy RK. Opioid tolerance and responsiveness: research findings and clinical observations. In: Gebhart GR, Hammond DL, Jensen TS, eds. Proceedings of the VII World Congress on Pain, Progress in Pain Research and Management, vol. 2. Seattle: IASP Press, 1994; 595–619.

53. Onghena P, Vanhoudenhove B. Antidepressant-induced analgesia in chronic non-malignant pain: a meta-analysis of 39 placebo-controlled studies. Pain 1992;49:205–220.

54. Fleischmann J. Calcium channel antagonists in the treatment of interstitial cystitis. Urol Clin North Am 1994;21:107–111.

55. Letourneau R, Pang X, Sant GR, Theoharides TC. Intragranular activation of bladder mast cells and their association with nerve processes in interstitial cystitis. Br J Urol 1996;77:41–54.

56. Pang X, Boucher W, Triadafilopoulos G, et al. Mast cell and substance P-positive nerve involvement in a patient with both irritable bowel syndrome and interstitial cystitis. Urology 1996;47:436–438.

57. Sluka KA, Willis WD, Westlund KN. Central control of peripheral joint inflammation and heat hyperalgesia. In: Gebhart GR, Hammond DL, Jensen TS, eds. Proceedings of the VII World Congress on Pain, Progress in Pain Research and Management, vol 2. Seattle: IASP Press; 359–371.

58. Bosheng Q, Pothoulakis C, Castagliuolo I, et al. Nitric oxide inhibits rat intestinal secretion by Clostridium difficile toxin A but not Vibrio cholerae enterotoxin. Gastroenterology 1996;111:409–418.

59. Andersson KE, Persson K. Nitric oxide synthetase and nitric oxide-mediated effects in lower urinary tract smooth muscles. World J Urol 1994;12:274–280.

60. Irwin P, Hammonds WD, Galloway NTM. Lumbar epidural blockade for management of pain in interstitial cystitis. Br J Urol 1993;71:413–416.

61. Gillespie L. Destruction of the vesicoureteral plexus for the treatment of hypersensitive bladder disorders. Br. J Urol 1994;74:40–43.

62. Gillespie L, Bray R. Levin N, Delamarter R. Lumbar nerve root compression and interstitial cystitis: response to decompressive surgery. Br. J Urol 1991;68:361–364.

63. Paice JA, Penn RD, Shott S. Intraspinal morphine for chronic pain: a retrospective, multicenter trial. J Pain Symptom Mgmt 1996;11:71–80.

CHAPTER 19

Management of Chronic Pelvic Pain

Ursula Wesselmann

Chronic pelvic pain is a common and debilitating problem that can significantly impair many aspects of the quality of life of women. Despite the challenge inherent in the management of chronic pelvic pain, many patients can be treated successfully. Effective treatment modalities are available to lessen the impact of pain and offer reasonable expectations of an improved functional status (1). The focus of this chapter is on chronic nonmalignant pelvic pain. Another very important issue, the management of malignant pelvic pain, is beyond the scope of this article. The reader is referred to other excellent reviews on this topic (2, 3). This chapter first reviews current knowledge of the pathophysiological mechanisms of chronic pelvic pain syndromes and then discusses the differential diagnosis and treatment of women, who suffer from chronic pelvic pain.

DEFINITION

Definitions of chronic pelvic pain are broadly based on duration, the anatomical and physical basis, or psychological characteristics of the pain (4). The International Association for the Study of Pain (IASP) defines chronic pelvic pain without obvious pathology as chronic or recurrent pelvic pain that apparently has a gynecological origin but for which no definitive lesion or cause is found (5). However, the IASP definition has not been widely used in the literature (6). This definition implies absence of pathology, which is not necessarily the case, and it also excludes cases in which pathology is present although not necessarily the cause of pain. The relationship of pain to the presence of pathology is often unclear in women with chronic pelvic pain. Women with chronic pelvic pain are a heterogeneous population, and therefore attempts to ascribe all cases to a particular cause undoubtedly fail (1, 6). Chronic pelvic pain can be continuous or cyclic. This chapter refers to chronic pelvic pain as pelvic pain in the same location for at least 6 months (1, 6). Most subacute (3 to 6 months' duration) and chronic (longer than 6 months' duration) pain

states begin with a nociceptive event or process, although that event may go unrecognized or unremembered (1).

EPIDEMIOLOGY

Overall, a woman has about a 5% risk of having chronic pelvic pain in her lifetime. However, patients with a previous diagnosis of pelvic inflammatory disease have a fourfold increased risk (approximately 20%) of chronic pelvic pain (7). It is estimated that 30 to 50% of the more than 45 million women of childbearing age in the United States suffer from dysmenorrhea or cyclic pain (8). In a Swedish study of 19-year-old women, 70% of women interviewed reported having had dysmenorrhea, with more than 50% reporting loss of time from work or school (9). In a recent study in the United States of 5263 eligible women aged 18 to 50 years, 14.7% reported chronic pelvic pain (10). Some 15% of these women with chronic pelvic pain reported time lost from work, and 45% reported reduced work productivity. These statistics are alarming, for they lead to the inescapable conclusion that pelvic pain severely impairs women's careers and quality of life (11). In the United States 10% of outpatient gynecological consultations are for chronic pelvic pain (12). In a recent review of published studies, Howard (13) found that 40% of laparoscopies were done for chronic pelvic pain. Chronic pelvic pain is listed as the indication for 12% to 16% of hysterectomies performed in the United States, accounting for approximately 80,000 procedures annually. Approximately 25% of women referred for evaluation of chronic pelvic pain have previously undergone a hysterectomy without the resolution of symptoms (14).

Estimated medical costs for outpatient visits for chronic pelvic pain in the United States are $881.5 million per year (10). The personal cost to the affected woman in terms of years of suffering, disability, marital discord, loss of employment, and unsuccessful medical intervention cannot be calculated so easily.

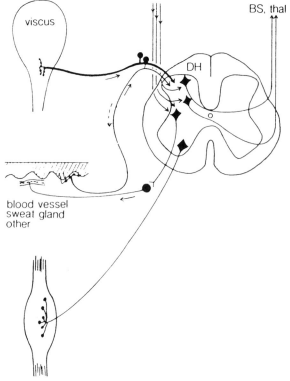

Figure 19.1. Referred visceral pain: observed phenomena and possible mechanisms. DH, dorsal horn; BS, brainstem; thal, thalamus. (Reprinted from Jänig W. Spinal visceral afferents, sympathetic nervous system and referred pain. In: New trends in referred pain and hyperalgesia. Vecchiet L et al., eds. 1993, 83–98, with kind permission of Elsevier Science-NL, Sara Burgerhartstraat 25, 1055 KV Amsterdam, The Netherlands.)

CHARACTERISTICS OF VISCERAL PAIN

Pelvic pain belongs to the category of visceral pain. Nowhere is the relationship of visceral pain to tissue damage less well understood than in the female pelvis; at least one third of patients with chronic pelvic pain have no obvious pelvic pathology (15). Pain arising from the viscera has long posed problems for the clinician. Persistent pain of visceral origin is a much greater clinical problem than that of skin, but the overwhelming focus of experimental work on pain mechanisms relates to cutaneous sensation. Until relatively recently, it was often assumed that concepts derived from cutaneous studies could be transferred to the visceral domain. However, there are several reasons to believe that the neural mechanisms involved in pain and hyperalgesia of the skin are different from the mechanisms involved in painful sensations from the viscera (16).

Visceral pain is a diffuse sensation that cannot be precisely localized. Pain originating in one viscus cannot be easily differentiated from pain originating in another viscus, which makes the differential diagnosis often very difficult. Visceral pain is often referred to segmentally related somatic structures (muscle, subcutaneous tissue, skin). Secondary hyperalgesia usually develops at the referred site (17). Pain of visceral origin is often associated with autonomic reflexes (nausea, increase in blood pressure). Possible mechanisms for these phenomena are sensitization of

spinal neurons, changes of balance between spinal circuits and descending control systems, viscerosympathetic reflexes, viscerosomatic reflexes, changes in regulation of peripheral microcirculation, and changes in retrograde axonal transport of afferent neurons (Fig. 19.1). Several psychophysical observations suggest that visceral inputs, like cutaneous inputs, are subject to sensitization: Many investigators have shown that patients suffering from functional bowel disorders exhibit exaggerated responses to distension of the esophagus, duodenum, and all portions of the colon (18). Repetitive distention of the sigmoid colon in normal patients leads to a significant increase in the reported area of referred sensation (19) (Fig. 19.2).

When treating a patient with chronic pelvic pain, it is important to consider all aspects of the pain syndrome, including the pain deep in the pelvic cavity (true visceral pain), pain referred to somatic structures (muscle, subcutis, and skin) and exaggerated autonomic reflexes associated with the chronic pain syndrome.

NEUROANATOMY OF THE PELVIC CAVITY

The visceral structures that may give rise to pain in the pelvic region in women belong to the genitourinary system (terminal part of the ureters, urinary bladder, pelvic urethra, ovaries, fallopian tubes, uterus, and upper vagina), the gastrointestinal system (sigmoid colon, rectum), and the associ-

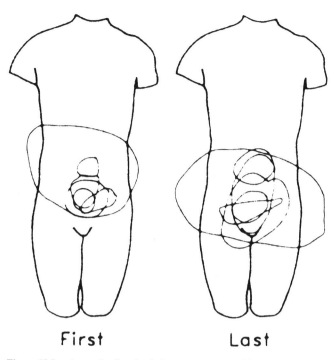

First   Last

Figure 19.2. Areas of referred pain in response to repetitive colonic distensions (60 mm Hg, 30 seconds) at 4-minute intervals in six subjects. The areas of referred sensation during the first and last (14th) colonic distensions are indicated by reproductions of subject drawings. Three patients had additional areas of referred sensation in the lower back and perineum (not shown). (Reprinted from Ness TJ et al. A psychophysiological study in humans using phasic colonic distension as a noxious visceral stimulus, Pain 1990; 43: 377–386, with kind permission of Elsevier Science-NL, Sara Burgerhartstraat 25, 1055 KV Amsterdam, The Netherlands.)

ated blood vessels and lymphatic structures (20). Viscera in the pelvic cavity receive afferent innervation by way of the autonomic nerve trunks. The visceral afferents that travel in the sympathetic nerve trunk have cell bodies in the thoracolumbar distribution, and those that travel with the parasympathetic fibers have cell bodies in the sacral dorsal ganglia. Both visceral sensory pathways are involved in visceral sensations and reflexes. These neural structures are the first of numerous relays of sensory neurons that transmit painful sensations from the pelvic cavity to the brain. Visceral information is processed by neurons in many laminae in the spinal cord gray matter, including laminae I, II, V to VII, and X. Ascending visceral spinal pathways include the dorsal columns and the spinothalamic and spinoreticular tracts (21). The spinothalamic tract terminates in the thalamic nuclei, from which information is then forwarded to the somatosensory cortex. The spinoreticular tract ends in the brainstem. Little is known about the destination of the dorsal column pathways for visceral pain. Recent research indicates that this pathway includes neurons in the nucleus gracilis and the ventral posterolateral nucleus of the thalamus (22). Perineal structures are somatically innervated through the pudendal nerve, which projects through the S2 to S4 nerve roots (23). Fig. 19.3 shows the innervation of the female reproductive organs.

SEX DIFFERENCES IN PAIN

Despite significant advances in pain research and clinical pain management, little effort has been devoted to exploring whether the same pain treatment strategies are effective for male and female patients. We are just beginning to realize the influence of the hormonal milieu on pain and the response to analgesic interventions in women and girls during different reproductive stages (24–26). Chronic pelvic pain is mainly a pain syndrome in women in their reproductive ages; rarely it is reported in preadolescent girls or—with new onset—in post-menopausal women, although pelvic pain syndromes can continue after a women has reached menopause or after all internal female reproductive organs have been removed. It therefore appears that women are particularly likely to develop chronic pelvic pain during certain chronobiological stages (25). More research in this area is needed (26).

CLINICAL FEATURES

Women with chronic pelvic pain syndromes complain about pain deep in the pelvic cavity, either unilateral, bilateral, or in the midline. The pain often radiates to the low back, anterior abdominal wall, buttocks, hips, perineal area, and anterior thighs. The pain syndrome can be exacerbated by walking or other postural changes. Many patients complain about associated symptoms, including dyspareunia and changes in bowel and urinary habits. Pain can be cyclic (related to the menstrual cycle), intermittent, or continuous.

Many of these patients are often anxious, depressed, and frustrated (27). They may have suffered for many years, but frequently have remained undiagnosed in spite of multiple physicians visits and having undergone extensive testing. Many women have had extensive pelvic surgery without relief of their symptoms (27).

DIFFERENTIAL DIAGNOSIS OF CHRONIC PELVIC PAIN

Chronic pelvic pain is often thought to have primarily gynecological origin. However, all other structures in the pelvic cavity, including the urinary tract and the lower gastrointestinal tract, have to be included in the differential diagnosis. Other origins to be considered include the musculoskeletal system and neurological and psychiatric problems. Table 19.1 lists the wide differential diagnosis of chronic pelvic pain. Localization of the source of pain is often difficult or inaccurate, because of the overlapping innervation pattern of the pelvic organs. It is important to understand that in many patients different etiologies of pelvic pain may not appear in pure form but rather in various mixtures with varying contributions to a woman's total discomfort (28–30). Given the large convergence of visceral input at the spinal cord level and in pelvic ganglia observed in electrophysiological experiments in animals (31–33), it would not be surprising if chronic pain in one pelvic organ could lead to the development of a chronic pain syndrome also in another area of the pelvis via altered central mechanisms. Close

—— Sympathetic   ⊏⊐ Parasympathetic   ▪▪▪▪ Somatic

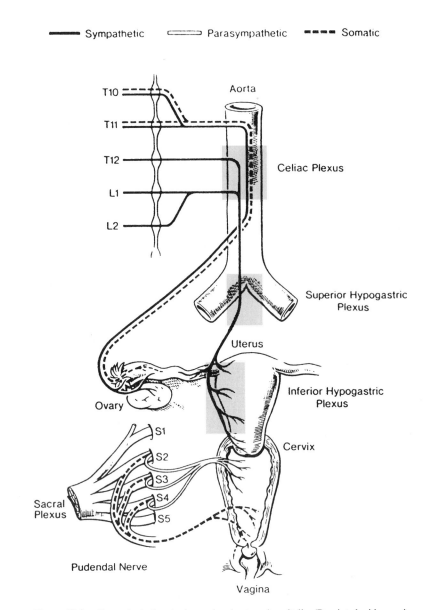

Figure 19.3. Gynecological pain, internal and external genitalia. (Reprinted with permission from Brose WG, Cousins MJ. Gynecologic pain. In: Coppleson M, et al., eds. Gynecologic oncology: fundamental principles and clinical practice. Edinburgh: Churchill Livingstone, 1992;1439–1479.)

attention to such detail is warranted in making a clinical diagnosis and designing a treatment plan (4).

For many years laparoscopy has been the routine tool in the investigation of chronic pelvic pain, because diagnosis based on history and physical examination is often inaccurate. Laparoscopy serves three important diagnostic functions: diagnostic confirmation, histological documentation, and patient reassurance (34). However, fewer than 50% of patients are helped by diagnostic or therapeutic laparoscopy, which indicates that laparoscopy is not the ultimate investigation or treatment for chronic pelvic pain (13). A study from the Netherlands (35) compared the use of laparoscopy during the initial evaluation of chronic pelvic pain with the use of an initial multidisciplinary evaluation without the routine use of laparoscopy. At 1 year of follow-up the multidisciplinary group showed a statistically significant improvement in general pain experience, disturbance of daily activities, and associated symptoms compared with the group receiving the laparopscopy-first approach. Pelvic pain is unique because a patient may have severe pelvic pathology such as adhesions or endometriosis with little or no pain. In contrast, another patient may have severe pain but minimal pelvic pathology (7).

PSYCHOSOCIAL FACTORS IN CHRONIC PELVIC PAIN

The literature examining psychological factors in pelvic pain has demonstrated a number of consistent findings. For

Table 19.1.   Causes of Chronic Pelvic Pain

Gynecological	Irritable bowel syndrome
Extrauterine	Neoplasia
Adhesions	Musculoskeletal, Neurological
Chronic ectopic pregnancy	Coccydynia
Chronic pelvic infection	Disk problems
Endometriosis	Degenerative joint disease
Residual ovary syndrome	Fibromyositis
Uterine	Hernias
Adenomyosis	Herpes zoster
Chronic endometritis	Low back pain
Leiomyomata	Levator ani syndrome (spasm of pelvic floor)
Intrauterine contraceptive device	Myofascial pain (trigger points, spasms)
Pelvic congestion	Nerve entrapment syndromes
Pelvic support defects	Osteoporosis (fractures)
Polyps	Scoliosis, lordosis, kyphosis
Urological	Strains, sprains
Chronic urinary tract infection	Other
Detrusor overactivity	Abuse (physical, sexual, prior or current)
Interstitial cystitis	Heavy metal poisoning (lead, mercury)
Stone	Hyperparathyroidism
Suburethral diverticulitis	Poryphyria
Urethral syndrome	Psychiatric disorders (depression, bipolar disorders, personality disorder)
Gastrointestinal	Psychosocial stress (marital discord, work stress)
Cholelithiasis	Sickle cell disease
Chronic appendicitis	Sleep disturbance
Constipation	Somatiform disorders
Diverticular disease	Substance abuse
Enterocolitis	Reflex sympathetic dystrophy
Gastric/duodenal ulcer	Tabes dorsalis
Inflammatory bowel disease	

Adapted with permission from Chronic pelvic pain. American College of Obstetricians and Gynecologists technical bulletin 223. Int J Gynecol Obstet 1996;54:59–68.

example, a lifetime prevalence of depression in women with chronic pain has been reported at 64%, compared with 17% of gynecological controls, and a current incidence of depression for 28% of chronic pelvic pain patients versus 3% for gynecological controls (36).

The prevalence of sexual and physical abuse among women with chronic pelvic pain is controversial. A history of sexual abuse has long been anecdotally associated with the development of a variety of medical symptoms (37), and that association appears to be particularly strong with chronic pelvic pain. Before basing assumptions upon the data presented, it is important to understand several methodological limitations inherent in the study of sexual trauma. Most of the studies have used retrospective, cross-sectional designs in which the evaluation of the physical complaint and the abuse history are taken concurrently (38). However, what is not known is the validity of retrospective recall of remote abuse events. Recollection of such remote events may be accurate in some individuals but in others may be subject to various recall biases. Furthermore, these studies may wrongly assume cause and effect between abuse history and the development of gynecological pain. Often sexual and physical abuse are symptoms of multiproblem families, characterized by chaos, alcohol and substance abuse, and general neglect that results in children not being adequately protected (38). Many studies

also have failed to use standardized measures to assess abuse and do not delineate among variables of importance such as age of onset of abuse, severity and duration of abuse, and the relationship of the perpetrator to the victim. Finally, it is important to recall the relatively high prevalence rates of sexual victimization in the general population, particularly at tertiary care sites in which many studies are conducted (38).

In controlled studies, the prevalence of childhood sexual victimization of patients with pelvic pain has ranged from 82% (39, 40) to 20% (41). This compares with rates of 23% for a control group of women receiving laparoscopy for infertility or tubal ligation (39, 40) and 13% among a nonpelvic pain comparison group (41). This large discrepancy may relate to varying assessment devices for determining sexual abuse history, one being rather stringent and the other designed to overcome amnesia. Most studies (36, 38, 42) report prevalence rates at around 58% compared with 30% for gynecological or pain controls.

Fewer studies have examined the relationship of physical abuse to chronic pelvic pain. Rapkin et al. (41) found a higher prevalence of physical abuse in general chronic pain patients than in those with pelvic pain complaints. Walling et al. (42) found that women with pelvic pain had higher lifetime prevalence rates of physical abuse than did women who were pain free (50% versus 30%) but no differences between chronic pelvic pain rates and those of chronic headache controls.

WORKUP OF THE PATIENT

An approach to patients with chronic pelvic pain is outlined in Table 19.2.

History

The diversity of possible causes makes a thorough history imperative. Many chronic pelvic pain patients have already had their histories taken repeatedly and may be frustrated to have to go through details of the history again. The history focuses on the nature, intensity, temporal pattern, location, duration, and radiation of the pain, as well as precipitating and relieving factors. A review of symptoms should include gynecological, gastrointestinal, urological, neurological, and musculoskeletal functions. Associated symptoms such as anorexia, constipation, and fatigue should be evaluated.

While taking the history, it is important to review in chronological order which physicians have been consulted, which diagnostic tests have been done, which therapeutic interventions have been tried, and what was the result of each intervention. A thorough review of all previous consultations and diagnostic and therapeutic interventions is imperative for deciding whether further diagnostic workup is required and what pain treatment plan is to be used.

Many women with chronic pelvic pain are in their reproductive ages (10). To be able to establish a treatment plan adjusted to the needs of the individual patient, it is important to address fertility concerns. Many women with chronic pelvic pain often have an impaired sexual life because of pain associated with intercourse. In patients with identifiable gynecological disease fertility may be reduced. Many pharmacological pain treatment approaches are not indicated, if the patient is interested in becoming pregnant soon.

Physical Examination

The physical evaluation is focused on the area of pain; it includes a general physical, neurological, musculoskeletal, and pelvic examination. Procedures during the physical examination that provoke or exacerbate the pelvic pain are carefully noted. Areas of hyperalgesia and trigger points are documented.

Psychological Interview

As in other chronic pain conditions, psychosocial and behavioral assessment is an essential part of the evaluation. A psychological interview, usually conducted by a psychologist or psychiatrist experienced in chronic pain management, should be part of the initial evaluation process (43, 44).

Further Consultations, Laboratory Data, and Diagnostic Tests

As stated earlier, the differential diagnosis of chronic pelvic pain is very wide. Before considering symptomatic pain man-

Table 19.2.   Approach to Patients with Chronic Pelvic Pain

Evaluation of Etiology
  History
    What diagnostic evaluations have been done?
    Are further diagnostic evaluations indicated?
    What pain treatments have been tried, and how well did they work?
    Is the patient receiving pain treatment, and does it reduce pain and improve the quality of life?
  Physical examination
  Psychological interview
  Discuss fertility concerns
Etiological treatment possible
  Start specific treatment
  Taper off symptomatic pain treatment as tolerated
Etiological treatment not possible
  Start symptomatic pain management

agement for chronic pelvic pain, determine the results of any consultations and tests that have already been done. Further laboratory studies and diagnostic tests depend on the history and physical examination and are tailored to the individual patient. Depending on the patient's symptoms, consultations with other specialists in gynecology, gastroenterology, urology, orthopaedics, neurology, or psychiatry maymight be indicated before a symptomatic pain treatment plan is established.

TREATMENT

Surgery

Surgical approaches to the treatment of pelvic pain used to be very common. However, since long-term success after surgical procedures is often disappointing when pelvic pain is the only indication for surgery (34, 45–47) and because of the uncertain role of endometriosis and pelvic adhesions in the etiology of chronic pelvic pain (48–52), nonsurgical treatment options should be explored first (1). Surgical therapy for chronic pain is limited to the treatment of surgically correctable etiologies (1). In patients who have chronic pelvic pain and a surgically correctable disorder, it is important for the physician and the patient to understand that the chronic pain syndrome may be improved but also may be unchanged or worsened by the procedure (48). Many patients with chronic pelvic pain have already undergone several surgical diagnostic and therapeutic procedures without any pain relief. In these patients further surgical procedures should be very carefully considered, since it is less likely that further surgery will result in pain relief after previous surgical approaches have already failed.

Pharmacological Therapy

Although chronic pelvic pain is common, very little is known about effective pharmacological treatment. Pharmacological symptomatic pain management for chronic pelvic pain should be considered after a thorough multidisciplinary evaluation has been completed and underlying disorders have been adequately excluded and or treated. Analgesic treatment can be started while further diagnostic workup is in progress. If an etiology of the chronic pain syndrome is found that requires therapy directed against the underlying disorder, symptomatic pharmacological therapy can be discontinued while treatment directed towards the underlying cause is instituted.

Several pharmacological classes of medications have been demonstrated to alleviate pain in patients with chronic pain syndromes (53, 54). These include: nonsteroidal anti-inflammatory drugs, antidepressants, anticonvulsants, local anesthetic antiarrhythmics, and opioids (Table 19.3). Most have been evaluated for the treatment of chronic neuropathic pain, central pain, and back pain (55). Very few case reports (14, 56, 57) or clinical trials (58) have focused on the treatment of women with chronic pelvic pain. The limited reports in the literature and our own experience at the Johns Hopkins University Blaustein Pain Treatment Center suggest that some pelvic pain syndromes can be successfully treated with medications commonly used to treat other chronic pain syndromes. Further clinical and basic science research in this area is urgently needed.

Although clinical trials and case reports on the pharmacological management of chronic pain syndromes provide general guidelines as to which drug to choose, we have no method to predict which drug is most likely to alleviate pain in a given individual patient. The goal of pharmacotherapy is to find a medication that produces significant pain relief with minimal side effects for an individual patient. It is important that the patient understands the limitations of this trial and error method of prescribing drugs. Adequate trials should be performed for each drug prescribed and only one drug should be titrated at a time, because the effects of a certain drug on pain scores can otherwise not be assessed. Since various medications can have different and selective effects on certain aspects of pain (deep pain in the pelvis, referred pain to musculature) it is important that the effects on each aspect of pain be carefully monitored. More than one treatment approach may be necessary to improve different aspects of the pain. The starting dose should always be the smallest available, and titration should occur at frequent intervals guided by pain scores and side effects. This requires frequent contact between the patient and the pain clinic during the titration period. Some side effects improve as the patient is taking the drug for several weeks, and it is important, if they are not intolerable, that the patient be guided through this period. Common reasons for inadequate medication trials are failure to titrate to an adequate dose and early termination of treatment due to side effects produced by increasing the dose too rapidly, starting at a high initial dose, or starting more than one drug at the same time (53, 55).

Regional Anesthesia

Regional anesthesia has been advocated as a diagnostic tool and therapeutic intervention for women with chronic pelvic pain (59). Over the past 7 years there has been new

Table 19.3. Pharmacologic Agents for Treatment of Chronic Pelvic Pain

Antidepressants
  Tricyclics
    Amytriptyline
    Nortriptyline
    Desipramine
    Doxepin
  Mixed reuptake inhibitors
    Venlafaxine
    Nefazodone
    Maprotiline
  Selective serotonin reuptake inhibitors
    Fluoxetine
    Trazodone
    Paroxetine
    Sertraline
Anticonvulsants, antiarrhythmics
  Sodium channel blockers
    Carbamazepine
    Phenytoin
    Lamotrigin
    Lidocaine
    Mexilitine
  Other Mechanisms of Action
    Valproic acid
    Clonazepam
    Gabapentin
Opioids
  Oral long-acting opioids
    Slow-release opioids
    Opioids with long half-life
  Transdermal opioids
    Fentanyl patch
  Epidural, intrathecal opioids
    Morphine
    Fentanyl
Other agents
  Nonsteroidal anti-inflammatory drugs

Adapted with permission from Rowbotham MC. Chronic pain: from theory to practical management. Neurology 1995;45(Suppl)9:S8.

interest in neurolytic superior hypogastric plexus blocks for the treatment of chronic pelvic pain associated with cancer (60, 61). The superior hypogastric plexus innervates the pelvic viscera via the hypogastric nerves. The hypogastric nerves carry sympathetic efferent nerve fibers and visceral afferent nerve fibers. Analgesia after neurolytic blockade of the superior hypogastric plexus may be due to interruption of the sympathetic outflow to the pelvic organs, as in sympathetically maintained pain syndromes (54), or interruption of the afferent pathways from the pelvic organs. Anecdotal reports have also described diagnostic superior hypogastric plexus blocks with local anesthetic and therapeutic blocks, either with local anesthetic (resulting in pain relief that lasted much longer—days or weeks—than expected from the half-life of the local anesthetic, as in patients with sympathetically maintained pain of the extremities) or neurolytic agents (59, 62) in patients with nonmalignant pelvic pain. Further controlled studies are necessary to assess the use of superior hypogastric plexus blocks for nonmalignant pelvic pain, especially the use of neurolytic blocks.

Pelvic pain may be due entrapment of the ilioinguinal, iliohypogastric, genitofemoral or pudendal nerves. Many of the patients in this category had surgery to the abdominal area in the past. Often the chronic pain syndrome can be managed by repeated local anesthetic nerve blocks to these nerves spaced over time (59).

Transcutaneous Electrical Nerve Stimulation

Transcutaneous electrical nerve stimulation therapy (TENS) can provide excellent pain relief for some patients without the side effects associated with pharmacological treatment. Numerous studies demonstrate that TENS is an effective and safe form of therapy in patients with primary dysmenorrhea (63–69). TENS has also been used successfully in patients with noncyclic chronic pelvic pain (1, 59).

Trigger Point Injections

Myofascial pain has been shown to respond to trigger point injections (70). Slocumb (71) and Ling and Slocumb (72) have used this technique to treat chronic pelvic pain. Patients with chronic pelvic pain typically have pain referred to somatic structures. Ling and Slocumb (72) reported high rates of pain relief (successful outcome in 84 to 100%) with local anesthetic injections into trigger points in the abdominal wall and sacral and vaginal areas.

Acupuncture

Acupuncture has been used through the centuries to control pain. However, acupuncture has not been systematically studied as a separate treatment component for chronic pelvic pain. Anecdotal reports in which acupuncture has been used as part of a multidisciplinary treatment approach indicate an effective role for the management of chronic pelvic pain (50, 57).

Neurosurgery

Presacral Neurectomy

The efficacy of presacral neurectomy and amputation of the uterosacral ligaments in the treatment of chronic pelvic pain has been debated since the early descriptions by Ruggi (73) and Jaboulay (74) in Europe and later in the United States (75). As medical therapy for pelvic diseases was advancing, there was a decline in these procedures. However, with the widespread use of laparoscopic surgery there has been a recent new interest in pelvic denervation for chronic pelvic pain. Reports in the literature regarding the pain relief achieved with these procedures are controversial. While some studies claim a high success rate (45, 76), others fail to prove that presacral neurectomy is effective (77). Better characterization of the patients who do and do not respond to these procedures may help to identify patients who can benefit from the procedure. Further research will show whether a diagnostic superior hypogastric plexus block can predict long-lasting pain relief from a surgical presacral neurectomy.

Decompression of Entrapped Nerves

Pudendal neurectomy has been advocated for patients whose pain is mainly in the perineal area. Several French studies suggest that up to 91% of patients referred to a pain clinic with perineal pain (78) have pudendal nerve entrapment. Surgical neurolysis and transposition eased the pain in 67% of the patients (79). The authors concluded that early diagnosis of nerve entrapment appeared to be the determining factor in improving results. Diagnostic pudendal nerve blocks with local anesthetic and electromyography and nerve conduction studies of the pelvic floor may help to confirm the diagnosis (80). Ilioinguinal, iliohypogastric (groin pain), or genitofemoral nerve (lower abdominal and perineal pain) entrapment may be secondary to surgical trauma in the area of the abdominal wall. Anecdotal reports have shown significant pain relief after neurectomy of these nerves (81).

Myelotomy

Recently limited midline myelotomy has been advocated for the relief of pelvic cancer pain following very promising results in a limited number of cancer patients (22). The aim of this procedure is to interrupt ascending nociceptive signals from the pelvic organs traveling in the medial part of the posterior column. However, before this irreversible procedure can be considered as one of the treatment options for patients with chronic nonmalignant pelvic pain, further research on the function of this pathway and the long-term consequences of its surgical interruption is necessary (82, 83).

Physical Therapy

Musculoskeletal dysfunction often contributes to the signs and symptoms of chronic pelvic pain, because visceral pain is referred to somatic structures. In some cases musculoskeletal pain can be the origin of the chronic pain syndrome (Table 19.1). Physical therapy can decrease musculoskeletal pain, and helps to improve mobility, and is an important aspect of a multidisciplinary approach to the treatment of chronic pelvic pain (84).

Psychological Therapies

In addition to symptomatic pain treatment, psychological treatment should be undertaken early on, since subclinical levels of depression should be treated at the earliest stages of the development of a painful disease (43). Furthermore, psychological factors may affect the success of any treatment, since patients who have chronic pain often remain anxious, are impatient, and have unrealistic expectations about a quick cure. Psychological techniques include relaxation techniques, biofeedback, psychotherapy, and group therapy (85).

A MULTIDISCIPLINARY APPROACH TO PAIN MANAGEMENT

Some of the greatest successes reported in the diagnosis and management of chronic pain have come from multidisciplinary approaches (86–88) (Table 19.4). Chronic pelvic pain is truly a multidisciplinary problem whose diagnosis and management require the concerted effort of a multidisciplinary team. In today's medical environment the time-consuming effort of a thorough history and physical examination and discussion of the pain management plan is often difficult (7). Although there are fewer studies on multidisciplinary approaches to the management of chronic pelvic pain than for other chronic pain syndromes, the available reports clearly show that chronic pelvic pain syndromes markedly improve when patients are enrolled in multidisciplinary treatment programs (14, 35, 50, 57, 89). Prior to a team approach, women with chronic pelvic pain syndromes often have drifted from one physician to another without a clear diagnosis and without much improvement, a frustrating process for the patients and their treating physicians and an expensive process for the health system. Given the clinical presentation of chronic pelvic pain, it is obvious that a multidisciplinary approach is likely to be more successful than a one-dimensional effort: patients with pelvic pain complain about pain deep in the pelvis; they usually present with referred pain to the musculature; and their pain usually affects many aspects of their life (work, recreational activities, sexual life). The multidisciplinary pain clinic, with input from pain specialists, anesthesiologists, neurologists, gynecologists, psychologists, physical therapists, urologists, gastroenterologists, and neurosurgeons, offers the opportunity to work simultaneously with the many contributing factors usually present in chronic pelvic pain problems. The treatment plan is tailored to the symptoms and needs of the particular patient. It is important to discuss with the patient at the beginning of her therapy her expectations and to define goals against which the success of the treatment can be measured. Outcome measures include a reduction in pain (ongoing and evoked pain), improved mood, increased participation in daily psychosocial activities at work and at home, and an improved sexual life. Although cures are uncommon, some pain relief can be provided to almost all patients using a multidisciplinary approach including pain medications, regional anesthesia, physical therapy, and psychological interventions, all the while exercising caution toward invasive and irreversible therapeutic procedures.

SUMMARY

The purpose of this chapter is to emphasize the need for an integrated, multidisciplinary approach to diagnosis and treatment of chronic pelvic pain syndromes. Chronic pelvic pain is a common problem among women. Women with chronic pelvic pain are a heterogeneous population, and therefore attempts to ascribe all cases to a particular cause invariably fail. The relation of pain to the presence of pathology is often unclear. The precise nature of the multidiscipli-

Table 19.4.   Multidisciplinary Approach to Women with Chronic Pelvic Pain

Etiologic treatment	Symptomatic pain relief
Gynecological	Pharmacological pain treatment
Urological	Regional anesthesia techniques
Gastroenterological	Physical therapy, TENS
Musculoskeletal	Trigger point injections
Neurological	Acupuncture
Other	Mental health care
	Surgery

nary approach varies with the human resources available. Nonetheless, the principles of a multidisciplinary approach are the same, no matter how large or small the number of participants. The recognition that chronic pelvic pain is of multifactorial originetiology may lead to more effective interventions and subsequent critical evaluation (6).

References

1. Chronic pelvic pain. ACOG technical bulletin 223. Int J Gynecol Obstet 1996;54:59–68.
2. Borsook D, Carr DB. Pain in gynecologic malignancy. In: Knapp RC, Berkowitz RS, eds. Gynecologic oncology. 2nd ed. New York: McGraw-Hill, 1993;451–467.
3. Brose WG, Cousins MJ. Gynecologic pain. In: Coppleson M, ed. Gynecologic oncology: fundamental principles and clinical practice. 2nd ed. Edinburgh: Churchill Livingstone, 1992.
4. Steege JF, Stout AL, Somkuti SG. Chronic pelvic pain in women: toward an integrative model. Obstet Gyn Surv 1993;48:95–110.
5. Merskey H, Bogduk N. Classification of chronic pain. Seattle: IASP Press, 1994.
6. Campbell F, Collett BJ. Chronic pelvic pain. Br J Anaesth 1994;73:571–573.
7. Ryder RM. Chronic pelvic pain. Am Fam Phys 1996;54:2225–2232.
8. Smith RP. Cyclic pelvic pain and dysmenorrhea. Obstet Gyn Clin North Am 1993;20:753–764.
9. Andersch B, Milson I. An epidemiologic study of young women with dysmenorrhea. Am J Obstet Gynecol 1982;144:655–660.
10. Mathias SD, Kuppermann M, Liberman RF, et al. Chronic pelvic pain: prevalence, health-related quality of life, and economic correlates. Obstet Gynecol 1996;87:321–327.
11. Unruh AM. Gender variations in clinical pain experience. Pain 1996;65:123–167.
12. Reiter RC. A profile of women with chronic pelvic pain. Clin Obstet Gynecol 1990;33:130–136.
13. Howard FM. The role of laparoscopy in chronic pelvic pain: promise and pitfalls. Obstet Gynecol Surv 1993;48:357–387.
14. Milburn A, Reiter RC, Rhomberg AT. Multidisciplinary approach to chronic pelvic pain. Obstet Gynecol Clin North Am 1993;20:643–661.
15. Rapkin AJ. Neuroanatomy, neurophysiology, and neuropharmacology of pelvic pain. Clin Obstet Gynecol 1990;33:119–129.
16. Gebhart GF. Visceral nociception: consequences, modulation and the future. Eur J Anaesth 1995;12:24–27.
17. Giamberardino MA, Vecchiet L. Experimental studies on pelvic pain. Pain Rev 1994;1:102–115.
18. Mayer EA, Gebhart GF. Functional bowel disorders and the visceral hyperalgesia hypothesis. In: Mayer EA, Gebhart GF, eds. Basic and clinical aspects of chronic abdominal pain. Amsterdam: Elsevier, 1993;3–28.

19. Ness TJ, Metcalf AM, Gebhart GF. A psychophysiological study in humans using phasic colonic distension as a noxious visceral stimulus. Pain 1990;43:377–386.

20. Bonica JJ. General considerations of pain in the pelvic and perineum. In: Bonica JJ, ed. The management of pain. 2nd ed. Philadelphia: Lea and Febiger, 1990;1283–1312.

21. Willis WD Jr, Coggeshall RE. Sensory mechanisms of the spinal cord. 2nd ed. New York: Plenum Press, 1991:456.

22. Hirshberg RM, Al-Chaer ED, Lawand NB, et al. Is there a pathway in the posterior funiculus that signals visceral pain? Pain 1996;67:291–305.

23. Renaer M. Chronic pelvic pain in women. New York: Springer Verlag, 1981.

24. Berkley KJ. Sex differences in pain. Behav Brain Sci 1997;20:371–380.

25. Berkley KJ. Female vulnerability to pain and the strength to deal with it. Behav Brain Sci 1997;20:473–479.

26. Wesselmann U. Gender differences: implications for pain management. Behav Brain Sci 1997;20:470–471.

27. Rapkin AJ. Gynecological pain in the clinic: is there a link with the basic research? In: Gebhart GF, ed. Visceral pain, progress in pain research and management. Seattle: IASP Press, 1995; 469–488.

28. Crowell MD, Dubin NH, Robinson JC, et al. Functional bowel disorders in women with dysmenorrhea. Am J Gastroenterol 1994;11:1973–1977.

29. Whitehead WE, Cheskin LJ, Heller BR, et al. Evidence for exacerbation of irritable bowel syndrome during menses. Gastroenterology 1990;98:1485–1489.

30. Walker EA, Gelfand AN, Gelfand MD, et al. Chronic pelvic pain and gynecological symptoms in women with irritable bowel syndrome. J Psychosom Obstet Gynecol 1996;17:39–46.

31. Wesselmann U. Untersuchungen der Impulsübertragung im Ganglion Mesentericum Inferius (Studies on the transmission of impulses in the inferior mesenteric ganglion). Dissertation, Medizinische Fakultät der Universität Kiel, West Germany. 1987:1–244.

32. Jänig W, Schmidt M, Schnitzler A, Wesselmann U. Differentiation of sympathetic neurons projecting in the hypogastric nerve in terms of their discharge patterns in cats. J Physiol 1991;437:157–179.

33. Cervero F. Sensory innervation of the viscera: peripheral basis of visceral pain. Physiol Rev 1994;74:95–138.

34. Parsons LH, Stovall TG. Surgical management of chronic pelvic pain. Obstet Gynecol Clin North Am 1993;20:765–778.

35. Peters AA, van Drost E, Jellis B, et al. A randomized clinical trial to compare two different approaches in women with chronic pelvic pain. Obstet Gynecol 1991;77:740–744.

36. Walker E, Katon W, Harrop-Griffiths J, et al. Relationship of chronic pelvic pain to psychiatric diagnoses and childhood sexual abuse. Am J Psychiatry 1988;145:75–80.

37. Kinzl JF, Traweger C, Biebl W. Family background and sexual abuse associated with somatization. Psychother Psychosom 1995;64:82–87.

38. Walker EA, Stenchever MA. Sexual victimization and chronic pelvic pain. Obstet Gynecol Clin North Am 1993;20:795–807.

39. Walker EA, Katon WJ, Neraass K, et al. Dissociation in women with chronic pelvic pain. Am J Psychiatry 1992;149:534–537.

40. Walker EA, Katon WJ, Hansom J, et al. Medical and psychiatric symptoms in women with childhood sexual abuse. Psychosom Med 1992;54:658–664.

41. Rapkin AJ, Kames LD, Darke LL, et al. History of physical and sexual abuse in women with chronic pelvic pain. Obstet Gynecol 1990;76:92–96.

42. Walling M, O'Hara MW, Reiter RC. Sexual abuse as a specific risk factor for chronic pelvic pain. XXI Annual Meeting, American Society of Psychosomatic Obstetrics and Gynecology, Charleston, SC, 1993 (abstract).

43. Skevington SM. The relationship between pain and depression: a longitudinal study of early synovitis. In: Gebhart GF, Hammond DL, Jensen TS. eds. Proceedings of the VII World Congress on Pain. Progress in Pain Research and Management, vol. 2. Seattle: IASP Press, 1994;201–210.

44. Elliot ML. Chronic pelvic pain: what are the psychological considerations. Am Pain Soc Bull 1996;6:1–4.

45. Lee RB, Stone K, Magelssen D, et al. Presacral neurectomy for chronic pelvic pain. Obstet Gynecol 1986;68:517–521.

46. Lichten EM, Bombard J. Surgical treatment of primary dysmenorrhea with laparoscopic uterine nerve ablation. J Reprod Med 1987;32:37–41.

47. Lichten EM. Three years experience with Luna: outpatient laser laparoscopic treatment of dysmenorrhea. Am J Gynecol Health 1989;5:144–147.

48. Carleson KJ, Miller BA, Fowler FJ Jr. The Maine Women's Health Study: 2. Outcomes of nonsurgical management of leiomyomas, abnormal bleeding, and chronic pelvic pain. Obstet Gynecol 1994;83:566–572.

49. Fukaya T, Hoshiai H, Yajima A. Is pelvic endometriosis always associated with chronic pain? A retrospective study of 618 cases diagnosed by laparoscopy. Am J Obstet Gynecol 1993;169:719–722.

50. Steege JF, Stout AL. Resolution of chronic pelvic pain after laparoscopic lysis. Am J Obstet Gynecol 1991;165:278–283.

51. Roseff SJ, Murphy AA. Laparoscopy in the diagnosis and therapy of chronic pelvic pain. Clin Obstet Gynecol 1990;33:137–144.

52. Soellner W, Huter O, Wurm B, et al. Longitudinal follow-up of chronic pelvic pain and occurrence of new symptoms 5 to 7 years after laparosopy. Am J Obstet Gynecol 1993;168:1645.

53. Galer BS. Neuropathic pain of peripheral origin: advances in pharmacologic treatment. Neurology 1995;45:S17–S25.

54. Wesselmann U, Raja SN. Reflex sympathetic dystrophy and causalgia. Anesth Clin North Am 1997;15:407–427.

55. Rowbotham MC. Chronic pain mechanisms and management. Neurology 1995;45(Suppl)9.

56. Beresin E. Imipramine in the treatment of chronic pelvic pain. Psychosomatics 1986;27:294–296.

57. Kames LD, Rapkin AJ, Naliboff BD, et al. Effectiveness of an interdisciplinary pain management program for the treatment of chronic pelvic pain. Pain 1990;41:41–46.

58. Walker EA, Roy-Byrne PR, Katon WJ, Jemelka R. An open trial of nortriptyline in women with chronic pelvic pain. Int J Psychiat Med 1991;21:245–252.

59. McDonald JS. Management of chronic pelvic pain. Obstet Gynecol Clin North Am 1993;20:817–838.

60. Leon-Casasola OA, Kent E, Lema MJ. Neurolytic superior hypogastric plexus block for chronic pelvic pain associated with cancer. Pain 1993;54:145–151.

61. Plancarte R, Amescua C, Patt RB, Aldrete JA. Superior hypogastric plexus block for pelvic cancer pain. Anesthesiology 1990;73:236–239.

62. Wechsler RJ, Maurer PM, Halpern EJ, Frank ED. Superior hypogastric plexus block for chronic pelvic pain in the presence of endometriosis: CT techniques and results. Radiology 1995;196:103–106.

63. Milsom I, Hedner N, Mannheimer C. A comparative study of the effect of high-intensity transcutaneous nerve stimulation and oral naproxen on intrauterine pressure and menstrual pain in patients with primary dysmenorrhea. Am J Obstet Gynecol 1994;170:123–129.

64. Walker JB, Katz RL. Peripheral nerve stimulation in the management of dysmenorrhea. Pain 1981;11:355–361.

65. Lundeberg T, Bondesson L, Lundström V. Relief of primary dysmenorrhea by transcutaneous electrical nerve stimulation. Acta Obstet Gynecol Scand 1985;64:491–497.

66. Mannheimer JS, Whalen EC. The efficacy of transcutaneous electrical nerve stimulation in dysmenorrhea. Clin J Pain 1985;1:75–83.

67. Santiesteban AJ, Burnham TL, George KL, et al. Primary spasmodic dysmenorrhea: the use of TENS on acupuncture points. Am J Acupunct 1985;13:35–42.

68. Neighbours LE, Clelland J, Jackson JR, et al. Transcutaneous electrical nerve stimulation for pain relief in primary dysmenorrhea. Clin J Pain 1987;3:17–22.

69. Dawood MY, Ramos J. Transcutaneous electrical nerve stimulation (TENS) for the treatment of primary dysmenorrhea: a randomized crossover comparison with placebo, TENS and ibuprofen. Obstet Gynecol 1990;75:656–670.

70. Travell J, Rinzler SH. The myofascial genesis of pain. Postgrad Med 1952;11:425–427.

71. Slocumb JC. Neurological factors in chronic pelvic pain: trigger points and the abdominal pelvic pain syndrome. Am J Obstet Gynecol 1984;149:536–543.

72. Ling FW, Slocumb JC. Use of trigger point injections in chronic pelvic pain. Obstet Gynecol Clin North Am 1993;20:809–815.

73. Ruggi C. La simpatectomia addominale utero-ovarica come mezzo di cura di alcune lesioni interne degli organi genitali della donna. Bologna: Zanichelli, 1899.

74. Jaboulay M. Le traitement de la nevralgie pelvienne par la paralysie du sympathique sacre. Lyon Med 1899;90:102–108.

75. Meigs JV. Excision of the superior hypogastric plexus (presacral nerve) for primary dysmenorrhea. Surg Gynecol Obstet 1939;68:723–732.

76. Zullo F, Pellicano M, DeStefano R, et al. Efficacy of laparoscopiclaparascopic pelvic denervation in central-type chronic pelvic pain: a multicenter study. J Gynecol Surg 1996;12:35–40.

77. Vercellini P, Fedele L, Bianchi S, Candiani GB. Pelvic denervation for chronic pain associated with endometriosis: fact or fancy? Am J Obstet Gynecol 1991;165:745–749.

78. Bensignor MF, Labat JJ, Robert R, Ducrot P. Diagnostic and therapeutic pudendal nerve blocks for patients with perineal nonmalignant pain. VIII World Congress on Pain 1996;56 (abstract).

79. Robert R, Brunet C, Faure A, et al. La chirurgie du nerf pudental lors de certaines algies perineales: evolution et resultats. Chirurgie 1993;119:535–539.

80. Beck R, Fowler CJ, Mathias CJ. Genitourinary dysfunction in disorders of the autonomic nervous system. In: Rushton DN, ed. Handbook of neuro-urology. New York: Marcel Dekker, 1994;281–301.

81. Harms BA, DeHaas DR, Starling JR. Diagnosis and management of genitofemoral neuralgia. Neurosurgery 1987;102:583–586.

82. Berkley KJ. On the dorsal columns: translating basic research hypotheses to the clinic. Pain 1997;70:103–107.

83. Gybels JM. Commissural myelotomy revisited. Pain 1997;70:1–2.

84. Baker PK. Musculoskeletal origins of chronic pelvic pain: diagnosis and treatment. Obstet Gynecol Clin North Am 1993;20:719–742.

85. Rosenthal RH. Psychology of chronic pelvic pain. Obstet Gynecol Clin North Am 1993;20:627–642.

86. Flor H, Fydrich T, Turk DC. Efficacy of multidisciplinary pain treatment centers: A meta-analytic review. Pain 1992;49:221–230.

87. Malone MD, Strube MJ. Meta-analysis of nonmedical treatments for chronic pain. Pain 1988;34:231–244.

88. Maruta T, Swanson DW, McHardy MJ. Three year follow-up of patients with chronic pain who were treated in a multidisciplinary pain management center. Pain 1990;41:47–53.

89. Gambone JC, Reiter RC. Nonsurgical management of chronic pelvic pain: a multidisciplinary approach. Clin Obstet Gynecol 1990;33:205–211.

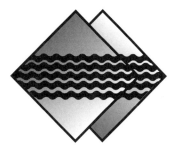

PART IV

Psychosocial Aspects

CHAPTER 20

Psychodynamics and Psychotherapy of the Chronic Pain Syndrome

Gerald M. Aronoff

INTRODUCTION

Relief of suffering has been the medical profession's primary objective throughout time. The past decade has witnessed a proliferation of theoretical approaches designed to be helpful for patients suffering from chronic pain and clinicians who treat this difficult problem. This chapter limits discussion to chronic nonmalignant pain. When pain remains intractable, the cause is often obscure and the time course variable, and the symptoms often evade conventional medical treatment.

Despite advances in biomedical technology, chronic pain often remains a medical enigma. Most treatment approaches to pain have been based on a dichotomy between physiological and psychological causes. This dualism greatly limits the treatment available to each patient. It reinforces the pursuit of relieving pain by isolating symptoms and treating target organs. Although this dichotomy has not been universally reversed, medical science has made significant contributions to the theory of pain as a multidimensional phenomenon influenced by neurological, physiological, psychological, social, ethnocultural, motivational, cognitive, and other factors (1).

Chronic pain is a biologically useless phenomenon that erodes productive human behaviors. However, many learn to cope with their ongoing discomfort without major change in their personal, social, or occupational roles. Others have a more difficult time coping and develop what is commonly called a chronic pain syndrome. It must be emphasized that chronic pain syndrome is not a diagnostic term but describes a clinical syndrome in which the persistent pain is associated with maladaptive and dysfunctional pain behaviors, poor coping, limitations in functional daily activities, frequently concurrent depressive signs and symptoms, and significant life disruption. Generally these individuals have had extensive diagnostic evaluation and all too often, excessive invasive therapeutic interventions. For some this has resulted in iatrogenic complications. For others, despite excellent medical care, symptoms are intractable. For all, there have been some behavioral consequences of their pain. That personality factors play a major role in defining the chronic pain patient is well accepted.

This chapter attempts to synthesize and review the existing body of knowledge pertinent to psychodynamic theory and techniques for treating chronic pain syndromes. In addition, it comments on alternative techniques for treating patients with intractable pain. In recent years psychoanalytical theory and psychodynamic psychotherapy have fallen into disfavor as a psychotherapeutic approach and are not emphasized in most psychiatric and clinical psychology training programs. Consequently many of the consultants who evaluate patients with chronic pain syndromes, having come from these training programs, do not have sufficient background to recognize the complexity of the chronic pain experience and the concurrent suffering, which not infrequently is rooted in conflict, trauma, or unmet needs in early life. Psychoanalytic and psychodynamic psychotherapy is costly, time consuming, and from a public health perspective not an efficient treatment approach. However, such psychotherapy may assist the clinician in understanding refractory and intractable symptoms in which the causation is obscure.

The role of pain in the personality reveals a complex configuration that can be viewed both psychodynamically and behaviorally. The clinical picture depends on the individual's psychological health. The manner in which pain operates at different levels of the personality is described, showing how it provides for relief from conflict and anxiety in a primary way and allows for manipulation of others secondarily (2).

PAIN AND THE ID, EGO, AND SUPEREGO

Psychoanalytical theory describes three sectors of the psyche: the id, or unconscious source of the person's primitive sexual and aggressive impulses; the superego, the partly conscious reflection of conscience and the rules of society; and the ego, similar to the self, a mediator with reality and manager of the psyche.

Sexuality, aggression, and dependency needs can be satisfied or frustrated by pain. The patient with chronic pain commonly has a pattern of masochistic behavior (3–5). Pain may gratify the need to suffer while passive-aggressively burdening another person, often a family member or a health care professional, with constant complaints of pain and demands for attention (3–7). The pain and disability can provide a sanction for dependent behavior; in this way, excessive dependency needs can be unconsciously gratified.

Superego problems in the pain-prone individual (5) reveal themselves in excessive guilt and the need for atonement. Engel (8) described a patient whose pain contributed positively to his overall adjustment, enabling him to succeed in business. When physicians found and treated the cause of his pain, the patient's functioning suffered considerably. Engel described how pain could be used to alleviate guilt and allow the person to function at a higher level. Pilowsky (7) agrees with Engel's formulation and adds that parents inflicting pain on their offspring form a cruel and unyielding superego with an associated chronic sense of guilt and low self-esteem, so that the perception of pain is a means of expiating guilt and reducing tension.

Clinical information supports the idea that chronic pain may be associated with a harsh superego development. Self-destructive behavior, such as suicide attempts, alcoholism, and masochistic relationships with abusive spouses, have been reported (3–5, 8–16). Many chronic pain patients suffered emotionally traumatic childhoods (17) and grew up with a family member who was severely ill or disabled (4). Patients with low-back pain were found to have histories of working intensely without the enjoyment of vacations for many years prior to their pain problem (10).

It is the task of the ego to cope with stress, and pain can be exacerbated when there is a breach in self-esteem (18). For example, a factory worker who has lost the use of an arm as a result of a painful injury not only loses his or her work but may also lose a sense of mastery and may be vulnerable to the reemergence of painful repressed affects, such as childhood depression and rage. These distressing feelings may be misperceived as a strictly physiological reaction. Furthermore, they may cause hypochondriacal processes, conversion reaction, or other psychic responses that can increase the pain and exacerbate the emotional breakdown.

Pain can be understood as it affects personal relations, as Sternbach (19) discussed in his depiction of pain games, wherein the goal for the patient is to frustrate family doctors and retain the pain. Szasz (20) elaborated on the interpersonal aspects of pain, stating that pain can be assessed in terms of communication manifested on three levels. In addition to the first intrapsychic level of signal interpreted by the ego as a threat to its integrity, the two interpersonal levels involve the communication of that threat to another person with indirect expression of need that cannot or will not be conveyed directly.

PAIN AS DEFENSE

Pain can be experienced as being ego alien (20–22) when the person separates it from the self, views the affected part of the body as "other," and converts "me" to "it." The person detaches the self from the pain experience (a dissociative defense to the pain) much as he or she avoids all threatening primitive affects, such as fear of annihilation. When pain persists, this process of detachment can intensify. The person may deny sensation, avoid social contact, withdraw, become isolated, and develop body image problems.

Muscle tension can serve as a defense against the emergence of feelings, according to Bernstein (23), who relates this to the frustration associated with uncovering oedipal issues. This phenomenon can be generalized to other situations in which the individual feels the need to suppress emotions.

Pilowsky (24) reports that pain can serve as a focal point to help the patient avoid other more salient problems. In this way physical pain can facilitate denial and repression of emotional conflict. He labels this excessive concern with pain and ill health as abnormal illness behavior.

PAIN AS PRIMITIVE EMOTIONAL EXPERIENCE

It is my opinion that pain can operate on a continuum of different levels of ego structure depending on the individual's psychological health. Szasz (20) referred to pain as an affect of undifferentiated pain anxiety: an ideational component and a diffuse physiological process. Arieti's (25, 26) concept of elementary first-order "protoemotions" of tension, fear, rage, and satisfaction are characteristic of the emotional communication of many chronic pain syndrome patients. At a similar level of differentiation is the psychological defense of denial common in chronic pain syndrome patients and more generally in psychosomatic patients. The alexithymic patient (27–29) described in the psychosomatic literature cannot comprehend his or her emotional reactions and only experiences inner sensory cues and motor activity. Here then is the lowest primitive level of defense and emotional experience.

Psychoanalytic concepts explain the psychology of chronic pain and assist in psychotherapy. Clinically, chronic pain syndromes can best be treated when psychotherapy is combined with the modification of secondary gains and reinforcement contingencies and resolution of dysfunctional cognitive distortions. Behavioral and cognitive-behavioral approaches to managing chronic pain are discussed in greater detail in Chapter 24.

PSYCHOTHERAPY

The literature concerning the psychotherapy of chronic pain provides a spectrum of approaches including the existential, psychodynamically oriented intrapsychic, interpersonal, behavioral, and cognitive-behavioral. In the office setting, none of the individual psychotherapies has proved as efficacious as individual and group psychotherapy provided in the structured therapeutic milieu of a multidisciplinary pain center. Merskey (30) and Aronoff (31) emphasize the high priority of treating the patient's pain as real, regardless of its cause. The existential reality requires acknowledgment and warrants serious attention because this brings about a more effective alliance. Even patients who initially resent the referral to a psychiatrist benefit from a positive attitude and a sympathetic, supportive style. Support can take the form of actively giving advice in a non-neutral, although tentative, fashion.

Psychodynamic understanding is crucial, according to Pinsky and Malyon (32), who are sensitive to the narcissistic regression of many patients. They help patients to integrate needs and drives and to achieve a sense of mastery. Because pain patients often are significantly concrete, lack verbal ability, and use operatory thinking, Pinsky and Malyon call these individuals dyslexithymic or hypothymic, derived from the term alexithymic coined by Sifneos (28) to describe psychosomatic patients, whose cognitive position may be defensive and therefore approachable through a trusting alliance with a psychotherapist. Pinsky and Malyon feel that rage or other strong emotions can be generated and more easily dealt with in group psychotherapy. Pinsky and Malyon (32) emphasize eclecticism: gestalt, analytical, psychodramatic, and reality-oriented techniques are used as overall approaches within an inpatient milieu. They focus on conflict recognition, evoking affects and extending cognition, and have an ego-oriented psychodynamic and existentialist method. A therapeutic program described by Sarno (33) consists of individual psychotherapy administered in a rehabilitation setting. In this program psychotherapy, which was viewed as critical, was directed toward accepting and expressing feelings, identifying behavior patterns, and learning to cope with stress.

Tunks and Mersky (34) emphasize the importance of supportive psychotherapy, in which the clinician establishes a trusting relationship, sharing compassion and empathy with the pain patient, who may be feeling very alone and isolated. Assistance with problem solving, information, advice, and reassurance become integrated into the treatment.

An interpersonal approach influenced by transactional analysis is favored by Sternbach (19), who applied this in a group setting. Because many pain patients show conflicting motivations about improving, Sternbach's technique focuses on these resistances. He describes and identifies character styles of confounder, professional, and addict. He treats the depression, stops the pain games, and helps patients with unmet needs that are expressed bodily. Sternbach sees the need for the patient to accept a psychological rehabilitation and believes that a behavioral and directive approach is more useful that Pinsky's inner-directed, insight-oriented one.

Cognitive techniques that identify irrational thinking have attracted some attention (12, 35). Underlying personal beliefs and distorted cognitions are directly addressed and restructured. The behavior modification of pain expression is practiced in most multidisciplinary pain units, including mine.

However, Fordyce (9) made the formal analysis, based on negatively reinforcing pain behavior while positively reinforcing healthy behaviors, such as physical activity, social interactions, realistic optimism, and plans for the future.

Cognitive-behavioral therapy has become increasingly popular since the mid 1980s and is perhaps the most widely used psychotherapeutic approach at multidisciplinary pain centers. Major contributions by Turk and Rudy (36) and Turk and Meichenbaum (37) emphasize that through a conditioned process patients develop altered and dysfunctional perceptions about themselves, their environment, and their future. The goal of treatment is to define the cognitive distortions and replace maladaptive styles and beliefs with more adaptive thoughts, feelings, and behaviors. Turk suggests that a comprehensive cognitive-behavioral approach is more likely to foster maintenance of treatment gains than other therapeutic options.

In the role of medical director at the Presbyterian Center for Pain Medicine, I evaluate patients for admission, coordinate the treatment program, and plan discharge. Although I have a background in psychodynamic psychiatry, I use a behavioral medicine approach in the pain treatment process. It is important, however, to emphasize that my professional identity is not primarily as a psychiatrist but rather as a board-certified pain medicine physician and also a psychiatrist. This is important, since virtually all of the patients referred to the pain center are referred for their chronic pain, not for their emotional difficulties. Patients and referring physicians must feel reassured that the physical symptoms will be acknowledged and that medical complaints will receive attention. However, patients must have confidence when the pain medicine physician's assessment indicates that no further diagnostic evaluation is indicated and that it will be therapeutic for them to participate fully in the pain management program and countertherapeutic to continue their pursuit for a cure. Some patients do need to learn to live with pain, and in our pain center it is the pain medicine physician who must assure them not only that it is possible but that there can be pain without suffering and that they can resume functional and productive lives. Adaptive coping behaviors, such as physical activity, social interactions, and future-oriented planning are positively reinforced. Chronic maladaptive pain behaviors, such as inactivity, attempts at gaining sympathy, medication dependencies, passivity, and helplessness are destabilized.

As treatment director, I coordinate psychiatric and psychological management with the help of three full-time PhD. clinical psychologists who are the individual and group psychotherapists; one of them is also the program director. I emphasize medical and psychological diagnoses, and the psychotherapists focus on intrapsychic dynamics, cognitive and behavioral change related to the adaptation to pain.

I (31) approach chronic pain as a complex psychosomatic process in which suffering is viewed as learned, goal-directed behaviors. Self-directed rage, denial, and displacement of affect; inadequate coping; inability to recognize, define, or adequately deal with life stresses; and tenuous support systems are all targets for psychotherapeutic treatments. Suffering is regarded as the emotional reaction to pain sensation and is felt to be amenable to change. Disability is viewed as a generally maladaptive process that can often be avoided or prevented and frequently is a product of learned helplessness as part of conditioned illness behavior. Psychotherapy is integrated into a medical diagnostic and therapeutic approach that is accepted by patients whose approach to their pain is through excessive somatization while minimizing psychic distress.

It is my premise that the optimal setting for the therapeutic process is a multidisciplinary pain center in which somatic therapies are juxtaposed with individual, group, and family psychotherapies in a specially structured milieu. In isolation, psychotherapy is generally ineffective in the treatment of chronic pain syndromes. Many patients entering the pain center have a primary medical diagnosis (or diagnoses) and one or more psychiatric diagnoses, the most common being a subtype of depression. In addition, some are found to have poor ego functioning. This may be related to the chronic pain process or indicate a premorbid process. In these patients the comprehensive pain program, through the therapeutic milieu and psychotherapies, is ego reconstructive. The staff are nurturing, positive role models who reinforce adaptive coping skills but not self-defeating maladaptive pain behaviors. They reinforce the therapeutic benefits of daily exercise, and, for some patients function as family substitutes, providing benevolent maternalism or paternalism in the place of previously dysfunctional relationships. Through inservice training the staff are made aware of and become sensitive to concepts of transference and countertransference, splitting, acting out behaviors, and defense mechanisms.

The clinical psychologists function individually and as a team, conducting individual and group psychotherapy with ego-oriented and psychodynamic aspects on the one hand coordinated with cognitive and behavioral aspects on the other. Other techniques include hypnosis, systematic relaxation training, and biofeedback. The first task of therapy is to establish an alliance with the patient and empathize with the struggle with pain. The psychologists acknowledge the depressive reaction that commonly accompanies chronic intractable pain. Dealing directly with the patient's resistance to a particular emotional event is usually fruitless and is likely to frustrate both patient and therapist. A more effective approach emphasizes character analysis. We investigate how a patient handles all emotional events rather than a specific situation. The patient's orientation to feelings in general is examined. This approach is also more acceptable to the patient, who may more easily gain insight about behaviors and gradually develop an awareness of the significance of feelings.

Developmental issues are discussed in an active and direct manner, but the emphasis is on present coping reactions. An undue focus on psychodynamics can be countertherapeutic when patients either blame their problems on the past or find explanations irrelevant. It becomes more important to explore how the patient's dependency needs were met when he or she

was functioning well and how the injury upset this balance than to focus on the origin of the dependent personality.

Pain center patients attend three types of psychotherapy groups. One group emphasizes affective release, another the identification and expression of conflict, and a third is didactic. Because the pain center program has limited duration, we do not have the luxury of time to work through resistance in the traditional manner. To assess motivation and provoke psychological movement, I use a direct and at times confrontational approach. This is extremely useful with patients whose major psychological defenses are somatization, denial, or projection. Often these patients become settled into a passive sick role of being taken care of and are maintained by worker compensation or medical disability. They do not recognize self-defeating, maladaptive behavior patterns or the secondary gain aspect of their pain.

Some confrontations occur in a group setting with other patients and staff present. This helps to clarify issues pertinent to a particular patient, which are often different from issues alleged by patients, and thereby reduces splitting. Some patients (often those with significant secondary gain) tend to view the confrontation as a threat to their highly prized disability status and angrily leave the pain unit when they are challenged. The secondary gain persists, as does their dependence on the health care delivery system.

Two examples of the use of this therapeutic approach are related in the case histories that follow.

CASE 1

A 35-year-old woman was admitted to the day treatment pain program with severe lower abdominal and suprapubic pain, recurrent episodes of cystitis, and painful bladder symptoms. She also had a recurrent *E. coli* infection. She had had extensive urological and gynecological evaluation and treatment, including multiple cystoscopies, pelvic examinations, anoscopy, and hydrodistention under anesthesia, all of which were essentially unremarkable. Significant medical history included partial hysterectomy with left oophorectomy and bladder suspension. She had been maintained on morphine sulfate (MS Contin) 30 mg three times a day, amitriptyline 50 mg at bedtime, gentamycin by self-catheterization three times daily, and oral antibiotics. Because of her ongoing pain and failure to respond to opioid therapy or trials of nerve blocks, she was referred to the comprehensive pain center.

Her developmental and psychosocial histories were extremely significant. She never knew her father and was raised by her mother until age 4, at which time the mother was ruled unfit "because of sexual, physical, and emotional abuse." The mother was diagnosed with bipolar disorder. The patient recalled at age 4 having her vagina probed with a knitting needle. From age 4 to 13 the patient lived with various relatives, and she vividly recalled repeated sexual abuse by multiple relatives and neighbors. She was raped at age 13. She then spent several years living on the street and at age 17 got pregnant. She went through this pregnancy essentially alone, without emotional support, and became a single parent. She had her first urinary tract infection (UTI) during the pregnancy and has had chronic UTIs since and pelvic pain in recent years in the context of major marital problems.

On mental status examination her facial expression was often inappropriate, with a tendency to close her eyes or avoid eye contact. She admitted to smiling inappropriately when feeling sad. Her mood was severely depressed with inappropriate affect. She acknowledged chronic suicidal ideation without plans but with past attempts. She had had psychiatric treatment, which she did not find helpful, and that included tricyclic antidepressant treatment. There was no evidence of a formal thought disorder, but she was assessed as having cognitive distortions regarding her self-perception and perception of others in her environment and of her future, all of which appeared to be distorted by her past traumas. She acknowledged feeling defective, unlovable, and worthless. She had associated feelings of helplessness and hopelessness. Her judgment was impaired, largely because of her depression and cognitive distortions. She began multidisciplinary treatment and at the end of 10 days was tapered from opioids and was actively participating in a functional restoration exercise program without interference by her pain. Emotionally, however, she was only marginally compensated, and in the context of a family psychotherapy session became enraged at her husband's lack of support, insensitivity to her pain, and refusal to accept or understand her chronic sexual dysfunction. That evening at home she made a suicide attempt (cry for help) by taking multiple medications. She came to the pain program in the morning but was unwilling to contract that she would ask for help if she again felt suicidal.

She was admitted to the psychiatric inpatient unit and stabilized, and she completed the pain program. She thrived in the supportive therapeutic milieu, was not given analgesic medication when she demonstrated pain behavior, and has remained off analgesic medication. She bonded emotionally with several patients and has continued friendships with them. She is learning to share her emotional distress, has less inappropriate acting out, and is less reliant on the health care system; her use of resources is markedly decreased. She continues on antidepressant (tricyclic and selective serotonin uptake inhibitor) medication and is in psychotherapy directed at her cognitive distortions and improving ego strength. She continues with chronic suicidal ideation and major marital problems, including ongoing sexual dysfunction in which she accedes to her husband's demands but hates "being touched," and still has a fragile facade of coping (although slowly improving). Other than the diagnosis of major depression, chronic, and dysthymic disorder, she met diagnostic criteria for pain disorder associated with psychological factors (admitting diagnosis was interstitial cystitis), and chronic pain syndrome. Factitious disorder with repeated UTIs possibly related to self probing was ruled out. Her borderline personality makes her prognosis somewhat guarded, and she continues feeling extremely needy and has limited ego strength and a low frustration tolerance. However, she is now aware of her emotional needs and believes that she was not only born to please others. Pain is no longer an issue; suffering, however, remains a problem.

CASE 2

A 51-year-old housewife and mother of two grown children was admitted with ilioinguinal neuralgia, chronic pain syndrome, and major depression. She had a complex medical history dating back 15 years. That was shortly after she relocated from a large Midwestern city where she had been socially prominent to a small southern town where she felt socially isolated. She began having gynecological problems, which at first were thought to be nonspecific, and the cause was obscure. She ultimately was given a diagnosis of endometriosis and eventually had a total abdominal hysterectomy with right salpingo-oophorectomy. Within hours of the surgery she developed a burning and pulling pain in the right inguinal region. This pain persisted for 14 years despite extensive diagnostic evaluation, all of which was unrevealing and nondiagnostic. She had hormonal therapy, exploratory surgery (with no evidence of adhesions), nerve blocks, and trigger point injections, without benefit.

For 2 years prior to this admission she had been homebound and severely depressed. Most of her time was spent in bed, and she only left the house to attend medical appointments. She was smoking nearly two packs of cigarettes a day. Medications on admission included fentanyl transdermal (Duragesic) patch 50 µg every 3 days, lorazepam 0.5 mg three times a day; aspirin, butalbital, and caffeine (Fiorinol) three times a day; atropine sulfate, hyoscyamine sulfate, scopolamine, and phenobarbital (Donnatol) as needed; metoclopramide (Reglan) 5 mg three times a day; and trimethobenzamide hydrochloride (Tigan) as needed. On admission her mental status was most notable for her appearing much older than her stated age; her hair was long and unkempt; she was wearing pajamas and a bathrobe; and she was both angry and extremely depressed. She agreed to treatment initially as an inpatient with the realization that had she not agreed she would have been placed involuntarily in the psychiatric unit. This was because her family was concerned that she was unable to care for herself and was a danger to herself as well as others, since her smoking in bed had already caused a fire.

Once admitted, she responded dramatically to the therapeutic milieu and staff support. Physical examination was most notable for point tenderness in the right inguinal region without radiation. Psychotherapeutically she initially responded with anger and hostility when she was asked to examine the rage she still felt toward her family for the geographical relocation years earlier and the realization that the entire family had thrived educationally, socially, and professionally while she allowed herself to become an invalid. She participated in individual and group psychotherapy, physical reconditioning, and functional restoration, which she initially found very difficult because of her limited endurance, weakness, excessive pain behaviors, and illness behaviors generally. Medication was tapered, and at the end of 3 weeks she was not complaining of pain and was off opioids, Fiorinal, Reglan, Tigan, and Donnatol. She refused to be tapered from the lorazepam. Because of her depression, pain, and insomnia she was placed on sedating tricyclic antidepressant medication. In addition she was taking sertraline 150 mg in the morning.

On her own she stopped smoking (and refused to consider use of nicotine patches). With her flight into health she began verbalizing some of her repressed anger. She left the pain program prematurely against medical advice. Although her inguinal pain has not returned as a complaint, after her premature discharge she called regularly with multiple somatic complaints ranging from headaches to general malaise, fever, and flulike symptoms, wanting to be seen in the office but unwilling to return to the pain program. She was again spending more time in bed during the day and consulting her primary care physician.

Her family has developed more insight into her somatizing and recognizes that for years they functioned as enablers. They are no longer willing to do so but feel very guilty about the patient's condition. Discharge diagnosis was (a) pain disorder associated with psychological factors, (b) chronic opioid dependence, and (c) major depression with psychotic features.

Both cases illustrate the importance of taking a very careful and extensive developmental and psychosocial history. Had this been done, neither of these patients would have been given their admitting diagnoses, the extensive diagnostic testing, nerve blocks and surgical procedures, nor would they have been maintained on opioids and multiple other medications. Unfortunately, the first patient, because of the multiple traumas in early life, was unable to progress appropriately through normal developmental stages necessary to form a healthy ego. She is insecure and feels defective, unlovable, and suspicious when people attempt to befriend her, and she has very limited ego resources. She continues to be depressed and chronically suicidal. Her husband, who is relatively uneducated, views psychotherapy as a waste of money and tells the children that their mother is depriving them of necessities because of her treatment. She no longer complains of pain but often views suicide as her best option. She is now in weekly psychotherapy, but her husband refuses marital or family therapy. She feels conflicted about remaining in the marriage but fears if she leaves she will lose custody of the children and she will then end her life.

The second patient was significantly less functional than the first at the time of admission. She was extremely regressed, had an invalid lifestyle, and was psychotically depressed and dependent on high-dose opioids and benzodiazepines. However, the long-term prognosis is significantly better than with the first patient for several reasons: (a) She

was raised in a healthier and more supportive nuclear family, in which she developed a healthier ego. (b) For a significant part of her life she had happiness and a sense of security. (c) She developed adaptive and functional interpersonal skills. (d) Her family, who are highly educated and secure in their professions, support her receiving psychiatric help. (e) She has financial resources that more easily allow her to implement a discharge treatment plan. However, the second patient is not motivated to take responsibility for getting on with life, which negatively affects the prognosis.

Both of these patients were treated in a therapeutic milieu that acknowledged their pain and suffering, attempted to understand the psychodynamics contributing to their symptoms, and used a cognitive-behavioral approach for treatment.

CONCLUSION

The psychodynamic literature pertinent to the chronic pain syndrome has been reviewed. Various psychotherapeutic styles have been discussed. Rarely is any one of these adequate in isolation to treat the difficult patient with intractable pain. Often it is optimal to structure a milieu in which pain behaviors can be integrated into this system. These cases illustrate that in approaching a chronic pain patient therapeutically, often it is more important to understand the patient in pain than merely the type of pain.

References

1. Aronoff GM, Evans WO. Evaluation and treatment of chronic pain at the Boston Pain Center. J Clin Psychiatry 1982;43:8, 2, 4–7.
2. Rutrick D, Aronoff GM. Combined psychotherapy for chronic pain syndrome patients at a multidisciplinary pain center. In: Aronoff GM, ed. Evaluation and treatment of chronic pain. Baltimore: Urban & Schwarzenberg, 1985;491–492.
3. Blumer D. Psychiatric considerations in pain. In: Rothman RH, Simeone FA, eds. Spine, vol 2. Philadelphia: Saunders, 1975.
4. Blumer D. Psychiatric and psychological aspects of chronic pain. Clin Neurosurg 1978;25:276–283.
5. Engel G. Psychogenic pain and the pain-prone patient, Am J Med 1959; 899–918.
6. Pilowsky I, Spence ND. Patterns of illness behavior in patients with intractable pain. J Psychom Res 1975;19:279–287.
7. Pilowsky I. Psychodynamic aspects of the pain experience. In: Sternbach RA, ed. Psychology of Pain. New York: Raven Press, 1978.
8. Engel G. Guilt, pain and success. Psychosom Med 1962;24:37–48.
9. Fordyce WE. Behavioral methods for chronic pain and illness. St. Louis: Mosby, 1979.
10. Gentry WD, Shows WD, Thomas M. Chronic low back pain: a psychological profile. Psychosomatics 1974;15:174–177.
11. Hackett TP. The pain patient: evaluation and treatment in Massachusetts General Hospital. In: Hackett TP, Cassem NH, eds. Handbook of general hospital psychiatry. St. Louis: Mosby, 1978.
12. Khatami M, Rush AJ. A pilot study of the treatment of out-patients with chronic pain: symptom control, stimulus control and social system intervention, Pain 1978;5:163–172.
13. Lowenstein R. A contribution to the psychoanalytic theory of masochism. J Am Psychoan Assoc 1924;5:197–234.
14. Melzack R. The McGill pain questionnaire: major properties and scoring methods. Pain 1975;1:277–299.

15. Merskey H. Pain and personality. In: Sternbach RA, ed. Psychology of pain. New York: Raven Press, 1978.

16. Stein M. Panel report: the problem of masochism in the theory and technique of psychoanalysis. J Am Psychoan Assoc 1956;14:526–538.

17. Swanson DW, Swenson WM, Maruta T, Floreen AC. The dissatisfied patient with chronic pain. Pain 1978;4:367–378.

18. Ramzy I, Wallenstein RS. Pain, fear and anxiety: a study in their interrelationships. Psychom Study Child 1958;23:147–189.

19. Sternbach RA. Pain patients: traits and treatment. New York: Academic Press, 1974.

20. Szasz TS. Pain and pleasure: a study of feelings. New York: Basic Books, 1975.

21. Bakan D. Disease, pain and sacrifice: toward a psychology of suffering. Chicago: University of Chicago Press, 1968.

22. Merskey H, Spear FG. Pain: psychological and psychiatric aspects. London: Balliere, Tindall & Cassell, 1967.

23. Bernstein A. A psychoanalytic contribution to the etiology of "back pain" and "spinal disc syndromes." J Am Acad Psychoan 1978;6:547–556.

24. Pilowsky I. Pain as abnormal illness behavior. J Hum Stress 1978;4:22–27.

25. Arieti S. The Intrapsychic self: feelings, cognitions and creativity in health and mental illness. New York: Basic Books, 1967.

26. Arieti S. Cognitive components in human conflict and unconsciousness motivation. J Am Acad Psychoan 1977;5:5–16.

27. Nemiah JC. Alexithymia: theoretical considerations. Psychother Psychosom 1977;28:199–206.

28. Sifneos PE. The prevalence of "alexithymic" characteristics in psychosomatic patients. Psychother Psychosom 1973;22:255–262.

29. Sifneos PE, Apfel-Savitz R, Frankel FI. The phenomenon of alexithymia: observations in neurotic and psychosomatic patients. Psychother Psychosom 1977;28:47–57.

30. Merskey H. Psychiatric aspects of the control of pain. In: Bonica JJ, Albe-Fessard DG, eds. Advances in pain research and treatment, New York: Raven Press, 1976.

31. Aronoff GM. A holistic approach to pain rehabilitation: the Boston Pain Unit. In: Ng LKY, ed. Research 36 Monograph Series. Washington: NIDA Research Monograph Series, May 1981;33–40.

32. Pinsky JJ, Malyon AK. The eclectic nature of psychotherapy in the treatment of chronic pain syndromes. In: Crue BL, ed. Chronic pain: further observations from City of Hope National Medical Center. New York: SP Medical & Scientific Books, 1979.

33. Sarno J. Chronic back pain and psychic conflict. Scand J Rehab Med 1976;8:143–153.

34. Tunks ER, Mersky H. Psychotherapy in the management of chronic pain. In: Bonica JJ, ed. The management of pain. Philadelphia: Lea & Febiger, 1990;1753–1754.

35. Turner JA, Romano JM. Cognitive behavioral therapy. In: Bonica JJ, ed. The management of pain. Philadelphia: Lea & Febiger, 1990;1711–1720.

36. Turk DC, Rudy TE. A cognitive-behavioral perspective on chronic pain: beyond the scalpel and syringe. In: Tollison DC, Satterwaite JR, Tollison JW, eds. Handbook of pain management. 2nd ed. Baltimore: Williams & Wilkins, 1994;136–151.

37. Turk DC, Meichenbaum D. A cognitive-behavioral approach to pain management. In: Wall PD, Melzack R, eds. Textbook of Pain. 2nd ed. London: Churchill Livingstone, 1989.

CHAPTER 21

Psychiatric Aspects of Nonmalignant Chronic Pain: A New Nosology

Gerald M. Aronoff

Chronic pain, a medical enigma, has become a major public health problem with serious consequences for the individual, family, and society. Apart from the human suffering, which is immeasurable, the economic loss from chronic pain is staggering. Approximately 30 million to 40 million Americans live with chronic pain (1). Chronic or recurrent headaches affect at least 40 million Americans; more than 65 million workdays are lost as a result of migraine alone. Chronic or recurrent low-back pain affects more than 15 million American adults with work-related injuries, causing 93 million workdays lost each year. The list goes on. In essence, chronic pain is said to cost the U.S. economy more than $100 billion a year (direct health care costs, disability, and lost productivity due to pain (2), and in a given year there may be 50 million adults on short- or long-term disability (3, 4).

My operational definition of pain is a complex, personal, subjective, and unpleasant sensory and perceptual experience that may or may not have any correlation with bodily injury or tissue damage. In the final analysis, chronic pain is what a patient says it is. Crue (5) emphasizes that chronic pain is more often perpetuated by central than by peripheral mechanisms.

CHRONIC PAIN SYNDROME

Unlike acute pain, which often is a symptom of an underlying disorder, is biologically useful, and is often relieved when the source of nociception is identified and removed, chronic pain syndromes often constitute the illness itself and serve no biological use. Many have taken issue with the diagnosis of chronic pain syndrome, and rightfully so. It is not a diagnostic but rather a descriptive term that connotes ongoing or persistent pain associated with dysfunctional and maladaptive pain behaviors, poor coping, self-limited daily activities, secondary emotional or behavioral disturbances, and significant life disruption. Frequently the subjective complaints are noted to be grossly in excess of objective findings. When used as a diagnosis, it is in error.

Although patients with chronic pain syndromes often present with several addictions or dependencies, opioids are generally contraindicated in the daily management of nonmalignant chronic pain disorders. Increasingly, however, it is now recognized that a subgroup of patients with chronic pain can be maintained on chronic opioid therapy. However, in general this group does not include those with chronic pain syndrome. Further discussion of this issue and guidelines for chronic opioid usage can be found in Chapter 32.

Numerous factors can influence chronic pain behavior. Among the most common are the implication of injury, probabilities of outcome, experience, ethnic and cultural differences, secondary gain, and the person's premorbid personality. There is no direct correlation between the extent of tissue damage from physical injury and the process referred to as suffering or the resulting disability.

Loeser's (7) model (Figure 21.1) for understanding chronic pain seems most appropriate because nociception and the resulting pain are often less important to the intractability of the symptoms and the extent of disability than are the suffering and pain behavior components. The numerous disciplines that have addressed the problem of chronic pain are unanimous in recognizing both the contribution of psychosocial factors to the disorder and the need for increased understanding of this enigma (8). One step in pursuit of this goal is to delineate a nosology that will take into account the psychosocial aspects of pain, provide a common language that can be understood by those who deal with the problem, and provide a context within which to understand the patient and the factors that contribute to the patient's pain.

With chronic pain syndromes there are often complex interactions between physical and psychological factors. These patients share many of the following characteristics: preoccupation with pain, strong and ambivalent dependency needs, feelings of isolation and loneliness, characterological masochism (meeting other people's needs at their own expense), inability to

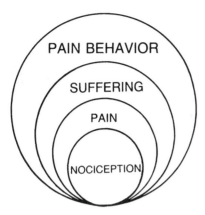

Figure 21. 1. Pain in the framework of sequential input. Suggested by Loeser (7).

take care of their own needs, passivity, lack of insight into patterns of self-defeating behavior, inability to deal appropriately with anger and hostility, and the use of pain as a symbolic means of communication (9). Chronic pain often is a conditioned psychosocioeconomic process in which personal gain may play an important role, especially in some situations resulting from occupational or other personal injuries.

Although psychodynamic and psychoanalytical concepts of chronic pain have contributed a great deal to the understanding of the process by which certain individuals are susceptible to disability from injuries or illness and to resulting chronic pain problems, these approaches have been less helpful in providing effective management tools. When psychoanalytical approaches to psychotherapy have been beneficial, the process was quite time consuming and costly. The techniques developed by behavioral psychologists have revolutionized the understanding of the most efficacious methods of dealing with chronic and intractable pain syndromes. Gratitude is owed to Fordyce (10, 11) and Sternbach (12, 13), among others; they were pioneers in discussing pain behavior, pain games, behavior modification in pain patients, and other interpersonal and psychosocial components of the pain process. More recently cognitive-behavioral techniques based on techniques by Turk and Rudy (14) and Turk and Meichenbaum (15) have been used.

In the chronic pain experience the suffering component is frequently magnified by psychopathology. In attempting to address issues related to diagnosis and treatment as well as impairment and disability the clinician must have a clear understanding of psychiatric nosology. The fourth edition of *Diagnostic and Statistical Manual of Mental Disorders* (DSM-IV) (16), published in 1994 by the American Psychiatric Association, was an attempt to improve the diagnostic taxonomy of mental disorders by classifying each diagnosis used with psychiatric patients in clinical, educational, and research settings.

Because many nonpsychiatric clinicians are unfamiliar with DSM-IV, its use is briefly described and several examples given later in this chapter. Each diagnostic entity is subdivided into five categories termed axes in the DSM-IV

nomenclature. As can be seen from Table 21.1, all axes except axis III, which designates the patient's general medical condition, pertain to psychological or social parameters.

There has been extensive clinical research indicating the tendency for affective or personality disorders to accompany intractable pain (17, 18), and it is gratifying to discover the number of DSM-IV diagnostic categories that include pain either as a diagnostic criterion or as a concomitant symptom (Table 21.2). The following section highlights these disorders, discusses pain within the context of each disorder, and suggests additional categories that I believe are relevant to an understanding of chronic pain syndromes.

SOMATOFORM DISORDERS

Somatoform disorders are those whose physical symptoms suggest a physical disorder for which there is evidence of underlying psychopathology but not demonstrable organic findings or known physiological mechanisms. "The symptoms must cause clinically significant distress or impairment in social, occupational, or other areas of functioning" (16). This category includes somatization disorder, undifferentiated somatoform disorder, conversion disorder, pain disorder, hypochondriasis, body dysmorphic disorder, and somatoform disorder not otherwise specified (16). In each of these disorders, symptom production is believed to be unintentional.

SOMATIZATION DISORDER

Somatization disorder is a chronic polysymptomatic disorder generally with onset early in life (before age 30). The somatic complaints are said to be clinically significant "if they result in medical treatments or cause significant impairment in social, occupational, or other areas of functioning" (16). Chiefly affecting women, their main feature is a repetitive or chronic concern with physical symptoms with a lack of physical findings to substantiate the subjective complaints. These persons tend to consult many physicians in an attempt to validate their symptoms and frequently have surgical procedures with negative disease findings. These patients are at high risk for prescription and nonprescription medication dependency and abuse, iatrogenic complications, and disability and should be managed conservatively unless there are clear signs or objective disease or injury warranting more aggressive treatment. DSM-IV notes comorbidity with major depressive disorder, panic disorder, and substance-related disorders as well as histrionic, borderline, and antisocial personality disorders. Diagnostic criteria are listed in Table 21.3.

CONVERSION DISORDER

There is little doubt that those said to have underlying hysterical personality patterns are more prone either to exaggerate their complaints or to present them melodramatically. However,

Table 21.1.   DSM-IV Multiaxial System

Axis 1
  Clinical disorders
  Other conditions that may be a focus of clinical attention
  Schizophrenia; somatoform disorders; mood disorders
Axis II
  Personality disorders, mental retardation
  Histrionic personality disorder; antisocial personality disorder
Axis III
  General medical conditions
  Adhesive arachnoiditis and back pain; diseases of the musculoskeletal
  system and connective tissue
Axis IV
  Psychosocial and environmental problems
  Interpersonal, occupational, legal, housing, and economic problems; problems
  with access to health care services; educational problems; problems related to
  the social environment; problems with primary support group
Axis V
  Global assessment of functioning
  Rate current or on admission, at discharge, and highest level past year
  90 = good functioning in all areas
  40 = major impairment in several areas

Table 21.2.   Emotional Disorders Associated with Chronic Pain Syndrome

A. Somatoform disorders
  1. Somatization disorder (previously referred to as either hysteria or Briquet's syndrome)
  2. Conversion disorder
  3. Pain disorder
  4. Hypochondriasis
  5. Undifferentiated somatoform disorder
  6. Body dysmorphic disorder
  7. Somatoform disorder not otherwise specified
B. Psychological factors affecting physical conditions
C. Malingering
D. Schizophrenia
E. Psychoactive substance use disorder

Table 21.3.   DSM-IV Diagnostic Criteria for Somatization Disorder

A. A history of many physical complaints beginning before age of 30 years that occur over several years and result in treatment being sought or significant impairment in social, occupational, or other important areas of functioning
B. Each of the following criteria must have been met, with individual symptoms occurring at any time during the course of the disturbance
  1. Four pain symptoms: a history of pain related to at least four sites or functions (e.g., head, abdomen, back, joints, extremities, chest, rectum, during menstruation, during sexual intercourse, during urination)
  2. Two gastrointestinal symptoms: a history of at least two gastrointestinal symptoms other than pain (e.g., nausea, bloating, vomiting other than during pregnancy, diarrhea, or intolerance of several foods)
  3. One sexual symptom: a history of at least one sexual or reproductive symptom other than pain (e.g., sexual indifference, erectile or ejaculatory dysfunction, irregular menses, excessive menstrual bleeding, vomiting throughout pregnancy.)
  4. One pseudoneurological symptom: a history of at least one symptom or deficit suggesting a neurological condition not limited to pain (conversion symptoms such as impaired coordination or balance, paralysis, or localized weakness, difficulty swallowing or lump in throat, aphonia, urinary retention, hallucinations, loss of touch or pain sensation, double vision, blindness, deafness, seizures; dissociative symptoms such as amnesia; or loss of consciousness other than fainting)
C. Either (1) or (2)
  1. After appropriate investigation, each of the symptoms in criterion B cannot be fully explained by a known general medical condition or the direct effects of a substance (e.g., a drug or abuse, a medication)
  2. When there is a related general medical condition, the physical complaints or resulting social or occupational impairment are in excess of what would be expected from the history, physical examination, or laboratory findings
D. The symptoms are not intentionally produced or feigned (as in factitious disorder or malingering)

Adapted with permission from American Psychiatric Association: Diagnostic and Statistical Manual of Mental Disorders, ed 4. American Psychiatric Association, Washington, 1994.

in no way do these statements imply that the patient's pain is not real or that it is not organically based. Working with these patients, it becomes apparent that their choice of descriptors for their pain usually involves emotionally laden and flamboyant language that often prejudices the clinician. Conversion symptoms are those that result from an emotional conflict, are not directly related to bodily disease, and are ultimately in accordance with the patient's concept of functional loss of a part rather than with actual anatomy and physiology. If these symptoms affect the body, they are called conversion symptoms. Comparable symptoms not affecting the body, such as hysterical loss of memory, are known as dissociative symptoms. Conversion symptoms commonly seen in the chronic pain population include pseudoseizure and other symptoms suggesting neurological disease without documented pathophysiology, such as paresthesias, coordination disturbances, and unexplained weakness. These symptoms are not under voluntary control, and symptom onset is generally sudden and preceded by extreme psychological stress. If symptoms become chronic,

these individuals are at risk for secondary impairments from prolonged inactivity (e.g., disuse atrophy and contractures).

A person with an underlying hysterical personality may not necessarily be expressing conversion symptoms, and likewise, not everyone with conversion symptoms has an underlying hysterical personality. Numerous studies of hysteria document the extremely high percentage of these psychiatric complaints that are associated with pain as a symptom (2, 19). In the most recent nosology of DSM-IV (Table 21.4), conversion disorder is not diagnosed when conversion symptoms are limited to pain; in such a case the term pain disorder associated with psychological factors should be used. In addition, one should differentiate conversion disorder from the more polysymptomatic somatization disorder described earlier.

PAIN DISORDER

Psychogenic pain disorders are fairly common among patients at pain centers. The primary clinical feature is the complaint of pain without adequate physical findings but associated with evidence of the causative role of psychological

Table 21.4.   DSM-IV Diagnostic Criteria for Conversion Disorder

A. One or more symptoms or deficits affecting voluntary motor or sensory function suggest a neurological or other general medical condition.
B. Psychological factors judged to be associated with the symptom or deficit because conflicts or other stressors precede the initiation or exacerbation of the symptom or deficit.
C. The symptom or deficit is not intentionally produced or feigned, as in factitious disorder or malingering.
D. The symptom or deficit cannot, after appropriate investigation, be fully explained by a general medical condition, by the direct effects of a substance, or as a culturally sanctioned behavior or experience.
E. The symptom or deficit causes clinically significant distress or impairment in social, occupational, or other important areas of functioning or warrants medical attention.
F. The symptom or deficit is not limited to pain or sexual dysfunction, does not occur exclusively during the course of somatization disorder, and is not better accounted for by another mental disorder.

Specify type of symptom or deficit:
   With motor symptom or deficit
   With sensory symptom or deficit
   With seizures or convulsions
   With mixed presentation

Reprinted with permission from American Psychiatric Association: Diagnostic and Statistical Manual of Mental Disorders, ed 4. American Psychiatric Association, Washington, 1994.

Table 21.5.   DSM-IV Diagnostic Criteria for Pain Disorder

A. Pain in one or more anatomical sites is the predominant focus of the clinical presentation and is sufficiently severe to warrant clinical attention.
B. The pain causes clinically significant distress or impairment in social, occupational, or other important areas of functioning.
C. Psychological factors are judged to have an important role in the onset, severity, exacerbation, or maintenance of the pain.
D. The symptom or deficit is not intentionally produced (as in factitious disorder or malingering).
E. The pain is not better accounted for by a mood, anxiety, or psychotic disorder and does not meet criteria for dyspareunia.

Subtypes
1. Pain disorder associated with psychological factors. This subtype is used when psychological factors are judged to have the major role in the onset, severity, exacerbation, or maintenance of the pain. In this subtype, general medical conditions play either no role or a minimal role in the onset or maintenance of the pain. This subtype is not diagnosed if criteria for somatization disorder are met.
2. Pain disorder associated with both psychological factors and a general medical condition. This subtype is used when both psychological factors and a general medical condition are judged to have important roles in the onset, severity, exacerbation, or maintenance of the pain.

Specifiers
1. Acute: if the duration of the pain is less than 6 months
2. Chronic: if the duration of the pain is 6 months or longer

Adapted with permission from American Psychiatric Association: Diagnostic and Statistical Manual of Mental Disorders, ed 4. American Psychiatric Association, Washington, 1994.

factors. It should be established that no other mental disorder is contributing to the disturbance. It is my impression that the premorbid personalities of these individuals commonly reveal evidence of neurotic functioning and less often, borderline personality organization preceding the trauma of an injury or painful medical illness. Subsequently the pain itself may become the focal aspect within that conflict (pain neurosis), as may financial compensation (compensation neurosis). Sometimes core issues are unmet dependency needs and both primary and secondary gain. The onset of symptoms commonly occurs shortly after physical trauma. The diagnosis of pain disorder must be made cautiously and periodically reexamined to rule out the possibility that the pain can be explained on an organic basis. If a specific treatment for a pain disorder is available and if the potential benefits to the patient outweigh the risks, that treatment should be suggested. If, however, invasive treatment offers no distinct advantage over conservative treatment and carries an increased risk, conservative treatments should be suggested. These patients characteristically overuse the health system, generally do not respond to multiple attempts at conventional treatments, and fairly commonly develop iatrogenic complications, including iatrogenic disability. They frequently develop a chronic pain syndrome, as described earlier in this chapter, in which they develop self-defeating and dysfunctional pain behaviors, learned helplessness, and a lifestyle of invalidism. These patients often refuse psychiatric or psychological consultation because they believe the cause is organic. Referral is often more successful in the context of a multidisciplinary pain center. Diagnostic criteria for pain disorder are listed in Table 21.5.

HYPOCHONDRIASIS

Hypochondriasis, a fascinated absorption and preoccupation with having a serious disease, is common among chronic pain patients. This is not to say that these persons may not have underlying organic disease and mechanical causes of pain but rather that their degree of somatic preoccupation becomes an obsession, they fail to be reassured by clinical or laboratory evaluations, and they remain fixated in their belief that they need more diagnostic tests and evaluations. They are at risk for iatrogenic complications.

Arguing with these persons and trying to dissuade them from their convictions is generally futile. The degree of their concern often causes significant psychosocial dysfunction. One must exclude true organic disease; however, the presence of true organic disease does not rule out coexisting hypochondriasis. These patients often have a gradual deterioration in relationships with their physicians, and when their symptoms persist, they become dissatisfied with their medical care and seek other medical opinions. Diagnostic criteria for hypochondriasis are listed in Table 21.6.

UNDIFFERENTIATED SOMATOFORM DISORDER

Undifferentiated somatoform disorder is diagnosed when (a) the physical symptoms or complaints are not explained by demonstrable organic findings or a known pathophysiological mechanism and are apparently linked to psychological factors or (b) there is not a full-symptom picture of somatization disorder. Criteria for diagnosis are listed in Table 21.7.

Table 21.6.   Diagnostic Criteria for Hypochondriasis

A. Preoccupation with fears of having or the idea that one has a serious disease, based on the person's misinterpretation of bodily symptoms.

B. The preoccupation persists despite appropriate medical evaluation and reassurance.

C. The belief in criterion A is not of delusional intensity (as in delusional disorder, somatic type) and is not restricted to a circumscribed concern about appearance (as in body dysmorphic disorder).

D. The preoccupation causes clinically significant distress or impairment in social, occupational, or other important areas of functioning.

E. The duration of the disturbance is at least 6 months.

F. The preoccupation is not better accounted for by generalized anxiety disorder, obsessive-compulsive disorder, panic disorder, a major depressive episode, separation anxiety, or another somatoform disorder.

Adapted with permission from American Psychiatric Association: Diagnostic and Statistical Manual of Mental Disorders, ed 4. American Psychiatric Association, Washington, 1994.

Table 21.7.   DSM-IV Diagnostic Criteria for Undifferentiated Somatoform Disorder

A. One or more physical complaints, for example, fatigue, loss of appetite, gastrointestinal or urinary complaints.

B. Either 1 or 2
  1. After appropriate investigation, the symptoms cannot be fully explained by a known general medical condition or the direct effects of a substance (e.g., a drug of abuse, a medication).
  2. When there is a related general medical condition, the physical complaint or resulting social or occupational impairment is in excess of what would be expected from the history, physical examination, or laboratory findings.

C. The symptoms cause clinically significant distress or impairment in social, occupational, or other important areas of functioning.

D. Duration of the disturbance is at least 6 months.

E. The disturbance is not better accounted for by another mental disorder (e.g., another somatoform disorder, sexual dysfunction, mood disorder, anxiety disorder, sleep disorder, or psychotic disorder).

F. The symptom is not intentionally produced or feigned (as in factitious disorder or malingering).

Adapted with permission from American Psychiatric Association: Diagnostic and Statistical Manual of Mental disorders, ed 4. American Psychiatric Association, Washington, 1994.

BODY DYSMORPHIC DISORDER

Originally called dysmorphobia, body dysmorphic disorder (BDD) affects a normal-appearing individual who has an imagined defect in appearance or whose overconcern with a slight physical anomaly causes significant distress or impairment in some important area of functioning. Important in making this diagnosis is the intensity of the overconcern, which can become an obsessive preoccupation. This diagnosis should not be used in people who have a concern (not found to be excessive) with a minor physical defect. The focus of concern can be any area of the body. Major depression and dysthymia are associated with this disorder but probably are complications rather than causes. Obsessive-compulsive disorder may also be associated with BDD.

Table 21.8.   DSM-IV Diagnostic Criteria for Body Dysmorphic Disorder

A. Preoccupation with an imagined defect in appearance. If a slight physical anomaly is present, the person's concern is markedly excessive.

B. The preoccupation causes clinically significant distress or impairment in social, occupational, or other important areas of functioning.

C. The preoccupation is not better accounted for by another mental disorder (e.g., dissatisfaction with body shape and size as in anorexia nervosa).

Adapted with permission from American Psychiatric Association: Diagnostic and Statistical Manual of Mental disorders, ed 4. American Psychiatric Association, Washington, 1994.

Unnecessary surgery is a noted complication (20). Criteria for diagnosis are listed in Table 21.8.

SOMATOFORM DISORDER NOT OTHERWISE SPECIFIED

Somatoform disorder not otherwise specified includes disorders with somatoform symptoms that do not meet the criteria for any specific somatoform disorder. Among these are disorders involving unexplained physical complaints (e.g., fatigue or body weakness) of less than 6 months' duration that are not due to another mental disorder. Also included are disorders with nonpsychotic hypochondriacal symptoms of less than 6 months' duration. Frequently there is associated anxiety or a depressive disorder.

PSYCHOLOGICAL FACTORS AFFECTING PHYSICAL CONDITION

In the third revised edition of *Diagnostic and Statistical Manual of Mental Disorders* (DSM-III-R) (21), psychological factors affecting physical condition described disorders that in the past had been referred to as either psychosomatic or psychophysiological. DSM-IV notes, "This category should be reserved for those situations in which the psychological factors have a clinically significant effect on the course or outcome of the general medical condition or place the individual at a significantly higher risk for an adverse outcome. There must be reasonable evidence to suggest an association between the psychological factors and the medical condition, although it may often not be possible to demonstrate direct causality or the mechanism underlying the relationship" (16). My experience indicates that a very common problem with pain patients is a tendency to suppress emotional expression and internalize feelings. The physiological expression of these tendencies is manifested in autonomic hyperactivity and muscle tension, both of which directly contribute to the pain. Although most categories of disease can be affected by psychological factors, some of the more common include tension and migraine headaches, angina pectoris, painful menstruation, sacroiliac pain, neurodermatitis, asthma, arthritis and fibromyalgia, peptic ulcers and other gastrointestinal conditions, and others. Diagnostic criteria are listed in Table 21.9.

Table 21.9.   DSM-IV Diagnostic Criteria for Psychological Factors Affecting Physical Condition

A. A general medical condition (coded on Axis III) is present.
B. Psychological factors adversely affect the general medical condition in one of the following ways:
   1. The factors have influenced the course of the general medical condition as shown by a close temporal association between the psychological factors and the development or exacerbation of or delayed recovery from the general medical condition.
   2. The factors interfere with the treatment of the general medical condition.
   3. The factors constitute additional health risks for the individual.
   4. Stress-related physiological responses precipitate or exacerbate symptoms of the general medical condition.

Adapted with permission from American Psychiatric Association: Diagnostic and Statistical Manual of Mental disorders, ed 4. American Psychiatric Association, Washington, 1994.

MALINGERING

Malingering, which is relatively uncommon, implies a conscious, intentional, and voluntary fabrication of a physical or psychological symptom for personal gain. To be classified as a malingerer, the person must be consciously feigning illness. Malingerers are often difficult to treat because the secondary gain or external incentives may be overwhelming (e.g., financial gain as in personal injury claims, work avoidance as in workers compensation claims or an aversion to the job, and attempts to obtain drugs by prescription rather than illicitly); frequently they feel they have more to gain by retaining the symptom than by relinquishing it. There is commonly a great deal of underlying psychopathology, and the primary treatment of malingering, if it is amenable to treatment at all, must be psychiatric. DSM-IV notes that under certain situations malingering may be adaptive behavior, for example feigning illness while a prisoner of war. In addition, I have evaluated persons who claimed the onset of illness or pain in the setting of a work incident (during a work slowdown as part of an economic recession) with the intent of receiving workers compensation in preference to being unemployed and possibly on welfare. The motivation was to provide for their families. There was no noted psychopathology. Yet because this was conscious, intentional, and voluntary, it was viewed as malingering. Diagnostic criteria are listed in Table 21.10.

SCHIZOPHRENIA

Patients with schizophrenia presenting to a pain center with primary pain complaints are uncommon, but they do exist. The pain is often discussed as part of a bizarre somatic delusion. A British study of 78 hospitalized schizophrenic patients found 29 to have pain complaints. Of these 13 had an appropriate physical cause; the remainder were thought to have psychogenic pain. The head, leg, and back were the most common sites. Complaints were most often described in sensory terms. The report summary indicated that patients with

Table 21.10.   DSM-IV Diagnostic Criteria for Malingering

A high index of suspicion of malingering should be aroused if any of the following is noted (15):
1. Medicolegal context of presentation (e.g., the person is referred by his or her attorney to the clinician for examination)
2. Marked discrepancy between the person's claimed distress or disability and the objective findings
3. Lack of cooperation during the diagnostic evaluation and in complying with the prescribed treatment regimen
4. The presence of an antisocial personality disorder

Adapted with permission from American Psychiatric Association: Diagnostic and Statistical Manual of Mental disorders, ed 4. American Psychiatric Association, Washington, 1994.

schizophrenia may have less pain than those with anxiety or depression, but they certainly do have pain from physical and psychological causes. The influence of phenothiazines on pain experience is uncertain (22). See DSM-IV for a detailed discussion of diagnostic criteria for schizophrenia.

PSYCHOACTIVE SUBSTANCE USE DISORDERS

Patients with chronic pain are often quite experienced in the use of medication. For some the pattern is sporadic and intermittent, with medications taken only by prescription from one primary physician; for others there are many physicians writing prescriptions, each unaware of the actions of their colleagues. Finally, still others receive medication from illicit sources outside of the medical system. Some persons' illicit drug use preceded the onset of their pain, and they hope to have this use legitimized by physicians. Other persons who never would have considered illicit drug use are faced with chronic pain and are unable to obtain legally what they feel is adequate medication. The problem is complex, and the physician is often in a compromised position in the midst of ethical dilemmas.

In DSM-III-R, the section on substance use disorders addresses the behavioral changes associated with use of substances that affect the central nervous system. "Nine classes of psychoactive substances were associated with both abuse and dependence: alcohol; amphetamines or similarly acting sympathomimetics; cannabis; cocaine; hallucinogens; inhalants; opioids; phencyclidine (PCP) or similarly active arylcyclohexylamines; and sedatives, hypnotics, or anxiolytics. Dependence (but not abuse) is seen with nicotine" (21). In DSM-IV caffeine is added to the list, and nicotine is now noted to have potential for dependence and abuse. Because of the availability of cigarettes and other nicotine-containing substances and the absence of a clinically significant nicotine intoxication syndrome, impairment in occupational or social functioning is not necessary for a rating of severe nicotine dependence. The definition of dependence is expanded from DSM-III-R to a "syndrome of clinically significant behaviors, cognitions, and physiologic symptoms that indicate loss of control of substance use and continued use of the substance despite adverse consequences" (16).

Table 21.11.   Diagnostic Criteria for Psychoactive Substance Dependence

A maladaptive pattern of substance use leading to clinically significant impairment or distress as manifested by three or more of the following, occurring at any time in the same 12-month period:

1. Tolerance, as defined by either of the following, is present.
   a. A need for markedly increased amounts of the substance to achieve intoxication or desired effect
   b. Markedly diminished effect with continued use of the same amount of the substance
2. Withdrawal, as manifested by either of the following is present.
   a. The characteristic withdrawal syndrome for the substance (refer to criteria A and B of the criteria sets for withdrawal from the specific substances)
   b. The same or a closely related substance taken to relieve or avoid withdrawal symptoms
3. The substance is often taken in larger amounts or over a longer period than was intended.
4. There is a persistent desire or unsuccessful efforts to cut down or control substance use.
5. A great deal of time spent in activities necessary to obtain the substance (e.g., visiting multiple doctors or driving long distances), use the substance (e.g., chain smoking), or recover from its effects.
6. Important social, occupational, or recreational activities are given up or reduced because of substance use.
7. The substance use is continued despite knowledge of having a persistent or recurrent physical or psychological problem that is likely to have been caused or exacerbated by the substance (e.g., current cocaine use despite recognition of cocaine-induced depression or continued drinking despite recognition that an ulcer was made worse by alcohol consumption).

Specifiers

Tolerance and withdrawal may be associated with a higher risk for immediate general medical problems and a higher relapse rate. Specifiers are provided to note their presence or absence.

With physiological dependence

This specifier should be used when substance dependence is accompanied by evidence of tolerance (criterion 1) or withdrawal (criterion 2).

Without physiological dependence

This specifier should be used when there is no evidence of tolerance (criterion 1) or withdrawal (criterion 2). In these persons substance abuse is characterized by a pattern of compulsive use (at least three items from criteria 3–7).

Course Specifiers (see DSM-IV for detailed description)

    Early full remission
    Early partial remission
    Sustained full remission
    Sustained partial remission
    On agonist therapy
    In a controlled environment

Adapted with permission from American Psychiatric Association: Diagnostic and Statistical Manual of Mental disorders, ed 4. American Psychiatric Association, Washington, 1994.

Noted is a pattern of repeated self-administration that usually results in tolerance, withdrawal, and compulsive drug-taking behavior (16). Diagnostic criteria are listed in Table 21.11.

It is emphasized in DSM-IV that neither tolerance nor withdrawal is necessary or sufficient for a diagnosis of substance dependence. Some persons (e.g., those with cannabis dependence) show a pattern of compulsive use without any signs of tolerance or withdrawal. Conversely, some postsurgical patients without opioid dependence may develop a toler-

Table 21.12.   DSM-IV Diagnostic Criteria for Psychoactive Substance Abuse

A. A maladaptive pattern of substance use leading to clinically significant impairment or distress, as manifested by one (or more) of the following occurring within a 12-month period
   1. Recurrent substance use resulting in a failure to fulfill major role obligations at work, school, or home (e.g., repeated absences or poor work performance related to substance use, substance-related absences, suspensions, or expulsions from school, neglect of children or household)
   2. Recurrent substance use in situations in which it is physically hazardous (e.g., driving an automobile or operating a machine when impaired by substance use)
   3. Recurrent substance-related legal problems (e.g., arrests for substance-related disorderly conduct)
   4. Continued substance use despite having persistent or recurrent social or interpersonal problems caused or exacerbated by the effects of the substance (e.g., arguments with spouse about consequences of intoxication, physical fights)
B. The symptoms have never met the criteria for psychoactive substance dependence for this substance

Adapted with permission from American Psychiatric Association: Diagnostic and Statistical Manual of Mental disorders, ed 4. American Psychiatric Association, Washington, 1994.

ance to prescribed opioids and have withdrawal symptoms without showing any signs of compulsive use (16).

PSYCHOACTIVE SUBSTANCE ABUSE

Substance abuse is a maladaptive pattern of intentional substance use or in the case of prescription psychoactive substances, misuse with resulting distress or impairment in persons not meeting criteria for substance dependence. The diagnosis of substance abuse is complicated by the unreliability of these patients' histories. Their objectives for making the medical appointment may be more geared to getting drugs than to getting appropriate treatment. Unless the clinician has a high index of suspicion, this diagnosis often is initially missed and is made later in treatment from the pattern of medication requests, phone calls to replace lost or stolen prescriptions, or calls from other physicians or pharmacies with notification of some irregularities or falsified prescriptions. Diagnostic criteria are listed in Table 21.12.

I would furthermore like to suggest that the DSM-IV criteria for psychoactive substance dependence are inappropriate to use with chronic pain patients as criteria for addiction. Addiction is a psychological and behavioral process that entails (*a*) loss of control over drug use, (*b*) compulsive drug use, and (*c*) continued use despite harm. I agree with the opinion of the American Society of Addiction Medicine in its conclusion that the DSM-IV criteria are not suitable for diagnosis of addiction when opioids are prescribed for treatment of pain because they rely too heavily on physical dependency and tolerance, which are physiological states anticipated in the opioid treatment of chronic pain. Only the DSM-IV criteria reflecting dysfunctional behaviors should be used in formulating any such diagnosis (22a).

I concur with the observation of Fishbain (19) that the DSM-IV substance use disorder work group appeared to ignore the concept of addiction as a diagnostic entity and that this creates difficulties in addressing addiction in chronic pain patients.

PROPOSED ADDITIONAL CATEGORIES

It is my opinion that although DSM-IV is a significant improvement on previous diagnostic and statistical manuals of mental disorders, it is perhaps incomplete in not providing categories adequate for including depression (as distinct from its present listing under mood disorders) or pain-prone disorder, both of which are extremely important concepts in understanding patients with pain disorders. It is hoped that consideration will be given to inclusion of these as part of the next edition of DSM.

DEPRESSION

Depression is the most common emotional disorder in patients with chronic pain syndromes (23). However, the complexity of the relation between chronic pain and depression is not addressed in the present DSM-IV classification system. Vegetative signs of depression are extremely common in chronic pain syndrome and for many patients, resolve in their entirety as the pain is effectively treated. Although the depression accompanying pain is often thought to be reactive to the pain process and life disruption, it is quite common to evaluate individuals whose depression preceded the pain or in whom the pain–depression relationship is unclear. Given this ambiguity, some clinicians diagnose major depression, and others, mood disorder due to a general medical condition.

Although the incidence of depression among pain patients is high, depressed mood is often masked and not readily apparent. Psychological tests, such as the Minnesota Multiphasic Personality Profile-2 (MMPI-2), McGill Pain Questionnaire (MPQ), Behavioral Assessment of Pain (BAP), and Profile of Mood States (POMS), may be useful adjuncts in understanding depression and in the attempt of clinicians to explain why certain behaviors persist. These pain behaviors may be a component of depressive spectrum illness, with the affect expressed somatically.

It is incumbent upon the clinician to recognize and distinguish functional from organic causes of depressive symptoms. These may range from dementing processes, some of which are not reversible, to the most readily reversible organic causes of depression and dementia, such as toxic states, endocrine or other metabolic disorders, and normal-pressure hydrocephalus. I have seen severely depressed patients with memory disturbance, often representing a pseudodementia that tends to disappear once the depression improves. In addition to clinical evaluation and routine psy-chological testing, it may be necessary to perform a complete neuropsychological battery of tests.

There is growing evidence that depression lowers pain tolerance, increases analgesic requirements, and in other ways adds to the debilitating effects of pain. Patients in pain often suffer from the vegetative signs of depression, including insomnia, appetite fluctuations with resulting obesity or malnutrition, diminished libido, and excessive use of alcohol or opioid and sedative-hypnotic medication. Patients usually attribute these problems to pain rather than depression, primarily because it is more socially acceptable to do so; it may also be a defensive use of somatization, denial, and repression.

Once the pain–depression–insomnia cycle is established, it becomes self-perpetuating and requires active intervention. It is increasingly recognized that tricyclic antidepressants may be useful in breaking this cycle (24). The clinical features of chronic pain with depression are listed in Table 21.13.

PAIN-PRONE DISORDER

Pain-prone persons, who were described initially by Engle (25) and more recently by Blumer (26), clearly form a major subgroup of patients with chronic pain syndromes. Blumer describes this entity as a variant of depressive disease with characteristic clinical, psychodynamic, biographical, and genetic features and strongly suggests that this is a different category from any mentioned in DSM-IV. Pain-prone persons often have quite characteristic developmental histories significant for stressful and often traumatic childhoods with many unmet dependency needs; a high incidence of emotional, physical, and/or sexual abuse; a personal or family history of illness including chronic pain or disability; and compulsive work records, perhaps working several jobs, which may insulate the individual from dealing with interpersonal or personal unresolved conflicts. These persons may function reasonably well without evidence of emotional or behavioral problems until they develop a pain problem as a result of an illness or injury. Their subjective complaints are often grossly disproportionate to the objective findings, and they do not respond to conventional approaches of medical, pharmacological, or surgical treatments. Having evaluated many of these persons, I believe that for them chronic pain is a way of saying, "Now it is my turn to be taken care of." This diagnosis is missed unless the clinician takes a very detailed developmental and psychosocial history. The clinical features of pain-prone disorders are listed in Table 21.14. Perhaps these features can provide the framework for future diagnostic criteria.

SUMMARY

Some of the more pertinent psychological aspects of non-malignant chronic pain have been discussed in the hope that nonpsychiatric clinicians may become familiar with the

Table 21.13.   **Clinical Features of Chronic Pain with Depression**

A. Depression may be reactive to pain or may precede pain.
B. The patient suffers from the symptoms of depression in DSM-IV:
   1. Poor appetite or significant weight loss (when not dieting) or increased appetite or significant weight gain
   2. Insomnia or hypersomnia
   3. Psychomotor agitation or retardation
   4. Loss of interest in or enjoyment of sex
   5. Social withdrawal
   6. Feelings of unworthiness, self-reproach, or excessive inappropriate guilt
   7. Recurrent thoughts of death, suicidal ideation, wishes to be dead, or suicide attempt
   8. Fearfulness or crying
C. The patient often denies psychological causes of depression and attributes depressive symptoms to pain.
D. Primary defenses are most often somatization, denial, and repression.
E. There is a decreased pain threshold.
F. There is a tenuous support system.
G. It is frequently associated with somatic preoccupation and hypochondriasis.
H. It is often associated with pain-prone disorder.

Table 21.14.   **Clinical Features of the Pain-Prone Disorder**

Somatic complaint
   Continuous pain of obscure origin
   Hypochondriacal preoccupation
   Desire for surgery
   Solid citizen
   Denial of conflicts
   Idealization of self and of family relations
   Ergomania (prepain): workaholism, relentless activity
Depression
   Anergia (postpain); lack of initiative, inactivity, fatigue
   Anhedonia: inability to enjoy social life, leisure, and sex
   Insomnia
   Depressive mood and despair
History
   Family and personal history of depression and alcoholism
   Past abuse by spouse
   Crippled relative
   Relative with chronic pain

Reprinted with permission of Blumer D, Heilbronn M. Chronic pain as a variant of depressive disease. J Nerv Men Dis 1982;170:3686.

nosology of the American Psychiatric Association in DSM-IV to improve communication in describing clinical syndromes. No one medical discipline has all the answers for this difficult group of patients. If this problem is to be addressed in a sensible way, it will be with medical and allied health professionals as a team with open channels of communication, so that evaluations are neither duplicated nor superfluous; at the same time, patients' needs are addressed and they receive the evaluations they deserve. Viewed from a public health perspective and in terms of preventive medicine, this is medically sound and ethically correct. One would anticipate retrospective studies in the future to show this.

Health care providers working with a different medical population have a responsibility to these patients to define, clarify, and present to them their problems accurately and in a manner comprehensible to them. For most of these patients, the days of being subtle have passed; the physician should be direct and if necessary confrontational. The goal, after all, is to help them with meeting their needs, not to allow them to continue to delude themselves that their problems are all physical. If they leave angrily because they do not want to hear what is said, it does not necessarily reflect our failure with them. Not all patients want assistance, nor can all patients be helped. In addition, the allied health care professionals involved in patient treatment have a responsibility to formulate—as well as possible—the impression of the patient's pain problem, not only from the medical, surgical, and pharmacological position, but also from the psychosocioeconomic perspective, because so often it is from these areas that the suffering, pain behavior, and disability arise.

References

1. Hendler N. Exaggerated pain caused by personality disorder: the histrionic personality versus the hysterical neurosis. In: Diagnosis and nonsurgical management of chronic pain. New York: Raven Press, 1981;64–97B.
2. Bonica JJ. The management of pain. Philadelphia: Lea & Febiger, 1990.
3. New approaches to treatment of chronic pain. National Institute of Drug Abuse Research Monograph 36. Washington: Department of Health and Human Services May 1981;vii.
4. Report on the Panel of Pain. National Institutes of Health Pub. 81–1912. Washington: NIH, 1980; 4–5.
5. Crue BL. Guest editor for issue on pain. Semin Neurol 1983;3(4).
6. Reference deleted.
7. Loeser J. In Stanton-Hicks M, Boas R, eds. Chronic low back pain. New York: Raven Press, 1982;145–148.
8. Merskey H. The effect of chronic pain upon the response to noxious stimuli by psychiatric patients. J Psychosom Res 8:405–419, 1.
9. Aronoff GM, McAlary PW. Pain centers: treatment for intractable suffering and disability resulting from chronic pain. In: Aronoff GM, ed. Evaluation and treatment of chronic pain. 2nd ed. Baltimore: Williams & Wilkins, 1992;416–429.
10. Fordyce WE. Operant conditioning in the treatment of chronic pain. Arch Phys Med Rehab 1973;54:399–408.
11. Fordyce WE. Behavioral methods for chronic pain and illness. St. Louis: Mosby, 1978.
12. Sternbach RA. Pain patients: traits and treatment. New York: Academic Press, 1974.
13. Sternbach RA. Chronic low back pain: the low back loser. Postgrad Med 1973;53:135–138.
14. Turk DC, Rudy TE. A cognitive-behavioral perspective on chronic pain: beyond the scalpel and syringe. In: Tollison DC, Satterwaite JR, Tollison JW, eds. Handbook of pain management. 2nd ed. Baltimore: Williams & Wilkins, 1994;136–151.
15. Turk DC, Meichenbaum D. A cognitive-behavioral approach to pain management. In: Wall PD, Melzack R, eds. Textbook of pain. ed 2. London: Churchill Livingstone, 1989.
16. American Psychiatric Association. Diagnostic and Statistical Manual of Mental Disorders. 4th ed. Washington: APA, 1994.
17. Perley, Guze S. The stability and usefulness of clinical criteria. N Engl J Med 1982;266:421–426.

18. Ward NG, Bloom VL, Dworkin S, et al. Psychobiological markers in coexisting pain and depression: towards a unified theory. J Clin Psychol 1982;43:8:32–41.

19. Fishbain D. DSM IV: implication and issues for the pain clinician. APS Bull 1995;5:6–18.

20. Maxmen JS, Ward NG. Essential psychopathology and its treatment. New York: Norton, 1995;297.

21. American Psychiatric Association. Diagnostic and Statistical Manual of Mental Disorders. 3rd ed revised. Washington: APA, 1987;169.

22. Watson GD, Chandarana PC, Mersky N. Relationships between pain and schizophrenia. Br J Psychol 1981;138:33–36.

22a. American Society of Addiction Medicine. Public policy statement of definitions related to the use of opioids in pain treatment. Adopted by the ASAM Board of Directors, April 16, 1997.

23. Aronoff GM, Evans WO. Evaluation and treatment of chronic pain at the Boston Pain Center. J Clin Psychol 1982;43:8:3–7.

24. Aronoff GM, Evans WO. Doxepin as an adjunct in the treatment of chronic pain. J Clin Psychol 1982;43:8:42–45.

25. Engle G. Psychogenic pain and the pain prone patient. Am J Med 1959;54:899–918.

26. Blumer D, Heilbronn M. Chronic pain as a variant of depressive disease. J Nerv Ment Dis 1982;170:381–406.

CHAPTER 22

A Guide for Psychological Testing and Evaluation for Chronic Pain

Ronald J. Kulich and William K. Baker

INTRODUCTION:

Psychological assessment is a necessary component of evaluation of the chronic pain patient. Psychosocial factors affect pain and disability. While pain centers and individual clinicians vary widely in their application of assessment tools, a standardized assessment protocol should be considered as a minimum standard of care when evaluating the chronic pain patient. While some insurance carriers continue to resist this component of evaluation, others are viewing early psychosocial assessment as a cost-effective intervention for patients who typically use multiple medical services. We recall one case in our pain center in which a nationally recognized HMO carrier sent a patient with preapproval for implantation of a spinal column stimulator, an intervention costing $15,000 to $25,000. Return-to-work rates at some institutions implanting this device have been as low as 10%. When the carrier was informed that a formal psychological screening was required, the adjuster explained that the policy would "not cover that." We proceeded with a formal psychological assessment nonetheless and determined that the patient was not a candidate because of a range of psychosocial issues and expectations on the part of the patient. We recommended a formal functional restoration rehabilitation program. This particular carrier became convinced of the potential savings and paid the hotel accommodations for this out-of-state patient. He was discharged with a return-to-work capacity within 6 weeks, with a total cost to the carrier of less than $6,000. At a savings of at least $9,000, this improved functional status for the patient.

The American Pain Society has sought to correct this problem, and many states are undertaking legislative efforts to enhance access to appropriate subspecialty pain services. Guidelines have been established for pain centers, and the role of psychological assessment has taken a prominent role (1). Others have proposed standards for psychological and disability assessment (2) and offered psychometric guidelines (3).

The following review offers the physician a template for performing many aspects of psychological assessment in a primary care setting, in some cases without formal psychological assessment. While the structure of a formal psychological assessment and selection of testing materials can vary widely, we also attempt to acquaint the reader with the most typical format and testing instruments employed by a psychologist specializing in chronic pain assessment.

DIFFERENTIAL DIAGNOSIS

Chronic pain is a multidimensional problem that surpasses a simple assessment of pain sensation. Psychological assessment of pain should be considered in the context of factors such as perception of disability, pain behavior, emotional response to pain, emotional precipitants to pain and disability, and the various social and financial antecedents and consequences (4). Psychological assessment first requires distinctions among acute pain, chronic pain, and chronic pain syndrome. A diagnosis of acute pain assumes identifiable nociception and a short time-limited course. Acute pain is "an unpleasant sensory and emotional experience arising from actual or potential tissue damage, or described in terms of such damage" (5). *Psychosocial concomitants rarely cause acute pain, although acute pain left untreated can lead to psychosocial sequelae.* Treatment is addressed by correcting the pathological process, often treating the pain with appropriate analgesics. Referral for comprehensive psychological assessment of acute pain is not usually required, although the role of adjunct psychological interventions with acute pain has been well documented (6). Chronic pain persists for several months and treatments may or may not ameliorate the condition, but the patient generally continues to function and does not undergo the multiple psychosocial and disability concomitants. Chronic pain syndrome is a complex multidimensional problem, defined by the Office of Disabilities of the Social Security Administration as "intractable pain of

6 months or more duration; marked alteration of behavior, with depression or anxiety; marked restriction in daily activities; excessive use of medication and frequent use of medical services; no clear relationship to organic disorder; and history of multiple, nonproductive tests, treatment, and surgeries" (5, 7).

Assuming that a diagnosis of chronic pain or chronic pain syndrome has been made, pain patients within this group should not be considered a homogenous population. A person's response to chronic pain may show substantial variability, and prior investigations have suggested that this may be a function of coping skills rather than tissue disease or damage, medical diagnosis, or location of the pain complaint. These distinct subgroups may require varying treatment interventions (8). Psychosocial factors may be discriminators within a chronic pain population, while site of the pain or diagnosis may fail to be relevant variables for differentiation.

When a referral is made for psychological assessment, a common assumption on the part of the patient and of many health care providers is that "they couldn't find anything; it must be psychological." Prior psychiatric classification systems and outdated psychoanalytical formulation have fostered the concept of a dichotomy between physical and environmental conditions, and the prejudice persists. Current definitions of pain assume a psychosocial role, and it is the task of psychological assessment to delineate this role.

GOALS OF PSYCHOSOCIAL ASSESSMENT FOR PAIN AND DISABILITY

The primary goals of psychological assessment include prediction of behavior and collection of data for structuring an effective psychological and medical treatment plan. The psychologist may also be asked to screen the patient for psychosocial factors that affect treatment outcome for specific medical treatments. Psychosocial assessment can establish the likelihood of returning to prior employment, likelihood of reinjury, or estimates of health care utilization (9). The assessment may establish risk of substance abuse or suicide or likelihood of compliance with proposed medical or psychological interventions.

Another focus of psychological assessment is the determination of deficits and abilities. Assessment of abilities and limitations can provide an end point status for resolving worker compensation or liability claims. Repeated measures also can be used to compare the patient's abilities and deficits before, during, and after treatment and provide data on cost effectiveness (7). Variables that may be expected to show change are depression, focus on somatic symptoms, sleep, job satisfaction, and/or perception of control over pain and disability. A *Diagnostic and Statistical Manual of Mental Disorders,* 4th edition (DSM-IV) psychiatric diagnosis may be assigned, as well as estimates of the patient's functional limitations (10). When return to work is planned, psychological factors also can be taken into account along with any necessary job site modifications. The Americans with Disabilities Act (11) allows for such psychosocial factors when evaluating employer compliance with federal guidelines.

EVALUATION AND MEASUREMENT OF PSYCHOSOCIAL FACTORS

Depression and Anxiety

Within acute pain populations, Magni (12) found 42% displaying a diagnosis of depression. The incidence of depression in chronic pain populations has been shown to be substantially higher, exceeding 80% (13), with reports showing more than 50% of chronic pain patients developing major depression. In these cases the incidence of recurrence is greater than 60%, with 15% of those patients dying by suicide (14). Studies consistently show a high correlation between scores on depression scales and presence of pain and disability behavior (15), but there is limited support for a causative relationship. Other studies show that depression predicts report of pain while pain predicts report of depression, with the latter more powerful than the former (16, 17). Holroyd et al. (15) reported depression scores elevated in chronic headache sufferers only when they were having headaches, while patients with constant chronic pain frequently complain of unremitting depression. Singer et al. (16) stated that with HIV-related pain, depression and increased disability are a consequence of the pain, while Bruehl and Carlson (17) reported that depression, anxiety, and life stressors were related to development of sympathetically maintained pain. If there is a causal relationship, the data suggest that individual differences play a role, and therefore a thorough assessment of physical and emotional functioning *before the pain set in* should be included in a comprehensive psychological evaluation.

Several investigators have attempted to reconceptualize the construct of depression accompanying chronic pain. In several studies the new constructs of "perceived life control" or "perceived life interference" controlled much of the variance, suggesting that manifestations of depression may be somewhat different in a chronic pain population from those in a psychiatric population (21, 22). In fact, chronic pain patients who have a history of depression prior to development of pain often assert that this depression is different and readily accept the less threatening and perhaps more valid descriptors of perceived loss of control. Cognitive distortions appear to be a major factor with the depressed chronic pain patient.

Evaluation of the patient's belief system is a major part of the assessment of a patient with chronic pain. Nonetheless, the formal criteria of DSM-IV (14) should be considered in an adequate assessment of the chronic pain patent. Tables 22.1 and 22.2 summarize the DSM-IV criteria and prevalence of depression.

The most frequently used self-report measure of depression is the Beck Depression Inventory (BDI), a brief self-report questionnaire composed of 21 items, of which the patient responds to a series of rank ordered statements. (23). While regularly employed as a component of psychological assessment, the BDI often is used in primary care settings as a brief screening instrument for affective symptoms. The BDI can be completed in 5 minutes, includes much of the DSM-IV content for affective disorders, and can be repeated on a weekly basis.

Table 22.1.   Diagnostic Criteria For Depression

Sleep
  Insomnia or hypersomnia
Interests
  Loss of interest or pleasure in activities
Guilt
  Excessive feelings of worthlessness, hopelessness, helplessness
Energy
  Fatigue or loss of energy
Concentration
  Diminished concentration ability, indecisiveness
Appetite
  Decreased appetite, > 5% weight loss or gain
Psychomotor
  Psychomotor retardation or agitation
Risk of suicide
  Suicidal ideation, plan, or attempt

Table 22.2.   Major Depression: Time Course and Prevalence

Major depression can follow a severe stressor, particularly a major medical trauma.
22–25% of those with a severe chronic medical condition are at risk.
At least 50% of persons with chronic persistent pain lasting > 6 months are at risk.
Major depression can occur at any age, while prevalence is only 2–3% in the
  general population.
Symptoms are daily and can be unremitting for more than 2 years.
15% die by suicide.
50–60% who have one episode will have a second, with 90% reoccurrence in
  those who have 3 episodes.
40% still have the symptoms a year after onset.

It is important to caution that self-report measures of depression such as the BDI may overestimate depression in the chronic pain population, in part because of the overlap of pain-related physiological symptoms and affective disorder symptoms (24-27). This problem is particularly evident with the elderly, in whom a range of physical symptoms may be present.

Other instruments that can be employed as rapid screening devices for depression include the Hamilton Rating Scale for Depression (HRS), a clinician-administered instrument (28), and the Zung Self-Rating Depression Scale (29). The Multidimensional Pain Inventory, a particularly useful instrument, is a relatively short, nonthreatening questionnaire that can be readily used on the physician's office (30). It contains an affective disorder subscale but lacks some of the critical symptom items present in the BDI.

The correlation of anxiety with chronic pain is well established, both as a contributor to symptoms and a consequence of acute pain, persistent pain, and related disability (6, 22, 31). Presence of anxiety symptoms before onset of back pain has been reported to be as high as 95%, although studies primarily have been prospective (32). Outcome studies of anxiety and pain also show a high correlation between measures of anxiety and depression (21, 22, 33, 34). From a psychophysiological standpoint, anxiety can lower the pain threshold, so that the patient interprets a range of sensations as painful and thereby comprises the self-report outcome from medical procedures.

The Brief Symptom Inventory (BSI) (35), the short version of the Symptom Check List (SCL-90), can be employed in a range of medical settings. The BSI contains items for anxiety, phobic anxiety, depression, and psychosis. Another relatively short scale is the Speilberger State/Trait Anxiety Inventory (STAI) (36). The state form has utility for repeated measures when changes in anxiety level are expected over time. Norms are available for chronic pain syndrome (37), and this relatively short scale has acceptable reliability and validity.

Pain Beliefs and Pain Coping Abilities

A patient's beliefs about pain and treatment and perception of disability are powerful predictors of functioning and disability. Patients who believe they can control their pain, avoid catastrophizing, and believe they are not severely disabled show greater improvement (38). Treatment compliance is related to the patient's beliefs about the potential efficacy of the treatment plan (39). The role of beliefs on positive outcome is well established, and distinguishing the effect of the placebo response for many invasive and noninvasive treatments is difficult. (40). Standardized questionnaires that categorize beliefs include the Survey of Pain Attitudes (SOPA), the Coping Strategies Questionnaire (CSQ), the Attributional Style Questionnaire (ASQ), and the Pain Beliefs and Perceptions Inventory (PBPI) (41–44). Health Care and Headache Locus of Control (LOC) scales address patients' beliefs about their sense of control over their pain (internal LOC), their belief that the health care provider can fix their problem, and the belief that they should relinquish control and responsibility to the doctor (external LOC), or their belief that their pain and limitations are random events unaffected by any internal or external influence (chance LOC) (45). Of course, the optimum belief is an internal locus of control rather than a focus that relegates the patient's life to control by the pain or the actions of health care providers. It is not surprising that chronic pain patients are much less likely to report control over their pain than medical clinic patients in acute pain, for whom the course of discomfort is predictable and effectively managed by pharmacological strategies.

With regard to perception of disability, other formal testing instruments include the Sickness Impact Profile (SIP). The most frequently cited self-report measure of disability, initially it was standardized on a general medical population (46–48). The SIP is a 136-item self-report checklist divided into composite psychosocial and physical scales. A perceived disability score is derived from the SIP; scoring is relatively easy; and it is a sensitive outcome measure. However, some have expressed concern over the SIP's ability to detect changes over time (49).

The Oswestry Disability Scale has also been widely used in physical therapy and occupational therapy settings (50), although Waddell and Turk (51) and others have suggested that the SIP may have a better factor structure and clinical utility. The Chronic Illness Problem Inventory (CIPI) (52) is an alternative to the SIP, particularly for patients with back pain, although studies examining predictive validity are not yet available. The Short Form-36 has grown in popularity as the major measure employed with medical outcomes research. Items address perception of disability, as well as social and perceived mental health functioning (53).

Somatization

The chronic pain patient's focus on symptoms can be a debilitating belief or behavior pattern, and the patient may seek out multiple concurrent treatments without benefit. The chronic disability and recurrent course of chronic pain may reinforce this somatic focus, with the patient's worry and somatic concern reinforced by multiple unsuccessful intervention strategies aimed at pain relief. Beliefs that the physician missed something or that an increase in pain is due to new tissue damage continues the cycle. Some patients qualify for a somatization disorder diagnosis when the complaints are not exclusive to pain. While suggestive and temporarily responsive to interventions due to placebo factors, these patients tend to have poor outcomes with the somatically focused interventions. Behavioral or rehabilitative interventions that specifically reinforce well behavior or positive cognitions incompatible with somatization have fared somewhat better, although long-term prognosis remains poor and management of the patient's health care-seeking behavior often becomes the focus of treatment. The DSM-IV (14) makes an effort to distinguish these patients from those with a diagnosis of pain disorder or chronic pain syndrome for this purpose. A summary of the criteria for somatization disorder is outlined in Table 22.3.

While Bacon et al. (54) reported that no one in their population met full DSM-IV criteria for somatization disorder, 25.8 % of chronic low-back pain patients reported a lifetime history of 12 or more somatic symptoms, as compared with 4.1% of controls. In fact, others have reported a much higher incidence of somatization disorder in the pain population, with some authors arguing that fibromyalgia and complex regional pain syndromes are manifestations of this disorder (55, 56). Major depression and alcohol dependence also were related to increased somatization.

The SCL-90 and its abbreviated version (BPI) have been used to assess somatization with chronic pain. Von Korff et al. (37), using the SCL-90, reported correlations with each of five pain conditions, while perceived health status was associated with back pain and headache. The Minnesota Multiphasic Personality Inventory (MMPI-2) has also been used to assess oversomatization, focusing on elevations on the Hypochondriasis and Hysteria subscales. However, most researchers argue that this instrument is sensitive to current somatization rather than possible long-standing somatization traits (57), and others report a change in these scales with rehabilitation treatment (58). Caution should be used in conclusions of oversomatization, since much of the item content on the scales may overlap with medical content.

It is debated whether somatization develops as a reaction to the pain or vice versa; that is, does the patient instead have

Table 22.3.   Diagnostic Criteria for Somatization Disorder

The patient has a pattern of recurring multiple clinically significant somatic complaints.

Complaints begin < age 30 and occur over several years; initial symptoms are often present in adolescence.

If they occur in the presence of a general medical condition, the physical complaints or resulting social or occupational impairment are in excess of what would be expected from the history, physical examination, or laboratory tests.

There must be a history of pain related to at least four sites (e.g., head, abdomen, back, joints, extremities, chest, rectum) or functions (e.g., menstruation, sexual intercourse, urination). There also must be a history of at least two gastrointestinal symptoms other than pain. Most persons with the disorder describe nausea and abdominal bloating. Vomiting, diarrhea, and food intolerance are less common. Gastrointestinal complaints often lead to frequent radiographs and can result in abdominal surgery that in retrospect was unnecessary. There must be a history of at least one sexual or reproductive symptom other than pain.

There must also be a history of at least one symptom other than pain that suggests a neurological condition.

The symptoms must not be feigned.

a premorbid history of personality characteristics that *result in* oversomatization or a pain-prone characteristic? Early developmental factors have not been shown to be reliable predictors of pain and disability (41, 59, 60).

Rehabilitation specialists have developed a classification termed symptom magnification syndrome, described as a "constellation of reports or displays of symptoms which control the environment to such a degree that the symptom behavior is maladaptive" (61). Clinical reports are replete with patients labeled as symptom magnifiers, and the term has been used inappropriately by insurance carriers as an indication of malingering and lack of motivation for rehabilitation.

A discussion of somatization rarely occurs without the concept of secondary gain (62). The gain, or positive reinforcement, relates to attention from significant others for pain behaviors, unconscious needs to be cared for, or financial motivation influencing disability behavior. A comprehensive discussion has ensued regarding the construct of secondary gain and the frequent abuse of this term as a pejorative (6, 10). Gallagher (63) proposes conceptualizing secondary gain from a biobehavioral perspective, suggesting that pain-related symptoms can be conditioned. The evaluation and treatment process should address reinforcing factors such as pain complaints, pain behaviors, and requests for medication, as well as psychophysiological and psychosocial processes influencing pain perception. The evaluation and treatment team should then adhere to a treatment plan through which pain self-management is reinforced and dysfunctional attitudes and behaviors are extinguished. The label "secondary gain" offers us little in this regard.

Long-Standing Behavior Patterns and Personality Coping Issues

The patient's lifelong behavior patterns and coping strategies are considered important in predicting a complicated treatment course with chronic pain, although the data are less than supportive from the standpoint of causative personality variables. There is little question that maladaptive behavior patterns and aberrant personality factors influence the patient's coping and ultimate effective medical management. Gatchel (58) reports that 51% of chronic pain patients met psychiatric diagnostic criteria for personality disorders. While this probably is an inflated number, many clinicians would argue that one destructive or manipulative patient is too many. While reviewing the criteria for various personality disorders is beyond the scope of this book, it is important to address the assessment of the patient with borderline personality characteristics. This diagnosis has been reported to occur in more than 30% of personality disorders. Many of these persons not only consume substantial medical services but also elicit the greatest negative affect from health care staff. A summary of this disorder is outlined in Table 22.4.

History of Sexual Abuse and/or Emotional Trauma

Sexual abuse and emotional trauma receive ongoing attention in the assessment of chronic pain (64–66). Bradley et al. (67) suggest a series of interview items adapted from the psychiatric literature. Reports imply that a higher proportion of victims of sexual abuse is found in chronic pain populations than the general population, although no studies demonstrate a causal link. No reports suggest that treatment of psychological sequelae associated with trauma result in improved pain reports or decreased disability, although case reports suggest that the effects of such abuse can predict a problematic treatment course. There does appear to be support for an adequate assessment of these factors, given the possibility of unnecessary medical interventions with this population.

Spouse, Family, and Cultural Factors

Much has been written about the role of the "significant other" in the evaluation of chronic pain (68–70). The earliest work by Block et al. (69) identified the oversolicitous spouse. One should be aware of the overprotective spouse, who makes statements such as reminding the patient to "take your medication," "lie down if you don't feel good," or "be careful; I'll do that for you." Block (69) found that the presence of a solicitous spouse in an interview setting resulted in an increase in overt pain behavior when the patient thought the spouse was observing the session. In contrast, patients with nonsolicitous spouses displayed increased pain behavior when they thought a ward clerk was observing. Hence it is possible that the patient gets attention for pain behavior and modifies the behavior accordingly, possibly with increased complaints and disability.

The Multidimensional Pain Inventory offers a scale for solicitousness (30). For full assessment of the patient the spouse should be present in at least a portion of the diagnostic interview. A spouse often can corroborate the veracity of the information supplied by the patient and provide additional

Table 22.4.   Diagnostic Criteria for Borderline Personality Disorder

A pervasive pattern of unstable and intense interpersonal relationships is present.
Marked impulsivity begins by early adulthood.
Frantic efforts to avoid real or imagined abandonment occur.
The patient is inappropriately angry even when faced with realistic time-limited separation, e.g., fury when someone who is important to him or her is just a few minutes late or must cancel an appointment.
Impulsive acts such as self-mutilating or suicidal behavior may be present.
Idealization of potential caregivers occurs, then switches abruptly to devaluing them, feeling that the other person doesn't care and is not "there" enough.
Changes are seen in the patient from needy supplicant for help to a righteous avenger of past mistreatment.
Substance abuse is common, and 8–10% of these persons commit suicide.

information on the patient's medical status, medication, alcohol use, or specific disability and pain behaviors. A family member's dissatisfaction or satisfaction with the patient's disability provides a basis for assessing prognosis or focus of treatment, and the family's willingness to support a treatment regimen is critical (9).

Cultural Factors

Although a number of investigators illustrate examples of ethnocultural differences, it remains difficult to extrapolate these data to the clinical assessment setting (71–73). Indeed, the majority of assessment instruments reviewed have been developed on white middle-class persons, so it is questionable whether they can be generalized to other populations. Given the paucity of cross-cultural studies addressing pain and disability, the clinician must carefully examine testing and interview data. Family members should be included in the assessment process to document the antecedents and consequences of pain and disability. Multidisciplinary team input by professionals familiar with the patient's cultural background should be considered. Just as cultural and economic incentives vary across settings, cultural differences severely impair the validity and generality of our assessments.

Job Satisfaction and Work Experience

While rehabilitation programs emphasize communication with the employer, medically oriented pain physicians tend to ignore this source of critical information. Work and personal history and the employer's impression of work habits and willingness to consider a return-to-work plan can be valuable aids in the determination of prognosis and shaping the treatment plan (74). Prior performance evaluation data can predict the patient's behavior in a treatment program or likelihood of repeating good or poor work behaviors. Consistencies or inconsistencies in background information can help to predict outcome and shape the treatment program. Lack of job satisfaction has been identified as a major predictor of reinjury with back pain (75). If work tasks or job tasks offer minimal opportunity for reinforcement and supervisor or work-task dissatisfaction is evident, an unsuccessful trial at return to work is likely (76). An adjuster may assert that the company does not owe the patient a job he likes, but the patient who must work in pain may perceive that such a job or other financial compensation is owed, and a successful return to work becomes elusive. Several standardized instruments attempt to address these issues. The Occupational Stress Inventory (OSI) (77) is a self-report inventory used with satisfactory reliability and validity in chronic pain settings. The scales on the OSI provide information about specific stressors at the work site, including information about the patient's perception of physical and psychosocial job demands.

Predicting successful return to work through psychological assessment is a frequently requested service by insurance carriers and treatment programs. Return-to-work rates range from 60 to 85%, depending on the treatment focus of a particular program and its selection criteria (76). The mere presence of any psychosocial concomitants of pain has been shown to predict poor outcome with invasive procedures such as spinal column stimulation. Conversely, outpatient pain rehabilitation and functional restoration programs that identify patients with psychopathology and then reinforce specific return-to-work goals and expectations have demonstrated high rates of return-to-work success (78).

LITIGATION AND FINANCIAL GAIN

Litigation is considered a predictor of disability, increased report of pain, disability, and treatment failure. Patients seeking compensation report greater distress, higher self-report of disability, and greater pain levels than nonlitigants. However, the relation between litigation and psychological distress variables remains complex. Tait et al. (79) report that patients who are working and litigating are more depressed than patients who are working but not litigating. However, an examination of their mean scores on the BDI fails to reveal other than mild mean levels of depression. Conclusions about conscious exaggeration of complaints or feigning illness cannot be drawn from these studies. In fact, the adversarial process of sustaining an injury in a work-related setting is itself a precipitant of distress, with distress contributing to pain and disability.

As the term malingering implies a conscious feigning of symptoms, usually for financial gain, the implication suggests volition on the part of the patient. A diagnosis of malingering remains difficult to support with objective evidence, since volition cannot be reliably measured. Chapman and Brena (80) report that "patterns of conscious failure to provide accurate self-report data" may suggest a diagnosis of malingering, although they consider that such conclusions should be made cautiously.

Clinicians often rely on observational data as their primary source of support for conclusions. Nonetheless, the chronic pain literature documents the reactive effect of observation on pain behavior (81). "Consistency" of self-report can be a function of anxiety, somatic concern, or operant factors which affect behavior. The examiner who does report a diagnosis of malingering, should include other sources of data,

such as the patient's history, observations made in a natural setting, reports of significant others, and history of inconsistencies or lack of reliability of the patient's self-report.

While malingering or conscious feigning of symptoms is rare, success with a given treatment intervention is often affected by issues of job satisfaction, fears of financial ruin, anger at others who may have "caused" their problem, or despair because the employer failed to call or make contact after the worker's injury. An effective treatment plan must necessarily involve everyone who influences the patient's treatment, including the attorney, insurance adjuster, rehabilitation nurse, and employer (82).

COMPONENTS OF THE FORMAL PSYCHOLOGICAL EVALUATION

Preparation for the Referral for Psychological Assessment

The psychological assessment should be an integral component of the pain assessment process, with the referring physician describing the psychological consultation not to see whether the pain is real, but rather to find the best fit between the individual and the treatment strategies. The patient should be offered assurance that psychological assessment is both typical and necessary in chronic pain. If affective symptoms are present, further assurance can be offered that more than 80% of chronic pain patients report depression symptoms, with these symptoms often being a good rather than poor prognostic indication of long-term positive outcome. Common other fears and negative cognitions often held by a pain patient may be reinforced by the medical treatments undertaken. Some of these typical beliefs or fears are included in Table 22.5.

Again, the primary focus of assessment is on the patient's current status rather than exploration of early developmental or various psychoanalytical constructs. The patient's current fears and expectations are likely to have the greatest influence on the outcome of the treatment regimen and likely are the more amenable to change.

The assessment setting offers the first step toward providing further assurance, and confidence in the clinician is enhanced when the psychologist is integrated into the medical setting. Guidelines from the Commission on Accreditation of Rehabilitation Facilities (83) encourage team evaluation at the site of the pain center, minimizing the patient's anxiety and fears of stigma.

Brief Screening and Outcome Assessment

Considerable data can be gathered by preassessment questionnaires, and standardized outcome assessment has rapidly become commonplace for most large medical settings. Outcome measures such as the SF-36 and SIP offer data from psychosocial and disability scales, although adequate standardization of these scales on pain populations is lacking (48, 53). The practicing physician can consider a short battery that

Table 22.5.   Fears and Negative Cognitions

"The doctor thinks it's in my head."
"The treatment didn't work; now he's dumping me [on the psychologist]."
"They must think I'm crazy."
"I won't get necessary surgery if I say the wrong thing."
"They think I'm an addict."
"Only weak people come here."
"I'll be asked about my childhood."
"They must think I'm addicted."
"What will my family (employer, etc.) think?"
"Who will see these records?"

Table 22.6.   Chronic Pain Interview Format

Identifying data
Current primary pain complaint and date of injury(s)
Additional pain complaints and/or somatic complaints
History of evaluation and treatment and effectiveness of prior treatments
Premorbid medical and psychiatric history
Concurrent medical and psychological treatments
Pain and/or disability behavior
Current versus prior functional status, anticipated sources of income
Recreational pursuits, activities of daily living
Spouse's work status (worker's compensation, disability,
    Social Security Disability Income)
Precipitants and consequences of pain
Attitudes toward health care providers, family, employer, insurance carrier
Family, employer, physician, attorney response to pain
Substance use history (smoking, alcohol, prescription and nonprescription drugs)
Current and past stressors, major life and developmental stressors, abuse history
Employment and education
Criminal and litigation history
Mental status
Current emotional status
Marital status
Personality
Social supports
Behavioral observations and pain behaviors, e.g., limping, callused or dirty
    hands, dress
Goals, motivation, and expectations

may provide valuable data for understanding some of the psychosocial concomitants present in the pain patient.

The Multidimensional Pain Inventory (MPI) (84) (as distinguished from the MMPI) can be particularly useful at the prereferral stage of assessment. The MPI is a 64-item face valid self-report inventory that has been standardized on a variety of pain populations. This relatively brief questionnaire is divided into three parts. The first addresses the patient's appraisal of pain, pain intensity rating, and the effects of pain on the patient's life. This includes a subscale addressing affective distress and perceived control over pain. The second relates to the patient's perception of the significant other's response to their pain and suffering, with a solicitousness scale addressing social factors that may influence report of pain and disability. The third relates to the patient's self-reported frequency of engagement in functional activity. These scales are particularly helpful for evaluation of self-report of function in discrete areas including household chores, outdoor work, activities away from home, and social activities. Administration can be completed in about 20 minutes, and items tend to be pain specific and lack "sensitive" subject matter. Computer scoring is inexpensive, with a program readily available for use with a small office computer. The printout provides a profile category, and these may assist the clinician in targeting treatment or screening patients for presence of psychosocial factors that influence outcome. The three subgroup profile classifications provided on the MPI are these:

1. Dysfunctional: These patients perceive their pain to be severe. They report significant pain interference in their lives, high levels of affective distress, and low levels of activity. They display more pain behaviors, use pain medications more frequently, spend more time in bed, and are more likely to be unemployed than other profile types (85).
2. Interpersonally distressed: These patients are characterized by a perception that their significant others are not understanding and supportive.
3. Adaptive coper: These patients perceive high levels of social support, low levels of pain and affective distress, low levels of perceived life interference, high levels of self-reported functional activities, and perceived control over their situation.

Other investigations have supported the taxonomy of the three subgroups (8), and studies have suggested that the classifications are not based on compensation or litigation status. The MPI appears to be the most promising instrument available for clinical assessment from a psychometric standpoint, although outcome studies remain lacking.

Other readily available evaluation-by-mail computerized assessment protocols should be used with some caution, particularly with extensive personality assessments. For example, some pain centers and medical practices have elected to mail patients the MMPI and then recommend psychological evaluation. The patient assumes that "I must have failed the test" and responds negatively to the suggestion for psychological assessment.

Pain assessment interview predictive validity and reliability of the psychological interview have received attention elsewhere in the general psychological literature, and clinical interview templates have appeared elsewhere in the pain literature (86, 87). Semistructured interview formats are similar in their content. Table 22.6 shows the template in current use in several pain center settings. Many of these items can be easily incorporated into the typical ongoing assessment undertaken by the primary care provider, although a comprehensive psychological assessment should address these areas as well.

Ratings of Pain Intensity

Pain intensity assessments have significant reliability, validity, and utility problems. Pain intensity reports change over time, and environmental factors influence the measurement of pain.

Nonetheless, there must be some rating of the patient's pain, and a patient rating appears to be a reasonable approach. The most common scales are the Visual Analog Scale (VAS) (88, 89) and the McGill Pain Questionnaire (MPQ) (90). The reliability and validity of average pain measures are improved by increasing the number of measurements. In order to obtain a reliable rating, Jensen and McFarland (91) recommend at least three measures of pain per day over 4 days. Extending ratings over more than 4 days did not improve validity and reliability, and they further recommended averaging multiple measures obtained over different times during the day and from different days. They also conducted a review of the maximum number of measurements needed in pain intensity measurement, concluding that 10- and 21-point scales provide sufficient levels of discrimination for chronic pain populations. Use of multiple measures is critical where pain is episodic, such as in chronic migraine.

The MPQ (90) and its 10 Pain Rating Index subclass (PRI) is one of the most widely used instruments. The MPQ can assist with differential diagnosis between various pain syndromes (91). Items have face validity, and clinicians have frequently reviewed individual item endorsements, for example while evaluating neuropathic versus myofascial pain. However, the MPQ and PRI subscale scores appear to be poor predictors of psychological disturbance within a chronic pain population.

OTHER FORMAL PSYCHOLOGICAL TESTING

The MMPI-2 (57) has received the most attention as a comprehensive personality instrument for assessing chronic pain, and no other instrument has received such extensive criticism. Riley et al. (92) reported a cluster analysis study showing the MMPI-2 interpretations to parallel MMPI interpretations, and complaints about the revised instrument essentially remain the same. Criticisms relate to the MMPI's focus on psychopathology, length of administration (about 2 hours), predictive value, overinterpretation by unskilled practitioners, and excessive reliance on computerized interpretive reports (93–96). Helmes and his associates (95, 96) have made the strongest criticisms of MMPI or MMPI-2 use and have suggested alternatives such as the Personality Assessment Inventory (PAI) (95). However, the literature lacks sufficient data on the PAI to suggest it as a reasonable replacement.

Despite the criticisms, research continues to support the MMPI-2 as a measure of pervasive coping difficulties. Elevations have been shown to correlate with affective disturbance and pain-related reduction in activities. Scale elevations suggesting oversomatization or personality coping problems are correlated with poor treatment outcome for behavioral and rehabilitation pain programs (97–99) and invasive procedures. While the presence of minimal psychological disturbance has been shown to reduce satisfactory outcome to as little as 18%, rigorous psychological screening for these costly procedures remains largely absent in most clinical settings. In fact, the MMPI has been used to screen for discectomy and spinal fusion, and one of the more recent studies by Spengler et al. (100) suggests that the MMPI may be a better predictor of

improvement than traditional medical measures such as a physical examination or radiological studies.

Observational Methods and Pain Behavior

The construct of pain behavior as a dependent variable has been appearing since the pioneering work by Fordyce and his colleagues (101, 102). A patient may achieve pain relief or social reinforcement if he performs in a certain manner (i.e., uses a hot pack, moans, or lies down). Intermittent reinforcement of the disability behaviors and learned avoidance of noxious stimuli increases disability. Overt pain behavior may be more prevalent in low-back pain than in facial pain (103), although other pain behaviors, such as medication use, complaints of pain, and visits to health care providers are present with other pain populations. Behavioral, operant, or rehabilitation-oriented treatment programs target well behaviors or behaviors incompatible with pain behaviors (104). It has therefore been reported that pain behavior suggests possible program candidacy.

Overt pain behavior scales measure behavior such as grimacing, limping, and complaints of pain (103, 104). More complex observational methods that require rater training and video assessment have fallen into disuse because of their complexity and cost. Nonetheless, measurement and reporting of observable behavior must be considered a component of a comprehensive assessment.

Pain Drawings

The utility of pain drawings has been questioned, since measures of psychopathology and pain drawings show only a weak relationship. Predictive validity is not supported, and pain drawing ratings have received limited use as outcome measures. Pain drawing may help to confirm the patient's location and quality of pain but may not be suitable as a psychological assessment instrument (105).

Projective Assessment Techniques

While we occasionally see use of projective methods with children (106), traditional projective assessment methods have not found their way into the armamentarium of psychologists who evaluate pain patients. No studies support predictive validity of tests such as the Rorschach, while projective testing still is used in occasional traditional assessment settings. Given these issues and the reluctance of pain patients to consider a psychological assessment, the use of projective techniques should be considered inappropriate at best.

Neuropsychological Testing

Neuropsychological testing, perhaps the most extensive of assessment protocols, typically is considered when there is a clear indication of cognitive or intellectual functioning deficits. While patients who have had a head injury or stroke are typical candidates, formal memory assessment and evaluation of higher level cognitive functions often are also considered in cases of whiplash or closed head injury. In many cases these reports are prepared for forensic use, with only occasional utility in a clinical setting if the patient displays more demonstrative deficits.

OTHER CRITICAL SOURCES OF INFORMATION

Rehabilitation Nurses, Adjusters, and Attorneys

There appears to be an explicit adversarial relationship between the patient and rehabilitation nurses, adjusters, and attorneys, with the physician generally siding with the patient. Nonetheless, each of these persons possess information on the patient's status and often it is they who have gathered the most thorough clinical record available for review. Adjusters and others involved in the patient's case may go to great lengths to document patient behavior that appears inconsistent with the patient's report to the physician, and communication with these persons only increases the chance of achieving a positive outcome with a difficult pain problem. In turn, the psychologist evaluating the case with possible forensic implications should solicit all sources of information available with appropriate releases from the patient. Patient self-report in the interview rarely is adequate. For example, we are reminded of a colleague who performed extensive testing, reviewed medical records, and accepted the patient's word that his concurrent alcohol and opioid use had not occurred for more than 5 years. An assertion was made that there were no psychological contraindications, and the patient considered that he should be considered a candidate for opioid maintenance. When testifying upon the patient's behalf at an industrial accident hearing, the psychologist was informed of the patient's driving under the influence convictions over the past several months, as well as the patient's anticipated incarceration. Although we can't possibly know everything about our patients, a candid conversation with the patient's attorney at the onset of evaluation might have provided the psychologist with some valuable data.

Prior Records

The first rule of psychological assessment is that past behavior is the best predictor of future behavior. Prior records can provide the physician with evidence of multiple previous complaints and health care-seeking behavior. History often known only to the patient's primary care physician can span the time prior to the onset of injury and pain, shedding light on adherence to prior treatment, history of somatization, psychiatric history, and/or history of substance abuse. These data can provide an excellent baseline from which to make current comparisons. Carriers also make available recent and past summaries from pharmacies, another source for determining prior or current medication treatments not reported by the patient.

SCREENING FOR MEDICAL INTERVENTIONS

Psychological testing as a means of screening for surgery has been used for more than 20 years, and the results of employing the MMPI with spinal surgery are well documented. A major problem lies with the overinterpretation or sole use of computer-generated profiles wherein the norms for the population being assessed are not considered. Efficacious psychological screening requires much more than simple self-report testing and estimates about "predictive" elevations on subscales. For example, if the chronic pain patient's goal of spinal surgery is to get back to work, reliability of work history, job satisfaction, and other factors that may keep the patient from achieving the stated goal should be assessed. An adequate understanding of the likely physical outcome of the procedure also must be in the repertoire of the psychologist and patient. For example, it is fairly common for a person seeking spinal surgery to anticipate that all of the back pain will go away, while the surgeon has attempted to emphasize an outcome directed at leg pain. Hence the reasons for the patient seeking the procedure are as important as the reasons for the physician undertaking the procedure. Similarly, screening for invasive procedures such as nerve blocks often is warranted.

A patient may ascribe substantial effect to a prior similar intervention, and a note by the prior anesthesiologist confirms the patient's claim of pain relief. In several cases an extended interview with the patient and the spouse, along with thorough review of prior records, revealed that the analgesic intake consistently increased immediately after each procedure, and the increases were maintained over an extended time. However, many patients adhere to an unshakable faith that only an invasive intervention can help, and the physician may unwittingly oblige regardless of predicable outcome (56). Again, much of this can only be ascertained with a more intricate psychological assessment. The question is not whether the patient has some underlying psychopathology but the extent to which mediating psychosocial factors are affecting outcome and whether those factors can be modified to maximize gain from the medical procedure.

The same issues exist for psychological screening for other procedures, including spinal column stimulation. For example, a review of the literature suggests that spinal column stimulation results in a relatively poor return-to-work rate, slightly more than 10%, for a range of possible reasons. Hence, it may not be realistic for the physician or patient to assume return to work will ensue, lest all parties be disappointed after completion of the rather expensive undertaking. Similarly, studies have not shown that opioid maintenance results in discernible improvements in function. Hence, the patient may achieve pain relief but may require intervention such as functional restoration if improvement in activity levels is expected. In turn, the patient should be rigorously screened from rehabilitation or functional restoration programs if his or her expectation lies solely with pain relief. We are reminded of the patient who stated that she was "pretty content with what I'm doing.

My relationship is better since I'm at home. I just need some relief of this pain." Again, the responsible psychological assessment should address a range of these issues.

CONCLUSIONS

While psychological assessment has been occurring since the development of pain treatment centers, established standards for assessment remain lacking. The past 10 years have shown an increase in the development of formal instruments, though issues of predictive validity, clinical utility, and cost have not been addressed. The following guidelines should be considered when designing an assessment protocol:

Determine the reasons for assessment, such as screening, establishing a pretreatment baseline, treatment planning, and disability determination.

Prepare the patient for assessment with appropriate introductory materials and instruments intended to reduce fear of the evaluation session.

Acquire data from all relevant sources whenever possible, including information that predates the development of the pain complaint.

Select instruments relevant to the particular pain population. This includes instruments with adequate psychometric properties and normative data.

Use computer-based interpretive systems cautiously.

Avoid drawing extensive conclusions from a single instrument.

Use an interview format and testing that address the range of problem areas with chronic pain, such as quality of life, perceived disability, cognitive distortions, long-standing coping deficits and skills, and influence of home and work on disability.

The practice of sending the patient for formal psychological testing persists, while the patient and clinician can achieve much more by a thorough assessment as outlined in this chapter. Many of the structured inventories and assessment approaches can also be effectively used in a primary care setting, and consultation with the psychologist can add more critical data for shaping a successful treatment plan.

References

1. International Association for the Study of Pain. Task force guidelines for desirable characteristics for pain treatment facilities. Seattle: IASP, 1991.
2. Mayer TG, Gatchel RJ. Functional restoration for spinal disorders: the sports medicine approach. Philadelphia: Lea & Febiger, 1988.
3. Dworkin SF, Whitney CW. Relying on objective and subjective measures of chronic pain: guidelines for use and interpretation. In: Turk DC, Melzack R, eds. Handbook of pain assessment. New York: Guilford Press. 1992;429–446.
4. Gamsa A. The role of psychological factors in chronic pain: 2. A critical appraisal. Pain 1994;57:17–29.
5. Carr DB, Jacox AK. Acute pain management guideline panel. In: Clinical practice guideline 1: acute pain management operative or medical procedures and trauma. AHCPR pub 92–0032. Washington: Department of Health and Human Services, 1992.

6. Williams DA. Acute pain management. In: Gatchel RJ, Turk DC, eds. Psychological approaches to pain management: a practitioners guide. New York: Guilford Press, 1996;55–77.
7. Deleted.
8. Jamison RN, Rudy TE, Penzien DB, Mosley TH Jr. Cognitive-behavioral classifications of chronic pain: replication and extension of empirically derived patient profiles. Pain 1994;57:277–292.
9. Turk DC, Rudy TE, Sorkin BA. Neglected topics in chronic pain treatment outcome studies: determination of success. Pain 1993;53:3–16.
10. Fishbain DA. Secondary gain concept: definition problems and its abuse in medical practice. Am Pain Soc J 1994;3:264–273.
11. American Medical Association guidelines. Guide to the evaluation of permanent impairment. 4th ed. Chicago: AMA, 1993.
12. Magni G, Moreschi C, Rigatti-Luchini S, Merskey H. Prospective study on the relationship between depressive symptoms and chronic musculoskeletal pain. Pain 1994;56:289–207.
13. Gamsa A, Vikis-Freibergs V. Psychological events are both risk factors in and consequences of chronic pain. Pain 1991;44:271–277.
14. Diagnostic and Statistical Manual of Mental Disorders. 4th ed. Washington: American Psychiatric Association, 1994.
15. Holroyd KA, France JL, Nash JL, Hursey KG. Pain state as artifact in the psychological assessment of recurrent headaches sufferers. Pain 1993;53:229–235.
16. Singer EJ, Zorilla C, Fahy-Chandon B, et al. Painful symptoms reported by ambulatory HIV-infected men in a longitudinal study. Pain 1993;54:15–19.
17. Bruehl S, Carlson CR. Predisposing psychological factors in the development of reflex sympathetic dystrophy: a review of the empirical evidence. Clin J Pain 1992;8:287–299.
18. Reference deleted.
19. Reference deleted.
20. Reference deleted.
21. Chapman CR, Cox GB. Anxiety, pain, and depression surrounding elective surgery: a multivariate comparison of abdominal surgery patients with kidney donors and recipients. J Psychosom Res 1977;21:7–15.
22. Gill KM, Ginsberg B, Muir M, et al. Patient-controlled analgesia in postoperative pain: the relations of psychological factors to pain and analgesic use. Clin J Pain 1990;6:137–142.
23. Turk DC, Okifuji A. Detecting depression in chronic pain patients: adequacy of self reports. Behav Res Ther 1994;32:9-16.
24. DeWilliams AC, Richardson PH. What does the BDI measure in chronic pain? Pain 1993;55:259–266.
25. Rudy TE. Multiaxial assessment of pain: multidimensional pain inventory. Computer program manual version 2.1 technical report. Pittsburgh: Pain Evaluation and Treatment Institute, 1989.
26. Turk DC, Rudy TE. The robustness of an empirically derived taxonomy of chronic pain patients. Pain 1990;43:27–36.
27. Perry F, Parker RK, White PE, Clifford A. Role of psychological factors in postoperative pain control and recovery with patient-controlled analgesia. Clin J Pain 1994;10:57–63.
28. Romano JM, Turner JA. Chronic pain and depression: does the evidence support a relationship? Psychol Bull 1984;97:18–34.
29. Steer RA, Beck AT, Garrison B. Applications of the Beck Depression Inventory. In: Sartorius N, Ban TN, eds. Assessment of depression. Heidelberg: Springer, 1985;123–142.
30. Kerns RD, Jacob MC. Assessment of the psychosocial context of the experience of chronic pain. In: Turk DC, Melzack R, eds. Handbook of pain assessment. New York: Guilford Press, 1992;235–253.
31. McCracken LM, Gross RT. Does anxiety affect coping with chronic pain? Clin J Pain 1993;9:253–259.
32. Polatin PB, Kinney RK, Gatchel RJ, et al. Psychiatric illness and chronic low back pain. Spine 1993;18:66–71.
33. Arniz A, Dressen L, DeJong P. The influence of anxiety on pain: attentional and attributional mediators. Pain 1994;56:307–314.
34. Arntz A, DeJong P. Anxiety, attention and pain. J Psychosom Res 1993;37:423–432.

35. Derogatis LR, Melisaratos N. The brief symptom inventory: an introductory report. Psychol Med 1983;13:595–609.

36. Spielberger CD. Manual for State-Trait Anxiety Inventory (Form Y). Palo Alto, CA: Consulting Psychologists Press, 1983.

37. VonKorff M, Dworkin SF, LeResche L, Kruger A. Epidemiology of temporomandibular disorders: TMJ pain compared to other common pain sites. In: Dubner R, Beghart GF, Bond MR, eds. Pain research and clinical management. Amsterdam: Elsevier, 1988:506–511.

38. Jensen MP, Turner JA, Romano JM, Karoly P. Coping with chronic pain: a critical review of the literature. Pain 1991;47:249–283.

39. Shutty MS Jr, DeGood DE, Tuttle DH. Chronic pain patients' beliefs about their pain and treatment outcomes. Arch Phys Med Rehab 1990;71:128–132.

40. Turner JA, Deyo RA, Loeser JD, et al. The importance of placebo effects in pain treatment and research. JAMA 1994;271:1609–1614.

41. Jensen MP, Karoly P. Self-report scales and procedures for assessing pain in adults. In: Turk DC, Melzack R, eds. Handbook of pain assessment. New York: Guilford Press, 1992;135–151.

42. DeGood DE, Shutty MS Jr. Assessment of pain beliefs, coping, and self efficacy. In: Turk DC, Melzack R, eds. Handbook of pain assessment. New York: Guilford Press, 1992;1992:214–234.

43. Cheatle MD, Brady J P, Ruland T. Chronic low back pain, depression, and attributional style. Clin J Pain 1990;6:114–117.

44. Williams DA, Robinson ME, Geisser ME. Pain beliefs: assessment and utility. Pain 1994;59:71–78.

45. Lipchik GL, Milles K, Covington EC. The effects of multidisciplinary pain management treatment on locus of control and pain beliefs in chronic non-terminal pain. Clin J Pain 1993;9:49–57.

46. Bergner M, Bobbitt RA, Carter WB, Gilson BS. The Sickness Impact Profile: development and final revision of a health status measure. Med Care 1981;19:787–805.

47. Brooks WB, Jordan JS, Divins GW, et al. The impact of psychological factors on measurement of functional status assessment of the Sickness Impact Profile. Med Care 1990;28:793–804.

48. Deyo RA. Comparative validity of the Sickness Impact Profile and shorter scales for functional assessment of low back pain. Spine 1986;11:951–954.

49. Deyo RA. Practice variations, treatment fads, rising disability: do we need a new research paradigm? Spine 1993;18:2153–2162.

50. Fairbank JCT, Couper J, Davies J B, O'Brien JP. The Oswestry Low Back Pain Disability Questionnaire. Physiotherapy 1980;66:271–273.

51. Waddell G, Turk DC. Clinical assessment of low back pain. In: Turk DC, Melzack R, eds. Handbook of pain assessment. New York: Guilford Press, 1992;1992:15–36.

52. Romano JM, Turner JA, Jensen MP. The chronic illness problem inventory as a measure of dysfunction in chronic pain patients. Pain 1992;49:71–75.

53. Carlsson J, Lars-Erik, A, Christion B, Sullivan M. Health status in patients with tension headache treated with acupuncture or physiotherapy. Headache 1990;9:593–599.

54. Bacon NM, Bacon SF, Atkinson JH, et al. Somatization symptoms in chronic low back pain patients. Psychosom Med 1994;56:118–127.

55. Bohr TW. Fibromyalgia syndrome and myofascial pain syndrome: do they exist? In: Weintraub MI, ed. Neurologic clinics: malingering and conversion reactions. Philadelphia: Saunders, 1995;365–384.

56. Ochoa JL, Verdugo RJ. Reflex sympathetic dystrophy: a common clinical avenue for somatoform expression. In: Weintraub M I, ed. Neurologic clinics: malingering and conversion reactions. Philadelphia: Saunders, 1995;351–364.

57. Keller LS, Butcher JN. Assessment of chronic pain patients with the MMPI-2. Minneapolis: University of Minnesota Press, 1991.

58. Gatchel RJ. Psychological disorders and chronic pain, cause-and-effect relationships. In: Gatchel RJ, Turk D C, eds. Psychological approaches to pain management: a practitioners guide. New York: Guilford Press, 1996:33–52.

59. Lynch ME. Psychological aspects of reflex sympathetic dystrophy: a review of the adult and pediatric literature. Pain 1992;49:337–347.

60. Merskey H, Lau CL, Russell ES, et al. Screening for psychiatric morbidity, the pattern of psychological illness and premorbid characteristics in four chronic pain populations. Pain 1987;30:141–157.

61. Matheson LN. Symptom magnification syndrome. In: Isemhagen SJ, ed. Work injury: management and prevention. Rockville, MD: Aspen, 1988:257–282.

62. King SA. Concept of secondary gain: how valid is it? Am Pain Soc J 1994;3:279–281.

63. Gallagher RM. Secondary gain in pain medicine: let us stick with biobehavioral data. Am Pain Soc J 1994;3:274–278.

64. Domino JV, Haber J D. Prior physical and sexual abuse in women with chronic headache: clinical correlates. Headache 1987;27:310–324.

65. Grunau RVE, Whitfield ME, Petrie JH, Fryer EL. Early pain experience, child and family factors as precursors of somatization: a prospective study of extremely premature and full term children. Pain 1994;56:353–359.

66. Wurtele SK, Kaplan GM, Keaimes M. Childhood sexual abuse among chronic pain patients. Clin J Pain 1990;6:110–113.

67. Bradley LA, Haile JM, Jaworski TM. Assessment of psychological status using interview and self-report instruments. In: Turk DC, Melzack R, eds. Handbook of pain assessment. New York: Guilford Press, 1992;193–213.

68. VonKorff M, Dworkin SF, LeResche L. Graded chronic pain status: an epidemiologic evaluation. Pain 1990;40:279–291.

69. Block AR, Kramer EF, Gaylor M. Behavioral treatment of chronic pain: the wife as a discriminative cue for pain behavior. Pain 1980;9:243–252.

70. Saarijarvi S, Rytokoski U, Karppi SL. Marital satisfaction and distress in chronic low back pain patients and their spouses. Clin J Pain 1990;2:148–152.

71. Bates MS, Edwards WT, Anderson KO. Ethnocultural influences on variation in chronic pain perception. Pain 1993;52:101–112.

72. Lipton JA, Marbach JJ. Ethnicity and the pain experience. Soc Sci Med 1984;19:1279–1298.

73. Wolff BB. Ethnocultural factors influencing pain and illness behavior. Clin J Pain 1985;1:23–30.

74. Fordyce WE, ed. Back pain in the workplace: management of disability in non-specific conditions. Seattle: IASP Press, 1995.

75. Mayer T, Gatchel R. Functional restoration for spine disorders: the sports medicine approach. Philadelphia: Lea & Febiger, 1988;122.

76. Kasl SV. Surveillance of psychological disorders in the work place: identifying and defining the issues. In: Keita GP, Sauter SL, eds. Work and well being: an agenda for the 1990's. Washington: American Psychological Association, 1992;73–95.

77. Occupational Stress Inventory. Odessa, FL: Psychological Assessment Resources, 1987.

78. Peters J, Large RG, Elkind G. Follow-up results from a randomized controlled trial evaluating in- and out-patient pain management programs. Pain 1992;50:41–50.

79. Tait RC, Chibnall JT, Richardson WD. Litigation and employment status: effects on patients with chronic pain. Pain 1990;43:37–46.

80. Chapman SL, Brena SF. Patterns of conscious failure to provide accurate self-report data in patients with low back pain. Clin J Pain 1990;6:178–190.

81. Block AR. Investigation of the response of the spouse to the chronic pain behavior. Psychosom Med 1981;43:415–422.

82. Weintraub MI, ed. Neurologic clinics: malingering and conversion reactions. Philadelphia: Saunders, 1995.

83. Standards Manual for Organizations Serving People with Disabilities. Tucson: Commission on Accreditation of Rehabilitation Facilities, 1993.

84. Kerns RD, Turk DC, Rudy TE. The West Haven-Yale Multidimensional Pain Inventory (WHYMPI). Pain 1984;23:345–356.

85. Turk DC, Wack JT, Kerns RD. An empirical examination of the "pain behavior" construct. J Behav Med 1985;8:119–130.

86. Getto CJ, Heaton RK, Lehman RA. PSPI: A standardized approach to the evaluation of psychosocial factors in chronic pain. Adv Pain Res Ther 1983;5:885–889.

87. Kulich RJ, Baker WK. Psychological evaluation in the management of chronic pain and disability. Curr Rev Pain 1997;1:116–125.

88. Huskisson EL. Visual analogue scales. In: Melzack R, ed. Pain measurement and assessment. New York: Raven Press. 1983;33–37.

89. Gramling SE, Elliott TR. Efficient pain assessment in clinical settings. Behav Res Ther 1992;30:72–73.

90. Melzack R. The McGill Pain Questionnaire: major properties and scoring methods. Pain 1975;1:275–299.

91. Jensen MP, McFarland CA. Increasing the reliability and validity of pain intensity measurement in chronic pain patients. Pain 1993;55:195–203.

92. Riley JL III, Robinson ME, Geisser ME, Wittmer VT. Multivariate cluster analysis of the MMPI-2 in chronic low back pain patients. Clin J Pain 1993;9:248–252.

93. Turk DC, Rudy TE. Toward the comprehensive assessment of chronic pain patients. Behav Res Ther 1987;25:237–249.

94. Trief PM, Yuan HA. The use of the MMPI in a chronic pain rehabilitation program. J Clin Psychol 1983;39:46–53.

95. Helmes E. What types of useful information do the MMPI and MMPI-2 provide on patients with chronic pain? Am Pain Soc Bull 1994;4:1–5.

96. Helmes E, Redden JR. A perspective on developments in assessing psychopathology: a critical review of the MMPI and MMPI-2. Psychol Bull 1993;113:453–471.

97. Naliboff BD, McCreary CP, McArthur DL, et al. MMPI changes following behavioral treatment of chronic low back pain. Pain 1988;35:271–277.

98. Guck T, Meilman P, Skultety F, Poloni L. Pain patients MMPI subgroups: evaluation of long term treatment outcome. J Behav Med 1988;11:159–169.

99. Swimmer GI, Robinson ME, Geisser ME. The relationship of MMPI cluster type pain, coping strategy and treatment outcome. Clin J Pain 1992;8:131–137.

100. Spengler DM, Ouelette EA, Battle M, Zeh J. Elective discectomy for herniation of lumbar disc. J Bone Joint Surg Am 1990;72:230–237.

101. Fordyce WE. Behavioral methods for chronic pain and illness. St. Louis: Mosby, 1976.

102. Fordyce WE, Roberts AH, Sternbach RA. The behavioral management of chronic pain: a response to critics. Pain 1985;22:113–125.

103. Keefe FJ, Dolan E. Pain behavior and pain coping strategies in low back pain and myofascial pain dysfunction syndrome patients. Pain 1986;24:49–56.

104. Keefe FJ, Gil KM. Behavioral concepts in the analysis of chronic pain syndromes. J Consult Clin Psychol 1986;54:776–783.

105. Greenough CG, Fraser RD. Comparison of eight psychometric instruments in unselected patients with back pain. Spine 1991;16:1068–1074.

106. Lollar DJ, Smits SJ, Patterson DL. Assessment of pediatric pain: an empirical perspective. J Pediatr Psychol 1982;7:267–277.

CHAPTER 23

A Cognitive Systems Approach to Treating Chronic Pain Patients and Their Families

Jeffrey B. Feldman, Leslie M. Phillips, and Gerald M. Aronoff

It is well established that the chronic pain experience is multidimensional, influenced by psychosocial factors and family systems (1–3). Therefore, it is paramount that physicians and other clinicians who treat chronic pain patients be familiar with these psychosocial and family influences. Indeed, it is quite possible to treat such patients correctly both medically and pharmacologically and have this treatment thwarted by incorrect beliefs about the pain or by dysfunctional family dynamics. For the chronic pain patient, the family environment is the primary one in which appropriate adaptation or maladaptation can occur, and as such families can be either physicians' best allies or their worst saboteurs. Those who treat chronic pain patients therefore need to be able to recognize cases in which family dynamics are contributing to maladaptation and refer such patients and their families for appropriate treatment (1).

Despite the literature supporting a family systems perspective in the rehabilitative treatment of chronic pain, individual treatment following a cognitive-behavioral model (4) remains the dominant paradigm. This model holds that pain-related cognitions and their resultant behaviors are the most important targets of rehabilitative chronic pain treatment (4). Given ample support for both the cognitive-behavioral and family systems models, it is necessary that those who treat chronic pain be well informed about both categories of influence on chronic pain, that is, family dynamics and pain-related cognitions and their associated behaviors.

This chapter examines both family systems and cognitive influences on chronic pain, providing a combined cognitive-systems conceptual framework with which to assess and treat chronic pain patients and their families. Patterns of dysfunction, cognitive beliefs, and family dynamics commonly seen in chronic pain patients are delineated. Guidelines by which to assess patients and determine appropriate treatment according to the degree of functional impairment, patterns of familial inter-

action, and pain-related beliefs are provided. Finally, the dynamics of treatment failure over the long term and the need to broaden intervention beyond the family system are discussed.

A COGNITIVE SYSTEMS APPROACH

In addition to appropriate medical workup of chronic pain patients, their beliefs about their pain, degree of life disruption, and familial interaction patterns also should be assessed. This is true particularly when patients are failing to show improvements with recognized effective medical and pharmacologic treatments. Cognitive-behavioral treatment focuses primarily on beliefs, or schemas, which are "internal maps" (5) by which individuals process, store, and act upon information (6). This therapy emphasizes a "collaborative empiricism" (6) whereby patient and therapist work together to identify and assess the validity of dysfunctional beliefs.

The importance of patient beliefs about chronic pain was demonstrated in a study by Jensen et al. (7), who found that patients' beliefs concerning their pain were better predictors of long-term rehabilitation success than were posttreatment activities, such as compliance with prescribed aerobic or strengthening exercises. Similarly, Lackner et al. (8) found self-efficacy beliefs were better predictors of task performance than were patients' judgments of their pain and potential injury. *Simply put, the best predictors of what patients could lift was what they believed they could lift.* These and related studies underscore the importance of pain-related schemas as influences on chronic pain.

However, the cognitive-behavioral perspective does not adequately address the importance of the family system (1). The family systems perspective that developed out of general systems theory holds that causation is bidirectional or circular rather than linear (9, 10). In the words of the family therapist Salvador Minuchin:

It [cognitive-behavioral therapy] presumes an action and a reaction, a stimulus and a response, or a cause and an effect. In the systems paradigm, every part of a system is seen as organizing and being organized by other parts. An individual's behavior is both caused and causative. A beginning or an end are defined only by arbitrary framing and punctuating. The action of one part is simultaneously the interrelationship of other parts of the system (11).

Given this, the focus of treatment is the family system as a whole (9). According to family systems theorists, families often develop maladaptive patterns of interaction that resist change, thus maintaining homeostasis (9, 11). However, healthy families adapt to both normal developmental changes in the family life cycle and to crises, such as acute or chronic illness. Thus families may have premorbid dysfunctional interactional patterns that are exacerbated by the presence of chronic pain, or they may be functioning adequately but fail to adapt to the crisis of chronic pain. Patterns of dysfunctional family interaction are detailed in the next section. Like faulty pain schemas, problematic family dynamics cast their own negative influence on chronic pain.

The cognitive-systems perspective proposed in this chapter recognizes the reciprocal relationship between pain schemas and the external systems by which they are influenced and that they in turn influence. Family systems help to create and maintain pain schemas, while these schemas interpret and shape family behavior patterns. Thus the assessment and treatment of chronic pain must take into account not only the faulty pain schemas but also the family and social systems that create and result from these schemas.

FAMILIES AND CHRONIC PAIN

The family is the social system of primary importance in generating and maintaining belief systems. While there are numerous approaches to the evaluation of families (1), we find it most useful to assess three dimensions: (*a*) the extent to which various family functions are being maintained, (*b*) the transactional patterns by which these are accomplished, and (*c*) the beliefs that support function or dysfunction. This is in keeping with our overall functional restoration approach and the cognitive-systems perspective previously described.

Family functions are carried out by subsystems of the family (i.e., spouse, parental, sibling subsystems), with members fulfilling roles and implicitly or explicitly assigned tasks (11). Table 23.1 provides a list of basic family functions. Families adapt to developmental stages and crises by changing roles and redistributing tasks. The influence of chronic pain on a family is readily assessed by determining the number of functions that are not continuing and/or the extent to which the member with chronic pain is exempted from such responsibilities. Often vocational functioning is limited or curtailed, with significant financial damage to the family. Less immediately, spiritual, social, recreational, and sexual activities are dis-

Table 23.1.   Family Functions

Financial support
Child rearing: caretaking, education, nurturance, playing, discipline
Domestic duties: housekeeping, cleaning, laundry, yard work, home maintenance
Feeding: shopping, cooking, washing dishes
Transportation: driving, vehicle maintenance
Emotional needs: intimacy, nurturance
Sexual needs
Spiritual needs
Relationships and responsibilities: extended family, friends
Social needs: friends, coworkers, business associates, organizations
Recreation: local, vacations

rupted, as is emotional support. Other family members, typically a spouse if present, take on the responsibilities of the person in pain without shifting his or her own role functions.

Family interaction patterns that support such dysfunction can be categorized as enmeshed, chaotic, or disengaged. *Enmeshed families have poorly defined boundaries* (11) *and are often solicitous of the member in pain.* In such families, if one person grimaces in pain, another winces. In this pattern family members frequently ask the member in pain, "How do you feel?" They are highly sympathetic and responsive to the individual's pain, asking what they can do to help, encouraging the individual to lie down or take medication, and taking on his or her usual family tasks. In this way, by providing attention and nurturance which might previously have been lacking and by exempting the person in pain from onerous or stressful tasks, they can be highly reinforcing of pain and pain behavior (4).

In contrast, disengaged families have rigid boundaries (11) *and largely withdraw from the person in pain.* Having accepted the person's inability to contribute to the family and meet spousal needs, family members attempt to maintain functioning without significant involvement of the individual in pain. Contact and communication are minimal, with problems in these areas often extant prior to the onset of the pain. In this way the pain can provide an excuse for distance between spouses whose relationship was already problematic.

It is also possible that over time, enmeshed patterns of interaction yield to disengagement in the face of prolonged frustration over being solicitous of the person in pain yet seeing him or her fail to improve. Both enmeshed and disengaged patterns are generally problematic for the family as a whole because other family members, typically the spouse, are overburdened by the responsibilities previously carried out by the person with pain. Their needs often are not being met, and they may feel dissatisfied and overwhelmed. In struggling to adapt, they may alternate between being solicitous and disengaged with the person in pain. Family functions may be delayed or simply not done by a spouse unaccustomed to doing them. Many women, for example, while feeling unable to do household chores complain about the inadequacy of the way it is done by the husband, further discouraging the husband from doing such activities. Family life simply becomes more chaotic and dysfunctional. This is the case particularly when family tasks were marginally or chaotically conducted before the onset of morbidity and when patterns of emotional intimacy were erratic and/or conflictual. *Chaotic families, therefore, may alternate between enmeshed and disengaged interactions, be unclear about role functioning, and be erratic in carrying out family tasks.*

Beliefs about people in pain, how they should be treated, and what should be expected of them underlie and reinforce dysfunctional patterns. Common dysfunctional beliefs about chronic pain and how a family member with such a condition should be treated are listed in Table 23.2. The individual beliefs listed in the table were delineated by Jensen and Karoly (12) through factor analysis of the items used in their Survey of Pain Attitudes. To these items we have added a list of corresponding family beliefs that reinforce the pain patients' beliefs and increase the likelihood of family dysfunction. These dysfunctional beliefs largely revolve around notions that hurt means harm, that rest and inactivity are the appropriate responses to pain, and that consequently family members should not expect the person in pain to do much. These beliefs also largely determine the interactions of such families. Many families believe that loving and caring for the person in pain should be expressed by constant care and solicitation regarding the pain and by verbal expressions of sympathy or nonverbal expressions of distress in response to the loved one's pain. Family members typically limit the patient's activities when they believe that the family member tends to overdo activities or can't be counted on to use reasonable caution. Another relatively common dysfunctional chronic pain dynamic occurs when a person, usually a spouse, champions the family member in pain against a seemingly unfeeling and indifferent medical system that can't seem to find the cause of the pain; the champion becomes the spokesperson or advocate for just how terribly the person in pain has been treated. The degree to which the family system adamantly and emotionally expresses such beliefs is one indication of how difficult they may be to change.

ASSESSMENT AND TREATMENT

Numerous issues should be considered in the assessment and treatment of chronic pain patients. These include adequacy of medical diagnosis, appropriateness of medication use, drug-seeking behavior, sleep interference, pain amplification, abnormal illness behavior, current and past psychological and psychiatric symptoms, and medical history, all of which are more fully discussed elsewhere in this volume (Chapters 5, 20, 21, 23, 24, 40). In this section we limit our focus to the assessment and treatment of dysfunctional patterns of behavior and thinking characteristic of chronic pain patients and their families. The cognitive systems approach, which evaluates family functioning, pain-related beliefs, and family interaction patterns, provides the conceptual framework. Intervention strategies based on mild, moderate, or severe impairment of the patient and family will be presented.

Table 23.2.   Cognitive Beliefs Concerning Pain

	Individual	Family
Control	The amount of pain I feel is completely out of my control.	We cannot expect him to control himself when he's in pain.
Disability	My pain would stop anyone from leading an active life.	We cannot expect her to contribute to the family.
Harm	If I exercise, I could make my pain problem much worse.	Don't allow him to be active: he could make himself worse.
Emotion	No matter how I feel emotionally, my pain remains the same.	That's not how she really feels; it's the pain speaking.
Medication	I will probably always have to take medication (for my pain).	Encourage him to take his pain medication when he hurts.
Solicitude	When I am hurting, people should treat me with care and concern.	She particularly needs our care and attention when she hurts.
Medical Care	When I find the right doctor, he or she will know how to reduce (cure) my pain.	We need to support his efforts to find the right doctor to cure him.

Categories of beliefs and examples of individual cognitions from the Survey of Pain Attitudes, Jensen & Karoly, 1991.

Functional Status

A major factor in determining the appropriate level of treatment is the extent to which the patient is maintaining prepain activities. The assessment of a person's functional status should include current work capacity, ability to conduct activities of daily living, functional tolerances (such as walking, sitting, and standing) and participation in social and leisure activities. A useful question in this regard is, "What is your typical day like currently, and how does it compare with a typical day before your pain began?" Assessment should further include overall evaluation of the family. Table 23.1 provides a list of family functions. The clinician should determine the degree to which these are being carried out and by whom. While such functions as work status and the carrying out of domestic chores are usually readily shared upon interview, others, such as the meeting of sexual and emotional needs, are less likely to be reported. It usually is worthwhile to interview both the patient and spouse to get their perspectives as well as to have a questionnaire that assesses the spouse's views concerning the patient and the pain's effect on the family (1). In general, the greater degree of impairment or degree of disparity between current and premorbid family functioning, the more aggressive and comprehensive the treatment needed. The interplay among the underlying belief systems of the patient and family, family interaction patterns, and patient dysfunction often requires an intensive team approach.

Further discussion categorizes patients according to mild, moderate, or severe levels of impairment. It should be understood that in clinical practice patients present along a continuum, without clear-cut distinctions between these levels of impairment.

Mild Impairment

Assessment of impairment must begin with careful biopsychosocial assessment, as noted in Chapters 5, 20, 21, and 40). If functioning is only mildly limited but the trend is toward decreasing activity on a pain-contingent basis, psychological or family intervention is indicated as an adjunct to appropriate medical care and prescribed physical or occupational therapy. While such intervention does not require the combined efforts of an interdisciplinary treatment team needed for more involved patients, treatment is most effective when providers work as a team with ongoing communication and common treatment goals.

Medical patients often resist referral to a psychologist or psychiatrist, particularly chronic pain patients, who frequently infer that the referring physician believes the pain is imaginary (4). A thorough explanation of the nature of the diagnosis is necessary. One must next clarify that all that should be done medically has been done despite the patient's ongoing pain. In other words, no further diagnostic tests or interventional procedures are warranted. Furthermore, one should emphasize that hurt is not going to cause harm and that patients can function with paced activity within medical restrictions.

Patients frequently react with anger to their perception that the physician is simply telling them they must just learn to live with it. Our general response is to normalize such anger and frustration, as well as the feelings of loss for one's former pain-free life. Feldman expresses to patients that telling someone to learn to live with chronic pain is like throwing someone into the ocean in a storm and saying, "Learn to swim." Most people need help if they are not to drown. Similarly, many patients can benefit from being taught the skills necessary to cope with chronic pain. Such coaching can best be done by a trained professional experienced in working with chronic pain. Furthermore, not only the patient but the family must mourn the loss of their prior pain-free life and make the significant changes necessary to cope with this chronic condition. Pointing out the family's functional difficulties (Table 23.1), the physician can, with benevolent authority (13), indicate that it is normal for the entire family to need professional help with the rehabilitation process.

Fixed beliefs and maladaptive family interactions are indications of resistance to adaptive coping with chronic pain. As previously noted, there is a relationship between level of functional impairment, the underlying belief systems, and the family dynamics of chronic pain patients. Table 23.2 lists commonly held pain-related beliefs. These may change or become more entrenched with time and reinforcement by family members. At an early stage the physician can evaluate the patient and family's response to explanations regarding diagnosis, how hurt will not cause harm, and recommendations for paced functional activity. Repeated requests for more diagnostic tests, referral to another specialist, or ongoing questioning concerning new medical developments at major medical centers are signs of cognitive resistance to change.

Patients or family members often simply say, "There must be something that can be done somewhere." Ongoing concern by family members that activity is making the patient worse and that rest and medication are the most appropriate ways to cope with pain are further warning signs. Such beliefs are almost certainly reinforced by the family's solicitous or protective responses and their sympathetic focus on the pain. Attempting to be supportive, close or enmeshed families generally contribute to the development of chronic pain syndrome. Enmeshed families need to be referred to a professional experienced in working with such patients and families before such patterns become entrenched.

Moderate Impairment

Patients evidencing moderate impairment are functioning at a significantly lower level than their premorbid state. They may still be working but most likely have given up many household chores and social and leisure activities. Patients frequently report that they are just making it through the day at work and then coming home and collapsing. Often finances are a problem because of decreased work capacity and/or medical costs. Sexual activity has generally decreased or ceased, adding to the strain on the marital relationship. Associated mood disturbance may develop, with the patient increasingly feeling loss of control.

Individual and family beliefs regarding the pain are likely to have progressively greater influence on the patient and family's behavior at the moderate level of impairment. Families may justify and even support the mood disturbance with the belief that he or she cannot be expected to control himself or herself when in pain (Table 23.2). Loss of functioning resulting from decreased activity may be interpreted by both the individual and family as indicating that the pain is getting worse. This may lead them to believe that there must be something the physicians have not found or that there has been a change in the underlying condition requiring further medical investigation. Family members feel that they are doing the right thing by supporting their loved one in advocating for his or her care and in "finding the right doctor." Families that tended toward enmeshment are likely to become more so in the face of the patient's progressive decline. Pain tends to be a frequent topic of conversation and subject of family focus. Family members are likely to have assumed many of the chores and responsibilities of the patient.

Alternatively, with some families the patient's credibility may come into question. This can occur when the family observes that the patient can do what he or she wants to do despite the pain but cannot do things that the spouse or other family members want him or her to do. Such perceptions can lead to an increasing frequency of angry "punishing responses" (14). This mounting frustration and anger can occur even when the reality of the pain is not at issue. The patient generally perceives family members as unsupportive, resulting in further passive-aggressive pain behavior. Increasingly disengaged or chaotic family interactions often ensue.

Moderately impaired chronic pain patients generally require an intermediate level of pain rehabilitation. This treatment involves an interdisciplinary team led by a physician experienced in working with chronic pain patients. Other disciplines usually include psychology, physical therapy, and nursing and may also include occupational therapy, exercise physiology, and vocational and pastoral counseling. Our intermediate program involves patient participation 4.5 hours a day, 2 days a week for 6 weeks. The treatment focuses on functional restoration and personal pain management. It involves a combination of structured physical reconditioning, instruction in pain management, and cognitive-behavioral psychological intervention. Through involvement in the treatment center and with an increasingly functional peer group of chronic pain patients, the individual is exposed to experiences and beliefs at variance with those supported in the family. The patient is encouraged to communicate changes fostered in the program to family members. In addition, goals are formulated to generate change in family functioning. Furthermore, family change is targeted through group education sessions and family conferences.

Severe Impairment

Patients with severe impairment usually are not working or have significant interference in vocational functioning. Typically they have ceased most social and leisure pursuits. They are doing few if any household chores, with the burden shifted to other family members. There is often a high degree of medical utilization, opioid dependence without adequate control of pain and suffering, and/or drug-seeking behavior. Sleep is highly disrupted, sexual activity has ceased, and there is a good deal of intrapersonal and interpersonal distress. Finances are usually strained, and there has been a severe degree of general life disruption for the patient and family.

The belief systems of patients and families experiencing severe impairment are correspondingly dysfunctional. Patients generally feel that the pain is in control of their life and develop a sense of helplessness and hopelessness. Family members often become resigned to such affective disturbance and develop a depressed family mood. Hurt is equated with harm, with the patient becoming progressively less functional and the family becoming increasingly resigned. Despite numerous medical consultations, there is a poor understanding of the pain condition, leading to continued doctor shopping and cure seeking.

The likelihood of dysfunctional family interaction patterns is quite high with this degree of functional impairment and distorted pain beliefs. Progressive enmeshment with frequent solicitude, nearly an exclusive pain focus, and an entrenched pattern of reinforcement of disability are common. Such enmeshment can actively sabotage treatment attempts. These families often develop an "us versus them" mentality. They generally are resistant if not openly hostile to treatment providers, especially those attempting to change the family's behavior. Alternative forms of resistance come from families who have become disengaged from the person in pain. They may cohabit with the individual but are emotionally and behaviorally estranged from him or her. In such cases the pain is viewed as the patient's problem, with overt resistance by other family members in involving themselves in his or her problem.

In cases of severe impairment a comprehensive pain rehabilitation program is the treatment of choice. This treatment also involves an interdisciplinary team of professionals coordinated by a physician experienced in both chronic pain management and a team approach. Treatment typically lasts all day, 5 days a week for 4 weeks. This may be done on an inpatient or outpatient basis, depending on the needs of the patient, with inpatients most frequently shifted to outpatient status as soon as clinically feasible. There are numerous indications for and goals of comprehensive treatment. These are discussed more fully in Chapter 40. From a cognitive systems perspective, the patient must be temporarily taken out of the dysfunctional family system and exposed to a different, more healthful system. The team and other patients who are further along in the rehabilitation process provide the model for the more healthful alternative system. Comprehensive treatment thus attempts to disrupt the homeostasis of the family system and expose the patient to an alternative system in which a new set of beliefs and behaviors are normative. Treatment necessarily begins with a focus on functional restoration by means of progressive exercise, which creates an experience at variance with the belief that hurt equals harm. The program also addresses faulty belief systems through cognitive-behavioral interventions, initially on an individual and later a family basis. This is done through family education sessions as well as individual family sessions that address the particular dysfunctional dynamics of the family. In summary, individual intervention is structured to create changes in thinking and behavior by extracting the patient from the family and exposing him or her to a functional system. Initial change in turn can reverberate through the rest of the family system, facilitated by programmatic interventions of team members as well as contact with other patient families.

CASE EXAMPLES
P. H.

P. H. was a 73-year-old divorced man referred for pain rehabilitation treatment by his oncologist. He had developed neuropathic pain secondary to cancer, which had been in full remission for more than 3 years. Prior to his referral for evaluation for pain rehabilitation, P. H. had another workup of the cancer that was entirely negative. He had also developed dependence on opiate analgesics during the cancer treatment, and at the time of his pain admission required high doses of such medication. The patient lived alone, but his adult children lived nearby and kept in frequent contact. Indeed, they voiced significant concerns about his continued ability to live independently and about his medication use. From the patient's viewpoint, his family initially supported him and continued to do so through the course of his cancer treatment. However, he currently viewed them as generally being unsupportive and inattentive. He resented their apparent indifference to his suffering as well as their stated concerns regarding his medication use. At least some of his family did indeed view the pain as psychogenic, or at least as a way for him to continue to get pain medications, and saw him as primarily chemically dependent. However, one particular member kept in frequent contact with him and did not doubt him but voiced concerns regarding his ability to live independently. This member tended to be solicitous of the patient and admitted feeling guilty if she did not maintain frequent contact.

The patient was admitted to a comprehensive pain rehabilitation program because he had continued severe pain in the absence of any active cancer, marked functional impairment, and significant medication dependency. He was initially treated as an inpatient to facilitate his opioid withdrawal and to assist with his self care. P. H. also had a significant comorbid depression, and antidepressant therapy was initiated. P. H.'s anger at his family became even more salient as he withdrew from the relatively high level of opioids. Counseling sessions with the patient and his family were initiated at this point. As the case was reviewed from the cognitive-systems perspective, it became clear that the family was initially quite solicitous of the patient but with the exception of the one member, gradually became disengaged. The initial family counseling sessions were designed to develop a common more healthful belief system regarding the pain, that is, that the pain was real but could be controlled without opiates, that hurt does not equal harm, and that the best way to cope with the pain is to focus on functional restoration. The pain was also reframed as a family problem and recovery a collective responsibility.

The patient's willingness to withdraw from opiates and work aggressively on his functioning did much to restore his credibility with disengaged family members. With this increased emotional support for his wellness, the patient was able to admit to the family that his medication use had become problematic, and that he had in part been using opiates for his depression. He further acknowledged using pain complaints to manipulate the family into spending more time with him. The family was able to plan time together rather than just see him in response to pain and to continue to support his wellness behavior. This included decreased solicitousness from the one member and replacement of this behavior with encouragement of independence and wellness. Ultimately the patient was able to return to independent living, stay off opiates, and continue to function well. He returned to a volunteer job he had held before the onset of his cancer and had weekly planned activities with his family.

This case illustrates the interaction between pain beliefs, family dynamics, and functional impairment in chronic pain. The functional restoration was necessary for him not only to improve himself physically but to develop the necessary self-efficacy and life data with which to modify his pain beliefs. However, the nature of the family dynamics were such that his

treatment gains would likely have been lost had he returned to the estrangement and manipulation that characterized his familial interactions.

A second case highlights the role of external sources in generating and perpetuating dysfunctional beliefs and creating disincentives to improved functioning.

B. C.

B. C. was a 43-year-old man evaluated by one of our pain center physicians because he had chronic back pain that began following a work-related fall 15 months earlier. The patient, a manager for a commercial real estate company, slipped and fell while making a business-related call. He reported falling flat on his back and hitting the back of his head upon impact. He described his pain as being constant and diffuse, encompassing his entire cervical, thoracic, and lumbar spine. He indicated that his pain level was constantly at least moderate and at times severe. He reported no pain in his legs, considerable difficulty with sleep secondary to his pain, and chest pain if he did not take alprazolam (Xanax).

B. C. had been extensively evaluated in southern California, where by his report he was told that while he did not have a surgical lesion, he had "eight herniated disks," some areas in which nerves were "crushed," and "severe arthritis." He reported being told by a physician that he had "enough injuries for three people to get disability." The patient further reported that upon physician recommendation he had spent 9 to 10 months in bed at different points since his injury. He had a trial of five or six epidural blocks that resulted in only intermittent and partial relief. He also reported attempting physical therapy at different times. He believed that the high level of medication he was on blocked the pain to such an extent that he greatly "overdid it," resulting in substantial increase in pain. It was our evaluating physician's assessment, after review of all records, prior scans, and a physical examination, that B. C. suffered from probable myofascial pain, was very deconditioned, and had developed a chronic pain syndrome with associated dysfunctional pain behaviors, poor coping, cognitive distortions, diminished activities of daily living, and global life disruption.

B. C. was a pleasant, intelligent, and articulate man who appeared to be sincerely seeking help. He described himself prior to injury as highly active and driven. Reportedly successful in his business, he was offered a higher-level position with another company prior to his injury. His premorbid personality style was confirmed by his wife, who reported in a family session later in treatment that when they met in high school she was very impressed by his take-charge manner. She described him as the leader of their neighborhood group of friends and indicated that he was a gifted athlete and that he always was a go-getter. Their marriage evolved to one of traditional roles, he working 10 to 12 hours a day and she staying at home with their children, who at the time of treatment were aged 9 and 4. B. C. described a strong sense of responsibility to his family and expressed feelings of guilt for what he had "put them through" since his injury. Concerned about his family's financial welfare, he had hired an attorney who was able to help him obtain Social Security disability. With the Social Security disability and worker's compensation payments, the family relocated to an area where the cost of living would be substantially less in an attempt to accept and cope with the disability.

B. C. reported significant symptoms of depression, feeling that he had "lost most of himself" since his injury. This was largely due to the patient's very high degree of perceived disability. On the Roland & Morris Disability Questionnaire (15) he endorsed all 24 items, indicating that his pain interfered with functioning in all areas of his life, limiting his ability even to dress himself. By comparison, the mean score of patients admitted to our program for comprehensive rehabilitation with chronic pain syndrome is 18. Probably reinforcing his sense of disability, despair, and anxiety was what he reported being told by his father, who had been disabled with back pain for a number of years: "You will get worse with time. Be very careful not to injure yourself more."

B. C. expressed a desire to be more functional despite his misgivings regarding the likelihood of improvement. He entered the comprehensive pain rehabilitation program initially on an inpatient basis. Though there were a number of setbacks, by the beginning of the third week he was able to drive himself 50 minutes from home, be on the treadmill for 24 minutes at his target heart rate, and do appropriate stretching and strengthening exercises. He began to consider the possibility of taking a job offered to him prior to his injury, believing that it would take about 6 more months of rehabilitation on his own after completion of the 4-week program to be able to consider it seriously.

In individual sessions B. C. spoke very highly of his wife in terms of her appearance, intelligence, and child-rearing skills. His major short-term goal was to be functional enough to take care of the children and some household tasks so that his wife could go out to work. He spoke with pride of her many skills and abilities and how she would easily be able to get a job. It took a while, though, for him to agree to schedule a conference with his wife. He ostensibly was protective of her time since she was busy with the children, chores, and job search and also because he did not want to further burden her because she had "been through so much already."

Mrs. C. presented as an intelligent woman who articulately expressed her concerns for her husband. Believing from experience that her husband tended to overdo things, she was concerned that he was being asked to do too much too soon. She had understandable concerns generated by the physicians they had seen earlier, his prior experiences in physical therapy, and the words of her father-in-law, that hurt would cause her husband harm. The fact that her husband was doing so much more on much less medication was not as impressive to her as his pain flare-ups, which were causing him "agonizing" sleepless nights. Explanations that pain often temporarily worsens in rehabilitation before people get better and that these flare-ups seemed to correspond to some impulsive overactivity on his part were met with skepticism. As her husband seemed to want to protect her from any demands the program might make on her, she wanted to protect him from program demands that might increase his pain. Their genuine concern for each other seemed to enmesh them in a dysfunctional homeostasis.

The opportunity to explore the possibility that Mrs. C. might also be resistant to change because of her newly elevated role in the family relative to her husband did not develop. The fact that the goals of the program would ultimately work counter to his case for continued disability was openly discussed with B. C. from the initial evaluation and throughout treatment. He thought that this would not be a problem until some time in the distant future. He was not prepared to jeopardize the financial welfare of his family, however. When he received notice of an upcoming hearing to reduce his benefits, he reported that he needed to leave the program. He evidently was advised by his attorney to discontinue the program and follow the advice of physicians who were more familiar to the attorney and supportive of B. H.'s case for disability benefits. In this way the disincentives of the system, the powerful voices advocating for and advising him, and his genuine concern for the welfare of his family overwhelmed the fragile beginnings he had made towards regaining a more functional life.

SYSTEMS BEYOND THE FAMILY

The treatment of chronic pain often fails because of multiple interacting systems that influence and inform patients and their families. While B. C. had only tentatively begun to move toward greater functioning, all too often even patients who make promising substantial changes in behavior and cognition do not maintain long-term gains. A cognitive-systems approach must therefore look at the external realities that influence patients and families, shaping the choices they make. Unless these external systems and the information they convey is accurately understood, judgments and decisions on the part of patients, families, physicians, and the treatment team will be flawed, distorted, incomplete, or inaccurate. Often the most important and problematic of these judgments and decisions involve return-to-work issues.

Return to work, while not the sole purpose of chronic pain rehabilitation, is often an integral part of a functional restoration approach. Treatment success or failure is increasingly judged, particularly in the eyes of third-party payers, by its ability to return patients to work or bring patients to maximum medical improvement, evaluate impairment, and bring closure to protracted workers compensation cases (13). Ability to return to work is generally judged by the patient's documented medical impairment and physical capacity. The literature on pain and work injuries repeatedly indicates, though, that psychosocial factors often are more important than physical factors in predicting who will report a work-related injury and who will successfully return to work (16–20). The literature does not find any single factor or specific cluster of factors as uniformly predictive of injury or return to work. Rather, many interacting factors on multiple system levels are involved in work-related injury and rehabilitation. A list of physical, psychosocial, environmental, and other system factors culled from the literature and our clinical experience is presented in Table 23.3. Full discussion of all of these factors is beyond the scope of this chapter; however, we can briefly mention the most frequently relevant that influence and inform the patient and family. These include the employer, the workers compensation system, physicians, and attorneys.

Assuming that individuals act according to their perception of their best interest, it is likely that patients will not have a return-to-work mind set if they believe that they will be reinjured, fired, or laid off upon returning to work and if financial incentives make disability a more attractive alternative. Patients report feeling hurt, disheartened, and angry when they do not hear from their supervisor or company representative after they are injured. This is so particularly if they worked at the company for a significant number of years. Even more problematic are employer statements of no limited duty or "can't take them back until they are fully recovered." Also, many patients verbalize an understanding of an unwritten rule that being laid off is significantly more probable following an injury claim (21). Furthermore, neither the employer nor the insurance carrier is generally willing to pay for education or retraining of the employee, although this policy prolongs payment of compensation benefits. The lack of a perceived viable alternative to disability is where rehabilitation most often fails (22).

The workers compensation system interacts with the employer and is an adversarial care system. Discussing this in relation to work-related injury, Bigos et al. (21) wrote, "The creation of the term industrial back pain apparently fostered the development of adversarial attitudes and expensive systems that have only worsened the burden by expanding costs without returning the injured worker to productivity. 'Adversarial help' seems, and mostly is, a contradiction in terms." It is our experience that employer human resource departments, insurance company personnel, and case managers often view injured workers with an adversarial mind set, presuming they are guilty of malingering (or at least embellishment) until proven otherwise. Sensing a negative attitude toward them and viewing their integrity as challenged, patients are often wary of the medical care they are directed toward. Viewing physicians as "company doctors," patients process information negatively, especially if they do not feel they are courteously treated or thoroughly examined. Through the negative lens of this adversarial schema, patients faced with persistent pain often do not believe everything that should be done for them has been done. Since what is desired is easily believed (22), patients seek physicians on their own who give them hope that they can be fixed through surgery. We often see patients who have been told by four or five physicians that surgery is not

Table 23.3.   Factors Influencing Chronic Pain and Return to Work

Physical
   Nature of injury
   Prior injuries, surgeries, treatment
   Other medical conditions
   Obesity
   Nicotine use
   Deconditioning
   Alcoholism, other addictions
Job related
   Time out of work
   Job demands
   Salary
   Wage replacement
   Job satisfaction
   Relationship with supervisor
   Relationship with coworkers
   Employer's commitment, flexibility
   Employment options
   Benefits
   Stress
   Commutation time and expense
Personal
   Age
   Education
   Transferable skills
   Personality variables
   Coping skills
   Personal values
   History of trauma or abuse
   Beliefs and understandings about injury and pain
   Fear of reinjury
   Anxiety
   Depression
   Marital and family situation
Other
   Perceived treatment by insurance company, rehab nurse, employer, physician
   Perceived adequacy of treatment
   Physician warnings and advice
   Attorney warnings and advice
   Union status
   Economic climate

appropriate but who cling to the belief that their pain will be cured by surgery because one physician gave them a 50% chance that they can be helped by surgery. Patients with such beliefs, embedded within a more general negative view of workers compensation, often perceive rehabilitation as a further extension of the adversarial arm of the insurance company. A recent patient responded to the first question on our intake questionnaire concerning the reason for his visit by stating, "The insurance company will not pay for the surgery I need." Attending physicians can be equally problematic in fostering disability. Patients report to us that they have been told by physicians such things as "You have a zero pound lifting restriction"; "Rehabilitation will only lead to injury"; "Your work days are over"; and as noted earlier, "You have enough wrong with your spine for three people to get disability."

Faced with an adversarial system in which they perceive themselves as unfairly treated and/or receiving inadequate

Chapter 23 Treating Chronic Pain Patients and Their Families 321

care, patients often turn to an attorney for assistance. Much controversy surrounds the issue of attorney involvement. Mundy et al. (24) report attorneys discouraging early return to work or modified duty. Cummings (22) stated that 90% of attorneys will not accept a case if the person wants to return to work. In contrast, Gallagher et al. (19), in an empirical evaluation of their patients, found that neither compensation status nor involvement of an attorney significantly improved prediction of return to work 6 months post discharge. While this may have been the case for their patients, we have found that when an attorney becomes involved in a case, it signals another step in an adversarial situation that often leads to greater cost and a poorer prognosis for successful rehabilitation.

From a cognitive-systems perspective we believe that to influence the beliefs and behaviors of patients we must be fully cognizant of the multiple interacting factors that affect patients and the sources of information fueling dysfunctional schemas. We cannot limit our lens to the individual or to the family systems level. Both cognitive and systems approaches require us to be aware of the interacting medical, legal, and occupational systems and the information they convey to the patient and family (3).

In contrast to the often indifferent, adversarial, and fragmented services for injured workers, which generate distrust, confusion, and ultimately greater cost, a consumer-oriented continuum of care is recommended. An admirable beginning toward a comprehensive customer service-oriented program for injured workers is health-care giant Columbia HCA's Florida Company Care initiative. Viewing both the employer and the injured worker as their customers, Company Care provides 24-hour emergency service to employees of contracted companies. Patients are seen in the same facility as those with private insurance, thereby reducing the "company doctor" perception. Patients are assigned a case manager and asked to complete a customer satisfaction survey. Sources of dissatisfaction are addressed, with every effort made to avoid an adversarial relationship. A follow-up appointment with patients is made in 3 days to assess recovery and address issues before they become problematic. Unless medically contraindicated, patients return to work, and arrangements with employers for modified duty are part of the original service contract. Injured workers are transported from their place of employment to their medical or physical therapy appointments by a Company Care vehicle. Since workers do not sit at home to "recover," disability behavior is not established and the potential for a disability mind set lessened. Patients who require physical therapy are referred to functionally oriented therapists who follow an established protocol of time-limited therapy. Patients who require assessment by a specialist see physicians from a panel who follow consensually established clinical protocols. In this way patients receive consistent messages from physicians reflecting the current best medical standards of care. Employers are viewed as both customers and partners, with efforts made to customize services to meet their needs. Education and injury prevention in addition to early intervention is emphasized. We have suggested further program development to identify and address the psychological factors that often underlie the "physical" injuries, especially for the approximately 10% of claimants who generate 80% of the costs in workers compensation (25–27).

SUMMARY

Chronic pain syndrome involves complex interactions among individuals in pain and the many people and social systems that influence and inform their beliefs. Of primary importance in this regard is the family, which can be a physician's best ally or worst saboteur in treatment. A cognitive-systems approach has been presented as a conceptual bridge between family systems and cognitive-behavioral treatment approaches. Using this perspective, one can assess the effect of chronic pain on the patient and family by evaluating the degree to which family functions are carried out and by whom, the cognitive beliefs of the patient and family members that support functioning or dysfunction, and the interaction patterns between family members. Guidelines for determining whether the patients should be treated in individual or family therapy or whether more comprehensive interdisciplinary treatment is warranted have been presented. It was argued that a comprehensive rehabilitation program is at times needed to initiate change in a patient enmeshed in a dysfunctional family homeostasis. It was further argued that all too often neither individual, family, nor program treatment is sufficient. The greatest barriers to successful rehabilitation tend to be the interacting occupational, medical, legal, and insurance systems, which can create adversarial relationships and/or disincentives to return to work. Only through changing these systems will we be able to reverse the suffering, dysfunction, and cost associated with chronic pain syndrome and our "disability epidemic" (13).

References

1. Kerns RD, Payne A. Treating families of chronic pain patients. In: Gatchel RJ, Turk DC, eds. Psychological approaches to pain management: a practitioner's handbook. New York: Guilford, 1996;283–304.
2. Kerns RD, Jacob MC. Assessment of the psychosocial context of the experience of chronic pain. In: Turk DC, Melzack R, eds. Handbook of pain assessment. New York: Guilford, 1994;235;253.
3. Goldberg PJ. The social worker, family systems, and the chronic pain family. In: Aronoff GM, ed. Evaluation and treatment of chronic pain. 2nd ed. Baltimore: Williams & Wilkins, 1992;465–474.
4. Turk DC, Meichenbaum DH, Genest M. Pain and behavioral medicine: a cognitive-behavioral perspective. New York: Guilford, 1983.
5. Lankton SR, Lankton CH. The answer within: a clinical framework of Ericksonian hypnotherapy. New York: Brunner/Mazel, 1983.
6. Beck AT, Rush AJ, Shaw BF, Emery G. Cognitive therapy of depression. New York: Guilford, 1979.
7. Jensen MP, Turner JA, Romano JM. Correlates of improvement in multi-disciplinary treatment of chronic pain. J Consult Clin Psychol 1994;62:172–179.
8. Lackner J, Carosella A, Feurstein M. Pain expectancies, pain and functional self-efficacy expectancies as determinants of disability in patients with chronic low back disorders. J Consult Clin Psychol 1996;64:212–220.

9. Hoffman L. Foundations of family therapy: a conceptual framework for systems change. New York: Basic Books, 1981.

10. Bateson G. Mind and nature. New York: E. P. Dutton, 1979.

11. Minuchin S, Rosman B, Baker L. Psychosomatic families: anorexia nervosa in context. Cambridge, MA: Harvard Unversity Press, 1978.

12. Jensen MP, Karoly P. Control beliefs, coping efforts, and adjustment to chronic pain. J Consult Clin Psychol 1991;59:431–438.

13. Aronoff G. Chronic pain and the disability epidemic. Clin J Pain 1991;7:330–338.

14. Kerns RD, Rosenberg R. Pain-relevant responses from significant others: development of a significant other version of the WHYMPI Scales. Pain 1995;61:245–250.

15. Roland M, Morris R. A study of the natural history of back pain: 1. Development of a reliable and sensitive measure of disability in low back pain. Spine 1983;8,141–144.

16. Bigos S, Battie M, Spengler, D, et al. A prospective study of work perceptions and psychosocial factors affecting the report of back injury. Spine 1991;16:1–6.

17. Bigos S, Battie M, Spengler, D, et al. A longitudinal, prospective study of industrial back injury reporting. Clinical Orthopaedics and Related Research 1992;279:21–34.

18. Lancourt J, Kettelhut M. Predicting return to work for lower back pain patients receiving worker's compensation. Spine 1992;17:307–310.

19. Gallagher RM, Williams RA, Skelly J, et al. Workers compensation and return to work in low back pain. Pain 1995;61:299–307.

20. Tate DG. Workers disability and return to work. Am J Phys Med Rehab 1992;71:92–96.

21. Bigos SJ, Baker R, Lee S. A definition and approach to helping the patient with a return to work predicament. Phys Med Rehab Clin North Am l993;4:109–123.

22. Cummings N. Psychotherapy and workers' compensation: golden opportunity or future disgrace? Workshop at the Brief Therapy Conference: Essence and Evaluation. Orlando, FL. Dec. 8–12, 1993; audiotape available from the Milton H. Erickson Foundation, Phoenix, AZ.

23. Reference deleted.

24. Mundy RR, Moore SC, Corey JB, Mundy GD. Disability syndrome: the effects of early vs. delayed rehabilitation intervention. Am Assoc Occup Health Nurs J 1994;42:379–383.

25. Spitzer WO. Scientific approach to the assessment and treatment of activity-related spinal disorders. Spine 1987;12 (Suppl):1.

26. Leavitt SS, Johnson TL, Beyer RD. The process of recovery: patterns in industrial back injury: costs and other quantitative measures of effort. Ind Med Surg 1971; 40:7.

27. Gatchel RJ, Polatin PB, Mayer TG, Gavey PD. Psychopathology and the rehabilitation of patients with chronic low back pain disability. Arch Phys Med Rehab 1994;75:666–670.

CHAPTER 24

Behavioral Management of Patients with Pain

Dennis C. Turk and Akiko Okifuji

In chronic pain, although pain may have begun with identifiable disease or injury, it persists beyond any expected period of healing, often for years. In a review of 65 studies of patients treated at multidisciplinary pain centers, the mean duration of pain exceeded 7 years. The prevalence of chronic pain and the myriad of problems associated with it have been well documented (1). Despite recent advances in the biomedical technologies that allow us to understand anatomical and physiological processes underlying many pain conditions, chronic pain continues to be a puzzle for health care providers. There are no treatments that consistently and permanently relieve chronic pain for all patients.

A person with chronic pain resides in a complex and costly world. The world is populated not only by patients but also his or her family members, health care providers, employers, and third-party payers (insurance companies, government). Chronic pain adversely affects these different persons in a range of ways. For example, family members feel increasingly hopeless and distressed as medical costs, disability, and suffering increase while income and treatment options decline. Health care professionals grow frustrated as treatment options are exhausted while the pain persists or even worsens. Employers, already resentful of growing workers compensation costs, have to manage decreased productivity. Third-party payers watch as health costs soar with repeated inconclusive diagnostic testing and failed treatment outcomes for the same chronic pain.

As the pain persists, those involved with the patient may begin to question the legitimacy of the complaints in the absence of objective biomedical findings. Some come to believe that the patient's complaints of pain are an attempt to gain attention, avoid undesirable activities, or seek disability compensation. Others may suggest that the pain is imaginary or the patient is outright malingering. In response to the skepticism, pain patients feel a strong need to prove the authenticity of their illness by increasing their complaints, which frequently results in doctor shopping and repeated laboratory tests and diagnostic procedures. Social isolation due to loss of work and withdrawal from social activities is common. Eventually pain becomes a central focus of life, leading to a redefinition of self-concept and social role.

Not knowing the mechanisms underlying unremitting pain is a source of considerable stress for pain patients. The labeling of their pain as chronic often leads to feelings of helplessness and a bleak future. Thus, it is hardly surprising to observe that patients experience a great deal of psychological distress, including feelings of self-preoccupation, demoralization, helplessness, frustration, anger, and depression. When viewed from this perspective, it becomes evident that assessment and treatment of chronic pain patients entail more than simple alteration of physiological pain pathways. As Melzack and Casey (2) suggest:

> The surgical and pharmacological attacks on pain might . . . profit by redirecting thinking toward the neglected and almost forgotten contributions of motivation and cognitive processes. Pain can be treated not only by trying to cut down sensory input by anesthetic blocks, surgical intervention . . . but also by influencing the motivational and cognitive factors (p 435).

In this chapter we discuss psychological perspectives of chronic pain. First we describe basic behavioral and cognitive paradigms and how those factors may contribute to the chronic pain experience. In the second part we discuss various treatment approaches that incorporate behavioral and cognitive methods. Note that the psychological treatments discussed in this chapter are not alternatives but important components of multidimensional treatment and rehabilitation programs that include biomedical and physical modalities.

PSYCHOLOGICAL FACTORS CONTRIBUTING TO CHRONIC PAIN

The importance of psychosocial and behavioral factors in the causation, severity, exacerbation, and maintenance of pain has been demonstrated repeatedly over the past quarter of a century (2, 3). The accumulated behavioral and cognitive research has facilitated understanding of chronic pain as a complex, multifactorial phenomenon. Treatments based on these psychological principles have been incorporated in more traditional rehabilitation programs.

Respondent Learning

Repeated pairings of pain and an event may produce a learned avoidance behavior through respondent learning, which has four primary components: unconditioned stimulus (US), unconditioned response (UR), conditioned stimulus (CS), and conditioned response (CR). A US is a stimulus capable of eliciting a UR in most persons. A UR is thus considered as a reflexive or innate response. Repeatedly pairing a US and a CS, which is a neutral stimulus, permits a CS alone to produce a response (CR) that is expected from the US (UR). In a simple example (Fig. 24.1) a patient feels pain every time he tries to exercise. Pain (US) elicits fear (UR). Exercise (CS) is paired with pain, and subsequently an attempt to exercise alone can elicit fear (CR).

Pain is quite salient as an unconditioned stimulus, capable of eliciting a range of negative emotional responses. Any neutral object or person may be associated with pain, and conditioned emotional responses may be acquired. For example, if a patient experiences pain (US) every time a physical therapist conducts a treatment session, fear or other negative emotional responses (UR) may result. An initially neutral object (exercise equipment) or person (physical therapist), paired repeatedly with pain experience, may elicit negative emotional responses from the patient. Table 24.1 shows the process of respondent conditioning.

A series of learning opportunities tend to result in higher learning and stimulus generalization. Sitting, walking, engaging in cognitively demanding work, social activity, sexual activity, and even thoughts about these activities may trigger anticipatory fear or other negative emotional responses. Subsequently, patients may display maladaptive responses to many objects, situations, or persons, including attempts to reduce conditioned emotional responses (negative emotional reactions) by avoiding those cues. According to this model, it is possible that the physical abnormality often observed in chronic pain patients, such as distorted gait and decreased range of motion, may actually be secondary to changes initiated in behavior through learning. With decreased activity, physical deconditioning increases the likelihood of experiencing pain upon even mild exercises, further prompting the person to avoid activities. Generalized avoidance of activities is likely to facilitate depression due to reduced level of positive reinforcement in life. The anticipation of suffering and avoidance of activities seem to contribute substantially to disability in chronic pain patients.

Operant Learning

A new era began in 1976, when Fordyce (3) proposed the principles of operant learning as a conceptual basis for understanding chronic pain. In the operant paradigm, behavior is assumed to be shaped and maintained by the nature of its consequence. Thus, the likelihood of behavior occurring in the future is determined by the consequence of that behavior in the past. If the behavior resulted in desired outcome, the behavior is likely to recur, whereas when consequences are undesirable, the probability of that behavior occurring again is diminished.

The central feature in the operant paradigm is observable behaviors. To understand chronic pain, therefore, Fordyce focused on behavioral manifestations of pain rather than pain per se. Manifestations of pain, or "pain behaviors," are considered as overt expressions of pain, distress, and suffering. In the acute pain situations, behaviors such as limping and avoiding physical activities are likely to be functional, preventing exacerbation of the symptoms, in particular, pain. However, when those overt behaviors result in a desirable consequence (i.e., are reinforced), those behaviors are likely to be maintained. For example, avoidance of physical activities in chronic pain (behavior) can be maintained by desirable consequences (reinforcer, e.g., sympathy from others) in the absence of nociceptive experience.

In addition, functional or "well" behaviors for chronic pain patients (e.g., physical activity, working) may not result in positive outcomes. Without reinforcement, well behaviors are not likely to be shaped and maintained. Table 24.1 displays the four types of reinforcement and their effects as postulated by the operant conditioning model. As we shall see, since the operant model of chronic pain is most concerned with overt behaviors, therapy based on the operant model consists of extinction of pain behaviors by withholding a desirable consequence and improvement in function by reinforcing well behaviors.

The primary difference between respondent learning and operant learning is that in operant learning, the consequence of behavior determines the likelihood of that behavior occurring again; by contrast, in respondent learning, the strength of pairing between a US and a CS is the most important factor. Despite the differences in mechanisms, operant learning and respondent learning seem to work together in maintenance of pain and inactivity. For example, avoidance of activity and resting, which result from conditioned fear and anticipated pain, are reinforced by the lack of pain experience.

Although the operant model of chronic pain has been extensively studied over the years, common misperceptions about it persist. For example, exhibition of pain behaviors by chronic pain patients is assumed always to be maladaptive, shaped and maintained *only* through contingencies of reinforcement. Although this assumption has rarely been challenged, data sug-

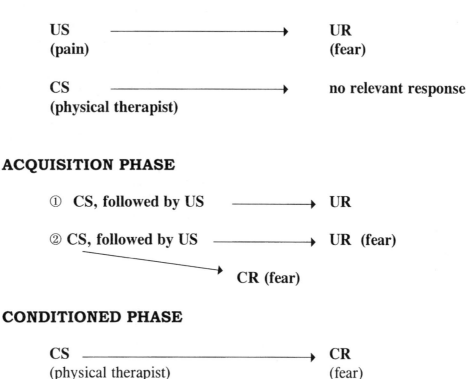

BEFORE THE CONDITIONING

US —————————————▶ UR
(pain)   (fear)

CS —————————————▶ no relevant response
(physical therapist)

ACQUISITION PHASE

① CS, followed by US —————————▶ UR

② CS, followed by US —————————▶ UR (fear)

CR (fear)

CONDITIONED PHASE

CS —————————————▶ CR
(physical therapist)   (fear)

Figure 24.1.   Respondent learning paradigm.

Table 24.1.   Operant Conditioning

Types of Conditioning	Consequence of Behavior	Probability of the Behavior Recurring
Positive reinforcement	Rewarding	⇑
Negative reinforcement	Withdrawing or avoiding something aversive	⇑
Punishment	Aversive	⇓
Punishment	Withdrawal of something rewarding	⇓

gest that factors other than operant learning may underlie exhibition of pain behaviors. In particular, biophysical findings and cognitive factors significantly predict the level of pain behaviors exhibited by chronic pain patients (4). Thus, thorough assessment is required to establish the function of pain behaviors and the clinical decision to modify them.

The concepts of secondary gain and symptom magnification are related to pain behaviors. Secondary gain is an "unplanned" behavioral process that is maintained because it presents fortuitous advantages. Similarly, symptom magnification may be reinforced by health care professionals. For example, the perception that health care professionals take pain complaints seriously is a heavily charged positive reinforcer for many chronic pain patients, especially for those whose complaints have been treated with suspicion. It is

unfortunately common that symptom magnification is viewed with disdain. Health care professionals often believe that patients have an ulterior motive of obtaining additional medications or disability payments. However, symptom magnification is not generally accompanied by awareness that those behaviors are being displayed but rather they may result from lack of attention. The old adage "the squeaky wheel gets the grease" is applied to complaints of pain, with greater attention given to more vociferous complaints and more dramatic pain behaviors.

Since overt pain behaviors are considered to be voluntary, chronic pain patients sometimes face accusations of being responsible for their own disability. It is important that pain behaviors not be considered as lack of motivation for getting well or malingering. Acquisition of any behaviors through associative learning is generally a gradual process, and pain behavior is no exception. That is, awareness of these behaviors as being reinforced is minimal or nonexistent. There is certainly no conscious deception on a patient's part but rather unintended performance of pain behaviors resulting from reinforcement contingencies. This should be separated from malingering, a *deliberate deception,* that is consciously motivated to achieve some desired outcome. It is commonly believed, especially among third-party payers, that a large proportion of chronic pain patients are malingerers, motivated to obtain financial gain. However, there is little support for this belief; on the contrary, feigning of chronic pain is rare (5).

Malingering, when it does occur, is usually readily detected by observation of patients' behaviors and physical examination.

Illness Behavior

A concept that is in some ways analogous to pain behavior is illness behavior. The major difference between the two concepts lies in the mechanisms that are believed to underlie the observed behavior. As noted, the operant paradigm postulates that behaviors are influenced by reinforcement contingencies (positive versus negative outcome), whereas illness behaviors are believed to be related to subjective appraisal processes.

Illness behavior is often considered synonymous with the sociological construct of the "sick role." However, the two concepts are not identical. The sick role is society's explicit norms and expectations regarding appropriate behaviors among those designated as ill (6). Society regards the sick role as a partially and conditionally legitimized state that a person may be granted, with the implicit assumption that the sick person accept that it is undesirable to be sick and recognize the obligation to cooperate with others for the purpose of achieving health as soon as possible. Furthermore, sick persons are expected to show clear evidence of having recognized this obligation by using the services of those whom the society regards as competent to diagnose and treat their illness. The sick role serves an important function for the patient; however, inactivity and overdependency of a patient on his or her spouse may become a core feature on which their marital relationship is based. In this sense the sick role may become maladaptive and the pain behaviors that are a feature of the sick role may be maintained.

The manner in which people monitor their bodies, respond to symptoms, and decide upon a remedial course of action was originally called illness behavior by Mechanic (7). The concept of illness behavior brings together all the psychological, social, and cultural influences on illness as well as the entire range of psychosocial consequences of being ill. People differ markedly, even with identical symptoms, in how frequently they complain about physical symptoms, in their propensity to visit physicians, and their response to the identical treatments. Often the nature of the patients' responses has little to do with their objective physical condition (7). For example, fewer than one third of those with clinically significant symptoms consult a physician (8).

People tend to notice bodily sensations when they depart from the ordinary baseline state. Because not all available information can be processed, some form of filtering is required. People whose affective states and physical functioning are changing attempt to make sense of what is happening by examining intuitive hypotheses about the seriousness of their problems and the need for attention (9, 10).

In their hypothesis testing, persons appraise new symptoms against prior experience as well as beliefs and expectations stored in memory. These representations of illness are based on the experiences of others and on general knowledge

(11). It is through a matching process of current state to established illness representations that people identify and evaluate symptoms, make interpretations of their causes and implications, and decide on types of help to seek.

Certain information is required to appraise symptoms accurately; yet in many instances only ambiguous and insufficient information is available. When information is vague or inadequate, it is more difficult to evaluate the likely outcome of various responses. Lazarus (12) noted, "The more ambiguous are the stimulus cues concerning the nature of the confrontation, the more important are general belief systems in determining the appraisal process." Most physical symptoms are ambiguous and thus are likely to be interpreted in light of preexisting beliefs. Misinterpretations of symptoms are likely to result in miscommunication between patients and health care providers. Thus, identification of specific appraisal processes can help account for a person's subjective presentation, and faulty attributions can become a target for therapeutic intervention.

Since originally described, the concept of illness behavior has been used in many ways. In the psychiatric literature it is frequently used with the modifier "inappropriate" or described as "abnormal illness behavior" (13). The latter phrase incorporates a rather arbitrary definition of abnormality with an emphasis on disability that is "disproportionate" to disease, a lifestyle that revolves around the illness role, and a perpetual search for additional medical care (14).

Abnormal illness behavior has been expanded in psychiatry to incorporate (a) mental disorders (e.g., hypochondriasis, somatoform disorders), (b) physical symptoms, (c) a dimension of behavior from denial to abnormal that is orthogonal to the extent of physical disability, and (d) a social explanation for maladaptive behavior (15, 16). The classification of abnormal illness behavior is made on the basis of a perceived discrepancy between the observed degree of somatic disease and the patient's reaction to it. Pilowsky (13) has defined abnormal illness behavior as the persistence of an inappropriate or maladaptive mode of perceiving, evaluating, and acting in relation to one's own state of health, despite the fact that a doctor or other appropriate social agent has offered a reasonable, lucid explanation of the nature of the illness and the appropriate management, based on a thorough examination and assessment of all parameters of functioning, including the use of special investigations when necessary, with a consideration for the sociocultural background. In an attempt to quantify and measure abnormal illness behavior, he developed an instrument, the Illness Behavior Questionnaire (17). However, the psychometric properties of the instrument have been seriously challenged (18, 19).

The concept of abnormal illness behavior assumes that the clinician's opinion is always accurate, that laboratory and other diagnostic tests are capable of identifying *all* sources of disease, and that there are objective criteria against which patients' responses can be contrasted. None of these assumptions, however, is warranted in all instances, particularly in the areas of chronic pain. However we wish to complete the assessment of a patient, it is rather grandiose to assume our own omnipotence. We are not omniscient, and thus we must not refer to "abnormal" illness behavior, which by definition assumes that we know what normal and abnormal responses should be.

Cognition

A great deal of research has been directed toward identifying cognitive factors that contribute to pain and disability. The basic assumption underlying these studies is that chronic pain patients are not passive receivers of sensory input but that they actively process information that determines coping with and adaptation to pain. Research has consistently demonstrated that patients' attitudes, beliefs, and expectations about their plight, themselves, their coping resources, and the health care system affect the reports of pain, activity, disability, and response to treatment. Some of the cognitive factors that have been found to be important in chronic pain are outlined in this section.

Beliefs about Pain

Clinicians working with chronic pain patients are aware that patients with similar pain histories may differ greatly in their beliefs about their pain. The cognitive model of chronic pain postulates that subjective interpretation of events, rather than objective characteristics of the event itself, influences behavior, emotion, and physiological responses. Even identical physical injury or disease can be experienced differently, depending on how persons attribute the underlying mechanisms of the damages. Thus, pain, when interpreted as signifying ongoing tissue damage or a progressive disease, is likely to produce considerably greater suffering and functional limitations than if it is viewed as a benign problem that is expected to improve with time.

To illustrate the importance of individual interpretations of symptoms and beliefs about pain, we can consider a person who wakes up one morning with a headache. A person who believes that the symptoms were caused by excessive alcohol consumption the night before probably does not experience high levels of emotional distress or autonomic activity. That interpretation may lead him or her to take a hot shower and two aspirins before going about the usual activities. This can be contrasted by the person who wakes up with a headache and recalls that his or her father reported similar symptoms just prior to his death from a brain aneurysm. In the latter case, the belief that the headache may be caused by a potentially lethal event may lead to increased emotional distress, heart rate, and muscle tension. This person may decide that he or she should immediately go to the emergency room. In both of these instances the same symptoms resulted in very different emotional states, activation of different physiological processes, and initiation of a different set of behavioral responses.

Certain beliefs may lead to maladaptive coping, greater disability, and suffering. Patients who believe their pain is likely to persist—is chronic—may feel helpless to do anything to alleviate it. As noted in the headache example mentioned earlier, their feelings and beliefs may exacerbate their suffering, which may in turn increase their physiological arousal and perceived pain. Thus a vicious circle is initiated. Over time these thoughts and feelings may maintain the pain and prolong disability. Patients who consider their pain to be an unexplainable mystery (20) may underestimate their ability to do anything to control pain and may continue to seek medical explanations rather than attempt to increase their coping efforts.

A person's beliefs, appraisals, and expectations seem to have a substantial role in determining functional limitations of chronic pain patients. For example, low-back pain patients often demonstrate poor behavioral persistence in various exercise tasks. Interestingly, their performance of those tasks tends to be independent of physical exertion or pain reports but rather is related to previous pain reports (21). These patients appear to believe that their ability to manage pain is poor, and they expect to have increased pain if they exercise. Thus, the rationale for their avoidance of exercise is not the presence of pain but their learned expectation of heightened pain and accompanying physical arousal that might exacerbate pain. If patients believe that disability is an inevitable reaction to their pain, that activity is dangerous, or that pain is an acceptable excuse for neglecting responsibilities, not surprisingly, their disability is likely to be maintained.

Once beliefs and expectations about a disease are formed, they become stable and are very difficult to modify. Patients tend to avoid experiences that could invalidate their beliefs, and they guide their behaviors in accordance with these beliefs even when the belief is no longer valid. Consequently, corrective feedback cannot be provided or obtained. For example, some muscular pain following activity may be caused by lack of muscle strength and general deconditioning, not by additional tissue damage. If one believes that pain indicates physiological abnormality, resting seems to be the best solution, and thus greater physical deconditioning and disability are likely to follow.

In addition to beliefs about capabilities to function despite pain, beliefs about pain per se appear to be important in understanding response to treatment, adherence to self-management activities, and disability. Successful rehabilitation appears to entail an important cognitive shift from believing in one's helplessness and passivity to resourcefulness and ability to function regardless of pain (1, 22).

Clearly, it is essential for patients with persistent pain to develop adaptive beliefs about impairment, pain, suffering, and disability and to deemphasize the role of experienced pain in their functioning. In fact, results from numerous treatment outcome studies have shown that changes in pain level do not parallel changes in other variables of interest, including activity level, medication use, return to work, rated ability to cope with pain, and pursuit of further treatment (23).

Self-Efficacy

Closely related to the sense of control is the concept of self-efficacy, or a personal conviction that one can successfully execute a course of action (i.e., perform required behaviors) to produce a desired outcome in a given situation (24). The self-efficacy expectation has been demonstrated as a major mediator of therapeutic change for chronic pain patients (25). Given sufficient motivation to engage in a behavior, a person's self-efficacy beliefs determine the choice of activities that the person will initiate, the amount of effort that will be expended, and how long the person will persist in the face of obstacles and aversive experiences.

Efficacy judgments are based on four sources of information regarding one's capabilities, listed in descending order of influence: (*a*) one's own past performance at the task of similar tasks, (*b*) the performance accomplishments of others who are perceived to be similar to oneself, (*c*) verbal persuasion by others that one is capable of performing, and (*d*) perception of one's own state of physiological arousal, which is in turn partly determined by prior efficacy estimation (24).

An experience of successful performance can be created by encouraging patients to undertake a relatively easy task in the beginning and gradually increasing the difficulty to match the difficulty of the desired behavioral repertoire. From this perspective the occurrence of coping behaviors is conceptualized as being mediated by the person's beliefs that situational demands do not exceed their coping resources. Research has consistently shown that improvement of physical performance tends to be accompanied by greater levels of self-efficacy beliefs (26, 27).

Catastrophizing

Catastrophizing—extremely negative thinking about one's plight and interpretation of even minor problems as catastrophes—appears to be a particularly potent way of thinking that greatly influences pain and disability. Several lines of research, both laboratory-based analog studies and clinical studies, indicate that catastrophizing is one of the most important determinants of how one reacts to pain. Those who spontaneously use catastrophizing self-statements tend to report greater pain than those do not (28). Turk et al. (1) concluded that "what appears to distinguish low from high pain tolerant persons in their cognitive processing, catastrophizing thoughts and feelings that precede, accompany, and follow aversive stimulation."

Coping

Self-regulation of pain and its effects depends on the person's specific ways of dealing with pain, adjusting to pain, and reducing or minimizing pain and distressed caused by pain—in short, coping strategies. Coping is assumed to be manifested by purposeful and intentional acts that are spontaneously employed. Coping strategies include decisions to act

with an intention of altering pain perception and ability to manage or tolerate pain. By employing coping strategies, a person improves the chance to continue everyday activities, thereby reducing functional limitations and enhancing the sense of control and self-efficacy.

Not all coping strategies are adaptive. Studies have found active coping strategies (i.e., efforts to function in spite of pain or to distract oneself from pain) to be associated with adaptive functioning, whereas passive coping strategies (i.e., depending on others for help in pain control and restricted activities) to be related to greater pain and depression. However, relative effectiveness of each active coping strategy is not well understood (29). As noted earlier, the most important factor in poor coping appears to be catastrophizing rather than differences in the nature of specific adaptive coping strategies. Moreover, the effectiveness of certain strategies may not be universal across all persons or across all situations. Interaction between coping strategies and personal and situational factors may be a critical factor in determining implementation of coping strategies.

HISTORICAL PERSPECTIVES OF CHRONIC PAIN

Unidimensional Models

Pain almost always follows damage to the body. Consequently, the earliest attempts to explain the mechanisms of pain assumed that there was an isomorphic relationship between physical damage and pain. According to these *somatogenic models* of pain, the presence and extent of pain should be explained by the degree of physical damage. Similarly, pain should be alleviated when the abnormality is corrected or the pain pathways are blocked. However, the presence of pain in the absence of identifiable physical disease or injury defies the model. The failure of the somatogenic model to explain chronic pain has prompted the other end of the dualistic view that persistent pain without organic abnormality must be driven by either psychological problems or motivation to receive secondary gain (e.g., disability payments)—a psychogenic perspective.

Research strongly suggests that regardless of the presence of injury or disease, neither the somatogenic nor the psychogenic model can fully explain chronic pain (30). The unidimensional models are at odds with the definition of pain proposed by the International Association for the Study of Pain (31), which emphasizes the involvement of both sensory and psychological processes in pain experience. This is not to say that physical and psychological factors do not influence pain but rather that by themselves, they are incomplete.

Toward Integration of Models

The first attempt to construct the integrative theoretical model of pain was proposed by Melzack and Wall (31). According to the influential gate control theory, emphasis is placed on the importance of integrating sensory, affective, and cognitive factors within the total experience of pain.

The cognitive-behavioral model of chronic pain attempts to extend the gate control model by including respondent and operant conditioning along with sensory-discriminative, motivational-affective, and cognitive-evaluative factors. The gate control model does not consider operant and respondent factors, as they are not directly related to the perception of pain but rather the maintenance of pain behaviors. The cognitive-behavioral model regards pain as a product of a complex perceptual process with the key emphasis on the patient's own subjective perspectives and feelings about his or her pain conditions, anticipation based on prior learned associations, and reinforcement contingencies (1). The cognitive-behavioral model considers pain experience as something more than a nociceptive event: the results of individual perception of sensory events that as noted earlier, could be influenced by a variety of cognitive and behavioral factors. Thus, in chronic pain it is the patient's perspective based on his or her idiosyncratic attitudes and beliefs that filter and interact reciprocally with emotional factors, social influences, behavioral responses, and sensory phenomena.

From the cognitive-behavioral perspective, people with persistent functional limitations due to pain are viewed as having negative expectations about their own ability to control motor skills without pain. Moreover, pain patients tend to believe that they have limited ability to exert any control over their pain. Such negative, maladaptive appraisals about the circumstance and personal efficacy may reinforce the experience of demoralization, inactivity, and overreaction to nociceptive stimulation. These cognitive appraisals and expectations are postulated as having an effect on behavior leading to reduced efforts and activity that may contribute to increased psychological distress (helplessness) and consequently physical limitations. If one accepts that pain is a complex subjective phenomenon that is uniquely experienced by each person, knowledge about idiosyncratic beliefs, appraisals, and coping repertoires become critical for optimal treatment planning.

It is also important that the influence of psychological factors not remain with the realm of psychological issues. Psychological factors affect not only behaviors, thoughts, and feelings but also physiological responses. For example, thinking of stressful events is known to increase muscle tension in the pain-affected areas (32). Physiological responses follow cognitive and behavioral activities. Indeed, the access to the physiological responses through cognition and behavior is the basic mechanism of behavioral techniques widely used in pain treatment.

Biomedical factors may have been influential in the original report of pain, but sensory factors play less and less of a role in disability over time, although deconditioning secondary to inactivity may exacerbate and maintain the problem. Inactivity also leads to increased focus on and preoccupation with the bodily sensations, particularly pain. These cognitive-attentional changes increase the likelihood of misinterpreting symptoms, overemphasizing symptom severity, and perceiving oneself as being disabled. Beliefs about the medicolegal system, health care system, employers, and personal support system are important, since they facilitate or disrupt the patient's sense of self-efficacy and become a basis for the patient's willingness to invest in treatment and accept personal responsibility in rehabilitation. Reduction of activity, fear of reinjury, unremitting pain, financial complications, and other environmental factors that support a pain patient's role can impede successful rehabilitation.

ASSESSMENT

To understand and appropriately treat a patient whose primary complaint is pain, an evaluation begins with a comprehensive history and a physical examination. Patients are usually asked to describe the parameters of pain: characteristics (e.g., stabbing, burning), locations, duration, and severity of pain. A standard medical approach to screen organic disease or injury, such as laboratory and diagnostic tests, must be readily available. However, it should be clear to readers by now that search for physical disease or injury is only a part of the story in assessment of patients with chronic pain.

In addition to the medical screening, an adequate pain assessment requires evaluations of the myriad psychosocial and behavioral factors that affect the individual and his or her experience of pain.. The primary purposes of the psychological assessment are twofold. First, understanding how thoughts, fears, levels and nature of dysphoric moods (i.e., anger, anxiety, depression), behaviors, and environmental factors (including interpersonal relationships) may contribute to the maintenance and exacerbation of pain is essential. Second, one must evaluate how living with chronic pain may be affecting those multiple factors. Needless to say, these two issues are not independent of each other; their reciprocal relationship is likely to facilitate a vicious circle of pain, functional limitation, and distress.

A number of assessment instruments are designed to evaluate patients' attitudes, distress, beliefs, and expectancies about themselves, their symptoms, and the health care system (33). Standardized assessment instruments have advantages over semistructured interviews for their ease in administration.

In using self-report inventories, one should take care not to overestimate the validity of the instruments, particularly if the instruments were standardized in nonpain populations. The presence of a certain symptom may mean one thing for a chronic pain patient and another for a pain-free individual. For example, a use of a standard cutoff point for inventories assessing depressive symptoms may overestimate the severity of depression in a pain patient because of the somatic complaints associated with pain (34, 35). Space does not permit a detailed examination of all pain assessment instruments; however, for a comprehensive discussion, see Turk and Melzack (36).

The self-report instruments should not be viewed as alternatives to interviews, which provide valuable data on how patients communicate their pain, distress, and suffering. These behaviors include verbal reports, paralinguistic vocalizations (e.g., sighs, moans), motor activity, facial expression, posturing, gesturing, and other behaviors designed to reduce pain (e.g., medication taking). Several observational methods to assess pain behaviors have been developed. For a review, see Keefe and Williams (37).

THERAPEUTIC INTERVENTIONS

The behavioral and cognitive principles discussed earlier have been applied to reduce pain, increase functioning, and help patients acquire adaptive coping skills. Following are brief descriptions of most commonly used behavioral and cognitive treatment methods in chronic pain.

Respondent Conditioning

The treatment of pain experience that was acquired through respondent learning is designed to decouple the association between stimuli and pain responses. The process generally involves breaking up of the US and CS; the presentation of CS is *not* followed by a CR. For example, a patient may tense the low-back area when asked to engage in a specific activity, contributing to the severity of pain. Behavioral techniques such as relaxation and biofeedback can act as a counter, an incompatible response, to muscle tension. Thus, relaxation in the presence of CS (e.g., the thought of engaging in the activity) is likely to interrupt the learned association between pain and the thought.

As in the acquisition of a response, repeated extinction trials are needed for successful breakup of the learned association. Substantial relapse may occur if the patient experiences the CR following the CS once again during the extinction stage. Clinicians should also be aware of the saliency of contextual cues. Objects and people in the context in which learning or unlearning occurs often become a part of the process. It is fairly common for patients to complain about the difficulties of executing the learned (or unlearned) skills outside of the clinic. To facilitate the generalization of the treatment effects, efforts should be made to identify what cues are salient in the patient's home environment. The treatment should include those cues and achieve reliable success in extinction of maladaptive responses.

Operant Conditioning

Treatment targets for the operant approach are frequencies of observable behaviors with the functional improvement as a primary goal. Behaviors must be made concrete and quantifiable. Targets for the increase are well behaviors, such as exercise tolerance. Increases in the frequency of certain behaviors are reinforced on schedule. Reinforcement can be performed in two ways: Positive reinforcement refers to the presentation of a consequence contingent on the behavior that one wishes to increase. In negative reinforcement, withdrawal of an aversive situation or object follows the exhibition of the target behavior. Occupational therapy and physical therapy are important components of an operant intervention because they emphasize increased activity levels.

Maladaptive behaviors become target behaviors, and the treatment should be directed toward reducing the frequency of such behaviors. Extinction of maladaptive behaviors can be accomplished in two ways: the presentation of an aversive consequence following the behavior (punishment) or the withdrawal of desirable consequences that have been reinforcing the behavior. The punishment does reduce the frequency of the target behavior; however, the aversive nature of punishment is likely to elicit negative feelings about the treatment, compromising motivation and rapport. One of the most commonly used strategies for the latter method is inattention (no responses will follow behaviors that used to elicit solicitous responses from others). Initially, ignoring pain behaviors may lead to an increase in these inappropriate behaviors in an effort to obtain positive reinforcement. However the pain behaviors are gradually extinguished in the absence of reinforcement, especially if positive attention is provided for well behaviors.

By extinction, one can change the nature of the reinforcement for pain behavior contingency. For example, "as needed" prescription of pain medication can be changed to a fixed time interval. In this way medication is time contingent, not pain contingent. The manipulation of the interval accomplishes the gradual tapering of undesirable medication intakes. Cairns and Pasino (38) demonstrated the effects of reinforcement and extinction. They showed that attention for activity and lack of attention for pain behaviors greatly increased the former and reduced the later. When the positive attention for activity was eliminated, patients reverted to their previous levels of inactivity.

One of the most important aspects of the operant treatment is the involvement of significant others, who tend to be the most potent reinforcer in a patient's natural habitat. Moreover, they are the best candidates for providing the generalization effects of learning from the treatment setting to the natural environment. In order to comply with the strict operationalization and reinforcement schedule, which are critical in reshaping of behaviors, operant treatment programs tend to require strict control over patients' environment, especially at the beginning of the rehabilitation. Indeed, many such programs are conducted on an inpatient basis. For the newly learned behaviors to be transferred to the patients' natural environment, their significant others must be included in the treatment, learn the principles of operant learning, and execute the consistent reinforcement contingencies across situations. Several studies have reported the data that support the effectiveness of operant-based rehabilitation programs for chronic pain (39–41).

Cognitive-Behavioral Treatment

In general, by the time patients with chronic pain come to a mental health professional, they have received multiple evaluations and a range of treatment provided by a host of health care professionals. A common feature across all patients is that the array of interventions did not adequately ameliorate their suffering. Thus, it is not surprising that when these patients are seen by a mental health professional, they are demoralized and frustrated and feel that their situation is hopeless, yet they continue to seek *the* cure for their suffering.

As noted earlier, the cognitive-behavioral model of pain acknowledges the importance of the ways cognitive variables interact with sensory, affective, operant, respondent, and physiological factors to form, maintain, and exacerbate the pain experience. Modification of maladaptive cognition requires some level of awareness. Cognitive-behavioral therapy is designed to help patients identify, evaluate, and correct maladaptive conceptualizations and dysfunctional beliefs about themselves and their predicament. Additionally, patients are taught to recognize the connections linking cognition, affect, behavior, and physiology along with their joint consequences. Patients are encouraged to become aware of and to monitor the ways that negative symptom-engendering or exacerbating thoughts and feelings may maintain and exacerbate maladaptive behaviors (Table 24.2).

A cognitive-behavioral therapist is concerned not only with the role of patients' thoughts in contributing to disability and to the maintenance and exacerbation of symptoms but also with the nature and adequacy of the patient's behavioral repertoire. The strategic plan of a cognitive-behavioral intervention is to facilitate patients' reconceptualizations of their plight. Patients initially believe that their illness is exclusively a medical problem. Most patients take a passive role in understanding their pain conditions with a belief that they have no personal control over pain and feel overwhelmed.

The cognitive-behavioral approach is designed to be optimistic, emphasizing both the effectiveness of the intervention and patients' ability to alleviate much of their suffering even if they cannot exert total control over their disease and physical limitations. Throughout the rehabilitation process, symptoms are reconceptualized so that patients come to view their situation as amenable to change by combined psychological and physical approaches (1).

Successful coping requires not only beliefs of efficacy but also successful execution of skills. The cognitive-behavioral treatment includes sessions in which patients are taught various behavioral and cognitive skills to reduce maladaptive pain responses. In the cognitive-behavioral treatment, these skills serve as feedback trials that provide an opportunity for patients to question, reappraise, and acquire self-control over maladaptive thoughts, feelings, behaviors, physiological responses, and adaptive skills. The goals of treatment are summarized in Table 24.3. Cognitive-behavioral treatment is composed of four interrelated phases: (*a*) reconceptualization,

Table 24.2.   Components of Cognitive-Behavioral Interventions

Problem-oriented

Educational (teach self-management, problem solving, coping, and communication skills)

Collaborative (patient and health care provider work together)

Makes use of in clinic and home practice to consolidate skills and identify problem areas

Encourage ventilation of feelings and then control of feelings that impair rehabilitation

Addresses the relation among thoughts, feelings, behavior, and physiology

Anticipation of setbacks and lapses; and teaching patients how to deal with these

Table 24.3.   Goals of a Cognitive-Behavioral Approach

Educate patients about the nature of pain and the relationships among pain, suffering, and disability.

Modify specific maladaptive thoughts, images, and feelings that are associated with emotional distress, such as exaggerated perception of imminent danger or loss, poor self-esteem (e.g., guilt), and anger (combat demoralization).

Teach patient to how and when to use coping techniques for specific challenges, e.g., symptom coping skills, problem solving for practical dilemmas, self-control and self-management skills to control emotional distress.

Foster a sense of self-efficacy and self-control as opposed to feelings and perceptions of helpless and hopelessness.

Teach patients to anticipate problems and to deal with them when they arise and thereby prevent relapse.

(*b*) skill acquisition of self-management strategies, (*c*) skill consolidation, and (*d*) generalization and maintenance.

Reconceptualization

Cognitive restructuring encourages people to identify and change stress-inducing thoughts and feelings associated with the pain. The crucial element in the successful treatment is bringing about a shift in the patient's repertoire from well-established, habitual, and automatic but ineffective responses. Cognitive restructuring helps foster the reconceptualization by making patients aware of the role of thoughts and emotions in potentiating and maintaining stress and physical symptoms.

Generally, the process of cognitive restructuring begins with a presentation of a situation or event that has provoked a pain-related response. The situation is dissected to identify key thoughts and feelings that follow a stressor and proceed the response. Then patients are encouraged to challenge the legitimacy of the thoughts: Was it true? Was it reasonable? Was it the only answer? Patients are told to gather evidence for or against their own automatic thoughts. Alternatives are identified, and the ways different patterns of thinking affect pain and feelings are evaluated.

Acquisition of Self-Management Skills

A wide variety of techniques have been shown to reduce pain, suffering, and disability. Some of these strategies are self-regulatory skills (e.g., relaxation, biofeedback, attention diversion) that allow pain sufferers to regulate their own physiological responses that may produce pain. Other self-management strategies are stress management skills (e.g., problem solving, behavioral rehearsals) that allow pain patients to manage the stress-inducing thoughts, behaviors, and emotions that trigger exacerbation and maintenance of pain along with maladaptive responses. With self-management strategies, instead of being a passive recipient of a medical intervention (e.g., medication, anesthetic nerve block), patients play an active role in learning and applying skills to manage the myriad of problems created by persistent pain.

Skill acquisition is a critical component in the cognitive-behavioral therapy. Techniques such as progressive relaxation, problem solving, distraction skills, and communication skills, to name only a few, are taught. Several publications have described in detail specifics of these techniques (1, 42).

Skill Consolidation

During the skill consolidation phase of the cognitive-behavioral treatment, patients practice and rehearse the skills that they have learned during the acquisition phase and apply them outside the clinic. The practice may start with the mental rehearsal, during which patients imagine using the skills in different situations. The therapist can use role playing, in which a patient rehearses learned skills in situations that mirror the home environment. In the role-playing sessions therapists may start with a relatively easy scene and make the role-playing scenario progressively more difficult. At times, the therapist and a patient exchange their roles because it provides an opportunity for the patient to observe alternative coping strategies. The importance of skill generalization through home practice cannot be overstated. When patients practice skills at home, it is useful to have them record their experiences, including any difficulties that arise. Once problems associated with using the newly acquired skills are identified, these become targets for further discussion.

Preparation for Generalization and Maintenance

To maximize the likelihood of maintenance and generalization of treatment gains, therapists focus on the cognitive activity of patients as they are confronted with problems throughout treatment (e.g., failure to achieve goals, plateaus in progress, recurrent stress). These events are employed as opportunities to teach patients to handle setbacks and lapses because they are probably inevitable parts of life and will occur after the termination of the treatment.

In the final phase of treatment, discussion focuses on possible ways of predicting and dealing with symptoms and related problems following treatment termination. It is helpful to assist patients to anticipate future problems, stress, and symptom-exacerbating events during treatment and to plan how to respond and cope with these problems.

CLINICAL EFFECTIVENESS AND COST EFFECTIVENESS

It is abundantly clear that there is no isomorphic relationship between tissue damage and pain report (43, 44). The acknowledgment of the multifactorial nature of chronic pain has facilitated the use of behavioral and cognitive-behavioral treatment within the rehabilitation framework. A wealth of evidence has demonstrated that multidisciplinary pain management problems are clinically more effective than traditional treatments in diverse pain problems, including arthritis (25), low-back pain (45), temporomandibular disorders (46), fibromyalgia (47), and chronic headaches (48). To date, more than 200 studies reporting on the efficacy of behavioral and cognitive-behavioral treatments for chronic pain patients have been published. The American Psychological Association (49) designated cognitive-behavioral treatment of chronic pain as one of only 20 areas for which there was good empirical support for the efficacy of clinical psychology.

On measures of pain reduction, improved mood, decrease in opioid medications, decline in the use of the health care system, increased activity, and return to work, multidisciplinary programs that include behavioral and cognitive-behavioral treatments have been shown to be highly effective (23). Moreover, when the results have been evaluated to determine the cost effectiveness, multidisciplinary programs that incorporate behavioral and cognitive-behavioral problems can save significant amounts of money in medical expenditures and indemnity costs (50). The projected savings are substantially greater than are realized by unimodal therapies such as surgery, nerve blocks, and physical therapy.

Several influential governmental and private agencies have acknowledged the importance of incorporating behavioral perspectives in assessment and treatment of chronic pain patients (e.g., Social Security Administration, Institute of Medicine, Commission on the Accreditation of Rehabilitation Facilities). Thus, the behavioral perspectives and approaches to treatment described are being acknowledged as essential in the successful rehabilitation of chronic pain patients.

References

1. Turk DC, Meichenbaum D, Genest M. Pain and behavioral medicine: a cognitive-behavioral perspective. New York: Guilford Press, 1983.
2. Melzack, R, Casey KL. Sensory, motivational and central control determinants of pain: a new conceptual model. In: Kenshalo D, ed. The skin senses. Springfield, IL: Charles C. Thomas, 1968;423–443.
3. Fordyce WE. Behavioral methods for chronic pain and illness. St. Louis: Mosby, 1976.
4. Turk DC, Okifuji A. Evaluating the role of physical, operant, cognitive, and affective factors in pain behavior in chronic pain patients. Behav Mod 1997;259–280.
5. Social Security Administration: Report of the Commission on the Evaluation of Pain. U. S. Department of Health and Human Services Pub. 64–031. Washington: U.S. Government Printing Office, 1987.
6. Parsons T. Social systems. London: Routledge and Kegan Paul, 1951.
7. Mechanic D. The concept of illness behavior. J Chron Dis 1962; 15:189–194.

8. White KL, Williams F, Greenberg BG. The ecology of medical care. N Engl J Med 1961;265:885.

9. Leventhal H. Behavioral medicine: psychology in health care. In: Mechanic D, ed. Handbook of health, health care, and the health professions. New York: Free Press, 1983;709–743.

10. Pennebaker J. The psychology of physical symptoms. New York: Springer-Verlag, 1982.

11. Turk DC, Rudy TE, Salovey P. Implicit models of illness. J Behav Med 1986;9:453–474.

12. Lazarus RS. Psychological stress and the coping process. New York: McGraw-Hill, 1966.

13. Pilowsky I. A general classification of abnormal illness behaviours. Br J Med Psychol 1978;1:131–137.

14. Wooley SC, Blackwell B, Winget C. A learning theory model of chronic illness behavior: theory, treatment, and research. Psychosom Med 1978;40:379–401.

15. Mayou R. Illness behavior and psychiatry. Gen Hosp Psychiatry 1989;11:307–312.

16. Pilowsky I, Spence ND. Patterns of illness behaviour in patients with intractable pain. J Psychosom Res 1975;19:279–288.

17. Main CJ, Waddell G. Psychometric construction and validity of the Pilowsky Illness Behavior Questionnaire in British patients with chronic low back pain. Pain 1987;9:13–25.

18. Stretton MS, Salovey P, Mayer JD. Assessing health concerns. Imagination. Cog Pers 1992;12:115–137.

19. Williams DA, Thorn BE. An empirical assessment of pain beliefs. Pain 1989;36:351–358.

20. Schmidt AJM. Performance level of chronic low back pain patients in different treadmill test conditions. J Psychosom Res 1985;29:639–645.

21. Jensen MP, Turner JA, Romano JM. Correlates of improvement in multidisciplinary treatment of chronic pain. J Consult Clin Psychol 1994;62: 172–179.

22. Flor H, Fydrich T, Turk DC. Efficacy of multidisciplinary pain treatment centers: a meta-analytic review. Pain 1992;49:221–230.

23. Bandura A. Self-efficacy: toward a unifying theory of behavior change. Psychol Rev 1977;84:191–215.

24. O'Leary A, Shoor S, Lorig K, Holman HR. A cognitive-behavioral treatment for rheumatoid arthritis. Health Psychol 1988;7:527–544.

25. Council JR, Ahern DK, Follick MJ, Kline CL. Expectancies and functional impairment in chronic low back pain. Pain 1988; 33:323–331.

26. Dolce JJ, Crocker MF, Moletteire C, Doleys DM. Exercise quotas, anticipatory concern and self-efficacy expectations in chronic pain: a preliminary report. Pain 1986;24:365–372.

27. Keefe FJ, Brown GK, Wallston DA, Caldwell DS. Coping with rheumatoid arthritis pain: catastrophizing as a maladaptive strategy. Pain 1989; 37:51–56.

28. Fernandez E, Turk DC. The utility of cognitive coping strategies for altering pain perception: a meta-analysis. Pain 1989;38:124–135.

29. Turk DC, Rudy TE. Toward the comprehensive assessment of chronic pain patients. Behav Res Ther 1987;25:237–249.

30. Merskey H. Classification of chronic pain: descriptions of chronic pain syndromes and definitions of pain terms. Pain 1986;(Suppl 3):S1–S225.

31. Melzack R, Wall PD. Pain mechanisms: a new theory. Science 1965;50:971–979.

32. Flor H, Turk DC, Birbaumer N. Assessment of stress-related psychophysiological responses in chronic back pain patients. J Consult Clin Psychol 1985;53:354–364.

33. DeGood DE, Shutty MS. Assessment of pain beliefs, coping, and self-efficacy. In: Turk DC, Melzack R eds. Handbook of pain assessment. New York: Guilford, 1992:214–234.

34. Romano J, Turner JA. Chronic pain and depression: does the evidence support a relationship? Psych Bull 1985;97:18–34.

35. Turk DC, Okifuji A. Detecting depression in chronic pain patients: the adequacy of self-reports. Behav Res Ther 1994;32:9–16.

36. Turk DC, Melzack R, eds. Handbook of Pain Assessment. New York: Guilford Press, 1992.

37. Keefe FJ, Williams DA. New directions in pain assessment and treatment. Clin Psychol Rev 1989;9:549–568.

38. Cairns D, Pasino JA. Comparison of verbal reinforcement and feedback in operant treatment of disability due to low back pain. Behav Ther 1977;8:621–630.

39. Fordyce WE, Fowler, RS, Lehmann JR, et al. Operant conditioning in the treatment of chronic pain. Arch Phys Med Rehab 1973;54:399–408.

40. Roberts AH, Reinhardt L. The behavioral management of chronic pain: long-term follow-up with comparison groups. Pain 1980;8:151–162.

41. Turner JA, Clancy S. Comparison of operant behavioral and cognitive-behavioral group treatment for chronic low back pain. J Consult Clin Psychol 1988;56:261–266.

42. Turk DC. Psychological aspects of pain. In: Expert pain management. Springhouse, PA: Springhouse, 1997:124–178.

43. Waddell G. A new clinical model for the treatment for low-back pain. Spine 1987;12:632–644.

44. Turk DC, Okifuji A, Scharff L. Chronic pain and depression: role of perceived impact and perceived control in different age cohorts. Pain 1995;61:93–101.

45. Nicholas MK, Wislon PH, Goyen J. Comparison of cognitive-behavioral group treatment and an alternative non-psychological treatment for low back pain. Pain 1992;48:339–347.

46. Turk DC, Zaki HS, Rudy TE. Effects of intraoral appliance and biofeedback/stress management alone and in combination in treating pain and depression in TMD patients. J Prosthet Dent 1993;70:158–164.

47. Goldenberg DL, Kaplan KH, Nadeau MG, et al. A controlled study of a stress-reduction, cognitive-behavioral treatment program in fibromyalgia. J Musculoskeletal Pain 1994;2:53–66.

48. Holroyd KA, Nash JM, Pingel JD, et al. A comparison of pharmacological (amitriptyline HCL) and nonpharmacological (cognitive-behavioral) therapies for chronic tension headaches. J Consult Clin Psychol 1991;59:387–393.

49. American Psychological Association Task Force on Promotion and Dissemination of Psychological Procedures. Training in and dissemination of empirically-validated psychological treatments: report and recommendation. Clin Psychol 1995;48:3–23.

50. Turk DC, Okifuji A. Efficacy of multidisciplinary pain centers: an antidote to anecdotes. In: Zenz M. ed. Balliere's Clinical Anesthesiology: International Practice and Research, in press.

APPENDIX

RESOURCES FOR PAIN THERAPY AND MANAGEMENT

Professional Societies

American Pain Society (APS)
4700 W. Lake Ave.
Glenview, IL 60025
847–375–4715
U.S. chapter, International Association for the Study of Pain (IASP)
L. E. Jones, B S
International Assoc. for the Study of Pain
N. E. 43rd St., Suite 306
Seattle, WA 98105
American Academy of Pain Medicine (AAPM)
4700 W. Lake Ave.
Glenview, IL 60025
847–375–4731

Journals

Pain. Journal of IASP; comes with membership. Dues on a sliding scale. Research journal. Published by Elsevier Science B. V., Amsterdam.
The Clinical Journal of pain. Journal of the American Academy of Pain Medicine. Published by Churchill Livingstone, Secaucus, NJ.
Journal of Pain and Symptom Management. Published by Elsevier, New York.

Books

The IASP has a press that publishes medical and scientific research texts on the nuances of pain specialty problems, such as headaches, complex regional pain syndrome, and pharmacology.
Guilford Press, 72 Spring St., New York, NY 10012 has multiple publications on pain therapy from a psychosocial, behavioral medicine perspective.

Patients' Resources

Managing Pain Before It Manages You, by M. Caudill. Guilford Press, NY, 1995. Patient workbook for pain management. Audiotape available through ISHK Bookservice, Cambridge, MA; 800–222–4745. Spanish edition available through Guilford Press, New York.
Taking Control of Your Headache: How to Get the Treatment You Need, by Paul N. Duckro, William D. Richardson, and Janet E. Marshall. Guilford Press, New York, 1995. A self-management guide for headache treatment.
Learning to Master Your Pain, by Robert N. Jamison. Professional Resource Press, Sarasota, FL, 1996.

The Chronic Pain Control Workbook, by E. M. Catalano. New Harbinger Publications, Oakland, CA, 1987. Patient information book for pain treatment and management.
The Arthritis Help Book, by Kate Lorig and James Fries. Addison Wesley, Reading, MA, 1990. A tested self-management program for coping with arthritis.
Societies and support groups for specific diagnoses such as fibromyalgia, interstitial cystitis, scoliosis, and chronic pain in general:
Endometriosis Association
8585 N. 76th Place
Milwaukee, WI 53223
414–335–2200

Interstitial Cystitis Association
P.O. Box 1553
Madison Square Station, New York, NY 10159
212–979–6057

National Chronic Pain Outreach Association, Inc.
7979 Old Georgetown Rd., Suite 100
Bethesda, MD 20814–2429
301–652–4948

American Chronic Pain Association
P.O. Box 850
Rocklin, CA 95677
916-632-0922

The American Fibromyalgia Syndrome Association, Inc.
6380 E. Tanque Verde Rd., Suite D
P.O. Box 31750
Tucson, AZ 85751–1750
520–733–1570

Also a resource for chronic fatigue syndrome and myofascial syndrome.
The Arthritis Foundation
1314 Spring St., N.W.
Atlanta, Georgia 30309
404–266–0795

National Scoliosis Foundation, Inc.
72 Mount Auburn St.
Watertown, MA 02172
617–926–0397

There is a growing number of Internet bulletin boards for fibromyalgia, cumulative trauma injury, and other chronic pain syndromes. Dr. Richard Chapman has linked many resources through the IASP website at http://weber.u.washington.edu/~cre/IASP.html.

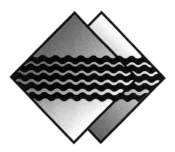

PART V

Special Populations

CHAPTER 25

Pain Associated with Advanced Malignancy, Including Adjuvant Analgesic Drugs in Cancer Pain Management

Richard B. Patt and Allen W. Burton

EPIDEMIOLOGY

The prospect of suffering from unrelieved pain is one of the most feared aspects of a cancer diagnosis for most patients and their families, yet only in recent years have the importance and value of effective management of cancer pain achieved a high degree of recognition both in academic environments and with the lay public (1, 2). There has been an historic commitment and interest in the dilemma of unrelieved cancer pain by pain specialists, most notably John Bonica (3), Kathleen Foley (4) and Victorio Ventafridda (5), that has served to engender today's rising level of recognition of this problem among the health care community.

Optimal management involves careful assessment, individualization of therapy, close follow-up and a proactive approach to treatment. Adequate control of pain can be achieved in the vast majority of patients with a rigorous and aggressive application of measures that are ultimately quite straightforward (6, 7).

Patients are reassured and symptoms are easier to control when it is articulated at the outset that pain is treatable and that symptom control is, along with anticancer therapy, one of the treatment team's priorities. Control of pain and related symptoms promotes an enhanced quality of life, improved functioning, better compliance and a means for patients to focus on those things that give meaning to life (8). In addition to their salutary effects on quality of life, mounting evidence suggests that good pain control influences survival (9, 10).

In spite of increased recognition of cancer-related pain as an important public health problem and numerous technological breakthroughs, pain associated with malignancy continues to be a significant clinical problem. Recent surveys reveal unacceptably high rates of unrelieved pain due to cancer (11, 12), even in developed nations. Thus, satisfaction of the mandate for the global application of available pain relief options remains elusive yet unquestionably important.

Prevalence of Cancer Pain

Cancer

Cancer is a ubiquitous disease that continues to be associated with high mortality rates despite ongoing research. An estimated 6.35 million new cases of cancer are diagnosed worldwide annually, half of which originate in developing nations (2). About 1.04 million new diagnosis of cancer are made annually in the United States alone (13). One of every five deaths in the United States is a result of cancer, which comes to about 1400 cancer-related deaths per day (14). That the incidence of cancer increases with age is particularly problematic given our rapidly aging population. Overall, cancer cure rates have not changed markedly over the past 4 decades: the overall 5-year survival rate for patients diagnosed with cancer in the United States is still only about 40 to 50% (15) and as a result of inadequate early detection, is less than one third worldwide (2). Cancer is the second most common cause of death in this country, and of every 10 deaths worldwide, 1 is due to cancer (2). The annual mortality rate is about 4.3 million worldwide and about 510,000 in the United States (13). Palliative treatment, which may extend survival, is often more successful than therapies with curative intent, and as a result there is an increasing trend for patients to have lingering advanced disease and chronic pain.

Cancer Pain

Together with anorexia and fatigue, pain is among the most common symptoms associated with cancer (16, 17). While the results of epidemiological studies vary, even recent studies continue to show that about two-thirds of patients have pain that is significant enough to require treatment during some phase of their illness. Significant pain is present in up to 25% of patients in active treatment and in up to 90% of patients with advanced cancer (11, 18-22).

Inadequately Controlled Cancer Pain

Despite its considerable prevalence, treatment has historically produced disappointing results, a trend that regrettably continues in most settings. A recent survey of members of the Eastern Cooperative Oncology Group (ECOG) assessed pain in 1308 outpatients with metastatic cancer. Of this group, 67% had pain during the week of the survey and 36% had pain that markedly impaired their ability to function (11). Bonica (2) conducted a survey of 2500 patients treated in developed nations that revealed an absence of satisfactory relief of pain in 50 to 80% of patients. In a survey of 1103 consecutive admissions to a U.S. acute-care cancer hospital, 73% of patients admitted to pain and 38% to severe pain (23). In another survey of 100 consecutive admissions to a U.K. hospice, 90 patients admitted to unrelieved pain persisting for the prior 4 weeks, and in 77 patients pain had been present for 8 weeks or more. Most patients in this series described their pain as severe or excruciating (24).

Horizons

These results are in stark contrast to cross-culturally validated surveys revealing that pain can be adequately controlled in 70 to 90% of patients by the application of relatively simple interventions when pain is targeted as a treatment outcome (25-28). Despite the availability of simple, cost-effective treatment (29), inadequately controlled pain remains a problem of epidemic proportions. This dilemma is especially compelling in developing nations that lack resources to provide for even the basic health needs of their citizenry (30).

Barriers to Change and Possible Solutions

In 1982 an interdisciplinary expert committee convened by the World Health Organization (WHO) developed a set of preliminary cancer pain management guidelines based on the concept of a three-step ladder approach to pharmacotherapy. This effort resulted in the publication of *Cancer Pain Relief,* a slim volume that by 1993 had been translated into 22 languages and distributed to more than 250,000 recipients, making it the most requested and second most translated of all WHO publications. Despite reliance on simple technology, widespread dissemination, and a subsequent revision of these guidelines (31), cancer patients in most parts of the world remain undertreated (32). While it is difficult to draw direct correlations between specific factors and adequacy of treatment, there is widespread agreement about the nature of these factors. That pilot studies using relatively simple interventions (e.g., oral analgesics and careful follow-up) have achieved favorable outcomes in the 70 to 90% range (25) suggests that the key to achieving more effective global cancer pain relief involves applying known technology more effectively rather than development of new medical technologies or drugs. In the largest prospective trial of the WHO method to date, Zech et al. (25) achieved favorable results in 76% of 2118 cancer patients treated over a 10-year interval.

The Wisconsin Cancer Pain Initiative has been working to improve the status of cancer pain control since 1986. A broad-based advocacy group, its seminal work inspired a grass-roots system of state cancer pain initiatives that has since been implemented in all 50 states. The Wisconsin group advanced the notion of classifying the impediments to optimal cancer pain according to whether they pertain to *(a)* the patient and family, *(b)* the health care team, or *(c)* the health care system (33-37). While a variety of such factors have been identified, authorities agree that so-called opiophobia, a reluctance to use opioids, largely because of exaggerated concerns of addiction and regulatory reprisal, exerts a potent influence at all levels and probably is the single most important impediment to better symptom control globally. Myths and misconceptions regarding the drug therapy of cancer pain that are commonly endorsed by health care providers are summarized in Table 25.1.

In general, in Western developed sectors, barriers are largely educational and attitudinal in nature, while in developed nations a multitude of resource and access problems are operant. For example, in Mexico and Indonesia, the unavailability of potent opioids remains a significant problem (38), while in Argentina treatment is constrained by insurers' failure to regard pain control and analgesics as being reimbursable. In Uganda, where war, famine, and the human immunodeficiency virus (HIV) epidemic are predominant concerns (39), the situation is even more compelling: only about 5% of cancer patients are recipients of even basic antineoplastic therapy, and there is essentially no pain management. Nevertheless, given that the overall awareness of the significance and treatability of cancer pain has never been higher, there is reason to hope that these barriers may be overcome (33).

Imperatives for Change

Cancer pain is widely acknowledged to exact a high toll on the well-being of the patient and his or her loved ones (8, 34). After incurability, cancer patients rank pain as the most fearful aspect of their illness (1), and of the range of symptoms associated with cancer, pain is reported as being the most distressing (2). However, notwithstanding a growing recognition that treating pain in the context of terminal illness is a moral imperative (35), health care's current emphasis on cost containment demands that additional arguments be marshaled to ensure continued funding and reimbursement. Fortunately, researchers have demonstrated that pain can usually be controlled effectively using straightforward, cost-effective therapies. Unfortunately, research that would directly link pain with survival benefit or various other morbidities is difficult to perform. Basic science work on the relation between pain, opioid therapy, and immune function (9) has provided preliminary suggestions that pain can kill, as has evidence from a recent controlled trial of celiac plexus block for pancreatic cancer that demonstrated significant survival benefit in treated patients (10). Indirect effects on survival may stem from the negative influence of pain on performance status. Performance status, as measured by the ECOG and Karnofsky

Table 25.1.   Myths and Misconceptions about Cancer Pain Management Prevalent among Health Care Providers

Tolerance to pain relief	Patients need increasing doses of medication because they enevitably become tolerant to pain relief.
Intolerance to adverse symptoms	Patients remain intolerant to adverse side effects of analgesics.
Adjuvant drugs	Relief of pain does not involve regimens of multiple classes of drugs and coanalgesics.
Parenteral drugs	Severe pain calls for the administration of parenteral drugs.
Addiction	Addiction is prevalent and dangerous.
Inevitable pain	Pain is an inevitable symptom of cancer and cannot be adequately relieved with drug treatment.
Ceiling dose	There is a ceiling dose above which the opioids cannot be prescribed.
Physical dependence	Patients remain physically dependent and will have withdrawl symptoms even with gradual tapering of dose.
PRN administration	The opioids should be prescribed on a PRN basis to manage cancer pain.
Low efficacy	Cancer pain cannot be managed effectively with analgesics.
Respiratory depression	Use of morphine to manage pain seriously depresses respiration and shortens life.
Prognosis	Use of potent opioids to manage cancer pain implies giving up on the patient.

Adapted with permission from Elliott TE, Murray DM, Elliott BA, et al. Physician knowledge and attitudes about cancer pain management: a survey from the Minnesota cancer pain project. Pain Symptom Management 1995;10:494–504.

Scales (Table 25.2), is a global rating of patients' overall functional status. When performance status is low, as is often the case when pain is severe, patients may find it difficult to comply with recommended antitumor therapy and may not be considered eligible for investigational anticancer therapies.

Although the physical aspects of pain are usually the most readily perceived and manageable components of the global suffering that characteristically accompanies a diagnosis of cancer, the equation of pain with physical discomfort is too simplistic. Dame Cicely Saunders, founder of the contemporary hospice movement, encouraged a more expansive view of pain with her use of the term total pain to include its psychological, emotional, and spiritual aspects, as well as the protean effects of uncontrolled pain on function and lifestyle (36). In this broader context, pain is viewed according to its potential to produce attendant dysfunction on a person's mood, sleep, nutrition, posture, sexuality: in short, quality of life (8, 37). While changes in the status of these markers of well-being are multifactorial, it has been demonstrated that alterations may return towards normal when pain is well controlled (8, 38). Thus, further benefits of good pain management often include improvements in nutrition, rest, and mood, all of which contribute to quality of life and have the potential to influence the outcome of antineoplastic therapy.

ASSESSMENT

Perspectives

The importance of the initial evaluation of the patient with cancer-related pain (Tables 25.3 to 25.6) cannot be overemphasized. Although the pain evaluation per se can be performed relatively rapidly, it is essential that this process be integrated with a detailed oncological, medical, and psychosocial assessment. The evaluation should address the pain, the patient, the disease, and the interrelationships among these factors. While no specific algorithmic approach to assessment has been universally accepted, the process usually consists of a detailed medical history with review of systems, a physical examination that emphasizes the neurological and musculoskeletal systems, a psychosocial assessment, and a review of the results of pertinent diagnostic studies (39). Because of the

Table 25.2.   Methods of Assessing Performance Status

ECOG		Karnofsky	
0	Fully active, able to carry on all predisease performance without restriction	100	Normal; no complaints, no evidence of disease
		90	Able to carry on normal activity; minor signs or symptoms of disease
1	Restricted in physically strenuous activity but ambulatory and able to carry out light or sedentary work (e.g., light housework, office work)	80	Normal activity with effort; some signs or symptoms of disease
		70	Cares for self; unable to carry on normal activity or to do active work
2	Ambulatory and capable of all self-care but unable to work; up and about more than 50% of waking hours	60	Requires occasional assistance but is able to care for most needs
		50	Requires considerable assistance and frequent medical care
3	Capable of only limited self-care, confined to bed or chair more than 50% of waking hours	40	Disabled, requires special care and assistance
		30	Severely disabled, hospitalization indicated; death not imminent
4	Completely disabled. Cannot carry on any self-care. Totally confined to bed or chair	20	Very sick; hospitalization necessary; active supportive treatment necessary
		10	Moribund; fatal processes; progressing rapidly
5	Dead	0	Dead

heterogeneous, dynamic, and multisystemic nature of cancer, patients with pain commonly present with complex and often mixed syndromes. For example, in a prospective evaluation of 2266 consecutive patients with cancer pain, Grond et al. (40) reported 30% of patients presenting with one, 39% with two, and 31% with three or more distinct pain syndromes and sites of pain. In addition, the underlying mechanisms of pain in this series were commonly mixed with nociceptive pain arising from bone and soft tissue in 35% and 45% of cases, respectively, and visceral and neuropathic pain in another 33% and 34% of patients, respectively.

Table 25.3.   Comprehensive Evaluation of the Patient with Cancer Pain

Review of medical record and radiological studies
Review of patient responses to any questionnaires
Discussion with referring physician, primary care provider, and/or oncologist
Introduction of clinician or team; patient orientation to facility
Psychosocial history
   Marital and residential status
   Employment history and status
   Educational background
   Functional status, activities of daily living
   Recreational activities
   Support systems
   Health and capabilities of spouse, significant other
Medical history (independent of oncological history)
   Coexisting systemic disease
   Exercise tolerance
   Allergies to medications and medication use
   Prior illnesses and surgery
Thorough review of systems (Table 25.4 and 25.5)
Oncologic history
   Prior malignancies
   Family history
   Diagnosis and evolution of disease
   Therapy and outcome, including side effects
   Patient's understanding of disease process, prognosis
Pain history (Table 25.6)
Physical examination
Team meeting if applicable
Determination of need for further studies
Formulate clinical impression (diagnosis)
Formulate recommendations (plan) and alternatives
Call oncologist and/or primary care provider if applicable
Exit interview
   Explain probable cause of symptoms
   If appropriate, discuss nature of disease
   Discuss prognosis for symptom relief
   Discuss management options
   Discuss specific recommendations
   Arrange for follow-up
   Dictate summary to referring and consulting physicians

Table 25.4.   Review of Systems (Symptom List)

Systemic, consistitutional	Gastrointestinal
Anorexia	Dysphagia
Weight loss	Nausea
Cachexia	Vomiting
Fatigue, weakness	Dehydration
Insomnia	Constipation
	Diarrhea
Neurologic	Psychological
Sedation	Irritability
Confusion	Anxiety
Hallucinations	Depression
Headache	Dementia
Motor weakness	
Altered sensation	Integument
Incontinence	Decubitus
	Dry, sore mouth
Respiratory	Genitourinary
Dyspnea	Hesitancy
Cough	Urgency
Hiccough	

Table 25.5.   Frequency of Symptoms in 275 Consecutive Patients with Advance Cancer

Symptom	Prevalence
Asthenia	90%
Anorexia	85%
Pain	76%
Nausea	68%
Constipation	65%
Sedation, confusion	60%
Dyspnea	12%

Reprinted with permission from Bruera E. Malnutrition and asthenia in advanced cancer. Cancer Bull 1991;43:387.

Table 25.6.   Elements of a Comprehensive Pain History

Premorbid chronic pain
Premorbid drug or alcohol use
Pain catalog (number and locations)
For each pain
   Onset and evolution
   Site and radiation
   Pattern (e.g., constant, intermittent, predictable)
   Intensity (best, worst, average, current) 0–10 scale
   Quality
   Exacerbating factors
   Relieving factors
   How the pain interferes
   Neurological and motor abnormalities
   Vasomotor changes
   Other associated factors
Current analgesics (use, efficacy, and side effects)
Prior analgesics (use, efficacy, side effects)

The initial evaluation serves several purposes and should be broad based: rather than limiting inquiry to the pain syndrome per se, the process should encompass evaluation of the person, his or her feelings and attitudes about pain and disease, family concerns, and the patient's premorbid psychological history (e.g., preexisting depressive or anxiety disorders, personality disorder, substance abuse) (41, 42). A recent study, for example, disclosed a 28% incidence of ongoing alcohol abuse in a cadre of patients with terminal cancer, of whom only 30% admitted to a prior history of alcohol abuse (43).

A compassionate but objective approach to assessment instills confidence in the patient and family that will be valuable throughout treatment. A thorough review of the patient's records and a detailed pain history help both to delineate the source of pain and to distinguish the degree to which the patient's complaints are related to nociceptive mechanisms versus psychological modulators. Learned pain behavior and prior analgesic use may make the presentation and management of patients with preexisting chronic nonmalignant pain and superimposed acute cancer pain especially complex (44).

The patient's self-report should be regarded as the primary source of information about pain, since it is in general considerably more accurate than the observations of health care providers and even loved ones. Neither behavioral observations nor vital signs should be used as substitutes for self-report, although they may serve an adjunctive and occasionally primary role in specific settings (e.g., preverbal children and developmentally disabled, comatose, and manipulative patients). Grossman et al. (45) described marked discrepancies between patient pain ratings and health care provider estimates, with the greatest discrepancies observed in patients reporting severe pain. Psychological testing is useful, although it must often be abbreviated in consideration of poor physical and emotional condition (46). The primary care physician or referring oncologist who has known the patient over time may be a source of valuable information and should be consulted personally.

Ideally, the consultation accomplishes more than simply rendering a diagnosis and treatment plan (47): it should also orient the patient, family, and referring physician to what can realistically be accomplished; should serve an educational function; and should ultimately reassure the patient. These goals have practical value: patients with an improved understanding of their medical condition and confidence in their health care providers are more compliant, tend to have better outcomes, and are probably less likely to use emergency services inappropriately (48-50).

Classification of Cancer Pain

A number of suggested schemata for classifying cancer pain have potential to aid in diagnosis and management.

Chronicity

One such classification is based on chronicity of symptoms. Acute pain is frequently associated with signs of sympathetic hyperactivity and heightened distress (51), particularly when it is incident related, as in the case of medical procedures such as bone marrow biopsy or lumbar puncture (52). Persistent (nonprocedural) acute pain has been characterized as a biological red flag, warning of ongoing tissue injury (53). Indeed, it is often temporally associated with the onset or recrudescence of primary or metastatic disease, and its presence should motivate the clinician to seek its cause aggressively. Acute pain further signals the need for treatment with potent analgesics that may resolve as antitumor therapy progresses (54).

In contrast, assessment and management of patients with chronic pain tends to be more complex (55, 56). Usually the source of pain has already been investigated and is known or suspected. The continued presence of symptoms implies that their cause cannot adequately be eliminated and suggests the need for some combination of palliation, adjustment, and acceptance. Having exceeded its value as a marker of injury, pain assumes the status of disease and may itself contribute

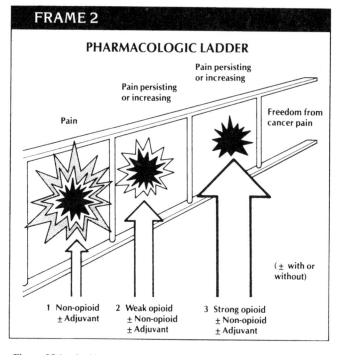

Figure 25.1. Ladder approach to cancer pain relief advocated by the World Health Organization. It relies primarily on pain intensity and to a lesser extent on pain mechanism as determinants of therapy. (Reprinted with permission of World Health Organization. Cancer pain relief. Geneva: WHO, 1986.)

markedly to a person's deterioration, both psychological and biological (57, 58). With time, biological and behavioral adjustment to symptoms occurs, and associated tachycardia, hypertension, pallor, and diaphoresis are typically blunted. Patients may appear stoic, with no outward signs of discomfort, or may display florid pain behavior (verbal signals; alterations in facial expression, gait, posture, and mood) (59). In either case, when physical signs are absent, care providers must guard against any tendency to minimize the importance of the patient's distress. Chronic pain with superimposed episodes of acute pain (i.e., breakthrough pain) (60) is probably the most common pattern observed in patients with ongoing cancer pain.

Intensity

Classification of cancer pain according to its intensity is clinically relevant for several reasons. The consistent use of measurements of pain intensity (discussed later) aids in reliable assessment of patients' progress and may serve as a basis for interpatient comparison when data are being gathered for research purposes. High pain scores should alert the clinician to the need for urgent or aggressive intervention. When drug treatment is being considered, the WHO-advocated analgesic ladder model (61) depicted in Figure 25.1 is usually applied. The severity of pain is the main determinant of the patient's place on the ladder, helping to determine whether the patient should receive a nonopioid analgesic, a so-called weak opioid (e.g., codeine, oxycodone), or a more potent opioid (e.g., morphine, hydromorphone) as initial treatment.

Pathophysiology

A general classification by pathophysiology distinguishes among nociceptive (somatic and visceral), neuropathic, and idiopathic, or so-called psychogenic, pain (62). These types of pain are discussed in Chapters 7 and 20–24. Shared characteristics and responsiveness to various therapeutic interventions have been observed within each category, and hence this classification is useful when formulating an initial approach to treatment. However, despite similarities in mechanism and causation, each pain problem must be regarded as a unique entity requiring an individualized plan that may have to be altered frequently. Factors that contribute to heterogeneity within a pathophysiological group include the nature and severity of the insult; overall physical, emotional, and psychological condition; and individual differences in the response to drugs and other treatment. Furthermore, in many patients the pain is the result of multiple interacting mechanisms and components (sensory, affective, cognitive, and behavioral), the sum of which contribute to a complex pain syndrome that often defies simple categorization (1).

Somatic Nociceptive Pain

Somatic pain is typically constant and well localized to the area of disease. Somatic pain is frequently characterized as aching, throbbing, sharp, or gnawing. It tends to be opioid-sensitive and amenable to relief by interruption of proximal pathways by chemical blockade when indicated.

Visceral Nociceptive Pain

Visceral pain originates from injury to sympathetically innervated organs (63). When pain is due to a lesion involving the abdominal or pelvic viscera, it is characteristically vague in distribution and quality and is often described as deep, dull, aching, dragging, squeezing, or pressurelike. When acute, it may be paroxysmal and colicky and can be associated with nausea, vomiting, diaphoresis, and alterations in blood pressure and heart rate. Mechanisms of visceral pain include abnormal distention or contraction of the smooth muscle walls (hollow viscera), rapid capsular stretch (solid viscera), ischemia of visceral muscle, serosal or mucosal irritation by algesic substances and other chemical stimuli, distention and traction or torsion on mesenteric attachments and vasculature, and necrosis (64). The viscera are, however, insensitive to simple manipulation, cutting, and burning (65). Visceral involvement often produces referred pain (66, 67) a phenomenon of pain and hyperalgesia localized to superficial and/or deep tissues often distant to the source of disease or injury. Examples include back pain of pancreatic or retroperitoneal origin, abdominal wall pain from peritoneal irritation, upper extremity pain of anginal origin, and phrenic nerve-mediated shoulder pain of hepatic origin.

Neuropathic Pain

Neuropathic pain is associated with aberrant somatosensory processes induced by injury to some element of the nervous system. Deafferentation pain, central pain, plexus avulsion, phantom pain, and sympathetically maintained pain are all subtypes of neuropathic pain (68). Sympathetically maintained pain in the cancer patient is exemplified by tumor invasion or irritation of the sympathetic chain, producing a reflex sympathetic dystrophy. This entity may accompany Pancoast's syndrome or lumbosacral plexopathy and is associated with causalgic, dysesthetic pain, often accompanied by typical vasomotor and dystrophic changes. Dysesthesias are usually experienced as discomfort and altered sensation, distinct from ordinary, familiar sensations of pain. Dysesthetic pain is variously described as burning, tingling, numbing, pressing, squeezing, and/or itching and is often extremely unpleasant, even intolerable. In addition to continuous pain there may be a component of superimposed intermittent shocklike pain most often characterized as shooting, lancinating, electrical, or jolting.

Neuropathic pain may be characterized by decreased responsiveness to standard analgesic therapies. In general, pain is less responsive to opioid therapy administered by standard or even neuraxial routes, commonly requiring higher doses that are often associated with side effects (69). There is a tendency in some instances for favorable response to a heterogeneous group of centrally acting medications called adjuvant analgesics or coanalgesics, agents developed for other purposes and only serendipitously observed to promote analgesia. These agents include the heterocyclic antidepressants, anticonvulsants, oral local anesthetics (sodium channel blockers), corticosteroids, N-methyl-D-aspartate (NMDA) blockers, and others. Dose-response relationship is often unpredictable, and trials of 3 to 4 weeks in doses titrated upward to tolerance are recommended.

Neuropathic pain may be more resistant to further denervation than nociceptive pain, whether accomplished by ablative surgery or chemical neurolysis. These approaches warrant caution because of their potential for ultimately increasing the pain. Ablative procedures may, however, result in short-term relief of pain, and so have somewhat greater merit in dying patients. Whenever possible, prognostic local anesthetic blocks should be performed prior to neuroablation, preferably repeatedly to rule out a placebo response. Sympathectomy often reliably reverses vasomotor changes, but long-term relief of pain is less common. Chronic electrical stimulation of deep brain structures and the spinal cord has been reported to produce long-term relief of pain in selected cases.

Person and Stage of Disease

Foley (4) devised a classification scheme (Table 25.7) based on patient type and stage of disease which she suggests is predictive of patients' response to therapy and hence may have utility as a guide to clinicians.

Table 25.7.   Predicted Features of Pain Based on Patient and Disease Characteristics

Pain Syndrome	Characteristics of Patients
Acute cancer-related pain	Patients tend to be hopeful
Related to diagnosis	Patients endure pain readily, often without seeking treatment
Related to treatment	Recurrence of pain can be devastating (identified with recrudescence of disease)
Chronic cancer-related pain	Psychological adaption or maladaption is established
Associated with treatment	Disease quiescent; overriding concern is with reestablishment of functional lifestyle
Associated with progression	Hopelessness, helplessness often predominate
Patients with preexisting chronic pain	Require intensive intervention and support; pain behavior established; accurate diagnosis essential
Patients with history of drug abuse	Difficult to evaluate and treat; risk of readdiction; risk of inadequate treatment; coordinate interdisciplinary resources (e.g., rehabilitation, social work)
Dying patients	Adequacy of treatment has greatest effect on patient and family; assure comfort at all costs

Adapted from Foley K.M. Treatment of cancer pain. N Engl J Med 1985;313:84-95.

Temporal Aspects of Pain

Despite efforts at classification, pain in the cancer patient is still an individual phenomenon, and successful treatment requires that management be tailored to the needs of the individual patient.

Constant Pain

Pain may be constant and unremitting, in which case it is most amenable to drug therapy administered around the clock, contingent on time rather than symptoms. This approach to management endeavors to prevent pain rather than treat it once it is established and is best accomplished by the around-the-clock use of long-acting analgesics or in selected cases, infusions of analgesics.

Breakthrough and Incident Pain

Despite the establishment of an effective preventive schedule, breakthrough pain is still a common phenomenon that must be anticipated and addressed. Breakthrough pain (60) is intermittent exacerbations of pain that occur spontaneously or in relation to specific activity. Breakthrough pain that is related to a specific activity, such as eating, defecation, socializing, or walking is referred to as incident pain. Breakthrough pain is best managed by supplementing the preventative around-the-clock regimen with analgesics with a rapid onset of action and a short duration. Once a pattern of incident pain is established, escape, or rescue, doses of analgesics can be administered in anticipation of the pain-provoking activity. When treatment by infusion therapy (subcutaneous, intravenous, epidural) has been elected, the addition of patient-controlled analgesia (PCA), which per-

mits patients to administer a preset amount of opioid at preset intervals, is an effective means to manage breakthrough and incident pain. Breakthrough pain that occurs consistently prior to the next scheduled dose of around-the-clock opioid is called end of dose failure (60) and is ideally managed by increasing the dose of the basal analgesic or reducing the intervals between doses.

Intermittent Pain

Pain that is intermittent and unpredictable in onset represents an extreme challenge to management. Around-the-clock dosing is likely to be unsatisfactory because analgesia is often inadequate during painful episodes and sedation usually supervenes during pain-free intervals. Intermittent pain is usually best managed by the administration as needed of an appropriately potent analgesic of rapid onset and short duration (e.g., immediate release morphine, hydromorphone, oxycodone) or if an alternate route is being used, the addition of PCA. When intermittent pain is well-localized, there may be a role for nerve block therapy, as well.

Cancer Pain Syndromes

Finally, the history, physical findings, and the results of radiological studies aid the practitioner in determining the specific pathological process that is present. Numerous distinct cancer pain syndromes have been recognized and described (Table 25.8)(22, 54). Mechanisms include obstruction of lymphatic and vascular channels, distention of a hollow viscus, edema, tissue inflammation, and necrosis. Severe symptoms are most often related to invasion of pain-sensitive structures by tumor mass.

Table 25.8.   Cancer Pain Syndromes

Bone invasion:

Presentation is variable; usually constant, often greatest at night and with movement or weight bearing; often a dull ache or deep, intense pain; may be associated with referred pain, muscle spasm, or when there is nerve compression, paroxysms of stabbing pain

Vertebral body invasion:

Often presents a severe local, dull, steady, aching pain; often exacerbated by recumbency, sitting, movement, and local pressure; may be relieved by standing; local midline tenderness may be present; associated nerve compression may produce radiating dermatomal pain and corresponding neurological changes; may be associated with epidural–spinal cord compression

Base of skull metastases:

Numerous specific syndromes described (middle fossa syndrome, jugular foramen syndrome, clivus metastases, orbital metastases, parasellar metastases, sphenoid sinus metastases, occipital condyle invasion, odontoid fractures); usually present with headache and a spectrum of neurological findings, especially involving cranial nerves; usually a late finding; may be difficult to diagnose radiographically

Nerve invasion:

Typically a constant, burning dysesthetic pain, often with an intermittent lancinating, electrical component; may be associated with neurologic deficit or diffuse hyperesthesia and localized paresthesia; muscle weakness and atrophy may be present in mixed or motor nerve syndromes

Leptomeningeal metastases, meningeal carcinomatosis:

Most common with primary malignancies of breast and lung, lymphoma and leukemia; headache is most common presenting complaint; characteristically unrelenting; may be associated with nausea, vomiting, nuchal rigidity, and mental status changes; associated neurological abnormalities may include seizures, cranial nerve deficits, papilledema, hemiparesis, ataxia and cauda syndrome; diagnosis confirmed with lumbar puncture

Spinal cord compression:

Pain almost always precedes neurological changes; urgent radiological workup required for rapid progression of neurological deficit, particularly motor weakness, or incontinence; early treatment may limit neurologic morbidity

Cervical plexopathy:

May result from local invasion by head and neck cancers or pressure from enlarged nodes; symptoms primarily sensory, experienced as aching preauricular, post-auricular, or neck pain

Brachial plexopathy:

Most commonly due to upper lobe lung cancer (Pancoast's syndrome), breast cancer, or lymphoma; pain is an early symptom, usually preceding neurological findings; usually diffuse aching in shoulder girdle, radiating down arm, often to the elbow and medial (ulnar) aspect of the hand; Horner's syndrome, dysesthesias, progressive atrophy, and neurological impairment (weakness and numbness) may occur; must differentiate from radiation fibrosis, which characteristically is less severe, less often associated with motor changes, tends to involve the upper trunks, and may be associated with lymphadema

Lumbosacral plexopathy:

May be due to local soft tissue invasion or compression; pain is usually presenting sign; may be referred to low back, abdomen, buttock, or lower extremity

Celiac plexopathy:

Usually relentless, boring, midepigastric aching pain radiating to midback; often relieved by fetal position and worse with recumbency

Chemotherapy-induced polyneurophathy:

Most common with vincristine, vinblastine, and cisplatin; may include jaw pain, claudication, and dysesthetic pain in the hands or feet

Postsurgical syndromes:

Most common after mastectomy, thoracotomy, radical neck dissection, nephrectomy and amputation; usually aching, shooting, or tingling in distribution of peripheral nerves (e.g., intercostalbrachial, intercostal, cervical plexus) with or without skin hypersensitivity

Osseous Invasion

Tumor infiltration of bone is cited as the most common cause of cancer pain (70) and is most often secondary to primary disease in the prostate, breast, thyroid, lung, or kidney (70, 71). Skeletal metastases are clinically evident in a third of patients with carcinoma and are found in two thirds of patients at autopsy (71). Although the majority of skeletal metastases do not produce pain (70, 72), pain from bony metastases can produce a variety of symptoms. When present, pain is usually constant but may be greatest at night and is often worse with movement or weight bearing. Patients may report a dull ache or deep, intense pain, and there may be referred pain, muscle spasm, or paroxysms of stabbing pain, particularly when bony lesions are accompanied by nerve compression. Painful bony metastasis in endocrine-resistant prostate cancer predicts a poor prognosis (73).

Since up to 50% decalcification must occur before osseous lesions are visible on plain radiographs (74), a bone scan (isotope scanning, scintigraphy) is preferred for detecting most bone metastases (70). In certain settings (primary bone tumors, thyroid cancer, multiple myeloma) plain films are considered to be more sensitive (39). In addition, since radioisotope scanning reflects the metastatic status of the bone and plain radiographs the net result of both new bone formation and old bone destruction, plain films may be valuable in patients with stabilized (burned out) metastases (75). Abnormal findings on scintigrams are not specific for malignant disease, and it is essential that they be interpreted together with other radiological studies and in the context of clinical findings. Neoplastic involvement must be differentiated from changes related to infection, trauma, or degeneration, because treatment differs, even in the patient with cancer. Scans may appear false-negative when lesions are predominantly osteoclastic, after radiation therapy, and when surrounding bone is diffusely involved with tumor, as is most likely to occur in patients with breast, lung, and prostate cancer (64). Additionally, the detection of osseous metastases in hidden sites (76) (T1 vertebral body, base of the skull, sacrum) may be difficult, particularly on plain films, because of overlying images of gas and normal bony structures.

Mechanisms of bone pain remain incompletely understood, but a biochemical explanation is attractive to explain how even small lesions can produce severe pain. Osseous metastases elaborate prostaglandin E_2 (PGE_2), which is hypothesized to contribute to pain by sensitization of peripheral nociceptors. Nonsteroidal anti-inflammatory agents and steroids are postulated to reduce pain from bony metastases via inhibition of the cyclo-oxygenase pathway of arachidonic acid breakdown, thus decreasing the formation of PGE_2. As deposits enlarge, stretching of the periosteum, pathological fracture, and perineural invasion contribute to pain, and requirements for analgesics increase. A recent study by Akakura et al. (73) suggests that onset of pain in bony metastasis may be attributable not to the extent of disease but to the rapidity of expansion of bone metastasis. Palliative radiation therapy is commonly successfully employed to relieve pain emanating from bony metastases. Hormonal therapy (chemotherapy, orchiectomy, hypophysectomy) often reduces bony pain in patients with hormonal dependent disease (breast, prostate), although the estrogen agent tamoxifen may increase pain transiently before it is relieved (tamoxifen flare) in a small proportion of patients (77).

Skull Metastases   Specific syndromes associated with metastatic spread of tumor to the base of the skull have been described by Greenberg et al. (78) and Elliot and Foley (79). Symptomatic metastases to the skull is usually but not always a late finding (78). The presenting complaint is usually headache, which is often followed by the onset of neurological abnormalities. Plain radiography and scintigraphy are often insufficient to make a reliable diagnosis. Supplementation with computed tomography (CT) (thin slices viewed as bone windows) is desirable to diagnose bony disease, while magnetic resonance imaging (MRI) and lumbar puncture are useful to evaluate the soft tissues and to detect leptomeningeal disease, respectively (79).

Vertebral Syndromes and Spinal Cord Compression   The bony spinal column is a frequent site of metastases, especially from tumors of the lung, breast, and prostate. Tumor invasion restricted to bone may result in severe local pain. Associated nerve compression tends to produce radiating pain and circumscribed neurological changes. Vertebral involvement may be associated with epidural-spinal cord compression that, if allowed to progress, is further associated with both pain and neurological impairment (paraplegia and quadriplegia) and is a major cause of morbidity.

Localized paraspinal, radicular or referred pain is usually the first sign of metastases to the bony vertebral column, usually preceding neurological changes by weeks. Cervical and lumbar involvement tend to produce unilateral symptoms, while thoracic involvement is often bilateral. Periosteal invasion is responsible for the dull, steady, aching pain that is frequently observed. Pain is often exacerbated by recumbency, sitting, movement, and local pressure and may be relieved by standing. Local tenderness of the bony spinal column and radicular pain in the cervical, thoracic, or upper lumbar regions, findings that are uncommon in nonmalignant neuromusculoskeletal disorders, should alert the clinician to consider vertebral involvement by tumor. Although invasion of the upper lumbar vertebrae is usually heralded by dull backache and/or radicular signs, pain may be localized to the sacroiliac joints or iliac crests, and thus radiological investigations of the lumbar spine should not be overlooked when these symptoms are present. In addition, invasion of the second cervical vertebra may result in referred pain to the occiput, and C7-T1 invasion may produce interscapular pain (80).

In the case of cord compression, pain almost always precedes neurological changes by weeks or days. Rapid progression of neurological deficit, particularly of motor weakness, or the appearance of urinary or fecal incontinence (or urinary retention) signals progressive epidural-spinal cord compression and warrants urgent intervention. Familiarity with the pertinent aspects of the clinical presentation and early diagnosis of spinal cord compression are warranted because the onset of this common disorder is heralded in almost all cases by pain, often independent of neurological findings, and early intervention is essential to limit neurological morbidity.

While surgical stabilization should be considered for cord compression, it is frequently not feasible. Decision making is complex, depending on probable life expectancy, severity and manageability of pain, tumor location, and the surgeon's experience. When appropriate, however, surgical stabilization may significantly reduce the mechanical pain associated with vertebral metastasis and can preserve or restore function. There is an excellent review on the topic by Gokaslan (81). In cases of severe debilitation, a limited surgical approach (posterolateral decompression without fusion) has been advocated by Weller and Rossitch (82).

Muscle Pain

It has only recently been recognized that muscle pain(cramps, myalgia, myofascial pain) is a much more common cause of nonmalignant pain than previously thought (83), and there is every reason to expect that it has been underdiagnosed in cancer patients as well (84). Underrecognition is probably due in part to the inability of standard radiographic techniques to document muscle injury, as well as the varied, sometimes vague, and usually nonneurological constellation of characteristic symptoms. Muscle cramps in the cancer patient are the subject of a recent excellent review (85).

Neural Invasion

Invasion or compression of somatic nerves by tumor is generally associated with constant, burning dysesthetic pain, often with an intermittent lancinating component. Diffuse hyperesthesia and localized paresthesia are common, and muscle weakness and atrophy may be present if the affected structure is a mixed or motor nerve. Pain attributable to nerve compression by tumor was diagnosed in 34% of patients referred to an anesthesiology-pain service, 40% in a tertiary care center, 20% in a neurology service, and 31% in a hospice (40, 86-88).

Plexopathies   Cervical plexopathy may result from local invasion by head and neck cancers or pressure from enlarged lymph nodes. Symptoms are primarily sensory in the distribution of the plexus and are typically aching preauricular, postauricular, or neck pain.

Brachial plexopathy (Pancoast's or superior sulcus syndrome) is associated most commonly with carcinoma of the lung (primary or metastatic) and breast, as well as lymphoma (89). Pain occurs in up to 85% of patients with brachial plexus invasion, usually as an early symptom, often preceding other neurological findings by up to 9 months (90, 91). Early recognition with referral for radiation therapy, surgery, or chemotherapy is essential to limit neurological morbidity, but unfortunately, a diagnosis is often delayed longer than 6 months (92).

The lower cord of the plexus (C8-T1) is affected most frequently, and pain is characteristically diffuse aching in the shoulder girdle with radiation down the arm, often to the elbow and medial (ulnar) aspect of the hand (89, 93). Dysesthesias, progressive atrophy, and neurological impairment (weakness and numbness) usually occur. Horner's syndrome is a common concomitant finding. Although less common, invasion of the upper plexus (C5-C6) may occur, usually with pain in the shoulder girdle and upper arm, radiating to the thumb and index finger. It can be difficult to differentiate brachial plexus abnormalities due to radiation fibrosis from those of tumor invasion because clinical findings are similar. Radiation-induced injury is more commonly associated with signs referable to dysfunction of the upper trunk (C5-C7 roots), including weakness of shoulder abduction and arm flexors. Pain is a less prominent finding after radiation injury and is more likely to be characterized as aching in the shoulder and tightness and heaviness in the upper arm accompanied by lymphedema (81), without a Horner's sign. Brachial plexus invasion is often associated with contiguous spread to the epidural space (94-96), and suspected brachial plexopathy requires a complete radiological evaluation with CT or MRI. If epidural extension is suspected, myelography may be indicated, depending on the MRI's quality.

Lumbosacral plexopathy due to local soft tissue invasion by tumor, lymphadenopathy, or compression from bony metastases occurs most commonly in association with tumors of the rectum, cervix, and breast and with sarcoma, and lymphoma. That pain is a valuable diagnostic sign is emphasized by the findings in one large study (97) in which pain was the presenting symptom in 70% of patients, followed only weeks or months later by the development of significant weakness and numbness. Pain was the only symptom in 24% of patients studied. Reflex asymmetry and mild sensory and motor changes, when present, were relatively early findings, and impotence and incontinence were relatively rare. In the same study, direct extension from local intra-abdominal disease was responsible for more than two thirds of cases, with metastatic disease accounting for a much smaller proportion. Pain may be local (85%), radicular (85%), or referred (44%) and is characteristically described as aching or pressurelike and only rarely as causalgic or dysesthetic (97). Depending on the level involved, pain is referred to the low back, abdomen, buttock, or lower extremity (97, 98). Suspected plexopathy must be differentiated from invasion of the spinal cord and cauda equina syndrome. Radiological investigations of the pelvis and lumbar spine and diagnostic nerve blocks are helpful to corroborate clinical findings. For sacrococcygeal plexopathy, plain films, CT, and scintigrams frequently demonstrate bony invasion of the sacral plates. If symptoms are permitted to progress unchecked, patients are likely to become immobile and depressed and are subject to increased risks of venous thrombosis, decubiti, and infection.

Leptomeningeal Metastases and Meningeal Carcinomatosis

Leptomeningeal metastases occur most commonly in patients with lymphoma, leukemia, and primary malignancies of the breast and lung. An 8 to 10% incidence was found in one autopsy study of patients with systemic cancer (99). Diffuse infiltration of the meninges by tumor has the potential to produce protean signs and symptoms. About 40% of patients have headache or back pain, presumably due to traction on the pain-sensitive meninges, cranial, and spinal nerves and/or raised intracranial pressure (100, 101). Headache, the most common presenting complaint, is characteristically unrelenting and may be associated with nausea, vomiting, nuchal rigidity, and mental status changes (101). Other neurological abnormalities include seizures, cranial nerve signs, papilledema, hemiparesis, ataxia, and cauda equina syndrome.

A diagnosis of leptomeningeal metastases is confirmed by analysis of cerebrospinal fluid (CSF), which reveals the presence of malignant cells and may also be remarkable for an increased opening pressure, raised protein, and decreased glucose (102). CT, MRI or myelogram is recommended to evaluate the extent of disease (68, 103). The natural history of patients with leptomeningeal metastases is gradual decline and death over 4 to 6 weeks, although survival is often extended to 6 months or more when treatment with radiation therapy and/or intrathecal methotrexate is instituted (104). Steroids are said to be useful in the management of headache (79).

Headache   Headache is a major but not invariable symptom of intracranial neoplasm (105), present in 60% of patients in one survey, half of whom classified headache as their primary complaint (106). Its pattern is not distinctive (107). Patients typically describe pain that is steady, deep, dull, and aching and that is rarely rhythmic or throbbing. It is usually intermittent and may be worse in the morning and with coughing or straining. Characteristically the intensity of pain is only moderate, rarely awakening patients from sleep and generally less than what is typically described in so-called benign headache syndromes. Symptoms often respond to simple measures including recumbency, the administration of aspirin or a steroid (108), and the application of cold packs. Symptoms often improve when radiation therapy is applied to treat the underlying malignancy (107, 109).

Cervicofacial Pain   The head and neck are richly innervated by contributions from cranial nerves V, VII, IX, and X and the upper cervical nerves. Analgesia may be difficult to achieve because of the erosive nature of many tumors and their location. Pain may arise from any of a variety of mechanisms, and as such, it varies in character. Mechanisms include soft-tissue ulceration, infection, and compression from adenopathy or tumor, mucositis, bony erosion, and nerve invasion. When cranial nerves and their branches are affected, symptoms may resemble those of trigeminal, glossopharyngeal, and/or intermedius neuralgia, with sudden, severe lancinating pain radiating to the face, throat or ear, respectively. Pain may be accompanied by altered sensation, trigger points, and impaired swallowing, breathing, and phonation.

Early consideration should be given to palliative radiation therapy. Depending on its underlying mechanism, pain may respond to treatment with the NSAIDs and opioids, anticonvulsants, antidepressants and/or antibiotics. Treatment with antibiotics should be considered when infection is present or suspected (110). Antibiotics should be considered not only for obvious infection but also as empirical therapy for suspected occult infection. Occult infection is especially likely when cancer or its therapies inhibit the bone marrow's capability of mounting a leukocytosis or if infection is difficult to diagnose because it is sequestered or there is anatomical distortion after surgery and radiation therapy. Neurolytic blocks, neurosurgery, and intraventricular opioids may be successful for pain that is otherwise intractable (111).

Pancreatic Cancer Pain

Pancreatic cancer pain has been well-characterized (112-114). Patients present most often with relentless, boring, midepigastric aching pain that radiates through to the midback and that is often relieved by the assumption of the fetal position and worsened by recumbency. While this presentation is common, other symptoms may be present, often because of related pathology, and distinguishing among these heterogeneous syndromes is essential to select the most appropriate form of management (113). The classic presentation mentioned here is most consistent with a likelihood of good outcome after celiac plexus block, while other symptoms suggest the need for alternative treatment and/or further diagnostic studies.

The optimal timing and application of the neurolytic celiac plexus block in pancreatic cancer pain is the subject of considerable debate. A recent prospective trial comparing NSAIDs and morphine with neurolytic celiac plexus block revealed significantly lower pain scores and opioid use for the first 4 and 8 weeks respectively after neural blockade, although quality of life did not improve significantly in either group (115).

Pain Due to Anticancer Therapy

As many as 20% of adults have pain caused directly by cancer therapy (116). This percentage is probably higher in the pediatric cancer population, especially considering the frequency with which painful diagnostic procedures (e.g.,

bone marrow biopsy, lumbar puncture) are required for the evaluation and treatment of leukemia and central nervous system (CNS) neoplasms (117).

Treatment-related pain problems are important because their appearance may be confused with more ominous pain syndromes associated with severe tumor recurrence or progression. Furthermore, when they are severe, compliance with recommendations for further antineoplastic therapy may be adversely affected, and they often pose particularly difficult management problems (118).

Chemotherapy

Oral mucositis, which usually occurs within 1 to 2 weeks of the initiation of chemotherapy, is most common with the use of methotrexate, doxorubicin, daunorubicin, bleomycin, etoposide, fluorouracil (5-FU), and dactinomycin (119). Mucositis may be more severe when these agents are used in combination with radiation therapy, especially for bone marrow transplantation. Treatment is with topical oral agents such as viscous lidocaine, oral hygiene (exclude candidiasis and other infections), diet adjustment, and potent opioid analgesics, often administered by PCA (120).

Painful polyneuropathy occurs most commonly with exposure to vincristine (motor and sensory involvement) and cisplatin (predominantly sensory involvement) (121). Symptoms may include jaw pain, claudication, and dysesthetic pain in the hands or feet. When detected early, symptoms often resolve upon reductions in dose. Symptomatic treatment consists of trials of the adjuvant analgesics (e.g., antidepressants, anticonvulsants), and in selected cases, opioids. The administration of steroids may be associated with pain due to several mechanisms, including avascular necrosis of the humeral and femoral joints, osteopenia, bone pain secondary to pathological fractures, and a pseudorheumatoid syndrome associated with rapid steroid withdrawal (122, 123).

Radiation Therapy

Radiation therapy may be associated with a variety of painful conditions, including oral mucositis, osteoradionecrosis, myelopathy, plexopathy, soft-tissue fibrosis, and the emergence of new secondary neurogenic tumors. When pain is due to neuropathic mechanisms, trials of the adjunctive analgesics may be beneficial.

Postsurgical Syndromes

Characteristic identifiable pain syndromes may follow mastectomy, thoracotomy, radical neck dissection, nephrectomy, and amputation. Recognition of these specific syndromes may help the clinician distinguish them from pain due to tumor recurrence. Interestingly, in a recent study (124) the incidence of post-mastectomy pain was higher after conservative surgery than modified radical mastectomy (33% versus 17%). In this same study 25% of patients experienced postoperative phantom breast pain. Another study by the same authors (125) on more than 500 postmastectomy patients revealed a 50% incidence of neuropathic postmastectomy pain, 25% of which was sufficiently severe to alter routine activities. Pain and altered sensation (allodynia) are often due to nerve entrapment (i.e., intercostobrachial and intercostal nerves). Treatment is with trials of adjuvant analgesics, opioids, nerve blocks, transcutaneous electrical nerve stimulation (TENS) and physical therapy, but often relief of symptoms is incomplete (125a-127).

Screening Instruments

Diverse instruments have been developed to obtain the variety of types of information that may be useful in assessing patients with cancer pain (128, 129). Most centers select items from this plethora of tools to form their own questionnaire, which ideally is completed by the patient prior to evaluation. The development and acceptance of a standard instrument would contribute to a better understanding of epidemiology and outcome and is a highly desirable goal. The Wisconsin Brief Pain Inventory (130, 131) and Memorial Pain Assessment Card (132) are becoming increasingly well-accepted and may emerge as standard tools for assessing cancer pain.

It is almost universally recommended that some form or forms of self-report constitute the foundation of pain assessment (45). While these may be complemented by behavioral, psychometric, and observational instruments, these adjuncts should not be relied upon exclusively. Several studies have demonstrated a relatively poor correlation between patients' and nurses' assessment of pain intensity (133, 134) and like results have been obtained when cancer patients' self-report was compared with physicians' observations (135). Similarly a comparison of the responses of cancer patients and their next of kin did not demonstrate uniformly high correlations (136). Especially noteworthy is a study by Grossman et al. (45) that revealed that the largest discrepancies between caregivers' and patients' reports occurred when pain was severe.

While a comprehensive battery of psychological testing is usually considered to be an appropriate component of the assessment of the patient with chronic nonmalignant pain, it is essential that testing of the cancer pain patient be brief and not excessively demanding.

Wisconsin Brief Pain Inventory

Completion of the BPI requires about 15 minutes, and it can be self-administered or used as an adjunct to the interview, apparently without affecting the reliability of results (131). It includes several questions about the characteristics of the pain, including its origin and the effects of prior treatments. In addition, the BPI incorporates two valuable features of the McGill Pain Questionnaire, a graphic representation of the location of pain and groups of qualitative descriptors. Severity of pain is assessed by a series of visual analog scales that score pain at its best, worst, and on average. Finally, the perceived level of interference with normal function (enjoyment of life, work, mood, sleep, general activity, walking, relations with others) is quantified with visual analog scales that are both numbered and labeled by the anchors "no interference" and "interferes completely." Preliminary evidence suggests that the BPI is cross-culturally valid (131) and is useful, particularly when patients are not fit to complete a more thorough or comprehensive questionnaire. Long and short forms are suitable for initial evaluation and follow-up, respectively.

Memorial Pain Assessment Card

The Memorial Pain Assessment Card is a simple, efficient, and valid instrument that provides rapid clinical evaluation of the major aspects of pain experienced by cancer patients (118). It is easy to understand and use and can be completed by experienced patients in less than 20 seconds. It consists of a two-sided 8.5×11-inch card that is folded so that four separate measures are created. It features scales intended for the measurement of pain intensity, pain relief, and mood and a set of descriptive adjectives. Its originators believe that it can help distinguish among pain intensity, pain relief, and global suffering or psychological distress (132).

Edmonton Staging System

One additional screening tool deserves mention because its intent and methodology are distinct from those of other instruments. The Edmonton staging system for cancer pain (137, 138), which is performed by the health care provider rather than the patient, was developed to predict the likelihood of achieving effective relief of pain in cancer patients. Patients are staged with an alphanumeric code in a fashion similar to the one used to characterize the clinicohistological status of tumors (139). The system's originators have provided validation that treatment outcome can be accurately predicted according to five clinical features (neuropathic pain, movement-related pain, recent history of tolerance to opioids, psychological distress, and a history of alcoholism or drug abuse). Staging requires only 5 to 10 minutes and requires no special skills. Its value lies in prospective identification of potentially problematic patients, further legitimizing clinical research on symptom control by introducing better standardization and improving our ability to assess critically the results of various therapeutic interventions in large populations of patients.

Assessment of Cancer Pain in Children

Developmentally appropriate pain assessment is an integral part of pediatric cancer pain therapy. Many child-specific tools have been developed over the past decade. They include Beyer's The Oucher, Eland's color scale-body outline, Hester's poker chip tool, McGrath's faces scale, and others (140-143). There is an excellent chapter on the subject by Beyer and Wells (144).

TREATMENT

The vast array of pain treatment options are best understood by recognizing that all potential therapies can ultimately be considered as pertaining to one of three overall strategies. A given therapy may relieve pain by modifying its source, interrupting its transmission, or modulating its influence at brain or spinal cord sites.

Antineoplastic Treatment

Ideally, cancer pain is managed by direct treatment of its underlying cause. Once elucidated, the pathological process responsible for pain can often be altered with surgical extirpation, external beam radiation therapy (targeted fractionated or single-dose therapy, hemibody or total body irradiation) (145, 146) radionuclides (e.g., strontium-89, samarium), chemotherapy (147), hormonal treatment (148), and even whole-body hyperthermia (149). Many patients are pleased to realize prompt and significant pain relief when their cancer responds to antitumor therapy. This is true especially for lymphoma treated with various chemotherapies and painful bone metastases, which often respond promptly and dramatically to local irradiation; in some settings it can be administered in a single, nonfractionated dose (150). Nevertheless, the majority of patients require some form of primary analgesic therapy, whether they are awaiting a tumoricidal response or because antitumor therapy has been maximized or is no longer applicable. Even when the goal of cure has been abandoned, further antitumor therapy should be considered when new symptoms arise or a change in the pain treatment strategy is planned. For rapid palliation of symptoms, as opposed to cure, radiation therapy is generally the most applicable of these modalities. Palliative antitumor measures have definite limitations with regard to efficacy, patient acceptance, and adverse effects, especially in patients with advanced disease. Finally, the decision to pursue antitumor therapy does not imply that analgesic drugs and other supportive therapy should be discontinued.

Pharmacological Management

Oral analgesics are the mainstay of therapy for patients with cancer pain. An estimated 70 to 90% of patients can be rendered relatively free of pain when straightforward guideline-based principles of pharmacological management are applied in a thorough, careful manner (4, 6, 7). The WHO's has developed a three-step ladder approach to cancer pain management that relies exclusively on the administration of oral agents (Fig. 25.1) and that is usually effective (21, 40, 151). For example, in a prospective evaluation of the WHO method, Zech et al. (25) observed good results in 76% of 2118 cancer patients treated over 10 years.

While pain can be managed in most patients with oral and transdermal agents alone, even through the terminal stages of illness, a small but important proportion of patients require

alternative forms of therapy (152). The role of more invasive forms of analgesia, ranging from parenteral analgesics to neural blockade and CNS opioid therapy, regrettably remains poorly defined, although it is widely recognized that the judicious application of such approaches is essential when more conservative therapies produce inadequate results.

Noninvasive routes (e.g., oral, transdermal, transmucosal) should be maintained as long as possible for reasons that include simplicity, maintenance of independence and mobility, convenience, and cost. Treatment has been markedly simplified by the introduction of controlled-release preparations of oral opioids (e.g., morphine sulfate [MS Contin, Oramorph, Kadian], oxycodone [Oxycontin]), and novel noninvasive approaches (e.g., transdermal fentanyl [Duragesic], oral transmucosal fentanyl citrate), and most important, the widespread acceptance of guideline-based therapies, as summarized here.

PRINCIPLES OF PHARMACOLOGICAL MANAGEMENT

Assessment

Comprehensive assessment ideally precedes initiation of therapy. Physiological determinants (the pain syndrome, the neoplastic process, associated symptoms, intercurrent medical conditions) and psychosocial determinants (beliefs, cultural milieu, economic status, family interactions) should be taken into account. A problem list and a set of realistic goals that are acceptable to the patient, family, and physician should be established, along with a treatment plan and contingencies. Treatment should be directed toward relief of total pain, which includes consideration of all aspects of function (e.g., disturbance of sleep, appetite, mood, activity, posture, and sexuality), and attention should be paid not only to physical but also to emotional, psychological, and spiritual aspects of suffering. Recommendations should include an explicit plan for reevaluation.

Nonsteroidal Anti-Inflammatory Drugs

Consider the regular (around-the-clock) administration of an NSAID as the sole treatment for mild pain or an NSAID combined with an opioid analgesic for moderate to severe pain (6, 7, 21). NSAIDs are particularly effective for pain of inflammatory and bony metastatic origin by virtue of interference with prostaglandin (PG) synthesis (70). Potential for benefits should be balanced against potential for toxicity (e.g., gastrointestinal (GI), genitourinary (GU), CNS, and hematological toxicity and masking of fever), considerations that are especially pertinent in the context of recent antitumor therapy and advanced age (153). Consider avoiding NSAIDs all together or instituting prophylaxis in patients predisposed to gastropathy. If prophylaxis is indicated, misoprostol appears to be the most effective protective regimen, as demonstrated by a study of 49 cancer patients randomized to receive either misoprostol or ranitidine along with high-dose diclofenac (200 to 300 mg/day). Patients underwent periodic endoscopy, which revealed a significantly lower incidence of gastroduodenal ulceration in misoprostol-treated patients (9% versus 39%) (154). The nonacetylated salicylates (sodium salicylate, choline magnesium trisalicylate) are associated with a favorable toxicity profile, since they fail to interfere with platelet aggregation, are rarely associated with GI bleeding, and are well tolerated by asthmatic patients (155, 156). A parenteral formulation of ketorolac is equianalgesic to low doses of morphine in some settings but is associated with the same range of side effects as oral NSAIDs (157). A new oral NSAID, bromfenac sodium (Duract) (158, 159) has recently been shown to provide analgesia that is comparable with treatment with oxycodone plus acetaminophen, but it is so far recommended only for short-term use.

In contrast to treatment with the opioid analgesics, NSAIDs are associated with a ceiling effect, above which dose escalations produce toxicity but no greater analgesia. However, the ceiling dose for a given drug differs from patient to patient, allowing some potential for dose titration. Regular (as opposed to intermittent) use promotes both anti-inflammatory and analgesic effects. Despite their apparent heterogeneity, the NSAIDs are in most respects clinically indistinguishable. Selection is based on the patient's prior experience, minor differences in toxicity, the clinician's experience, schedule, and cost. When efficacy is poor, the clinician may consider rotating to another NSAID, usually from a different biochemical class. Although evidence from controlled trials is insufficient to support this practice, it is clear that for a given patient, clinical response differs among various agents (interindividual variability), and there is recent evidence that various classes of NSAIDs may exert their anti-PG effects on different subtypes of cyclo-oxygenase (160), the enzyme primarily responsible for PG degradation.

"Weak" Opioids

When NSAIDs provide insufficient relief, are contraindicated, or are poorly tolerated or when pain is severe at presentation, the addition or substitution of a so-called weak opioid (i.e., codeine, hydrocodone, dihydrocodeine, oxycodone preparations) is recommended as an analgesic of intermediate potency (Table 25.9) (6). Almost exclusively formulated as combination products, these agents are weak only insofar as the inclusion of aspirin, acetaminophen, or ibuprofen results in a ceiling dose above which the incidence of toxicity increases. The nomenclature "opioids conventionally used to treat moderate pain" is now endorsed in preference to "weak opioids" in recognition of the fact that when equianalgesic dosing is applied, the potency of the opioid per se is not a clinically important distinguishing feature of this class of drugs. For example, there is now available a sole-entity prepa

ration of oxycodone that, when prescribed in sufficient doses, is effective for even severe pain (161), since the ceiling effect imposed by the aspirin or acetaminophen is absent. Likewise, fentanyl, although up to 100 times as potent as parenteral morphine, is rendered clinically useful by using a dosing schedule in a microgram rather than milligram range.

While the weak opioids are appropriate for mild or intermittent pain, practitioners often rely excessively on these agents, frequently continuing their use after they are no longer effective in an ill-advised attempt to avoid prescribing more potent opioids that are also more highly regulated. Propoxyphene is rarely appropriate for the management of cancer pain because of its low potency (162), and codeine is considerably emetogenic and constipating relative to its analgesic potency. Oxycodone, now available not only as a combination product (Percocet, Percodan) but also as a sole-entity preparation (Roxycodone) and in a slow-release formulation (Oxycontin), is considerably more potent than codeine and may be the most useful drug in this class. The potency of hydrocodone and dihydrocodeine preparations (Lortab, Vicodin) is between that of codeine and oxycodone (163). These agents have the perceived advantage of not requiring triplicate prescriptions (DEA Class C-III versus C-II), although the clinician must be cautious not to exceed the usual recommended dose of acetaminophen (4 to 5 g/day) as opioid requirements increase.

"Potent" Opioids

When combinations of codeinelike drugs and NSAIDs provide insufficient analgesia or when pain is severe at presentation, therapy should progress to include more potent opioid analgesics in a ladder fashion (Fig. 25.1) (21). Morphine, hydromorphone, transdermal fentanyl, and oxycodone are appropriate first-line agents for the institution of basal analgesia (Tables 25.9 and 25.10). Methadone, although inexpensive, and to a lesser extent levorphanol are usually reserved for special circumstances because their half-lives are long and unpredictable, introducing the potential for accumulation, especially in the presence of advanced age and altered renal function (164). Less potent analgesics should not be summarily excluded, since NSAIDs may provide additive or synergistic analgesia, and codeinelike preparations may be useful for breakthrough or incident pain. Opioids should initially be introduced in low doses, since the early development of side effects will impair compliance, but they should be rapidly titrated to effect.

Individualization

Pharmacological therapy should be individualized in light of the specific characteristics and needs of each patient (165). Dose response and side effects vary widely with physiological and behavioral factors (e.g., age, drug history, extent of disease) (166, 167). Effective doses often dramatically exceed

Table 25.9.   Comparison of Opioid Agonists Used in Cancer Pain Management

Generic Name	Trade Name	Route	Equivalent Dose[a]	Duration (Avg Range)
Morphine	Various	IM	10 mg	3–4 hr
	MSIR; etc.	Oral	20–30 mg	3–4 hr
	Various	Rectal	5 mg	4 hr
Controlled release morphine	MS Contin Oramorph	Oral	30 mg	12–8 hr
Hydromorphone	Dilaudid	Oral	7.5 mg	3–4 hr
		IM	1.5 mg	3–4 hr
Oxymorphone	Numorphan	IM	1 mg	3–6 hr
		Rectal	5-10 mg	4–6 hr
Meperidine	Demerol	Oral	300 mg	3–6 hr
		IM	75 mg	3–4 hr
Heroin	Diamorphine	IM	5 mg	4–5 hr
		Oral	60 mg	
Methadone	Dolophine	IM	20 mg	4–8 hr
		Oral	10 mg	4–8 hr
Levorphanol	Levodromoran	IM	2 mg	4–8 hr
		Oral	2 mg	4–8 hr
Oxycodone controlled release	Various	Oral	30 mg	3–6 hr
	Oxycontin	Oral	30 mg	12 hr
Transdermal fentanyl	Duragesic	TID	—[b]	72 hr

[a]Compared with 10 mg parenteral morphine.
[b]See Table 25.10.

Table 25.10.   Dosage Equivalency for Transdermal Fentanyl[a]

Oral Morphine[b] (mg/24 hr)	IM Morphine[c] (mg/24 hr)	Transdermal Fentanyl (μg/hr)
45–134	8–22	25
135–224	23–37	50
225–314	38–52	75
315–404	53–67	100
405–494	68–82	125
495–584	83–97	150
585–674	98–112	175
675–764	113–127	200
765–854	128–142	225
855–944	143–157	250
945–1034	158–172	275
1035–1124	173–187	300

Courtesy of Janssen Pharmaceutical (modified by author).
[a]Package insert; hourly dose based on 24 hour morphine equivalents.
[b]Conversion from oral morphine: based on a *conservative* analgesic activity ratio of 60 mg oral morphine to 10 mg IM morphine (6:1 oral to parenteral conversion ratio rather than the widely accepted 3:1 ratio). As a result, converting from oral morphine to transdermal fentanyl using this chart, while generally quite safe, may result in underdosing of up to half of patients, who will require rapid upward titration to achieve analgesia.
[c]Conversion from IV or IM morphine: an analgesic activity ratio of 10 mg IM morphine to 100 μg IV fentanyl was used to derive the equivalence of parenteral morphine to transdermal fentanyl. *These recommendations tend to be reliable.*

guidelines recommended in standard texts (10 mg intramuscularly, 30 mg by mouth), which for the most part are derived from experience with acute or postoperative pain in opioid-naive individuals.

Dosing Guidelines

The correct dose of an opioid for the management of cancer pain is the one that effectively relieves pain without inducing unacceptable side effects. The starting dose is gradually and steadily titrated upward until either pain control is achieved or side effects occur. If side effects ensue before adequate pain relief is established, they are treated aggressively in an algorithmic fashion. Other strategies that can be employed (e.g., opioid rotation, anesthetic interventions) are discussed later.

Side Effects

Constipation and miosis are the only two opioid-mediated effects to which significant tolerance appears never to develop. Thus, opioid-induced constipation is sufficiently common that it should almost universally be treated prophylactically. Usually a combined mild laxative and softener (Senokot-S) is prescribed when opioid therapy commences (168) along with instructions for a sliding-scale regimen that provides progressively stronger cathartics until a regular bowel habit ensues. An osmotic agent (e.g., lactulose) is the usual second-line agent of choice for refractory constipation. The evaluating clinician should remain alert for bowel obstruction and fecal impaction, which may present as spurious diarrhea because of the leakage of liquid stool around a distal fecal plug. Impaction is confirmed by manual rectal examination, and its occurrence leaves no alternative to manual disimpaction, which is time consuming and unpleasant and usually requires strong analgesics. Finally, unrecognized constipation can contribute to nausea and vomiting.

Opioid-mediated nausea and sedation occur in up to half of patients first exposed to an opioid and after dose increases. These symptoms usually resolve spontaneously with continued opioid use, and thus patients should be reassured and encouraged to adhere to their prescribed regimen of analgesics. Patients who are not routinely apprised of these features mistake side effects for allergy. For nausea and/or vomiting, a major tranquilizer (e.g., haloperidol, prochlorperazine, chlorpromazine) administered orally or rectally is the usual agent of first choice, especially when cost is a consideration (169). A properistaltic agent (e.g., metoclopramide) is appropriate when gastric stasis is suggested by nausea, bloating, and early satiety. Scopolamine is particularly useful for vertiginous nausea (i.e., amplified by walking). Commonly used as an adjunct to emetic chemotherapies, ondansetron (Zofran) can be considered for refractory nausea but is usually avoided because of its cost. Dronabinol, an oral agent containing active elements of marijuana, and corticosteroids are other treatments for refractory nausea. Sedation that fails to improve with time can often be managed effectively with a psychostimulant such as methylphenidate or dextroamphetamine (170).

When side effects are refractory to pharmacoreversal, consideration should be given to a trial of a similar alternative opioid analgesic, since side effects are often idiosyncratic and may not be triggered by agents that are in other respects quite similar. A prospective study of 100 consecutive inpatient pain consultations conducted at a tertiary care cancer center revealed that 80% of patients required a change in drug or route of administration, for convenience (31%), to diminish side effects (25%), or as a transition to the oral route once pain control was achieved (19%) (171). Finally, in patients with amenable pain syndromes, the presence of refractory side effects is an indication to consider other more invasive therapeutic modalities (discussed later).

Follow-Up

Once an acceptable drug regimen has been established, adequacy should be periodically reassessed. A prospective study of 100 consecutive inpatient pain consultation patients at a tertiary care cancer center revealed that 182 changes in 80 patients in drug type or route of delivery were required over 14 weeks (172). Patients are often reluctant to request more potent analgesics because of fear of addiction. Increased drug requirements related to progression of disease and the development of

physical tolerance should be anticipated. Tolerance is most frequently manifested by decreased duration of analgesics.

Education and Potential for Addiction

Patient and family education, an essential element of a successful pain relief program, is ideally accomplished through the combined efforts of physicians and nurses. Patients commonly maintain deeply rooted fears of addiction that are culturally reinforced. The distinctions among addiction (psychological dependence), physical dependence, and tolerance should be explained. Tolerance, the need for increasing dosages over time to maintain a desired effect, and physical dependence, a state characterized by the onset of characteristic withdrawal symptoms when a drug is precipitously stopped or a specific antagonist is administered, are biophysiological phenomena that are inevitable and should be regarded as pharmacological effects (Table 25.11). They are unrelated to addiction and need not impede analgesic therapy: since the patient usually develops tolerance to most side effects as well as to analgesia, doses can usually be increased to counter tolerance; should opioid therapy become unnecessary, patients are generally able to discontinue use without problems when a gradual taper is instituted.

Addiction is a psychobehavioral phenomenon with possible genetic influences characterized by overwhelming drug use, nonmedical drug use, and continued use despite the presence or threat of physiological or psychological harm. In contrast to tolerance and physical dependence, which are inevitable with chronic use, true addiction is an extremely rare outcome of medical therapy. The main exception involves patients with a history of drug abuse, who pose significant risks of developing patterns of aberrant drug use.

Schedule

Because sympathetic arousal occurs and even potent analgesics may be ineffective if analgesics are withheld until pain becomes severe, a time-contingent schedule for the administration of analgesics is generally preferred to symptom-contingent administration. With prolonged administration on demand, patterns of anticipation and memory of pain become established and may contribute to suffering, even during periods of adequate analgesia. Around-the-clock administration of appropriate analgesics maintains more even therapeutic blood levels and decreases the likelihood of intolerable pain (Fig. 25.2)(173).

Basal Analgesia

Compliance and overall quality of analgesia are enhanced by the regular administration of long-acting opioid analgesics for basal pain control, supplemented by a short-acting opioid analgesic administered as needed (escape, or rescue, doses) for breakthrough and incident pain. In con-

Table 25.11   Contemporary Description of Penomena Historically Associated with Addiction

Phenomena	Etiology	Definition	Incidence	Management
Physical dependence	Physiological, pharmacological	Withdrawal syndrome if Opioids abruptly stopped or naloxone administered	Almost invariable	Avoid by gradual taper
Tolerance[a]	Physiological, pharmacological	Increased dose required to achieve Analgesia[b]	Almost invariable	Reestablish analgesia with upward titration
Addiction (psychological dependence)	Psychological; questionable genetic influences	Nonmedical use despite harm	Rare (1%)	Identify; multidisciplinary management
Withdrawal abstinence syndrome)	Physiological, pharmacological	Characteristic signs and symptoms[c]	Almost invariable	Avoid, reverse with opioids

[a]Although inevitable to some degree, current thinking posts this phenomenon as considerably less severe than previously thought, recognizing instead that dose increases in cancer patients are most likely due to disease progression.

[b]Patients develop tolerance to most adverse effects, especially nausea and sedation, but slowly if at all to constipation and miosis.

[c]Characteristic signs and symptoms include lacrimation, diaphoresis, rhinorrhea, pupillary dilation, gooseflesh, muscle tremor, nausea, vomiting, abdominal cramping, diarrhea, raised heart rate, respiratory rate and blood pressure, chills, hyperthermia, flushing, yawning, restlessness, irritability, anorexia, disturbed sleep, and generalized body aches.

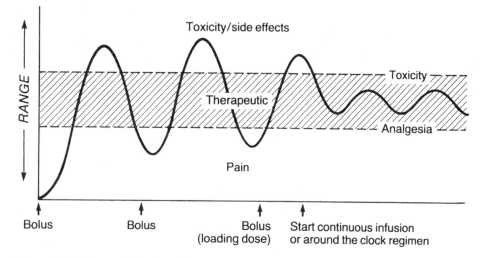

Figure 25.2.   The potential for alternating bouts of toxicity and pain often associated with standard as-needed dosing. Note the transition to continuous infusion and reductions in peak and trough levels. Similar effect occurs with institution of controlled-release oral opioids or transdermal fentanyl administered around the clock.

temporary practice, preferred basal analgesics include transdermal fentanyl, controlled-release morphine, and oxycodone preparations (174), which are available in a wide range of doses but cannot be broken, crushed, or chewed, and transdermal fentanyl. Transdermal fentanyl (Fig. 25.3) is best reserved for the management of relatively stable basal pain (discussed later). When these agents are poorly tolerated, methadone or levorphanol may be prescribed, but careful monitoring is required, particularly in elderly patients, to prevent accumulation and overdose, a risk that is greatest during the initial phase of treatment (164).

Escape, or Rescue, Doses

A drug of relatively high potency, short onset, and brief duration, such as immediate-release morphine, hydromor-phone, or oxycodone, is selected for as-needed administration to manage exacerbations of pain (60). These agents should be prescribed at intervals based on their expected duration of action, usually every 2 to 4 hours as needed. Patients should be instructed to maintain careful records that accurately reflect their analgesic use. When breakthrough medications are used more than 2 to 3 times over 12 hours consistently, the dose of the basal, long-acting analgesic may be increased. If incident pain is a significant problem, the patient should be instructed to take the breakthrough dose in anticipation of pain-provoking activity. A new formulation of oral transmucosal fentanyl citrate (Fig. 25.4) has been shown to produce meaningful relief of breakthrough pain within 5 minutes of initiating consumption, an onset that mimics intravenous administration, despite the noninvasive character of this therapy (175).

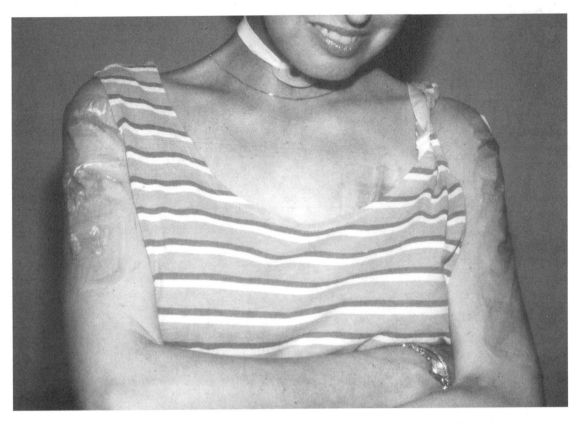

Figure 25.3.   Patient using transdermal fentanyl for the around-the-clock management of stable basal pain.

Adjuvant Analgesics

Selected patients benefit from treatment with adjuvant agents, which are discussed in detail later in this chapter. In general, these agents are mechanism specific, and use should be based on a specific indication.

Oral and Transdermal Routes

When possible, analgesics should be administered orally or by a similarly noninvasive route (transdermal, rectal, transmucosal) to promote independence and mobility and for ease of titration. In the presence of a functional, intact GI system, once dose is adjusted to account for hepatic first-pass effect, oral administration provides analgesia that is as effective as parenteral (but not spinal) administration.

Alternative Routes

When pain control is inadequate with oral analgesics or the oral route is contraindicated, consideration should be given to alternative means of drug delivery. A recently introduced formulation of transdermal fentanyl provides steady plasma levels of analgesic for 72 hours following a single application of a 25, 50, 75, or 100 µg/hour patch (Table 25.10), once treatment is established (176). The surface area of the patch is directly proportional to the administered dose of fentanyl. The system's rate-controlling membrane regulates drug release at a slower

rate than average skin flux, ensuring that the delivery system rather than the skin is the main determinant of absorption. Of all of the factors with the potential to influence the rate of absorption of transdermal fentanyl, temperature is most important, so patients should be warned against applying heating pads and such devices. Although low levels of fentanyl can be detected in the bloodstream just an hour after administration, a consistent, near-peak level is not obtained for 12 to 18 hours after treatment is initiated. Patients need to be cautioned that pain relief will accrue over the first day of treatment, and they should be provided with rescue doses of short-acting analgesics during this interval. In addition, as a result of the formation of a skin depot of drug, effects persist for 12 to 18 hours following removal of the patch, so that adverse effects may require prolonged treatment. Although the transdermal fentanyl system was originally studied predominantly in the perioperative setting, its ultimate approval was limited to the management of chronic pain. Conversion schemes are conservative, so that up to half of patients dosed according to the product's package insert require rapid upward titration. Because of the lag between dose and response, transdermal fentanyl analgesia is best suited for patients with relatively stable dose requirements and is particularly useful when the oral route is contraindicated.

The rectal route is reliable for short-term use except in the presence of diarrhea, fistulae, or other anatomical abnormalities. Rectal administration is usually avoided in older children and in conditions that increase pain when patients are positioned for suppository insertion. Morphine and hydromor-

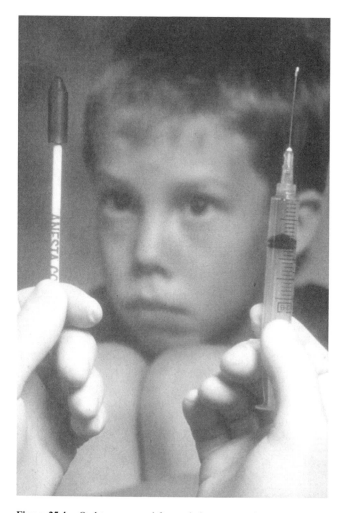

Figure 25.4. Oral transmucosal fentanyl citrate, a novel means of delivering fentanyl across the mucous membranes of the mouth for rapid onset relief of breakthrough pain.

phone are available in rectal preparations, and oxymorphone hydrochloride (Numorphan) rectal suppositories provide 4 to 6 hours of potent analgesia (177). Rectal methadone has been shown to be safe and effective but must be compounded by a manufacturing pharmacist (178).

Other options include continuous subcutaneous or intravenous infusions of opioids by means of a portable pump, intravenous or subcutaneous PCA, and intrathecal or epidural opioids administered via an externalized catheter or internalized pump. New means of administering opioids being explored include mucous membrane (sublingual and transnasal), transdermal, and respiratory absorption (179).

Alternative Drugs and Drugs to Avoid

The clinician should maintain familiarity with the pharmacological profiles of a variety of opioids (Tables 25.9 and 25.10) and should consider drug substitution when a patient exhibits tolerance to the analgesic effects or intolerance to the side effects of standard analgesics. When converting between drugs or routes, half to two-thirds of the calculated equianal-

gesic dose of the new drug is usually recommended as a starting dose (6); it is titrated rapidly as needed.

The chronic administration of meperidine, especially orally, is contraindicated. Administered chronically, all opioids may produce some degree of myoclonus, but the accumulation of normeperidine, a metabolite, may lead to frank seizure activity, especially when renal function is impaired (180).

Agonist-antagonist and partial agonist opioids should generally be avoided for a variety of reasons, the most important of which is the presence of a ceiling effect, or dose above which toxicity but not analgesia increases. With the usual exception of buprenorphine, these agents may precipitate withdrawal, and their administration complicates the usually inevitable eventual transition to pure agonist agents. Pentazocine (Talwin), the only one of these agents widely available orally, is associated with a high incidence of hallucinations and confusion, and buprenorphine is not easily or reliably reversed by naloxone.

Alternative Therapies

Adequate pain relief cannot always be achieved through pharmacological means alone (181). Initial screening should identify patients in whom behavioral or psychological modalities may be employed successfully. Relaxation and imagery training significantly reduce pain scores in patients who have mucositis during bone marrow transplant (182). When comprehensive trials of pharmacological therapy have failed, consideration should be given to alternative modalities, including additional antitumor therapy, neural blockade, CNS opioid therapy, neurosurgical options, and rarely, electrical stimulation (183, 184).

Adjuvant Analgesics

The term adjuvant has been used in the context of various medical disorders to refer to a so-called helper therapy. Usually added to a primary therapeutic intervention that depends on an alternative mechanism for its efficacy, the aim of generic adjuvant therapy is to elicit an additive or synergistic effect or to diminish the toxicity of the primary therapy. The term adjuvant is used in the context of pain management and palliative care in two related but distinct ways. The first, which is probably less useful because it is too broad, posits an adjuvant drug as one that meets one of three criteria: it enhances opioid-mediated analgesia, diminishes opioid-mediated side effects, or improves other symptoms associated with cancer (52). The second, more useful definition is a heterogeneous group of medications originally developed for purposes other than relief of pain that have been observed to promote analgesia in *specific* clinical settings. We rely on this latter construct in discussing the adjuvant analgesics.

While a large variety of drugs are purported to possess adjuvant properties, only a limited number reliably relieved pain in controlled or partially controlled trials. Some cancer patients with pain benefit, usually from the addition of corticosteroids; selected antidepressants, usually tricyclic; anticonvulsants; amphetamines; and more rarely, NMDA antagonists; α-adrenergic antagonists; antihistamines, and phenothiazines. It is important to note these points: *(a)* Not every agent belonging to each component drug class appears to possess analgesic properties. *(b)* Even agents with confirmed analgesic properties relieve only specific types of pain derived from specific selected conditions. *(c)* Even then, pain relief does not accrue in all affected patients.

The adjuvant analgesics differ from opioid analgesics in important general ways. Opioids are all-purpose analgesics; that is, no matter what clinical condition is being treated, if administered in an adequate dose, they always produce some degree of pain relief. Although some conditions appear to be less opioid responsive than others, the clinician can count on achieving some degree of analgesia if an opioid is administered in a sufficient dose, although regrettably, in less opioid-responsive conditions, escalating side effects may eclipse the utility of analgesia, rendering opioid therapy unacceptable. In contrast, responses to adjuvant analgesics are more binary: depending on the nature of the clinical condition being treated (and perhaps other more obscure variables) treatment may or may not elicit pain relief. Most recognized adjuvants are especially likely to be effective for various types of neuropathic pain.

A second fundamental difference relates to the dose-response curve: even when adjuvants are clearly effective, the nature of the dose-response relation is fundamentally different from that of the opioids. The relation between dose and response is usually relatively linear for opioids, even though, depending on the responsiveness of the pain, the slope of the line describing the dose-response relation may be shallow or steep. In contrast, even should an adjuvant produce a desirable effect, there is no certainty that raising the dose will enhance analgesia or that if a response occurs, it will be proportionate or replicable. These features of the adjuvants dictate the development of novel study methodologies, as exemplified by a trial of transdermal clonidine conducted by Byas-Smith et al. (185) that used a two-stage enriched enrollment design. By identifying likely responders to the study drug in its first phase and excluding nonresponders from the study's second phase, this design was able to detect clinical responses that would not have been apparent had a less stratified population been subject to study.

Sequential Drug Trials

While sequential drug trials for refractory pain have long been performed informally, this concept has been refined in light of an improved understanding of neuropathic pain and adjuvant analgesics. The recognition that neuropathic pain often fails to respond adequately to the routine administration of opioids and often responds in a binary fashion (no response or partial response) to many adjuvants *titrated over time* underlies the contemporary concept of sequential trials. Patients with amenable pain syndromes are informed that a

quick fix is unlikely and are apprised of the likelihood that their pain may respond to treatment with one of a variety of related drugs pertaining to distinct classes of adjuvant agents. It is further communicated that the behavior of each of the multiple agents that possesses the potential to provide a salutary effect is such that likely candidates are best initiated singly in low doses and titrated upward over time until analgesia is achieved, side effects supervene, or the agent under trial can be excluded and a new trial can be commenced (186). This process of knowledge-based trial and error, typically characterized by multiple trials, inadequate starting doses, gradual dose escalation, and a high frequency of bothersome but reversible side effects, can be extremely frustrating for the chronic pain patient, especially in the absence of preparation. Furthermore, it is often too time consuming for the patient with acute or progressive cancer pain and a limited expectancy of life. This necessitates consideration of alternative approaches, such as anesthetic or neurosurgical interventions and escalation of opioid doses into ranges associated with side effects; concomitant aggressive titration of agents (e.g., antiemetics, psychostimulants) is targeted at overcoming side effects. Not only are representatives of distinct classes of drugs considered when designing a sequential trial (e.g., antidepressants, anticonvulsants), but similar agents belonging to the same drug class (e.g., amitriptyline, nortriptyline, desipramine) are appropriate for inclusion because of variability of response across time and from person to person.

Antidepressants

The efficacy of selected antidepressants as analgesics per se, independent of their effects on mood and nighttime sleep, has been demonstrated mostly in noncancer models, although utility has been demonstrated for some agents in cancer patients as well (187-192). That antidepressants characteristically induce analgesia in responders with doses generally considered insufficient to relieve depression argues for a direct, independent underlying mechanism of effect. In addition, although onset is not immediate, analgesia is generally established more rapidly than are antidepressant effects (typically 3 to 7 days versus 14 to 21 days). The operant mechanism for antidepressant-mediated analgesia presumably relates to increased circulating pools of norepinephrine and serotonin induced by reductions in the postsynaptic uptake of these neurotransmitters. Another mechanism that may contribute to analgesia is suggested by the observation that the coadministration of at least amitriptyline and clomipramine increases plasma morphine levels (193).

Although heterocyclic is the technically correct term to describe the subset of antidepressants that appear to have the greatest utility as analgesics, the term tricyclic antidepressant is still in common use because most are tertiary amines. The most compelling indication for tricyclic antidepressant therapy remains variants of neuropathic pain (e.g., postherpetic neuralgia, central pain, diabetic neuropathy), although recent trials have demonstrated efficacy for disorders that include headache, arthritis, chronic low-back pain, and psychogenic pain (186).

Amitriptyline and to a lesser extent imipramine remain the most extensively studied of these agents, and as a result they are the usual first choices of academically-based pain specialists. Although usually relatively innocuous, side effects are especially prominent with these agents. Since amitriptyline and imipramine are respectively metabolized to nortriptyline and desipramine, agents with superior side effect profiles, many authorities, especially in private practice, advocate the latter two agents as drugs of first choice. Data from controlled clinical trials support the use of amitriptyline, nortriptyline, desipramine, imipramine, doxepin, maprotiline, and clomipramine. Trazadone, while sedating and thus potentially helpful for sleep disturbances, appears to have limited value as an analgesic. Interestingly, despite their efficacy for depression and generally favorable side effect profiles, the newer selective serotonin reuptake inhibitors (SSRIs) such as fluoxetine (Prozac), paroxetine (Paxil), and sertraline (Zoloft) overall appear to be less effective for treating pain than are the heterocyclic antidepressants. Obviously, if pain is a secondary manifestation of depression, the SSRIs and other antidepressants may be beneficial in therapeutic doses.

The main indication for treatment with the heterocyclic antidepressants is neuropathic pain that is relatively constant and unrelenting and that is not predominantly intermittent, lancinating, jabbing, or shocklike. Paroxysmal neuropathic pain may also be treated effectively with tricyclic antidepressants but is often first treated with an anticonvulsant. As noted, tricyclic antidepressants have also been used successfully in headache and other syndromes, and thus a trial in nearly any cancer pain syndrome that has not responded favorably to primary analgesics is justified.

Usually amitriptyline, nortriptyline, or desipramine is started at 10 to 25 mg nightly and gradually titrated upward, usually to a range of 50 to 125 mg and occasionally higher, until toxicity occurs or analgesia is established. Dry mouth, constipation, drowsiness, and dysphoria are the most prominent of a wide range of side effects, although more serious, usually anticholinergic side effects may occur (e.g., urinary retention, cardiac dysrhythmias). Unlike the side effects of opioid therapy, the development of tolerance is less robust, and side effects are less readily reversible. As a result, if side effects are more prominent than analgesia, the offending agent is usually discontinued and a pharmacological analog or a drug from another class is started. Although not as reliably analgesic as the tricyclic antidepressants, the newer SSRIs may be preferred for the fragile elderly, patients predisposed to developing serious anticholinergic side effects, patients whom multiple trials of tricyclics have failed because of side effects, and when depression is a prominent comorbidity. Usual starting doses of the SSRIs are the same as are suggested for the management of depression (fluoxetine 20 mg, paroxetine 20 mg, sertraline 50 mg), administered as a single morning dose to take advantage of their propensity for mild stimulation of activity.

Anticonvulsants and Baclofen

Ample but predominantly anecdotal reports on the efficacy of carbamazepine for the nonsurgical treatment of trigeminal neuralgia (tic douloureux) (194) carbamazepine, phenytoin, valproate, clonazepam, and most recently gabapentin, alone or in combination with the tricyclic antidepressants, have led to successful use of these agents to treat neuropathic pain (195). Most authorities consider them as drugs of first choice for neuropathic pain that resembles classic trigeminal neuralgia, that is, predominantly paroxysmal, jabbing shocklike pain. Anticonvulsants are also usually considered a second-line therapy for relatively steady, constant neuropathic pain when tricyclic antidepressants are poorly tolerated, ineffective, or only partially effective (186). Anticonvulsants presumably relieve pain in these settings as a result of their ability to dampen ectopic foci of electrical activity and spontaneous discharge from injured nerves, in a manner analogous to their salutary effects in seizure disorders. Carbamazepine therapy has been most thoroughly documented, and thus, in the absence of contraindications, it is usually considered the drug of first choice (196). The most toxic of the anticonvulsants used to treat pain, carbamazepine is associated with idiosyncratic hepatotoxicity (rare) and bone marrow depression (incidence of up to 2%), and thus is avoided in patients with liver metastases or bone marrow depletion and in those receiving cytotoxic therapy. Used chronically, carbamazepine therapy requires monitoring of complete blood counts (CBC) and liver function tests every 2 to 3 months. Ataxia, confusion, dizziness, and nausea are relatively common with upward dose titration, and thus carbamazepine is also best avoided in the fragile elderly, especially combined with other psychotropic agents. Clonazepam in doses of 0.5 mg twice a day is often well tolerated by patients who have had or are at risk for side effects with carbamazepine, phenytoin and valproate. Carbamazepine is usually started at 100 mg twice a day and titrated up to 300 to 400 mg four times a day while awaiting an analgesic response or toxicity. Failure of one anticonvulsant does not appear to predict outcome for trials of an alternative agent.

Gabapentin (197) is a new anticonvulsant that according to anecdote may be highly efficacious for neuropathic pain, especially when lancinating, although controlled trials have not yet been reported. Felbamate, another new anticonvulsant, is known to interact with NMDA receptors, but its use is probably only rarely warranted because of concerns about the development of aplastic anemia (198). Although it is a γ-aminobutyric acid (GABA) agonist and not an anticonvulsant, baclofen, with or without carbamazepine, has been reported to be effective for lancinating ticlike neuropathic pain. Baclofen is usually started at 5 mg twice or three times a day or and may be titrated up to 30 to 90 mg/day, as tolerated. The other main role for baclofen in pain management is as an intrathecal infusion for spasticity, especially if it is due to spinal cord injury and multiple sclerosis (199).

Oral Local Anesthetics

Because of historical accounts of transient relief of pain after intravenous infusions of local anesthetics, oral and rectal analogs already in use as antiarrhythmics have been exploited for relief of neuropathic pain (200, 201). Although oral tocainide and rectal flecainide have been used with some success, the agent of choice from this group, especially in the United States, is mexiletine, which is usually regarded as a second- or third-line agent for continuous or intermittent neuropathic pain disorders. The oral local anesthetics block sodium channels and presumably relieve pain by mechanisms similar to those invoked to explain anticonvulsant-mediated analgesia. Mexiletine is usually started at 150 mg/day and titrated upward to a maximum dose of 300 mg three times a day. Up to 40% of patients may discontinue therapy because of side effects, the most common of which are nausea and vomiting.

Amphetamines

While the most widely accepted use for amphetamines in palliative care is as a means to reverse opioid-mediated sedation (202), research suggests that dextroamphetamine and methylphenidate (Ritalin) possess analgesic properties (203) and are excellent antidepressants. Unlike classic antidepressants, their effect on mood is usually apparent with the first dose. Furthermore, prior to the introduction of SSRIs, methylphenidate developed an excellent record of safety in geriatric patients with refractory depression. Arrhythmias are almost nonexistent, and instead of inducing anorexia, these agents typically have a paradoxical effect of increasing appetite by enhancing alertness. Nervousness and agitation, the most common adverse effects, usually respond to dose reductions. Agitated delirium may occur in patients with coexisting psychiatric disorders, brain metastases, or metabolic disturbances, all of which are precautions to use. Methylphenidate is typically started at 10 mg on awakening and 5 mg with the noon meal, after which titration to effect is instituted. Because of its short half-life, patients are usually able to sleep well at night, especially if they have become more active as a result of increased alertness. D-Amphetamine can be administered on a similar schedule, and an extended-release formulation is available for both agents.

Corticosteroids

The efficacy of corticosteroids as treatment for acute pain resulting from raised intracranial pressure (ICP) and spinal cord compression is well-established. In addition, these agents have been administered empirically for a variety of cancer pain syndromes with good results (204). Pain relief is presumably related to reduced peritumoral edema and inflammation with consequent relief of pressure and traction on nerves and other pain-sensitive structures, although beneficial effects on mood,

appetite, and weight also may indirectly contribute to improved subjective pain reports. Improvements in pain are often rapid and dramatic but usually depend on continued administration. While results may be maintained in a proportion of patients, benefits are often short-lived, leveling off in a few weeks, presumably because of the replacement of edema by tumor growth in patients with aggressive disease. A trial of oral steroids may be beneficial in any patient with pain that appears to be predominantly due to spread of bulky tumor (e.g., selected patients with pelvic, rectal, esophageal, or hepatic tumor deposits or invasion of the brachial and lumbosacral plexus). Dexamethasone is the usual drug of choice because it has less potent mineralocorticoid effects. While a variety of side effects and complications can result from even acute steroid administration (e.g., diabetes mellitus, psychosis), serious problems usually arise only from chronic use. As a result, in the presence of progressive cancer, when a trial produces beneficial results, it is reasonable to maintain use without tapering (205). While most patients note improvements in mood when steroid therapy is commenced, a small proportion have dysphoria and even florid psychosis. Interestingly, one such episode does not appear to predict similar reactions on reexposure. The optimal dose of steroids, both for oncological emergencies (e.g., raised ICP, cord compression) and chronic pain is not known. For the former, 100 mg dexamethasone intravenously is administered initially in some institutions, followed by intravenous maintenance. The large bolus dose produces severe but transient perineal burning (ants in one's pants) via an unknown mechanism. For the management of nonemergency pain, oral doses of 2 to 6 mg dexamethasone three or four times a day are common.

N-methyl-D-Aspartate Antagonists

The NMDA receptor has recently been described and implicated in the transmission of pain. Although research on various agents with antagonist activity at the NMDA receptor is under way, ketamine, a partial NMDA antagonist, is the only available agent that appears to mediate pain by this nonopioid mechanism. It has long been used as an intravenous anesthetic agent, and subanesthetic doses have been administered for prolonged periods with fair success in a small number of patients with refractory neuropathic cancer pain (206, 207). Because of side effects and the risk of complications, ketamine infusion should be regarded as a treatment of desperation reserved for rare use until additional experience has been reported.

α$_2$-Adrenergic Antagonists

The centrally acting antihypertensive clonidine has been observed to promote analgesia for neuropathic pain when administered near the neuraxis. Epidural administration has recently received U.S. Food and Drug Administration (FDA) approval, and trials of intrathecal clonidine are under way. In a prospective randomized study of 38 patients with severe cancer pain (208) that persisted despite large doses of spinal opioids, the addition of epidural clonidine was associated with significant improvement in 45% of patients overall and 56% of patients with neuropathic pain. Hypotension during the initiation of treatment and rebound hypertension during withdrawal are the main potential risks of treatment.

Other Purported Adjuvants

Despite lack of data from controlled trials, antihistamines, benzodiazepines, and antipsychotics have been used, mostly historically, in efforts to enhance analgesia. While these agents have clear roles for primary indications other than pain (anxiolysis, antiemesis), with few exceptions they are not reliably associated with analgesia and thus should not be relied on as substitutes for opioid analgesics.

In contrast to other neuroleptics, methotrimeprazine reliably produces dose-related analgesia that is comparable with opioid-mediated analgesia. Controlled trials have confirmed analgesia that is comparable with that achieved with parenteral morphine in postoperative, labor, and cancer pain (209, 210). Its analgesic potency is similar to or slightly less than that of parental morphine (equianalgesic ratio of 3:2), and like morphine, it has no apparent ceiling effect. Methotrimeprazine is considerably more sedating and less emetogenic than morphine, and because of its propensity to produce orthostatic hypotension, treatment is usually reserved for nonambulatory patients. Disadvantages include the lack of an oral preparation, limited availability, and high cost. Methotrimeprazine is an excellent option when a potent nonopioid is required in a bed-bound patient, especially when sedative effects are desired. A retrospective survey of 675 patients treated at St. Christopher's Hospice (211) revealed that 12% of patients had received methotrimeprazine for agitation, nausea, or pain. Treatment duration ranged from 1 to 240 days (mean 12), with usual doses ranging from 12.5 to 50 mg every 4 to 8 hours, with some patients requiring 75 to 100 mg doses. Treatment for agitation, which had not responded to chlorpromazine, was judged effective in 94% of patients. Sedation was reported in 56% of patients but necessitated discontinuation in only about 5%.

Although clinical lore perpetuates the hypothesis that the butyrophenones have utility as primary or adjuvant analgesics, these beliefs have been confirmed by neither controlled trials (212) nor by survey data (213). Proponents advocate trials for rectal tenesmus, bladder tenesmus, neuropathic pain, and whenever suffering or psychological distress is prominent.

A careful review of the literature reveals insufficient evidence to support the contention that the benzodiazepines have meaningful analgesic properties in most circumstances (214). Although treatment with the benzodiazepines may reduce

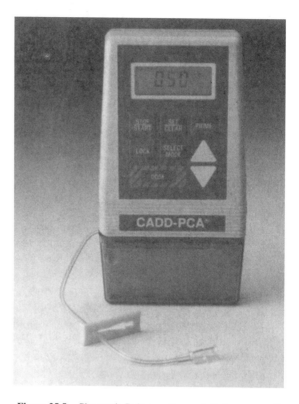

Figure 25.5. Pharmacia Deltec continuous infusion pump with patient-controlled analgesia, suitable for the home-based delivery of subcutaneous, intravenous, and epidural infusions. This is just one of an assortment of the reliable battery-powered portable devices available.

complaints of pain, this appears to be an indirect effect of their psychotropic properties rather than true analgesia. Thus the use of benzodiazepines should be discouraged except in extremely specific settings. Clinical experience suggests a possible role for short-term use to manage acute muscle spasm, use as an anxiolytic when stress appears to influence reports of pain, and use for lancinating neuropathic pain as a part of sequential trials, in which case clonazepam and alprazolam are the agents of choice. They should probably not be considered as first-line choices even for these indications, since benefits are often eclipsed by the cognitive impairment, physical and psychological dependence, worsening depression, the risk of overdose, and other side effects.

Continuous Subcutaneous Infusion of Opioids

The continuous subcutaneous infusion (CSCI) of opioids, which is common, is an excellent option for patients whose medical condition precludes the use of the oral route or whose pain is poorly controlled despite large doses of oral opioids (152, 179). Treatment is best initiated in the hospital setting but is readily adaptable to the home. A variety of infusion pumps (Fig. 25.5) are portable, battery-driven, and inexpensively leased, and they feature sophisticated alarm systems.

To initiate a CSCI of opioid, the 24-hour dose of parenteral drug is summed. If the patient's drug regimen includes oral analgesics, conversion tables are used (Tables 25.9 and 25.10) to calculate the equianalgesic parenteral dose of opioid (usually morphine or hydromorphone). The total daily dose of parenteral drug is divided by 24 and the pump is set accordingly. Tissue irritation is minimized when volumes under 1 to 2 mL are prescribed, a practice that is facilitated by ordering an appropriately concentrated formulation of the opioid. The pump's tubing is primed with drug and attached to a 27-gauge pediatric butterfly needle that is inserted subcutaneously and taped flush to the patient's skin. Any subcutaneous site can be used, although the infraclavicular fossa and chest wall are frequently selected to facilitate easy ambulation (Fig. 25.6). The infusion site is checked twice daily for signs of irritation and is changed weekly or as needed.

Absorption of subcutaneously administered opioids is rapid, and steady-state plasma levels are generally approached within an hour (215). Most parenteral opioids are suitable for CSCI, although morphine and hydromorphone are used most commonly and meperidine, methadone, and pentazocine should be avoided because of the potential for tissue irritation. Physician orders should provide for rescue doses of drug adequate to counter incomplete analgesia. One method is to order subcutaneous injections equal to the hourly dose to be administered every 1 to 2 hours as needed. At the end of 24 hours the infusion is increased by the sum of the recorded rescue doses. If analgesia is adequate but side effects, usually oversedation, are prominent, the infusion rate may be halved and titrated upward as needed.

Continuous Intravenous Infusion of Opioids

Indications for opioids administered by continuous intravenous infusion (CII) are similar to the indications for CSCI, although CSCI is preferred in the home care setting unless a permanent vascular access device (Hickmann, Broviac) is already in place (216). Indications include intolerance of the oral route because of GI obstruction, malabsorption, opioid-induced emesis, dysphagia, or the requirement for large numbers of pills. Other indications include a prominent bolus effect with intermittent injections, the necessity for rapid titration, and requirements for bolus injections that exceed nursing capabilities. Although CII is used frequently during the terminal phases of illness (217), imminence of death per se is not a valid indication for its use. In the presence of anxiety, CII should not be used as a substitute for counseling or sedation.

CII should not be regarded as a panacea for chronic cancer pain, as studies indicate that it is ineffective in up to one third of patients (218). Unless its limitations are realized, the complaints of patients whose pain control is inadequate despite treatment may not be taken seriously. Therapy with CII can be accomplished successfully with a variety of opioids, although the bulk of experience is with morphine. Meperidine should be avoided because of the possibility of

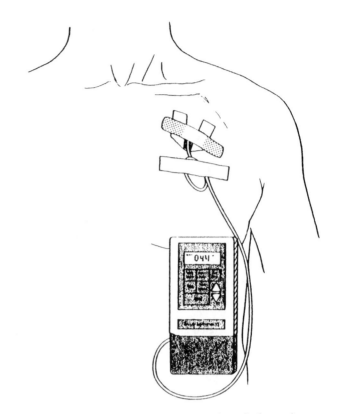

Figure 25.6. Placement of a subcutaneous butterfly for continuous bedside infusion of opioids.

CNS toxicity related to accumulation of normeperidine. A flow-calibrated infusion device with alarm features is used to deliver medications. PCA is an excellent option but is reserved for patients with the capacity to understand and use this modification correctly. Recommended procedures for the selection of drugs and dosage are essentially the same as with CSCI therapy. Dosage is adjusted upward until pain relief is adequate or side effects become intolerable. There is no ceiling dose, and indeed the administration of hourly doses as high as 500 mg morphine equivalents have been documented without problems (152). Escape doses of a short-acting opioid with rapid onset should be used to counter breakthrough pain, and adjuvant drugs (antiemetics, laxatives, amphetamines) should be prescribed judiciously to counter opioid-mediated side effects. Nursing requirements are stringent, consisting mainly of frequent monitoring of vital signs, particularly after the administration of loading boluses.

Behavioral Pain Management

A variety of behavioral pain management techniques (hypnosis, relaxation, biofeedback, sensory alteration, guided imagery, and cognitive strategies) have been used in patients with cancer (219). Relaxation and imagery training significantly reduce visual analog scale scores in patients who have mucositis during bone marrow transplant (220). Behavioral intervention entails instruction in specific skills that with practice the patient can use independently or with supervision to enhance the effectiveness of other methods of pain relief.

Like most adjuvant therapies, these techniques are applied as needed. Patients with well-controlled pain are rarely sufficiently motivated to learn these techniques, while at the opposite extreme, those with very severe pain are also typically not good candidates because of functional limitations in their capacity to learn new skills (34). Training in behavioral pain management training is probably most effective for patients who have no significant psychological or psychiatric problems (34) and in insightful psychology-minded patients.

Acceptance improves when the distinction between behavioral pain management and psychotherapy is clear and when the decision to institute behavioral methods is understood not to reflect a belief that pain is psychogenic. Treatment is more difficult with confusion or when concentration is impaired by either the primary disease or intercurrent drug therapy.

As with other specialized techniques for pain management, the availability of trained experts is a limiting factor. Nurses, volunteers, and hospice workers have adopted behavioral pain management techniques, and investigators have shown that in other areas of symptom control (e.g., nausea) when properly trained, nonpsychologists can use these modalities successfully.

Intraspinal Analgesia

The benefits of neuraxial *anesthesia* (the administration of local anesthetics into the epidural or intrathecal space) are well-known for patients with acute pain related to labor, surgery, and postoperative recovery. In general, this approach to pain relief is not applicable to patients with chronic cancer pain because effects are nonselective: reduction in pain is accompanied by motor weakness, sensory anesthesia, and interference with sympathetic activity, which can cause hypotension that precludes home use. In contrast, neuraxial *analgesia* is achieved by the epidural or intrathecal administration of an opioid. Pain transmitted by Aδ and C fibers, which corresponds to most oncological pain, may be dramatically relieved but in a highly selective fashion with an absence of motor, sensory, and sympathetic effects (221, 222), making these modalities highly adaptable to the home care environment (223-225).

The principle underlying CNS opioid therapy is that introducing minute quantities of opioids in close proximity to their receptors (substantia gelatinosa of the spinal cord) (226) achieves high local concentrations. As a result, in properly selected patients, analgesia is often superior to that achieved when opioids are administered by other routes, and since the absolute amount of drug administered is reduced, side effects are minimized. Opioid-induced mental obtundation and so-called narcotic bowel syndrome (pseudo-obstruction) (227) are sometimes reversed in conjunction with marked improvements in comfort at much lower overall doses.

The CNS can be accessed via an intrathecal, epidural, or intraventricular approach, although the intraventricular route is

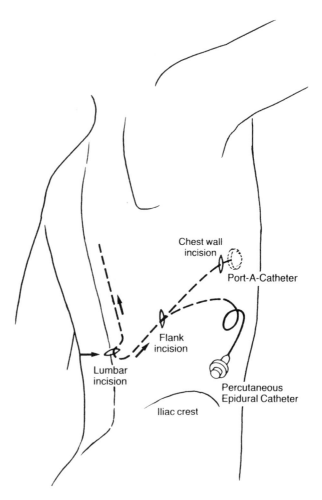

Figure 25.7. Implanted epidural or intrathecal catheter placed through a small lumbar incision, then tunneled subcutaneously to be either externalized for epidural use or attached to a port for intrathecal use.

used infrequently, primarily for intractable head and neck pain, and then usually when an access device (Ommaya reservoir) is already in place (228). The institution of intraspinal opioid therapy requires the participation of an anesthesiologist or neurosurgeon familiar with techniques of screening, implantation, and maintenance as well as a home care system that is adaptable and innovative. Perhaps the most important aspects of intraspinal opioid therapy are its reversibility and the reliability and simplicity of advance screening measures to confirm efficacy. Screening can generally be accomplished on an outpatient basis by observing the patient's response either to a morphine infusion via a temporary percutaneous epidural catheter or a series of single-shot intrathecal injections. Simple procedures requiring 5 to 15 minutes, screening injections are associated with minimal discomfort and are generally well tolerated even by ill patients. If improved pain control and reduced side effects are sufficiently profound to warrant more prolonged therapy, temporary catheters are usually, within a period of days to weeks, replaced with a permanent implanted catheter (modified Hickman or Broviac catheter; Fig. 25.7) because of concerns about infection and catheter migration (229).

Intraspinal opioid therapy is sufficiently new that guidelines for administration and selection of route, drug, and protocol are still emerging. A lumbar epidural catheter has been the most widely accepted means of access to the CNS, particularly among anesthesiologists, although implantable intrathecal systems have advantages in specific settings (230). Chronic administration of epidural opioids can be accomplished by intermittent boluses administered by the patient, family members, or nursing personnel or more commonly by continuous infusion via a standard PCA portable infusion pump connected to the epidural port. Continuous infusion is the preferred means of administration because intervals of pain between injections are avoided and because of the impression that the development of tolerance is delayed. Interestingly, although epidural opioid analgesia was developed to avoid problems associated with local anesthetic administration, combinations of epidural opioids and dilute local anesthetic agents have been determined to be safe and are often beneficial for pain that is refractory to opioids alone (231).

Subarachnoid catheter placement is an alternative to epidural administration. Opioid requirements are less than with epidural administration because of more direct access to the CNS. Morphine may be administered via an implanted subcutaneous port or an infusion device implanted within the subcutaneous tissue of the anterior abdominal wall. The prototype system (Infusaid, Shiley) uses a Freon-driven pump, initially developed for intra-arterial hepatic chemotherapy, that is about the size and shape of a hockey puck. A 50-mL reservoir is filled percutaneously every 14 to 21 days, and a constant volume of drug (2 to 4 mL/day) is infused continuously (232). Alterations in dosage are accomplished by replenishing the reservoir with an opioid of the appropriate concentration or by bolus administration through a separate port. The inconvenience of fixed-rate delivery is compensated by significantly lower upfront equipment costs. The more sophisticated SynchroMed system manufactured by Medtronic (Fig. 25.8) incorporates microprocessor technology to facilitate alterations in infusion rates noninvasively via a laptop computer and telemetry (233). Although its reservoir capacity is limited to 18 mL, a wide range of delivery rates allows refills to be scheduled every 1 to 2 months. The Algomed or PAR (patient-activated reservoir) (Fig. 25.9), also manufactured by Medtronic, is a newer system recently approved in Australia, Europe, and Latin America and now in U.S. clinical trials. It may be ideally suited for cancer patients for its simplicity, reduced cost, and reliance on demand dosing. Essentially a modified ventricular shunt system, its features include a 50-mL reservoir and a patient-activated valve implanted beneath the skin overlying the ribs and delivering 1 mL boluses as often as every hour.

Although the upfront costs of fully implantable intrathecal systems range from about $10,000 to $25,000, suprisingly, these systems are ultimately extremely cost effective for patients with indolent disease and life expectancies exceeding 6 months (234, 235). Economy over time arises from reduced

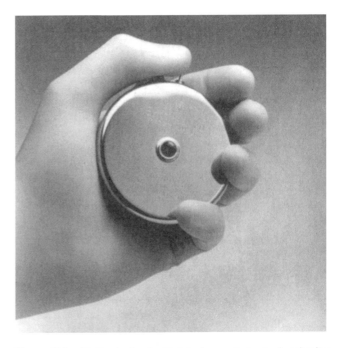

Figure 25.8. Medtronic SynchroMed hockey puck-sized microcircuitry-controlled pump usually implanted subcutaneously.

nursing and pharmacy charges and especially the absence of the need for a leased portable external pump. Unfortunately, relative to epidural systems, the efficacy of subarachnoid analgesia is often limited, as only epidural systems can accommodate sufficient concentrations of local anesthetic to achieve dermatomal hypalgesia, a decided benefit for refractory neuropathic and movement-related pain.

Side effects (e.g., respiratory depression, nausea, vomiting, pruritus, urinary retention, dysphoria), while common for intraspinal opioids administered to opioid-naive patients, are extremely rare in opioid-tolerant individuals (221).

Nerve Blocks

Local Anesthetic Blockade

Local anesthetic injections (Table 25.12) can be broadly classified as being applicable for diagnostic, prognostic, and/or therapeutic purposes (236, 237). Diagnostic blocks help to characterize the underlying mechanism of pain (nociceptive, neuropathic, sympathetically mediated) and to discern the anatomical pathways involved in pain transmission (238). Although valuable information may be obtained, especially in the setting of chronic pain, in which time is a less urgent matter, such procedures cannot pinpoint causation with certainty and should never be used to form a conclusion regarding the degree to which the pain is "real." Their main indication is as a preliminary intervention conducted prior to a therapeutic nerve block or other definitive therapy. The same diagnostic nerve block may provide prognostic information as well, roughly simulating the effects anticipated to accompany

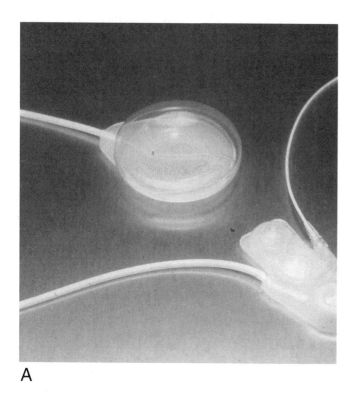

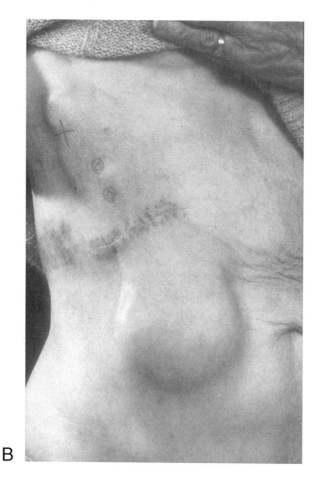

Figure 25.9. Investigational Algomed infusion device, a fully implantable patient-activated system for intrathecal opioid therapy. **A.** Implantable components of the device. **B.** An emaciated patient after implantation.

Table 25.12.   Indications for Local Anesthetic Blocks for Cancer Pain

Diagnostic block
Prognostic block
Pain emergency
Muscle spasm
Premorbid chronic pain
Treatment-related pain
Tumor-induced reflex sympathetic dystrophy
Continuous infusion for chronic pain

the more prolonged blockade associated with neurolysis (239). Careful interpretation of the results of a prognostic block helps the clinician determine the potential for subsequent neurolysis to relieve pain, and in addition provides the patient an advance opportunity to learn about the side effects that may accompany treatment. Patients often grasp the relation between a prognostic and therapeutic block when plain language is used to liken their conduct to taking a new car out on a test drive before buying it. While results often have good predictive value, they are not entirely reliable.

While therapeutic local anesthetic blocks are widely used for pain of nonmalignant origin, they play a more limited role in the treatment of cancer pain (239, 240). The main limitation of local anesthetic blockade in the setting of cancer pain is the typically transient nature of attendant pain relief. Therapeutic injec-

tions of local anesthetics, with or without corticosteroids, into trigger points, subcutaneous foci of localized muscle spasm, may provide lasting relief of myofascial pain (241). Such minor procedures can be administered at the bedside but are often are most efficacious when administered in a series coupled with physical therapy. They are particularly useful when muscle spasm arises as a result of prolonged bed rest and for pain that follows thoracotomy, mastectomy, or radical neck dissection. More diffuse subcutaneous injections of local anesthetic may have a salutary effect near the sites of greatest pain in patients with acute herpes zoster or postherpetic neuralgia. Local anesthetics are also often used with intralesional or perineural injections of corticosteroids as a means to help verify correct anatomical placement and for temporary interruption of pain and muscle spasm. While epidural injections of local anesthetic-steroid combinations are unlikely to provide lasting relief for back pain due to progressive neoplastic lesions, they may be effective for vertebral compression fractures, especially those that are due to osteopenia induced by steroid therapy. Local anesthetic injections administered in a series may contribute to lasting pain relief in the setting of posttraumatic sympathetically maintained pain (e.g., reflex sympathetic dystrophy or complex regional pain syndromes) (242). Although infrequent, such symptoms may arise as a result of tumor invasion of nervous system structures (e.g., brachial or lumbosacral plexopathy), in which case either local anesthetic blockade of the stellate ganglion or lumbar sympathetic chain has been used with some success to relieve pain (243, 244). Finally, local anesthetic blocks administered either in a series or continuously via a catheter may have a role in the pain emergency (245) to provide respite from pain and distress and to facilitate accurate assessment and the formulation of a long-term plan.

Neurolytic Blockade

Neurolytic blocks have played an important role in the management of intractable cancer pain and remain a primary focus of the anesthesiologist with specialized training in pain management (246) ideally complemented by the support offered by a multidisciplinary team. In general these techniques are reserved for patients with malignant pain that is severe and is expected to persist. Most techniques are appropriate for pain that is well localized and neither widely disseminated nor generalized. Neurolytic blocks, like other invasive modalities, are considered when pain persists despite thorough trials of aggressive pharmacological management or when drug therapy produces unwanted and uncontrollable side effects. Careful selection of the proper procedure and attention to technical detail substantially limit the incidence of side effects and unwanted neurological deficit. The important features of patient selection are listed in Table 25.13.

Both from a historical perspective and in contemporary practice, most neurodestructive techniques entail chemical neurolysis, that is, the injection of alcohol or phenol near a nerve or nerves to destroy a portion of the targeted nerve, to interrupt the transmission of impulses for a prolonged interval. Nervous structures may be affected indiscriminately, and thus great care must be exercised to ensure pain relief without unwanted motor or autonomic dysfunction. Neither chemical, thermal, nor surgical interruption of nerves reliably produces *permanent* relief of pain because of axonal regrowth and/or the development of deafferentation pain. These factors, together with the risk of accidental damage to nervous and nonnervous structures, limit the application of ablative procedures to patients with severe intractable pain and a limited expectancy of life. Cryoanalgesia produces a more selective lesion (247) but is more often associated with an unacceptably short duration of action, making it a more appropriate option for nonmalignant pain. Radiofrequency-generated thermal lesions are another effective means of inducing therapeutic nerve injury that has stimulated increasingly intense interest in recent years. While results are more discrete and controllable than those achieved with chemical blockade, anesthesiologists are not routinely familiar with this technology, and it may be unavailable because of equipment costs; so chemical techniques still predominate. Independent of technique, ultimately careful selection of the proper procedure and attention to technical detail are the most important factors limiting the incidence of side effects and unwanted neurological deficit.

Table 25.13.   Patient Selection for Neurolysis

Pain is severe
Pain is expected to persist
Pain cannot be modified by less invasive means
Pain is well-localized[a]
Pain is well-characterized[b]
Pain is not multifocal[c]
Pain is of somatic or visceral origin[d]
Limited life expectancy[e]

[a]Blocks are usually most effective when the topographical extent of pain is limited. The main exceptions are sympathetic blocks, which typically provide relief for relative diffuse visceral pain. In addition, epidural neurolysis may be considered for segmental pain distributed over several dermatomes. Pituitary ablation also has potential applications for disseminated pain emanating from osseous metastases, especially in patients with breast or prostate cancer.
[b]The main exception is visceral pain, which is often vague and difficult for patients to define clearly.
[c]Pituitary destruction may be considered for disseminated pain due to osseous metastases, especially in patients with breast or prostate cancer. Other forms of neurolysis may be cautiously considered, with the goal of eliminating the most severe pain and controlling secondary pain with opioids.
[d]Although temporary pain relief can often be achieved with local anesthetic blocks, in general neuropathic pain is less likely to respond favorably to neurolysis. Not an absolute contradiction.
[e]Requires carefully individualized decision making. In general, problems such as differentiation pain and transience are minimized when selection is limited to patients with predicted life expectancy of less than a year. Less destructive or more discrete techniques (cryoablation, radiofrequency thermoablation) can be considered more liberally in patients with long life expectancies.

While well-controlled studies are lacking, large clinical series report significant relief of pain in an average of 50 to 80% of patients, with the best results obtained when studies include patients who have received multiple blocks. Overall, significant complications are reported usually in fewer than 5% of patients (248-250). Optimal results require the judicious use of fluoroscopic and sometimes CT guidance to verify needle placement and the application of simple but essential adjuncts such as careful aspiration, the use of a nerve stimulator, the administration of test doses of local anesthetic, and eliciting paresthesias.

Neurolytic Agents

Alcohol and phenol are the only agents commonly used to produce chemical neurolysis in contemporary practice, although ammonium sulfate and chlorocresol are still occasionally advocated (251). The histopathological sequelae of neurolysis are discussed in detail elsewhere (251).

Ethyl alcohol is commercially available in 1- and 5-mL ampules as a pungent, colorless solution that can be readily injected through small-bore needles and that is hypobaric with respect to CSF. For peripheral and subarachnoid blocks, alcohol is generally used undiluted (referred to as 100% alcohol, dehydrated alcohol, or absolute alcohol), while a 50% solution is often used for celiac plexus block. If left exposed to the atmosphere, highly concentrated alcohol is diluted by absorbed moisture. Alcohol injection is typically followed by intense burning pain and occasionally almost imperceptible erythema along the target nerve's distribution. Although often only partially blunted by prior injections of local anesthetic, pain immediately after alcohol injection lasts just a few minutes, rendering it less distressing to informed patients. Denervation and pain relief sometimes accrue over a few days following injection.

Injectable phenol must be prepared by a pharmacist, but it has a shelf life of about a year when refrigerated and kept from light. Authorities have advocated various concentrations of phenol ranging from 3 to 15% prepared with saline, water, glycerine, and various radiological dyes. Phenol is relatively insoluble in water, and as a result concentrations in excess of 6.7% cannot be obtained at room temperature without adding glycerine to increase its solubility in water. Phenol mixed in glycerine is hyperbaric with respect to CSF but is so viscid that even when warmed, it is difficult to inject through needles smaller than 20 gauge. Phenol characteristically exhibits a biphasic action: its initial local anesthetic effect produces subjective warmth and numbness that usually give way to chronic denervation over a day's time. Hypalgesia after phenol injection is typically not as dense as after alcohol, and quality and extent of analgesia may fade slightly within the first 24 hours of administration.

Although it is widely held that neuroma formation is more common when peripheral blocks are performed with alcohol rather than with phenol, most authorities feel that alcohol and phenol are in most respects interchangeable. This is true especially because neuroma formation and attendant neuralgic pain rarely if ever follow subarachnoid or sympathetic neuroablation. The relative indications for alcohol versus phenol are discussed elsewhere in greater detail (252).

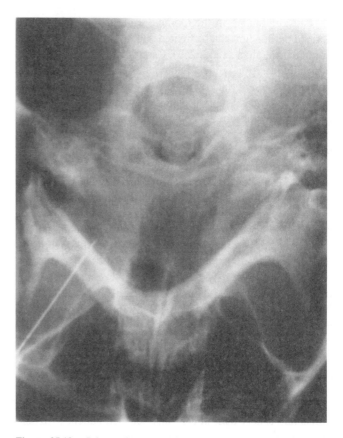

Figure 25.10. Submental vertex radiographic view of base of the skull demonstrating needle tip impinging on foramen ovale for alcohol Gasserian ganglion block. Lateral views are also required to determine that needle tip is advanced sufficiently far.

Peripheral Nerve Blocks

Peripheral nerve blocks have a limited but important role in the management of cancer pain (253). Blockade of multiple adjacent nerves is often required because of overlapping sensory fields. Careful patient selection is essential to avoid motor weakness when mixed nerves are targeted. Neuroma formation and posttreatment dysesthesias are the main impediment to the more liberal use of peripheral neurolytic blocks in patients with a long life expectancy.

Neoplastic head and neck pain remains a therapeutic challenge because of the tendency for tumors in these regions to invade locally and because of the rich sensory innervation of rostral structures. Physiological splinting, a strategy that is normally unconsciously adopted, is often ineffective because symptoms that aggravate pain (swallowing, eating, coughing, and movement of the head) are involuntary. The outcome of neural blockade may be adversely affected by anatomical distortion induced by prior surgery or radiation therapy and by the potential for tumor invasion or radiation fibrosis to reduce contact between the neurolytic agent and targeted nervous tissue. Nevertheless, in well-selected patients blockade of the involved cranial and/or upper cervical nerves is very useful. Blockade of the trigeminal nerve within the foramen ovale at

the base of the skull (Fig. 25.10) or of its branches may be beneficial for local pain. Even when pain is limited to the distribution of a single division of nerve V, when tumor progression is anticipated, it is preferable to extend the field of analgesia prophylactically by blocking the Gasserian ganglion in its entirety (254). In some cases blockade of cranial nerve IX or X or upper cervical nerves may be required for complete relief. Bilateral destruction of the glossopharyngeal and vagus nerves is not recommended because of potential interference with swallowing mechanisms and protective airway reflexes. When intractable craniocervical pain is not amenable to neural blockade, intraspinal opioid therapy by means of an implanted cervical epidural catheter (255) or intraventricular opioid therapy may be considered (256). A recent report details favorable outcomes in patients treated with high cervical subarachnoid infusions of dilute bupivacaine (257). Intractable hiccoughs (singultus) is also amenable to nerve block therapy. Unilateral phrenic nerve block has been performed under these circumstances with excellent results (236). Prior to performance of a neurolytic phrenic nerve block or surgical crush, the results of a prognostic block with local anesthetic must be carefully evaluated to assure adequacy of ventilatory function.

Pain originating in the thoracic wall, abdominal wall, or parietal peritoneum can be treated with multiple paravertebral or intercostal blocks (252, 253). Careful attention to the depth of needle insertion renders pneumothorax uncommon. Injections of the appropriate sacral nerve roots within their foramina relieve perineal pain in patients with normal urinary and GI function with minimal risk of sphincter disturbance (258). Neurolytic injections of other peripheral nerves are sometimes attempted, but generally only after local anesthetic injection has confirmed that reduction in pain is possible without decrement in motor function. When preexisting motor dysfunction is present or the involved limb is rendered useless by intractable pain (e.g., due to plexus invasion, pathological fracture) neurolytic block of the brachial plexus or its branches is a further option (259, 260). Although theoretically motor loss should occur routinely after psoas compartment block, we have treated nearly a dozen patients with instillations of 10 to 12% phenol and have observed not only little or no attendant paresis but usually improved function as a result of less splinting.

Central (Neuraxial) Neurolytic Blockade

Subarachnoid (intrathecal) injections of alcohol or phenol continue to play an important role in the management of intractable cancer pain in carefully selected patients. Advantages include a high proportion of good results in well-selected patients, ease of performance with minimal requirements for equipment, minimal or no requirements for hospitalization, duration of pain relief that is generally adequate for preterminal patients, ease of repetition when indicated, suitability for aged or debilitated patients, and a low complication rate when proper technique is observed. Unfortunately, training in this technique is available in only a limited number of centers.

Lytic neuraxial block produces pain relief by chemical rhizotomy. Since alcohol and phenol destroy nervous tissue indiscriminately (261, 262) exquisite attention to the selection of the injection site, volume and concentration of injectate, and selection and positioning of the patient are essential to avoid neurological complications. Most authorities agree that neither alcohol nor phenol offers a clear advantage except insofar as variations in baric properties facilitate positioning of the patient (263, 264). Except for perineal pain, alcohol is usually preferred, since most patients are unable to lie on their painful side, as is required for intrathecal phenol neurolysis.

Many reports of large uncontrolled series of patients treated with intrathecal rhizolysis have appeared in the medical literature. Results are difficult to compare because of variations in selection of patients, extent and type of underlying neoplasm, injection techniques, and criteria for assessing outcome. In an analysis of 13 published series documenting treatment of more than 2500 patients Swerdlow (265) reported that 58% of patients obtained "good" relief; "fair" relief was observed in an additional 21%, and in 20% of patients "little or no relief" was noted. Average duration of

relief is estimated at 3 to 6 months (236), with a wide range of distribution. Reports of analgesia persisting 1 to 2 years are fairly common (265).

Complication rates should be low with proper attention to detail and when repeated blocks with small volumes are performed in preference to a single treatment with a large volume of drug. In representative series using alcohol (n = 252) and phenol (n = 151), a total of 407 and 313 blocks were performed respectively (266, 267). In these two series, neither motor weakness nor fecal incontinence occurred, and of 8 patients with transient urinary dysfunction, incontinence persisted in just 1.

Subarachnoid neurolysis can be performed at any level up to the midcervical region (Fig. 25.11), above which the risk of drug spread to medullary centers and the potential for cardiorespiratory collapse increases (268). Blocks in the region of the brachial outflow are best reserved for patients with preexisting compromise of upper limb function. Similarly, lumbar injections are avoided in ambulatory patients, as are sacral injections in patients with normal bowel and bladder function. Hyperbaric phenol saddle block is relatively simple and is particularly suitable for many patients with colostomy and urinary diversion.

Epidural phenol neurolysis is an alternative for patients with pain of moderately extensive anatomical distribution (269). Until recently, epidural neurolysis was performed infrequently. Results were inferior to those obtained with subarachnoid blockade (265), presumably because the dura acts as a barrier to diffusion, resulting in limited contact between the drug and targeted nerves. There has been a resurgence of interest in epidural neurolysis related to improved results associated with modifications in technique (270). These require inpatient admission; they involve placing an indwelling catheter for serial neurolysis performed over several days. In contrast to subarachnoid administration, epidural instillation of neurolytics may be associated with lower incidences of motor weakness, headache, and meningeal irritation (265), but spread is much less predictable and treatment is performed at a limited number of centers.

Sympathetic Blockade

Unlike somatic nerve blocks, repeated local anesthetic injections of the sympathetic system are more likely to produce prolonged relief of pain by interrupting reflex mechanisms (242, 243). When local anesthetic sympathetic blocks provide only temporary relief or when clinical findings suggest visceral or sympathetically-mediated pain, consideration of chemical sympathectomy is warranted.

Celiac Plexus Block

Celiac plexus block continues to be one of the most efficacious and common nerve blocks employed in patients with cancer pain (236). It has great potential for relieving upper abdominal and referred back pain secondary to malignant

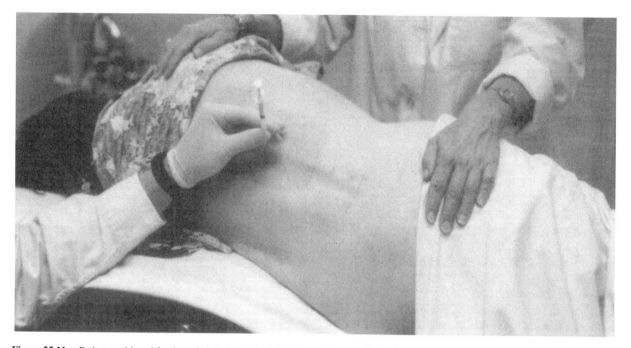

Figure 25.11.   Patient positioned for thoracic intrathecal alcohol injection. The vertebral column at the level of the injection site has been rendered least dependent by placement of padding and/or table tilt, and the patient is simultaneously tilted anteriorly. These maneuvers are intended to limit spread of hypobaric alcohol to the posterior (sensory roots) that correspond to the dermatomes affected by pain.

neoplasms involving structures derived from the foregut (distal esophagus to mid-transverse colon, liver, biliary tree, and adrenal glands). The most common indication for celiac axis block is pancreatic cancer, which contrary to traditional teaching, is frequently associated with painful rather than painless jaundice (271). Celiac axis block is most commonly performed by positioning needles bilaterally within the retroperitoneum by a posterior percutaneous approach. Despite the proximity of major organs (aorta, vena cava, kidneys, pleura) and the requirements for a large volume of neurolytic (50 mL of 50% alcohol) complication rates are uniformly low (271, 272), although some complications are serious. In contemporary practice most authorities consider radiological guidance mandatory to verify needle placement (273). Traditionally fluoroscopy has been used, but CT guidance is increasing in popularity because vascular structures, viscera, and masses can be visualized. Alternative approaches include injection under direct vision at the time of laparotomy (274), transaortic injection (275), and an anterior approach similar to that used for pancreatic biopsy (276).

Although studies have been criticized for methodological deficiencies (277), 85 to 94% incidence of good to excellent relief of pain has been obtained in large series of patients undergoing one or more neurolytic celiac plexus blocks for pain from pancreatic cancer per se (276), or a variety of intra-abdominal neoplastic conditions (278). In a series of 136 patients, analgesia was present until the time of death in 75% of cases, and in an additional 12.5% pain relief was maintained for more than 50% of survival time (272). A recently published randomized double-blind, placebo-controlled study of intraoperative celiac neurolysis demonstrated that treated

patients had not only improved pain control, reduction in opioid use and improved function but also statistically significant improvement in survival (10). Another recent prospective trial comparing treatment with NSAIDs and morphine versus neurolytic celiac plexus block revealed significantly lower pain scores and reduced drug consumption for 4 and 8 weeks after block, respectively (109).

Cervicothoracic, or Stellate Ganglion, Block

Repeated local anesthetic injections of the sympathetic outflow to the head, neck, and arm often provide persistent relief of sympathetically maintained pain, and because of their documented ease and safety, the latter are preferred to neurolytic injections. Stellate ganglion neurolysis is hazardous because of the close proximity of other important structures (brachial plexus, laryngeal nerves, epidural and subarachnoid space, vertebral artery) and the potential for injury because of inaccurate needle placement. If local anesthetic injections have been documented to provide temporary relief of pain, surgical extirpation of the ganglia may be considered, or neurolysis may be performed cautiously using radiological guidance and small volumes of injectate (279).

Lumbar Sympathetic Ganglia, Superior Hypogastric Plexus, and Ganglion Impar

When trials of local anesthetic blocks have been shown to provide temporary relief of pain, neurolysis of the lumbar sympathetic chain with phenol may be undertaken. Lumbar sympathetic block is most applicable for pain in the lower extremities due to lymphedema or reflex sympathetic imbalance (236), although it has also been applied for rectal and pelvic pain (237). Superior hypogastric plexus block (280) (Fig. 25.12) is generally preferred for intractable chronic pelvic or rectal pain of neoplastic origin. In contrast to subarachnoid injection, risks of bowel, bladder, and motor dysfunction with either lumbar sympathetic or hypogastric block, even when performed bilaterally, are extremely low, particularly with radiological guidance. Preliminary experience with presacral blockade of the small unpaired ganglion impar (ganglion of Walther) at the junction of the sacrum and coccyx (Fig. 25.13) suggests efficacy for sympathetically mediated anal or genital pain (281).

In the first published study of superior hypogastric block (280), 28 patients with intrapelvic neoplasms or radiation enteritis were studied, and all had significant or complete relief of pain with no complications. In all but 2 patients with pain due to neoplasm, relief persisted until death (3 to 12 months). De Leon-Casasola et al. (282) achieved similar results in another study of 26 cancer patients with severe (10 of 10 intensity) intractable pelvic pain: 70% had satisfactory relief (less than 4 of 10 intensity) and the remaining patients, moderate relief (4 to 7 of 10). Complications were not observed, and no patients with satisfactory relief required repetition at 6 months. Superior hypogastric plexus block, which requires fluoroscopic guidance, is essentially a modification of lumbar sympathetic block with needles directed more caudally, ultimately to lie just beyond the sacral promontory.

Ganglion Impar (Ganglion of Walther)

The ganglion impar is a solitary retroperitoneal structure at the level of the sacrococcygeal junction that marks the termination of the paired paravertebral sympathetic chains. Although the anatomical interconnections of the ganglion impar are rarely described in any detail, even in the anatomy literature, the sympathetic component of perineal pain syndromes appears to derive at least in part from this structure. The first report of interruption of the ganglion impar for the relief of perineal pain appeared in 1990 (281). Of 16 patients, 8 with advanced cancer and burning, tenesmic pain involving the perineum, anus, and genitalia had complete, durable relief of pain, and the remainder had significant reductions in pain. Blocks were repeated in two patients with further improvement. No complications occurred, and follow-up, which depended on survival, was carried out for 14 to 120 days. The technique entails the use of a 20- or 22-gauge spinal needle that is manually bent near its hub at about 30°. The needle is introduced through the anococcygeal ligament with its concavity oriented toward the concavity of the sacrum and coccyx. Under fluoroscopic guidance the needle is advanced until its tip lies near the anterior surface of the junction of the sacrum and coccyx, posterior to the rectum where injection takes place.

Other Interventions

Transcutaneous electrical nerve stimulation (TENS) is a noninvasive means of reducing pain that entails the application of low-voltage electrical stimulation over a painful site by means of a portable beeper-sized power source attached to ECG electrodes. TENS is most often used as an adjunct to other more reliably effective modalities, since it rarely relieves pain entirely and appears to be partially dependent on the placebo response (283). The risk-benefit ratio of spinal cord stimulation does not appear to warrant its use in patients with cancer pain (284). Deep brain stimulation is a highly

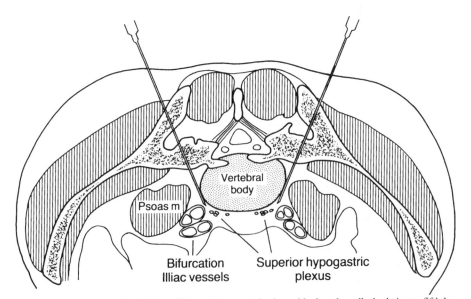

Figure 25.12.   Cross-sectional view of bilateral hypogastric plexus block and needles' relation to fifth lumbar vertebra, psoas muscle, and iliac vessels.

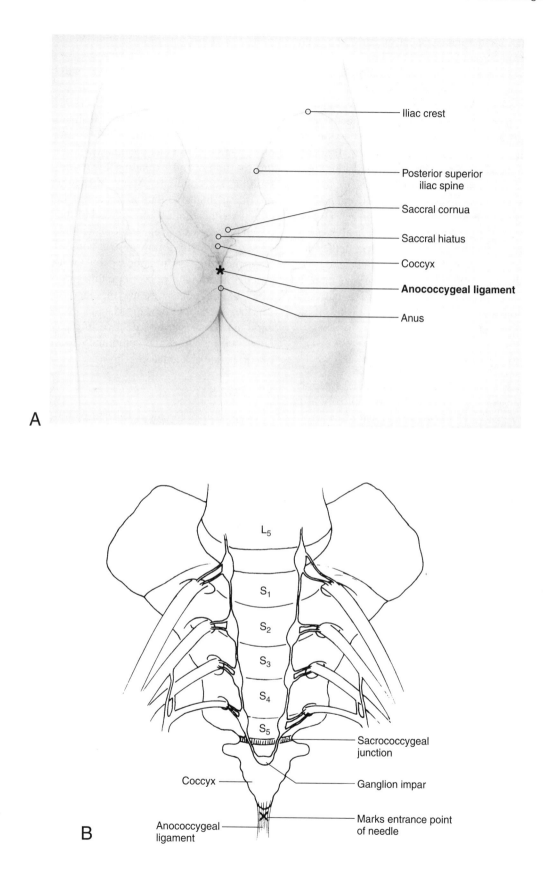

Figure 25.13.   Blockade of the ganglion impar for the relief of sympathetically mediated anorectal and genital pain. A. External landmarks. B. Internal landmarks.

promising approach for the management of intractable pain (285). It entails stimulation of areas of the brain with dense populations of opioid receptors, producing profound analgesia, apparently mediated by endorphins. Pituitary ablation is another useful technique that is still not widely available. It entails destruction of the gland by means of the injection of a small quantity of alcohol through a needle positioned transnasally under light general anesthesia (286). Pituitary lysis is remarkably effective in relieving pain originating from disseminated bony metastases, particularly secondary to hormone-dependent tumors (breast and prostate). Commissural myelotomy has been reported to be efficacious in cancer pain refractory to more conservative therapy (287). Finally, percutaneous cordotomy produces a thermal lesion within the substance of the spinal cord and reliably relieves unilateral truncal and lower limb pain (288). As with pituitary ablation, it necessitates a high degree of skill and expertise, but pain relief is often profound and the rigors of a major neurosurgical procedure are avoided.

Home-Based and Hospice Care

Hospice is often incorrectly regarded as a place people go to die (289). Hospice is best regarded conceptually as a philosophy of care that is a "a blend of clinical pharmacology and applied compassionate psychology" (290). Contemporary hospice care originated in the United Kingdom, where treatment is still often provided in an institutional setting, much like a hospital or nursing home. In the United States hospice care has developed primarily as a home-based service, with a minority of institutions offering short inpatient stays to stabilize refractory symptoms and to provide respite for overwhelmed families. For it to be effective, it is essential that clinicians providing pain management for oncology patients be familiar with local hospice resources, many of which provide essential physician education about care near the end of life, a subject that is still underemphasized in postgraduate training.

The guiding therapeutic principles of home-based pain management are in most respects similar to those that apply to ambulatory and inpatient pain management. Differences generally relate to a recognition that further curative therapy is futile rather than that care is being provided at home. No compromise in quality of care based on where it is delivered is justified. This is not to say that equivalent care is rendered; it usually is not. Rather, the nature of care tends to differ according to the considerations that cause the selection of the home as the place of treatment in the first place.

Hospice care is comfort oriented, focusing specifically on alleviating symptoms rather than necessarily treating their underlying cause or causes. As a result, the need for laboratory investigations, from interventions as minor as blood tests to more sophisticated tests such as MRI, is limited. The deci-

sion to perform any investigation should be subjected to a simple but key inquiry: will the results of the test alter symptoms or provide information that will help improve the patient's well-being?

Factors that influence the selection of home treatment are advanced, incurable disease, realization and acceptance of the appropriateness of palliative care (care directed at preserving comfort and the quality of life rather than at curing the tumor and extending life), and a desire to die in familiar surroundings. Many difficulties associated with providing intensive palliative care at home can be reconciled by education and orientation of the family. They must be encouraged to keep accurate records, to be extremely observant and to follow instructions; their access to the physician must be unimpeded by the demands of a busy practice. Fortunately, to bridge this gap, health care institutions, that is, home care nursing, laboratory, and pharmacy services, have been developed to act as the physician's eyes, ears and hands. To be effective, the physician must learn about the resources the community has to offer and make maximal use of them.

SUMMARY

Regrettably, chronic and acute pain occur in a high frequency of cancer patients. If inadequately addressed by the clinician, pain and other distressing symptoms may interfere with primary antitumor therapy and markedly detract from the quality of life of patients, family members, and care providers. While a strong focus on pain control is important independent of disease stage, it is a special priority in patients with advanced disease who are no longer candidates for potentially curative therapy.

While rarely eliminated altogether, pain can be controlled in the vast majority of patients, usually with the careful application of straightforward pharmacological measures combined with diagnostic acumen and conscientious follow-up. In the small but significant proportion of patients whose pain is not readily controlled with noninvasive analgesics, a variety of alternative measures, when selected carefully, are also associated with a high degree of success. An increasingly large cadre of clinicians have come to recognize that far from an exercise in futility, caring for patients with advanced irreversible illness can be a highly satisfying endeavor that is usually met with considerable success. Thus, no patient should ever wish for death as a result of inadequate control of pain or other symptoms, and clinicians need never communicate overtly or indirectly that nothing more can be done. Comprehensive cancer care is best regarded as a continuum that commences with prevention and early detection, focuses intensely on curative therapy, and ideally is rendered complete by a seamless transition to palliation and attention to quality of life.

References

1. Ahles TA, Blanchard EB, Ruchdeschel JC. The multidimensional nature of cancer-related pain. Pain 1983;17:277-288.
2. Bonica JJ, Ekstrom JL. Systemic opioids for the management of cancer pain: an updated review. Adv Pain Res Ther 1990;14:425-446.
3. Bonica JJ. Cancer pain: a major national health problem. Cancer Nurs 1978;1:313.
4. Foley KM. Treatment of cancer pain. N Engl J Med 1985;313:84.
5. Ventafridda V. Continuing care: a major issue in cancer pain management. Pain 1989;36:137-143.
6. American Pain Society. Principles of analgesic use in the treatment of acute pain and chronic cancer pain. 3rd ed. Skokie, IL: APS, 1992.
7. Jacox A, Carr DB, Payne R, et al. Management of cancer pain: clinical practice guideline 9. Agency for Health Care Policy and Research pub. 94-0592. Rockville, MD: ACHPR, 1994.
8. Ferrell BR, Wisdon C, Wenzl C. Quality of life as an outcome variable in management of cancer pain. Cancer 1989;63:2321.
9. Liebeskind JC. Pain can kill. Pain 1991;44:3-4.
10. Lillemoe KD, Cameron JL, Kaufman HS, et al. Chemical splanchnicectomy in patients with unresectable pancreatic cancer. Ann Surg 1993;217:447-457.
11. Cleeland CS, Gonin R, Hatfield AK, et al. Pain and its treatment in outpatients with metastatic cancer. N Engl J Med 1994;330:592-596.
12. Von Roenn JH, Cleeland CS, Gonin R, et al. Physician attitudes and practice in cancer pain management. Ann Intern Med 1993;119:121-126.
13. Silverberg E, Boring CC, Squires TS. Cancer statistics, 1990. CA Cancer J Clin 1990;40:9.
14. American Cancer Society. Cancer facts and figures: 1994. Atlanta: ACS, 1994.
15. American Cancer Society. Cancer facts and figures: 1989. Atlanta: ACS, 1989.
16. Walsh TD. Oral morphine in chronic cancer pain. Pain 1984;18:1.
17. Bruera E. Malnutrition and asthenia in advanced cancer. Cancer Bull 1991;43:387.
18. Bonica JJ. Management of cancer pain. Rec Res Cancer Res 1984;89:13.
19. Daut RL, Cleeland CS. The prevalence and severity of pain in cancer. Cancer 1982:50;1913.
20. Mumford JW, Mumford SP. The care of cancer patients in a rural South Indian hospital. Pall Med 1988;2:157.
21. World Health Organization. Cancer Pain Relief. Geneva: WHO, 1986.
22. Portenoy RK. Cancer pain: epidemiology and syndromes. Cancer 1989;63:2307.
23. Brescia FJ, Adler D, Gray G, Ryan MA. A profile of hospitalized advanced cancer patients. J Pain Symptom Manage 1990;5:221.
24. Twycross RG, Fairfield S. Pain in far-advanced cancer. Pain 1982;14:303.
25. Zech DFJ, Grong S, Lynch J, et al. Validation of the World Health Organization guidelines for cancer pain relief: a 10-year prospective study. Pain 1996;63:65-76.
26. Takeda F. Preliminary report from Japan on results of field testing of WHO draft interim guidelines for relief of cancer pain. Pain Clin 1986;1:83-89.
27. Ventafridda V, Tambutini M, Carceni A, et al. A validation study of the WHO method for cancer pain relief. Cancer 1987;59:850.
28. Toscani F, Carini M. The implementation of the WHO guidelines for the treatment of advanced cancer pain in a district general hospital in Italy. Pain Clinic 1989;3:37.
29. Swerdlow M, Stjernsward J. Cancer pain relief: an urgent problem. World Health Forum 1982;3:325-330.
30. Ventafridda V, De Conno FD. Status of cancer pain and palliative care worldwide. J Pain Symptom Mgmt 1996;12:79-143.
31. World Health Organization Expert Committee. Cancer pain relief and palliative care. Geneva: WHO, 1990;3-75.
32. Jadad AR, Browman GP. The WHO analgesic ladder for cancer pain management: stepping up the quality of its evaluation. JAMA 1995;274:1870-1873.
33. Angarola RT. Availability and regulation of opioid analgesics. Adv Pain Res Ther 1990;6:513.
34. Angarola RT, Wray SD. Legal impediments to cancer pain treatment. Adv Pain Res Ther 1989;11:213.
35. Cleeland CS. Barriers to the management of cancer pain. Oncology 1987;12 Suppl: 19-26.
36. Cleeland CS, Cleeland LM, Dar R, et al. Factors influencing physician management of cancer pain. Cancer 1986;58:796-800.
37. Pinkert T. The view from the public health service. J Pain Symptom Mgmt 1988;3:S9.
38. Allende S, Carvell HC. Mexico: status of cancer pain and palliative care. J Pain Symptom Mgmt 1996;12:121-123.
39. Merriman A. Uganda: status of cancer pain and palliative care. J Pain Symptom Mgmt 1996;12:141-143.
33. Soebadi RD, Tejawinata S. Indonesia: status of cancer pain and palliative care. J Pain Symptom Mgmt 1996;12:112-113.
34. Cleeland CS. The impact of pain on the patient with cancer. Cancer 1984;54:2643-2645.
35. Duffy JC. Keynote address: a call to action. J Pain Symptom Mgmt 1988;3:S6-S8.
36. Saunders C. The management of terminal illness. London: London Hospital Medical Publications, 1967.
37. Mor V. Cancer patients' quality of life over the disease course: lessons from the real world. J Chron Dis 1987;40:535.
38. McMillian SC, Williams FA, Chatfield R, et al. A validity and reliability study of two tools for assessing and managing cancer pain. Oncol Nurs Forum 1988;15:737-744.
39. Edeiken J, Karasick D. Imaging in cancer. CA Cancer J Clin 1987;37:239.
40. Grond S, Zech D, Diefenbach C, et al. Assessment of cancer pain: a prospective evaluation in 2266 cancer pain patients referred to a pain service. Pain 1996;64:107-114.
41. Buchanan J, Millership R, Zalcberg J, et al. Medical education in palliative care. Med J Aust 1990;152:27.
42. Twycross R. Palliative care: a compulsory issue. In: Lipton S et al, eds. Adv Pain Res Ther, vol 13. New York: Raven Press, 1990;297.
43. Seifert L, et al. The frequency of alcoholism among patients with pain due to terminal cancer. J Pain Symptom Mgmt 1995;10:599-603.
44. Reddy SK, Weinstein SM. Medical decision making in a patient with a history of cancer and chronic non-malignant pain. Clin J Pain 1995;11:242-246.
45. Grossman SA, Sheidler VR, Swedeen K, et al. Correlation of patient and caregiver ratings of cancer pain. J Pain Symptom Mgmt 1991;6:53-57.
46. Copp LA, Anderson VC, Brown MJ, et al. National institutes of health consensus panel: integrated approach to the management of pain. J Pain Symptom Mgmt 1987;2:35-44.
47. Portenoy R. Management of pain in patients with advanced cancer. Res Staff Phys 1987;33:59.
48. Lacroix JM. Low back pain factors of value in predicting outcomes. Spine 1990;15:495.
49. Cohrn RS, Ferrer-Brechner T, Pavlov A, et al. Prospective evaluation of treatment outcome in patients referred to a cancer pain center. In: Fields HL et al., eds. Adv Pain Res Ther, vol 9. New York: Raven Press, 1985;655.
50. Tollison CD. Patient education influences pain recovery. Pain Mgmt 1991;4:9.
51. Sternbach RA. Pain: a psychophysiological analysis. New York: Academic Press, 1968.
52. Jay S, Elliot C, Ozolins M, et al. Behavioral management of children's distress during painful medical procedures. Behav Res Ther 1985;23:513.

53. Sternbach RA. Acute versus chronic pain. In: Wall PD, Melzack R. Textbook of pain. 2nd ed. Edinburgh: Churchill Livingstone, 1989;242.

54. Foley KM. Cancer pain syndromes. J Pain Symptom Mgmt 1987;2:S13-S17.

55. Sternbach RA. Pain patients: traits and treatments. New York: Academic Press, 1974.

56. Black RG. The chronic pain syndromes. Surg Clin North Am 1975;55:4.

57. Saunders C. The philosophy of terminal care. In: Saunders C, ed. The management of terminal malignant disease. London: Edward Arnold, 1984;232.

58. Tunks E. Is there a chronic pain syndrome? Adv Pain Res Ther 1990;13:257.

59. Sanders S. Behavioral assessment and treatment of clinical pain: appraisal and current status. In: Hersen M, Eisler RM, Miller PM, eds. Progress in behavior modification. New York: Academic Press, 1979;249-291.

60. Portenoy RK. Breakthrough pain: definition and management. Oncology 1983;3:25-29.

61. World Health Organization. Cancer Pain Relief. Geneva: WHO, 1986.

62. Payne R. Cancer pain: anatomy, physiology and pharmacology. Cancer 1989;63 (Suppl):2266.

63. Newman PP. Visceral afferent functions of the nervous system. London: Arnold, 1974.

64. Procacci P, Maresca M. Pathophysiology of visceral pain. Adv Pain Res Ther 13;1990;123.

65. Newman PP. Visceral afferent functions of the nervous system. London: Arnold, 1974.

66. Kellgren JH. Somatic simulating visceral pain. Clin Sci 1939;4:303.

67. Cervero F. Visceral pain. In: Dubner R, Gebhart GF, Bond MR, eds. Proceedings of the VI World Congress on Pain. Amsterdam: Elsevier, 1988;216.

68. Tasker RR, Dostrovsky JO. Deafferentation and central pain. In: Wall PD, Melzack R. Textbook of pain. 2nd ed. Edinburgh: Churchill Livingstone, 1989;154.

69. Jacobson L, Chabal C, Brody MC. Relief of persistent postamputation stump and phantom limb pain with intrathecal fentanyl. Pain 1989;37:317.

70. Galasko CSB. Skeletal metastases. London: Butterworths, 1986;99.

71. Enneking WF, Conrad EU III. Common bone tumors. Clin Symp 1989;41:1.

72. Pollen JJ, Schmidt JD. Bone pain in metastatic cancer of the prostate. Urology 1979;13:129.

73. Akakura K, Akimoto S, Shimazaki J. Pain caused by bone metastasis in endocrine-therapy-refractory prostate cancer. J Cancer Res Clin Oncol 1996;122:633-7.

74. Foley KM. Pain syndromes in patients with cancer. Adv Pain Res Ther 2;1979:59.

75. Thrupkaew AK, Henkin RE, Quin JL III. False negative bone scans in disseminated metastatic disease. Radiology 1974;113:383.

76. Kanner R. Diagnosis and management of pain in patients with cancer. Basel: Karger, 1988.

77. DeVita VT Jr, Hellman S, Rosenberg SA, eds. Cancer: principles and practice of oncology, 3rd ed. Philadelphia: Lippincott, 1989;1252.

78. Greenberg HS, Deck MDF, Vikram B, et al. Metastases to the base of the skull: clinical findings in 43 patients. Neurology 1981;31:530.

79. Elliot K, Foley KM. Neurologic pain syndromes in patients with cancer. Crit Care Clin 1990;6:393.

80. Payne R. Pharmacologic management of bone pain in the cancer patient. Clin J Pain 1989;5(Suppl):S43.

81. Gokaslan ZL. Spine surgery for cancer. Curr Opin Oncol 1996;8:178-181.

82. Weller SJ, Rossitch E Jr. Unilateral posterolateral decompression without stabilization for neurologic palliation of symptomatic spinal metastasis in debilitated patients. J Neurosurg 1995;82:739-744.

83. Travell J. Myofascial trigger points: clinical view. Adv Pain Res Ther 1;1976:919.

84. Abrams SE. The role of non-neurolytic blocks in the management of cancer pain. In: Abrams SE, ed. Cancer pain. Boston: Kluwer, 1989;67.

85. Siegal T. Muscle cramps in the cancer patient: causes and treatment. J Pain Symptom Mgmt 1991;6;84.

86. Patchell RA, Posner JB. Neurologic complications of systemic cancer. Neurol Clin 1985;3:729.

87. Gilbert MR, Grossman SA. Incidence and nature of neurologic problems in patients with solid tumors. Am J Med 1986;81:951.

88. Twycross RG, Lack SA. Symptom control in far advanced cancer: pain relief. London: Pitman, 1983.

89. Kori SH, Foley KM, Posner JB. Brachial plexus lesions in patients with cancer: 100 cases. Neurology 1981;31:45.

90. Foley KM. Brachial plexopathy in patients with breast cancer. In: Harris JR, Hellman S, Henderson IC, et al., eds. Breast diseases. Philadelphia: Lippincott, 1987.

91. Scott JF. Carcinoma invading nerve. In: Wall PD, Melzack R. Textbook of pain. 2nd ed. Edinburgh: Churchill Livingstone, 1989;598.

92. Yacoub M, Hupert C. Shoulder pain as an early symptom of Pancoast tumor. J Med Soc N J 1980;77:583.

93. Batzdorf U, Brechner VL. Management of pain associated with the Pancoast syndrome. Am J Surg 1979;137:638.

94. Cascino TL, Kori S, Krol G, et al. CT scan of the brachial plexus in patients with cancer. Neurology 1983;33:1553.

95. Kanner RM, Martini N, Foley KM. Epidural spinal cord compression in Pancoast syndrome (superior pulmonary sulcus tumor): clinical presentation and outcome. Ann Neurol 1981;10:77.

96. Foley KM. Overview of cancer pain and brachial and lumbosacral plexopathy. In: Foley KM, ed. Management of Cancer pain. New York: Memorial Sloan Kettering Cancer Center, 1985;25.

97. Jaekle KA, Young DF, Foley KM. The natural history of lumbosacral plexopathy in cancer. Neurology 1985;35:8-15.

98. Pettigrew LC, Glass JP, Maor M, et al. Diagnosis and treatment of lumbosacral plexopathy in patients with cancer. Arch Neurol 1984;41:1282.

99. Posner JB, Chernik NK. Intracranial metastases from systemic cancer. Adv Neurol 1978;19:579.

100. Olson ME, Chernik NL, Posner JB. Infiltration of the leptomeninges by systemic cancer: a clinical and pathologic study. Arch Neurol 1930:122.

101. Wasserstrom WR, Glass JP, Posner JB. Diagnosis and treatment of leptomeningeal metastases from solid tumor: experience with 90 patients. Cancer 1982;49:759.

102. Schild SC, Wasserstrom WR, Fleischer M, et al. Cerebrospinal fluid biochemical markers of central nervous system metastasis. Ann Neurol 1980;8:597.

103. Lee YY, Glass JP, Geoffray A, et al. Cranial computed tomographic abnormalities in leptomeningeal metastases. AJNR Am J Neuroradiol 1984;5:559.

104. Glass JP, Foley KM. Carcinomatous meningitis. In: Harris JR, Hellman S, Henderson IC, et al., eds. Breast diseases. Philadelphia: Lippincott, 1987;497.

105. Kunkle EC, Hernandez RR, Wolff HG. Studies on headache: the mechanisms and significance of headache associated with brain tumor. Bull N Y Acad Med 1942;18:400.

106. Rushton JG, Rooke ED. Brain tumor headache. Headache 1962;2:147.

107. Zimm S, Wampler GL, Stablein D, et al. Intracerebral metastases in solid tumor patients: natural history and results of treatment. Cancer 1981;48:384.

108. Guitin PH. Corticosteroid therapy in patients with brain tumor. Natl Cancer Inst Monogr 1977;46:151.

109. Black P. Brain metastasis: current status and recommended guidelines for management. Neurosurgery 1979;5:617.

110. Bruera E, MacDonald RN. Intractable pain in patients with advanced head and neck tumors: a possible role for local infection. Cancer Treat Rep 1986; 70:691-92.

111. Patt RB, Jain S. Management of a patient with osteoradionecrosis of the mandible with nerve blocks. J Pain Symptom Mgmt 1990;5:59-60.

112. Foley KM. Pain syndromes and pharmacologic management of pancreatic cancer pain. J Pain Symptom Mgmt 1988;3:176.

113. Reber HA, Foley KM, eds. Pancreatic cancer pain: presentation, pathogenesis and management. J Pain Symptom Mgmt 1988;3:163.

114. Ihse I. Pancreatic pain. Br J Surg 1990;77:121.

115. Kawamata M, Ishanti K, Ishikawa K, et al. Comparison between celiac plexus block and morphine treatment on quality of life in patients with pancreatic cancer pain. Pain 1996;64:597-602.

116. Foley KM. Pain syndromes in patients with cancer. Med Clin North Am 1987;71:169.

117. Miser AW, Miser JS. The treatment of cancer pain in children. Pediatr Clin North Am 1989;36:979.

118. Campa JA, Payne R. Pain syndromes due to cancer. In: Patt RB, ed. Cancer pain. Philadelphia: Lippincott, 1993;41-56.

119. Shubert MM, Sullivan KM, Morten TH, et al. Oral manifestations of chronic graft-versus-host disease. Arch Intern Med 1984;144:1591.

120. Carl W. Oral and dental care of patients receiving radiation therapy for tumors in and around the oral cavity. In: Carl W, Saka K, eds. Cancer and the oral cavity. Chicago: Quintessence, 1986;167.

121. Young DF, Posner JB. Nervous system toxicity of chemotherapeutic agents. In: Vinken PJ, Bruyn GW, eds. Handbook of Clinical Neurology, vol 9. Neurological manifestations of systemic diseases, part II. Amsterdam: North Holland, 1989;91.

122. Ihde DC, DeVita VT. Osteonecrosis of the femoral head in patients treated with intermittent combination chemotherapy (including corticosteroids). Cancer 1975;36:1585.

123. Rotstein J, Good RA. Steroid pseudorheumatism. Arch Intern Med 1957;99:545.

124. Tasmuth T, von Smitten K, Kalso E, et al. Pain and other symptoms during the first year after radical and conservative surgery for breast surgery. Br J Cancer 1996;74:2024-2031.

125. Tasmuth T, von Smitten K, Hietanen P, et al. Pain and other symptoms after different treatment modalities of breast cancer. Ann Oncol 1995;6:453-9

125a.Vecht CJ, Van de Brand HJ, Wajer OJ, et al. Post-axillary dissection in breast cancer due to lesion of the intercostobrachial nerve. Pain 1989;38:171.

126. Watson CP, Evans RJ, Watt VR, The post-mastectomy pain syndrome and the effect of topical capsaicin. Pain 1989;38:177.

127. Eija K, Tasmuth T, Neuvonen PJ. Amitriptyline effectively relieves neuropathic pain following treatment of breast cancer. Pain 1995;64:293-302.

128. Chapman CR, Casey KL, Dubner R, et al. Pain measurement: an overview. Pain 1985;22:1.

129. Williams CR. Toward a set of reliable and valid measures for chronic pain assessment and outcome research. Pain 1988;35:239.

130. Daut RL, Cleeland CS, Flannery RC. Development of the Wisconsin brief pain questionnaire to assess pain in cancer and other diseases. Pain 1983;17:197.

131. Cleeland CS. Assessment of pain in cancer. Adv Pain Res Ther 16;1990:47.

132. Fishman B, Pasternak S, Wallenstein S, et al. The Memorial pain assessment card: a valid instrument for the evaluation of cancer pain. Cancer 1987;60:1151.

133. Van der Does AJW. Patients' and nurses' ratings of pain and anxiety during burn wound care. Pain 1989;39:95.

134. Choiniere M, Melzack R, Girard N, et al. Comparisons between patients' and nurses' assessment of pain and medication efficacy in severe burn injuries. Pain 1990;40:143.

135. Peteet J, Tay V, Cohen G, et al. Pain characteristics and treatment in an outpatient cancer population. Cancer 1986;57:1259.

136. O'Brien J, Francis A. The use of next-of-kin to estimate pain in cancer patients. Pain 1988;35:171.

137. Bruera E, MacMillan K, Hanson J, et al. The Edmonton staging system for cancer pain: preliminary report. Pain 1989;37:203.

138. Bruera E, Schoeller T, Wenk R, et al. A prospective multicenter assessment of the Edmonton staging system for cancer pain. J Pain Symptom Mgmt 1995;10:348-355.

139. American Joint Committee for Cancer Staging and End Result Reporting. Manual for Staging of Cancer. Chicago: AJCC, 1977.

140. Beyer J, Aradine C. Content validity of an instrument to measure young children's perceptions of the intensity of their pain. J Pediatr Nurs 1986;1:386.

141. Eland J. Eland color scale. In: McCaffery M, Beebe A, eds. Pain: clinical manual for nursing practice. St. Louis: Mosby, 1989.

142. Hester N, Foster R, Kristensen K. Measurement of pain in children: generalizability and validity of the pain ladder and the poker chip tool. In: Tyler D, Krane E, eds. Advances in pain research and therapy: pediatric pain, vol 1. New York: Raven Press, 1990;79.

143. McGrath PA. Pain in children: nature, assessment, and treatment. New York: Guilford, 1990.

144. Beyer JE, Wells N. Assessment of cancer pain in children. In: Patt RB, ed. Cancer pain. Philadelphia: Lippincott, 1993;57-84.

145. Mauch PM, Drew MA. Treatment of metastatic cancer to bone. In: Devita VT, ed. Cancer: principles and practice of oncology. ed 2. Philadelphia: Lippincott, 1985;2132-2141.

146. Salazar OM, Da Motta NW, Bridgman SM, et al. Fractionated half-body irradiation for pain palliation in widely metastatic cancers: comparison with single dose. Int J Radiat Oncol Biol Phys 1996;36:49-60.

147. Estes NC, Morphis JG, Hornback NB, et al. Intraarterial chemotherapy and hyperthermia for pain control in patients with recurrent rectal cancer. Am J Surg 1986;152:597-601.

148. Mellette SJ. Management of malignant disease metastatic to the bone by hormonal alterations. Clin Orthop 1970;73:73-78.

149. Faithfull NS, Reinhold HS, Van Den Berg AP, et al. The effectiveness and safety of whole body hyperthermia as a pain treatment in advanced malignancy. In: Erdmann W, Oyama T, Pernak MJ, eds. Pain clinic. Utrecht: VNU Science, 1985.

150. Price P, Hoskin PJ, Easton D, et al. Prospective randomized trial of single and multifraction radiotherapy schedules in the treatment of painful bone metastasis. Clin Oncol 1989;1:1989;1:56-62.

151. Jadad AR, Browman GP. The WHO analgesic ladder for cancer pain management: Stepping up the quality of its evaluation. JAMA 1995;274:1870-1873.

152. Bruera E. Subcutaneous administration of opioids in the management of cancer pain. In: Foley K, Ventafridda V, eds. Recent advances in pain research, vol 16. New York: Raven Press, 1990;203-218.

153. Schlegel SI, Paulus HE. Nonsteroidal and analgesic use in the elderly. Clin Rheum Dis 1986;12:245.

154. Valentini M, Cannizzaro R, Poletti M. Nonsteroidal antiinflammatory drugs for cancer pain: comparison between misoprostol and ranitidine in prevention of upper gastrointestinal damage. J Clin Oncol 1995;13:2637-2642.

155. Rothwell KG. Efficacy and safety of a non-acetylated salicylate, choline magnesium trisalicylate in the treatment of rheumatoid arthritis. J Int Med Res 1983;11:343.

156. Leonards JR, Levy G. Gastrointestinal blood loss from aspirin and sodium salicylate tablets in man. Clin Pharmacol Ther 1973;14:62.

157. Buckley MMT, Brogden RN. Ketorolac: a review of its pharmacodynamic and pharmacokinetic properties and therapeutic potential. Drugs 1990;39:86-109.

158. McQuay HJ, Carroll D, Frankland T, et al. Bromfenac, acetaminophen, and placebo in orthopedic postoperative pain. Clin Pharmacol Ther 1990;47:760-766.

159. Carroll D, Frankland T, Nagle C, McQuay H. Oral bromfenac 10 and 25 mg compared with sublingual buprenorphine 0.2 and 0.4 mg for postoperative pain relief. Br J Anaesth 1993;71:814-817.

160. Needleman P, Isakson PC. The discovery and function of COX-2. J Rheumatol 1997;24 (Suppl)49:6-8.

161. Kalso E, Vainio A. Morphine and oxycodone hydrochloride in the management of cancer pain. Clin Pharmacol Ther 1990;47:639-46.

162. Cooper SA, Beaver WT. A model to evaluate mild analgesics in oral surgery patients. Clin Pharmacol Ther 1976:20;241.

163. Hopkinson JH III. Vicodin: a new analgesic: clinical evaluation of efficacy and safety of repeated doses. Curr Ther Res 1978;24:633-645.

164. Ettinger DS, Vitale PJ, Trump DL. Important clinical pharmacologic considerations in the use of methadone in cancer patients. Cancer Treat Rep 1979;63:457.

165. Ferrer-Brechner T. Rational management of cancer pain. In: Raj PP, ed. Practical management of pain. Chicago: Year Book Medical, 1986;312-328.

166. Kaiko RF, Wallenstein SL, Rogers AG, et al. Sources of variation in analgesic responses in cancer patients with chronic pain receiving morphine. Pain 1983;15:191-200.

167. Cleeland CS, Tearnan BH. Behavioral control of cancer pain. In: Holzman AD, Turk DC, eds. Pain management. New York: Pergamon Press, 1986;193-212.

168. Twycross RG, Harcourt JMV. The use of laxatives at a palliative care center. Palliat Med 1991;5:27.

169. Baines M. Nausea and vomiting in the patient with advanced cancer. J Pain Symptom Mgmt 1988;3:81-85.

170. Bruera E, Chadwick S, Brenneis C, et al. Methylphenidate associated with narcotics for the treatment of cancer pain. Cancer Treat Rep 1987;71:67-70.

171. Cherny NJ, Chang V, Frager G, et al. Opioid pharmacotherapy in the management of cancer pain. Cancer 1995;76:1283-1293.

172. Deleted.

173. Paalzow LK. Pharmacokinetic aspects of optimal pain treatment. Acta Anaesthesiol Scand Suppl 1982;74:37-43.

174. Kaiko RF. Controlled-release oral morphine for cancer-related pain: the European and North American experiences. Adv Pain Res Ther 1990;16:171.

175. Fine PG, Marcus M, De Boer AJ, Van der Oord B. An open label study of oral transmucosal fentanyl citrate (OTFC) for the treatment of breakthrough cancer pain. Pain 1991;45:149-153.

176. Miser AW, Narang PK, Dothage JA, et al. Transdermal fentanyl for pain control in patients with cancer. Pain 1989; 37:15-21.

177. Cole L, Hanning CD. Review of the rectal use of opioids. J Pain Symptom Mgmt 1990;5:118-126.

178. Ripamonti C, Zecca E, Brunelli C, et al. Rectal methadone in cancer patients with pain: a preliminary clinical and pharmacokinetic study. Ann Oncol 1995;6:841-843.

179. Bruera E, Ripamonti C. Alternate routes of administration of narcotics. In: Patt RB, ed. Cancer pain. Philadelphia: Lippincott, 1993;161.

180. Kaiko RF, Foley KM, Grabinski PY, et al. Central nervous system excitatory effects of meperidine in cancer patients. Ann Neurol 1983; 13:180-185.

181. Patt R, Jain S. Recent advances in the management of oncologic pain. In: Stoelting RK, Barash PG, Gallagher TJ, eds. Advances in anesthesiology, vol 6. Chicago: Year Book Medical, 1989;355-414.

182. Syrjala KL, Donaldson GW, Davis MW, et al. Relaxation and imagery and cognitive-behavioral training reduce pain during cancer treatment: a controlled clinical trial. Pain 1995;63:189-198.

183. Watling CJ, Payne R, Allen RR, Hassenbusch S. Commissural myelotomy for intractable cancer pain: report of two cases. Clin J Pain 1996:12:151-156.

184. Hassenbusch SJ, Stanton-Hicks M, Covington EC. Spinal cord stimulation versus spinal infusion for low back and leg pain. Acta Neurochir 1995;64S:109-115.

185. Byas-Smith MG, Max MB, Muir J, Kingman A. Transdermal clonidine compared to placebo in painful diabetic neuropathy using a two-stage 'enriched enrollment' design. Pain 1995;60:267-274.

186. Portenoy RK, Kanner RM. Nonopioid and adjuvant analgesics. In: Portenoy RK, Kanner RM, eds. Pain management: theory and practice. Philadelphia: Davis, 1996;219-247.

187. Watson C, Evans R, Reed K, et al. Amitriptyline versus placebo in postherpetic neuralgia. Neurology 1982;32:671-673.

188. Kishore-Kumar R, Max MB, Schafer SC, et al. Desipramine relieves post-herpetic neuralgia. Clin Pharmacol Ther 1990;47:305-372.

189. Panerai AE, Monza G, Mouilia P, et al. A randomized, within-patient, crossover, placebo-controlled trial on the efficacy and tolerability of the tricyclic antidepressants chlorimipramine and nortriptyline in central pain. Acta Neurol Scand 1990;82:34-38.

190. Sindrup SH, Ejlertsen B, Froland A, et al. Imipramine treatment in diabetic neuropathy: relief of subjective symptoms without changes in peripheral and autonomic nerve function. Eur J Clin Pharmacol 1989;37:151-53.

191. Sindrup SH, Gram LF, Skjold T, et al. Clomipramine vs desipramine vs placebo in the treatment of diabetic neuropathy symptoms: a double-blind cross-over study. Br J Clin Pharmacol 1990;30:683-691.

192. Walsh TD. Controlled study of imipramine and morphine in chronic pain due to cancer. Proc Am Soc Clin Oncol 1986;5:237.

193. Vantafridda V, Bianchi M, Ripamonti C, et al. Studies on the effects of antidepressant drugs on the antinociceptive action of morphine on plasma morphine in rat and man. Pain 1990;43:155-162.

194. Sweet WH. Treatment of trigeminal neuralgia (tic douloureux). N Engl J Med 1986;315:174-177.

195. Hatangdi VS, Boas RA, Richard EG. Postherpetic neuralgia: management with antiepileptic and tricyclic drugs. Adv Pain Res Ther 1976;1:1:583-587.

196. Swerdlow M. The use of anticonvulsants in the management of cancer pain. In: Erdmann W, Oyamma T, Pernak MJ, eds. The pain clinic. Utrecht: VNU Science, 1985.

197. Rosner H, Rubin L. Gabapentin adjunctive therapy in neuropathic pain states. Clin J Pain 1996;12:56-58.

198. Rho JM, Donevan SD, Rogawski MA. Mechanisms of the anticonvulsant felbamate: opposing effects on N-methyl-D-aspartate and gamma aminobutyric acid-A receptors. Ann Neurol 1994;35:229-234.

199. Ordia JI, Fischer E, Adamski E, Spatz EL. Chronic intrathecal delivery of baclofen by a programmable pump for the treatment of severe spasticity. J Neurosurg 1996;85:452-457.

200. Dejgard A, Petersen P, Kastrup J. Mexiletine for treatment of chronic painful diabetic neuropathy. Lancet 1:1988;9-11.

201. Lindstrom P, Lindblom U. The analgesic effect of tocainide in trigeminal neuralgia. Pain 1987;28:45-50.

202. Bruera E, Chadwick S, Brenneis C. Methylphenidate associated with narcotics for the treatment of cancer pain. Cancer Treat Rep 1987;71:120.

203. Forrest WH Jr, Brown BM Jr, Brown CR. Dextroamphetamine with morphine for the treatment of postoperative pain. N Engl J Med 1977;13:712-715.

204. Shell H. Adrenal corticosteroid therapy in far-advanced cancer. Geriatrics 1972;27:131-141.

205. Bruera E, Roca E, Cedaro L, et al. Action of oral methylprednisolone in terminal cancer patients: a prospective randomized double-blind study. Cancer Treat Rep 1985;69:751-754.

206. Mercadante S, Lodi F, Sapio M, et al. Long-term ketamine subcutaneous continuous infusion in neuropathic cancer pain. J Pain Symptom Mgmt 1995;10:564-567.

207. Yang CY, Wong CS, Chang JY, Ho ST. Intrathecal ketamine reduces morphine requirements in patients with terminal cancer pain. Can J Anaesth 1996;43:379-383.

208. Eisenach JC, DuPen S, Dubois M, et al. Epidural clonidine analgesia for intractable cancer pain. Pain 1995;61:391-399.

209. Beaver WT. A comparison of the analgesic effects of methotrimeprazine and morphine in patients with cancer. Clin Pharmacol Ther 1966;7:436-446.

210. Lasagna RG, DeKornfeldt TJ. Methotrimeprazine: a new phenothiazine derivative with analgesic properties. JAMA 1961;178:887-890.

211. Oliver DJ. The use of methotrimeprazine in terminal care. Br J Clin Pract 1979;39:339-340.

212. Judkins KC, Harmer M. Haloperidol as an adjunct analgesic in the management of postoperative pain. Anaesthesia 1982;37:1118-1120.

213. Hanks GW, Thomas PJ, Trueman T, Weeks E. The myth of haloperidol potentiation. Lancet 1983;2:523-524.

214. Patt RB, Reddy S. The benzodiazepines as adjuvant analgesics. J Pain Symptom Mgmt 1994;9:510-514.

215. Nahata MC, Miser AW, Miser JS, et al. Analgesic plasma concentrations of morphine in children with terminal malignancy receiving a continuous subcutaneous infusion of morphine sulfate to control severe pain. Pain 1987;18:109-114.

216. Bruera E, Ripamonti C. Adjuvants to opioid analgesics. In: Patt RB, ed. Cancer pain. Philadelphia: Lippincott, 1993;185-194.

217. Portenoy R. Continuous intravenous infusion of opioid drugs. Med Clin North Am 1987;71:233-241.

218. Portenoy RK, Moulin DE, Rogers A, et al. Intravenous infusions of opioids in cancer pain: clinical review and guidelines for use. Cancer Treat Rep 1986;70:575-581.

219. Mount BM. Psychological and social aspects of cancer pain. In: Wall PD, Melzack R, eds. Textbook of pain. Edinburgh: Churchill Livingstone, 1984;460-471.

220. Syrjala KL, Donaldson GW, Davis MW, et al. Relaxation and imagery and cognitive-behavioral training reduce pain during cancer treatment: a controlled clinical trial. Pain 1995;63:189-198.

221. Cousins MJ, Mather LE. Intrathecal and epidural administration of opioids. Anesthesiology 1984;61:276-310.

222. Yaksh TL. Spinal opiates: a review of their effect on spinal function with an emphasis on pain processing. Acta Anaesthesiol Scand 1987;31(Suppl 85):25.

223. Smith DE. Spinal opioids in the home and hospice setting. J Pain Symptom Mgmt 1990;5:175.

224. Boersma FP, Buist AB, Thie J. Epidural pain treatment in the northern Netherlands: organizational and treatment aspects. Acta Anaesthesiol Belg 1987;38:213.

225. Crawford ME, Andersen HB, Augustenborg G, et al. Pain treatment on outpatient basis using extradural opiates: Danish multicenter study comprising 105 patients. Pain 1983;16:41.

226. Snyder SH. Opiate receptors in the brain. N Engl J Med 1977;296:266-271.

227. Patt RB, Jain S. Long term management of a patient with perineal pain secondary to rectal cancer. J Pain Symptom Mgmt 1990;5:127-128.

228. Roquefeuil B, Benezech J, Blanchet P, et al. Intraventricular administration of morphine in patients with neoplastic intractable pain. Surg Neurol 1984;21:155-158.

229. DuPen SL, Peterson DG, Bogosian AC, et al. A new permanent exteriorized epidural catheter for narcotic self-administration to control cancer pain. Cancer 1987;59:986.

230. Waldman S, Leak D, Kennedy D, Patt RB. Intraspinal opioid analgesia in the management of oncologic pain. In: Patt RB, ed. Cancer pain. Philadelphia: Lippincott, 1993;285-328.

231. Du Pen S, Kharasch ED, Williams A, et al. Chronic epidural bupivacaine-opioid infusion in intractable cancer pain. Pain 1992;49:293-300.

232. Coombs DW, Saunders RL, Harbaugh R, et al. Relief of continuous chronic pain by intraspinal narcotics infusion via an implanted reservoir. JAMA 1983;250:2336.

233. Penn RD, Paice JA, Gottschalk W, et al. Cancer pain relief using chronic morphine infusions: early experience with a programmable implanted drug pump. J Neurosurg 1984;61:302.

234. Bedder MD, Burchiel KJ, Larson A. Cost analysis of two implantable narcotic delivery systems. J Pain Symptom Mgmt 1991;6:368.

235. Hassenbusch SJ, Bedder M, Patt RB, Bell GK. Current status of intrathecal therapy for nonmalignant pain management: clinical realities and economic unknowns. J Pain Symptom Mgmt 1997;14:S36-S48.

236. Bonica JJ. Management of pain. Philadelphia: Lea & Febiger, 1953.

237. Cousins MJ. Anesthetic approaches in cancer pain. Adv Pain Res Ther 16;1990:249-273.

238. Raj PP, Ramamurthy S. Differential nerve bock studies. In: Raj PP, ed. Practical management of pain. Chicago: Year Book, 1986;173-177.

239. Abram SE. The role of nonneurolytic nerve blocks in the management of cancer pain. In: Abram SE, ed. Cancer pain. Amsterdam: Kluwer, 1989;67-75.

240. Porges P. Local anesthetics in the treatment of cancer pain. Recent Results Cancer Res 1984;89:127.

241. Travel JG, Simons DG. Myofascial pain and dysfunction: the trigger point manual. Baltimore: Williams & Wilkins, 1983.

242. Payne R. Neuropathic pain syndromes, with special reference to causalgia and reflex sympathetic dystrophy. Clin J Pain 1986;2:59-73.

243. Gerbershagen HU. Blocks with local anesthetics in the treatment of cancer pain. In: Bonica JJ, Ventafridda V, eds. Adv Pain Res Ther, vol 2. New York: Raven Press, 1979;311-323.

244. Warfield CA, Crews DA. Use of stellate ganglion blocks in the treatment of intractable limb pain in lung cancer. Clin J Pain 1987;3:13.

245. Patt RB, Manfredi P. Cancer pain emergencies. In: Parris WCV, ed. Principles and practice of cancer pain management. Newton, MA: Butterworths;4-77.

246. Swerdlow M. History of neurolytic block. In: Racz GB, ed. Techniques of neurolysis. Boston: Kluwer, 1989;1.

247. Evans PJD. Cryoanalgesia. Anaesthesia 1981;36:1003-1013.

248. Hay RC. Subarachnoid alcohol block in the control of intractable pain: report of results in 252 patients. Anesth Analg 1962;41:12-16.

249. Perese DM. Subarachnoid alcohol block in the management of pain of malignant disease. Arch Surg 1958;76:347-354.

250. Papo I, Visca A. Phenol subarachnoid rhizotomy for the treatment of cancer pain: a personal account of 290 cases. In: Bonica JJ, Ventafridda V, eds. Adv Pain Res Ther, vol 2. New York: Raven Press, 1979;339-346.

251. Lipton S. Neurolysis: pharmacology and drug selection. In: Patt RB, ed. Cancer pain. Philadelphia: Lippincott, 1993;343-358.

252. Patt RB. Peripheral neurolysis and the management of cancer pain. Pain Digest 1992;2:30-42.

253. Doyle D. Nerve blocks in advanced cancer. Practitioner 1982;226:539-544.

254. Madrid JL, Bonica JJ. Cranial nerve blocks. In: Bonica JJ, Ventafridda V, ed. Adv Pain Res Ther, vol 2. New York: Raven Press, 1979;463-468.

255. Waldman SD, Feldstein GS, Allen ML, et al. Cervical epidural implantable narcotic delivery systems in the management of upper body pain. Anesth Analg 1987;66:780-782.

256. Lobato RD, Madrid JL, Fatela LV, et al. Intraventricular morphine for intractable cancer pain: rationale, methods, clinical results. Acta Anaesthesiol Scand 1987;31:68-74.

257. Appelgren L, Janson M, Nitescu P, Curelaru I. Continuous intracisternal and high cervical intrathecal bupivacaine analgesia in refractory head and neck pain. Anesthesiology 1996;84:256-72.

258. Robertson DH. Transsacral neurolytic nerve block: an alternative approach to intractable perineal pain. Br J Anaesth 1983;55:873-875.

259. Mullin V. Brachial plexus block with phenol for painful arm associated with Pancoast's syndrome. Anesthesiology 1980;53:431-433.

260. Kaplan R, Aurellano Z, Pfisterer W. Phenol brachial plexus block for upper extremity cancer pain. Reg Anesth 13:58-61.

261. Peyton Wt, Semansky EJ, Baker AB. Subarachnoid injection of alcohol for relief of intractable pain with discussion of cord changes found at autopsy. Am J Cancer 1937;30:709.

262. Smith MC. Histological findings following intrathecal injections of phenol solutions for relief of pain. Br J Anaesth 1963;36:387-406.

263. Swerdlow M. Intrathecal neurolysis. Anaesthesia 1978;33:733-740.

264. Katz J. The current role of neurolytic agents. Adv Neurol 1974;4:471-476.

265. Swerdlow M. Subarachnoid and extradural blocks. Adv Pain Res Ther 2;1979:325-337.

266. Hay RC. Subarachnoid alcohol block in the control of intractable pain. Anesth Analg 1962;41:12-16.

267. Stovner J, Endresen R. Intrathecal phenol for cancer pain. Acta Anaesthesiol Scand 1972;16:17-21.

268. Holland AJC, Youssef M. A complication of subarachnoid phenol blockade. Anaesthesia 1979;34:260-262.

269. Dobrogowski J, Marian K. Epidural neurolytic block in cancer patients. In: Erdmann W, Oyama T, Pernack MJ, eds. Pain Clinic I. Utrecht: VNU Science, 1985;51-54.

270. Racz GB, Heavner J, Haynsworth R. Repeat epidural phenol injections in chronic pain and spasticity. In: Lipton S, Miles J, eds. Persistent pain, vol 5. Orlando: Grune & Stratton, 1985;157-179.

271. Thompson GE, Moore DC, Bridenbaugh PO, et al. Abdominal pain and celiac plexus nerve block. Anesth Analg 1977;56:1-5.

272. Brown BL, Bulley CK, Quiel EC. Neurolytic celiac plexus block for pancreatic cancer pain. Anesth Analg 1987;66:869-873.

273. Jain S. The role of celiac plexus block in intractable upper abdominal pain. In: Racz GB, ed. Techniques of neurolysis. Boston: Kluwer, 1989;161.

274. Flanigan DP, Kraft R. Continuing experience with palliative chemical splanchnicectomy. Arch Surg 1978;113:509-511.

275. Ischia S, Luzzani A, Ischia A, et al. A new approach to the neurolytic block of the coeliac plexus: the transaortic technique. Pain 1983;16:333-341.

276. Matamala AM, Lopez FV, Martinez LI. Percutaneous approach to the celiac plexus using CT guidance. Pain 1988;34:285-288.

277. Sharfman WH, Walsh TD. Has the efficacy of celiac plexus block been demonstrated in pancreatic cancer pain? Pain 1990;41:267-271.

278. Jones J, Gough D. Coeliac plexus block with alcohol for relief of upper abdominal pain due to cancer. Ann R Coll Surg Engl 1977;59:46-49.

279. Racz GB, Holubec JT. Stellate ganglion phenol neurolysis. In: Racz GB, ed. Techniques of neurolysis. Boston: Kluwer, 1989;133-143.

280. Plancarte R, Amescua C, Patt R, et al. Superior hypogastric plexus block for pelvic cancer pain. Anesthesiology 1990;73:236.

281. Plancarte R, Amescua C, Patt RB. Presacral blockade of the ganglion impar (ganglion of Walther). Anesthesiology 1990;73:A751.

282. De Leon-Casasola OA, Kent E, Lema MJ. Neurolytic superior hypogastric plexus block for chronic pelvic pain associated with cancer. Pain 1993;54:145-151.

283. Ventafridda V, Sganzerla EP, Fochi C, et al. Transcutaneous nerve stimulation in cancer pain. Adv Pain Res Ther 1979;2:509-515.

284. Meglio M, Cioni B. Personal experience with spinal cord stimulation in chronic pain management. Appl Neurophysiol 1982;45:195-200.

285. Young RF, Brechner T. Electrical stimulation of the brain for relief of intractable pain due to cancer. Cancer 1986;57:1266-1272.

286. Lahuerta J, Lipton S, Miles J, et al. Update on percutaneous cervical cordotomy and pituitary alcohol neuroadenolysis: an audit of our recent results and complications. In: Lipton S, Miles J, eds. Persistent pain, vol 5. New York: Grune & Stratton, 1985;197-223.

287. Watling CJ, Payne R, Allen RR, Hassenbusch S. Commissural myelotomy for intractable cancer pain: report of two cases. Clin J Pain 1996;12:151-156.

288. Lipton S. Percutaneous cordotomy. In: Wall PD, Melzack R, eds. Textbook of pain. New York: Churchill Livingstone, 1984;632-638.

289. Smith JL. Care of people who are dying: the hospice approach. In: Patt R, ed. Cancer pain management: a multidisciplinary approach. Philadelphia: Lippincott, 1993;543-52.

290. Doyle D. Education and training in palliative care. J Palliat Care 1987;2:5.

CHAPTER 26

Breakthrough Pain

Richard B. Patt and Neil Ellison

INTRODUCTION

The temporal aspects of pain and the presence and nature of breakthrough pain are fundamental to the clinician's understanding and effective management of cancer pain. While the existence and importance of these phenomena are well accepted by clinicians, observations about their nature are predominantly empirical (1). The clinical importance of the temporal features of pain is evidenced by the development of an entire new lexicon surrounding associated concepts. Because the clinical focus on these largely empiric phenomena is new, the terms used to refer to the clinically relevant temporal features of pain, although in common use, remain imprecisely and in some cases vaguely defined (1).

TEMPORAL CHARACTERISTICS OF PAIN

The temporal characteristics of pain can be described as consisting of (*a*) the presence or absence of pain at a given moment, (*b*) its intensity or severity at a given moment, and (*c*) its tempo, the rate and pattern of change in intensity and severity over short and long intervals. Both acute and chronic pain consists of series of related events that occur over time, and thus pain can be broadly classified as constant or intermittent. Chronic pain is usually a relatively constant phenomenon punctuated by intermittent exacerbations. The constant, unrelenting component of chronic pain has been variously called baseline or basal pain. Superimposed intermittent exacerbations of pain (changes in tempo from baseline), which have come to be called breakthrough pain, have recently become a focus of intense clinical interest.

The International Association for the Study of Pain (IASP), long active in establishing a taxonomy for painful disorders, has suggested an alphanumeric coding system aimed at assisting clinicians and investigators in comprehensively classifying painful disorders (2, 3). Arguably unwieldy,

it recommends classification along the following five axes: region, system, temporal characteristics, intensity, and causation. While the temporal classifications suggested by the IASP may have important implications for researchers by virtue of their breadth, their implications for the clinician managing cancer pain and pertinence to the concept of breakthrough pain remain uncertain.

BREAKTHROUGH PAIN

Breakthrough Pain versus Uncontrolled Pain

Breakthrough pain implies a component of baseline or basal pain that is under relatively stable control. On this basis breakthrough pain should be distinguished from poorly controlled baseline pain, the pain emergency, and so-called crescendo pain.

Poorly controlled baseline pain is characterized by relatively consistent high levels of pain interrupted by erratic fluctuations in severity. Exacerbations of pain observed in these settings are best considered as being distinct from breakthrough pain, which by current definitions occurs in the context of basal pain that is at least moderately well controlled. This is an important distinction, since poorly controlled baseline pain is best managed by adjusting the dose and/or schedule of regularly administered analgesics, rather than a strategy that targets the exacerbations.

Although ill-defined, the pain emergency is best viewed as an acute condition of mounting pain that occurs either de novo or in the context of a history of well-controlled pain (4, 5). Breakthrough pain differs from the pain emergency in that its cause is usually known, so symptomatic treatment is usually warranted. A pain emergency mandates a diagnostic evaluation aimed at identifying the cause of pain, which if correctable may suggest an appropriate treatment strategy that may limit morbidity and even mortality. Examples of pain emergencies include pain due to bowel obstruction, pathological fractures, and epidural spinal cord compression. Crescendo pain (6) is probably best regarded as a subacute pain emergency characterized by progressive, unrelenting increases in pain severity. It is usually described in the context of a history of stable pain due to cancer, most often in dying patients. Crescendo pain implies the need to treat mounting basal pain, usually with rapidly titrated doses of opioids administered parentally by continuous infusion and supplemental nurse- or patient-administered boluses. In contrast to breakthrough pain, treatment is directed at the entirety of the pain experience rather than just exacerbations. Crescendo pain in a dying patient is associated with special management considerations that may include the use of various alternative routes, anesthetic or neurosurgical interventions, and even terminal sedation (6).

Classification

The concept of breakthrough pain is relatively new, and only recently have there been efforts to define and characterize breakthrough pain in the medical literature. Thus, current definitions and ideas about what constitute the salient features of breakthrough pain are still developing. Breakthrough pain can be characterized in several ways. The most pertinent feature may be the nature of any precipitating factors, since additional nomenclature and therapeutic strategies have arisen around these phenomena. Breakthrough pain that occurs with a relatively consistent temporal relation to specific activities has come to be called incident pain. Breakthrough pain that occurs at predictable intervals just prior to the next scheduled dose of an analgesic drug is end-of-dose failure. Finally, breakthrough pain that appears to be idiosyncratic and unrelated to either activity or scheduled doses of analgesics is typically called either spontaneous or idiopathic breakthrough pain or simply breakthrough pain. This classification is clinically important because treatment recommendations for breakthrough pain depend on whether it has features of incident pain or end-of-dose failure or is spontaneous or idiopathic. Although there is little apparent support in the literature, at least one recognized cancer pain authority advocates a different classification that regards breakthrough pain as a subset of incident pain (1).

Other features of breakthrough pain, while clinically important, remain even less well characterized. Portenoy and Hagen (7) suggest that the evaluation of breakthrough pain should take into account its (a) relation to a fixed opioid dose, (b) temporal characteristics, (c) precipitating events, (d) predictability, (e) pathophysiology, and (f) causation. These phenomena are explored more fully later in the chapter.

Relation to Fixed Opioid Dose

Cancer pain is typically composed of variable components of basal and breakthrough pain, with the main exception being acute procedure-related pain (e.g., lumbar puncture, bone marrow biopsy, venipuncture), which has been recognized to be particularly important in children (8). Most guidelines recommend that the treatment of chronic cancer pain that is sufficiently severe to warrant the use of opioid analgesics be undertaken with the concomitant use of two pharmacokinetically distinct preparations of opioid analgesics. Typically, once pain is stabilized, a relatively long-acting agent (e.g., oral controlled-release [CR] morphine, oral CR oxycodone, transdermal fentanyl) is prescribed on a time-contingent or around-the-clock basis to counter basal pain, and an agent with a relatively rapid onset of action and short duration of effect (e.g., immediate release [IR] morphine, oral hydromorphone, oxycodone) is prescribed on a symptom-contingent basis or as needed. In this context, doses of the short-acting opioid are called rescue doses or escape doses, and their frequency is used to gauge the need to adjust the dose of basal analgesic.

When treatment includes a basal analgesic administered around the clock, breakthrough pain may or may not be temporally related to the fixed opioid analgesic regimen. Breakthrough pain that is related to the around-the-clock dosing regimen usually occurs with greater frequency near the end of a dosing interval (end-of-dose failure), in which case it typically has a more gradual onset and generally lasts longer than pain that is unrelated to the dosing interval of opioids (9). The incidence and severity of end-of-dose failure usually correlates with the adequacy of around-the-clock dosing regimens prescribed for the management of basal pain. End-of-dose failure is typically more prevalent and severe either when basal (around-the-clock) analgesics are prescribed in inadequate doses or when the interval between administrations is excessive. In contrast to other types of breakthrough pain, the management of end-of-dose failure is best approached by modifying the dose or schedule of long-acting around-the-clock opioids (9).

Temporal Characteristics

Breakthrough pain can be characterized by temporal features that include its rapidity of onset, duration, and frequency. The onset of breakthrough pain has been classified as sudden, or paroxysmal, and gradual. Sudden or paroxysmal episodes have been arbitrarily defined as those that arise within less than 3 minutes, while gradual onset breakthrough pain establishes itself more slowly. The duration of breakthrough pain has been characterized arbitrarily as brief (seconds to 20 minutes) or sustained (longer than 20 minutes). When such pain occurs very frequently and/or for sustained intervals, it is probably best regarded as a recrudescence of basal pain rather than as breakthrough pain. Preliminary studies characterize breakthrough pain as a highly heterogenous phenomenon, and thus its frequency appears to be highly variable.

Precipitating Events

As noted, breakthrough pain may be spontaneous or may be precipitated by a recognizable event (incident pain or precipitated pain). Precipitated pain may be volitional (induced by an action subject to some control, such as movement, swallowing, or coughing) or nonvolitional (caused by events that are subject to less control, such as flatulence, myoclonic jerking, or anxiety). Breakthrough pain associated with volitional activity is commonly called incident pain.

Predictability

The concepts of predictable pain and precipitated pain are closely related to that of incident pain, although these terms are not synonymous. Predictable pain refers to the notion that especially with coaching, many patients can correlate the occurrence of breakthrough pain with precipitating events. While precipitated pains are usually predictable, not all precipitated pains are predictable, as for example with pain related to involuntary movement in patients with myoclonus. Seemingly spontaneous pain is in some cases actually somewhat predictable, especially when associated with environmental cues. On appreciating such cues (e.g., stress) patients can often can often be taught to reliably predict episodes of breakthrough pain (9).

Pathophysiology

A pathophysiological classification of pain that distinguishes among somatic nociceptive, visceral nociceptive, and neuropathic pain has become widely accepted (10) and is clinically relevant to breakthrough pain. Pain of somatic nociceptive origin emanates from injury to nonneurological, nonvisceral connective tissues, such as muscle, bone, skin, ligaments, and joints, and is often described by patients in familiar terms that include sharp, stabbing, dull, and achy. Prototypical examples of somatic nociceptive pain include soft-tissue trauma, postoperative pain, bone metastases, and pathological fractures. Pain of visceral nociceptive origin originates from injury to hollow or solid viscera, is often diffuse, and is characteristically described as vague, dull, dragging, or pressurelike. Examples include labor pain, bowel obstruction, and pain due to liver capsule distention. Somatic and visceral nociceptive pain originate with activation of peripheral A delta and C nociceptors by noxious mechanical, chemical, or thermal stimuli. Impulses are conveyed along classically described neuroanatomical pain-conducting pathways that include the dorsal horn of the spinal cord, the contralateral spinothalamic tract, the thalamus, and subcortical and cortical structures and are modulated by both biochemical and cognitive mechanisms. Somatic and visceral nociceptive pain typically responds robustly and in a relatively linear manner to treatment with opioid analgesics.

Neuropathic pain follows obvious or subclinical injury to elements of the peripheral or central nervous system and is often but not invariably associated with abnormal neurological findings ranging from reproducible sensory or motor deficits to subjectively abnormal dysesthetic (from the Latin, "bad feeling") sensations. The latter may include paresthesias, hyperalgesia, hyperpathia, allodynia, and hyperesthesia (3, 11, 12). In contrast to nociceptive pain, neuropathic pain is often described as a bizarre or foreign experience for which there is no familiar frame of reference. It is typically described in terms that

include tingling, numb, burning, or shocklike (lancinating). Prototypical conditions associated with neuropathic pain include diabetic neuropathy, herpes zoster, brachial plexopathy, spinal cord injury, peripheral nerve compression, and phantom limb pain. The mechanisms that underlie the development and maintenance of neuropathic pain are less clearly understood than those that contribute to nociceptive pain. They include the propagation of abnormal sensations to the central nervous system, plasticity, and windup phenomena. Neuropathic pain may be less opioid responsive than nociceptive pain, and in contrast to nociceptive syndromes often responds favorably to treatment with adjuvant analgesics (e.g., antidepressants, anticonvulsants, oral local anesthetics) (13). Neuropathic pain has been further categorized as central pain or deafferentation pain, depending on whether the causative injury involves the peripheral or central nervous system, respectively, although this distinction has fallen out of favor because of the perception that it has few practical therapeutic implications (12).

Causation

The causation of breakthrough pain in cancer patients may be related directly to the tumor (e.g., bone metastasis, nerve compression), cancer treatment (14) (e.g., postmastectomy pain, osteoradionecrosis, polyneuropathy after chemotherapy) or premorbid chronic disorders (e.g., discogenic low back pain).

Prevalence

Since breakthrough pain has only been recently recognized as a distinct clinical entity, few studies describe it in detail, and its prevalence is thus difficult to ascertain, although numerous researchers refer to the number of patients with breakthrough pain as an incidental finding in the course of studies evaluating other aspects of cancer pain (15–17). Portenoy and Hagen (7) are the only investigators who have formally conducted a prospective evaluation of breakthrough pain in cancer patients. Breakthrough pain has not been formally evaluated in populations of patients with pain of nononcological causes.

Table 26.1 summarizes selected available data on the incidence of breakthrough pain and its subtypes. Due to the absence of acceptance for a formal, detailed definition of breakthrough pain, the use of different methodologies (e.g., inclusion criteria, treatment algorithms, (Fig 26.1) frequency of assessment) and diversity among study populations, the data reported here provide only a rough estimate of prevalence. This paucity of data and its diversity emphasize the critical need for more extensive studies of breakthrough pain that use standard methodologies.

Studies Explicitly Evaluating Breakthrough Pain Phenomena

To date, studies conducted by Portenoy and Hagen (7) and Bruera et al. (18) provide the best estimates of prevalence, since

Table 26.1.　Prevalence of Breakthrough Pain in Patients with Cancer

Author	Population	No. of Pts. Evaluated	No. of Pts With Breathrough Pain
Hayes et al (16)	Adult cancer patients with stable chronic severe pain who were receiving either controlled or IR hydromorphone	48	40 (84%)
Mercadante et al (68)	Patients with advanced lung cancer	52	12 (24%)
Ashby et al (69)	Adult inpatients with advanced cancer pain	20	19 (95%)
Bruera et al (70)	Patients with advanced cancer	118	23 (19%)
Mercandante et al (71)	End stage cancer patients with severe pain who were not regularly treated by opioids	98	30 (31%)
Portenoy and Hagen (59)	Adult cancer inpatients referred to a pain service	70	41 (63%)
Kerr et al	Patients with poorly controlled cancer pain	18	15 (83%)

they were specifically intended to characterize breakthrough pain and because both prospectively evaluated consecutive referrals to a cancer pain consultation service. Portenoy and Hagen (7) reported a 63% overall incidence of breakthrough pain in their study population. Bruera's report, which limited itself to the evaluation of incident pain, revealed a much lower incidence, 19%. Even when Portenoy's data are adjusted to exclude breakthrough pain of other origins, the incidence of (incident-type) breakthrough pain varied nearly threefold (55% versus 19%). The most obvious probable explanations for this large disparity relate to differences in (a) the characteristics of the populations studied, (b) eligibility criteria, and (c) operational definitions for pain phenomena. Portenoy and Hagen screened all adult inpatients referred to a cancer pain consultation service over a 3-month period, while Bruera et al. considered all patients admitted to a palliative care unit over a period of 9 months. Patients recruited from a palliative care unit differ from patients hospitalized at a comprehensive cancer center in important ways (19). A particularly pertinent difference as regards incident pain, for example, relates to the likelihood that patients in a palliative care unit are less ambulatory and are thus less likely to have pain with movement. Another explanation for the lower incidence observed by Bruera's group was their use of "well-controlled" pain as an entry criterion in contrast to Portenoy's use of "baseline pain of moderate intensity or less," a feature that stipulates less stable pain control, a probable predictor of breakthrough pain. In addition, their use of different definitions for incident pain should have contributed to differences in outcome. The variation of reported prevalence may also be attributable to other more obscure characteristics of the study population, since neither group provided a thorough description of demographics and other patient characteristics (e.g., activity levels, ambulatory status, life expectancy, and

performance status). Finally, both studies evaluated relatively small numbers of patients, presumably with a wide range of types of cancer pain, and it is probable that patients with different primary malignancies, patterns of disease spread, and underlying mechanisms of pain experience different patterns or types of breakthrough pain. Mercadante (20) drew attention to these issues in a commentary on the Portenoy study and further emphasized the need for more controlled studies of breakthrough pain phenomena. He argued that a definition of breakthrough pain that stipulates baseline pain of moderate or less intensity but imposes no limits on the frequency or duration of breakthrough pain episodes is contradictory, since very frequent or prolonged exacerbations detract from baseline control. In addition, he argued specifically the need to control for confounding variables, including ambulatory and performance status, extent of disease, and survival prognosis.

Other Studies

Reporting on 184 evaluable consecutive consultations for cancer pain, Banning et al. (22) noted that 172 patients (93%) had exacerbations of pain with movement (incident pain) and that 124 (67%) reported that pain interrupted their sleep. After 1 to 2 weeks of treatment, movement-related pain had resolved in about a third of the 131 affected patients available for reevaluation. The severity of incident pain was rated as mild, moderate, and severe by 27 (21%), 20 (15%), and 36 (27%) of the 131 reevaluated patients, respectively.

Mercadante et al. (23) evaluated 98 opioid-naive outpatients with severe or intolerable cancer pain in the course of a trial intended to determine the influence of pain mechanism, analgesic responsiveness, and "incidental pain" on the outcome of treatment with the World Health Organization (WHO) ladder methodology. Although the investigators' criteria for incident pain were not specifically defined, patients appeared to have been stratified according to the presence of a prominent component of breakthrough pain. Overall, 30% of their 98 patients had breakthrough pain: about half of the 16 patients who responded favorably to a trial of NSAIDs had incident pain, as opposed to only 12% of the 58 patients whom NSAIDs failed and who responded favorably to a trial of opioids and as opposed to two thirds of the remaining 24 patients whom trials of opioids and NSAIDs had failed.

In the course of prospectively evaluating the mechanistic aspects of pain in hospice inpatients, Ashby et al. (19) recorded the incidence and severity of "breakthrough pain events" in 20 patients over a mean of 21 days. Breakthrough pain was observed in all but one patient, at a mean frequency of 0.37 events per day (range 0 to 2.5 events per day).

In a pilot study of oral transmucosal fentanyl citrate (OTFC) for the management of breakthrough pain, Fine et al. (24) evaluated 10 inpatients with advanced cancer over a 2-day interval. Although patients' baseline regimen of opioids was not reported, their median visual analog pain intensity was 60 of 100. Patients experienced a mean of 2.1 episodes of breakthrough pain per day, all between 7:00 AM and 7:00 PM.

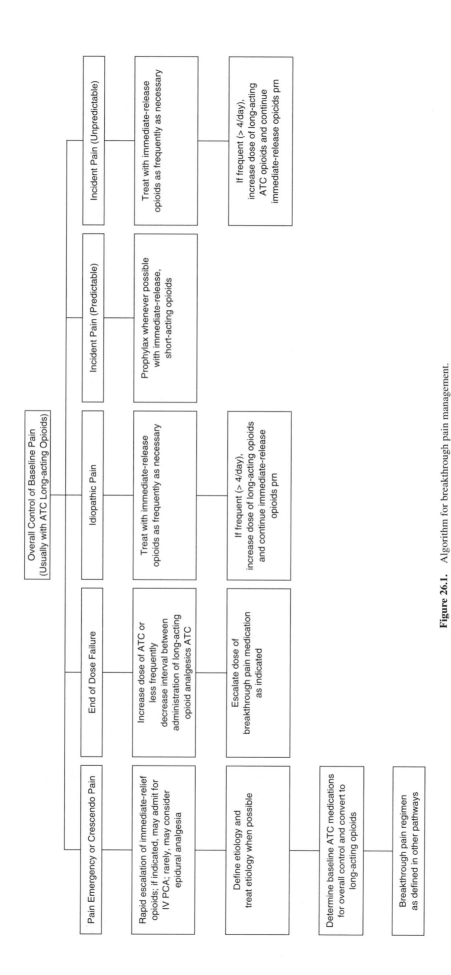

Figure 26.1. Algorithm for breakthrough pain management.

Detailed Results of Studies Explicitly Evaluating Breakthrough Pain Phenomena

To date, Portenoy and Hagen's (7) study most carefully characterizes breakthrough pain. (Table 26.2). They evaluated all adult inpatients referred to a pain service at a comprehensive cancer center over a 3-month period. Of this cadre of 90 patients, 70 met their criteria for stable dosing (dose increases of no more than 20% per day for 48 hours), of whom 63 met their criteria for well-controlled pain (pain of moderate intensity or less). Of these 63 patients with stable dosing and well-controlled pain, 41 (63%) met the study's criteria for the presence of breakthrough pain (temporary flares of severe or excruciating pain) and were surveyed regarding the nature of the breakthrough pain they had had over the prior 24 hours.

Some 55% of pain episodes met criteria for incident pain, and 29% met criteria for end-of-dose failure. End-of-dose failure and incident pain (mixed breakthrough pain) were concomitantly present in 43% of pain episodes, and 45% of episodes were idiopathic. Three quarters of episodes appeared to be directly related to tumor activity, with most of the remainder presumed to be due to antitumor therapy. Breakthrough pain appeared to be mediated by a variety of underlying mechanisms, and almost all episodes occurred in the same location as patients' baseline pain. The median number of breakthrough pains over a 24-hour period was 4 (range 1 to 3600 pains), and about one fourth of patients identified more than one distinct type of breakthrough pain. Breakthrough pain arose rapidly (less than 3 minutes) in 43% of patients and more gradually (more than 3 minutes) in the remainder. The median duration of breakthrough pain was 30 minutes, and 41% of episodes were both rapid of onset and brief. Data on duration are presumably influenced by the use of rescue doses; the 30-minute median duration observed is consistent with the usual latency to effect of standard analgesics.

Bruera et al. (18) reported their observations on the incidence and nature of incident pain in the context of an open trial of the use of methylphenidate to counter opioid-mediated sedation. In contrast to Portenoy and Hagen's study (7), this report's scope was limited to the subset of patients with incident-type breakthrough pain, and further, presumably since its focus was evaluating a therapeutic intervention, it provided fewer details on pain characteristics. Bruera's group screened 118 consecutive admissions to an inpatient palliative care unit, all of whom had advanced cancer and pain. They identified 23 patients (19%) with "severe incident pain," of whom 14 were ultimately evaluable. The authors defined incident pain as spontaneous or provoked "severe" acute exacerbations of pain occurring against a background of "good" opioid-mediated pain control. All patients were receiving oral or subcutaneous morphine or hydromorphone in fixed doses administered around the clock. Incident pain appeared to be due to bone metastases in 12 of 14 patients (86%) and was presumed to be related to chest wall invasion and inguinal adenopathy in the remaining 2 patients. Movement appeared to be respon-

Table 26.2. Characteristics of 51 Breakthrough Pain Episodes in 41 Hospitalized Cancer Patients*

Presumed (General) Etiology	
Related to neoplasm	39 (75%)
Related to treatment	10 (20%)
Unrelated to neoplasm or treatment	2 (4%)
Presumed Mechanism	
Somatic	17 (33%
Visceral	10 (20%)
Neuropathic	14 (27%)
Mixed	10 (20%)
Location	
Site Same as Baseline Pain	49 (96%)
Site Distinct From Baseline Pain	2 (4%)
Precipitants	
No precipitant (spontaneous)	23 (45%)
Precipitated (incident) Pain	28 (55%0
Volitional	22 (43%)
Nonvolitional	6 (12%)
Relation to Fixed Dose Opioid	
End-of-Dose Failure	15 (29%)
No apparent relationship	36 (71%)
Specific Etiology	
End-of-Dose Failure, No Precipitant	6 (12%)
Precipitant, No End-of-Dose Failure	9 (18%)
End-of-Dose Failure + Precipitant	22 (43%)
Idiopathic	14 (27%)
Onset and Duration	
"Paroxysmal" onset (< 3 minutes)	22(43 %)
"Gradual" onset (< 3 minutes)	29 (47%)
Duration less than 20 minutes	21 (41%)
Median duration	30 minutes
Range of duration	1–240 minutes
Paroxysmal onset + Brief Duration	21 (41%)
Number of Episodes per 24 Hours	
Median	4 episodes/24 hr
Range	1–3600 /24 hr
1-3 episodes/24 hr	15 patients (37%)
4-6 episodes/24 hr	14 patients (34%)
7-10 episodes/24 hr	7 patients (17%)
> 10 episodes/24 hr	5 (12%)
Maximum episodes	1 per minutes (with cough)
Number of Distinct Breakthrough Pains	
1 Type of Breakthrough Pain	32
2 Distinct Types of Breakthrough Pain	8
3 Distinct Types of Breakthrough Pain	1

*Portenoy RK, Hagen NA. Breakthrough pain: Definition, prevalence and characteristics. Pain 1990;41:273–81

sible for provoking pain in all cases: pain was precipitated by sitting in 2 patients, standing and walking in 2 others, and unspecified movement in the remaining 10 patients (71%).

Results of Studies Serendipitously Evaluating Breakthrough Pain

As noted, numerous cancer pain studies designed to assess various other aspects of cancer pain refer serendipitously to the incidence and management of breakthrough pain. Although such studies cannot be expected to provide as reliable or detailed data as those designed specifically to investigate these phenomena, in virtue of the overall paucity of applicable data, selected results are summarized briefly here.

In addition to its clinical significance, the incidence of breakthrough pain has been adopted by clinical researchers as an indirect reflection of analgesic efficacy, especially in the context of studies that evaluate long-acting or CR formulations of opioids. Although the primary intent of these studies is not to evaluate breakthrough pain, the use of breakthrough pain incidence as a primary outcome measure suggests their data may be meaningful. However, cautious interpretation of their results is warranted, since most do not clearly define breakthrough pain other than as the need for unscheduled doses of opioids. The main limitation of such studies, though, is that by limiting their scope to highly discrete populations, they fail to depict the global phenomenon of breakthrough pain. In the interest of ensuring homogeneity among groups and limiting confounding variables, entry is usually limited to patients with "stable" pain (characteristically defined as fewer than 2 or 3 episodes of breakthrough pain daily), usually as established during a pretest stabilization period.

Several dose equivalency and proportion studies have compared the time-contingent administration of various oral formulations of CR and immediate-release morphine. Their results suggest that patients with well-controlled pain who are treated in closely supervised settings by expert clinicians may experience as few as 0.2 to 0.48 daily episodes of breakthrough pain (15, 25–28).

Studies of other CR opioid preparations administered to populations with stable cancer pain yield similar results. Hays et al. (16) evaluated the twice-daily administration of oral CR hydromorphone versus administration of IR hydromorphone every 4 hours in 48 patients with chronic cancer pain and reported an average of one episode of breakthrough pain per day. In the course of comparing a new formulation of CR morphine suppositories with morphine given subcutaneously every 4 hours to 23 patients with chronic cancer pain taking "stable" doses of analgesics (no more than 3 episodes of breakthrough pain per day), Bruera et al. (29) reported a mean of 1.2 daily episodes of breakthrough pain in both treatment arms.

As would be expected, drug evaluations in medical populations with less stable pain typically reveal higher incidences of breakthrough pain. A study of a new preparation of CR codeine given every 12 hours conducted in 30 patients with chronic nonmalignant pain of at least moderate severity revealed an average of 3.6 episodes of daily breakthrough pain compared with about six daily episodes during placebo plus rescue treatment (30). During the evaluation of transdermal fentanyl in 10 home hospice patients with pain due to advanced metastatic cancer, Herbst and Strause (31) reported that 1 of 10 and 2 of 6 patients had in excess of two episodes of breakthrough pain per day at weeks 2 and 4, respectively, despite adjustments in the transdermal dose. In a double-dummy crossover comparison of intravenous and subcutaneous hydromorphone infusions conducted in 15 hospitalized cancer patients with "stable" but severe pain (732 oral MS equivalents per day) a mean of five rescue doses was used over each of the investigation's 48-hour study intervals, independent of route of administration (17). In a similar study comparing continuous subcutaneous hydromorphone supplemented with either nurse boluses or patient-controlled anesthesia (PCA) boluses, patients with advanced cancer experienced a mean of 1 and 0.36 daily episodes of breakthrough pain, respectively (32).

MANAGEMENT

Although several guidelines address the global management of cancer pain, specific evidence-based guidelines for treating breakthrough pain have not been promulgated. General recommendations for treating breakthrough pain can be found in the literature, but optimal management remains largely empirical (1).

The WHO (33) has recommended a general framework for managing cancer pain based predominantly on pharmacotherapy that has been widely accepted. It employs a primary strategy of matching analgesic potency with pain intensity (NSAIDs for mild pain and various opioids for moderate to severe pain) and secondarily recommends basing drug selection on the presumed mechanisms of pain (NSAIDs and opioids for nociceptive pain and adjuvants for neuropathic pain). Breakthrough pain, however, is not specifically addressed. Guidelines developed more recently by the U.S. government's Agency for Health Care Policy and Research (AHCPR) (34) endorse the principles of the WHO guidelines and go on to recommend the administration of regularly scheduled analgesic doses (i.e., around the clock), as well as additional rescue doses as needed for breakthrough pain. The AHCPR guidelines do not provide specific recommendations for selecting drugs or drug doses to treat breakthrough pain. Researchers have, however, reported on the clinical outcomes of series of patients whose breakthrough pain has been managed with various protocols (Table 26.1). Although expert recommendations have evolved from these experiences, further research of a more focused nature is indicated to establish evidence-based guidelines.

Regimens

Oral and Transdermal Opioids

Reliance on oral (33–35) and transdermal (34) administration of opioids is recommended for the management of chronic cancer pain when possible. These routes of administration are preferred because they promote independence and minimize illness conviction, do not require special nursing and pharmacy care, and are convenient and cost effective. Single-entity pure opioid agonists with relatively short latencies to onset and brief durations of action are typically recommended to treat breakthrough pain in patients whose basal pain is controlled with scheduled doses of long-acting oral or transdermal opioids. Available agents include IR oral morphine, hydromorphone, and oxycodone provided either as tablets or elixir. Of these, IR morphine is most commonly prescribed. Oral morphine is considered the drug of choice for both around-the-clock and rescue analgesia for pain due to cancer because of its short half-life, linear pharmacokinetics, widespread availability, and long history of successful use (36).

Parenteral Opioids

Because of its cost, invasiveness, and increased requirements for nursing and pharmacy interventions, parenteral administration of opioids is typically reserved for specific indications that include compromised gastrointestinal function (e.g., chronic nausea and vomiting, dysphagia, xerostomia, obstruction, malabsorption, coma) and acutely unstable pain. The chronic administration of parenteral opioid analgesics is most commonly undertaken with morphine or hydromorphone. Morphine appears to be used most commonly for the same reasons it is preferred for oral administration. Hydromorphone is usually selected when there is a history of intolerance to morphine or, because it is more soluble than morphine, for high-dose subcutaneous administration. Once reserved for inpatient use, recent experience suggests that fentanyl citrate (37) and even sufentanil (38) are safe and effective alternatives for chronic use as well. Due to ease of administration, the subcutaneous route has emerged as the parenteral route of choice for chronic administration, except when an indwelling intravenous catheter is already present (39).

Constant infusions are usually supplemented with rescue doses administered in response to patient demand (PCA). Due to logistical considerations, constant infusions of an opioid are almost exclusively supplemented with rescue doses of the same agent. Rescue doses are typically expressed as a percentage of the fixed hourly administration rate. Most infusion devices suitable for the administration of analgesics possess a feature that restricts the minimum interval between patient-administered boluses (lock-out interval) that is subject to physician control.

The frequency and amount of parenteral rescue doses provided in clinical practice is contingent on available technology. For example, as a result of the ready availability of high-tech infusion devices in acute hospital settings, recommendations for rescue doses in inpatients typically use very short lock-out intervals, often as brief as 10 or 15 minutes. Simpler, less costly infusion devices are typically used in hospice and home care, which explains recommendations that favor longer intervals between administrations in these settings. These pragmatic considerations are also probably responsible for numerous reports describing the use of continuous parenteral infusions that rely on frequent adjustments of the continuous rate to maintain comfort in lieu of the provision of breakthrough or patient-administered doses.

Reviews of continuous parenteral infusions supplemented by PCA or nurse-administered boluses recommend the provision of rescue doses ranging from 50 to 200% of the hourly

infusion rate at intervals ranging from every 15 minutes to every 2 hours (39–43) (Table 26.1). For example, using rescue doses equal to 25% of the hourly infusion rate, Swanson et al. (44) reported effective pain relief in 95% of 117 ambulatory cancer patients managed with intravenous or subcutaneous PCA opioids. Vanier et al. (45) used rescue doses of subcutaneous hydromorphone equal to the hourly infusion rate provided as often as every 60 minutes.

INCIDENT BREAKTHROUGH PAIN AS A PREDICTOR OF POOR OUTCOME

Recent systematic efforts have been made to prospectively identify pain states, which predict poorer response to pharmacological therapy than would otherwise be expected. This line of inquiry is important to help the clinician prospectively identify patients at risk for treatment failure, allowing for the early mobilization of appropriate interdisciplinary resources. In addition, identifying well-defined problem pain scenarios should allow better integration and comparison of data generated by different investigators and should facilitate the development of clinical practice protocols.

Most authorities agree that breakthrough pain, and in particular incident pain, especially associated with movement, is among the subset of problem pain syndromes. Bruera et al. (46) have demonstrated pilot validity for an alphanumeric staging system, the Edmonton Staging System for Cancer Pain, that is similar to that used to grade the clinicohistological status of tumors (47). The Edmonton system prognosticates the likelihood of treatment failure (Table 26.3). Incident pain is among the seven clinical features of pain predicting that conventional management will be associated with a poor outcome. In a discussion of opioid nonresponsive pain, Hanks and Justins (48) and Hanks (49) likewise distinguish incident (bone) pain as an important (relatively) nonopioid responsive pain syndrome, citing the ineffectiveness of standard breakthrough dose regimens of morphine. In a carefully conducted prospective study of the characteristics of pain in patients with lung cancer, Mercadante et al. (23) distinguished incident pain as the only clinical feature that reliably correlated with treatment failure.

In a separate study, Mercadante et al. (23) endeavored to determine the influence of pain mechanism, responsiveness to various analgesics, and the presence of incidental pain (pain with movement) on the success of pharmacotherapy. His group prospectively evaluated 130 outpatients referred for "severe" or "intolerable" cancer pain who were opioid naive at the time of consultation. The study applied the WHO pharmacological ladder and established a relatively homogeneous study population by limiting its evaluation to those 98 patients who lived for about 2 months (45 to 75 days) after evaluation. The study stratified patients according to a positive or negative response to sequential trials of NSAIDs and opioids, apparent pain mechanism, and the presence or absence of incidental pain. Of these factors, only the presence of incidental pain correlated with treat-

Table 26.3.   Features Purported to Predict the Outcome of Pharmocotherapy

Study	Positive Predictive Factors
Ashby et al, 1992 (69)	Incident (movement-related) breakthrough pain
Bruera et al, 1992 (70)	Incident (movement-related) breakthrough pain, neuropathic pain, tolerance, history of alcohol or drug abuse, psychological distress
Mercadante et al, 1992 (71)	Incident (movement-related) breakthrough pain
Mercadante et al, (68)	Incident (movement-related) breakthrough pain

Study	Factors That Were Not Significantly Predictive
Ashby et al, 1992 (69)	Neuropathic pain
Bruera et al, 1992 (70)	Opioid dose, delirium
Mercadante et al, 1992 (71)	Neuropathic pain
Mercadante et al, 1994 (68)	Neuropathic pain

ment outcome. When findings were controlled to eliminate the influence of analgesic response and pain mechanism, only 50% of patients with incident pain achieved good pain control compared with an 80% incidence of favorable outcome in patients without incident pain.

CLINICAL SIGNIFICANCE OF BREAKTHROUGH PAIN

The assessment and management of breakthrough pain must be considered within the context of the overall pain management strategy, and interventions should be individualized accordingly. Based on its heterogeneous nature, various patterns of breakthrough pain demand different clinical responses. Severe, distressing, or frequent breakthrough pain should be identified and aggressively managed. However, some degree of breakthrough pain is probably inevitable, and when mild or infrequent, such episodes are often well tolerated and manageable.

Whether or not eliminating breakthrough pain is even feasible, the preservation of infrequent, low-level breakthrough pain may in some cases be desirable. To the degree that its frequency and severity guide clinical decisions, breakthrough pain can be regarded as having a teleological purpose. Most important, the frequency and timing of breakthrough pain have come to be relied on as a critical determinant of the need to adjust the dose and timing of regularly scheduled analgesics. A changing pattern of breakthrough pain may indirectly gauge of the adequacy of rehabilitation, as pain often predictably increases with heightened activity. Slowly mounting breakthrough pain may reflect the development of tolerance or indolent tumor progression, while new sites or sudden increases in pain may alert the clinician to the need to consider rapid tumor progression or new metastases.

The management of breakthrough pain and its relation to the dose of around-the-clock analgesic influences not only pain relief but also the incidence and severity of adverse effects. Opioid therapy rarely eliminates pain. The overriding goal of therapy is to achieve the most favorable balance possible between comfort and side effects.

Notwithstanding the need to individualize therapy, the literature has begun to yield evidence for critical thresholds of

pain intensity that are statistically associated with meaningful changes in functional status and quality of life. Large differences in interference with quality of life domains as pain intensity scores move from the mild (1 to 3) to moderate (4 to 6) and severe (7 to 10) ranges have been demonstrated. Unfortunately, the literature provides little support for "ideal" breakthrough pain scenarios, and trials comparing global efficacy, adverse effects, and satisfaction in patients stratified by pain tempo are needed.

CONTEMPORARY MANAGEMENT

Portenoy and Hagen (7) have proposed that the management of breakthrough cancer pain should reflect reliance on four principles: (a) comprehensive assessment, including evaluation of the characteristics, causation, and pathophysiology of pain, along with the relation of the pain to the patient's overall clinical status; (b) consideration of the underlying cause of pain; (c) optimizing the analgesic regimen (e.g., adjustment of the around-the-clock regimen), and (d) the provision of rescue doses based specifically on the nature and type of breakthrough pain that is present.

By elucidating the causes of pain, a comprehensive evaluation may suggest therapeutic interventions, such as chemotherapy, radiotherapy, radionuclides, or surgical excision or stabilization, that may resolve pain or simplify its pharmacological management (50). For example, external beam irradiation or strontium-89 may improve breakthrough pain that is due to bone metastases, and surgical or physiatric stabilization may decrease breakthrough pain due to pathological fracture. Likewise, palliative anesthetic or neurosurgical options may be indicated for specific troublesome pain syndromes such as abdominal pain due to pancreatic cancer (51) or localized rib pain (52). In addition, assessment may identify environmental and psychological mediators of pain that can be addressed with behavioral or rehabilitative interventions (53).

Although the literature supports opioids as the treatment of choice for breakthrough pain, other agents have important adjunctive roles in specific settings. Pain of neuropathic origin may be less responsive to opioids than nociceptive pain (54) and often responds favorably to the addition of a variety of adjuvant analgesics from classes that include antidepressants and anticonvulsants (13). Corticosteroids have been reported to be effective in patients with poorly controlled pain due to bone metastases or plexopathy (29, 55, 56), and agents such as laxatives, antiperistaltic drugs, and spasmolytics that can modify provocative factors are helpful in specific settings. Finally, despite similar pharmacodynamic properties, the efficacy and side effect profiles of opioids differ idiosyncratically among patients, and as a result, substitution of one opioid agonist for another may improve pain control (57).

Optimal opioid management of breakthrough pain is contingent on its specific features. Breakthrough pain that appears to be temporally related to scheduled doses of long-acting opioids is usually best managed by adjusting the dose or schedule of the primary analgesic (9). The therapeutic response to this strategy helps confirm the presence or absence of end-of-dose failure as an explanation for breakthrough pain. If such adjustments are met with unremitting new side effects, consideration may be given to a trial of an alternative around-the-clock opioid.

In contrast to end-of-dose failure, other types of breakthrough pain are typically best managed by adjusting the demand component of opioid therapy (rescue or escape doses). Both incident pain and idiopathic breakthrough pain are usually managed with the administration as needed of rescue doses of short-acting opioids (i.e., IR morphine, hydromorphone, or oxycodone). Selection among these drugs is empirical, but except in the case of methadone, levorphanol and transdermal fentanyl, which have no readily available short-acting oral counterparts, it is generally preferred to initially use a short-acting formulation of the long-acting around-the-clock agent (36). By convention, the selection of the initial dose of rescue medication reflects the dose of the basal analgesic (7). Initial rescue doses equal to 5 to 15% of the total daily opioid intake every 2 to 4 hours appear to be safe and generally effective (58). Optimal outcome is ultimately achieved by adjusting the timing and dose of the rescue drug based on patient self-report of efficacy and side effects.

When incident pain is relatively predictable, rescue doses are provided prophylactically about 30 minutes in advance of the pain-provoking activity (59). When unanticipated breakthrough pain occurs, the rescue dose should be taken as soon after onset as possible, independent of the timing of the basal dose. If these strategies are unsuccessful, consider a trial of an alternative short-acting opioid or a change in the route of administration. Breakthrough pain that is predictable, infrequent, mildly or moderately intense, or slow to develop can often be managed effectively with oral analgesics such as IR morphine, hydromorphone, or oxycodone. Breakthrough pain that is severe or that occurs unpredictably, frequently, or precipitously may not be adequately relieved with available oral agents. Although intravenous and subcutaneous opioids are pharmacokinetically well suited for labile and/or severe breakthrough pain, these advantages are offset by their invasiveness.

Incident pain is presumably especially difficult to treat successfully because opioid requirements vary dramatically over short intervals. Doses of opioids required to treat pain during periods of rest are typically inadequate when activity increases, and conversely, doses required to ease movement-related pain may produce sedation and other side effects when the provocative activity ceases (1, 12, 48, 61).

Oral Transmucosal Fentanyl Citrate: An Emerging Intervention Specific for Breakthrough Pain

The availability of a variety of long-acting formulations of opioid analgesics has made the basal component of chronic cancer pain easier to manage effectively than in the past. However, fewer alternatives for managing breakthrough pain exist. The shortcomings of current methods for managing breakthrough pain have already been discussed. Although cancer pain treatment guidelines recommend using a rescue dose to treat breakthrough pain (34), this review identified no research, even of the case series type, that evaluated a drug specifically for its use as a rescue medication for cancer pain, with one single exception. OTFC, a new formulation of an established opioid analgesic, has been evaluated on a pilot basis for breakthrough pain (62, 63). In addition, recently completed extensive controlled research on the use of OTFC as a specific remedy for breakthrough pain confirms its safety and demonstrates superior efficacy to routine oral agents in cancer patients receiving concomitant therapy with transdermal and CR oral opioids for basal pain (data on file, Anesta Corp., Salt Lake City; Patt RB, Payne R, Chou C, et al., unpublished data, 1996).

Fentanyl citrate is a potent opioid agonist that has been widely used as an intravenous adjunct to anesthesia since its introduction into clinical practice in the early 1960s. Over the past decade the applications for fentanyl have expanded to include analgesia for minor procedures outside the operating room, postoperative PCA, and especially for cancer pain and intravenous, subcutaneous, and epidural analgesia. A transdermal preparation of fentanyl citrate used mostly to treat cancer pain was released in the United States in 1991 and is now available in more than a dozen countries.

OTFC is a new dosage form that is commercially available in the United States for specific indications and that is undergoing clinical trials specifically for the management of incident and breakthrough pain in cancer patients (66). It is a noninvasive means of delivering the potent opioid fentanyl through the oral mucosa, facilitating rapid absorption into the circulation and analgesia of relatively fast onset and short duration. The duration of analgesia is slightly prolonged as a result of a small proportion of fentanyl that is swallowed and subjected to hepatic first-pass effect. The availability of fentanyl in a lozenge form allows for easy self-administration and permits patients to titrate dose to an effective level of analgesia.

In a recent study, OTFC was used to treat breakthrough pain in patients with advanced cancer (33). Patients were given OTFC 10 to 15 μg/kg four or five times a day over 2 days for breakthrough pain. Patients reported a significant reduction in pain along with an increased sense of well-being. Onset of significant analgesia typically occurs within 5 minutes of beginning consumption of a unit and peaks about 30 minutes later. Patients required no additional rescue medication while using OTFC. The results of this study suggest that OTFC may be useful for the management of breakthrough pain caused by cancer.

CONCLUSION

Careful assessment is essential for optimal cancer pain management. As part of that assessment, the clinician should determine the pain's temporal features and should seek to identify the presence and characteristics of breakthrough pain. An understanding of the tempo of pain will aid the clinician in establishing a judicious treatment regimen.

Although the clinical importance of breakthrough pain has been repeatedly emphasized, this and other concepts related to the temporal aspects of pain have only recently been addressed in the medical literature. Recent survey data have begun to provide a clearer understanding of the prevalence and characteristics of breakthrough pain in cancer. Research on the effectiveness and limitations of current treatment strategies is lacking (1). More studies are needed to clarify characteristics, determine prevalence, explore treatment strategies, and determine the influence of breakthrough pain on the cancer patient's quality of life.

References

1. McQuay HJ, Jadad AR. Incident pain. Cancer Surv 1994;21:17–24.
2. IASP Subcommittee on Taxonomy. Classification of chronic pain. Pain 1986;(Suppl 3):S1–S225.
3. Bonica JJ. The management of pain. 2nd ed. Definitions and taxonomy of pain. Philadelphia: Lea & Febiger, 1990;18–27.
4. Clark JL, Kalan GE. Effective treatment of severe cancer pain of the head using low-dose ketamine in an opioid-tolerant patient. J Pain Symptom Mgmt 1995;10:310–314.
5. Patt RB, Manfredi P. Cancer pain emergencies. In: Parris WCV, ed. Principles and practice of cancer pain management. Butterworths, in press.
6. Coyle N, Adelhardt J, Foley KM, Portenoy RK. Character of terminal illness in the advanced cancer patient: pain and other symptoms during the last four weeks of life J Pain Symptom Mgmt 1990;5:83–93.
7. Portenoy RK, Hagen NA. Breakthrough pain: definition, prevalence and characteristics. Pain 1990;41:273–81.
8. Schechter NL. Pain in children with cancer. Adv Pain Res Ther 1990;16:57–71.
9. Portenoy RK, Hagen NA. Breakthrough pain: definition and management. Oncology 1989;Suppl:25–29.
10. Payne R. Cancer pain: anatomy, physiology and pharmacology. Cancer 1989;63 (Suppl):2266.
11. Tasker RR, Dostrovsky JO. Deafferentation and central pain. In: Wall PD, Melzack R, eds. Textbook of pain. 2nd ed. Edinburgh: Churchill Livingstone, 1989;154.
12. Patt RB. Classification of cancer pain syndromes In: Patt RB, ed. Cancer pain. Philadelphia: Lippincott, 1993;3–22.
13. Bruera E, Ripamonti C. Adjuvants to opioid analgesics In: Patt RB, ed. Cancer pain. Philadelphia: Lippincott, 1993;143–159.
14. Campa, Payne. In: Patt RB, ed. Cancer pain. Philadelphia: Lippincott, 1993.
15. Portenoy RK, Maldonado M, Fitzmartin R, et al. Oral controlled-release morphine sulfate: analgesic efficacy and side effects of a 100-mg tablet in cancer pain patients. Cancer 1989;63:2284–2288.
16. Hays H, Hagen N, Thirlwell M, et al. Comparative clinical efficacy and safety of immediate release and controlled release hydromorphone for chronic severe cancer pain. Cancer 1994;74:1808–1816.
17. Moulin DE, Kreeft JH, Murray-Parsons N, Bouquillon AI. Comparison of continuous subcutaneous and intravenous hydromorphone infusions for management of cancer pain. Lancet 1991;337:465–468.
18. Bruera E, Fainsinger R, MacEachern, Hanson J. The use of methylphenidate in patients with incident cancer pain receiving regular opiates: a preliminary report. Pain 1992;50:75–77.
19. Ashby MA, Fleming BG, Brooksbank M, et al. Description of a mechanistic approach to pain management in advanced cancer: preliminary report. Pain 1992;51:153–161.
20. Mercadante S. What is the definition of breakthrough pain? Pain 1991;45:107.
21. Reference deleted.
22. Banning A, Sjøgren P, Henriksen H. Treatment outcome in a multidisciplinary cancer pain clinic. Pain 1991;47:129–134.
23. Mercadante S, Maddaloni S, Roccella S, Salvaggio L. Predictive factors in advanced cancer pain treated only by analgesics. Pain 1992;50:151–155.
24. Fine PG, Marcus M, DeBoer AJ, et al. An open label study of oral transmucosal fentanyl citrate (OTFC) for the treatment of breakthrough cancer pain. Pain 1991;45:149–55.
25. Finn JW, Walsh TD, MacDonald N, et al. Placebo-blinded study of morphine sulfate sustained-release tablets and immediate-release morphine sulfate solution in outpatients with chronic pain due to advanced cancer. J Clin Oncol 1993;5:967–972.
26. Deleted.
27. Walsh TD, MacDonald N, Bruera E, et al. A controlled study of sustained-release morphine sulfate tablets in chronic pain from advanced cancer Am J Clin Oncol 1992;15:268–272.
28. Deschamps M, Band PR, Hislop TG, et al. The evaluation of analgesic effects in cancer patients as exemplified by a double-blind, crossover study of immediate-release versus controlled-release morphine J Pain Symptom Mgmt 1992;7:384–392.
29. Bruera E, Fainsinger R, Spachynski K, et al. Clinical efficacy and safety of a novel controlled-release morphine suppository and subcutaneous morphine in cancer pain: a randomized evaluation. J Clin Oncol 1995;13:1520–1527.
30. Arkinstall W, Sandler A, Goughnour B, et al. Efficacy of controlled-release codeine in chronic non-malignant pain: a randomized, placebo-controlled clinical trial. Pain 1995;62:169–178.
31. Herbst LH, Strause LG. Transdermal fentanyl use in hospice home-care patients with chronic cancer pain J Pain Symptom Mgmt 1992; 7:S54–S57.
32. Bruera E. Subcutaneous administration of opioids in the management of cancer pain. Adv Pain Res Ther 1990;16:203–218.
33. World Health Organization: Cancer Pain Relief. Geneva: WHO, 1986.
34. Jacox A, Carr DB, Payne R, et al. Management of cancer pain. Clinical practice guideline 9. AHCPR Pub 94–0592. Rockville, MD: Agency for Health Care Policy and Research, 1994.
35. Portenoy RK. Practical aspects of pain control in the patient with cancer. CA Cancer J Clin 1988;38:327–352.
36. Foley KM. Diagnosis and treatment of cancer pain. In: Jolleb AI, Fink DJ, Murphy GP, eds. American Cancer Society textbook of clinical oncology. Atlanta: ACS, 1991;555–575.
37. Miser AW, Dothage JA, Miser JS. Continuous intravenous fentanyl for pain control in children and young adults with cancer. Clin J Pain 1987;3:152–157.
38. Paix A, Coleman A, Lees J, et al. Subcutaneous fentanyl and sufentanil infusion substitution for morphine intolerance in cancer pain management Pain 1995;63:263–269.
39. Portenoy RK. Continuous intravenous infusion of opioid drugs. Med Clin North Am 1987;71:233–241.
40. Lindley C. Overview of current development in patient-controlled analgesia. Support Care Cancer 1994;2:319–326.
41. Coyle N, Cherny NI, Portenoy RK. Subcutaneous opioid infusions at home. Oncology 1994;8:21–37.
42. Storey P, Hill HH, St Louis RH, Tarver EE. Subcutaneous infusions for control of cancer symptoms. J Pain Symptom Mgmt 1990;5:33–41.
43. Bruera E. Subcutaneous administration of opioids in the management of cancer pain. Adv Pain Res Ther 1990;16:203–218.
44. Swanson G, Snith J, Bulich R, et al. Patient-controlled analgesia for chronic cancer pain in the ambulatory setting: a report of 117 patients. J Clin Oncol 1989;1903–1908.
45. Vanier MC, Labrecque G, Lepage-Savary D, et al. Comparison of hydromorphone continuous subcutaneous infusion and basal rate subcutaneous infusion plus PCA in cancer pain: a pilot study. Pain 1993;53:27–32.
46. Bruera E, MacMillan K, Hanson J, et al. The Edmonton staging system for cancer pain: Preliminary report. Pain 1989;37:203.
47. American Joint Committee for Cancer Staging and End Result Reporting. Manual for staging of cancer. Chicago: AJCC, 1977.
48. Hanks GW, Justins DM. Cancer pain: Management. Lancet 1992;339:1031–1036.
49. Hanks GW. Opioid-responsive and opioid-non-responsive pain in cancer. Br Med Bull 1991;47:718–731.
50. Gonzales GR, Elliott KJ, Portenoy RK, Foley KM. The impact of a comprehensive evaluation in the management of cancer pain. Pain 1991;47:141–144.
51. Patt RB, Black RG, Reddy SK. Neural blockade for abdominopelvic pain of oncologic origin. Cancer Bull 1995;47:52–60.

52. Patt RB, Reddy S. Spinal neurolysis for cancer pain: Indications and recent results. Ann Acad Med Singapore 1994;23:2–6.

53. Syrjala KL, Donaldson GW, Davis MW, et al. Relaxation and imagery and cognitive-behavior training reduce pain during cancer treatment: a controlled clinical trial. Pain 1995;63:189–198.

54. Portenoy RK, Foley KM, Inturissi C. The nature of opioid responsiveness and its implications for neuropathic pain: new hypothesis derived from studies of opioid infusions. Pain 1990;43:273–286.

55. Ettinger AB, Portenoy RK. The use of corticosteroids in the treatment of symptoms associated with cancer. J Pain Symptom Mgmt 1988;3:99–103.

56. Bruera E, Roca E, Cedaro L, et al. Action of oral methylprednisolone in terminal cancer patients: a prospective randomized double-blind study. Cancer Treat Rep 1985;69:751–754.

57. de Stoutz ND, Bruera E, Suarez-Almazor M. Opioid rotation for toxicity reduction in terminal cancer patients. J Pain Symptom Mgmt 1995;10:378–384.

58. Portenoy RK. Cancer pain management. Semin Oncol 1993b;20 (Supp1):19–35.

59. Portenoy RK, Hagen NA. Management of breakthrough pain. Prim Care Cancer 1991;May:24–27.

60. Deleted.

61. Hanks GW: Opioid-responsive and opioid-non-responsive pain in cancer Br Med Bull. 1991;47:718–31.

62. Ashburn MA, Fine PG, Stanley TH. Oral transmucosal fentanyl citrate for the treatment of breakthrough cancer pain: a case report. Anesthesiology 1989;71:615–617.

63. Fine PG, Marcus M, DeBoer AJ, et al. An open label study of oral transmucosal fentanyl citrate (OTFC) for the treatment of breakthrough cancer pain. Pain 1991;45:149–55.

64. Deleted.

65. Deleted.

66. Ashburn MA, Fine PG, Stanley TH. Oral transmucosal fentanyl citrate for the treatment of breakthrough cancer pain: a case report. Anesthesiology 1989;71:615–17.

67. Deleted.

68. Mercadante S, Armata M, Salvaggio L. Pain characteristics of advanced lung cancer patients referred to a palliative care service. Pain 1994;59:141–145.

69. Ashby MA, Fleming BG, Brooksbank M, et al. Description of a mechanistic approach to pain management in advanced cancer: preliminary report. Pain 1992;51:153–161.

70. Bruera E, Fainsinger R, MacEachern, Hanson J. The use of methylphenidate in patients with incident cancer pain receiving regular opiates: a preliminary report. Pain 1992;50:75–77.

71. Mercadante S, Maddaloni S, Roccella S, Salvaggio L. Predictive factors in advanced cancer pain treated only by analgesics. Pain 199250:151–155.

CHAPTER 27

Continuous Care of Cancer Pain Patients

Ricardo Ruiz-López

Happiness demands not only complete goodness but a complete life. In the course of life we encounter many reverses and all kinds of vicissitudes…nobody calls a man happy who suffered fortunes like this and met a miserable end. Aristotle: *Ethics* (1).

During the past decades there has developed a great effort to inform clinicians about the new trends and modalities of the treatment of acute and chronic pain. In the medical literature a high prevalence of undertreated pain has been reported in the various clinical situations, including family medicine, surgery, oncology, emergency units, burn units, and pediatric wards.

In regard to cancer patients, undertreatment of pain is not merely an educational problem; it can reflect a deficiency of the programs of care. The inadequate understanding of the psychosocial problems, symptomatic control, and coordination of patient's care can decrease quality of life, and health system barriers can interfere with effective pain control in patients with cancer. Thus, this chapter will cover the following topics:

Definition of quality of life
The structure and functions of the pain and palliative care team
The education of patient and relatives in cancer pain management
Cancer pain and palliative care: the continuum of hospital-hospice-home

DEFINITION OF QUALITY OF LIFE

The concept of quality of life was introduced as one of the goals of medical treatment in the late 1970s through some surveys in the United States (2–4). This concept emerges from the development of Western health policies over the past 50 years from restoring welfare to objectives related with psychosocial needs. The World Health Organization's (5) definition of health as "a state of complete physical, mental and social well being and not merely the absence of disease" focuses on the issue of the wholeness of life and the importance of the psychosocial component. While some definitions include such terms as happiness and satisfaction as being important aspects, others mention that measures of sociopersonal or quality of life should include physical, social, and emotional function, attitudes to illness, and personal features of patients' daily life, including family interactions and the cost of illness (6). Some definitions of quality of life treat it as related to the individual's own perception, emphasizing the breadth of the term as covering many aspects of life (7). When applied to cancer pain patients, it should consider different clinical dimensions providing a framework in which physical—toxicity, physical impairment, body image and function—psychological, social, spiritual, cultural, and philosophical factors interact in a specific way and individually to the patient, changing with the evolution of the disease.

Therefore, quality of life measures the difference, at a particular period of time, between the hopes and expectations of the individual and the individuals' present experience (8, 9). According to Calman (9) four stages of action are required to modify the quality of life:

1. Assessment and definition of the problems and priorities of the individual.
2. Planning of care with the patient's full involvement. This step requires full discussion with the patient and family and requires insight by the patient into the dynamics of the situation.
3. Implementation of the action plan, by either the patient or the caring team. This goal may be accomplished by improving physical symptoms, altering the

psychological status, or reducing the expectation of the individual while still retaining hope.

4. Evaluation of the results of intervention and reassessment of the problem.

During the past decade medical ethical considerations on the consequences of developments of health care and medical oncology have led to the general assumption in Western societies that promoting the quality of life and alleviating suffering are almost as important as preserving life. Moreover, the increasing concerns about economic growth and development of health care and the perception that health care policies are determined on the basis of cost-benefit analysis give a solid groundwork for the implementation of multidisciplinary, interdisciplinary teams for the management of patients with advanced diseases, whose quality of life is considered the principal goal of medical therapy.

STRUCTURE AND FUNCTIONS OF THE PAIN AND PALLIATIVE CARE TEAM

Specialized care of persons with cancer and other irreversible diseases has undergone major changes during the past 3 decades. Although the concept of medical effectiveness can be greatly modified by physicians' attitudes and environmental issues, the organizational issues and philosophy of a modern pain and palliative care team are not dissimilar to those postulated by Bonica (10) in his early work, when he stated that "complex pain problems can be treated more effectively by a multidisciplinary, interdisciplinary team, each member of which contributes with his or her specialized knowledge and skills to the common goal of making a correct diagnosis and developing the most effective therapeutic strategy."

The development of the hospice movement over the past 50 years has provided interdisciplinary care to patients and families at home, establishing inpatient units for palliative care in local hospitals or in specialized institutions. In either type of setting, the multidisciplinary, interdisciplinary team plays a major role, providing medical treatment and psychosocial support and attending the spiritual needs to patients and their families (11–13).

The Multidisciplinary Team

Care of the cancer pain patient must be active and continuous, addressed to the family unit. It should attend physical, psychological, social, and spiritual needs, supporting work done by a multidisciplinary and interdisciplinary team, as the multiple issues faced by patients and their families usually exceed the expertise of a single practitioner or caregiver.

In this type of team, members with diverse training share the main goal of improving the quality of life of the patient and interact as a group of individuals with the common purpose of working together. Each member has his or her own expertise and training and makes decisions within that area of responsibility. Teamwork does not mean joining health care workers together in one room, nor is it the same as collaboration. Information must be the key issue for interaction of members and must be shared by the vehicle of the clinical record (14-16).

Structure

The structure of the multidisciplinary team varies with the development of the program of care, its objectives and goals, the availability of resources, and the type of setting, be it home, hospice, or hospital. The patient and family should be considered as members of the team.

Physician

The most important challenge and the first to be considered is the relief of pain and other symptoms. Thus, the physician plays a central role in the team. The physician must be competent in general medicine, know the principles and practice of hospice care, and understand malignant disease and any other disease represented in the patient population, such as AIDS and degenerative neurological diseases. Ideally, he or she should have a specific training in palliative medicine and skills of pain management, including surgical and anesthesiological procedures. This assertion suggests that a team must be composed of physicians from a wide variety of specialized backgrounds, such as anesthesiology, neurosurgery, oncology, psychiatry, internal medicine, and family medicine, among others.

Physicians may play various roles, including managing pain and symptoms in an individual patient, being responsible for medical assessment and coordination, training and supporting the multidisciplinary team, and ensuring coordination of care of the individual patient. Other physicians may act only as consultants, being coordinated by the attending physician of the patient.

Psychologist

The role of the psychologist is to perform a first evaluation of the patient and family status, focusing on personal problems of illness, disability, and impending death. He or she must deal with the patients' and relatives emotional needs. The psychologist should cover the patients' and family understanding of diagnosis, prognosis, and expectations, the strengths and resources available to the family, the problems precipitated by the terminal illness, past losses and the way they were handled, particular cultural factors, and expectations and plans for the future. The psychologist should help the team when there is dysfunction within the family and participate in patients' symptom control by teaching and assessing relaxation techniques, imagery, distraction techniques, and coping strategies.

Nurse

The nurse is the team member who will most visit the patient and family, at home or in an institution. His or her role begins with attention and information about the details of physical care: bathing, control of odor, pressure areas, mouth care, bladder care, bowel care, diet, and fluids. Other responsibilities include organizing the patient's environment to minimize loss of control, observing what brings comfort and relief, reporting response to medical treatments or secondary effects, and instructing the patient and family about the medication plan.

Social Worker

The social worker's goals are to help the patient to develop skills to deal with the social problems of illness, disability, and impending death; to link the patient with the community; and to establish practical aid for peer support.

Chaplain

A sympathetic chaplain who is a skilled listener is a key team member. Sometimes the patient has feelings of guilt for past events, a sense of meaninglessness, and a sense of life as unjust and unfair. Faith may be questioned. The role of chaplain is listening, facilitating recollection, dealing with regrets, spiritual counseling, and helping the patient prepare for what lies ahead. For patients with a tradition of religious rituals and sacraments, this member of the team can be very important. Therefore, pastoral counseling should be made available and pastoral care members should develop information about community resources that provide spiritual care and support.

Physical Therapist

Rather than attempting to improve function, the goal of the palliative care physiotherapist is to plan activity oriented to maximizing the patients' diminishing resources. This can be accomplished by active or passive range of motion exercises in the bedridden patient to prevent contractures and improve circulation, massage to relax aching muscles, treatment of lymphedema, instruction in transfers or positioning, and the use of physical therapies for the alleviation of pain.

Occupational Therapist

The occupational therapist's role is to maintain autonomous functions such as self-care needs, including grooming, feeding, dressing, moving about, and so on. He or she also assesses the functions with which the patient needs assistance and those that can still be performed with autonomy. He or she should provide adaptive equipment or functional splints, changing treatments in accordance with the patient's status. In the inpatient setting the focus of the occupational therapist on leisure can help to restore a sense of normal living through introduction of corrective measures to help the patient adapt residual capacities to maintain activities of daily living.

Volunteer

Volunteers' roles vary according to the patient's setting, although the focus is to improve the quality of life, to provide a supportive presence that may facilitate communication, and to assist with the normal activities of daily living. Volunteers should be carefully selected and specifically trained by the pain and palliative care team.

EDUCATION OF PATIENT AND RELATIVES IN CANCER PAIN MANAGEMENT

Teaching patients and their relatives about the issues is an essential feature of cancer pain management and palliative care. Health care professionals in a palliative care team must have adequate skills to enable the patient with an irreversible disease to live at his or her maximum potential until death, promoting education to regain independence and to improve the quality of life.

Characteristics of Education

Early Intervention

If the needs of the person with advanced disease are addressed at the early stages of the disease, the problems associated with the eventual progression of the disease will be fewer, and later distress may be decreased.

Participation of the Multidisciplinary Team

Poor symptom control and inadequate understanding of psychosocial problems are the major difficulties for very sick patients and their families. Because physical, emotional, psychological, and spiritual problems must be addressed, participation of the various disciplines that integrate a modern palliative care team is essential for developing a coordinated program of education (17, 18).

Communication

Effective communication is an important part of the therapy. In treating patients with advanced stages of incurable diseases it is mandatory to provide intelligible and coherent information to the patient and relatives, focusing on the development of basic listening skills in the health care professionals (Table 27.1). Fluent communication between physicians and nurses is essential for good patient care, and it is important to avoid specialist language or jargon that may give little help to the patient's problems (19, 20, 20a). Thus,

Table 27.1. Communication with the Cancer Pain Patient

Fluent communication
Basic listening skills
Specific communication tasks of palliative care
   Breaking bad news
   Therapeutic dialogue
Communicating with the family and with other professionals

the palliative care team should use a common language, in terms not only of idiomatic expression but of well-developed skills in verbal and nonverbal communication.

Essential Information

Information presented orally to the patient should be supplemented with written material. Booklets, graphic representations, written counseling, and videotapes may help in daily activities as well as alleviate patients' fears and uncertainty about the therapy and the progression of the disease (21-27).

Continuity

When possible, patients should have the opportunity to end their lives in the place most appropriate to them and their families. If there is a possibility of movement between different settings, continuity of education must be guaranteed to the patient by the palliative care team (11, 29). Nowadays, the lack of experience of death in the family determines the place of most deaths. Whereas a century ago 90% of deaths occurred in the home, for the past few decades more than 65% (with regional variations) occur in hospital or institutions. The resulting disruption of family support requires an educational effort by the team.

Content

Information about the Use of Analgesic Drugs

Understandable information about pain, pain assessment, symptoms related to the disease, and the use of drugs for symptomatic alleviation must be given to patients and relatives. Written information should address major barriers to effective pain management, the use of opioid analgesics, and concepts about addiction and tolerance to allay patients' unfounded fears (Table 27.2) (30). The literature indicates that to have the desired effect, information should be presented more than once, and because patients seek information from multiple sources, in more than one way (22–26, 30a, 30b).

Adjunct Medications

Patients and relatives should be encouraged to remain active and to participate in self-care when possible. Written instructions for treating constipation must be available, as must simple pharmacological aids, by written consent in

Table 27.2. Information about the Use of Morphine

What is morphine and how does it work?
Morphine? Does that mean I am at the end of the road?
Doesn't morphine speed things up, make you die sooner?
Will morphine take the pain away completely?
If I take morphine now, will there be anything stronger for me when the pain gets worse?
Wouldn't it be better to keep off morphine until things become really unbearable?
Will I need bigger and bigger doses to control the pain?
How long can I go on taking morphine?
Will I become addicted?
What are the differences among morphine in solution, morphine tablets, and the other routes?

Modified from Twycross R G, Lack S A. Therapeutics in terminal cancer. 2nd ed. London: Churchill Livingstone, 1990.

case of insomnia or anxiety not relieved by initial pharmacological prescription.

Nonpharmacological Management

Detailed information must stress the importance of nonpharmacological interventions as adjuncts to analgesics with demonstration, if available, of physical modalities, such as heat, cold, massage, and transcutaneous nerve stimulation; psychological interventions, including relaxation, imagery, and distraction; and occupational therapies.

Guidelines for the Use of Medical Technology

Patients and their families may have difficulty in understanding and remembering the details of functioning of medical equipment, such as use of pumps, care of dressings and catheters, portable suction machines, and so on. Written instructions, especially in the domestic setting, must be provided to patients' relatives to avoid problems and guarantee collaboration with the home care team.

Peer Support Groups

Information about programs of self-help and mutual support should be available to patients and relatives if there is any established in their community. Support networks can also help patients to maintain social identity and provide emotional support, material aid, and access to information (31, 32).

Written Plan for Continuous Care

Doctors should communicate the discharge plan to ensure continuity in pain management and palliative care to patients, especially when the patient is being transferred from one health care setting to another, such as being discharged from a hospital to a hospice or nursing care facility. In that case, specific instructions must be written to contact the members on call during the night and weekends to ensure continuity of care.

Factors that Contribute to Effectiveness

Cooperation with the Patient's Relatives

The attitude of the relatives to pain relief with opioids and other therapies is crucial for the outcome of the treatment. A prejudiced attitude on their part may cause anxiety in the patient. It is invaluable to inform and instruct the relatives and make sure that they participate in decisions with the patient.

Cross-Cultural Issues

Special consideration should be given to the fact that there are many pitfalls and much danger of miscommunication in dealing with persons from other cultural backgrounds (32–34). Today, many communities and cities are composed of groups of people from different countries or stemming from different sociocultural settings. Even within rural areas of the same country, cultural differences abound and intergenerational cultural gaps are frequent. The professional palliative care team must pay much attention to the mentioned features in order to achieve effectiveness.

Psychosocial Assessment

Patients with cancer commonly have psychological damage as a result of their illness. Available data suggest that the incidence of pain, depression, and advanced delirium all increase with higher levels of physical debilitation and advanced illness. Psychological assessment is required to evaluate symptoms of depression and to investigate risk factors that predispose cancer patients to depressive or anxiety disorders that should receive specific treatment (32, 33). Assessment of the family and social environment is required to adapt educational issues to each individual situation and to define operational strategies with the interdisciplinary care team (35).

Ongoing Monitoring of the Patient

Traditional clinical settings cannot adequately serve the needs of the patient and relatives regarding easy access to the care team for education and/or information. The dynamic nature of symptoms in cancer and the increasing tendency to offer palliative care at the home and in outpatient settings demand innovative methods of symptom management. In this way, a consultation telephone hotline can be a good way to fulfill the requirements for ongoing monitoring of the patient.

CANCER PAIN AND PALLIATIVE CARE: THE CONTINUUM HOSPITAL-HOSPICE MODEL

One of the most challenging tasks of care in cancer pain is to ensure specialized services throughout the different settings where the patient will be managed during the course of the disease. Most patients need specialized care in two or more settings, as there is an increasing movement in the industrialized countries to enable the person with advanced disease to live until death at his or her own maximal potential, letting patients end their lives in the setting most appropriate to them and their families. Therefore, a major objective of care in cancer pain management is to help the patient reach the limit of his or her physical and mental capacities with the highest autonomy in the environment wherever possible. The provision of continuity of care in such terms is conditioned by the availability of resources and mainly by an effective communication within the team, the patient, and the family (Fig. 27.1).

The place of death and quality of care are among the most important concerns for the patient and family. Until the nineteenth century people died where they had spent their life or where they wished to. In the last century, because of different conceptual assumptions, Western society has changed the place for dying from home to the hospital, which in many cases is not the place preferred by the patient. In the United Kingdom in 1965, 63% of deaths took place in the hospital, whereas 73% did in 1987. In the United States in 1957 70% died in the hospital. In Italy 72% of patients died in hospital in 1986 and 67% in 1990. In Israel at present, 29% of terminal patients die in hospital, 41% at home, and 31% at institutions for chronic diseases. In Western Australia the availability of home care services has allowed 70% of patients die at home. If the patients are asked where they wish to spend the last days of their lives, the majority answer home.

Hospital

Since the nineteenth century, technology and industry have developed enormously, and life expectancy has doubled. In the twentieth century the hospital setting has become a place designed to recover health and manage treatable diseases. Healing and prolongation of life have been assumed its main objectives. There seems to be no time or space for patients who won't get well. On the other hand, society seems to be trying to eliminate death from its style of life, and the dying person is sent to the hospital to keep him or her far from the center of the family.

Nowadays the hospital setting has to be considered as one important step for the multidisciplinary team in some circumstances. The hospital is the place where specific palliative therapies can be administered, such as radiation therapy or transfusions, and to manage symptoms of difficult control such as pain. In some cases an admittance to the hospital is needed to perform a surgical procedure to alleviate pain, such as nerve blocks. Delirium sometimes requires admittance to hospital to make a quick and correct diagnosis of its causes and to treat them if possible. Severe dyspnea coming from pleural effusion or other causes can require thoracocentesis in hospital. Difficult ulcers (paraneoplasic vasculitic syndromes), ischemic complications, or other

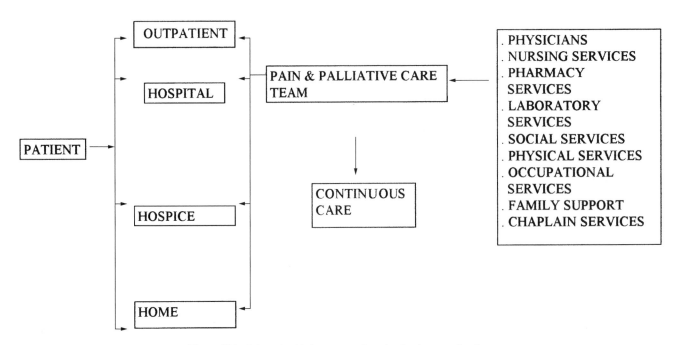

Figure 27.1 Pain and palliative care services, levels of care, and patients.

miscellaneous conditions can be more effectively controlled in a hospital setting. In any case, the hospital stay should not be prolonged.

Other causes of admission to hospital can arise in the family, such as poor coping or extreme anxiety, as well as distressing symptoms such as severe dyspnea, neoplastic ulcers, or agony. Finally, the patient who lives alone and has no means to acquire a caregiver sometimes requires admittance to the hospital or a hospice institution. The patient may decide to stay in the hospital due to his own will.

The best way to achieve good results without the disadvantages of a hospital setting for a terminal cancer patient is to create in local hospitals a palliative care unit (PCU). Some hospitals have a PCU, which avoids many of the problems of the traditional hospital model. The team must be trained in the treatment and control of the advanced disease and in the integral care of patient and family to be able to resolve problems that appear during the disease. They must have communication skills; loss of communication usually means that the patient merely becomes a care receiver instead of an active participant in the decision taking. The team must have time to dedicate to the patient and families. The PCU team has to become familiar to the patient. The atmosphere must be adequate to make possible some degree of independence and maintain privacy. Usually the hospital is a hostile place for the patient, who ignores hospital regulations. Also, privacy during family conferences is important, and a special room for this purpose is desirable, avoiding discussions in the corridor. The PCU must have special equipment but not sophisticated technology. The concept "nothing more can be done" must be abandoned, and inadequate therapeutic attempts or prolongation of agony should be avoided (36–38).

Hospice

The first hospice where modern medicine in a rational and scientific basis was applied to terminal patients was St. Christopher's Hospice in London (Table 27.3). The human component was not forgotten, and pain management was one of the bases. It was the beginning of palliative care as we know it today, and the hospice movement has been expanded all over the world (13, 14). The main purpose of the hospice is to take care of the human being who is ill with no possibility of healing. Its principal objective is to treat to the patient as a whole, making him or her and the family participate in decision taking. The major principles in the hospice setting are the following: symptom control; rehabilitation; attention to psychological and spiritual needs; allowing the patient and family to choose where to live the final phase of the disease and where to die; maintaining good communication between the members of the team, including the patient and his family; and giving support during agony, providing accessibility to staff and enough time to comfort the patient (36–38, 40, 43).

Home

The home setting offers several advantages for patients, who maintain the social and familial role, employs their time as they wish to their own rules, and develops personally satisfactory eating and sleeping habits. Changing those habits in the final days of life can lead to suffering and stress. Furthermore, patients at home keeps their privacy, can go on with occupational activities, and are in a familiar environment. The family is more satisfied by the active participation in the caregiving and respect to the patient's wishes.

Table 27.3.   List of Elements Brought Together at St. Christopher's Hospice

Beds integrated in local community
Development and monitoring of symptom control
Family support
Bereavement service
Home care
Research and evaluation
Education and training

Saunders C, Bains M. Living with dying: the management of terminal disease. Oxford, UK: Oxford University Press, 1983.

Table 27.4.   Home Care in Cancer Pain Management: Critical Issues

24-hour specialized care available
Patient and relatives taught about the disease
Information about home remedies
Appropriate technological support
Written information on the use of medication

Home care as a part of continuous care in the cancer patient benefits the health system, as the number of hospital admittances and length of stay decrease, and provides quality of care according to modern ethical rules. For a patient to be kept at home some conditions must be fulfilled: 24-hour specialized care by the palliative care team; teaching the patient and relatives about all issues related to the illness and its complications; information about home remedies for the appropriate management of pain and other symptoms, appropriate technological support for medical equipment, and written information about the use of medication (Table 27.4). The patient and family must be assured that admittance to an institution is available if the clinical situation becomes uncontrolled. Care of the patient's family after the death of the patient by means of a bereavement program is crucial. If a family shows specific difficulties at the immediate phase of death, referral to community peer support groups or specialized counseling must be given.

References

1.   Aristotle. Ethics. Harmondsworth, UK: Penguin Books, 1976.
2.   Aaronson, NK, Beckmann J, eds. The quality of life of cancer patients. New York: Raven Press, 1987.
3.   Andrews FM, Withey SB. Social indicators of well-being. New York: Plenum Press, 1976.
4.   Campbell A, Converse PE, Rodgers WL. The quality of American life. New York: Sage, 1976.
5.   World Health Organization. Constitution. Geneva: WHO, 1948.
6.   Spitzer WO, Dobson AJ, Hall J, et al. Measuring the quality of life of cancer patients: a concise QL-index for use by physicians. J Chron Dis 1981;34:585–597.
7.   Krupinsky J. Health and the quality of life. Soc Sci Med 1980;14:203–211.
8.   Calman KC. Definitions and dimensions of quality of life. In: Aaronson N K, Beckman J, eds. The quality of life of cancer patients. New York: Raven Press, 1987;1–9.
9.   Calman KC. The quality of life in cancer patients: an hypothesis. J Med Ethics 1984;10:124–127.
10.   Bonica JJ. General clinical considerations (including organization and function of a pain clinic). In: Bonica JJ, ed. Recent advances in pain. Springfield IL: Charles C. Thomas, 1974;274–298.
11.   Ventafridda V. Continuing care: a major issue in cancer pain management. Pain 1989;36:137–143.
12.   Parkes CM, Parkes J. Hospice versus hospital care: reevaluation after ten years as seen by surviving spouses. Postgrad Med J 1984;60:120–124.
13.   Saunders C, Baines M. Living with dying: the management of terminal disease. Oxford, UK: Oxford University Press, 1983.
14.   Saunders CMS. Terminal care. In: Weatherall D J, Ledingham J G G, Warrell DA, eds. Oxford textbook of medicine. Oxford, UK: Oxford University Press, 1983;2881–2813.
15.   Doyle D. A home care service for terminally ill patients in Edinburgh. Scot Health Bull 1991;49:12–21.
16.   Doyle D, Hanks GWC, MacDonald N, eds. Oxford textbook of palliative medicine. Oxford, UK: Oxford University Press, 1993.
17.   Jacox A, Carr DB, Payne R, et al. Management of cancer pain. Clinical practice guideline 9. Agency for Health Care Policy and Research pub. 94–0592. Rockville, MD: U.S. Public Health Service, March 1994.
18.   Di Mola G. Le cure palliative: Approccio assistenziale ai malati terminali. Milano: Fondazione Floriani, 1992.
19.   Earnshaw-Smith E. Dealing with dying patients and their relatives. Br Med J 1981; 282: 1779.
20.   Questions and answers about pain control: a guide for people with cancer and their families. American Cancer Society and the National Cancer Institute, 1992.
20a.   Buckman R. Communication in palliative care: a practical guide. In: Doyle D, Hanks GWC, MacDonald N, eds. Oxford textbook of palliative medicine. Oxford, UK: Oxford University Press, 1993;47–61.
21.   Ferrell BR, Rhiner M, Ferrell BA. Development and implementation of a pain education program. Cancer 1993;72 (11 Suppl):3426–3432.
22.   Cancer pain can be relieved: a guide for patients and families. Madison: Wisconsin Cancer Pain Initiative, 1989.
23.   Jeff asks about cancer pain: a booklet for teens about cancer pain. Madison: Wisconsin Cancer Pain Initiative, 1990.
24.   Dolore da cancro e cure palliative. Collana rapporti tecnici 804. Ginevra: Organizzazione Mondiale de la Sanità, 1990.
25.   Manual of care for terminally ill cancer patients. Tokyo: Ministry of Health and Japan Medical Association, 1989.
26.   Facing forward: a guide for cancer survivors. US Department of Health and Human Services, 1990.
27.   Teamwork: the cancer patient's guide to talking with your doctor. National Coalition for Cancer Survivorship, 1991.
28.   Reference Deleted.
29.   Ward SE, Goldberg N, Miller-McCauley V, et al. Patient-related barriers to management of cancer pain. Pain 1993;52:319–324.
30.   Twycross RG, Lack SA. Therapeutics in terminal cancer. 2nd ed. London: Churchill Livingstone, 1990.
30a.   Hanks GW, Hoskin, PJ. Opioid analgesics in the management of pain in patients with cancer: a review. Palliat Med 1987;1:1–25.
30b.   Regnard CFB, Davies A. A guide to symptom relief in advanced cancer. Manchester: Haigh & Hochland, 1986.
31.   Walker KN, MacBride A, Vachon ML. Social support networks and the crisis of bereavement. Soc Sci Med 1977;11:35–41.
32.   Schneidman ES. Some aspects of psychotherapy with dying persons. In: Garfield CA, ed. Psychosocial care of the dying patient. New York: McGraw-Hill, 1978.
33.   Bond MR. Psychologic and emotional aspects of cancer pain. In: Bonica JJ, Ventafridda V, eds. Advances in pain research and therapy. New York: Raven Press, 1979;2:81–88.
34.   Reference deleted.
35.   Houts PS. Home care guide for cancer: how to care for family and friends at home. American College of Physicians, 1994.

36. Saunders CMS. Foreword. In: Doyle D, Hanks GWC, MacDonald N, eds. Oxford textbook of palliative medicine. Oxford: Oxford University Press, 1993; v–viii.

37. Soigner et accompagner jusqu'am bout: soulager la souffrance. Paris: Ministry of Social Affairs and Employment, 1986.

38. Zimmerman JM. Hospice: complete care for the terminally ill. 2nd ed. Baltimore: Urban & Schwarzenberg, 1986.

39. Reference deleted.

40. The management of pain in the terminal stage of life. Stockholm: Swedish National Board of Health and Welfare, 1989.

41. Reference deleted.

42. Reference deleted.

43. Hillier ER, Lunt B. Goal setting in terminal cancer. In: Twycross RG, Ventafridda V, eds. The continuing care of terminal cancer patients. Oxford: Pergamon Press, 1979.

CHAPTER 28

Management of Pain in HIV-Infected Persons

Edward Lor and John Stansell

INTRODUCTION

The introduction of new combination antiretroviral strategies (highly active antiretroviral therapy, or HAART), improved prophylaxis of opportunistic infections, and maturation of the acquired immunodeficiency syndrome (AIDS) epidemic have combined to produce remarkable reductions in progression to end-stage human immunodeficiency virus (HIV) disease and death among HIV-infected persons over the past 2 years. Yet no one can say how long this interval of improved outcomes will be sustained. The emergence of resistance to the protease inhibitors and the nonnucleoside reverse transcriptase inhibitors suggests that these benefits of primary antiretroviral therapy may be fleeting. Certainly no patient with symptomatic HIV disease or with an AIDS diagnosis has yet survived to lead a normal life. Patients with symptomatic HIV disease now and in the foreseeable future can be expected to face progressive debilitation and eventual death as a consequence of their infection and immunocompromise. Pain is often an unavoidable part of AIDS and advanced HIV disease. Nothing is extraordinary about the kind of pain that AIDS patients have. However, the incidence, severity, and multiplicity of sources of pain makes treating the discomfort of AIDS a vexing task. Although each AIDS patient has unique pain control needs, this chapter attempts to paint a broad picture of the issues and treatments confronting the clinician caring for the AIDS patient.

PAIN AND THE AIDS PATIENT

Pain is the constant companion of many persons with AIDS or advanced HIV disease. Half or more of AIDS patients complain of pain that impairs their quality of life. The incidence of pain syndromes increases with progressive immunocompromise. Estimates of the incidence of pain among HIV-infected persons range from 25 to 30% among HIV-symptomatic

persons, 50 to 60% of AIDS patients, and 50 to 75% of hospitalized AIDS patients to nearly everyone in the final stages of AIDS-related illness. Moreover, the number of sites of pain tend to increase as AIDS-related immunodysfunction progresses. The terminally ill AIDS patient rarely suffers from a single site of discomfort; rather, multiple sites and sources of pain are the general rule. Thus diffuse arthralgias and myalgias so frequently the source of discomfort for AIDS patients may be joined by the pain of visceral distention due to lymphoma, mycobacterial disease, or the lancinating pain of neuropathy. Most of these pain syndromes can be directly attributed to the ravages of the virus itself or the untoward side effects of treatments directed against HIV or its attendant opportunistic infections or malignancies. There is usually little contribution from non-HIV-related sources. Thus, the incidence and the intensity of the pain afflicting these patients can be likened to that of cancer patients.

Any of several cofactors or comorbidities may influence the expression of pain in HIV-infected persons. Certainly substance abuse may complicate the expression of pain and its treatment. Interestingly, the few studies evaluating HIV-infected substance abusers found no significant differences in number of reports of pain or the intensity of reported pain from those of HIV-infected persons without a history of substance abuse. Despite this, substance abusers were far less likely to receive adequate treatment for their pain syndromes. The perception of drug-seeking behavior appeared to form a barrier to the effective treatment of disease-related discomfort for this group of HIV-infected persons (1). Similarly, HIV-infected persons with a history of psychiatric disorders are likely to be undertreated for their pain syndromes, because the patient may be unable to convince the medical provider of the validity of reported pain or to communicate a lack of treatment effect or both. Furthermore, depression, which frequently accompanies progressive HIV disease, can fundamentally affect the severity of reported pain. HIV-infected persons who rank high on depression measurement tools tend to report more intense pain. Similarly, social factors can also influence the incidence and intensity of pain. Isolation from friends, lovers, and family can increase reported pain, although these factors can be hard to isolate from depression. Finally, financial concerns may influence the reports of pain, particularly when these financial concerns threaten the livelihood of dependents.

Despite the recognition of the significant harm pain works upon the quality of life of HIV-infected persons, the primary and specialty care providers who manage these patients are woefully remiss in providing adequate analgesia to meet the demands of pain control for these patients. McCormack et al. (1a) found 60 to 70% of AIDS patients reported severe pain. However, 40% of those reporting such pain were receiving no treatment, and only 60% of those receiving treatment found the analgesia adequate to control pain. Similarly, Breitbart et al. (1b) described the analgesia offered HIV-infected patients in severe pain (8 to 10 on a 10-point scale). Some 25% received no therapy; 40%, nonsteroidals only; and only 6% received strong opioids for pain relief. What, then, are the reasons for the failure to recognize and treat pain in HIV-infected persons? Roughly, these reasons can be broken down into two categories: patient- and physician-related barriers.

Patient-Related Barriers

Every physician recognizes the patient who despite all evidence to the contrary insists that he or she adheres to all prescribed therapy. Not really intending to deceive, the patient is simply attempting to please the physician, to be a "good patient." Similarly, HIV-infected patients may be reluctant to admit to pain, particularly if they believe the physician has negative feelings about those seeking pain control. Conversely, the patient may be reluctant because of a belief that such complaints are a sign of weakness. We have found this latter case to be particularly prominent among women with families. They do not wish to give an impression that their ability to parent is in any way compromised. Patients may have a heightened fear of opioid use, particularly in the age of combination therapy. Rather than risk drug interaction or intolerance, they may eschew the use of analgesia completely. Furthermore, the usually unwarranted fear of addiction prevents many patients from seeking pain relief. A prior episode of increasing tolerance to analgesia may play in to this fear. Sedation or the fear of impairment of mental faculties leads some patients not to seek or to refuse treatment for pain. This seems true particularly for persons who continue employment despite progressive HIV disease. Finally, a small number of patients refuse treatment because of a real or imagined fear of crime. We have seen this patient-related barrier to pain control most frequently in homeless or unstably housed HIV-infected persons. Those living on the streets or in shelters may indeed be at increased risk for assault and injury if in possession of opioid pain relievers.

Physician-Related Barriers

The foremost barrier to effective management of HIV-related pain by a treating physician is ignorance. Failure to understand the prevalence of pain in AIDS patients or an inadequate grasp of the essentials of pain management in this patient population are likely the greatest physician-related barriers to effective pain control in HIV-infected persons. Misconceptions about the potential for abuse or the risk of addiction can be included in the lack of understanding that may impair effective pain control. These irrational fears of habituation should never be allowed to stand in the way of effective palliative care for the terminally ill AIDS patient. Recently concern about the interaction of analgesics with the protease inhibitors or nonnucleoside reverse transcriptase inhibitors has become a potential barrier to pain management in some HIV-infected patients. Clinicians must be constantly aware of the goals of therapy and focus upon the overall quality of life while prescribing medications to prolong quantity of life. Finally, fractionation of care among several medical providers may lead to miscommunication and misunderstanding. This may result in prejudice against the legitimate analgesia needs of the HIV-infected patient. This is true particularly when dealing with patients who are frequently undertreated for the pain of AIDS or cancer-women, injection drug users, the less educated, or persons with severe pain. The value of a single, involved medical provider who understands a patient and his or her pain threshold cannot be overstated.

SELECTION OF ANALGESIC THERAPY

The selection of analgesic therapy is based on the interplay of the intensity of each patient's pain and current analgesic therapy. Pain intensity can be measured on a written or verbal number rating scale (1c, 2). Pain that is rated 5 or higher on a scale of 0 to 10 can interfere with the quality of life and is defined as substantial pain (3). Pain ratings of 1 to 4 correspond to mild pain; 5 to 6, to moderate pain; and 7 to 10, to severe pain. The three-step analgesic ladder of the World Health Organization (WHO) uses these three categories of pain to guide analgesic drug therapy (4) (Figure 28.1).

Patients receiving no analgesic therapy who have mild to moderate pain should be treated with nonopioid analgesic drugs (step 1). These drugs include acetaminophen, aspirin, and other nonsteroidal anti-inflammatory drugs (NSAIDs). The dose of the nonopioid analgesic should be maximized if possible before a step 2 opioid analgesic is added. The dose of acetaminophen should not exceed 4 g/day to prevent liver damage (5). Patients taking any NSAID should be monitored for gastropathy, renal failure, hepatic dysfunction, and bleeding (6). The risk of bleeding problems can be minimized by using nonacetylated salicylates, such as choline magnesium trisalicylate, which do not interfere with platelet function (7). Gastric distress maybe ameliorated by the use of a histamine H_2 antagonist or sucralfate (8). Misoprostol is also effective in preventing asymptomatic NSAID-induced gastric ulceration (9).

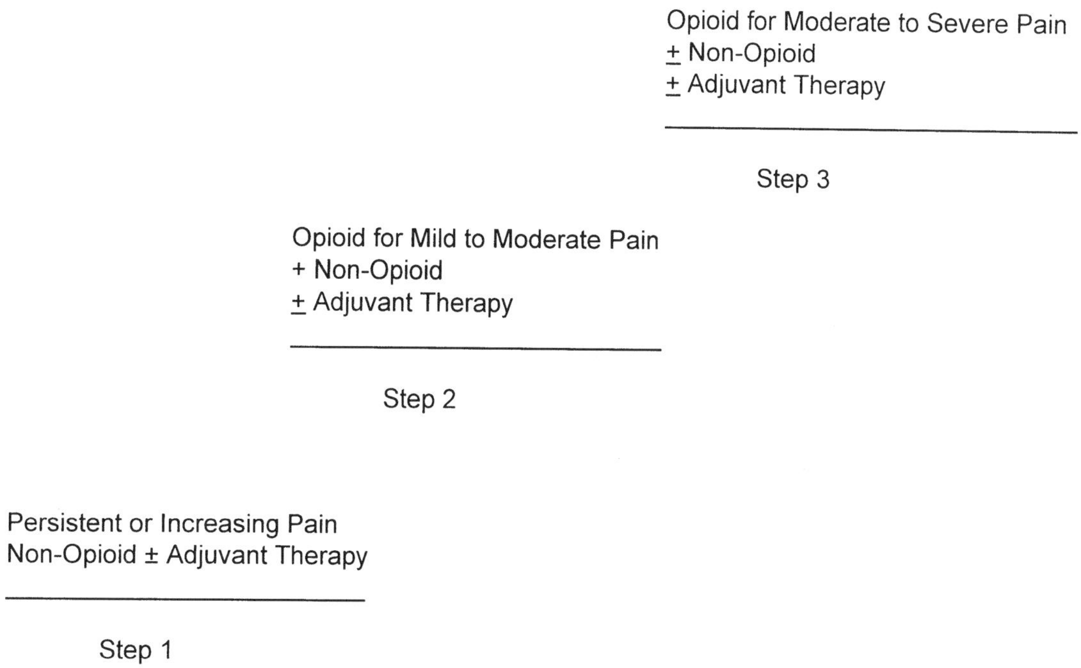

Opioid for Moderate to Severe Pain
± Non-Opioid
± Adjuvant Therapy

Step 3

Opioid for Mild to Moderate Pain
+ Non-Opioid
± Adjuvant Therapy

Step 2

Persistent or Increasing Pain
Non-Opioid ± Adjuvant Therapy

Step 1

Figure 28.1   Three-step analgesic ladder of the World Health Organization (4).

The step opioids used to treat moderate pain include codeine, dihydrocodeine, hydrocodone, oxycodone, and propoxyphene. Step 2 opioids may be restricted to the treatment of moderate pain because of dose-limiting side effects or because they are prepared in fixed combinations with nonopioid analgesics. Propoxyphene is not recommended for routine use because of its long half-life and the risk of accumulation of norpropoxyphene, a toxic metabolite (10). The value of codeine is limited by the increasing incidence of side effects at doses above 1.5 mg/kg of body weight (11). Oxycodone is available as a short-acting tablet and a sustained release tablet, which may allow greater flexibility and usefulness.

Step 3 opioids, commonly prescribed for the relief of moderate to severe pain, include morphine, oxycodone, hydromorphone, and fentanyl. These opioids should be used one at a time to capitalize on idiosyncratic differences in patient's responses (12, 13). Morphine is the most commonly used to control severe pain because of its wide availability, varied formulations, and well-characterized pharmacological properties (10, 14). Sustained-release formulations of morphine for oral administration at 8- or 12-hour intervals are the mainstay of the control of chronic cancer pain because of the ease of their administration and titration (15, 16). Hydromorphone's advantage is that it is six times as soluble in aqueous solutions as morphine and five times as potent (17). Fentanyl transdermal patches can control chronic stable pain for up to 72 hours for those who cannot tolerate oral medications (18). Methadone and levorphanol may also be considered for relief of severe pain but are not recommended for initial therapy because of their long half-lives and the risk of drug accumulation (10, 11).

Opioids not recommended for use in the control of moderate to severe pain include meperidine, buprenorphine, pentazocine, butorphanol, dezocine, and nalbuphine. Meperidine should not be used because it has a short half-life and its metabolite, normeperidine, can cause seizures (10, 14). Partial opioid agonists such as buprenorphine offer limited benefit because of their low maximal efficacy. Above a certain dose adverse effects outweigh analgesic benefits (10, 14). Mixed opioid agonist-antagonists such as pentazocine, butorphanol, dezocine, and nalbuphine are not recommended because of their low maximal efficacy and their potential to reverse analgesia and to cause physical withdrawal by patients already receiving an agonist, such as morphine or methadone (10, 14). There is no one optimal or maximal dose of a step 3 opioid analgesic drug (10, 11, 14). The appropriate dose is one that relieves the patient's pain throughout its dosing interval without causing unmanageable adverse effects. The initial dose should be based on the patient's level of pain and the efficacy of prior analgesic therapy. Subsequent therapy should be based on assessment of the efficacy of therapy, with dosage titrated upward as needed. When switching from one opioid analgesic drug to another, one must know the equianalgesic equivalences between one drug and another and between one route and another (14).

ROUTE OF ADMINISTRATION

Most patients with chronic pain should receive oral analgesic therapy, because it is simpler, easier to use, and less expensive than parenteral administration (10, 19). If a patient cannot swallow tablets or liquids, morphine concentrates and soluble

Table 28.1.   Equlanalgesic Dosing Table for Opioids

Step 2	Approximate Oral Dose	Approximate Parenteral Dose	Starting Dose >50kg (oral)	Starting Dose <50kg (oral)
Codeine	130 mg q 3–4 hr	75 mg q 3–4 hr	60 mg q 3–4 hr	0.5–1 mg/kg q 3–4 hr
Hydrocodone with acetaminophen (Vicodin, Lortab)	30 mg q 3–4 hr	Not available	10 mg q 30–4 hr	0.2 mg/kg q 3–4 hr
Oxycodone with acetaminophen (Roxicet, Percocet, Percodan) plain tablets or sustained-release tablets (oxycontin)	30 mg q 3–4 hr	Not available	10 mg q 3–4 hr	0.2 mg/kg q 3–4 hr
Step 3				
Morphine (Roxanol) Sustained-release tablets (MS Contin, Oramorph)	30 mg q 3–4 hr	10 mg q 3–4 hr	30 mg q 3–4 hr	0.15 mg/kg q 3–4 hr
Hydromorphine (Dilaudid)	7.5 mg q 3–4 hr	1.5 mg q 3–4 hr	6 mg q 3–4 hr	0.03–0.08 mg/kg q 3–4 hr
Methadone	20 mg q 8 hr	10 mg q 8 hr	20 mg q 8 hr	0.2 mg/kg q 8 hr
Levorpanol (Leo-Dromoran)	4 mg q 8 hr	2mg q 8 hr	4 mg q 8 hr	0.04 mg/kg q 8 hr
Fentanyl (Sublimaze) transdermal patch (Duragesic) Oral Transmucosal (Oralet)	Not available	0.1 mg continuous IV infusion or 25 mg q 72 hr transdermal	200 mg	200 mg

tablets can be administered sublingually or as a suppository (10, 11, 14). These routes may have their limitation due to frequency of administration (e.g., every 3 to 4 hours). Fentanyl can be administered via an oral transmucosal system or transdermal for patients unable to tolerate oral administrations (19). Hydromorphone may also be administered rectally via suppository (19). Subcutaneous or intravenous administration of morphine, hydromorphone, or fentanyl is preferred to transdermal administration of fentanyl in patients unable to take oral medications for 24 to 48 hours, patients with frequent episodes of incidental pain, and patients with acute, severe pain in which injections or infusions facilitate an escalating dosage. Since bioavailability of parenteral and oral opioids differs (Table 28.1), dosages must be changed when routes are switched. Patient-controlled analgesia (PCA) pumps may expedite pain relief. Intramuscular opioid therapy is not recommended, because it is painful and hard for family caregivers to administer (19).

APPROPRIATE DOSING INTERVALS

Analgesic drugs should be scheduled at intervals that prevent the recurrence of pain and minimize the number of daily doses. The appropriate dosing interval is determined by the opioid used and the route of administration. The analgesic effects of short-acting oral opioids (i.e., morphine, hydromorphone, or oxycodone) begin within 30 minutes of administration and can last up to 4 hours (10, 11). In patients given controlled-release formulation (morphine or oxycodone), peak effects maybe felt in 3 to 4 hours and may last up to 12 hours (20, 21).

The analgesic effect of transdermal fentanyl begins approximately 12 hours after application of the patch, peaks in 24 to 48 hours, and lasts for about 72 hours (18). If the analgesic effect of transdermal fentanyl does not last for 72 hours, the dose should be increased or the patches reapplied every 48 hours. In patients given morphine or hydromorphone subcutaneously, analgesia begins within 10 to 15 minutes and lasts 3 to 4 hours (10). In patients given these opioids intravenously, pain relief should begin within 5 minutes and last for 1 to 2 hours (10).

PREVENTION AND RESCUE

As in all patients with chronic pain, the goal of treating chronic pain in the AIDS patient is not only pain relief but also pain prevention for sustained analgesia (10, 11, 14). In most cases, after the patient has been given a few doses of medication on an as-needed (prn) basis to allow an effective dose to be determined, around-the-clock dosing can be instituted. Supplemental reduced doses of analgesic drugs should be available to patients for breakthrough pain due to activity, stress, or progressive disease (23). Furthermore, the total dose of an as-needed rescue mediation available in a specific interval should be equal to the regular dose given during the interval.

Pain prevention is also an appropriate goal in the treatment of acute moderate to severe pain that is expected to last more than 24 hours. Resolution of the source of the acute pain should be anticipated with regular downward dose titration if the pain is well controlled without the need of additional analgesics. Initial therapy of acute pain that is not expected to last more than 24 hours can consist solely of treatment as needed.

Table 28.2.   Most Commonly Used Anti-Inflammatory Agents

	Dosage Form	Dosage Range	Adverse Effects, Comments
Acetaminophen (Tylenol)	Tablets, capsules, elixir, suppositories	650–1000 mg q 4–6 hr (max 4 g/day)	Monitor liver enzymes; chronic alcoholics may be at increase risk for hepatotoxicity. Does not cause GI ulceration, bleeding; no effects on platelets
Ibuprofen (Motrin)	Tablets, suspension	400–800 mg q 6–8 hr (max 3200 mg/day)	Gastric distress, GI bleeding, ulceration, diarrhea, vomiting, dizziness, renal dysfunction, fluid retention
Indomethacin (Indocin)	Capsules, suppositories, suspension	25–50 mg q 6–12 hr (max 200 mg/day)	See Ibuprofen; also, drowsiness, dizziness, mental confusion, GI distress frequent in doses >100 mg/day
Naproxen (Naprosyn)	Tablets, suspension	250–500 mg q 8–12 hr (max 1500 mg/day)	See Ibuprofen; interstitial nephritis, and nephritic syndrome have been reported

Table 28.3.   Adjuvant Drugs Used in Combination with Analgesic Drugs

Tricylicic antidepressant	25–150 mg q hs	Dry mouth, dizziness, postural hypotension, blurred vision, urinary retention, extrapyramidal syndrome, constipation
Amitriptyline (Elavil)	25–200 mg q hs	
Desipramine (Norpramin)	25–150 mg q hs	
Nortriptyline (Pamelor)		
Carbamazepine (Tegretol)	200–400 mg bid–tid	Therapeutic level 4–12 µg/mL, drowsiness, ataxia, nausea, vomiting, dizziness, bone marrow suppression
Gabapentin (Neurontin)	300 mg tid	Nausea, vomiting, gastrointestinal upset, drowsiness, ataxia
	1800 mg tid	
Clonazepam (Klonopin)	0.5–6 mg tid	Drowsiness, ataxia, mental status changes
Mexiletine (Mexitil)	150–300 bid–tid	Tremor, ataxia, drowsiness, confusion, nausea, vomiting, anorexia
Baclofen (Lioresal)	10–20 mg bid–qid	Drowsiness, ataxia, nausea, vomiting

MANAGEMENT OF ADVERSE EFFECTS OF ANALGESICS

Pain prevention must be accompanied by the prevention of adverse effects. Unavoidable adverse effects require specific therapy and may require a trial of other opioids (24) or anesthesiological or surgical intervention. All patients receiving around-the-clock opioid therapy need regular laxative therapy, such as a stool softener and a bowel stimulant (i.e., docusate sodium and sennosides) (25). Opioid-associated nausea is often caused by constipation but may require treatment with centrally acting antiemetic drugs such as prochlorperazine or haloperidol (10, 11, 14). Sedation and cognitive impairment can usually be managed by allowing time for tolerance to develop after therapy is initiated or the dose is escalated and by the use of opioid-sparing, nonsedating drugs in combination with analgesic agents (Tables 28.2 and 28.3) (10, 11, 14). Persistent sedation and cognitive dysfunction due primarily to opioid analgesia can be reduced by dose reduction, switching to another opioid, or the use of caffeine (26), methylphenidate (27) or stronger sympathomimetics. Opioid-induced myoclonic jerks may be managed by dose reduction, switching to another opioid, or the use of clonazepam (28). Appropriate titration of opioid dosage rarely results in respiratory depression or cardiovascular collapse (10, 14). If life-threatening complications occur, naloxone should be administered and subsequent doses of opioids should be withheld or reduced (10, 11, 14).

ADJUVANT THERAPY

Adjuvant drug therapy enhances the analgesic efficacy of opioids, treats concurrent symptoms that exacerbate pain, and produces independent analgesia for specific types of pain. The early use of adjuvant drugs is aimed at optimizing the patient's comfort and function by preventing or reducing the toxic effects of opioids. The agents most commonly used in adjuvant therapy for chronic pain are NSAIDs, tricyclic antidepressants, and anticonvulsant agents.

NSAIDs are effective in the treatment of pain from bone metastasis, soft-tissue infiltration, arthritis, serositis, and recent surgery (11). Beyond their value as step 1 nonopioid analgesics, NSAIDs can enhance the efficacy of opioid analgesics in patients with inflammatory based pain.

Tricyclic antidepressant drugs are used at the first-line adjuvant therapy for neuropathic pain and may also improve underlying depression and insomnia (10, 29). Amitriptyline is the most widely used drug of this class, but its sedative and anticholinergic adverse effects may be dose limiting (29, 30). Desipramine and nortriptyline cause less sedative and anticholinergic adverse effects. Low doses of these agents should be administered at night to maximize tolerated doses and efficacy. Serum drug levels can be used to assess compliance, detect altered metabolism, and minimize toxicity. Venlafaxine (31) has shown some promise as an adjuvant for neuropathic pain.

An anticonvulsant drug can be useful in patients with neuropathic, lancinating, or ticlike pains (10, 11, 14, 32, 33) and may be added to a tricyclic antidepressant drug for neuropathic pains that are incompletely relieved by several days or weeks of full dose antidepressant therapy. An anticonvulsant may be used alone in patients who cannot tolerate antidepressant drug therapy. Carbamazepine (33, 34), gabapentin (35, 36), and clonazepam (37) are the anticonvulsants most commonly used for neuropathic pain.

Patients with neuropathic pain not responding to maximized doses of either a tricyclic antidepressant or an anticonvulsant and those who cannot tolerate these drugs may benefit from the use of mexiletine (38, 39) or baclofen (40). Other drugs possibly used as an adjuvant for neuropathic pain based on anecdotal reports are lamotrigine (41) and flecainide.

DRUG-DRUG INTERACTIONS

Polypharmacy is a reality in treating HIV infection. There are various mechanisms of drug-drug interactions, including alterations in drug absorption, inhibition or induction of the cytochrome P-450 system, alterations in renal elimination, and pharmacodynamic interactions. Since the advent of protease inhibitors and nonnucleoside reverse transcriptase inhibitors (NNRTI), the cytochrome P-450 system is probably one of the most important causes of drug-drug interactions (42) (Tables 28.4 and 28.5). The specific cytochrome P-450 isoenzymes that are affected by each agent determine the agents that may interact with the protease inhibitor or NNRTI (43). For an individual patient, these interactions are often difficult to predict, since enzymes are not affected to the same degree with various drugs. There is also variation from person to person. Specific dosage recommendations are often not available. Monitoring patients carefully is the key to managing drug interactions (44).

28.4.   Drug–Drug Interactions with Protease Inhibitors

Protease Inhibitors	Analgesics	Antidepressants	Other Drugs
Ritonavir (Norvir)	Fentanyl	Amitriptyline	Mexiletine
	*Meperidine	Desipramine	Carbamazepine
	Methadone	Nortriptyline	
	*Propoxyphene		
Saquinavir (Invirase)			*Carbamazepine
Indinavir (Crixivan)			Carbamazepine
Nelfinavir (Viracep)			Carbamazepine

*Indicated drug should not be used with specific medication. Other drugs should be used with additional caution, dosage adjustment, or monitoring for either toxicity or reduced efficacy.

Table 28.5.   Nonnucleoside Reverse Transcriptase Inhibitors

Protease Inhibitor	Other Drug
Delavirdine (Rescriptor)	*Carbamazepine
Nevirapine (Viramune)	

*Indicated drug should not be used with specific medication. Other drugs should be used with additional caution, dosage adjustment, or monitoring for either toxicity or reduced efficacy.

References

1. Breitbart W, Rosenfeld B, Passik S, et al. A comparison of pain report and adequacy of analgesic therapy in ambulatory AIDS patients with or without a history of substance abuse. Pain 1997;72:235–243.

1a. McCormack J, Li R, Zarowny D. Inadequate treatment of pain in ambulatory HIV patients. Clin J Pain 1993;9:279–283.

1b. Breitbart W, Rosenfeld BD, Passik SD, et al. The undertreatment of pain in ambulatory AIDS patients. Pain 1996;65:243–249.

1c. Au C, Loppinzi CL, Dhodapicar M, et al. Use of a verbal pain scale improves the understanding of oncology in-patient pain intensity. J Clin Oncol 1994;12:2751–2755.

2. Fishman B, Pasternak S, Wallenstein SL, et al. A valid instrument for the evaluation of cancer pain. Cancer 1987;60:1151–1158.

3. Serlin RC, Mendoza TR, Nakamura Y, et al. What is cancer pain, mild, moderate or severe? Grading pain severity by its interference with function. Pain 1995;61:277–284.

4. Cancer pain relief and palliative care: Report of a WHO Expert Committee. WHO Tech PEP Ser 1990;804:1–73.

5. Strom BL. Adverse reactions to over the counter analgesics taken for therapeutic purposes. JAMA 1994;272:1366–1367.

6. Eisenberg E, Berkey CS, Carr BD, et al. Efficacy and safety of nonsteroidal anti-inflammatory drugs for cancer pain: a meta-analysis. J Clin Oncol 1994;12:2756–2765.

7. Stuart JJ, Pisico EJ. Choline magnesium trisalicylate does not impair platelet aggregation. Pharmatherapeutics 1981;2:547–551.

8. Hollander D. Gastrointestinal complications of non-steroidal anti-inflammatory drugs: prophylactic and therapeutic strategies. Am J Med 1994;96:274–281.

9. Valentin M, Cannizaro R, Poletti M, et al. Non-steroidal anti-inflammatory drugs for cancer pain: comparison between misoprostol and ranitidine in prevention of upper gastrointestinal damage. J Clin Oncol 995;13:2637–2642.

10. Twycross R. Pain relief in advanced cancer. London: Churchill Livingstone, 1994.

11. Levy MH. Pharmacologic management of cancer pain. Semin Oncol 1994;21:718–739.

12. Galer BJ, Cone N, Pasternak GW, Portenoy RF. Individual variability in the response to different opioids: report of five cases. Pain 1992;49:87–91.

13. MacDonald N, Der L, Allan S, Champion P. Opioid hyperexcitability: The application of alternate opioid therapy. Pain 1993;53:353–355.

14. Cherny NI, Portenoy RF. The management of cancer pain. CA Cancer J Clin 1994;44:2263–2303.

15. Thirwell MP, Sloan PA, Maroun JA, et al. Pharmacokinetics and clinical efficacy of oral morphine solution and controlled-released morphine tablets in cancer patients. Cancer 1989;63(Suppl):2275–2283.

16. Finn JW, Walsh TD, MacDonald N, et al. Placebo-blinded study of morphine sulfate solution-release tablets and immediate-release morphine solution in outpatients with chronic pain due to advance cancer. J Clin Oncol 1993;11:973–978.

17. Roy SD, Flynn GL. Solubility and related physiochemical properties of narcotic analgesics. Pharm Res 1988;5:580–586.

18. Payne R. Transdermal fentanyl: suggested recommendations for clinic use. J Pain Symptom Mgmt 1992;7(Suppl):S40–S44.

19. Principles of analgesic use in the treatment of acute pain and chronic Pain. 4th ed. Skokie, IL: American Pain Society, 1995.

20. Thirwell MP, Sloan PA, Maroun JA, et al. Pharmacokinetics and clinical efficacy of oral morphine solution and controlled-release morphine tablets in cancer patients. Cancer 1989;3(Suppl):2275–83.

21. Sunshine A, Olson NZ, Colon A, et al. Onset and duration of analgesia for controlled release vs. immediate release oxycodone alone or in combination with acetaminophen in postoperative pain. Can Pharmacol Ther 1995;57:137 (abstract).

22. Deleted.

23. Portenoy RF, Hagen NA. Breakthrough pain: definition, prevalence and characteristics. Pain 1990;41:73–81.

24. De Stutz ND, Bruera E, Suarez-Almazor M. Opioid rotation for toxicity reduction in terminal cancer patients. J Pain Symptom Mgmt 1995;10:378–384.

25. Levy MH. Constipation and diarrhea in cancer patients. Cancer Bull 1991;43:412–422.

26. Sanynok, J, Yaksh TL. Caffeine as an analgesic adjuvant: A review of pharmacology and mechanisms of action. Pharmacol Rev 1993;45:43–85.

27. Bruera E, Brennels C, Paterson AH, MacDonald RN. Use of methylphenidate as an adjuvant to narcotic analgesics in patients with advance cancer. J Pain Symptom Mgmt 1989;4:3–6.

28. Eisele JH, Grigsby EJ, Dsa G. Clonazepam treatment of myoclonic contractions associated with high-dose opioids: case report. Pain 1992;49:231–232.

29. Watson CPN. Antidepressant drugs at adjuvant analgesics. J Pain Symptom Mgmt 1994;9:392–405.

30. Potter WZ, Rudorfer MV, Manji J. The pharmacologic treatment of depression. N Engl J Med 1991;325:633–642.

31. McQuay HJ, Tramer M, Nye BA, et al. A systematic review of antidepressants for neuropathic pain. Pain 1996;68:217–227.

32. McQuay HJ. Pharmacological treatment of neuralgic and neuropathic pain. In: Hanks GW, ed. Cancer survey series: advances and prospects in clinical, epidemiological and laboratory oncology, vol 7, no 1. Pain and cancer. Oxford, UK: Oxford University Press, 1988: 141–159.

33. Galer BA. Neuropathic pain of peripheral origin: Advances in pharmacologic treatment. Neurology 1995;45(Suppl 9):S17–S25.

34. Wilton TD. Tegretol in the treatment of diabetic neuropathy. S Afr Med J 1974;48:869–871.

35. Mellick GA, Mellicy LB, Mellick LB. Gabapentin in the management of reflex sympathetic dystrophy. J Pain Symptom Mgmt 1995; 10:265–266.

36. Rosner H, Rubin L, Kestenbaum A. Gabapentin adjunctive therapy in neuropathic pain stress. Clin J Pain 1996;12:56–58.

37. Reddy S, Patt RB. Benzodiazepines as adjuvant analgesics. J Pain Symptom Mgmt 1994;9:510–514.

38. Dejgard A, Peterson P, Kastrup J. Mexiletine for treatment of chronic pain diabetic neuropathy. Lancet 1988;1:9–11.

39. Fross RD. Mexiletine, an oral local anesthetic for treatment of neuropathic pain. Neurology 1992;42(Suppl 3):152 (abstract 96P).

40. Fromm GH. Ballopen as a adjuvant analgesic. J Pain Symptom Mgmt 1994;9:500–509.

41. Mackin GA. Medical and pharmacological management of upper extremity neuropathic pain syndrome. J Hand Ther 1997;10:96–109.

42. Aeschliman J, Tyler L. Understanding drug interactions associated with CYP enzymes. (University of Utah Drug Information Service) Adverse Drug Reaction News 1996;9:1–8.

43. Van Cleef GF, Fisher EJ, Polk RE. Drug interaction potential with inhibitors of HIV protease. Pharmacotherapy 1997;17:774–778.

44. Tseng LT, Folsy MM. Management of drug interactions in patients with HIV. Ann Pharmacother 1997;31:1040–1058.

CHAPTER 29

Assessment and Management of Patients with Sickle Cell-Related Pain

Richard Payne

SICKLE CELL HEMOGLOBINOPATHIES: BASIC CONCEPTS

Sickle cell anemia was identified in the Unites States by Herrick (1), who observed sickle-shaped red blood cells (RBCs) in an anemic African-American medical student in Chicago. Pain is a cardinal feature of this disease, which is caused by an abnormal hemoglobin that is inherited in an autosomal recessive manner (2, 3).

Normal adult hemoglobin contains two α- and two β-globin protein chains (HbA$^{\alpha2}\beta_2$). Sickle hemoglobin (HbSS$^{\alpha2\beta2\ 6\ glu\rightarrow val}$) consists of two normal α-chains, and the substitution of glutamic acid for valine in the sixth amino acid position of the β-chain. As a result of this single amino acid substitution, this altered hemoglobin polymerizes into rigid tubules and assumes a sickled appearance in the presence of deoxygenated blood. These sickled cells are more rigid and become trapped in small capillaries and occlude the microcirculation, causing pain, infarction, and end organ failure (4). Also, abnormal interactions between the sickled erythrocyte and the endothelial cell surface have been implicated as an important component of the pathogenesis in the vaso-occlusive crises (VOC) (5).

By contrast, fetal hemoglobin (hemoglobin F, or HbF) contains two α- and two γ-globin protein chains (α_2,γ_2). This, the predominant hemoglobin in the fetus, persists into the first few months of life. HbF inhibits the polymerization of deoxyhemoglobin S (6); therefore, the clinical manifestations of sickle cell disease does not occur until several months after birth, when HbF declines to less than 30% of total hemoglobin. In addition, therapies that increase the production of HbF, such as hydroxyurea administration, are now known to be important in the treatment of sickle cell anemia (7, 8).

In parts of Africa and the Mediterranean basin, 20 to 40% of the population is homozygous recessive for the sickle cell gene and thus have the disease. The hemoglobin S genotype may impart some protection against malaria (9), and this is cited as the teleological explanation for its presence and persistence in man. Estimates are that about 0.2% of African-Americans have sickle cell anemia and about 8% are heterozygotes, having the HbSA genotype, or the sickle cell "trait". The HbSA phenotype is almost always asymptomatic except in high altitudes, in which oxygen tension is low (9). Approximately 1 in 500 African-American and 1 in 1000 Hispanic-American newborns have sickle cell anemia (9).

CLINICAL CHARACTERISTICS OF DISEASE

Pain and Associated Complications

Although pain characterizes sickle cell disease, there is much variability in the timing, severity, and frequency of painful occurrences. In general, approximately 20% of patients have pain only rarely; 60% have one or two episodes each year; and 20% have more than two episodes of pain per month, and are considered severely affected. In the adult population, the typical VOC is a relatively unpredictable event that occurs within periods of relative good health and well-being. Pain is usually present in the bone, chest, and abdomen. Children may have a particular complication, sickle cell dactylitis, most likely caused by avascular necrosis of the marrow, producing painful swelling in the hands and feet. Dactylitis may be precipitated by cold (10), and almost never occurs after 4 or 5 years of age. Recurrent splenic infarction in children will produces abdominal pain, and when the spleen is destroyed, there is a specific vulnerability to pneumococcal infections (11).

Other manifestations of the disease in children and adults include aplastic and megaloblastic crises, sequestration crises (i.e., sudden massive pooling of RBCs, especially in the spleen), hemolytic crises, osteomyelitis (especially *Salmonella typhinurium*), priapism, renal failure, jaundice, and hepatomegaly, ischemic leg ulceration, stroke, and a host of other ischemic manifestations in every organ (9).

Table 29.1.   Factors Influencing Frequency of Vaso-occlusive Crises

Increased frequency of vaso-occlusive crises
  Cold weather
  Young men (15–25 years old)
  Pregnancy, especially third trimester
Decreased frequency of vaso-occlusive crises
  Presence of α-thalassemia[a]
  Elevated Hb F levels (> 30% total hemoglobin)
  RBC membrane polymorphisms (inhibit aggregation to vascular endothelium) (15)

---

[a]Thalassemia is another type of hemoglobinopathy in which there is a defect in the synthesis of one or more globin chains. (14)

Table 29.2.   Causes of Death in Patients with Sickle Cell Anemia

Causes of Death
  Pulmonary fat embolism
  Acute multiorgan system failure
  Acute chest syndrome
  Renal failure
  Seizures
Factors Associated with Risk of Early Death
  Persistent leukocytosis
  Depressed Hb F levels

Pain associated with VOC can be quite severe. Ballas et al. (12) measured pain by visual analogue scales in 23 patients admitted for 60 VOC episodes (12). The average admission pain score was 9.5 cm on a 10-cm scale, and the most frequent sites of pain were back, legs, knees, arms, chest, and abdomen. These findings are consistent with surveys in other adult populations in which bone pain alone or in combination with abdominal visceral pain was the most common site of pain. For example, in a survey of 117 adult patients with sickle cell anemia, 47 had bone pain alone, 36 had bone and visceral pain, and only 6 patients did not report any pain during the 32-month period of the survey (13). I also reported a case of a 29-year-old man who required doses of morphine up to 40 mg/hour during a 6-day VOC episode (13), confirming that severe pain and relatively high opioid doses are required for treatment by some patients. A one month-long survey of 8 inpatient admissions for VOC (representing 9 VOC episodes) found that the episode averaged 7.9 days (range 2 to 22 days) and patients required an average dose of 459.8 mg intravenous morphine sulfate equivalents per day (range 30 to 890 mg/day) for treatment of pain. Factors that appear to precipitate VOC and modify the number of episodes over time are listed in Table 29.1 (14).

The acute chest syndrome is an important variant or complication of a VOC (16, 17). This syndrome consists of chest wall pain, with or without fever, and a pulmonary infiltrate. Usually no infection is discoverable, and recently lung or rib infarction, with associated pleuritis and chest splinting has been cited as an important cause of this sometimes fatal syndrome. An association between acute chest syndrome and increased mortality in children receiving morphine infusions has been reported (18), and many experts view acute chest syndrome as an ominous finding during a VOC. The development of chronic lung disease is also increased in patients with repeated episodes of the acute chest syndrome.

A recent large national study identified the incidence and risk factors for acute chest syndrome (17). This study evaluated 3,751 patients over at least 2 years, representing more than 19,000 patient-years of observations, and found the incidence of acute chest syndrome to be higher in children than in adults, and in patients with HbSS disease than in HbSC disease. There is an inverse correlation between HbF levels and incidence of the acute chest syndrome. Adults with acute chest syndrome had a higher mortality rate than does who did not.

The *judicious* use of opioids with care to avoid hypoventilation and the exacerbation of intravascular sickling secondary to low oxygen saturation is particularly important in this circumstance. Aggressive respiratory treatments, especially the use of incentive spirometry to minimized and treat pulmonary atelectasias, has been advocated as an effective way to manage this syndrome (16).

Life Expectancy and Causes of Death in Sickle Cell Anemia

Advances in supportive care have increased the likelihood of survival for most patients with sickle cell anemia. The median survival of patients with sickle cell anemia increased from 14.3 years in 1973 to 42 to 48 years in the 1990s (14, 19). The widespread use of penicillin and pneumococcal vaccines to prevent and treat the *Streptococcus pneumoniae* sepsis, which can disseminate in asplenic persons, is acknowledged to be a major cause of this increased survival. In fact, before the widespread use of these two agents in the 1970s, 20% of the deaths of sickle cell patients came in the first 2 years of life, many related to infectious complications.

A recent study investigating the natural history of sickle cell disease in the United States evaluated 3764 patients aged less than 1 year to 65 years and studied the circumstances of death in 209 adult patients (19). The sickle hemoglobinopathy variant, HbSC (HbSC$^{[\alpha2\ \beta2\ 6\ glu\rightarrow lys]}$) is associated with a longer life expectancy than was HbSS, 60 to 68 years in the former versus 42 to 48 years in the latter. Causes of death are listed in Table 29.2. A third of deaths occurred during a VOC in the absence of otherwise life-threatening organ failure, and 18% of all deaths were a result of subacute or chronic organ failure, usually renal or hepatic (19). Adult patients with more than three VOC episodes per year had only a 50% chance of survival to age 40, whereas patients with fewer than one VOC episode per year had a 50% chance of survival to age 55 (19).

MANAGEMENT OF PAIN IN SICKLE CELL ANEMIA

Management of Acute Pain in Vaso-Occlusive Crises

A flow chart illustrating the management of patients with VOC in sickle cell diseases is listed in Figure 29.1. Standard

treatment approaches to the management of a VOC episode include intravenous hydration, oxygen inhalation, and parenteral analgesics (opioids and non-opioids). Although "standard" protocol in most emergency rooms and hospitals calls for intravenous hydration, some experts have argued that this is unnecessary, since most patients are not dehydrated at the

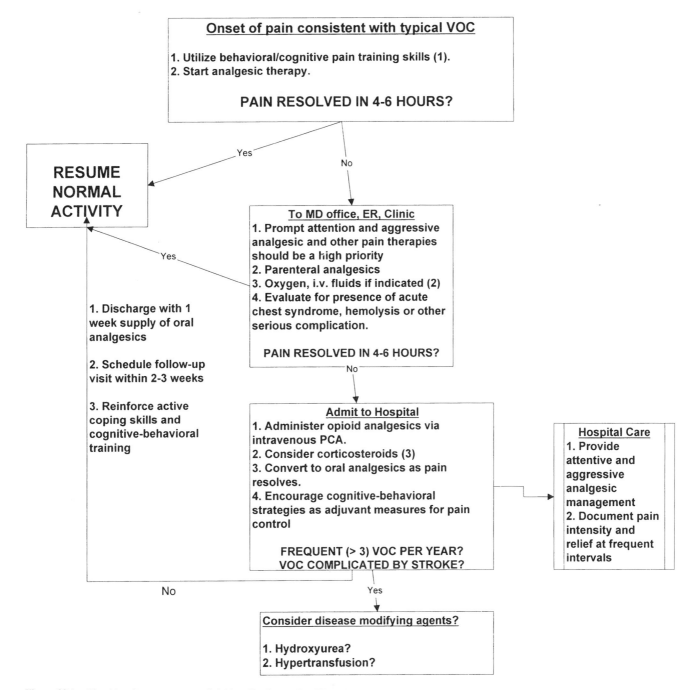

Figure 29.1   Algorithm for management of sickle cell pain. (1) See Gil et al. (20) for discussion of cognitive-behavioral therapies for sickle cell pain. (2) A recent controlled trial indicates that 50% oxygen inhalation did not decrease duration of pain, analgesic consumption, or length of hospitalization (21). (3) A recent controlled trial evaluated the effect of methylprednisolone added to intravenous opioids versus placebo and intravenous opioids and showed that the steroid-treated group had shorter duration of VOC (22).

initiation of the VOC episode. However, an intravenous line is often needed for the administration of parenteral analgesics for rapid titration of opioid analgesics when pain is severe. Recent papers have argued that acute and chronic sickle cell pain should be managed according to principles similar to those for management of cancer pain (2, 3, 23). In fact there are many similarities and dissimilarities between sickle cell and cancer-related pain, as noted in Table 29.3.

Oral Opioids in the Management of Acute and Chronic Sickle Cell-Related Pain

Oral morphine administration has been advocated for the management of acute pain in sickle cell anemia (25) as a way to control pain without the need for emergency department visits or even inpatient admission. Brookoff and Polomono (23) reported on the use of intravenous and oral morphine protocol in an emergency department. They observed that the need for inpatient admissions decreased by 44%, and the number of repeat emergency department visits decreased by 67%. This protocol provided for the initiation of intravenous morphine followed by oral controlled-release morphine. This treatment strategy was modeled after treatment paradigms for cancer pain (23). Similarly, Conti (26) et al. also reported a reduction in emergency department visits following the institution of a oral morphine analgesic protocol for acute sickle cell management (26).

Teresi et al. (27) reported a randomized controlled trial in which oral sustained-release morphine was compared with continuous intravenous morphine using a double-dummy technique to maintain double blinding and showed that the therapies were comparable in a small number of inpatients being treated for acute pain. Larger prospective trials are needed to confirm the role of oral analgesics in the management of acute VOC in the home and hospital emergency department or clinic.

GUIDELINES FOR ANALGESIC USE IN ACUTE AND CHRONIC SICKLE CELL PAIN

Pharmacological management of sickle cell pain is similar to cancer pain management, and the three-step analgesic ladder and other basic guidelines for pharmacological management of pain are entirely applicable (28). Because bone pain is a particularly prominent feature of VOC, much interest has centered on the use of nonsteroidal anti-inflammatory analgesics, especially ketorolac tromethamine, which can be administered parenterally. However, a controlled trial in which patients were randomized to ketorolac 60 mg intramuscular versus placebo (with meperidine rescue doses available in either arm) could not demonstrate a difference in meperidine use between the placebo and ketorolac group (29). Although it is still widely used, there is much evidence that meperidine is associated with signs of central nervous system excitability, including seizures, in the sickle cell population, just as in the cancer population. In fact, given the degree of renal impairment associated with sickle cell anemia, these

Table 29.3.   Comparison of Sickle Cell and Cancer Pain Patients

Similarities
  Clinical models of acute and chronic pain in man
  Opioid analgesics accepted medical therapy
  Pain often an indicator of disease severity
Differences
  Nearly lifelong experience of pain and exposure to opioid analgesics in patients with sickle cell anemia
  High frequency of episodic (often emergency department) care in sickle cell anemia
    Pain management may occur less often by consistent provider in sickle cell patients
    Cancer patients often have defined clinical services, specific inpatient floors and nursing staffs, and a relatively small number of house staff and attending staff who are involved with care
  Sickle cell pain affecting almost exclusively African-American and other minority populations
    Race and ethnicity may influence analgesic prescribing (24)
  No consensus on the value of chronic maintenance opioid therapy in sickle cell pain, unlike the case with cancer pain, in which this is accepted medical practice

patients may be even more vulnerable to the accumulation of normeperidine, which is eliminated by renal excretion (30).

Once patients are admitted to the hospital, many experts recommend the use of intravenous opioid administration via patient-controlled analgesia (PCA) (Fig. 29.1). Schecter et al. (31) and Shapiro et al. (32) have reported on the use of PCA opioids for the management of VOC. Schecter administered morphine as a 0.1 mg/kg loading "bolus" dose, followed by 0.3 to 2.5 mg doses every 15 minutes by patient activation of the drug infusion pump. Shapiro studied 96 episodes of PCA treatments in 46 patients. The hourly dose of morphine was 0.09 mg/kg, and patients averaged 5.4 attempts on the day of maximum use (32). Shapiro noted that 14 of the 46 patients (30%) reported problems with PCA use, and 11 patients expressed overt dissatisfaction with its use. However, the sense of control imparted by PCA delivery and the elimination of "negotiations" over drug dosing and confrontations over the use of opioid medications, make this mode of analgesic delivery quite appealing, and it should be considered as first line therapy.

Many patients come into the emergency department (or some sickle cell centers have day hospital facilities) for treatment of pain and are discharged to home without admission to the hospital if their pain can be controlled. The day hospital offers a substantial advantage for many patients, particularly if it provides a means for the patient to be seen by physicians who know them, and who have expertise in the management of sickle cell disease.

The role of other analgesic agents and routes of delivery is less well established. For example, many sickle cell patients have movement-related bone pain. This type of breakthrough pain is difficult to manage, particularly when it occurs in ambulatory patients without access to fast-acting parenteral opioids. Recently the administration of transmucosal fentanyl (the opioid agonist fentanyl is embedded in a sweetened lozenge on a stick and sucked by the patient) has been shown to provide rapid (within 5 to 15 minutes) onset of action (33). This type of drug delivery system may be appropriate for some opioid-tolerant sickle cell patients in whom incident pain is a major problem, so that fast onset of opioid action is desired, and in whom the drug can be used safely because of chronic administration of opioids has produced tolerance to the respiratory depressant effects. On the other hand, epidural opioid administration may avoid or minimize sedation and mental clouding that occurs with systemic opioid administration; the pain of VOC is usually diffuse or multifocal and its duration unpredictable; therefore, epidural opioids are seldom appropriate for the management of acute VOC. The role of behavioral and other psychological therapies for chronic pain in sickle cell anemia has been established (20), although the efficacy of these approaches in acute pain is less clear.

MANAGEMENT OF CHRONIC PAIN AND OTHER COMPLICATIONS OF SICKLE CELL DISEASES

Hydroxyurea Treatment

Levels of HbF above 20% of total hemoglobin appear to protect against polymerization of deoxygenated hemoglobin and thus appear to be antisickling (34). Azacitidine and hydroxyurea (HU) increase intracellular HbF concentrations. A recent randomized controlled trial comparing HU with placebo in 299 symptomatic patients demonstrated that HU was an effective therapy in sickle cell anemia for patients with frequent (more than 3) VOC per year (7). The study was terminated early when it became apparent that the HU group had a statistically significant decrease in number of VOC episodes, including the time to first and second VOC; number of episodes of acute chest syndrome; and the number of transfusions compared with placebo (7). The total dose of HU ranged from 0 to 35 mg/kg per day. The long-term safety of HU is not certain as its chronic use is problematic because of its possible teratogenic effects when used by pregnant women and the increased risk of malignancy.

Blood Transfusion for Cerebrovascular Complications

Recently the National Heart, Lung, and Blood Institute (NHLBI) of the National Institutes of Health (NIH) issued a clinical report announcing that blood transfusions have been shown to decrease the incidence of stroke in high-risk patients with sickle cell disease (35). This controlled trial, known as the Stroke Prevention Trial in Sickle Cell Anemia (STOP), was terminated 16 months early because the benefits of hypertransfusion became apparent in comparison to the control group. In this study 130 children aged 2 to 16 years who were judged to be at high risk for stroke because of abnormal cerebral circulation determined by transcranial Doppler studies were randomized to receive blood transfusions every 3 to 4 weeks to maintain their sickle hemoglobin levels below 30% of the total hemoglobulin. The control group who received best supportive care. After a year, the rate of stroke in the hypertransfusion group was 90% less than in the control group. Of course, blood

Table 29.4.   Prevalence of Substance Abuse in Sickle Cell Anemia Patients

Study	Results
Brozovick et al. (37)	No addiction in 600 adult patients
Vichinsky et al. (38)	Drug "addiction" in 3/101 patients
	Drug "dependence" in 7/101
Payne (13)	"Suspected" drug abuse in 9/114
	"Definite" drug abuse in 5/114

transfusions carry the risk of transmission of blood-borne infections, hypersensitivity reactions, and iron overload, so that this therapy can only be recommended only for children at risk for this devastating complication.

Bone Marrow Transplantation

Recently, allogeneic bone marrow transplantation was shown to be "curative in young patients with symptomatic sickle cell diseases" (36). In this study, 22 children under 15 years of age who had HLA-matched siblings received an allogeneic bone marrow transplant after pretreatment with busulfan, cyclophosphamide, and antithymocyte globulin. These children had clinically significant disease with high morbidity, including stroke (12 children), chest syndrome (5 children), and frequent VOC (5 children); 20 of the patients survived, with a mean follow-up of 23.9 months (range 10 to 51 months), and 16 of these 20 patients had "stable engraftment" of donor RBCs. Thus, a survival of 91% was reported at the 4-year end of the study, with an "event-free" survival of 73% reported. Although the results of this clinical trial are exciting, it must be emphasized that the patients who participated were very severely affected, and therefore the risks of bone marrow transplantation could be justified more readily than in general. Thus the applicability of these results to a larger population of less severely affected individuals with sickle cell disease is not clear.

PREVALENCE OF SUBSTANCE ABUSE DISORDERS IN SICKLE CELL ANEMIA

A major factor in the management of pain in sickle cell disease is the fear of iatrogenic addiction and the prevalence of coexisting substance abuse disorders in certain segments of the affected population. However, very few data have been published in this area. The perspective of most emergency department physicians and house staff is distorted by the small number of frequent users of the hospital services, which reinforces a perception that many patients, especially young black men and boys, with this disorder are drug seeking. However, as noted in Table 29.4, the prevalence of substance abuse disorders in sickle cell patients appears to be grossly exaggerated, especially if one considers iatrogenic substance abuse. A major problem in this area is the use of appropriate definition of addiction and substance abuse disorders. A detailed discussion of these definitions is beyond the scope of this chapter but is addressed by Portenoy and Payne (39).

Many patients exhibit behaviors that raise concerns regarding the possibility of substance abuse (39). These behaviors include excessive complaining about pain, hoarding medications, unsanctioned dose escalations, and the use of medications for unapproved indications (e.g., for sleep or sedation rather than analgesia). However, one must be very cautious when attributing these behaviors to addiction because of the common occurrence of *undertreatment* of pain in sickle cell, cancer, and other medical populations (39a, 40). In fact, the term pseudo-addiction has been used to describe *apparent* drug-seeking behaviors, such as those described in Table 29.2, in patients that are actually caused by inadequate control of pain (41). These behaviors may diminish when adequate pain management is provided, which supports the contention that pain avoidance, rather than drug-seeking activities, is the major motivation for these actions. In summary, it appears that the risk of true iatrogenic addiction in sickle cell anemia is no greater than the risks of this complication in any other medical illness.

References

1. Herrick JB. Peculiar elongated and sickle-shaped red corpuscles in a case of severe anemia. Arch Intern Med 1910;6:517.
2. Patt R, Payne R. Pain management. In: Beutler E, Lictman MA, Coller BS, Kipps TJ, eds. Williams hematology. 5th ed. New York: McGraw-Hill, 1995;203–208.
3. Payne R. Pain management in sickle cell anemia. Anesthesiol Clin North Am 1997;15:2.
4. Evans E, Mohandas N, Leung A. Static and dynamic rigidities of normal and sickle erythrocytes: major influence of cell hemoglobin concentration. J Clin Invest 1984;73:477–88.
5. Bunn HF. Pathogenesis and treatment of sickle cell disease. N Engl J Med 1997;337:762–769.
6. Sewehand LS, Johnson CS, Meiselman HJ. The effect of fetal hemoglobin on the sickling dynamics of SS erythrocytes. Blood Cells 1983;9:147–166.
7. Charache S, Terrin ML, Moore RD, et al. Effect of hydroxyurea on the frequency of painful crises in sickle cell anemia. N Engl J Med 1995;332:1317–1322.
8. Goldberg MA, Brugnara C, Dover GJ, et al. Treatment of sickle cell anemia with hydroxyurea and erythropoietin. N Engl J Med 1990;323:366–372.
9. Beutler E. The sickle cell disease and related disorders. In: Beutler E, Lictman MA, Coller BS, Kipps TJ, eds. Williams hematology. 5th ed. New York: McGraw-Hill, 1995;616–650.
10. Delengowski A, Stevens MCG, Padwick M, Serjeant GR. Observations on the natural history of dactylitis in homozygous sickle cell disease. Clin Pediatr 1981;20:311.
11. Powars DR. Natural history of sickle cell disease: the first ten years. Semin Hematol 1975;12:267.
12. Ballas SK. Pain measurement in hospitalized adults with sickle cell painful episodes. Ann Clin Lab Sci 1993;23:358–61.
13. Payne R. Pain management in sickle cell disease: rationale and technique. Ann NY Acad Sci 1989;565:189–206.
14. Diggs LM. Anatomic lesions in sickle cell disease. In: Abramson H, Bertles JF, Wethers DL, eds. Sickle cell disease: diagnosis, management, education and research. St Louis: Mosby, 1973;189–229.
15. Reference deleted.
16. Rucknagel DL, Kalinyak KA, Gelfand MJ. Rib infarcts and acute chest syndrome in sickle cell diseases. Lancet 1991;337:831–833.
17. Castro O, Brambilla DJ, Torrington B, et al. The acute chest syndrome in sickle cell disease: incidence and risk factors. Cooperative Study of Sickle Cell Disease. Blood 1994;84:643–649.
18. Cole TB, Spinkle RK, Smith SJ, Buchanan GR. Intravenous narcotic therapy for children with severe sickle cell pain crises. Am J Child 1986;140:1255–1259.
19. Platt OS, Brambilla DJ, Rosse WF, et al. Mortality in sickle cell disease: life expectancy and risk factors for early death. N Engl J Med 1994;330:1639–1644.
20. Gil K, Phillips G, Webster DK, et al. Experimental pain sensitivity and reports of negative thoughts in adults with sickle cell disease. Behav Ther 1995;26:273–293.
21. Zipursky A, Robieux IC, Brown EJ, et al. Oxygen therapy in sickle cell disease. Am J Ped Hematol Oncol 1992;14:2;22–28.
22. Griffin TC, McIntire D, Buchanan GR. High-dose intravenous methylprednisolone therapy for pain in children and adolescents with sickle cell disease. N Engl J Med 1994;33:733–737.
23. Brookoff D, Polomano R. Treating sickle cell pain like cancer pain. Ann Intern Med 1992;116:364–368.
24. Reference deleted.
25. Friedman EW, Webber AB, Osborn HH, Schwartz S. Oral analgesia for treatment of painful crisis in sickle cell anemia. Ann Emerg Med 1986;7:787–791.
26. Conti C, Tso E, Browne B. Oral morphine protocol for sickle cell crisis pain. Md Med J 1996;45:33–35.
27. Teresi ME, Wicklund BM, McMillan SK, et al. Comparison of controlled-release oral morphine to continuous morphine infusions in the control of pain in sickle cell crises. Am J Pain Mgmt 1994;4:62–66.
28. Jacox A, Carr D, Payne R. New clinical-practice guidelines for the management of pain in patients with cancer. N Engl J Med 1994;330:169–173.
29. Wright SW. Meperidine and ketorolac in the treatment of painful sickle cell crises. Ann Emerg Med 1992;21:925–28.
30. Tang R, Shimomura S K, Rotblatt M. Meperidine-induced seizures in sickle cell patients. Hosp Formulary 1992;764–772.
31. Schecter NL, Berrier FB, Katz SM. The use of patient-controlled analgesia in adolescents with sickle cell pain crises: a preliminary report. J Pain Symptom Mgmt 1988;3:109–113.
32. Shapiro BS, Cohen DE, Howe CJ. Patient-controlled analgesia for sickle cell-related pain. J Pain Symptom Mgmt 1993;8:22–28.
33. Payne R. Dose titration trials of oral transmucosal fentanyl citrate (OTFC) for the management of breakthrough pain in cancer patients. American Pain Society meeting, New Orleans, October 1997 (abstract).
34. Noguchi CT, Rodger GP, Serjeant G, Schecter AN. Levels of fetal hemoglobin necessary for treatment of sickle cell disease. N Engl J Med 1988;318:96–99.
35. Anonymous. Reducing sickle cell strokes. JAMA 1997;278:1227.
36. Walters MC, Patience M, Leisenring W, et al. Bone marrow transplantation for sickle cell disease. N Engl J Med 1996;335:369–376.
37. Brozovick MC, Davies SC, Yarumian A, et al. Pain relief in sickle cell crises. Lancet 1986;1:320–321.
38. Vichinsky EP, Johnson PR, Lubin RB. Multidisciplinary approach to pain management in sickle cell disease. Am J Pediatr Hematol Oncol 1982;4:328–33.
39. Portenoy RK, Payne R. Acute and chronic pain. In: Lowinson JH, Ruiz P, Millman RB, Langrod JG, eds. Substance abuse: a comprehensive textbook. 3rd ed. Baltimore: Williams & Wilkins, 1997;563–589.
39a. Newman RG. The need to re-define addiction. N Engl J Med 1983;18:1096–1098.
40. Cleeland CS, Gonin R, Hatfield AK, et al. Pain and its treatment in outpatients with metastatic cancer. N Engl Med 1994;330:592–594.
41. Weissman DE, Haddox JD. Opioid pseudo-addiction: an iatrogenic syndrome. Pain 1989;36:363–366.

CHAPTER 30

Pain Management in Elderly Patients

F. Michael Gloth III

PAIN IN THE ELDERLY AS A CHALLENGE

Almost all physicians encounter patients with pain. Amazingly, few medical schools provide formal didactic sessions on pain management. Medical students are more likely to receive formal instruction on Chagas' disease (which is unlikely to be seen in the career of the average physician in the United States) than in palliative care, which is likely to be needed by many of our patients. Probably the most distressing of symptoms for patients and caregivers is pain. It can be extremely frustrating for physicians and other health care providers, who have entered the field of medicine to help relieve suffering, to fail to provide adequate pain management for their patients. Unfortunately, this is all too often the case.

Some 25 to 50% of community-dwelling elderly people suffer from major pain problems. The prevalence of pain in the nursing home is 45 to 80%, and the prevalence of analgesic use is 40 to 50%. One of the primary risk factors for inadequate pain control is advanced aged. Clearly, pain is an important problem in elderly patients. Most have at least one chronic disease or disorder. Arthritis, hypertension, heart disease, visual difficulties, cerebrovascular disease, or diabetes is found in at least 10% of the population 65 years and older. In many patients, multiple medical problems complicate their overall treatment. The management of pain in the older population is further complicated by age-related alterations in physiological factors, pharmacodynamics of drug distribution and metabolism, and pain perception. These factors, combined with the adverse effects that can occur with pain medications, make prescribing an analgesic for the aged patient in pain a daunting task indeed.

Some other reasons identified for inadequate pain management in older patients include inadequate pain assessment by health care professionals, physicians' reluctance to prescribe opioids, and inadequate knowledge of pain management. Patients' reluctance to report pain or reluctance to take opioid medication also help to explain inadequate cancer pain management.

PAIN ASSESSMENT

All too often intervention for pain is initiated without measuring the level of pain or discovering whether the pain has improved. Imagine prescribing an antihypertensive medication without monitoring blood pressure. Prescribing an analgesic without monitoring the benefit through an accepted pain scale is analogous. Unfortunately, few pain scales have been adequately standardized for frail, elderly patients. I have found visual analog scales and those that use descriptive terms like "lancinating" to be of little use in a population that frequently has compromised cognition or visual acuity or a limited education. I have had good success with the Functional Pain Scale (FPS) (Table 30.1), which has been validated in a frail elderly population. This scale incorporates three levels of assessment. Pain is rated as tolerable or intolerable. Pain that is reported as intolerable should be considered an urgent matter and further evaluation and intervention rendered immediately, with frequent follow-up to assure improvement into the "tolerable" range as rapidly as possible. There is also a functional component. Some patients are likely to rank pain at the highest level, especially if they are apprehensive over receiving adequate pain medication. With the FPS, if a patient says the pain is a 5, it cannot be based on the functional component. This portion of the scale adds an objective component to the assessment. Finally, the 0 to 5 scale does present a means of monitoring change (responsiveness). Ideally all patients should reach a 0 to 2 level, preferably 0 or 1.

Table 30.1.   Functional Pain Scale

0, No pain
1, Tolerable and doesn't prevent any activities
2, Tolerable but does prevent some activities
3, Intolerable but patient can use telephone, watch TV, or read
4, Intolerable and patient cannot use telephone, watch TV, or read
5, Intolerable and patient cannot verbally communicate because of pain

This table may be reproduced for clinical purposes.

Pain Perception

Elderly patients are underrepresented in most pain studies. Studies that included primarily elderly people measured nociception based on threshold levels of mechanical, electrical, or thermal stimuli. With the exception of some skin sensation, which changes with age, it is not clear that nociception changes. The sensory processes seem to be the same, but report bias changes with age. For example, pain tolerance decreases and the frequency of pain complaints increases with age. Certain types of visceral pain may differ in old versus younger patients. Silent myocardial infarction seems more common in elderly patients, and the "surgical abdomen" may present without leukocytosis or marked pain. Headache is less common in elderly patients; however, when it occurs, the cause is often more serious than that in younger patients. Temporal arteritis, cervical osteoarthritis, depression, congestive heart failure, subdural hematoma, and electrolyte disturbances rank high among the differential diagnoses of headache in the elderly. As a person ages, a change in the willingness to label noxious stimuli as painful occurs. For these reasons, communication between physician and patient becomes very important for adequate pain control.

Metabolic Changes

Age-related alterations in creatinine clearance (usually with normal serum creatinine levels due to decreases in muscle mass) are important because of the resultant diminished rate of clearance for some medications. Drug distribution usually is different in older patients from that in younger ones because of changes in blood flow to organs, protein binding, and body composition that occur with aging. Whereas relative reductions in total body water and lean body mass are present, body fat usually increases. Thus, a water-soluble drug can be expected to have lower volume of distribution but increased early plasma concentrations in elderly patients than in younger ones. Conversely, lipid-soluble drugs (e.g., diazepam) tend to have a larger distribution. Thus, not only for analgesics but for adjuvant medication as well, consideration of the lipophilic nature of medication may lead to change of agent or dosage for seniors with a higher portion of body fat and less water content.

Affective and Cognitive Components

Depression is another entity in elderly patients that is often overlooked and that requires consideration when managing a patients with pain. Investigation of the association between depression and pain complaints in elderly patients has revealed that initial control of depression greatly facilitates pain management. It is important not to fall into the trap of thinking that the pain itself is the sole cause of depression and that controlling the pain will eliminate the depression. Depression must be treated aggressively, for without such treatment, pain management will remain elusive. Because tricyclic antidepressants, such as nortriptyline and desipramine, also may be useful in neuropathic pain, such agents should be considered when such pain develops.

Issues such as secondary gain, mental focus, experience, and anxiety also should be taken into account. A patient who receives a visit from his or her daughter every time he or she has pain is likely to have a powerful secondary gain from the pain that makes pain management much more difficult. Secondary gain must be identified and appropriate measures taken to remove it or to develop a strong incentive with a secondary gain from pain relief. For example, the daughter who visits the mother in the nursing home stays longer when there is pain relief and makes an effort to make additional visits between painful episodes, minimizing or removing the secondary gain from the pain.

The patient who has little to consider other than pain is also more difficult to control. The soldier in battle who is wounded may not notice the pain until after the melée has ended and attention can be directed to the wound. In part, it is for this reason that hospice care often involves distraction therapy. Patients who are lying in bed with their focus on little else other than their next pain pill may be given music or book tapes or even tapes of the waves crashing on the seashore to change the mental focus away from the pain. While pain diaries may be helpful, the constant question "Are you in pain?" makes it difficult not to focus on pain. Such questioning in and of itself may make pain control more difficult. It is preferable, therefore, to focus on function or other goals in general. For example, one develops a goal of improving comfort to a level that allows the patient to get to the bedside commode or to the bathroom or to walk in the hallway. Questioning can focus on function, such as "Were you able to get to the bathroom today?" or "Were you able to walk in the hall?"

Experience also can have significant influence. Either personal experience or experience of another may play a role in how we adapt to pain. The apprehension of some patients who have seen a family member suffer through a similar illness (for example a previous cancer course in which hospice was not instituted) may make pain management much more difficult. Anxiety itself can augment a pain response, and it is for this reason that combining agents such as hydroxyzine with an opioid has led to better pain control. Unfortunately, some anxiolytics, such as hydroxyzine, are associated with anticholinergic effects that may lead to mental status change, orthostatic hypotension, and an increased risk of falls. Such agents therefore should generally be avoided in the old patient.

TREATMENT

As is true with most clinical situations, appropriate treatment of pain starts with a proper history, including the onset, duration, description, and any affective and cognitive components involved in the pain. A thorough physical examination is also in order because older persons often present with relatively subtle findings as manifestations of very serious disease. Removal of the underlying cause or providing a cure for the source of pain is ideal, but even in the circumstance of removing an inflamed gall bladder or appendix, one must deal with the postoperative pain resulting from the surgical wound. In other scenarios such as some cancers, there is no cure and the focus is solely on palliation. It is helpful to break treatment down into pharmacological and nonpharmacological interventions.

Nonpharmacological Interventions

Nonpharmacological interventions include cold, which can suppress tissue damage. Cold and warmth lead to the release of endogenous opioids, as do other interventions such as transcutaneous electrical nerve stimulation (TENS) and acupuncture. Other interventions, such as relaxation techniques, biofeedback (particularly with vascular headaches), or hypnosis, may be useful. One should not overlook the importance of physical and occupational therapy, which offer a variety of modalities including the use of braces or splints, changes in biomechanics, and exercise itself, all of which have been demonstrated to improve pain. Nerve blocks and tumor site radiation may also be helpful in a variety of pain settings.

Pharmacological Interventions

Pharmacological interventions can be broken down into nonopioid and opioid therapies. With all pharmacological interventions, a patient who cannot afford the medication is likely not to be compliant or to sacrifice other important aspects of health care, such as nutrition, to control the pain. A health plan that covers medications in the hospital but not on an outpatient basis may lead to excellent pain control in the acute care setting, with inadequate pain management once the patient is discharged from the hospital.

Another issue is that on average a 70-year-old takes seven different medications and the addition of analgesics to a complex medication regimen may lead to drug interactions when because of age and comorbidity it is difficult enough to anticipate adverse events associated with even a single drug.

Nonopioid Drugs

Nonopioid drugs are generally the first line of therapy. Some agents that should be considered include acetaminophen. This is a relatively safe drug in the elderly. It should be remembered, however, that acetaminophen appears in many combination products, and it is important to establish whether the patient has hepatic disease or is taking other drugs that are metabolized through the liver. Vigilance regarding both prescription and nonprescription medications that contain acetaminophen is important. For example, a patient who is prescribed two Tylox (oxycodone with 500 mg of acetaminophen) every 6 hours, will end the day with 4 g of acetaminophen. This is the ceiling for analgesic benefit. Higher doses are not associated with better analgesia but only with increased incidence of adverse events. Should the patient go to the medicine cabinet because of inadequate pain management and take two extra-strength Tylenols for breakthrough pain even twice in a 24-hour period, he or she would have taken 6 g of acetaminophen, the dose after which one worries about toxicity. Certainly, if alcohol is a factor, caution with medications that have large amounts of acetaminophen becomes even more important. Nevertheless, acetaminophen is generally very well tolerated in the elderly and has stood up well against nonsteroidal anti-inflammatory drugs, which have a much worse gastrointestinal side effect profile and may be considerably more dangerous in the elderly. Nonsteroidal anti-inflammatory drugs all have concerns related to hypertension and renal effects. Agents that seem to have a better safety profile based on clinical trials and theoretical advantages include nabumetone 1000 to 1500 mg as a single or divided dose and etodolac, which is available in immediate- or extended-release form. Both of these agents have clinical trials that have demonstrated less gastric erosion by endoscopy than other nonsteroidal anti-inflammatory drugs. Nabumetone is not secreted in the bile acid and does not seem to have the platelet inhibition that occurs with many other nonsteroidal anti-inflammatory drugs. Etodolac theoretically has its advantage because of inhibition of cyclo-oxygenase 2 (involved in the production of prostaglandins associated with inflammation) with relatively less inhibition of cyclo-oxygenase 1 (associated with the production of cytoprotective prostaglandins in the gut) in therapeutic dosing ranges. Newer agents under development have much greater cyclo-oxygenase 2 than cyclo-oxygenase 1 selectivity. Neither of these two nonsteroidal anti-inflammatory agents comes in a liquid form, and when a liquid agent is needed, choline magnesium trisalicylate should be considered. It also has few problems with regard to platelet aggregation, and it may have some advantages with regard to gastrointestinal toxicity. Unlike aspirin, however, choline magnesium trisalicylate does not announce toxicity with tinnitus. The antiprostaglandin activity of nonsteroidal anti-inflammatory drugs has been touted as the basis for these agents being effective, particularly in metastatic bone pain.

Other agents that have received attention with regard to metastatic bone pain include radionuclides (e.g., strontium-89 and samarium-153 lexidronam) and the bisphosphonates (e.g., pamidronate). Radionuclides are recommended in metastatic bone pain when survival is anticipated to exceed 3 weeks and other more conventional treatments have failed. Radionuclides take about a month before they are effective. In only about 10% of cases are radionuclides effective without additional adjuvant medication to control pain. When they are effective, the benefit should last up to 6 months. Most patients require more than a single treatment, and each treatment costs more than $2000.

Bisphosphonate therapy has gained attention for treatment of metastatic bone pain. Recently the U.S. Food and Drug Administration (FDA) approved pamidronate 90 mg intravenously every month for skeletal pain associated with multiple myeloma or breast cancer. Of the bisphosphonates, pamidronate has been studied the most extensively. Administration should be over 3 to 4 hours to minimize associated adverse events, which usually come in the form of transient flulike symptoms. Hypocalcemia and temporary lymphocyte suppression have also been seen. Other available bisphosphonate agents, such as etidronate, alendronate, and tiludronate, in doses recommended for Paget's disease have probable benefit in metastatic bone pain, as well.

Vitamin D deficiency, which is likely in patients who are elderly and homebound, especially in the presence of antiepileptics or fat malabsorption syndromes, should also be recognized as a potential cause of either deep musculoskeletal pain or superficial light pressure pain. Vitamin D deficiency, of course, has been associated with fractures, which are a significant source of pain. Research has demonstrated that perhaps more than a third of nursing home subjects who have been confined indoors for more than 6 months and are over age 65 and more than half of such community-dwelling subjects are likely to suffer from vitamin D deficiency. Because a single treatment of 100,000 IU is likely to restore a patient to normal vitamin D status and resolve pain associated with deficiency of this vitamin, one does not want to overlook this cause of pain.

Tramadol also helps control pain, and except in a substance-abuse population, it should have a low tolerance problem and may be beneficial for a variety of types of pain. It is important to start low with this medication and gradually increase it; even at the maximal dose of 100 mg every 6 hours, the equianalgesic effect does not exceed a 60-mg dose of controlled-release morphine. Like acetaminophen, which is manufactured by the same company, the mechanism for analgesia is not fully understood with tramadol. There is exceedingly weak (-receptor binding, and this by no means accounts for the bulk of its analgesic effect.

Topical agents are also available for site-specific pain. Capsaicin has been demonstrated to be particularly useful in neuropathy. One should start with the lowest dose (0.025% every 6 hours). The use of a topical spray such as Solarcaine may diminish the burning sensation that some people feel when capsaicin is applied without interfering with its efficacy. Because capsaicin interferes with the reuptake of substance P, it should be used on a schedule of every 6 hours. Skipping doses permits reaccumulation of substance P and thus a return of pain.

Other agents, such as tricyclic antidepressants, some antiepileptics (e.g., clonazepam, carbamazepine, gabapentin,

and phenytoin), and mexiletine have also been recommended for neuropathic pain. Most of these agents are effective in doses below those needed for the treatment of depression or seizures. For cancer pain the World Health Organization and the Agency for Health Care Policy and Research have recommended that if there is no response to nonopioids initially, the next step should be to use opioids.

Opioids

When prescribing opioids it is important to recognize a number of myths that are pervasive in both the medical and lay communities and that have given morphine and other opioids a stigma among both prescribers and patients. Even chronic use of morphine to control pain rarely leads to addiction. It is important to recognize the difference between physiological dependence or tolerance, both of which are likely to develop, and addiction, which has a psychological component wherein a person craves a medication, places himself or herself in harm's way, and engages in self-destructive behavior to acquire a drug.

The elderly patient may contribute to the high incidence of undertreated pain because of concerns or fears about adverse effects or addiction with pain medications, including medications not associated with the potential for addiction. This fear is not based on fact because the addiction risk is low (less than 0.1%) when analgesics are used for acute pain in patients who are not substance abusers. Of course, for the patient with a terminal illness who requires potent analgesics for comfort in the final days of life, addiction is irrelevant.

Tolerance to adverse events, including nausea and emesis, is also likely to develop, and indeed a person who has nausea and vomiting on morphine is likely to have those symptoms resolve as tolerance develops over the course of a few days to weeks. It is therefore important to work on palliating the nausea and vomiting through antiemetic medications, rather than trying different opioids. Changing the dose (usually decreasing it) also may help. Unlike nonopioid medications, the opioids have no ceiling, that is, dosing can continue to be increased as tolerance develops or pain worsens. The limitation is reached when an opioid comes in a combined preparation that includes a nonopioid with a ceiling on analgesic efficacy. Most opioids can also be given in liquid form or through alternative administration routes. Some adverse events, such as pruritus, may be associated with receptor binding, and the use of a more potent opioid (e.g., oxycodone or hydromorphone in place of morphine) may be a remedy or may augment other interventions to control such adverse events.

The one adverse event associated with opioids that can be expected to persist is constipation, and it is important when using opioids to make sure that the patient has good bowel hygiene with adequate hydration. A bulk fiber product emphasizing mobility is appropriate. A senna product is often helpful because its colonic receptor binding may make it particularly useful with opioid-induced constipation. When chronic cathartics must be used, an agent such as sorbitol (70%, 20 mL by mouth twice each day), may be particularly beneficial because it is well tolerated without long-term effects on the gastrointestinal tract and is relatively low in cost.

In the elderly it is useful to start with a short-acting opioid and rapidly switch to a controlled-release formulation, with emphasis on regular dosing schedules. Solely "as-needed" dosing should be avoided. Rather, such dosing should be employed only for rescue of breakthrough pain. If demand dosing is used three times in a regular dosing schedule, consider increasing the amount or frequency of the regular dosed medication. It is helpful to think of "prn" as standing for "pain relief negligible," keeping in mind that regular dosing uses less opioid and provides better pain relief. It is important to inform patients, however, that they may refuse a regularly scheduled medication if they don't need it or if they are developing undesired side effects. Such refusals and the reasons for them must be immediately relayed to the attending physician.

Patient-controlled analgesia (PCA), whether oral or parenteral, can be most beneficial in a cognitively intact population, offering the likelihood of the best pain control in conjunction with the least amount of opioid needed to control pain. PCA need not only be with subcutaneous, intravenous, or other type of high-tech pumping system. Oral medications employing a long-acting agent such as morphine (oral dose required is usually about three times the parenteral dose needed for the same duration) (Table 30.2) or oxycodone in conjunction with a similar short-acting agent can also be used.

It makes sense to change types and routes of administration as infrequently as possible. For this reason, controlled-release agents such as oxycodone or morphine are used more frequently, with the same agent in the short-acting form used for breakthrough pain. This simplifies conversion to controlled-release medications, since one can convert directly by adding up the amount of short-acting medication taken over a given period and increasing the controlled-release medication concomitantly. For example, a patient who uses 30 mg of short-acting morphine every 4 hours can be anticipated to require 90 mg of controlled-release morphine every 12 hours. It is common to start at doses that are too low, and there should be a low threshold for increasing medication by 50 to 100% when pain relief is inadequate. Thus a patient who gets inadequate pain control from 60 mg of controlled-release morphine every 12 hours should have the dose increased to 90 to 120 mg every 12 hours. Some people metabolize the medication more quickly, and should they have adequate pain relief for 8 hours and then get breakthrough pain, the solution is to increase the frequency of dosing to every 8 hours from every 12 hours. Controlled-release morphine or controlled-release oxycodone should never be taken more frequently than every 8 hours. If breakthrough pain occurs in 3 to 4 hours, the recommendation is to increase the amount of medication, maintaining the same dosing schedule. It is also helpful to recognize that some older persons metabolize medica-

Table 30.2.   Approximate Equianalgesic Dosing

Opioid	Parenteral Dose	Controlled-Release Oral Dose	Immediate-Release Oral Dose
Morphine	4 mg q4 h	30–40 mg q12h	10 mg q3–4h
Fentanyl patch	25–50 µg/hr	NA	NA
Oxycodone	NA	30 mg q12h	10 mg q4h
Hydromorphone	0.5 mg q4h	NA	3 mg q4h
Codeine	48 mg q4h	NA	100 mg q4h
Meperidine	30 mg q4h	NA	80–100 mg q3h

tion more slowly and may need less frequent dosing at surprisingly low quantities of opioids, such as 15 to 30 mg of controlled-release morphine every 24 hours. Most opioids are available as liquids. Many can also be given as rectal suppositories. Although not formulated as such, both controlled-release morphine and controlled-release oxycodone have been used as suppositories with clinical benefit. Additional caution is warranted with administration of controlled-release oxycodone in this manner, because absorption may be increased by 30%. Regardless, few patients tolerate rectal suppositories for long, and this route should be used only when needed on a temporary basis.

Meperidine should be avoided in the elderly because of increased risk of seizures (normeperidine is a metabolite that accumulates beyond the analgesic duration of meperidine and lowers seizure threshold) when used chronically, an association with falls, increased likelihood of sedation and psychotomimetic activity, and poor oral absorption. The combination with a product such as hydroxyzine, which is anticholinergic and can be associated with orthostatic hypotension and confusion, compounds the danger. Other agents that are antagonistic to the µ-receptor are less desirable, given the high prevalence of depression among people with chronic pain and the advantage of the euphoric component that occurs when the µ-receptor is bound. There is no role for agonist-antagonist agents that avoid µ-binding. Remember, other agents, such as nonsteroidal anti-inflammatory drugs, amphetamines (including methylphenidate, which may also have utility in the setting of depression), and other nonopioid analgesics, may be useful adjuvants to the opioids, improving tolerance and pain resolution.

Transdermal fentanyl patches should generally be avoided in old persons because of fluctuating absorption based on body temperature and difference in subcutaneous fat and water in elderly compared to younger, more studied populations. The fentanyl patch may be useful when oral medication cannot be administered and subcutaneous or other routes that require special pumping devices are too cumbersome. An opioid-naive person, however, should never be started on more than 25 µg per hour. Fentanyl takes approximately 8 hours to achieve peak serum levels, and removal of the patch still leaves a subcutaneous reservoir of active drug, which has a half-life of approximately 18 hours.

The opioids alone may not adequately control neuropathic pain at doses that allow good quality of life, and the use of agents such as nortriptyline, clonazepam, carbamazepine, phenytoin, gabapentin, tramadol, mexiletine, and others have reports of benefits for neuropathic pain. Other nonpharmacological techniques, such as TENS, acupuncture, nerve blocks, and irradiation, also may be useful, depending on the cause of the pain.

The main issue is to follow patients closely in the first few days following a change in the pain regimen so that serious adverse events can be avoided, and just as important, so that pain can be relieved as quickly as possible. In the terminally ill patient the stages of dying often resemble opioid toxicity, and the use of an opioid antagonist, such as naloxone, is rarely necessary. If naloxone is to be used in a person chronically taking opioids, it is important to recognize that this can induce agonizing withdrawal. Naloxone should not be used in the manner described in the Physicians Desk Reference (0.4 mg), but rather dilute the ampule of naloxone with 10 mL of normal saline (0.04 mg/mL), and give 1 mL intravenously every 5 minutes until **partial** reversal occurs. Because of the short half-life of naloxone, this procedure may have to be repeated.

The cause of certain adverse reactions associated with centrally acting analgesics has been distinguished by differentiating the receptors (μ, κ, δ) to which specific agents bind. Table 30.3 lists some of the receptors, examples of drugs that bind to each, primary locations, and actions. As research progresses, it seems likely that we may synthesize agents that promote analgesia without the adverse effects that are common to today's agents.

Selection of a particular opioid analgesic should be based on receptor action and route of administration. Of course, the nature of the pain also should be considered. Neuropathic pain is not as responsive to opioids as is pain of other causation.

Morphine has a greater affinity for μ-receptors than other receptors. The euphoria from the μ-opioid binding action of morphine is particularly useful for reducing anxiety and may have additional mechanisms for managing pain. Tolerance to sedation, respiratory depression, and emesis develop before tolerance to analgesia, so an agent like morphine may be better tolerated if the dose is gradually titrated. Because codeine also acts at the μ- and κ-receptors, precautions and benefits are similar to those of morphine. About 10% of people lack an enzyme necessary to metabolize codeine and thus the analgesic effect of codeine does not work for them. Morphine at equianalgesic doses would be preferable for them.

Meperidine is converted to normeperidine, which is not metabolized as quickly as the parent compound. For this reason, normeperidine concentrations can accumulate, often causing adverse neuropsychiatric effects (e.g., anxiety, irritability, seizures). This accumulation combined with the poor bioavailability of meperidine make it unsuitable for controlling pain in elderly patients that is expected to last more than 1 or 2 days.

Levorphanol and methadone have greater affinities for κ- than μ-receptors. The half-life exceeds the duration of analgesia; consequently, excessive sedation and respiratory depression may result. These agents are poor choices in elderly patients. Because long-acting oral morphine and morphinelike centrally acting analgesics are available, there is little reason to use methadone even in terminally ill patients with chronic pain.

Pentazocine and similar agents (e.g., buprenorphine) have agonist and antagonist properties. Their effects are related to agonism at one or more opioid receptors and to antagonism at another. There is an association with a psychotomimetic action and severe withdrawal from μ-receptor opioids. The elderly may be particularly susceptible to mental status changes, in part because of the greater prevalence of diseases affecting cognitive function in this population. The combination products incorporating an opioid receptor agonist and a different receptor antagonist have not been shown to be free of addiction potential and have not been demonstrated in rigorous trials to have any advantage; in fact they may have considerable disadvantage compared with centrally acting opioid analgesics that do not have antagonistic properties.

Urinary retention is a complication of centrally acting analgesics and may be an issue in elderly men with benign prostatic hypertrophy. Just as the sphincter of Oddi can be affected by opioid analgesics, an effect on the urethral sphincter with resultant bladder retention may occur with such agents as well. For this reason, it is important to query patients regularly about urinary retention.

One should be careful to evaluate suspected adverse events thoroughly. Oftentimes reactions are misinterpreted as side effects from medication when such is not the case at all. For example, a patient who has been in pain for a long time may fall asleep from exhaustion once pain is finally relieved. All too often this is mistaken as a side effect of morphine. If respirations are found to be 12 breaths per minute or greater, the sleep is unlikely to be attributable to the opioid. Other clues such as miosis should be present when opioid receptors are filled.

It is estimated that dementia occurs in approximately 5% of the population 65 years and older; after age 85, this figure increases to more than 20%. In many instances, disorientation increases when the patient is moved to a different environment. The hospital undoubtedly qualifies as a different environment. It is relatively common for previously undetected dementias to manifest themselves following an overnight stay in the hospital even in the absence of infection or use of centrally acting medication.

Route of Administration

In the elderly the route of administration is an even greater consideration than in younger persons, because of changes in skin integrity and gastrointestinal absorption and motility. For this reason, centrally acting analgesics are available in many formulations, including tablets, capsules, suppositories, drops, intravenous solutions, and more recently, transdermal patches. Fentanyl patches have become popular but should be used with caution for the reasons noted earlier.

Table 30.3.   Differentiation of Opioid Receptors

Receptor	Example	Location	Actions
μ	Morphinelike opioids	Periaqueductal gray Rostroventral medulla Medial thalamus Dorsal horn of spinal cord (supraspinal analgesia)	Respiratory depression, euphoria, miosis
κ	Pentazocine	Spinal cord, deep cortex	Sedation, miosis, psychotomimetic effects
δ	Enkephalins	Limbic, dorsal horn	hypotension, miosis

Adjuvant Analgesics

Tricyclic antidepressants (e.g., amitriptyline) have been used successfully to manage various types of neuropathies, which may result from metabolic disease, infections, intraoperative nerve injury, or local tissue invasion of a tumor mass. Pain management can usually be achieved with doses below those necessary to control depression. Unfortunately, the role of tricyclic antidepressants in pain management is limited by their anticholinergic effects (increased noradrenergic and serotonergic neurotransmission). Although these effects (e.g., constipation, blurred vision, dry mouth, urinary retention, sedation) are a cause for concern in a patient of any age, the elderly patient may be at greater risk for such effects because of preexisting conditions such as glaucoma and benign prostatic hypertrophy. Additional adverse effects of tricyclic antidepressants may include cardiac effects, particularly arrhythmia, cognitive changes, and orthostatic hypotension, which may result in falls. All can have potentially detrimental effects in the frail, elderly patient.

Antiepileptic medications also are used to manage selected types of pain, including trigeminal neuralgia (or glossopharyngeal neuralgia), which is fairly common in elderly patients. Carbamazepine may be effective when administered initially at 100 mg orally twice daily and increased to 800 mg per day as needed. If carbamazepine is ineffective, phenytoin or clonazepam is a good alternative. The greatest concern with antiepileptics in elderly patients is their propensity to cause falls and interfere with vitamin D metabolism, which is a particular concern in the homebound elderly.

INITIATING ANALGESIC THERAPY IN ELDERLY PATIENTS

General guidelines for prescribing analgesics to elderly patients are outlined in Table 30.4. A principal rule with the elderly is to begin at a low dose and to proceed slowly with changes. The specific drug regimen is important in maintaining adequate pain control. As-needed scheduling of a medication should be used only when the medication is not anticipated to be needed. Anxiety associated with the early onset of pain and delay in taking an analgesic inevitably leads to exacerbations in pain and greater difficulty in obtaining control. In these circumstances, larger doses of analgesics are required and the fre-

Table 30.4.   Guidelines for Prescribing Analgesics for Elderly Patients

Obtain complete medical history
  Concurrent medications
  Prior adverse reactions
  Concomitant illnesses
Resist prescribing without a diagnosis
Begin with low doses (often less than the minimum recommended dose) and increase slowly
Emphasize medicinal debridement
  Continually review medications, including over-the-counter drugs
  Decrease or remove medications when indicated

quency of adverse reactions can be expected to increase. PCA appears to be more effective at controlling pain than regular dosing of analgesic medications. A study by Egbert and colleagues (Suggested Reading list) revealed that patients receiving PCA required fewer doses of analgesics and had less pain than patients receiving regularly scheduled nurse-administered intramuscular centrally acting analgesics (i.e., opioid agents).

Adverse drug reactions affect the elderly at more than twice the frequency as with younger subjects, and they increase as the number of medications increases. A person taking six medications is 14 times as likely to have an adverse reaction as a younger one on the same number of medications. Therefore, any new medication to be added to the drug regimen of an elderly patient should be carefully considered.

Along with potential problems of starting new medications, an older person who is hospitalized may have toxicity due to a sudden improvement in compliance. For example, I have seen patients who cut down on the number of pills without notifying their health care provider. Upon entering the hospital, medications are given as prescribed. In some circumstances the reduction on the patient's part was based on toxic symptoms. In an acutely ill person, with the addition of other medications, the adverse symptoms may become even more pronounced.

The prudent physician carefully evaluates an older patient who demonstrates a mental status change while in the hospital. Infections, such as pneumonia or those occurring in the urinary tract, may present solely as a change in mental status and improve rapidly when appropriate antibiotic therapy is initiated. Additionally, the older patient may suffer from impaired hearing, vision, and mobility, which may be further compounded by the nature of surgical procedures. Such circumstances may induce alterations in mental status and misperceptions of reality.

Finally, multispecialty pain clinics or consultation with colleagues in other disciplines when such pain clinics are not available should occur in any circumstance when pain control is not achieved or when the clinician is uncomfortable with the pain management.

CONCLUSION

In general with the geriatric population, the rule for dosing is begin low and go slow. Inappropriate use of opioids has been a tremendous obstacle in palliative care, because of both reluctance to use them and inappropriate prescribing. Pain is not a situation in which an intervention can be prescribed and the patient asked to call back in a week. Most interventions provide relief in hours to minutes. The use of some assessment tool to evaluate the level of pain and whether there has been a change is important. Monitoring for adverse events is also critical. Patients need to know what to expect and when to expect it. Keep the lines of communication open and communicate often, especially in the beginning of a regimen.

Suggested Reading

Anderson S, Worm-Pederson J. The prevalence of persistent pain in a Danish population. In: Proceedings of the V World Congress on Pain. Pain Suppl 1987;4:S332.

Avorn J. Biomedical and social determinants of cognitive impairment in the elderly. J Am Geriatr Soc 1983;31:137–143.

Birren JE, Shapiro HB, Miller JH. Influence of salicylate upon pain sensitivity. J Pharmacol Exp Ther. 1950; 100:76–81.

Bradley JD, Brandt KD, Katz BP, et al. Comparison of an antiinflammatory dose of ibuprofen, an analgesic dose of ibuprofen, and acetaminophen in the treatment of patients with osteoarthritis of the knee. N Engl J Med 1991;325:87–91.

Clark WC, Mehl L. Thermal pain: a sensory decision theory analysis of the effect of age and sex on various response criteria, and 50% pain threshold. J Abnorm Psychol 1971;78:202–212.

Cleeland CS, Gonin R, Hatfield AK, et al. Pain and its treatment in outpatients with metastatic cancer. N Engl J Med 1994;330:592–596.

Crook J, Rideout E, Browne G. The prevalence of pain complaints among a general population. Pain 1984;18:299–314.

Egbert AM, Parks LH, Short LM, Burnett ML. Randomized trial of postoperative patient-controlled analgesia vs intramuscular narcotics in frail elderly men. Arch Intern Med 1990;150:1897–1903.

Ferrell BA. Pain management in elderly patients. J Am Geriatr Soc 1991;39:64–73.

Ferrell BA, Ferrell BR, Osterweil D. Pain in the nursing home. J Am Geriatr Soc 1991;39:64–73.

Gennis V, Garry PJ, Haaland KY, et al. Hearing and cognition in the elderly. Arch Intern Med 1991;151:2259–2264.

Gloth FM, Burton JR. Autopsies and death certificates in the chronic care setting. J Am Geriatr Soc 1990;38:151–155.

Gloth FM III, Lindsay JM, Zelesnick LB, Greenough WB III. Can vitamin D deficiency produce an unusual pain syndrome? Arch Intern Med 1991;151:1662–1664.

Golden WE, Lavender RC, Metzer WS. Acute postoperative confusion and hallucinations in Parkinson disease. Ann Intern Med 1989;111:218–222.

Gordon RS. Pain in the elderly. JAMA 1979;241:2491–2492.

Green DM, Swets J A. Signal detection theory and psychophysics. New York: Wiley, 1966.

Gustafson Y, Brännström B, Berggren D, et al. A geriatric-anesthesiological program to reduce acute confusional states in elderly patients treated for femoral neck fractures. J Am Geriatr Soc 1991;39:655–662.

Doyle D, ed. Oxford textbook of palliative medicine. 2nd ed. Oxford, UK: Oxford Medical, 1997.

Harkins SW, Chapman CR. The perception of induced dental pain in young and elderly women. J Gerontol 1977;32:428–435.

Harkins SW, Warner MH. Age and pain. Ann Rev Gerontol Geriatr 1980; 1:121–131.

Hoskin PJ, Hanks GW. Opioid agonist-antagonist drugs in acute and chronic pain states. Drugs 1991;41:326.

Hospice/palliative care training for physicians. Unipac I–VI. Gainsville, FL: American Academy of Hospice and Palliative Medicine, 1996.

Hyman SE, Cassem NH. Pain. In: Rubenstein E, Federman D D eds. Scientific American medicine. 11 Neurology XIV 1994;12.

Jacox A, Carr DB, Payne R. New clinical guidelines for the management of pain in patients with cancer pain: special report. N Engl J Med 1994;330: 651–655.

Jacox A, Carr DB, Payne R, et al. Management of cancer pain: clinical practice guidelines 9. AHCPR Pub. 94–0592. Rockville, MD: Agency for Health Care Policy and Research, March 1994.

Klein LE, German PS, Levine DM, et al. Medication problems among outpatients: a study with emphasis on the elderly. Arch Intern Med 1984;144:1185–1188.

Lau-Ting C, Phoon WO. Aches and pains among Singapore elderly. Singapore Med J 1988;29:164–167.

Meyers FH, Jawetz E, Goldfien A. Review of medical pharmacology. 7th ed. Los Altos, CA: Lange Medical, 1980;269–273.

Mumford JM. Pain perception threshold and adaptation of normal human teeth. Arch Oral Biol 1965;10:957–968.

NIH Consensus Development Conference. The treatment of sleep disorders of older people: consensus statement. From NIH in cooperation with Gardiner-Caldwell SynerMed, Califon, NJ 07830.

Nolan L, O'Malley K. Prescribing for the elderly: 1. Sensitivity of the elderly to adverse drug reactions. J Am Geriatr Soc 1988;36:142–149.

Parmelee PA, Katz IR, Lawton MP. Relation of pain to depression among institutionalized aged. J Gerontol 1991; 46:P15–P21.

Portenoy RK, Bruera E. Topics in palliative care, vol 1. Oxford, UK: Oxford Medical, 1994.

Porter J, Jick H. Addiction rate in patients treated with narcotics. N Engl J Med 1980;302:123.

Roy R, Michael T. A survey of chronic pain in an elderly population. Can Fam Phys 1986;32:513–516.

Sack KE. Update on NSAIDs in the elderly. Geriatrics 1989;44:71–90.

Saunders C, Baines M, Dunlop R. Living with dying: a guide to palliative care. 3rd ed. Oxford, UK: Oxford Medical, 1995.

Schumacher GA, Goodell H, Hardy JD, et al. Uniformity of the pain threshold in man. Science 1940;92:110–112.

Sherman D, Robillard E. Sensitivity to pain in the elderly. Can Med Assoc J 1960;83:944–947.

Shock NW, Greulich RC, Andres R, et al. Normal human aging: the Baltimore longitudinal study of aging. NIH Pub 84–2450. Washington: US Government Printing Office, 1984.

Seidl LG, Thornton GF, Smith JW, Cluff LE. Studies on the epidemiology of adverse drug reactions: 3. Reactions in patients on a general medical service. Bull Johns Hopkins Hosp 1966;119:299–315.

Steel K, Gertman PM, Crescenzi C, Anderson J. Iatrogenic illness on a general medical service at a university hospital. N Engl J Med 1981;304:638–642.

Tinetti M, Speechley M, Ginter SF. Risk factors for falls among elderly persons living in the community. N Engl J Med 1988; 314:1701–1707.

Tucker MA, Andrew MF, Ogle SJ, et al. Age associated change in pain threshold measured by transcutaneous neuronal electrical stimulation. Age Ageing 1989;18:241–246.

Uhlmann RF, Larson EB, Rees TS, et al. Relationship of hearing impairment to dementia. JAMA 1989;261:1916–1919.

Uhlmann RF, Teri L, Rees TS, et al. Impact of hearing loss on mental status testing. J Am Geriatr Soc 1989;37:223–228.

Van Nostrand JF, Furner SE, Suzman R, eds. Health data on older Americans: United States, 1992. National Center for Health Statistics. Vital Health Stat 3(27), 1993.

Warren JW, Tenney JG, Hoopes JM, et al. A prospective microbiological study of bacteriuria in patients with chronic indwelling urethral catheters. J Infect Dis 1982;146:719.

Woodrow KM, Friedman GD, Siegelaub MS, et al. Pain tolerance: differences according to age, sex and race. Psychosom Med 1972; 34:548–556.

Zenz M, Willweber-Strumpf A. Opiophobia and cancer pain in Europe. Lancet 1993;341:1075–1076.

CHAPTER 31

Management of Chronic Pain in the Patient with Substance Abuse

Henry U. Lu, Steven D. Passik, and Russell K. Portenoy

INTRODUCTION

Nearly a third of the United States population have used illicit drugs, and an estimated 6 to 15% have a substance use disorder of some type (1-3). As a result of this high prevalence, problems related to abuse and addiction are encountered commonly among those who seek treatment for acute or chronic pain.

Chemical dependency is a heterogeneous set of disorders. The issues surrounding the management of pain are likely to vary among those who are actively abusing illicit drugs, alcohol, or prescription drugs; those in drug-free recovery; and those in methadone maintenance programs. The problems presented by patients who are actively abusing vary with the favored drug, the frequency of use, and the types of physical or psychosocial comorbidities. To assess and manage pain, clinicians must understand the basic concepts in addiction medicine and the specific concerns posed by these diverse groups of patients.

DEFINING ABUSE AND ADDICTION IN THE CLINICAL SETTING

The nomenclature applied to substance abuse and addiction is highly problematic. Tolerance and physical dependence are commonly confused with abuse and addiction, and all definitions applied to medical patients are typically extrapolated from addict populations without medical illness. This nomenclature must be clarified for clinical populations, including those with pain (4) (Table 31.1).

Tolerance

Tolerance is the reduction in a drug effect over time (or the need for a higher dose to maintain an effect), which is induced by exposure to the drug (5, 6). The term cannot be applied if an

Table 31.1. Proposed Terminology of Substance Abuse

Term	Definition
Physical dependence	Pharmacologic property of some drugs defined solely by abstinence syndrome on abrupt dose reduction, discontinuation of dosing, or administration of an antagonist drug
Tolerance	Diminution of one or more drug effects, either favorable or adverse, caused by exposure to the drug; may be pharmacologic or associative (related to learning)
Substance abuse	Use of a substance in a manner outside of sociocultural conventions; according to this definition, all use of illicit drugs, as well as use of a licit drug in a manner not dictated by convention (e.g., according to a physician's orders)
Addiction	Commonly used term not in current psychiatric nosologies; can be taken to mean aberrant use of a substance in a manner characterized by loss of control, compulsive use, and continued use despite harm

Reprinted with permission from Passik SD, Portenoy RK. Substance abuse issues in palliative care. In: Berger A, Portenoy RK, Weissman D, eds. Supportive oncology. Philadelphia: Lippincott-Raven, 1998;514.

explanation for declining effects unrelated to drug exposure, such as progression of a tissue-damaging lesion, can be discerned.

Clinicians and patients alike commonly express concern that tolerance to analgesic effects may compromise the benefits of opioid therapy and lead to the requirement for progressively higher and ultimately unsustainable doses. Additionally, the development of tolerance to the reinforcing effects of opioids and the consequent need to increase doses to regain these effects has been speculated to be an important element in the pathogenesis of addiction (7). In contrast to these expectations, an extensive clinical experience has not confirmed that tolerance causes substantial problems in the clinical setting (8, 9). Although tolerance to a variety of opioid effects can be reliably observed in animal models (10), and tolerance to nonanalgesic effects, such as respiratory depression and cognitive impairment, occurs routinely in patients (11), analgesic tolerance does not usually interfere with the clinical efficacy of opioid drugs. Numerous surveys have demonstrated that most patients find an effective dose that remains stable for long periods. Dose escalation, when it is required, usually reflects progression of a painful lesion (12-18) and cannot therefore be attributed to tolerance. Analgesic tolerance is rarely the driving force for dose escalation.

Clinical observation also fails to support the conclusion that tolerance is a substantial contributor to the development of addiction. It is widely accepted that addicts without a medical disorder may or may not have any of the manifestations of analgesic tolerance, and the occasional opioid-treated patient who presents findings consistent with analgesic tolerance typically does so without evidence of abuse or addiction.

Physical Dependence

Physical dependence is defined solely as an abstinence syndrome (withdrawal) following abrupt dose reduction or administration of an antagonist (5, 6, 19). Physical dependence is unapparent unless abstinence is induced. There is no evidence that the physiological changes that underlie the phenomenon are a problem as long as abstinence is avoided.

There is great confusion among clinicians about the differences between physical dependence and addiction. Some incorrectly consider the terms to be synonymous and others believe that physical dependence, that is, the potential for abstinence syndrome, is a necessary component of addiction (20, 21). The latter belief rests on the idea that the avoidance of withdrawal symptoms creates behavioral contingencies that result ultimately in addiction (7). This perceived association between physical dependence and addiction has not been supported by experience acquired during opioid therapy for chronic pain. Physical dependence does not preclude the uncomplicated discontinuation of opioids during multidisciplinary pain management of nonmalignant pain (22), and opioid therapy is routinely stopped without difficulty in cancer patients whose pain disappears following effective antineoplastic therapy. Indirect evidence for a fundamental distinction between physical dependence and addiction is even provided by animal models of opioid self-administration, which have demonstrated that persistent drug-taking behavior can be maintained in the absence of physical dependence (23).

Thus, the stigmatizing labels "addict" and "addiction" should never be used to describe patients who are only perceived to have the capacity for an abstinence syndrome. These patients must be labeled "physically dependent." Use of the word "dependent" alone is also unacceptable because it fosters confusion between physical dependence and psychological dependence, a component of addiction. For the same reason, the term "habituation" should not be used.

Definition of Abuse

The term substance abuse is also stigmatizing and subject to confusion. It is best applied to any drug use that falls outside of social or cultural norms (24, 25). According to this definition, any use of an illicit drug is abuse. The use of alcohol or a licit drug can be labeled abuse only by comparison with current norms of use (discussed later).

Definition of Addiction

The confusion in the nomenclature applied to addiction is exemplified by the fourth edition of *Diagnostic and Statistical Manual of Mental Disorders* (DSM-IV) of the American Psychiatric Association (21). DSM-IV eschews the term addiction and instead offers definitions of substance abuse and substance dependence (Table 31.2). The criteria for substance abuse are focused on the negative psychosocial sequelae of drug use, and the criteria for substance dependence highlight chronicity and add the dimensions of physical dependence and tolerance. These criteria were developed in reference to substance abusers without pain. Although substance dependence is meant to be used in a manner synonymous with addiction, the reference to tolerance and physical dependence is inappropriate and precludes the use of this terminology in patients who are prescribed abusable drugs for legitimate purposes and develop either tolerance or physical dependence as expected consequences of therapeutic drug use (26).

Any definition of addiction that includes phenomena related to physical dependence or tolerance cannot be applied to clinical populations, including those with pain. A better definition of addiction notes that it is a chronic disorder characterized by "the compulsive use of a substance resulting in physical, psychological or social harm to the user and continue use despite that harm" (25). This definition appropriately emphasizes that addiction is fundamentally a psychological and behavioral syndrome. The necessary characteristics are *(a)* loss of control over drug use, *(b)* compulsive drug use, and *(c)* continued use despite harm.

The concept of aberrant drug-related behavior is a useful first step in applying this definition to clinical populations. A broad range of drug-taking behaviors may be considered problematic by prescribers and may indicate the development of addiction (Table 31.3). True addiction is only one of several possible explanations for such behavior, however, and it is valuable to consider the larger differential diagnosis (Table 31.4). For example, the challenging diagnosis of pseudoaddiction must be considered if the patient is reporting distress associated with unrelieved symptoms. This term was coined to depict the distress and drug seeking that can occur in the context of unrelieved cancer pain (27).

Table 31.2.   Definitions of Substance Dependence and Substance Abuse

Substance dependence

A maladaptive pattern of substance abuse, leading to clinically significant impairment or distress, as manifested by three or more of the following occurring at any time in the same 12-month period.

A. Tolerance, as defined by either of the following:
  1. A need for markedly increased amounts of substance to achieve intoxication or desired effect.
  2. Markedly diminished effect with continued use of the same amount of the substance.

B. Withdrawal, as manifested by either of the following:
  1. The characteristic withdrawal syndrome for the substance.
  2. The same (or close related) substance is taken to relieve or avoid withdrawal symptoms.

C. The substance is often taken in larger amounts or over a longer period than was intended.

D. There is a persistent desire or unsuccessful efforts to cut down or control substance use.

E. A great deal of time spent in activities necessary to obtain the substance (e.g., visiting multiple doctors or driving long distances), use the substance, (e.g., chain-smoking), or recover from its effects.

F. Important social, occasional, or recreational activities are given up or reduced because of substance use.

G. The substance use is continued despite knowledge of having a persistent or recurrent physical or psychological problem that is likely to have been caused or exacerbated by the substance (e.g., current cocaine use despite recognition of cocaine-induced depression, or continued drinking despite recognition that an ulcer was made worse by alcohol consumption)

Substance abuse

A maladaptive pattern of substance abuse leading to clinically significant impairment or distress, as manifested by one (or more) of the following, occurring within a 12-month period.

A. Recurrent substance use resulting in a failure to fulfill major role obligations at work, school, or home, (e.g., repeated absences or poor work performance related to substance use; substance related absences; suspensions, or expulsions from school; neglect of children or household).

B. Recurrent substance use in situations in which it is physically hazardous (e.g., driving an automobile or operating a machine when impaired by substance use)

C. Recurrent substance-related legal problems (e.g., arrests for substance-related disorderly conduct).

D. Continued substance use despite having persistent or recurrent social or interpersonal problems caused or exacerbated by the effects of the substance (e.g., arguments with spouse about consequences of intoxication, physical fights).

E. The symptoms have never met the criteria for Substance Dependence for this class of substance.

Reprinted with permission from American Psychiatric Association. Diagnostic and Statistical Manual for Mental Disorders. 4th ed. Washington: APA Press, 1994.

Table 31.3.   Spectrum of Aberrant Drug-Related Behaviors That Raise Concern about the Potential for Addiction

More suggestive of addition
  Selling prescription drugs
  Prescription forgery
  Stealing or drugs from others
  Injecting oral formulations
  Obtaining prescription drugs from nonmedical sources
  Concurrent abuse of alcohol or illicit drugs
  Repeated dose escalation or similar noncompliance despite multiple warnings
  Repeated visits to other clinicians or emergency rooms
    without informing prescriber
  Drug-related deterioration in function at work, in the family, or socially
  Repeated resistance to changes in therapy despite evidence
    of adverse drug effects
Less suggestive of addition
  Aggressive complaining about the need for more drugs
  Drug hoarding during periods of reduced symptoms
  Requesting specific drugs
  Openly acquiring similar drugs from other medical sources
  Occasional unsanctioned dose escalation or other noncompliance
  Unapproved use of the drug to treat another symptom
  Reporting psychic effects not intended by the clinician
  Resistance to a change in therapy associated with tolerable adverse effects
  Intense expressions of anxiety about recurrent symptom

Reprinted with permission from Portenoy RK. Opioid therapy for chronic nonmalignant pain: current status. In: Fields HL, Liebeskind JC, eds. Progress in pain research and management, vol. 1. Pharmacological approaches to the treatment of chronic pain: new concepts and critical issues. Seattle: IASP Press, 1994;247-287.

Table 31.4.   Differential Diagnosis for Aberrant Drug-Related Behaviors

Addiction (substance dependence disorder)
Pseudoaddiction
Psychiatric disorders associated with impulsive or aberrant drug taking
Personality disorders, including borderline and psychopathic
  personality disorders
Depressive disorders
Anxiety disorders
Encephalopathy with confusion about appropriate therapeutic regimen
Criminal intent

These categories are not mutually exclusive.
Reprinted with permission from Passik SD, Portenoy RK. Substance abuse issues in palliative care. In: Berger A, Portenoy RK, Weissman D, eds. Supportive oncology. Philadelphia: Lippincott-Raven, 1998;519.

The cardinal feature is that the aberrant behaviors disappear when an effective analgesic intervention is administered.

Alternatively, impulsive drug use may indicate another psychiatric disorder, diagnosis of which may have therapeutic implications. Occasionally, aberrant drug-related behavior appears to be causally related to a mild encephalopathy, with confusion about the appropriate therapeutic regimen, and rarely, problematic behaviors indicate criminal intent. These diagnoses are not mutually exclusive.

Issues in the Assessment of Aberrant Drug-Related Behavior

The identification and assessment of aberrant drug-related behavior are, therefore, the prerequisites to the diagnosis of addiction in patients who are treated for pain. This assessment can be particularly challenging if a history of substance abuse is reported. Patients with this history highlight the importance of several other concerns, including *(a)* the need for assessment over time, *(b)* the problem of undertreatment, *(c)* the sociocultural influence on the definition of aberrancy, and *(d)* the importance of disease-related variables.

Need for Assessment over Time

It may be difficult to interpret aberrant behavior and apply appropriate diagnostic labels until sufficient time has passed to allow repeated observations and evaluate medical and psychosocial characteristics. Astute psychiatric assessment is essential and may require evaluation by consultants who can clarify the interactions among unrelieved pain, personality factors, and psychiatric illnesses. The complexity of these interactions may be greatest in the population of active substance abusers (28). Some patients self-medicate their symptoms of anxiety or depression, insomnia, or even problems of adjustment (such as boredom due to diminished ability to engage in usual activities and hobbies). Others have characteristic pathology, such as borderline personality disorder, that may underlie the use of prescribed drugs in a chaotic and impulsive manner that regulates inner tension, expresses anger at doctors or significant others, or ameliorates chronic emptiness or boredom.

The Problem of Undertreatment

Clinical observation suggests that the inadequate management of symptoms may be an impetus for aberrant drug-related behaviors. Undertreatment is prevalent even in those with cancer or AIDS (29, 30), for whom opioid therapy is widely considered appropriate. When medically ill patients have a history of substance abuse and are undertreated, the diagnosis of addiction versus pseudoaddiction can be very challenging. Indeed, some of these patients appear to return to illicit drug use as means to self-medication, at least in part, and others adopt patterns of behavior (e.g., manipulation or aggressive behaviors) that generate great concerns about the possibility of true addiction. Unrelieved pain complicates the interpretation of aberrant behaviors in all patients and is a particular concern in the management of pain in those with a history of substance abuse.

Sociocultural Influences

By definition, the use of an illicit drug or the use of a prescription drug without a medical indication is abuse. If either type of drug is used in a compulsive manner that continues despite harm to the user or others, a diagnosis of addiction may be appropriate (Table 31.1). These definitions are consonant with the social and cultural norms of drug taking.

When a drug is prescribed for a legitimate medical purpose, there may be less certainty about behaviors that may be characterized as aberrant and diagnosed as abuse or addiction. Although the aberrancy of some behaviors, such as prescription forgery and the intravenous injection of an oral formulation, would not be argued, many other behaviors are less clear-cut. For example, is it aberrant for the patient with unre-

lieved pain to consume a few extra doses of a prescribed opioid, particularly if this behavior was not specifically prohibited by the clinician? Is it aberrant to use an opioid drug prescribed for pain as a nighttime hypnotic?

The ability to categorize such questionable behaviors as outside social or cultural norms also presupposes certainty about the parameters of normative behavior. In the area of prescription drug use, no empirical data define these parameters. If a large proportion of patients are discovered to engage in a specific behavior, such as the occasional use of extra doses, it may be normative, and judgment about deviance would be influenced accordingly.

The importance of social and cultural norms in turn raises the inevitable possibility of bias. Bias against a social group can influence the willingness of clinicians to label a questionable drug-related behavior as aberrant when performed by a member of that group. Clinical observation suggests that this type of bias is common in the assessment of drug-related behaviors of patients with substance abuse histories. Questionable behaviors by such patients may be promptly labeled as abuse or addiction, even if the drug abuse history was in the remote past.

Disease-Related Variables

The core concepts used to define addiction may also be problematic as a result of changes associated with chronic pain. Deterioration in physical or psychosocial functioning, mood disturbances, and family disruption related to pain may be difficult to separate from the morbidity associated with drug abuse. This may particularly complicate efforts to evaluate the concept of use despite harm, which is critical to the diagnosis of addiction. Prolonged observation, tapering or discontinuation of the drug, and concurrent therapies may in some cases be needed to clarify the degree to which the drug was the problem.

RISK OF ABUSE AND ADDICTION DURING PAIN TREATMENT IN POPULATIONS WITH CURRENT OR REMOTE DRUG ABUSE

With appropriate definitions of abuse and addiction, it is possible to examine the true risks associated with the therapeutic use of abusable drugs, including the use of opioids to treat acute or chronic pain. There is very little empirical information about this risk in patients with a current or remote history of substance abuse. Although anecdotal reports suggest that successful long-term opioid therapy of cancer pain or chronic nonmalignant pain is possible in some cases (31-35), it is also likely that the risk of aberrant drug-related behaviors during treatment with an abusable drug is higher in this population.

Categories of Substance Abusers

Based on anecdotal observations, it may be hypothesized that patients with a history of drug abuse can be divided into categories with prognostic importance. Important subpopulations include those with a remote history of opioid abuse, those with a history of opioid abuse who are in methadone maintenance treatment, and those actively abusing opioid drugs (36). To this scheme it may be reasonable to add other groups, such as patients with a remote or present history of addiction to alcohol, nonopioid illicit drugs (e.g., cocaine), or nonopioid prescription drugs (e.g., benzodiazepine). Patients who are participating in 12-step or other drug-free recovery programs may also be distinguished. These distinctions may be relevant indicators of the types of problems likely to occur during pain therapy. For example, a small retrospective study (31) suggested that all of these groups were at relatively high risk for inadequate pain management, but only those who were actively abusing could not reliably achieve adequate symptom control once they were treated aggressively by pain service personnel. An anecdotal report observed that even a remote history of abuse can stigmatize a patient and complicate pain treatment (32).

Generalizations developed from clinical experience may fail to prepare clinicians for the vagaries of practice, in which the experience of pain itself or the existence of various comorbidities can alter responses in an unpredictable way. This variability demands a comprehensive assessment of each case. This assessment must characterize the drug abuse history, identify salient comorbidities, and provide a detailed evaluation of the pain.

MANAGEMENT OF PAIN IN POPULATIONS WITH CURRENT OR REMOTE DRUG ABUSE

Taking a Substance Use History

Clinicians often avoid asking patients about drug abuse for fear that patients will be offended, become angry, or feel threatened. Often clinicians expect that the patients will not respond truthfully. These attitudes reduce the likelihood of truthful communication and increase the problems associated with the monitoring of therapy over time. The clinician must be nonjudgmental when taking the patient's history of substance use and anticipate defensiveness on the part of the patient. It can be helpful to mention that patients often misrepresent their drug use for valid reasons, including fear of stigmatization, mistrust of the interviewer, or concern about undermedication.

The clinician must be inquisitive and knowledgeable about drug abuse. The use of street names for drugs should be avoided unless the clinician is certain his or her knowledge of the names in use is current. The interview should include a review of all drugs taken, including the chronology of use over time, the current frequency of use, and triggers that initiate use. One helpful interview technique, known as the pyramid approach, begins with general questions about the role of substances in the patient's life, beginning with licit ones such as caffeine and nicotine. It then proceeds to more specific questions about illicit substances.

It is very important to inquire about the desired effects of all drugs used. This question can often lead to very valuable information about comorbid mood disturbances, unrelieved symptoms, and the degree to which the patient perceives that pain precipitates or perpetuates problems with drug use. The answers may provide a key to helping patients with control of symptoms they find particularly noxious and diminish the need for drugs of abuse.

Additional efforts may be required for comprehensive assessment of the pain and substance use history. It may be necessary to obtain all medical records, contact other health care providers, or contact pharmacies to assess drug-taking behavior. A request for a urine toxicology study at the time of initial evaluation may be informative (discussed later).

Role of Opioid Therapy

Opioids are first-line treatment for acute pain and chronic cancer pain, and there is growing recognition that these drugs should be used early in chronic pain associated with other incurable progressive diseases, such as AIDS. In all populations in which opioids are accepted medical therapy, the treatment of patients with a history of substance abuse requires a system for monitoring drug-taking behavior that is appropriate for the perceived level of risk. Treatment may be routine if the risk is perceived to be low. This might be the case if drug abuse occurred in the remote past. If the risk is perceived to be high, however, an intensive monitoring system would be appropriate (discussed later).

The long-term treatment of chronic nonmalignant pain with opioid drugs continues to be controversial. In populations with pain and substance abuse, there is neither a large and reassuring clinical experience nor empirical data that confirm the safety and efficacy of opioid therapy. Clinicians must exercise caution in recommending opioid trials to such patients. Generally, the use of opioid therapy for chronic nonmalignant pain should not be initiated if the patient is an active substance abuser, and such treatment should be offered to those with remote history of significant abuse or addiction only by experienced clinicians who can provide skilled assessment and monitoring over time.

Issues in Drug Selection

In studies of former addicts, agonist-antagonist opioids have less abuse potential than the pure agonist drugs. This characteristic may be important in a population with a history of substance abuse. These drugs have never been shown to yield better outcomes, however, and their capacity to cause withdrawal when given to patients who are physically dependent on a pure agonist drug contraindicates their use in patients with substantial opioid exposure. An agonist-antagonist drug should not be administered, therefore, to a patient receiving methadone or a patient with a history of polysubstance abuse, who may be physically dependent on opioids. These agonist-antagonist opioids also have a ceiling dose for analgesia, further limiting their utility for long-term therapy.

There is clinical lore, based on anecdotal observations, that links the risk of addiction to specific drug characteristics, including short half-life, rapid rise in plasma concentration following administration, and intravenous route of delivery. Although these characteristics do not appear to be relevant to the abuse liability in patient populations without substance abuse, it may be prudent to consider them when treating those with a history of drug abuse. If a pure agonist drug is selected for chronic therapy, there is no disadvantage to the use of a long-acting preparation, and it is possible on theoretical grounds that the slower onset and decline of effects associated with these drugs reduces the risk of aberrant drug-related behaviors. Accordingly, it is appropriate to consider oral methadone, oral controlled-release or sustained-release opioid formulations, and transdermal opioid formulations as preferred drugs for long-term opioid therapy in patients with histories of substance abuse. For pain that is moderate but exceeds the maximal efficacy of nonsteroidal anti-inflammatory drugs, the use of lower doses of the long-acting opioids or the use of tramadol may be preferable if there is concern about the use of the short-acting analgesics conventionally used for pain of this type (such as acetaminophen-codeine preparations). Tramadol is a unique opioid compound that has been demonstrated to have a relatively low abuse potential.

Given the dual role of methadone as a treatment for opioid addiction (37) and an analgesic (38-41), clinicians who manage patients with substance abuse histories and are considering opioid therapy must understand the pharmacology of this drug (42, 43). The use of methadone for the management of opioid addiction is subject to federal regulation. Prescribers must have a specific license; treatment for most patients is based on a single dose per day; and the parameters for acceptable monitoring are closely defined. When it is used as an analgesic, however, no special license is required; therapy almost always requires multiple doses per day; and monitoring can be undertaken in a manner consistent with conventional medical practice.

The differences in the dosing of methadone for its two indications are striking. Abstinence can be avoided and opioid craving can be reduced with a single daily dose. This is consistent with the long elimination half-life of this drug. Analgesic effects after a dose, however, are usually much briefer than would be expected given the half-life. Indeed, one double-blind study demonstrated that the duration of analgesia after a single dose of methadone is comparable to that of morphine, a short half-life opioid (44). Although there are exceptions, most patients appear to require a minimum of four doses per day to achieve sustained analgesia with methadone.

Patients who are receiving methadone maintenance as a treatment for opioid addiction can be administered methadone as an analgesic outside the guidelines of an addiction treatment program. This typically requires a substantial change in therapy, including dose escalation and multiple daily doses. Although the management of such a change does not pose difficult problems from a pharmacological perspective, it can create considerable stress for the patient and the clinicians involved in the treatment of the addiction disorder. Some patients express a lack of confidence in the analgesic efficacy of methadone because the drug has been labeled as addiction therapy rather than a pain therapy. Others wish to continue the morning dose for addiction even if treatment during the rest of the day uses the same drug at an equivalent or higher dose. Some physicians who work at methadone clinics are willing to stay involved and prescribe opioids, including methadone, outside the program, and others wish to relinquish care. The decisions concerning analgesics in such patients must be made individually, following a detailed assessment.

Issues in Drug Administration and Monitoring

Individualization of Dose

Successful opioid therapy depends on individualization of the dose without regard to its size. This important guideline can be problematic in persons with histories of substance abuse. Although it may be appropriate to exercise caution in prescribing abusable drugs to these persons, the decision to forego the principle of dose individualization may increase the likelihood of undertreatment. The unrelieved pain that results can increase the likelihood of aberrant drug-related behaviors. Although these behaviors may be best understood as pseudoaddiction, they often confirm clinicians' fears and encourage even greater caution in prescribing.

Impact of Tolerance

Although analgesic tolerance is seldom a problem in the clinical setting, it is nonetheless true that patients who are actively abusing drugs may have sufficient tolerance to influence the response to prescribed drugs. Although one survey failed to identify any difference in the need for postoperative analgesics between those with and those without a substance abuse history (45), anecdotal experience suggests that some actively abusing patients who are given an opioid for therapeutic purposes do require relatively high initial doses or rapid dose escalation to establish or retain therapeutic effects. Similarly, clinical observation suggests that some patients receiving methadone maintenance require relatively high opioid doses to treat acute pain and relatively rapid dose escalation at the start of therapy to identify a useful dose for chronic pain management. From a practical perspective, the clinician must be cautious in estimating the degree to which tolerance may be operating but also cognizant of the potential need for higher doses.

Recognizing Specific Drug Abuse Behaviors

As noted previously, patients who are prescribed abusable drugs must be carefully monitored over time for the development of aberrant drug-related behaviors, using a system of monitoring appropriate to the perceived level of risk. If there is a high level of concern about such behaviors, monitoring may require relatively frequent visits, regular assessment of significant others who can provide observations about patients' drug use, and periodic urine drug screens.

Urine drug screening can facilitate the early recognition of aberrant drug-related behaviors in patients who have been actively abusing drugs in the recent past. Urine should be screened for both illicit and licit but unprescribed drugs. The patient should be fully informed about this approach, which should be explained as a method of monitoring that can be reassuring to the clinician and thereby facilitate aggressive symptom-oriented treatments. The patient should also be apprised of the clinician's response to positive screens. This response usually entails increasing the monitoring procedures for continued treatment, including greater frequency of visits, smaller quantities of prescribed drugs, and so on. In the case of repeated violations, referral for concurrent drug rehabilitation may be the most appropriate course. If the abuse is extreme, ongoing analgesic treatment cannot be justified.

In some cases the approach to monitoring may best be accomplished through the use of a written contract. This contract, which is kept in the medical record, defines the drug regimen, explicitly states the responsibilities of both the patient and the clinician, and stipulates the consequences of aberrant drug use. These guidelines should include specific reference to the methods that will be used to renew prescriptions and the response to the report of lost or stolen drugs.

Patients who protest the use of urine drug screens or contracts may be unwilling or unable to enter a collaborative relationship in which the clinician can be confident of responsible drug taking by the patient and the patient can be confident that the clinician will respond to unrelieved symptoms with aggressive therapies. Such patients may not be candidates for treatment with abusable drugs.

Other Aspects of Patient Monitoring and Education

Patients must be given detailed instructions about the parameters of responsible drug taking. The goal is to prevent the use of illicit drugs, if possible, and to eliminate abuse of the prescribed drug regimen. Patients suspected of aberrant drug use must be seen frequently. Weekly visits are common initially. Frequent visits help establish close ties with staff, allow evaluation of both symptom control and addiction-related concerns, and allow the prescription of small quantities of drugs, which may diminish the temptation to misuse and provide an incentive for keeping appointments.

For patients who are considered to be at high risk for aberrant behavior, the clinician's response to "lost" prescriptions, requests for early refills, and other aberrant behaviors should be decided in advance, to the extent possible, and clearly explained to the patient. There can be no prescription renewals if appointments are missed. The patient should be told that dose changes require prior contact with the clinician or designee. It may be useful to reassure the patient that dose escalation of drugs used for symptom control is common and acceptable, if the clinical evaluation supports this course and the patient deals with the need for a change in drug regimen without relying on aberrant behaviors.

The rigidity of the plan to deal with "lost" prescriptions or the need for early refills due to unsanctioned dose escalation again depends on the clinician's assessment of the degree of abuse. In some cases, it is appropriate to stipulate at the outset that early refills for prescription loss will not be provided unless the patient presents a police report that documents the event. In other cases, it may be sufficient to inform the patient that the behavior is unacceptable and may lead to an inability to provide uninterrupted treatment. Subsequent decisions about the response to aberrant behavior can then be based on observation of the patient's response to these guidelines.

To avoid conflicts after hours or during holiday periods, clinicians who cover for the primary care giver must be informed about the guidelines that have been established for each patient with a history of abuse. Again, the restrictions should be made more or less stringent based on the level of concern about aberrant behaviors.

Some patients are so concerned about the potential for addiction or readdiction that compliance with therapy is threatened. It is ironic that some patients actually prefer rigid guidelines because of an enhanced sense of control over drugs. In discussing the need for compliance, it is also important to have the patient realize that there is a risk of readdiction associated with uncontrolled pain or other symptoms. Counseling can also help patients identify possible triggers to drug and alcohol abuse that they may encounter during treatment and develop strategies for avoiding illicit drug use or uncontrolled use of prescribed drugs at those times.

Treatment of Comorbid Psychiatric Disorders

Psychiatric comorbidity, including personality disorders (e.g., borderline, antisocial), depression, and anxiety disorders, is relatively high in patients with substance abuse histories (28). The treatment of anxiety and depression can increase the patient's comfort and possibly diminish the likelihood of relapse. For these reasons, early psychiatric consultation should be considered when significant psychiatric impairment is observed.

The Role of Drug Recovery Programs

Some patients can be referred to a drug recovery program as a means to curtail drug abuse during treatment for pain. Patients can document their attendance at groups to further reassure the clinician about the effort to comply with therapy. Patients who enter a program and are given a sponsor may allow the physician or designee to contact the sponsor, who may also help support the clinical plan. This type of contact also helps to prevent the patient's ostracism by others in the program if controlled prescription drugs are needed.

Although there may be clear benefits for the patient who can successfully use a drug recovery program while receiving abusable drugs as prescribed therapy, there are potential problems. Some of these programs endorse drug-free recovery in very strong terms, and it may not be possible for the patient to maintain comfortable contacts while using opioids or other prescription drugs. The response of those in the program to a request for dose escalation may be quite different from that of the clinician, and this disparity may compound the patient's stress or lead to underreporting of symptoms.

The Role of Multidisciplinary Pain Programs

Multidisciplinary pain programs offer effective multimodality treatment for selected patients with chronic pain. The structure of these programs may or may not be optimal for patients with a history of substance abuse. It should not be assumed that the traditional multidisciplinary pain management program has the expertise necessary to manage these clinical problems. The decision to refer a patient with chronic pain to such a program must be based on a careful assessment of both the patient and program. The balance between treatment for drug abuse and treatment for pain and disability must be appropriate for the needs of the patient.

Role of Addiction Medicine Specialists

In some cases, the combined efforts of an addiction medicine specialist and pain specialists can provide optimal care for the patient with pain and a history of substance abuse (46). A treatment strategy that is jointly developed may increase the likelihood that control over drug use can be maintained while interventions are provided to enhance comfort and function (47).

CONCLUSION

Patients with a remote or current history of substance abuse who require therapy for pain pose numerous problems in assessment and management. Clinicians must recognize the heterogeneity of this population and understand the complexity of the interface between the therapeutic use of abusable drugs for symptom control and the multifaceted nature of abuse and addiction. Important issues include assessment of symptoms and drug-taking behaviors, difficulties in maintaining symptom control, management of drug use and prevention of drug abuse, education and communication between the treatment team and other clinicians, and the need to address the unique fears of patients who may be stigmatized by a history of socially unacceptable behavior. Research in these areas has only recently begun. Practical management as yet is based largely on clinical experience and anecdotal observations.

References

1. Colliver JD, Kopstein AN. Trends in cocaine abuse reflected in emergency room episodes reported to DAWN. Publ Health Rep 1991;106:59–68.
2. Groerer J, Brodsky M. The incidence of illicit drug use in the United States, 1962–1989. Br J Addiction 1992;87:1345–1351.
3. Regier DA, Meyers JK, Dramer M, et al. The NIMH epidemiologic catchment area program. Arch Gen Psychiatry 1984;41:934–958.
4. Passik SD, Portenoy RK. Substance abuse issues in palliative care. In: Berger A, Portenoy RK, Weissman D, eds. Supportive oncology. New York: Lippincott, 1989;8:513–529.
5. Dole VP. Narcotic addiction, physical dependence and relapse. N Engl J Med 1972;286:988–992.
6. Martin WR, Jasinski DR. Physiological parameters of morphine dependence in man-tolerance, early abstinence, protracted abstinence. J Psychiatr Res 1969;7:9–17.
7. Wikler A. Opioid dependence: mechanisms and treatment. New York: Plenum Press, 1980.
8. Portenoy RK. Opioid tolerance and efficacy: basis research and clinical observation. In: Gebhardt G, Hammond D, Jensen T, eds. Proceedings of the VII World Congress on Pain. Progress in Pain Research and Management, vol. 2 Seattle: IASP Press, 1994;595–619.
9. Foley KM. Clinical tolerance to opioids. In: Basbaum AI, Besson JM, eds. Towards a new pharmacotherapy of pain. Chichester, UK: John Wiley & Sons, 1991:181–203.
10. Ling GSF, Paul D, Simantov R, Pasternak GW. Differential development of acute tolerance to analgesia, respiratory depression, gastrointestinal transit and hormone release in a morphine infusion model. Life Sci 1989;45:1627–1636.
11. Bruera E, Macmillan K, Hanson JA, MacDonald RN. The cognitive effects of the administration of narcotic analgesics in patients with cancer pain. Pain 1989;39:13–16.
12. Twycross RG. Clinical experience with diamorphine in advanced malignant disease. Int J Clin Pharmacol Ther Toxicol 1974;9:184–198.
13. Kanner RM, Foley KM. Patterns of narcotic drug use in a cancer pain clinic. Ann N Y Acad Sci 1981;362:161–172.
14. Chapman CR, Hill HF. Prolonged morphine self-administration and addiction liability: evaluation of two theories in a bone marrow transplant unit. Cancer 1989;63:1636–1644.
15. France RD, Urban BJ, Keefe FJ. Long-term use of narcotic analgesics in chronic pain. Soc Sci Med 1984;19:1379–1382.
16. Portenoy RK, Foley KM. Chronic use of opioid analgesics in nonmalignant pain: report of 38 cases. Pain 1986;25:171–186.
17. Urban BJ, France RD, Steinberger DL, et al. Long-term use of narcotic-antidepressant medication in the management of phantom limb pain. Pain 1986;24:191–197.
18. Zenz M, Strumpf M, Tryba M. Long-term opioid therapy in patients with chronic nonmalignant pain. J Pain Symptom Mgmt 1992;7:69–77.
19. Redmond DE, Krystal JH. Multiple mechanisms of withdrawal from opioid drugs. Ann Rev Neurosci 1984;7:443–478.
20. World Health Organization. Technical report 516: Youth and drugs. Geneva: WHO, 1973.
21. American Psychiatric Association. Diagnostic and Statistical Manual for Mental Disorders. 4th ed. Washington: APA, 1994.
22. Halpern LM, Robinson J. Prescribing practices for pain in drug dependence: a lesson in ignorance. Adv Alcohol Subst Abuse 1985;5:184–197.
23. Dai S, Corrigal WA, Coen KM, Kalant H. Heroin self-administration by rats: influence of dose and physical dependence. Pharmacol Biochem Behav 1989;32:1009–1015.
24. Jaffe JH. Current concepts of addiction. Res Publ Assoc Res Nerv Ment Dis 1992;70:1–21.
25. Rinaldi RC, Steindler EM, Wilford BB, Goodwin D. Clarification and standardization of substance abuse terminology. JAMA 1988;259:555–557.

26. Sees KL, Clark HW. Opioid use in the treatment of chronic pain: assessment of addiction. J Pain Symptom Mgmt 1993;8:257–264.

27. Weissman DE, Haddox JD. Opioid pseudoaddiction: an iatrogenic syndrome. Pain 1989;36:363–366.

28. Khantzian EJ, Treece C. DSM-III psychiatric diagnosis of narcotic addicts: recent findings. Arch Gen Psychiatry 1985;42:1067–1071.

29. Breitbart W, Rosefeld BD, Passik SD, et al. The undertreatment of pain in ambulatory AIDS patients. Pain 1996;65:239–245.

30. Cleeland C, Gonin R, Hatfield A, et al. Pain and its treatment in outpatients with metastatic cancer. N Engl J Med 1994:330:592–596.

31. Macaluso C, Weinberg D, Foley KM. Opioid abuse and misuse in a cancer pain population. J Pain Symptom Mgmt 1988;3:S24 (abstract).

32. Gonzales GR, Coyle N. Treatment of cancer pain in a former opioid abuser: fears of the patients and staff and their influence on care. J Pain Symptom Mgmt 1992;7:246–249.

33. Dunbar SA, Katz NP. Chronic opioid therapy for nonmalignant pain in patients with a history of substance abuse: report of 20 cases. J Pain Symptom Mgmt 1996;11:163–171.

34. Portenoy RK. Chronic opioid therapy in non-malignant pain. J Pain Symptom Mgmt 1990;5 (suppl):S46–62.

35. Kennedy JA, Crowley TJ. Chronic pain and substance abuse: a pilot study of opioid maintenance. J Subst Abuse Treat 1990;7:233–238

36. Foley KM. The treatment of cancer pain. N Engl J Med 1985; 313:84–95

37. Lowinson JH, Marion IJ, Joseph H, Dole VP. Methadone maintenance. In: Lowinson JH, Ruiz P, Millman RB, eds. Substance abuse: a comprehensive textbook. Baltimore: Williams & Wilkins, 1992;550.

38. Fainsinger R, Schoeller T, Bruera E. Methadone in the management of cancer pain: a review. Pain 1993;52:137–147.

39. De Conno F, Groff L, Brunelli C, et al. Clinical experience with oral methadone administration in the treatment of pain in 196 advanced cancer patients. J Clin Oncol 1996;14:2836–2842.

40. Gardner-Nix JS. Oral methadone for managing chronic nonmalignant pain. J Pain Symptom Mgmt 1996;11:321–328.

41. Thomas Z, Bruera E. Use of methadone in a highly tolerant patient receiving parenteral hydromorphone. J Pain Symptom Mgmt 1995; 10:315–317.

42. Inturrisi CE, Colburn WA, Kaiko RF, et al. Pharmacokinetics and pharmacodynamics of methadone in patients with chronic pain. Clin Pharmacol Ther 1987;41:392–401.

43. Hunt G, Bruera E. Respiratory depression in a patient receiving oral methadone for cancer pain. J Pain Symptom Mgmt 1995;10:401–404.

44. Grochow L, Sheidler V, Grossman S, et al. Does intravenous methadone provide longer lasting analgesia than intravenous morphine? A randomized, double blind study. Pain 1989;38:151–157.

45. Kantor TG, Cantor R, Tom E. A study of hospitalized surgical patients on methadone maintenance. Drug Alcohol Depend 1980; 6:163–173.

46. Wesson DR, Ling W, Smith DE. Prescription of opioids for treatment of pain in patients with addictive disease. J Pain Symptom Mgmt 1993; 8:289–296.

47. Sees KL, Clark HW. Opioid use in the treatment of chronic pain: assessment of addiction. J Pain Symptom Mgmt 1994;9:74.

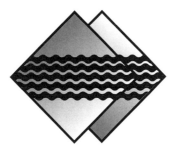

PART VI

Pharmacological Aspects

CHAPTER 32

Pharmacological Management of Chronic Pain: A Review

Gerald M. Aronoff and Rollin M. Gallagher

INTRODUCTION

Relief of pain and suffering has been the objective of the medical profession throughout history. Despite advances in treatment technology, however, pain often remains a medical enigma. Traditional management has generally encompassed such options as bed rest, physical therapy, nerve blocks, surgery, and medication. The purpose of this chapter is to discuss the role of medications in the treatment of nonmalignant chronic pain.

The use of pharmacological agents for pain relief is described in the Eber, Berlin, and Smith papyri from the 16th century. In Hellenic Greece, Hippocrates gave great attention to pain and distinguished between intense pain that cannot be controlled and pain that proper treatment can allay. In the 2nd century, Galen conducted experiments that led him to theorize about the causes of pain. He concluded that pain was the lowest conscious sensation (1).

In Europe, the Dark Ages saw a stagnation in the growth of knowledge about pain. Because pain was considered to be an act of God, its elimination was believed to be a sin. However, in Persia during the 10th century, Avicenna described 15 varieties of pain and speculated about the various bodily disturbances that produced them. It was not until the 15th century that Western medicine openly discussed the use of opium, belladonna, mandrake, and cold packs for the treatment of pain (2).

As late as 1628, Harvey still believed that the heart was where pain was felt. Descartes in the same period considered pain to be conducted by nerves to the brain directly. This seemed to predate the later specificity theories of Muller (3), Latze and Dallenbach (4), and von Frey (5). It was not until the late 1800s that Erb and Luckey (6), Goldscheider (7), and others proposed the pattern theory of pain. Finally, in the middle of the 20th century, a modern understanding of pain emerged, with the work of Hardy, Wolff and Goodell, Beecher, and Wall and Melzack showing the neurophysiological complexities of the pain experience (1, 2). A growing body of evidence indicates that pain itself can be considered a disease process that is self-perpetuating, causing both morphological and physiological changes in the central nervous system (CNS) and that new systems of classification based upon this pathology are indicated (8). Developing pharmacological interventions that specifically target these processes is in the near future of pain medicine (8, 9). A solid appreciation of the complex peripheral and central neurophysiology of nociception, pain perception, and pain modulation, which earlier chapters discuss in detail, and of the principles of behavioral pharmacology forms the basis for the rational and effective use of pharmacological agents for chronic pain.

PAIN PERCEPTION, PAIN BEHAVIOR, AND REINFORCEMENT

Pain and the relief of pain powerfully modify behavior. Because pain hurts and is unpleasant, people go to great lengths to ablate or minimize it or to avoid conditions that precipitate it. Thus, drugs and other treatments that promise to modify pain, even when unproved or of questionable validity, have great salience in human society. When the well-developed desire for pain relief is combined with the natural human tendency to experiment to solve problems, physicians are arguing against powerful human motivations when trying to dissuade a patient from trying new treatments.

Drugs that reduce pain powerfully reinforce drug-seeking behavior. These drugs are readily available and historically successful in treating our various aches and pains; hence the highly prevalent use of over-the-counter pain remedies such as NSAIDs, which act primarily in the periphery to reduce nociception. Centrally acting remedies also abound, although they may not be promoted as analgesics per se. Alcohol, marijuana, and opiates are well-known examples of ancient remedies for pain and suffering still used widely today. These drugs powerfully influence emotions and behavior as well as pain perception. Figure 32.1 presents a simplified model of the interaction of pain perception, pain behavior, and medications (10). Medications influence this model in several ways:

- Inhibit prostaglandin synthesis and secondary activation of nociceptors (e.g., the NSAIDs)
- Stabilize neuronal membranes to reduce ectopic nerve impulse generation and neuropathic pain (e.g., anticonvulsants and probably the tricyclic antidepressants)
- Reduce the suffering of pain (e.g., the opioid analgesics)
- Modify emotional and behavioral responses to pain that may perpetuate nociception or worsen pain perception (e.g., antidepressants, by treating secondary depression or anxiety, may improve patients' ability to comply with pain management instructions, including regimens in exercise, pacing, relaxation, and medication)

So closely related are pain and emotions that separating the analgesic effects from the emotional and behavioral effects of certain drugs may be difficult. This close relation forms the basis for the rational use of centrally acting drugs in chronic pain disorders.

THE CLINICAL PHARMACOLOGY OF CHRONIC PAIN: GENERAL PRINCIPLES

The successful use of medications for chronic pain depends upon careful clinical reasoning founded upon a working knowledge of the phenomenology and physiology of pain syndromes and the specific clinical actions of these drugs. Gallagher and Pasol (10) have outlined 10 general principles that usefully guide the practitioner to rational choices when prescribing medication.

1. *Make safety a priority when treating nonmalignant chronic pain.* The principles of efficacy, expediency, and cost follow. Consider drug and disease interactions. Benzodiazepines (BZDs) must be used cautiously, particularly in the elderly and those operating machinery, because they increase the risk of falls and accidents. Consider other serious risks, such as gastrointestinal (GI) bleeding from NSAIDs or liver disease from long-term high-dose acetaminophen (Tylenol). Ironically, opioids have fewer deleterious and toxic side effects or drug or disease interactions than most other medications used for pain. The literature does not substantiate the long-held belief that opioids are deleterious for patients in pain, particularly when used judiciously within a comprehensive pain program (10–12). Unfortunately, in a misguided effort to avoid exposure to opioids, toxic doses of ineffective drugs may be used in a futile effort to control pain. Undertreatment of pain and suffering may lead to unnecessary impairment, disability, stress, immunological compromise and secondary medical and psychiatric disorders.

2. *Make efficacy a priority when treating a terminally ill patient with pain.* Physicians and patients together may choose to risk using combinations of drugs in higher and higher doses to obtain relief of pain and suffering, enabling a patient to be more functional. However, the physician must continuously reevaluate the risk-benefit ratio of dosing. Unnecessarily high doses in an attempt to ablate pain without regard for untoward physiological, cognitive, emotional, and behavioral effects may worsen outcomes in terms of functional losses such as valuable interpersonal time with family and friends and inability to complete one's affairs.

3. *Review potential interactions with medical conditions and with other medications.* The physician should carefully review potential interactions of analgesics with

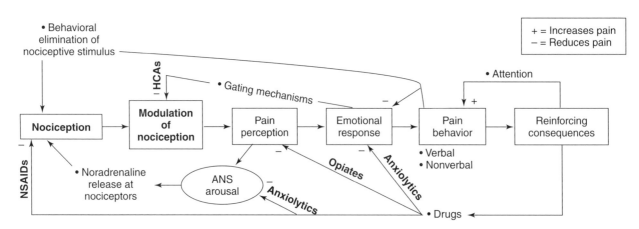

Figure 32.1 Biobehavioral dimensions of pain. ANS, autonomic nervous system; HCA, heterocyclic antidepressant; NSAID, nonsteroidal anti-inflammatory drug. (Reprinted with permission from Gallagher RM, Pasol E. Psychopharmacologic drugs in the chronic pain syndromes. Curr Rev Pain 1997;1:137–152.)

illnesses causing pain (e.g., diabetes with neuropathy, cancer, or rheumatoid arthritis) or comorbid with pain, particularly when treating older patients and those with chronic medical illness. For example, avoid heterocyclic antidepressants (HCAs) in postatrioventricular (A-V) node conduction disturbance and use them cautiously in urinary retention. The plethora of medications taken by chronically ill and elderly populations may interact with analgesics. Changing metabolism and secondarily, serum levels may lead to toxicity or alterations in the therapeutic activity of medications.

4. *Selectively choose drugs for pain disorder and comorbid psychiatric disorder according to efficacy and specific mechanism.* The efficacy of medication in chronic pain syndromes has been difficult to establish because of methodological problems such as poorly defined populations for study (e.g., low back pain that can be caused by any of several mechanisms), longitudinal designs of insufficient duration (e.g., most studies are less than 3 months), and inadequate outcome measures (e.g., subjective pain relief rather than functional improvement). Despite these problems, as we shall discuss, the efficacy of individual drugs in well-defined conditions, many with known receptor-based mechanisms, has been supported in the literature and should help guide psychotropic drug choice.

5. *Balance side effect profile against efficacy.* For example, in a patient with radicular low-back pain in whom weight loss may be critical for functional outcome, amitriptyline, which is effective in neuropathic pain, also may cause considerable weight gain. Choose another drug, such as nortriptyline.

6. *Consider drugs' effects on the efficacy of other analgesics.* For example, although BZDs are known to be excellent drugs for calming acute anxiety states associated with pain, they may interfere with opioid analgesia.

7. *Consider behavioral effects when prescribing.* Know the effects of a drug on critical neuropsychological functions, such as learning, memory, and psychomotor performance, that are critical to outcome in rehabilitation yet often not considered when prescribing. BZDs interfere with memory and learning and disinhibit negatively conditioned behavior. These effects are particularly problematic in pain rehabilitation, which relies on the premise that patients will learn new coping skills. What is the abuse liability of a drug? Diazepam's rapid onset of action makes abuse more likely than with clonazepam. What are a drug's behavioral consequences? To avoid unpleasant withdrawal, a patient dependent on regular doses of a short-acting sedative such as alprazolam or butalbital in Fiorinal and Fioricet may develop secondary drug-seeking pain behavior, sometimes manifesting as pain symptoms.

8. *Select combinations of medications from different classes.* Consider appropriate combinations of medication to influence the various nociceptor and neurotransmitter systems of pain perception: nociception, transmission of nociception, pain perception, suffering, pain modulation and pain behavior, as outlined in Figure 32.1, and their neurophysiological substrates. The traditional strategy of staying with one or two very familiar drugs in each class is often ineffective in chronic pain, no matter what its cause. One must be willing to try drugs of different classes in combination and also different drugs within the same class. The clinical problem of herniated lumbar disc suggests the importance of this principle. Thus, for a patient with an acute disc and radicular leg pain without surgical indications, the following medication combinations may be useful:

- *To reduce the inflammatory response and related nociception at the site of the herniation:* Ibuprofen 400 to 800 mg three or four times a day. If ineffective in 5 to 7 days, change to another NSAID. Consider epidural steroids.

- *To reduce pain perception, related CNS arousal, and secondary noradrenaline release at nociceptive sites leading to sensitization of nociceptors:* Acetaminophen with codeine 30 mg, 1 or 2 tablets every 4 hours as needed to control moderate to severe pain. When not effective, successively try hydrocodone/APAP (Vicodin), hydrocodone bitartrate with acetaminophen (Lorcet 10/650), and acetaminophen with oxycodone (Percocet) as increasing opioid analgesic potency is required. Increase the potency of opioid rather than the number of pills to avoid acetaminophen toxicity. If longer-term opioid use is required, use longer-acting opioids such as methadone, morphine sulfate (MS Contin), or transdermal fentanyl patches until control is achieved. Treat episodic anxiety with a short-acting BZD, say lorazepam 0.25 to 0.5 mg, and train in behavioral and relaxation techniques.

- *To reduce neuropathic pain and to restore disturbed sleep:* nortriptyline, titrating upward from 10 mg at bedtime every 5 to 7 days until effects or antidepressant levels are reached. Maintain for a 3-week trial. If idiosyncratic effects occur, switch to another HCA. If side effects are intolerable, consider a serotonin-specific reuptake inhibitor (SSRI) (probably paroxetine) or an anticonvulsant.

- If any one of these agents is ineffective or creates intolerable or bothersome side effects, systematically substitute another agent. Change only one drug at a time so as to assess which drug and at what dose is effective. Institute behavioral pain management techniques simultaneously.

9. *Establish a reliable method of monitoring pain and activity levels.* Diaries should be used to establish baseline pain levels prior to treatment and to monitor the patient's response to treatment. Instructions are provided during the first visit, and charts are reviewed at subsequent clinic visits to reinforce diary keeping and the

patient's responsibility for their outcome. Diaries provide detailed information about factors that worsen or alleviate pain, about the patient's behavior, and about the effects of medication and other interventions. Daily diaries help identify critical points at which use of short-acting medication, physical methods (e.g., icing and stretching), or behavioral methods (e.g., pacing and relaxation) may change the pain pattern and course of treatment.

10. *Avoid irrational polypharmacy.* When patients report unrelieved or increased pain, in their eagerness to alleviate suffering, physicians may prescribe higher doses or a new drug without considering other factors that might affect the outcome. Physicians should consider the possibility of untoward drug interactions, side effects, toxicity, and behavioral effects and also investigate the possibility that either disease progression or nondisease factors, such as a change in activity or stress, may be responsible for nonresponse or an increase in pain. The reinforcement paradigm of Figure 32.1 helps explain this tendency. Well-established unconscious operant pain behaviors powerfully induce medication prescription. Our social role as physicians creates enormous pressure to relieve pain and suffering with prescriptions, a behavior that is positively reinforced by grateful and approving patients and by their continued business. Not prescribing elicits punishing disapproval from the patient; therefore we tend to prescribe rather than doing nothing. *Keep in mind that almost any new intervention, including a new medication, may have an initial placebo effect: the patient will actually feel better despite there being no specific pharmacological advantage to the medication prescribed.* Also, "doing something" reinforces the therapeutic bond and fulfills the expectations of the physician and patient in the sick role. Both may relax when on this familiar turf, whereas when the physician withholds medication, both may feel punished: the patient deprived and symbolically unloved and the physician tense and guilt-ridden.

What are some useful clinical strategies to minimize the tendency to polypharmacy? *First, medication trials should be carefully planned after adequate data gathering.* The database prior to starting drugs should include the following:

- A complete medical and pain history
- A selective physical and mental status examination
- A comprehensive formulation of the clinical problem, including an assessment of the various types of pain (e.g., nociceptive, neuropathic); hypotheses about mechanisms perpetuating pain (e.g., deconditioning, sleep disturbance, depressive illness, poor adherence to indicated treatment); medical problems (including comorbid psychiatric disorder); and psychosocial factors that might influence treatment
- A diagnostic list, including pain diagnoses, hypothesized mechanisms (e.g., neuropathic, inflammatory, myofascial), and associated other medical problems, including, critically, psychiatric disorders

- A baseline record of pain levels and fluctuations using the pain diaries, usually for at least a week

Second, do not assume that every pain needs a pharmacological response or that flare-ups necessarily require new or more medication. Often other interventions, including physical (e.g., icing, TENS, and stretching), behavioral (e.g., relaxation training with and without biofeedback, pacing, cognitive restructuring and stress management), and trigger point therapies (e.g., spray and stretch with ethyl chloride) can be quite effective in controlling pain. If psychological symptoms occur, do not assume that a psychiatric disorder (e.g., major depression, panic disorder) is present requiring a full therapeutic trial of psychotropic medication. Often reassurance, brief support, and cognitive-behavioral techniques will suffice.

Third, select medication based on careful formulation of the type of pain, the mechanisms perpetuating pain, and any comorbid or secondary psychiatric disorder. Figure 32.2 proposes a general algorithm for drug selection.

Fourth, close follow-up, every 1 to 2 weeks but occasionally several times weekly, may be necessary to establish optimum dosing for a medication and to minimize noncompliance. Thus medication is given a full therapeutic trial. A common problem is inadequate dosing and compliance. For example, HCAs, commonly used and effective in neuropathic pain, are often stopped before effective doses are reached. Instead of appropriately titrating the dose upward, the tendency is to add another medication.

MEDICATIONS USED FOR CHRONIC PAIN

Peripherally Acting Medications

The first category of medications to be discussed are those useful with pain related to inflammation. Thermal and chemical nociceptors involve prostaglandin receptors on nerve endings. The nociceptive process can be generated from a multitude of sources. In most pathophysiological conditions, however, inflammation causes thermal stimulation, edema causes pressure, and such autocoids as serotonin, bradykinin, histamine, and other substances released from injured tissues initiate the nociceptive process.

Anti-Inflammatory Agents

Aspirin and Acetaminophen

Despite the proliferation of NSAIDs on the market, aspirin continues to be widely used for early treatment of chronic pain because of its low cost and efficacy (13–15). The appropriate dosage for nonarthritic pain is related to aspirin's ceiling effect at approximately 1000 mg. Halpern notes that the optimal dose may be less than the 600-mg oral dose commonly used and that higher doses of aspirin do not increase the therapeutic effects, although at oral doses above 1 g toxicity increases dramatically (16). In the treatment of mild to moderate pain, aspirin is generally given every 3 to 4 hours.

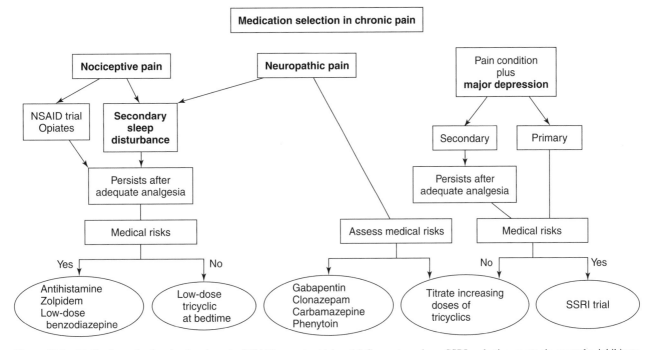

Figure 32.2   Medication selection in chronic pain. NSAID, nonsteroidal anti-inflammatory drug; SSRI, selective serotonin reuptake inhibitors. (Reprinted with permission from Gallagher RM, Pasol E. Psychopharmacological drugs in the chronic pain syndromes. Curr Rev Pain 1997;1:137–152.)

To avoid toxicity, the interval between doses should be increased as the dose itself is increased. As the dose increases, so does the half-life, from 3 or more hours with 300 mg to 9 hours with 2 g, while urinary excretion decreases (17). Toxicity from aspirin may carry its own warning signal, tinnitus, although this is not always present. Possible difficulties with excessive doses of aspirin over a long time are CNS damage and salicylate poisoning. Furthermore, aspirin must be taken with care by people with such GI problems as gastritis, peptic ulcer disease, and other ulcerative conditions of the stomach. Angioedema, rhinitis, nasal polyposis, and bronchial asthma are also contraindications and complications. Less common toxic effects include abdominal pain, nausea, shock, tinnitus, acid-base disturbances, and respiratory alkalosis. Luckily, these side effects are relatively rare, and even the more common complications afflict fewer than 5% of the overall population. However, approximately 10% of adverse drug reactions in U.S. hospitals are aspirin related. It may well be that this high percentage reflects the high usage of aspirin compounds.

Aspirin does not generally cause liver damage in healthy adults, but it may exacerbate preexisting liver disease. It may also exacerbate already diminished kidney function, especially among the elderly, by causing further renal impairment, such as diminished glomerular filtration and decreased renal tubular secretion, leading to the retention of toxic levels of salicylate. The toxicity appears to be related to tissue rather than blood levels. The margin of safety for aspirin is said to be relatively high when compared with other nonsteroidal antiinflammatory drugs (NSAIDs). Aspirin also increases prothrombin time and inhibits the second phase of platelet aggregation (15).

Salicylates can cause pathological cochlear changes and deafness, but this ototoxicity is generally reversible. Tinnitus is not always a reliable indicator of toxicity. Salicylate dosages may also be monitored by serum levels. When aspirin is used in high doses for rheumatoid arthritis, supplementation with vitamin C should be considered. Aspirin occasionally causes an iron deficiency anemia and may precipitate aplastic anemia in the elderly (18).

Some people cannot tolerate aspirin for a variety of reasons. For them, acetaminophen is often a substitute. This drug is rapidly absorbed from the GI tract, reaches a peak plasma concentration within 30 minutes to 2 hours after ingestion, and is primarily metabolized by the liver. Liver damage has been described with the ingestion of more than 10 to 15 g; 25 g or more is said to be a potentially fatal dose for adults (18). Whereas aspirin is antipyretic and anti-inflammatory, acetaminophen does not have anti-inflammatory properties. This reduces its usefulness, although its analgesic and antipyretic capabilities are equal to those of aspirin and the ceiling dosage is the same. As with aspirin, acetaminophen should be used with caution by people taking anticoagulants. In addition, taking HCAs or BZDs along with acetaminophen may lead to hypersensitivity, hepatitis, or cholestasis. There are also interactions when acetaminophen is taken with antibiotics or indomethacin (18, 19).

Other Anti-Inflammatory Agents

A number of drugs in addition to aspirin fall within the class of medications for which the primary actions seem to be caused by the inhibition of prostaglandin synthesis. The ability of these compounds to induce general analgesia and to relieve the pain associated with inflammatory processes is now well established. Indeed, studies have shown that in some circumstances these agents have a potency comparable with that of the opioids. Their usefulness in such conditions as rheumatoid arthritis and osteoarthritis is equally well established. In general, they may provide symptomatic improvement for ankylosing spondylitis, but they do not generally alter the natural course of the disease.

Contraindications to the use of NSAIDs are the same as those generally noted for aspirin. They may cause gastritis, gastric bleeding, and peptic ulcer in some patients, especially those with a history of peptic ulcer disease. Alcoholism, smoking, and concurrent steroid use may pose additional risk factors. With NSAIDs the incidence of GI irritation is similar to that of aspirin, approximately 2 to 10% with occasional use and 30 to 50% with high-dosage regular use. A recent study shows that the prophylactic use of famotidine at 40 mg twice a day reduced the incidence of duodenal ulcers from 13 to 2% and of gastric ulcers from 20 to 8% (20). Lower doses (20 mg twice a day) reduced duodenal but not gastric ulcers. Mild changes of liver function test results may occur in about 15% of patients taking NSAIDs. These elevations may stabilize, progress, or be transient despite continued therapy. Allergic reactions may occur with any of these agents. As with aspirin, the other NSAIDs may induce asthmatic attacks in susceptible individuals. It is estimated that in the United States, approximately 10% of the population are aspirin intolerant. Symptoms include nasal polyposis, bronchial asthma, and skin reactions (17). In a person known to be intolerant to aspirin or another NSAID, there is increased risk to subsequent NSAID trials.

Special advice must be given to certain patients for whom NSAIDs are prescribed. In children, for example, toxic reactions may occur at lower dosages than those that would produce similar toxicity in an adult. Because these agents alter platelet aggregation, patients with coagulation disorders (e.g., hemophilia and some forms of malignancy with bleeding diathesis) must be carefully monitored when these drugs are administered. Patients requiring warfarin type of anticoagulants, heparin, sulfonamides, sulfonylurea, or hydantoins should be observed for signs of toxicity when concurrently taking NSAIDs. When prescribing these drugs for the elderly, lower dosages may have to be considered because of the greater possibility of inducing hepatic and renal toxicity (17). NSAIDs can reduce the antihypertensive effect of propranolol and other β-blockers, inhibit the natriuretic effect of furosemide, and inhibit renal lithium clearance.

Acute interstitial nephritis and renal failure associated with prostaglandin depletion are well-known complications of NSAIDs. In the presence of preexisting renal insufficiency, renal function should be carefully monitored and smaller doses should be used, because the reduced excretion increases the half-life of these drugs and may exacerbate already diminished renal functioning, precipitating overt renal decompensation (17). Peripheral edema has been observed in some patients.

Therefore NSAIDs, especially those with high sodium content, should be used cautiously in patients with hypertension, fluid retention, or heart failure (17).

Diflunisal

One of the major advantages of diflunisal, a salicylic acid derivative, is that it has a plasma half-life of 8 to 12 hours, and therefore the frequency of administration can be only two to three times a day. It has anti-inflammatory and general analgesic actions but is not recommended as an antipyretic.

Indomethacin

Indomethacin has become an accepted part of the rheumatologist's armamentarium and is useful also as an antipyretic in Hodgkin's disease. Indomethacin is said to be more effective than aspirin for conditions such as ankylosing spondylitis, osteoarthritis, acute gout, pleurisy, pericarditis, and pericardial effusion. Complications and toxicity with this drug are common, affecting up to 50% of those receiving therapeutic dosages. About 20% of these patients are forced to discontinue the medication. It is also a general analgesic, but its side effects often prevent its use for noninflammatory pain. Indomethacin's interactions include enhancement of the action of anticoagulants and possible cardiac toxicity when used with thyroid medications (17).

Sulindac

An analog of indomethacin, sulindac was synthesized as a result of a search for a compound as effective as indomethacin but less toxic. It has a long duration of action, 16 hours, and is often useful for a long-term anti-inflammatory treatment, since the dosing can be accomplished twice daily.

Diclofenac Sodium

Diclofenac sodium is a phenylacetic acid with established anti-inflammatory and analgesic effects. Its indications include the treatment of rheumatoid arthritis, osteoarthritis, and ankylosing spondylitis. It is rapidly absorbed from the GI tract, with peak plasma levels reached in 2 to 3 hours. Despite its relatively short half-life, diclofenac sodium diffuses into and persists in synovial fluid for 4 to 24 hours, although it has not been established that diffusion into the joint plays a role in the drug's effectiveness. As with other NSAIDs, the most frequent side effects are GI related. Compared with other NSAIDs, diclofenac sodium has a high therapeutic index based on analgesic and anti-inflammatory effects (21).

Phenylbutazone and Oxyphenbutazone

The butazones are effective anti-inflammatory drugs for the treatment of ankylosing spondylitis, acute gout, bursitis, capsulitis, peritendinitis, and other arthropathies. However, because of the potentially severe adverse effects (agranulocytosis and aplastic anemia) their use should be limited to short-term intervention with close monitoring for evidence of bone marrow failure (22). The butazones are also contraindicated in patients with peptic ulcer disease, congestive heart failure, and hypertension and in patients with reduction in granulocytes (16).

Azapropazone

Azapropazone is a pyrazole derivative with a spectrum of activity similar to that of phenylbutazone but without its severe toxicity. In contrast to many of the NSAIDs, 62% of azapropazone is excreted unchanged in the urine. In patients with renal impairment, the dosage should be reduced and the patient monitored carefully (22).

The Propionic Derivatives

The most widely used NSAIDs in U.S. clinical practice are the propionic derivatives represented by ibuprofen, naproxen, fenoprofen, ketoprofen, and flurbiprofen. In addition to their effect on prostaglandin synthesis, they are thought to affect the histamine and kinin systems of inflammation mediation. Side effects include nonspecific edema and GI irritation. These drugs have a wider margin of safety than indomethacin. In addition to their application to inflammatory conditions, they are now approved by the U.S. Food and Drug Administration (FDA) for noninflammatory painful conditions, although their mechanism of action is not clear. These drugs are also used for menstrual cramps, the proposed mechanism being reduction of prostaglandin levels in menstrual fluid (23). Long-acting preparations of these medications (e.g., naproxen) may improve patient compliance through a more convenient dosing schedule of once or twice daily dosing.

Naproxen and Naproxen Sodium

Naproxen and naproxen sodium are rapidly absorbed from the GI tract, with peak plasm levels attained at 1 to 2 hours. Mean plasma half-life is 13 hours, making it appropriate for twice-daily dosing. These drugs are recommended for mild to moderate pain and for the treatment of primary dysmenorrhea and are also indicated for the treatment of rheumatoid arthritis, osteoarthritis, ankylosing spondylitis, tendinitis, bursitis, and acute gout. Multiple studies (18, 24, 25) suggest a favorable long-term GI profile. This is related to rapid dispersion, reducing exposure of the gastric mucosa to the concentrated drug, and to its lactose-free content, which eliminates the risk of GI side effects associated with lactose intolerance.

Pyranocarboxylic Acid

Etodolac is a pyranocarboxylic acid NSAID that exhibits analgesic, anti-inflammatory, and antipyretic properties. Its indications include the management of pain and acute and long-term use in the management of osteoarthritis. Unlike other NSAIDs, which significantly suppress gastric and duodenal prostaglandins, contributing to undesirable gastric side effects, etodolac apparently selectively spares cytoprotective prostaglandins in the gastric mucosa. This has been suggested as a possible mechanism for the gastric safety of etodolac (26, 27).

Opioid Analgesics

The first mention of the poppy as a sedative anodyne is in Eber's papyrus of the 16th century. However, the first specific reference to the use of poppy juice was found in the writing of Theophratus in the 3rd century. Paracelsus (1493–1591) is credited with the repopularization of opium in Europe and indeed was called Dr. Opiatus. In 1803, Serturner isolated and described morphine. Its use spread, and it became so widely available that morphinism was a major problem for Civil War soldiers (28).

With severe acute pain, cancer pain, and postoperative pain, the use of opioid analgesics is usually appropriate. In these situations, physicians' reluctance to use opioids because of fear of causing physical dependence and tolerance is generally inappropriate. Twycross has emphasized that in a cancer pain population, increasing requirements for opioid analgesia generally do not represent tolerance but rather progression of the disease (29). It should also be noted that the dosage of an opioid frequently can be decreased through balanced analgesia with adjuvants and peripherally acting nonopioid analgesics. Judicious use of these drug combinations not only can enhance analgesia but can also diminish adverse side effects and treat symptoms other than pain (10, 13). Nonpharmacological pain management techniques of proven efficacy (30) should also be employed to reduce suffering and improve analgesic efficacy (12, 31–33). Unfortunately, training in these techniques is often considered as a last resort, when frequent practice and long use leads to better efficacy (30).

Although there is no doubt that the opioids are often the drugs of choice for severe acute pain and chronic cancer pain, in our opinion their use in chronic nonmalignant pain must be selective (10–12, 33). As recently as 10 years ago, one of the outcome measures for a successful multidisciplinary pain center was the percentage of patients "successfully" weaned and maintained off opioids during follow-up. In retrospect, we can say that many of these patients had not done well prior to their admission when they were taking opioids and therefore, justification of the medication taper was not difficult. However, with today's knowledge and hindsight, many pain medicine practitioners believe that a disservice has been done to a small group of patients who would have benefited from long-term opioid treatment but for whom some practitioners have dogmatically refused to prescribe opioids. This issue should be revisited.

Much has been learned, especially from clinical studies and treatment of cancer pain. We now know that in appropriately selected patients, opioids have low morbidity (perhaps less than NSAIDs), and a low addiction potential. Although tolerance occurs in some cases, generally patients become tolerant to bothersome side effects more than to analgesic effects. Evidence from cancer studies suggests that when patients are clinically stable on a certain opioid dose and then request a dose escalation, it may be more related to progression in their disease than to tolerance. When principles from the World Health Organization (WHO) analgesic ladder paradigm (34) are followed appropriately, combining NSAIDs, adjuvants, and opioids, we can manage the vast majority of patients with severe chronic pain.

A subgroup of the nonmalignant pain population can be treated effectively with long-term opioids (35–40) (Table 32.1). These persons, who have a well-documented medical condition as the cause of their pain, have attempted alternative techniques of pain management and are being carefully monitored by a physician. In general, either these patients did not respond to treatment with nonopioid analgesics, adjuvants, or alternative techniques of pain management (e.g., physical therapy, psychotherapy, relaxation therapy, and pain center therapy) or they receive added benefit from the selective use of opioids in combination with these other medications and treatment. In addition, it should be demonstrated that these patients remain functional while receiving opioid analgesics but attempts to taper the medications result in diminished function, impairment in overall activities of daily living, and increased

Table 32.1.   Guidelines for Maintenance Opioid Use in Chronic Nonmalignant Pain

---

Documented medical condition as the cause of the pain.

Prior systemic therapeutic trials of alternative pain control regimens (analgesics, adjuvants, psychosocial interventions, appropriate medical treatments, and behavioral approaches) have been unsuccessful.

Documentation that nonopioid treatments have resulted in (a) inadequate analgesia impairing functional ADL and (b) continued suffering.

Prior to initiating opioid maintenance, nonalgologists should (a) obtain consultation with an algologist or (b) consult with a specialist in management of the specific problem being treated. Consultation report should document occurrence with opioid treatment.

Document detailed discussion of short- and long-term effects and risks. Signed informed consent is suggested.

One physician should be responsible for writing prescriptions (which should be on a time-contingent rather than pain-contingent basis) and monitoring clinical progress. Recommended initial frequency of appointments is at least monthly. Patients must be seen and records must show reason for continuing opioids.

Documentation that maintenance opioids improve analgesia, functional ADL, and diminish suffering.

Use lowest clinically effective opioid dose. Peripherally acting nonopioids and adjuvants used concurrently may allow lower doses of opioids.

A history of substance dependence or abuse is a precaution.

Any evidence of drug-seeking behavior, obtaining opioids from multiple sources, or frequent requests for dose escalation without documentation of significant worsening of the clinical condition should be a cause for careful review and reconsideration of maintenance opioid use.

ADL, activities of daily living.

suffering. With balanced analgesics, they can remain active and productive with diminished pain and suffering. When this occurs, they do not exhibit significant pain behaviors. When it does not occur, some find alternative ways to obtain the medication they need for pain control. It has been suggested that this behavioral pattern should not be viewed as addiction but rather as pseudoaddiction related to inadequate treatment (40). There is little evidence that exposure to opioids in patients with painful conditions leads to true addiction unless predisposing factors, such as prior substance abuse, are present (41, 42). Patients with a history of substance abuse or dependence, significant psychopathology, or excessive environmental stressors contributing to their pain and suffering in general should only cautiously, if at all, be maintained on opioids for nonmalignant pain. It must be emphasized that most chronic pain syndrome patients can be effectively managed without the regular daily use of opioid analgesics. Yet in patients carefully selected for opioid maintenance, addiction is rarely a clinical problem.

Opioid Agonists

Opioids can be classified as agonists, agonist-antagonists, and antagonists. In this section only the agonist and agonist-antagonist groups will be discussed, since the antagonist drugs are not analgesics. The opioid agonists have generally similar clinical effects when given at equianalgesic doses. The differences among the individual drugs are important because a patient may have an adverse reaction to one of the opioids but not to others. Usually the reason for choosing one agonist rather than another is that one confers some advantage, for instance in route of administration or in the time action of the agent. However, at equianalgesic dosages the reasons for choosing one agonist over another are the specific adverse effects of a particular opioid for an individual patient and the differences in oral absorption or time action of analgesic effect (28).

The use of opioids in pregnancy may result in neonatal withdrawal symptoms. This may be a special problem with longer-acting opioids, such as methadone, because the abstinence syndrome may be delayed until after the infant leaves the hospital. Also, the physician must be cognizant of the possibility that long-term exposure to systemic opioids may have some adverse effect on the CNS development and weigh that possibility against the adverse effects in the infant of poorly controlled pain in the mother.

The agonists are useful in relieving anxiety, which normally accompanies severe pain. At usual clinical dosages the emotional reaction to the pain is changed, and it is believed that this may be due largely to the action of the agonists on the limbic system. Other central nervous system effects include analgesia, drowsiness, mood changes, mental clouding, and on occasion, respiratory depression.

The major toxic effects of the agonist opioids are vomiting and respiratory depression. In the supine patient, therapeutic doses of agonists do not generally have significant effects on blood pressure or cardiac rate and rhythm. However, these substances do cause vasodilation; therefore, one must watch for orthostatic hypotension and syncope. Opioids also cause a marked decrease in contractility in the small and large intestine, often resulting in constipation. Morphine is the standard with which other opioid agonists are often compared. Table 32.2 highlights some of the comparative characteristics of opioid agonists.

Studies have found that with postoperative pain, 10 mg of D-amphetamine combined with morphine is twice as potent as morphine alone, and a combination of 5 mg of D-amphetamine is 1.5 times as potent as morphine alone (43). It has also been found that in proportion to its dose, D-amphetamine generally improves performance that has been diminished by morphine. Researchers have discovered that a potent, common, nonsedating analgesic can be produced by a combination of the well-absorbed oral opioid anileridine with amphetamine. A dose of 25 mg of anileridine plus 5 mg of D-amphetamine taken orally leads to an analgesic equivalent to approximately 12 to 15 mg of injectable morphine (44).

The agonist-antagonist group consists of pentazocine, butorphanol, nalbuphine, and buprenorphine. The raison d'être for this class of drugs is not that they provide better analgesia than the agonist opioids but rather that they were thought to have a much lower incidence of physiological dependence (44). Having said this, we note that although it is somewhat less than that of the agonist drugs, there is a definite abuse potential, and the possibility of a withdrawal syndrome should be recognized after chronic use (13).

One of the more worrisome side effects of pentazocine is the incidence of psychotomimetic effects. The incidence of these seems to be reduced (although still present) with the newer members of this class, and in clinical trials this is described as approximately 1%. Caution must be exercised with these medications. Patients should not have taken opioids for a period depending on the half-life of the opioid, as the agonist-antagonist drug precipitates an abstinence syndrome.

When the physician now considers the use of opioids in a chronic pain patient, the advent of long-acting opioid preparations has changed the equation considerably. Long-acting morphine and oxycodone enable the patient to reach a steady state while avoiding the fluctuations in blood levels, and therefore fluctuating pain control, that characterize the clinical use of short-acting opioids. The side effect burden of these medications appears to be lower as well. Methadone has long been the drug of choice for chronic pain and is effective for many patients; however, its use carries the burden of its pharmacokinetics; its analgesic effects last 4 to 8 hours, but its half-life is far longer, with the result that toxic levels can accumulate as a patient and physician attempt to reach an analgesic steady state. Generally, in chronic pain patients physicians should avoid using meperidine (Demerol) because of the toxicity of its principal metabolite, normeperidine, and pentazocine because of its psychotomimetic effects and its lower efficacy than that of pure agonists.

In the context of a rehabilitation focus for patients with chronic pain, a concern about the use of opioids while driving or using other dangerous machinery has been expressed. The effects of opioids on performance has been exaggerated. In fact there is good evidence that patients habituate to the sedative and psychomotor effects of opioids (41), whereas they do not habituate to the negative effects of pain on task performance (45). It appears that pain is more deleterious than opioids on functional performance!

In summary, we have learned that (*a*) nociceptive pain is most opioid responsive, (*b*) neuropathic and central pain less but variably responsive, and (*c*) psychologically maintained pain is generally nonresponsive to and inappropriate for chronic opioid treatment. As always, optimal management of the patient with chronic pain depends on comprehensive assessment, and we still have much to learn about identifying which patients are most appropriate for opioids.

Table 32.2.   Drug-Drug Interactions with HCAs

Drug	Effect
SSRIs	Serotonin toxicity
MAOIs	MAOI crisis
Cimetidine	Inhibition of metabolism, increasing blood
Methylphenidate	levels and toxicity of HCAs
Acetaminophen	
Oral contraceptives	
Chloramphenicol	
Isoniazid	
MAOIs	
Disulfiram	
Disulfiram	Psychosis and confusional state
Guanethidene	Blockage of neuronal reuptake
Propranolol	
Clonidine	
Methyldopa	Agitation, tremor, tachycardia
Thiazides	Decreased HCA effect, augmented hypotension
Acetozolamide	
Cardiazam	Decreased cardiac conduction, prolonged QT
Quinidine	interval
Procainamide	
Warfarin	Increased bleeding
Neuroleptics	Increased HCA effect, ventricular arrythmias, sedation
Psychostimulants	Blocked HCA metabolism, increased cardiotoxicity
Cyclobenzaprine (Flexeril)	Synergistic effect
Halothane anesthetics	Tachycardia, synergistic anticholingeric effect
Testosterone	Psychosis
Opiates	Potentiate analgesia, synergistic anticholinergic effects
Benzodiazepines	Sedation, confusion, increased suicide risk, impaired motor function
Alcohol	
Propanolol	Agitation, tremor, tachycardia
Anticholinergic drugs	Increased anticholinergic toxicity
Anticonvulsants	Induction of heptic metabolism decreasing HCA levels
Valproate	Increased HCA levels
HCAs	Increased Dilantin levels, decreased carbamazepine levels

Antidepressants and Anticonvulsants

Centrally active drugs such as antidepressants and anticonvulsants are commonly used medications in chronic pain and are considered first-line drugs in the treatment of neuropathic pain and to treat psychiatric comorbidity. These medications affect pain experience through four distinct but often complementary clinical actions (10). First, these drugs are known to be effective *adjuvants to opiate analgesia,* and they constitute an integral part of the three-step analgesic ladder recognized by the WHO in 1990 (34). Second, certain of these drugs possess *independent analgesic efficacy* for specific pain disorders within the present classification of chronic pain, particularly neuropathic pain. Third, these drugs have *psychotropic effects on psychiatric syndromes,* such as depression, anxiety, and sleep disorders, that frequently accompany pain disorders and exacerbate pain-related disability. Fourth, these drugs may be used to treat *troublesome physiological symptoms,* such as sleep disturbance or muscle spasm, that often accompany pain and may contribute considerably to the disability associated with chronic pain states.

Antidepressants in Chronic Pain

Antidepressants are probably the psychotropic drugs most commonly prescribed for chronic pain. A meta-analysis of 39 placebo-controlled double-blind studies of the effectiveness of antidepressants in chronic pain indicated that antidepressants are significantly more effective than placebo in reducing pain in chronic pain patients (46). In this study, the average chronic pain patient receiving an antidepressant had less pain than 74% of the patients who received placebo. This effect appears to be consistent with a direct analgesic activity of the medication that is independent of antidepressant activity. However, because of the relatively uneven methodologies of the studies, the applicability of these findings to chronic pain in general is questioned (12, 47). The multiple physical and psychosocial factors that may confound or interact with antidepressant response must be controlled for, either through sampling strategies or in analyses, to establish these effects (48, 49). Antidepressants may be clinically effective in chronic pain through one or more of several mechanisms:

1. *Direct analgesic effect:* These medications are thought to modulate pain perception through activity on noradrenergic and serotonergic neurophysiological systems that descend from the midbrain to the dorsal horn (50). Like certain anticonvulsants, inhibition of sodium channel activity in the neuronal membrane may contribute to their analgesic properties in neuropathic pain.
2. *Amelioration of comorbid psychiatric disorder.* Depressive illnesses may worsen pain perception, interfere with coping, and contribute additional morbidity (51). In this category, effects on pain may be through either of two mechanisms: first by the

treatment of masked depression that is causing the pain symptom (52); and second by the treatment of manifest depression that enables the patient to tolerate the pain better (53). Panic disorder also specifically responds to antidepressants.
3. *Reduction of pain-related symptoms,* such as changes in appetite and sleep, that contribute to morbidity and disability (12).
4. *Potentiation or enhancement of opioid analgesia* (54, 55). This probably results from a combination of the first three mechanisms.

Pain defined by region, mechanism, or description may respond to specific medication. However, controlled, standardized trials comparing antidepressants with other medications and with each other in specific conditions are lacking.

Heterocyclic Antidepressants

First-generation HCAs (e.g., amitriptyline, imipramine, and doxepin) have been the most widely used for the management of chronic pain, alone or comorbid with depression. In studies of neuropathic pain, HCAs have demonstrated an analgesic effect even when depression is controlled for or patients with depressive illness are excluded from the study (56, 57). HCAs have been reported to relieve lancinating pain as well as constant pain (58, 59). The hypothesis that myofascial pain may be an expression of deafferentation neuralgia (54) suggests that these medications may be used successfully in diverse myofascial disorders.

Most studies of HCAs report on older drugs, such as amitriptyline, imipramine, and doxepin, which consistently show an analgesic effect. However, the problematic side effect burden of amitriptyline related to its anticholinergic and antihistaminergic activity has led to comparative studies of other tricyclics. Desipramine, which has far fewer side effects, may approach the efficacy of amitriptyline for relief of neuropathic pain. Both amitriptyline and desipramine block norepinephrine reuptake; their effectiveness compared with that of SSRIs, such as fluoxetine, suggested to investigators that norepinephrine reuptake blockade contributed to the analgesic effect of antidepressants. Nortriptyline, with activity in both noradrenergeric and 5-hydroxytryptamine (5-HT) systems, and like desipramine with a lower side effect profile than amitriptyline, also seems effective, and blood levels can be reliably obtained.

In summary, the clinical pharmacology literature and clinical experience suggest that the HCAs constitute useful treatment for central deafferentation and neuropathic pain, particularly when the pain is prominently dysesthetic or burning. A trial of antidepressants may be useful in any patient with primary neuropathic pain and certainly should be considered when pain has responded inadequately to standard pharmacological management with NSAIDs and/or opioids. Unlike HCA's antidepressant effect, which may require several weeks, these drugs may relieve pain within a few days. However, pain relief may not occur for 1 to 3 weeks and may require titration to higher doses, often at the same level for depression, for some patients (10, 50).

Side effects of HCAs

The usefulness of HCAs in chronic pain patients is limited somewhat by troublesome side effects, by problematic interaction with other medications, and by their potential for deleterious effects on medical problems other than chronic pain. These effects reflect each drug's profile of receptor affinities such as anticholinergic, antihistaminic H_1 and H_2, adrenergic, and serotoninergic (10). HCAs commonly produce a benign race in heart rate, particularly desipramine because of its stronger norepinephrine reuptake blockade effect, and dry mouth and constipation. Orthostatic hypotension can be dangerous, particularly in cardiac patients or elderly patients, because of the risk of fractures from falls. Urinary retention can be problematic in the elderly.

Drug-Drug Interactions of HCAs

Dangerous interactions occur particularly with monoamine oxidase inhibitors (MAOI crisis) and SSRIs (serotonin toxicity). These and other HCA interactions are shown in Table 32.2.

Drug-Disease Interactions of HCAs

HCAs are contraindicated with post—A-V node conduction disturbance; they may lower the seizure threshold; and they may have a hypoglycemic effect. Rarely they precipitate narrow-angle glaucoma.

Selective Serotonin Reuptake Inhibitors

SSRIs specifically inhibit the neuronal reuptake of serotonin with little other receptor activity. Because these drugs have little anticholinergic and antihistamine activity compared with the HCAs, their side effect profile and risk of problematic interactions with other drugs and medical illnesses is minimal. Despite the purported role of serotonin in pain modulation, a clear-cut analgesic role for the SSRIs has not been empirically established. Even so, fluoxetine showed analgesic activity in experimental animal pain models (60) and chronic pelvic pain, and case reports suggests its utility in the management of headache (61), fibrositis (62), diabetic neuropathy (63), and phantom limb pain (54). However, these studies did not control for depression. Paroxetine (Paxil) is effective in the treatment of neuropathic pain (64). Both fluvoxamine and mianserin were more effective than placebo in chronic tension type headache; however, fluvoxamine, the SSRI, was more effective than mianserin in the nondepressed patients, suggesting that the therapeutic activity of fluvoxamine was unrelated to a direct effect on depression (65).

The most common side effects of SSRIs include agitation, anxiety, sleep disturbance, tremor, sexual dysfunction, and headache. Rarely, SSRIs have been associated with extrapyramidal-like symptoms, arthralgias, lymphadenopa-

thy, inappropriate antidiuretic syndrome, agranulocytosis, and hypoglycemia. SSRIs interact with MAOIs, causing the life-threatening central serotonin syndrome manifested by abdominal pain, diarrhea, sweating, fever, tachycardia, elevated mood, hypertension, altered mental state, delirium, myoclonus, increased motor activity, irritability, and hostility. Severe manifestations of this syndrome can include hyperpyremia, cardiovascular shock, and death. SSRIs are essentially devoid of type 1 A antiarrhythmic effect of HCAs, nor do SSRIs have any α–adrenergic antagonistic effect; therefore they rarely are associated with orthostatic hypotension. Sertraline, fluoxetine, and paroxetine are relatively free of interactions with CNS depressants such as BZDs, alcohol, barbiturates, and lithium. Combining paroxetine or fluvoxamine with anticoagulants such as warfarin increases bleeding time; therefore, anticoagulants must be adjusted. Fluvoxamine potentiates the effects of diazepam, terfenadine, astemizole, theophylline and warfarin. SSRIs in combination with HCAs generally increase HCA levels.

The relatively benign side effect and toxicity profiles of SSRIs compared with HCAs favor their use when there is no therapeutic advantage to using the HCAs or the HCAs are relatively contraindicated because of risk (e.g., cardiac conduction defects, potential for suicide, seizures).

Atypical Antidepressants

Bupropion (Wellbutrin), *trazodone* (Desyrel), *nefazodone* (Serzone) and *venlafaxine* (Effexor) are so-called atypical antidepressants that may be useful in chronic pain (10). Trazodone has little intrinsic analgesic activity but has been used for comorbid depression and to induce sleep. It has the disadvantage of association with priapism, which although it is rare, makes its use unacceptable to many men. Bupropion, nefazodone, and venlafaxine have not been studied in pain. Bupropion has the advantages of low side effect profile, including low sexual impairment, unique mechanism of action (good for treatment-resistant depressions), and short half-life, which avoids buildup in geriatric patients. Significantly increased seizure risk in at-risk" patients and slightly increased risk in normal patients merits avoiding peak plasma levels by prescribing multiple divided doses.

Venlafaxine and nefazodone are two newer antidepressants that have not been studied for their analgesic properties. Venlafaxine, like HCAs, affects norepiniphrine and 5-HT systems and so may have analgesic properties as well; it has fewer side effects and minimal drug interaction risk, and it does not build up in geriatric patients. Its major problems include increased diastolic blood pressure (usually at doses over 300 mg/day), nausea (tolerance develops in 2 to 6 weeks) twice-daily dosing requirement, and variable final dosing. It is the drug of choice for severe melancholic or geriatric depression (18). Nefazodone, a phenylpiperazine similar to trazodone, has fewer anticholinergic side effects than the HCAs and is less likely to impair sexual functioning than either HCAs or SSRIs. It has a potentially lethal interaction with the commonly used antihistamines terfenadine (Seldane) and astemizole (Histamil) because it inhibits their hepatic metabolism.

Choosing an Antidepressant

The SSRIs have largely replaced the HCAs as first-line drugs for depression. However, the unproven efficacy of SSRIs for pain makes selection of an antidepressant more complicated in pain patients. Figure 32.2 (10) outlines Gallagher's simple algorithm for choosing antidepressants in populations of chronic pain patients with and without comorbid depression. For any one patient, the choice of the most appropriate antidepressant trial may be confounded by the complex interaction of factors that determine efficacy. Positive effects must be weighed against the potential for negative effects. Optimal judgment requires a specific knowledge of the pharmacology, efficacy, and side effect profile of the medications themselves and the clinical evaluation of the patient, including a detailed knowledge of the following factors: *the characteristics of the medication; the phenomenology of the pain syndrome; any other medical problems; the use of other medications; any comorbid psychiatric disorder; and the psychological characteristics of the patient.*

Pain medicine lacks clinical algorithms based upon controlled clinical trials comparing the efficacy of one antidepressant with another in specific pain syndromes. However, the evidence for efficacy of HCAs is better established than for SSRIs. Therefore, if there are no medical contraindications, HCAs are preferable in a clinical trial. Choice of medication requires knowledge of side effects and drug and disease interactions.

Neuropathic pain (e.g., radiculopathy, causalgia, diabetic neuropathy) alone may respond to HCAs. The favorable side effect profile of nortriptyline and desipramine increases patients' acceptance of titration to higher doses. Desipramine is much less expensive than nortriptyline but more expensive than amitriptyline. Start with low doses, such as nortriptyline 10 mg, desipramine 25 mg, or amitriptyline 25 mg and titrate weekly up to antidepressant doses if necessary until relief or side effects intervene. If *myofascial pain* or *inflammatory pain* is part of a more systemic clinical syndrome such as fibromyalgia, which is often associated with evidence of CNS disorder such as sleep disturbance and depression, a trial of HCAs may be warranted. *Migraine headache* prophylaxis with HCAs or SSRIs may be effective (66); however, newer abortive approaches, such as self-administered sumatriptan or dihydroergotamine mesylate (DHE), which have strong serotonin agonist activity, often successfully prevent progression of headache to a full-blown incapacitating migraine (67) while avoiding the risks and side effects associated with regularly taking HCAs. Combining injected abortive approaches such as sumatriptan or DHE with SSRIs and HCAs must be done cautiously for fear of precipitating serotonin toxicity.

Other medical problems, such as cardiac conduction disturbance, particularly post—A-V node blocks, are a precaution to HCAs. In patients with heart disease, risk factors, or old age, if a trial of HCAs is warranted, obtain an electrocardiogram (ECG) prior to starting these and monitor ECG as doses are titrated. SSRIs such as paroxetine, fluoxetine, and sertraline are reasonable choices for a trial. Use HCAs cautiously in the context of medical problems that they may worsen, such as orthostatic hypotension and urinary retention. Antidepressants may lower the insulin needs of diabetics. HCAs, particularly maprotiline, may lower seizure threshold.

Comorbid psychiatric disorder often complicates pain disorder (68, 69) and influences treatment outcome. Since a pain medicine evaluation often overlooks psychiatric disorders, such as depressive illness, the clinician must actively screen for them repeatedly during the course of treatment (69). Depression appears to lower pain threshold and tolerance (70), increase analgesic requirements, and in other ways add to the debilitating effects of pain. Many patients in pain have insomnia and fatigue, which are also extremely common vegetative symptoms of depression. Patients usually attribute insomnia to pain rather than depression because pain is the more socially acceptable malady (17). It is difficult to distinguish cause and effect within the pain—depression—insomnia cycle, but once the cycle is established, it becomes self-perpetuating and requires active intervention. If comorbid *major depression (MDD)* exists, antidepressants should be titrated to therapeutic levels for depression over 2 to 3 weeks. SSRIs (fluoxetine 20 mg, paroxetine 20 mg, sertraline 50 mg) should be given for 2 weeks to assess response, and then titrated appropriately. HCAs usually start with nortriptyline 25 mg at bedtime or desipramine 50 mg at bedtime and increase to 75 mg and 150 mg respectively over about 10 days, monitoring side effects. (Lower doses are used for geriatric populations.) Give the dose about 3 weeks to work and monitor serum levels for therapeutic range.

MDD is often overlooked in medical practice (71, 72), and when diagnosed, often inadequately treated (73). In pain populations the diagnosis of MDD can be difficult and unreliable because of denial or response bias (patients not reporting symptoms when asked because of fears of stigma) and confounding of the physical symptoms of MDD, such as sleep disturbance and fatigue, by pain, medical problems, or medications (69). Several common errors may lead to inadequate treatment of comorbid MDD (10, 73): (*a*) *choosing a medication not effective for MDD (e.g., diazepam); (b) underdosing with an effective medication; (c) ineffectively managing side effects, causing noncompliance; (d) stopping medication too soon.* If MDD occurs with neuropathic pain, HCAs are the drug of choice but must be titrated to antidepressant doses, usually higher than needed for neuropathic pain alone. For MDD in the absence of neuropathic pain, SSRIs are the drug of choice because their low side effect profile, fewer interaction problems, and better acceptance make adequate dosing more likely. When physicians are uncomfortable with treating

MDD, they should have a low threshold for psychiatric consultation or referral because of the physical, psychological, and social morbidity associated with untreated depression (74).

The timing of depression relative to onset of pain, the type of depression, and whether or not there is a personal or family history of depression may influence treatment choice. In a recent study of depression in chronic myofascial facial pain patients and their families and in controls and their families, Dohrenwend et al. (75) showed that pain patients with late-onset depressive illness have rates of prepain depression and rates of depression in first-degree relatives that are equivalent to those of pain patients without depression and controls without depression; in other words, it appears that depression in these myofascial pain patients is not familial and that other nonfamilial mechanisms, such as learned helplessness (76), must be considered. What are treatment implications of this finding for pain patients? In some chronic pain patients who first present with major depression after the onset of pain-related disability, depressive symptoms respond well to effective control of pain without using antidepressants (10, 12). Particularly if the depressive symptoms are relatively mild, if there is no family history, and if medical cautions exist, we may delay using antidepressants for 2 weeks to evaluate response to effective pain treatment. However, the risks associated with this procedure (e.g., untreated depression leading to poor pain treatment outcome and higher risk for chronic disability and suicide) are sufficiently high so that the general clinician without considerable experience should seriously consider appropriate psychiatric consultation.

Suicide is always a risk in patients with depression, a risk heightened by the suffering and chronicity of intractable pain. The salience of this issue is heightened by our contemporary heated debate on physician-assisted suicide. The risks of antidepressant medications differ. If taken in overdose, HCAs have far greater potential for successful suicide than do SSRIs. *Yet the key to preventing suicide is identification of depression early in its course and rapid and effective treatment combined with effective pain management.* Consultation with a psychiatric colleague is essential, and hospitalization must be considered.

In all cases of depression, appropriate psychotherapies (e.g., cognitive-behavioral and interpersonal) should be added to medications for even greater benefit, perhaps in conjunction with behavioral pain management training. When medical problems or a patient's beliefs preclude medication, the clinician must rely on psychotherapeutic treatments; but in the latter instance, the clinician should continue trying to help patients overcome the cognitive distortions and negative emotions that prevent them from using medication.

In patients with comorbid *panic disorder,* antidepressants can very effectively block panic attacks, often at doses lower than in major depression. BZDs can *temporarily* provide control of symptomatic anxiety but should be replaced by anxiety control training (30, 32) to avoid other problems (see section on antianxiety medications).

A patient's reluctance to accept antidepressant treatment, for example because of religious beliefs, can impede successful outcome. The clinician should explore the patient's ideas and beliefs to identify misunderstanding about the nature of pain and depression and to educate about the mechanism of action of these drugs. When physicians prescribe antidepressants for neuropathic pain, even in the absence of depression, patients may believe that the physician is suggesting that depression is causing pain; they may become defensive and even overtly hostile because of negative experience, such as an insurer's earlier efforts to discredit the patient by attempting to establish psychological causation to avoid financial responsibility. In fact, among disabled low-back pain patients with equal spinal pathology, those with more psychological distress (elevated depression score on the MMPI) are likely to be judged as less severely impaired even when they are not (77). Thus the physician must explain when antidepressants are being used as analgesics or to treat comorbid depression and why, and that depression is a common and expected complication of chronic disabling pain. Also, they must explain that depression does not invalidate nociceptive or neuropathic pathology or their suffering, nor does it mean that the pain is imaginary or caused by depression or that depression is caused by personal weakness.

Figure 32.2 presents simple, rational clinical guidelines for treating depression, pain, and insomnia in persons with chronic pain (10). To regulate sleep, low doses of sedating HCAs (e.g., doxepin or amitriptyline) are preferable to BZDs; zolpidem (Ambien) is our choice for episodic stress-related sleep-onset insomnia. We do not generally use HCAs for regional myofascial low-back pain unless seeking antidepressant or sedating effects. Antidepressant trials should be considered in any patient whose pain has responded inadequately to standard pharmacological management with opioids, particularly malignant pain. We advise titrating from low doses, to which some will respond, to the higher doses customarily used for depression. Analgesics benefits may not occur until after 1 to 3 weeks.

Anticonvulsants in Chronic Pain

Anticonvulsants, widely accepted in the management of chronic neuropathic pain, particularly lancinating, burning, and dysesthetic pain, are postulated to cause their analgesic effect primarily by suppressing ectopic neuronal discharges. Spontaneous aberrant electrical activity has been recorded from different levels of the neuraxis in experimental models of nerve injury, also found in patients with chronic neuropathic pain (78–81). Phenytoin (Dilantin), carbamazepine (Tegretol), valproic acid (Depakote), and clonazepam (Klonopin) suppress spontaneous neuronal firing (82). Phenytoin reduces cortical responses to paired stimuli and decreases posttetanic potentiation (83). The anticonvulsant effect of carbamazepine may be mediated by the so-called peripheral BZD receptors in the brain and possibly also through the potentiation of adenoreceptors and stabilization of sodium channel ion neurons; this latter effect may also mediate its analgesic effects in chronic pain. Anticonvulsants have been used in chronic neuralgias, sometimes in combination with an HCA (84). Multiple clinical studies suggest that carbamazepine (85–87), phenytoin (88–90), clonazepam (91) and valproic acid (58, 92) are useful in pain management. Several studies have documented the successful use of anticonvulsants for cancer-related neuropathic pain caused by neural invasion by tumor, radiation fibrosis, and surgical scarring (93); these drugs have also been used successfully in postherpetic and deafferentation neuralgias (94). The clearest indications for anticonvulsants are lancinating neuropathic pain and chronic dysesthetic pain. With the exception of gabapentin, their potentially toxic interactions with other medications and their toxic and side effect burden (14, 95, 96) restricts their general use to patients not responding to other medications, except in the case of trigeminal neuralgia, for which carbamazepine in the drug of first choice.

Gabapentin, a drug initially developed as an adjunct to anticonvulsant therapies (47, 97), is now being widely used in various pain conditions, particularly in neuropathic pain. Its immediate and widespread acceptance is based upon clinicians' reports of efficacy for complex regional pain syndrome 1 (RSD) (98) and neuropathic pain disorders (99) and its relative safety and low side effect profile (47, 100, 101). Unlike other anticonvulsants, gabapentin has no documented long-term toxicity, active metabolites, hepatic enzyme induction, or major drug interactions (97). Side effects are minimal, dose-dependent, and similar in description to those of other anticonvulsants (e.g., sedation, disequilibrium, ataxia, and nausea). Gabapentin is recommended as a first-choice drug for neuropathic pain, particularly when there is a potential for HCA-related side effects or toxic drug-disease or drug-drug interactions (10). Dosing regimens are not established empirically. Clinical experience suggests a regimen starting at 100 mg twice a day and titrating by 100-mg increments every 5 days, switching to a 300-mg capsule when appropriate. Some practitioners (D. Longmire, personal communication, 1996) have reported success at doses between 1500 and 3600 mg.

Carbamazepine has been used successfully to treat trigeminal neuralgias and other neuropathic pains, but its side effect burden and toxicity are problematic (10). Its slow absorption from the GI tract is enhanced by food, and it is protein-bound, metabolized through hepatic microsomal P450 cytochrome oxidase and the mitochondrial β-oxidation system, and excreted by the kidneys. Hepatic enzyme induction decreases serum half-life from about 15 to 20 hours at 3 weeks to about 12 hours during long-term administration. Dose-related side effects of carbamazepine include leukopenia, lethargy, double vision, cognitive changes, elevated liver function findings, hyponatremia, nausea and vomiting, fluid retention, and neurological symptoms including diplopia, blurred vision, fatigue, nausea, vertigo, nystagmus, and ataxia. Usually these symptoms are reversible with dose reduction. Idiosyn-

cratic effects include aplastic anemia, hepatic failure, Stevens-Johnson syndrome, rash, leukopenia, thrombocytopenia, hyponatremia, syndrome of inappropriate antidiuretic hormone secretion (SIADH), and conduction abnormalities such as Stokes-Adams syndrome. Fatalities have been associated with hepatic failure, exfoliative dermatitis, pancreatitis, and blood dyscrasias such as agranulocytopenia and aplastic anemia. Carbamazepine's teratogenic effects, especially during the first trimester, include neural tube defects, craniofacial defects, and hypoplasia of the fingernails. Carbamazepine may be toxic when combined with HCAs, possibly because of its structural similarity to imipramine. The starting dose of carbamazepine is 50 mg twice a day titrated within 2 to 3 days to 100 mg twice a day. Doses may be increased up by 200 mg per week until the optimum response is obtained, with the normal dose range being between 600 and 1600 mg a day. Obtain plasma levels in 1 or 2 weeks, checking serum levels 10 days to 3 weeks after achieving a maintenance dose to assure that autoinduction has not lowered serum levels. Monitor complete blood count and platelets at the start of therapy, weekly for 4 weeks, monthly thereafter during the next 6 months, and every 1 to 3 months thereafter. Serious blood dyscrasias develop suddenly, usually within the first 6 months, and are heralded by symptoms such as fever, infections, and sore throat, bruising, and petechiae. Patients should be instructed to report these immediately. Monitor liver function tests and bilirubin monthly for 2 to 3 months, then every 4 months thereafter. Asymptomatic LFT elevation, leukopenia, or thrombocytopenia can be managed with dose reductions and may spontaneously resolve. Hyponatremia occurs with 6 to 31% of patients. Monitor serum levels when combining carbamazepine with other medications, especially verapamil, erythromycin, fluoxetine, cimetidine, isoniazid, and propoxyphene. Alcohol, reserpine, phenobarbital, primidone, and valproic acid lower serum levels, and carbamazepine lowers serum levels of doxycycline, warfarin, and theophylline and potentiates vasopressin.

Valproic acid's starting dose is 250 mg once or twice daily, titrating by increments of up to 250 mg/week while monitoring blood levels. Therapeutic doses range from 250 to 1000 mg per day, divided in 3 doses, with a therapeutic level between 50 and 100 µg/mL. Valproic acid can be used as an adjunct to other anticonvulsants, such as phenytoin and BZDs, as well as with antidepressants; however, these combinations require careful monitoring of serum levels, prothrombin time (PT), and partial thromboplastin time (PTT), particularly with warfarin and NSAIDs. Prior to initiating a trial with valproic acid, baseline hepatic function should be tested, and serum levels must be monitored throughout treatment. Abrupt withdrawal in epileptic patients is contraindicated. Valproate may potentiate the CNS effects of alcohol and MAOIs and increase blood levels and toxicity of phenobarbital, primidone, and phenytoin. Valproic acid has been associated with exfoliative dermatitis such as Stevens-Johnson syndrome, hypotension, cardiovascular collapse, arrhythmias, depression, confusion, tremors, headaches, peripheral neuropathy, hepatic dysfunction, and GI symptoms of nausea, vomiting, constipation, and abdominal cramps. Hematological effects include thrombocytopenia and leukopenia.

Phenytoin is used for neuropathic pain at a dose range of 100 to 250 mg 2 to 4 times daily while monitoring for therapeutic blood levels between 10 and 20 µg/mL, with therapeutic effects occurring 3 to 5 days after initial treatment. Serum levels increase with the use of BZDs, chloramphenicol, dicumarol, disulfiram, tolbutamide, salicylates, halothane, cimetidine, and alcohol. Reserpine, carbamazepine, and calcium-containing antacids impede absorption. Phenytoin diminishes the effects of corticosteroids, warfarin, anticoagulants, quinidine, digoxin, and furosemide.

Clonazepam, a long-acting BZD often used as an anticonvulsant and for anxiety, may be an effective adjuvant in chronic pain management, particularly for chronic neuropathic pain. Its analgesic activity is probably related to a combination of its effect on the GABA-A receptor and secondary effects on autonomic arousal and pain perception, as well as additional analgesic properties possibly related to its anticonvulsant properties. It is used primarily combined with other analgesics such as opioids, NSAIDs, and antidepressants (10), with the usual dose 0.5 to 2 mg and a range between 0.25 mg and 10 mg daily. Peak plasma levels occur 1 to 2 hours after a single dose without active metabolites. Abrupt discontinuation precipitates withdrawal symptoms, although they are not as severe as with other BZDs without active metabolites but with shorter half-lives, such as alprazolam and lorazepam. Symptoms of withdrawal consist of anxiety, nervousness, diaphoresis, restlessness, irritability, fatigue, light-headedness, tremors, insomnia, and weakness. Liver function tests should be checked periodically. If a trial of clonazepam is not successful within 2 to 4 weeks, a discontinuation by progressive dose reduction of approximately 25% per week is recommended. Clonazepam should be used cautiously with other sedatives, particularly in combination with opioids because of the risk of respiratory suppression; its effects are antagonized by flumazenil. Clonazepam and lithium together may be neurotoxic.

Neuroleptics in Chronic Pain

Neuroleptic medications, often called antipsychotics, have four potential uses in chronic pain patients (10). They are the drug of choice when pain is part of a *delusional system.* In major depression with psychosis, neuroleptics may be used initially to treat psychosis while antidepressant treatment such as with HCAs and/or SSRIs or with electroconvulsive therapy progresses. If pain is a delusional symptom of a schizophrenic disorder, neuroleptics may be maintained long-term. Since the disturbance is primarily psychiatric, these patients are best treated by a psychiatric team, similar to an internist treating diabetes with neuropathy in consultation with pain specialist. Neuroleptics are useful when patients with chronic pain lose control of *anger.* Patients with chronic pain are often caught in irrational bureaucracies that are not responsive to their real needs for financial support and timely, effective treatment. These patients can become angry and threatening. Neuroleptics, most commonly the phenothiazines and butyrophenones, may be helpful as *adjunctive medication* in a variety of chronic or episodic pain syndromes. Their regular use is restricted by their side effect profile and significant risk for toxicity, such as tardive dyskinesia. Low-potency neuroleptics such as the phenothiazines are more prone to cause sedation, orthostatic hypotension, and anticholinergic side effects. High-potency neuroleptics, such as haloperidol and fluphenazine, are more prone to cause extrapyramidal symptoms, such as dystonia and parkinsonism, best managed with benztropine (Cogentin) and antihistamines such as diphenhydramine (Benadryl). Some intractable akathisias have been treated with β-blockers. Rarely neuroleptic use is complicated by *neuroleptic malignant syndrome,* a dangerous condition manifested by rigidity, fever, and autonomic instability. Management consists of physiological supportive therapy, discontinuation of neuroleptic, and in some cases bromocriptine and dantrolene. Long exposure to neuroleptics may induce tardive dyskinesia. Neuroleptics lower the seizure threshold. Phenothiazines should be avoided in patients who take MAOIs and should be used cautiously with antihypertensives, opiates, barbiturates, antihistamines, atropinic medications, and anticholinergic drugs such as HCAs.

Because of design problems in many studies showing efficacy and the problem of toxicity with regular use, neuroleptics are secondary adjuvant analgesic drugs, most useful for managing acute agitation or psychotic symptoms and for controlling nausea and vomiting. Their use as adjuvant analgesics has been limited to intractable neuropathic pain that has failed to respond to the use of antidepressants, anticonvulsants, and antianxiety agents in combination with opioids. Neuroleptics such as haloperidol are the mainstay for managing agitated delirium in hospitalized patients. The selection of a neuroleptic as an adjuvant is based upon the therapeutic needs of the individual patient. If a low-potency neuroleptic has been chosen, an ECG should be run and liver function tests obtained because of the potential for low-potency neuroleptics to cause cholestatic jaundice. Start with the lowest dose possible, titrating slowly while evaluating clinical response and side effects; for example, start the high-potency neuroleptic haloperidol (Haldol) at 0.5 mg two or three times a day and the low-potency neuroleptic chlorpromazine at 10 to 25 mg two or three times a day. In all cases, review potential medication interactions, particularly in combination with anticonvulsants and antidepressants. Once acute agitation is controlled, refer for psychiatric consultation before committing to longer-term use.

Psychostimulants in Chronic Pain

Stimulants increase central release of norepinephrine, dopamine, and serotonin and may be serotonin agonists. They increase arousal and decrease fatigue in normal adults and are used to treat apathy in disorders such as geriatric depression and dementia and for narcolepsy. Amphetamines increase analgesia and decrease sedation both in animals and humans (10). In postsurgical patients, they potentiate morphine analgesia with a single dose (43). Side effects caused by α- and β-adrenergic activity include increased systolic and diastolic blood pressure and reflexive slowing of heart rate. Large doses may cause cardiac arrhythmias. Side effects include GI disturbance, urinary hesitancy, anorexia, dryness of mouth, hypertension, tachycardia, insomnia, restlessness, agitation, confusion, dysphoria, and delirium. Amphetamines inhibit the cytochrome P450 enzyme system, raising blood levels of HCAs, neuroleptics, and other medications metabolized by P450. Interaction with other medications, such as phenylpropanolamine used as a decongestant, may produce hypertension. Psychostimulants may increase the hypotensive effect of guanethidine; decrease metabolism of anticoagulants, anticonvulsants, and heterocyclic antidepressants; cause hypertensive crisis with MAOIs; and lower the seizure threshold. Because of potential for abuse and addiction, careful drug monitoring is mandatory.

Caffeine increases the analgesic effect of aspirin and acetaminophen by 40% in postpartum pain (102) and is typically used in over-the-counter preparations. Caffeine, amphetamine, and cocaine induce an increased sense of well-being, energy, alertness, concentration, self-confidence, motivation for work, a desire to talk to people, and reduced sleepiness. Caffeine is safe and effective when used in the recommended dosage of 100 to 200 mg not more than every 3 to 4 hours (10). Tolerance to caffeine develops; symptoms of withdrawal after abrupt cessation include headache, drowsiness, yawning, decreased energy and alertness, difficulty concentrating, a diminished sense of well-being and contentment, decreased sociability and talkativeness, flulike symptoms, headache, blurring of vision, and impaired psychomotor performance. Acute and chronic caffeine intoxication (caffeinism) causes anxiety, insomnia, and cardiovascular and GI symptoms. Caffeine should be eliminated in patients with anxiety disorder, insomnia, palpitations, tachycardia, arrhythmia, hernia, ulcers, and pregnancy.

Cocaine potentiates morphine analgesia by blocking the reuptake of serotonin (28) and is used in combination with opioids for cancer pain, primarily as a local and regional anesthetic in the oral and nasal cavity (31). Cocaine's cardiovascular toxicity, high abuse liability, and very short half-life of approximately 40 minutes regardless of the route of administration limit its use in pain management (28).

Clinical Use of Psychostimulants

Psychostimulants are most commonly prescribed to alleviate the sedative effect of opioid administration for pain in advanced *malignancy*. Amphetamines have been useful in combination with morphine for severe postoperative pain and in the management of spasmodic torticollis. Occasionally they are used to promote energy, initiative, and mood in depressed patients when conventional antidepressants are not helpful. In

these cases, methylphenidate treatment is usually started at 2.5 mg at 8:00 AM and at noon. The dosage gradually increases for several days until therapeutic objectives are achieved or side effects such as overstimulation, anxiety, insomnia, paranoia, or confusion intervene. Typically, effective doses are less than 30 mg per day, although some patients require up to 60 mg. Methylphenidate doses are maintained for 1 to 2 months, after which many patients can be successfully withdrawn (10). The recommended dose range for dextroamphetamine is 5 to 20 mg a day. Chronic use of high doses can lead to personality changes, paranoid psychosis, psychological and physical dependency, withdrawal symptoms, mild fatigue, and depression. Contraindications to stimulants include anxiety disorders, paranoid disorders, schizophrenia, hyperthyroidism, seizures, arrhythmias, uncontrolled hypertension, and angina. The daily oral dose range for methylphenidate is 10 to 40 mg a day.

Anti-Anxiety Agents in Chronic Pain

Anxiety, a psychological state associated with stress and ubiquitous in acute pain and anxiety disorders, is frequently comorbid with chronic pain. Stress and anxiety play an important role in precipitating and perpetuating pain. Several related mechanisms may explain the efficacy of anxiolytic medications (10). (*a*) *Pain causes anxiety and the stress response;* reducing anxiety in pain states may prevent the negative psychophysiological sequelae of these states (described later). (*b*) *Anxiety causes autonomic nervous system (ANS) arousal, leading to skeletal muscle tension;* this mechanism is thought to be at least partially responsible for the precipitation and perpetuation of episodic muscle spasm post injury and for muscle contraction (tension) headaches associated with psychological and/or biomechanical stress. Symptoms of myofascial pain syndromes may worsen with anxiety. (*c*) *Ectopic firing of injured nerves causes neuropathic pain, precipitating muscle tightening and vulnerability to spasm, particularly when anxiety activates muscle tension. (d) ANS arousal activates vasomotor changes that liberate nociceptive algogens at the site of injury. (e) ANS arousal liberates noradrenaline at the site of injury, which by increasing the sensitivity of nociceptors lowers the threshold for pain perception. (f) Pain-related anxiety activates psychophysiological and functional disorders such as irritable bowel syndrome, chest pain, and headache. (g) Anxiety interferes with effective cognitive and behavioral coping.*

Benzodiazepines

BZDs are commonly prescribed in both acute and chronic pain states, often incorrectly. Their reputation for inducing dependency and abuse overshadows the more clinically important problem of behavioral toxicity. Understanding this latter problem, which is generally overlooked by physicians, is key to their successful use in chronic pain states (10, 12). These drugs depress presynaptic release of serotonin and excite GABA (103). Their analgesic effects in acute pain are attributed to reductions in anxiety, tension, and insomnia. Diazepam and midazolam reduce postoperative pain (3, 104). BZDs can be useful for short-term management of acute musculoskeletal pain.

The efficacy of BZDs in cancer pain and chronic nonmalignant pain appears to be limited (103). Clonazepam and alprazolam may be beneficial for certain chronic pain conditions, most notably neuropathic pain (103, 105). We have successfully used clonazepam, a BZD often used as an anticonvulsant, in treating trigeminal neuralgia, paroxysmal postlaminectomy pain, and posttraumatic neuralgias. Physicians often prescribe BZDs for sleep problems that frequently accompany chronic pain. They are not recommended for regular and frequent use in sleep disorders because of tolerance, dependency, and cognitive effects. BZDs may also be useful for the management of *comorbid anxiety disorder*, such as generalized anxiety disorder. Alprazolam and clonazepam have been most thoroughly studied for use in panic disorder, and the former may have some antidepressant properties. BZDs other than clonazepam play a limited role in chronic pain management. Their long-term use is not fully accepted because of the potential for dependence and because they may interfere with opioid analgesia.

The *neurobehavioral toxicity* of BZDs is clinically salient. They impair memory and psychomotor performance and are associated with increased incidence of falls, a particular problem for those with musculoskeletal disorders. A more insidious effect, inhibiting new learning, may prove to be particularly deleterious during pain rehabilitation because of the importance of the ability to learn the new cognitive and motor coping skills that are prerequisite to functional recovery and return to work (12, 106, 107).

The longer the half-life of a BZD and its active metabolites, the greater the risk of cumulative side effects such as sedation, amnesia, psychomotor impairment, and ataxia with risk for falls. 3-Hydroxy compounds with short half-lives and a lack of active metabolites, such as oxazepam (Serax), lorazepam (Ativan), alprazolam (Xanax), triazolam (Halcion), and temazepam (Restoril), have less potential for accumulation. Those with longer elimination half-lives, such as diazepam (Valium), chlordiazepoxide (Librium), clorazepate (Tranxene), prazepam (Centrax), and flurazepam (Dalmane) are more likely to cause cumulative toxic effects, a particular problem in the medically compromised patient and the elderly. A single dose of a BZD with a very short half-life, such as triazolam or midazolam, may produce confusion and amnesia, particularly in patients with organic brain disease. Patients taking regular doses of short-acting BZDs are subject to withdrawal symptoms that may be accompanied by seizures and other symptoms, including tinnitus, amnesia, psychosis, delirium, rebound anxiety, panic, headache, dizziness, diaphoresis, myalgias, tremors, and muscle twitching. BZDs potentiate other sedatives, such as alcohol, opioids, barbiturates, phenothiazines, MAOIs, and volatile anesthetics, causing sedation, confusion, and psychomotor impairment; they also potentiate opioid-caused respiratory depression. Doses should be adjusted down for elderly patients and those with renal, liver, CNS, or pulmonary disease. Cimetidine increases BZD levels. Anticonvulsants and adrenal steroids decrease BZD levels. BZDs are contraindicated in sleep apnea. Toxicity from BZDs may be antagonized with the use of flumazenil 0.2 to 1 mg.

Antihistamines, such as hydroxyzine and diphenhydramine, are commonly used to sedate patients in acute pain; they may also be used for anxiety or sleeplessness, often to avoid BZDs, at doses ranging from 25 to 50 mg intramuscularly or 25 to 100 mg by mouth. These drugs do not produce physical dependence.

We avoid using barbiturate preparations such as Fiorinal and Fioricet because their short-acting barbiturate, butalbital, is addictive and may cause transformational headaches. Also, other more effective interventions are available. Carisoprodol (Soma), a sedative marketed for its muscle-relaxing properties, may be useful in patients with recurrent muscle spasm; doses are usually 350 mg two to four times a day, but it is also addicting.

Buspirone, an antianxiety agent unrelated to the BZDs, does not interact with the GABA receptor system. It has a strong affinity for serotonin ($5HT_{1A}$) receptors in vitro and a moderate affinity for dopamine receptors in the brain. However, its anxiolytic mechanism is not well known. Buspirone's principal use is for chronic anxiety, particularly generalized anxiety disorder. Buspirone is ineffective in single doses, taking about 2 weeks for full therapeutic effects to occur. In contrast to the BZDs, buspirone does not sedate, impair motor function, interact with other sedative hypnotics, develop tolerance, produce drug dependency, potentiate alcohol, or suppress sedative withdrawal (96). There is no drug rebound, as is found with short-acting BZDs, and it has little if any abuse liability.

Choosing an Anxiolytic or Sedative

Consider clonazepam for patients with *neuropathic pain* if they cannot tolerate or do not respond to HCAs. Starting doses may be 0.25 to 0.5 mg at bedtime or twice a day, titrating up carefully while watching for sedation. For patients with *acute anxiety* due to breakthrough pain we tend to use hydroxyzine 25 to 50 mg or lorazepam 0.25 to 0.5 mg because of its short half-life and reliable intravenous, intramuscular, and oral absorption. Buspirone, starting at 5 mg twice a day and titrating to 10 mg three times a day to 15 mg four times a day, may be helpful for *chronic anxiety*. Behavioral methods of anxiety control (32) are preferable to regular long-term use of BZDs, which can be used as a backup system for breakthrough anxiety. When regular BZD use is warranted, we use clonazepam starting at 0.25 to 0.5 mg at bedtime; higher doses may produce sedation and mental changes. We avoid regular use of high-potency, short-acting BZDs such as alprazolam, which are associated with dangerous withdrawal and are often not clinically effective when used several times daily for long periods. Because of these drugs' short duration, patients cannot go for more than a few hours without having breakthrough anxiety and/or withdrawal symptoms, a pattern that induces multiple daily dosing and psychological dependency.

Capsaicin, a topical analgesic cream, has been used for the treatment of postherpetic neuralgia, arthritis, diabetic neuropathy, causalgia, and reflex sympathetic dystrophy syndrome (14, 16). Studies suggest that capsaicin renders the skin insensitive to pain by depleting and preventing a reaccumulation of substance P in peripheral sensory neurons (16). There are no known systemic side effects or drug interactions with topically applied capsaicin cream, making it potentially helpful for older patients who may have coexisting diseases and often take concomitant systemic medications. The initial enthusiasm for capsaicin, as for most new pain treatments that are often considered a panacea when introduced, has been tempered by its failure to cure pain. But it has its place alongside the many other pharmacological and nonpharmacological techniques in the armamentarium of the physician treating pain disorders.

A recent report suggests that calcitonin is useful in the treatment of phantom limb pain (85, 108). Patients receiving 100 IU of calcitonin intravenously over 5 minutes experienced immediate pain relief. This is encouraging, considering the difficulty in treating phantom pain (109).

The antiarrhythmic drugs lidocaine and tocainide have been shown to be useful in the treatment of the pain of diabetic peripheral neuropathy, trigeminal neuralgia, and Dercum's disease (adiposis dolorosa) (110). With lidocaine, a 5 mg/kg dose was administered by intravenous infusion over 30 minutes. Significant benefit was obtained and lasted 3 to 21 days.

Antispastic Medication

Many patients with chronic pain syndromes are maintained on centrally acting antispastic medication. These include drugs of the mephenesin class, BZDs, baclofen, and dantrolene. The mephenesin class is perhaps the most widely prescribed of the muscle relaxants currently available. There are no well-controlled studies in which the relative safety and efficacy of these compounds are compared. The mechanism of action of this class is poorly understood. The most prominent action is to depress polysynaptic reflexes preferentially over monosynaptic reflexes. Significant muscle relaxation appears to be achieved only with considerable sedation. It is difficult to determine whether these are true relaxants or sedative drugs. Their use should be discouraged in view of newer and more effective agents (10, 14).

The mechanism of action of quinine is to increase the refractory time of the muscle so that the response to multiple stimulations is reduced. This particular property seems to make it useful for special types of muscle cramps, such as nocturnal leg cramps, which is the most frequent use. The dose is 200 to 300 mg before retiring. With some patients,

only a brief trial of quinine therapy is required to provide relief from muscle cramps. Even large dosages may fail to give relief to others.

The three most effective antispastic medications are baclofen, dantrolene, and diazepam. From a clinical viewpoint, baclofen appears to act on presynaptic mechanisms rather than postsynaptic γ-aminobutyric acid (GABA) receptors, as does diazepam. Furthermore, baclofen may act preferentially in part to reduce the release of excitatory transmitters, possibly including substance P, from nociceptive afferent nerve endings, those coming from the skin and elsewhere, which tend to produce flexor reflexes when activated. It has also been demonstrated that baclofen produces a dose-dependent, stereospecific, antinociceptive effect in the intact animal, suggesting that baclofen may be useful in pain syndromes unrelated to flexor spasms (104).

A number of studies comparing baclofen and diazepam report that their overall antispastic effects are comparable. However, baclofen is usually preferred, at least initially, because it is much less likely to produce sedation or to reduce residual voluntary power. Similarly, baclofen does not produce generalized muscle weakness, as does dantrolene. It also differs from dantrolene in that it appears to produce essentially no abnormalities of other organ systems, such as the liver. Therapy begins with half a 10-mg tablet twice a day to be increased by half a tablet every 3 days to a usual maximum of two tablets four times a day. Occasionally 100 to 150 mg per day is useful. In many patients 5 or 10 mg four times a day is sufficient. Abrupt withdrawal of baclofen should be avoided because it often produces a temporary rebound in the number and severity of flexor spasms and in a few patients may precipitate temporary hallucinations.

Therapeutic blood levels of baclofen are considered to be 80 to 400 ng/mL. A 40-mg dose in healthy subjects produces levels remaining above 200 ng/mL for 8 hours. The serum half-life of baclofen is 3 to 4 hours. The use of baclofen may be limited by its adverse effects, which include drowsiness, insomnia, dizziness, weakness, and mental confusion.

Although dantrolene does reach the CNS, its primary action is peripheral. It appears to reduce muscle tension through a direct effect on the contractile mechanism. It is said to produce pronounced skeletal muscle relaxation without affecting coordination or neuromuscular transmission. A number of placebo-controlled clinical trials have demonstrated its efficacy in relieving spasticity due to cerebrovascular damage, spinal cord lesions, multiple sclerosis, or cerebral palsy. In the few studies in which dantrolene has been compared with diazepam, the drugs have been said to have approximately equal efficacy. Theoretically, if the two agents have equal efficacy in patients with certain types of spasticity, dantrolene may be useful for those in whom the sedative side effects of diazepam are more of a problem, such as the elderly and persons with CNS lesions or other disorders of cerebral function. Simultaneous use of dantrolene and diazepam (and perhaps also baclofen) may control the troublesome symptoms of spasticity better than either drug alone, with smaller doses and fewer side effects (104).

Dantrolene may be hepatotoxic; therefore, therapy with this agent should be continued only if it can be shown clearly that dantrolene itself offers considerable benefit. Its major drawback is provoking generalized weakness because it acts peripherally on skeletal muscle. Patients begin therapy with one 25-mg tablet daily; dosage can initially be increased by one tablet twice a day, but this is rarely indicated. If no definite benefit is demonstrable within 6 weeks or within 2 weeks of reaching the maximum tolerated dosage if adjustments in dosage have taken longer than 6 weeks, therapy should be discontinued (104).

BZDs directly potentiate the action of GABA. Some studies show that diazepam is useful alone or as adjunct therapy for spasticity, especially in patients with lesions affecting the spinal cord and occasionally in patients with cerebral palsy. There is no convincing evidence that diazepam is better than either baclofen or dantrolene. Diazepam is probably not as effective as baclofen in patients who primarily have intermittent, painful flexor spasms. Studies show few demonstrable differences between diazepam and baclofen with various types of spasticity, except that the incidence of unwanted side effects such as somnolence, dizziness, and increased muscular weakness is markedly higher with diazepam (111).

Many clinicians treating intractable chronic pain are dismayed by the frequency with which the BZD drugs are prescribed for chronic pain patients with concurrent depression (10). Lipman (112) has noted that BZDs increase anger and hostility when given over 8 weeks. This can be an adverse response for this already difficult population of chronic pain sufferers. It has been suggested that one of the mechanisms by which the BZDs and the barbiturates adversely affect pain is by action on the neurotransmitters. It is suggested that BZDs deplete serotonin, often adding to depression, paradoxical rage, habituation, disrupted sleep, and hangovers due to alterations of stage 3 and 4 sleep and rapid eye movement (REM) sleep. It has also been suggested that the BZDs inhibit serotonin release, and theoretically they may increase pain perception as well (104). These theories, combined with our clinical experience, suggest that this class of medication should not be used for long-term treatment of chronic pain.

Diazepam is said to be useful in the treatment of various nonspastic types of involuntary muscle activity, such as those seen in tetanus, stiff-person syndrome, or local muscle spasms of various traumatic causes. For elderly patients or patients with major symptoms of higher CNS dysfunction, the initial dose should not exceed 2 mg per day, and increments must be made extremely cautiously. In the treatment of spasticity, intramuscular or intravenous diazepam is occasionally useful in the treatment of acute low-back muscle spasm. Because its common side effects include drowsiness, light-headedness, weakness, fatigue, dizziness, vertigo, and ataxia, diazepam must be used cautiously in patients who are receiving other CNS active medications or alcohol, the side effects of which tend to be additive.

Botulinum toxin type A (BTX-A), a neurotoxin, has proved safe and effective in the treatment of strabismus, blepharospasm, and seventh nerve disorders. Intramuscular injection of BTX-A produces highly specific cholinergic neuromuscular blockade that is useful in treating abnormal muscle movement and spasticity, as well as pain due to involuntary or excessive muscle contraction. In a recent review Raj (114) discussed BTX-A in the treatment of various focal dystonias, including cervical dystonia or torticollis and writer's cramp (occupational dystonias). BTX-A is also noted to be effective in treating pain associated with upper motor neuron disorders, including stroke, traumatic brain injury, cerebral palsy, multiple sclerosis, and Parkinson's disease (115). Raj notes that use of BTX-A in many clinical settings in which pain is associated with muscle contraction represents an important new treatment modality that may prove more cost effective than invasive and irreversible surgeries, better tolerated than systemic pharmacotherapy, for pain, and highly valuable as an aid in achieving the overall objectives of physical therapy.

SUMMARY

Some of the more common medications considered useful in the treatment of chronic pain have been discussed. The practitioner should begin medication trials with the least potent medication capable of alleviating the patient's symptoms, with an eye to minimizing side effects and avoiding toxicity. After successful control is achieved, self-control techniques should be added to help reduce dose requirements (10, 12, 30, 32, 112). Patients should be periodically reassessed for their need to maintain dose, and reliance on daily pharmacotherapy should be reduced or discontinued when feasible if the patient can maintain functioning. No medication is entirely benign, and patients should not be given prescriptions for indefinite periods without monitoring. In all instances the physician should ask the same fundamental question as when administering any treatment, namely, do the potential benefits of treatment outweigh the risk? Any significant morbidity associated with treatment should be discussed with the patient, who should ultimately decide whether or not to use a specific medication.

References

1. Todd EM. Pain: historical perspectives. In: Crue BL, ed. Chronic pain. New York: SP Medical & Scientific Books, 1979.

2. Bonica JJ. Introduction. In: Bonica JJ, ed. Pain: research publications association for research in nervous and mental disorders, vol 58. New York: Raven Press, 1980.

3. Muller J. Handbuch der Physiologie des Menschen, vol 2. Baly W, translator. London: Taylor & Walton, 1840.

4. Latze, Dallenbach KM. Pain: history and present status. Am J Psychol 1939;52:331–347.

5. Von Frey M. Bertrage zur physiologie des schmerzsennes. Ber Verhandl Koneg Sachs Ges Wess Leipzeg 1984;46:185–196; 288–296.

6. Erb, Luckey GWA. Some recent studies of pain, Am J Psychol 1985;7:109.

7. Goldscheider A. Du spezifesche Energre der Gefiihlsnerven der Haut. Monatsschr Prakt Dermatol 1984;3:282.

8. Bennett GJ. Chronic pain due to peripheral nerve damage: an overview. In: Fields HL, Leibeskind JC, eds. Progress in pain research and management, vol 1. Seattle: IASP Press, 1994;51–59.

9. Price D, Mao J, Mayer DJ. Central mechanisms of normal and abnormal pain states. In: Fields HL, Leibeskind JC, eds. Progress in pain research and management, vol 1. Seattle: IASP Press, 1994;61–84.

10. Gallagher RM, Pasol E. Psychopharmacologic drugs in the chronic pain syndromes. Curr Rev Pain 1997;1:138–152.

11. American Pain Society and the American Academy of Pain Medicine. Joint Statement on the Use of Opioids in Intractable Pain. 1996.

12. Gallagher RM, Woznicki M. Low back pain rehabilitation. In: Stoudemire A, Fogel BS, eds. Medical psychiatric practice, vol 2. APA Press, 1993.

13. American Medical Association Drug Evaluations. 5th ed. Chicago: AMA, 1983.

14. Amoi S. The pain handbook. St. Louis: Mosby, 1995.

15. Baskin SI, Smith L, Hoey LA, et al. Age-associated changes of responses to acetylsalicylic acid. Pain 1981;2:18.

16. Halpern IM. Analgesic and antiinflammatory medications. In: Tollison CD, ed. Handbook of chronic pain management. Baltimore: Williams & Wilkins, 1989;57.

17. Aronoff GM, Evans WO. Handbook on the rational use of medication for pain, New York: DellaCorte, 1987.

18. Martin FW. Hazards of medications. Philadelphia: Lippincott, 1971.

19. Canalese J, Gimson AES, Davis M, Williams R. Factors contributing to mortality in paracetamol-induced hepatic failure. Br Med J 1981;282:1992;01.

20. Taha AS, Hudson N, Hawkey CJ, et al. Famotidine for the prevention of gastric and duodenal ulcers caused by steroidal anti-inflammatory drugs. N Engl J Med 1996;334:1434–1439.

21. Maier R, Menasse R, Riesterer L. The pharmacology of diclofenac sodium (Voltarol). Rheumatol Rehabil 1979;(Suppl 2):1121.

22. Dewson DD, Mather IE. Nonsteroidal antiinflammatory agents. In: Raj PP, ed. Practical management of pain. Chicago: Year Book, 1986;523–524.

23. Alvin PE, Lett IF. Current status of the etiology and management of dysmenorrhea in adolescence. Pediatrics 1982;70:516–525.

24. Luggen ME, Gartside PS, Ness V. Nonsteroidal antiinflammatory drugs in rheumatoid arthritis: duration of use as a measure of relative value. J Rheumatol 1989;18:1565–1569.

25. Van Den Ouweland FA, Corstens FNM, Van DePutte LBA. Gastrointestinal blood loss during treatment with naproxen for rheumatoid arthritis. Scand J Rheumatol 1987;18:365–370.

26. Dvorwik D, Lee DKN. Possible mechanisms for the gastric safety of etodolac. J Musculoskel Med 1991;8(Suppl 4):S47–S53.

27. Russell RI, Sturrock RD, Tana AS. Endoscopic studies of patients treated with etodolac. J Musculoskel Med 1991;8(Suppl 4):S60–S64.

28. Jaffe J, Martin WRP. Opioid analgesics and antagonists. In: Gillman AG, Goodman LS, Gilman A, eds. The pharmacological basis of therapeutics. ed 6. New York: MacMillan, 1980.

29. Twycross RG. Morphine and diamorphine in the terminally ill patient. Acta Anesthesiol Scand Suppl 1982;74:128–134.

30. Gallagher RM. Behavioral and biobehavioral treatment in chronic pain: perspectives on the evidence of effectiveness. Mind-Body Med 1997;2: (in press).

31. Jacox A, Carr DB, Payne R, et al. Management of cancer pain. Clinical practice guideline 9. AHCPR Pub 94–0592. Rockville, MD: Agency for Health Care Policy and Research, March 1994.

32. Gallagher RM, McCann W, Hughes J, et al. The behavioral medicine service: an administrative model for biopsychosocial teaching, research and clinical care. Gen Hosp Psychiatry 1990;12:283–295.

33. Sanders SH, Rucker KS, Anderson KO, et al. Clinical practice guidelines for chronic non-malignant pain syndrome patients. J Back Musculoskel Rehab 1995;5:15–120.

34. World Health Organization. Cancer pain relief and palliative care. WHO Technical Report Series 804. Geneva: WHO, 1990;1–75.

35. Mayne GE, Brown M, Arnold P, Moya F. Pain of herpes zoster and postherpetic neuralgia. In: Raj RP, ed. Practical management of pain. Chicago: Year Book, 1986.

36. Portenoy RK. Chronic opioid therapy in nonmalignant pain, J Pain Symptom Manag 1990;5 (Suppl):4661.

37. Portenoy RK. Chronic opioid therapy for persistent noncancer pain: can we get past the bias? APS Bull 1991;1:1, 45.

38. Portenoy RK. Chronic opioid therapy in nonmalignant pain. J Pain Symptom Manag 996l;5 (Suppl):S46–S62.

39. Portenoy RK, Foley KM. Chronic use of opioid analgesics in nonmalignant pain: report of 38 cases. Pain 1986;25:171–186.

40. Savage SR. Long-term opioid therapy: Assessment of consequences and risks. J Pain Symptom Manag 1996;11:274–286.

41. Zaczny JP. A review of the effects of opiates on psychomotor and cognitive functioning in humans. Exp Clin Psychopharmacol 1995;3:432–466.

42. Zacny JP. Should people taking opioids for medical reasons be allowed to work and drive. Addiction 1996;91:1581–1584.

43. Forrest WH et al. Dextroamphetamine with morphine for the treatment of postoperative pain. N Engl J Med 1977;296:712–715.

44. Webb SS, Smith GMP, Evans WO, Webb NC. Toward the development of a potent nonsedating oral analgesic. Psychopharmacology 1978;60:2528.

45. Crombez G, Eccleston C, Baeyens F, Eelen P. Habituation and the interference of pain with task performance. Pain 1997;70:149–154.

46. Onghena P, Van Houdenhove B. Antidepressant-induced analgesia in chronic non-malignant pain: a meta-analysis of 39 placebo-controlled studies. Pain 1991;49:205–219.

47. Goa KL, Sorkin EM. Gabapentin: a review of its pharmacological properties and clinical potential in epilepsy. Drugs 1993;3:46.

48. Goodkin K, Guillian CM. Antidepressants for the relief of chronic pain: do they work? Ann Behav Med 1989;11:83–101.

49. Walker EA, Sullivan MD, Stenchever MA. Use of antidepressants in the management of women with chronic pelvic pain. Obstet Gynecol Clin North Am 1993;20:743–751.

50. Max M. Antidepressants as analgesics. Progress in pain research and management, vol 1. Seattle: IASP Press, 1994.

51. France RD. The future of antidepressants: treatment of pain. Psychopathology 1987;20(Suppl 1):99–113.

52. Blumer D, Heilbron M. Chronic pain as a variant of depressive disease: the pain-prone disorder. J Nerv Ment Dis 1982;170:381–406.

53. Aronoff GM, Evans WO. Doxepin as an adjunct in the treatment of chronic pain. J Clin Psychiatry 1982;43(8/Sec 2):4245.

54. Ventafridda V, Bonezzi C, Caraceni A, et al. Antidepressants for cancer pain and other painful syndromes with deafferentation component: comparison of amitriptyline and trazodone. Ital J Neurosci 1987;8:579–587.

55. Botney M, Fields HL. Amitriptyline potentiates morphine analgesia by direct action on the central nervous system. Ann Neurol 1983;13:160–164.

56. Matthew NT. Prophylaxis of migraine and mixed headache: a randomized controlled study. Headache 1981;21:105–109.

57. Max MB, Culnane M, Schafer SC, et al. Amitriptyline relieves diabetic neuropathic pain in patients with normal and depressed mood. Neurology 1987;37:589–596.

58. Raftery H. The management of postherpetic pain using sodium valproate and amitriptyline. J Irish Med Assoc 1959;72:399–407.

59. Watson CPN, Chipman M, Reed K, et al. Amitriptyline versus maprotiline in post-herpetic neuralgia: a randomized, double-blind, crossover trial. Pain 1992;48:29–36.

60. Hynes MD, Lochner MD, Bemisk, et al. Fluoxetine, a selective inhibitor of serotonin uptake, potentiates morphine analgesics without altering its discriminative stimulants properties or affinity for opioid receptors. Life Sci 1985;36:2317–2323.

61. Diamond S, Frietag FG. The use of fluoxetine in the treatment of headache. Clin J Pain, 1989;5:200–201.
62. Geller SA. Treatment of fibrositis with fluoxetine. Am J Med 1989;87:594–595.
63. Theesen KA, Marsh WR. Relief of diabetes neuropathy with fluoxetine DILP 1989;23:572–574.
64. Sindrup SH, Gram LF, Brosen K, et al. The selective serotonin reuptake inhibitor paroxetine is effective in the treatment of diabetic neuropathy symptoms. Pain 1990;42:135–144.
65. Manna V, Bolino F, DiCicco L. Chronic tension type headache, depression and serotonin: therapeutic effects of fluvoxamine and mianserin. Headache 1994;34(1)44–49.
66. Bank J. A comparison study of amitriptyline and fluvoxamine in migraine prophylaxis. Headache, 1994;34(8)476–478.
67. Pramond R, Saxena and Peer T. Felt-Hansen. Sumatriptan-migraine: The headache. New York: Raven Press, 1993;329–341.
68. Atkinson JH. Psychopharmacologic agents in the treatment of pain syndromes. In: Tollison CD, ed. Handbook of chronic pain management. Baltimore: Williams & Wilkins, 1989;69–99.
69. Gallagher RM, Moore P, Chernoff I. The reliability of depression diagnosis in chronic low back pain: pilot study. Gen Hosp Psychiatry 1995; 17:399–413.
70. Krass S, Gallagher RM, Myers P, Friedman R. Pain threshold and sensitivity in depressed and non-depressed patients with chronic back pain. Proceedings of the Annual Meeting of the American Pain Society. November 1996.
71. Wells KB, Golding JM, Burnham MA. Psychiatric disorder in a sample of the general medical population with and without chronic medical conditions. Am J Psychiatry 1988;145:976–981.
72. Depression Guideline Panel. Depression in primary care, vol 1. Detection and diagnosis. Clinical practice guideline 5. AHCPR Pub 93–0551. Rockville, MD: Agency for Health Care Policy and Research, 1993.
73. Depression Guideline Panel. Depression in Primary Care, vol 2. Treatment of major depression. Clinical Practice Guideline 5.AHCPR Pub 93–0551. Rockville, MD: Agency for Health Care Policy and Research, 1993.
74. Wells KB, Golding JM, Burnham MA. The functioning and well-being of depressed patients: results from the Medical Outcomes Study. JAMA 1989;262:914–919.
75. Dohrenwend B, Marbach J, Raphael, Gallagher RM. Why is depression comorbid with chronic facial pain? A family study test of alternatives hypotheses. Proceedings of the annual meeting of the American Pain Society, 1995.
76. Seligman MEP. Helplessness: On depression, development, and death. San Francisco: WH Freeman, 1975.
77. Gallagher RM, Williams B, Skelly J, et al. Worker's compensation and return-to-work in low back pain. Pain 1995;61:299–307.
78. Loeser JD, Ward AA, White LE. Chronic deafferentation of human spinal cord neurons. J Neurosurg 1968;29:4850.
79. Nashald BE, Wilson WE. Central pain and irritable midbrain. In: Crue B, ed. Pain and suffering. Springfield, IL: Charles C. Thomas, 1970;95.
80. Nysfrom B, Hagbarth KE. Microelectrode recording from transmitter nerves in amputees with phantom limb pain. Neurosci Lett 1981;27:211–216.
81. Tasker RR, Dostrovsky JO. Deafferentation and central pain. In: Wall PD, Melzack R, eds. Textbook of pain. New York: Churchill Livingstone 1989;154–180.
82. Maciewicz R, Bouckoms A, Martin JB. Drug therapy of neuropathic pain. Clin J Pain 1985;1:39–49.
83. Englander RN, Johnson RSN, Brickley JJ, Nanna GR. Effects of antiepileptic drugs on thalamocortical excitability. Neurology 1977;27:1134–1139.
84. Swerdlow M. Anticonvulsant drugs and chronic pain (CW Book). Management of cancer pain. Clin Neuropharmacol 1984;7:51–82.
85. Dunsker SB, Mayfield FN. Carbamazepine in the treatment of flashing pain syndrome. J Neurosurg 1976;45:49–51.
86. Nicol CF. A four year double blind trial of carbamazepine in facial pain. Headache 1969;9:54–57.
87. Elliot F, Little A, Mebrandt W. Carbamazepine for phantom limb phenomena. N Engl J Med 1956;295:678.
88. Canton FK. Phenytoin treatment of thalamic pain. Br Med J 1972;2:590.
89. Chadda VS, Mathur MS. Double blind study of the effect of diphenylhydantoin sodium in neuropathy. J Assoc Phys India 1978;26:403–406.
90. Ellenberg M. Treatment of diabetic neuropathy with diphenylhydantoin. N Y State J Med 1976;68:295:618.
91. Caccia MR. Clonazepam in facial neuralgia and cluster Ha: clinical and electrophysiological study. Eur Neurol 1975;13:560–563.
92. Peiris JB, Perera GLS, Devendra SV, Lionel NOW. Sodium valproate in trigeminal neuralgia. Med J Aust 1980;2:278.
93. Bruera E, Nauigante A, Barugel M, et al. Treatment of pain and other symptoms in cancer patients: patterns in a North American and South American hospital. J Pain Symptom Manag 1990;5:78.
94. Monks R. Psychotropic drugs. In: Bonica JJ, ed. The management of pain. Philadelphia: Lea & Febiger, 1990;1677.
95. Taub A, Collins WF. Observations on the treatment of denervation dysesthesia with psychotropic drugs: postherpetic neuralgia, anesthesia dolorosa, peripheral neuropathy. Adv Neurol 1974;4:309–315.
96. Maxmen JS, Ward NG. Psychotropic drugs: fast facts. New York: Norton, 1995.
97. Chadwick D. Gabapentin. Lancet 1994;343:89–91.
98. Mellick GA, Mellicy LB, Mellick LB. Gabapentin in the management of reflex sympathetic dystrophy. J Pain Symptom Manag 1995; 10:265–266.
99. Rosner H, Rubin L, Kestenbaum H. Gabapentin adjunctive therapy in neuropathic pain states. Clin J Pain 1996;12:56–58.
100. Andrew J, Chadwick D, Bates D. Gabapentin in partial epilepsy. Lancet 1990;335:1114–1115.
101. Melick GA, Seng ML. The use of gabapentin in the treatment of reflex sympathetic dystrophy and a phobic disorder. Am J Pain Manag 1995;5:7–9.
102. Laska EM, Sunshine A, Zighelboim I, et al. Effect of caffeine on acetaminophen analgesia. Clin Pharmacol Toxicol 1983;33:4, 498–509.
103. King SA, Strain JJ. Benzodiazepine use by chronic pain patients. Clin J Pain 1990;6:143–147.
104. Singh PN, Sharma P, Gupta PK, Pandey K. Clinical evaluation of diazepam for relief of post operative pain. Br J Anesth 1981;53:831–836.
105. Fernandez F, Adams F, Holmes VF. Analgesic effect of alprazolam in patients with chronic, organic pain. J Clin Psychopharmacol 1987;7:167–169.
106. Mayer TG, Gatchel RJ, Mayer H, et al. A prospective two-year study of functional restoration in industrial low back pain. JAMA 1987; 258:1763–1768,
107. Hazard RG, Genwich JW, Kalish SM, et al. Functional restoration with behavioral support: a one year prospective study of patients with chronic low back pain. Spine 1989;14:157–161.
108. Martens RA, Martens S. The milk sugar dilemma: living with lactose intolerance. East Lansing, MI: MeoiEd Press, 1987.
109. Zrbanec D, Spaventi S. Effect of calcitonin on the skeleton and bone pain in patients with osteolytic metastases. Acta Med Iugoslav 1987;41:33–42.
110. Kastrup J, Peterson P, Dejgard A, et al. Intravenous lidocaine infusion: a new treatment of pain in diabetic neuropathy. Pain 1987;28:69–75.
111. Young RR, Delwaide PM. Spasticity. I and II. N Engl J Med 1981; 304:2833, 9699.
112. Lipman RS. Pharmacotherapy of anxiety and depression. Psychopharmacol Bull 1981;17:3, 91–103.
113. Aronoff GM, Evans WO. Evaluation and treatment of chronic pain at the Boston Pain Center. J Clin Psychiatry 1982;43:(8/Sec 2):49.
114. Raj P. Botulinum toxin in the treatment of pain associated with musculoskeletal hyperactivity. Curr Rev Pain 1997;1:403–406.
115. Tsui JKC. Botulinum toxin as a therapeutic agent. Pharmacol Ther 1996;72;13–24.

CHAPTER 33

Nonsteroidal Anti-Inflammatory Analgesics and Their Combinations with Opioids

William T. Beaver

During the past 20 years, an important development in the management of acute pain with analgesic drugs has been the emergence of nonsteroidal anti-inflammatory analgesics that are clearly more effective than optimal doses of aspirin or acetaminophen and that compare favorably not only with combinations of aspirin or acetaminophen with narcotics but even, in some cases, with strong injectable opioids. These drugs have already proved particularly effective in dental pain, postoperative pain, and pain associated with acute musculoskeletal trauma. They have revolutionized the treatment of dysmenorrhea. Many provide longer pain relief than any of the conventional oral analgesics.

Unfortunately, for many types of pain the utility of these agents has not as yet been adequately explored through controlled studies. In particular, excluding studies in rheumatic disease, there are relatively few trials of these drugs in chronic pain that meet even the minimum criteria for a well-controlled clinical trial of analgesic efficacy. The few studies that do exist are mainly single-dose studies in cancer pain (1), and there is a virtual absence of studies in the typical pain clinic population of patients with nonmalignant chronic pain. Furthermore, while the results of available *single-dose* studies comparing analgesics in chronic pain are generally consistent with the results of single-dose studies of the same drugs in other pain models, there are very few controlled *repeat-dose* analgesic studies in any pain model, and the legitimacy of extrapolating estimates of comparative efficacy on repeated dosing across pain models is unknown.

This chapter focuses on the comparative analgesic efficacy of nonsteroidal anti-inflammatory drugs (NSAIDs) and their combinations with opioids, but some of the salient adverse effects associated with their use are also considered. When possible, efficacy comparisons are based on studies in chronic pain, but as noted earlier, the analgesic efficacy of many NSAIDs and their combinations has been studied adequately only in acute pain. There are numerous papers and guidelines for the treatment of pain reviewing the use of NSAIDs as analgesics (2–10), as constituents of analgesic combinations (11–15), and in the treatment of cancer pain (3, 15–24).

MECHANISMS OF ANALGESIC ACTION

Aspirin was introduced into medicine by Dreser and Hofmann in 1899, and after a century of use, the complete picture of the mechanisms of its various therapeutic actions remains unclear (25). In the early 1960s, using a cross-perfusion model in the dog, Lim et al. (26) provided evidence for a peripheral mechanism of analgesia for both aspirin and acetaminophen while confirming morphine's site of action in the central nervous system (CNS). A decade later Vane and his coworkers (27–31) established the importance of the inhibition of the arachidonic acid cascade as the most likely mechanism for the antipyretic, analgesic, and anti-inflammatory actions of aspirin and other NSAIDs, as well as the mechanism for several of their more prominent adverse effects.

The classical schema for the mechanism of the peripheral analgesic effect of NSAIDs is initiated by tissue injury, the primary cause of inflammation and pain, which produces arachidonic acid as a result of the action of phospholipase A_2 on phospholipids released from disrupted cell membranes. This arachidonic acid serves as a substrate for the cyclo-oxygenase (COX) pathway, which leads to the production of prostacyclin, prostaglandins, and thromboxanes. Prostaglandin E_2. (PGE_2) and prostacyclin contribute to the development of inflammatory erythema and pain. However, these prostanoids do not seem to activate nociceptors directly as pain mediators but rather cause hyperalgesia by sensitizing the pain nerve endings to both mechanical stimuli and other chemical mediators, such as bradykinin and histamine. NSAIDs exert their anti-inflammatory and analgesic actions by blocking COX at the site of tissue injury in the periphery, while their antipyretic effect can be attributed to blockade of the PGE_2 formation in the hypothalamus that is caused by the release of interleukin-1 by bacterial and viral infections (32). As would be expected for a structurally diverse class of drugs with a spectrum of therapeutic and adverse effects as extensive as that of the NSAIDs, subsequent research and clinical experience during the past 15 to 20 years have shown that the mechanisms of their anti-inflammatory and analgesic effects are considerably more complex than is depicted in this classical schema and that many factors influence their therapeutic and adverse effects.

There is a consensus among rheumatologists that the *average* efficacy of available NSAIDs is about the same for the various indices of antirheumatic effect when these drugs are administered at usual doses to groups of patients in the treatment of rheumatoid arthritis or osteoarthritis (33–37). However, there is evidence that among *individual* patients there is substantial variation in therapeutic response to individual NSAIDs (33, 35). The determinants of this variability are unknown, although individual differences in pharmacokinetics have been suggested.

Physicochemical and pharmacokinetic factors have substantial influence on both similarities and differences in the therapeutic and adverse effects of NSAIDs (6, 33, 35, 38). Almost all NSAIDs are bound about 99% to plasma albumin and are weak organic acids (pK_a 3 to 5). Protein binding favors their migration into inflamed tissue, where they are released and concentrated following degradation of the transporting protein. The relatively acidic environment of the extracellular space in inflamed tissue favors formation of the undissociated, un-ionized, lipid-soluble NSAID, which penetrates the cell membrane, dissociates, and becomes trapped intracellularly in its ionic form (6, 33, 38). This accounts for very high concentrations of NSAIDs in inflamed joints and other sites of inflammation relative to most other tissues. Unfortunately, from the standpoint of adverse effects, ion trapping also favors accumulation of NSAIDs intracellularly in the stomach wall, kidney, and liver (6, 38).

There are still only very limited data relating NSAID plasma levels to analgesic effect, although this is an area of active investigation. The plasma half-life correlates in a general way with duration of analgesic action, but this correlation is not good enough to allow accurate prediction of optimal dosing intervals from plasma half-life data alone. Drug accumulation in inflamed (injured) tissue in part explains why the duration of action of NSAIDs with shorter half-lives, such as ibuprofen, is longer than would be predicted from their plasma half-life (6).

The pharmacokinetics of some NSAIDs (most of the arylpropionic acids, or "profens," ketorolac, and etodolac) is complicated by the existence of two optical isomers or enantiomers that contain an asymmetrical or chiral carbon atom (33, 35, 39). It is the S enantiomers that inhibit COX, but only naproxen is marketed as the pure S enantiomer; the others are available only as racemic mixtures containing equal amounts of the active S and the inactive R isomers. To complicate matters further, ibuprofen and fenoprofen undergo substantial unidirectional chiral inversion of the R to S form in the liver, while ketoprofen and flurbiprofen are minimally inverted in man (39). There are theoretical reasons the pure S enantiomer of NSAIDs might be preferable to the racemates, but there is thus far little evidence that this is a clinically important issue.

Potentially more important in understanding the mechanistic differences among NSAIDs for therapeutic and adverse effects was the discovery that there are at least two COX isoenzymes, COX-1 and COX-2 (25, 32, 37, 40–43). COX-1 is the constitutive enzyme that is normally present in most tissues and is responsible for physiological regulation or homeostasis in housekeeping functions such as regulating renal blood flow, gastroprotective effects in the stomach, and the function of vascular endothelium and platelets (32, 40). COX-2, on the other hand, is "the inducible form of the enzyme, expressed in endothelial cells, macrophages, synovial fibroblasts, mast cells, chondrocytes and osteoblasts after tissue trauma, and therefore plays an important role in [pain and] inflammation" (40).

Theoretically, an NSAID that preferentially inhibited COX-2 and exerted little or no effect on COX-1 might be devoid of adverse effects on the GI tract, the kidney, and platelets, while maintaining analgesic and anti-inflammatory efficacy. However, assay of the relative specificity of NSAID inhibition of COX-1 and COX-2 depends on species; tissue; and whether the assay is performed on isolated enzymes, disrupted cells, whole cells, or in vivo (32, 41), and there is some evidence that both COXes play a physiological role (41). Furthermore, there are no *highly* selective COX-2 inhibitors in clinical use, and the analgesic efficacy of marketed, even moderately selective COX-2 inhibitors is poor or uncertain, while all have been associated with some reports of gastrointestinal (GI) perforation, ulceration, and bleeding on long-term use. Newer, highly selective compounds are under development, but their efficacy must be clearly defined and their GI safety must be demonstrated in long-term studies (32, 41, 44).

NSAIDs have a number of actions that do not depend on the inhibition of COX but that may be mechanistically important for their analgesic and anti-inflammatory effects (25, 33, 40). Arachidonic acid is also metabolized by the lipoxygenase pathway to leukotrienes, and some NSAIDs can block this pathway to varying degrees. NSAIDs interfere with a number of membrane-associated cell processes, including G protein-mediated signal transduction, and they also inhibit neutrophil and macrophage function, including the release of many mediators of inflammation.

Dissociation between the Analgesic and Anti-Inflammatory Effect of NSAIDs

While the antirheumatic efficacy of usual doses of NSAIDs is similar, there are substantial differences among NSAIDs in their analgesic efficacy, and there is poor correlation between anti-inflammatory and analgesic activity (38, 40, 42). This has been demonstrated both in animal experiments and in controlled clinical trials of analgesic efficacy in a number of human pathological pain models. While pharmacokinetic factors can account for some of these differences, many of the differences are probably due to the fact that "NSAIDs exert their analgesic effect not only through peripheral inhibition of prostaglandin synthesis but also through a variety of other peripheral and central mechanisms" (40). In particular, attention has been directed to the effect of NSAIDs on nociceptive processing in the CNS (38, 40, 42, 43, 45–47). Malmberg and Yaksh (46) have shown that NSAIDs exert a direct spinal action by blocking the hyperalgesia induced by the activation of spinal glutamate and substance P receptors. "Some NSAIDs, in addition to their effects on prostaglandin synthesis, also affect the synthesis and activity of other neuroactive substances believed to have key roles in processing nociceptive input within the dorsal horn. . . .These other actions, in conjunction with the inhibition of prostaglandin synthesis, may synergistically augment the effects of NSAIDs on spinal nociceptive processing" (42).

ADVERSE EFFECTS OF NSAIDS

Gastrointestinal Toxicity of the NSAIDs

From the standpoint of morbidity and mortality, GI adverse effects undoubtedly constitute the most important group of NSAIDs' adverse effects. Indeed, GI ulceration, perforation, and hemorrhage (collectively referred to as NSAID gastropathy) are more worrisome than all other NSAID adverse effects combined (48).

Although it had been known for several decades that aspirin ingestion often produces gastric erosions and occult blood loss and less frequently, peptic ulceration with perforation and massive hemorrhage (4), it was only with the proliferation and extensive prescribing of nonsalicylate NSAIDs in the 1970s and 1980s that the seriousness and magnitude of NSAID gastropathy was appreciated (33, 35, 37, 41, 48–67). In 1988, the U.S. Food and Drug Administration (FDA) required the following class labeling in the warnings section of the package insert for all NSAIDs:

"Risk of G.I. ulcerations, bleeding, and perforation with NSAID therapy: Serious gastrointestinal toxicity such as bleeding, ulceration, and perforation can occur at any time, with or without warning symptoms, in patients treated with NSAIDs. Although minor upper gastrointestinal problems, such as dyspepsia, are common, and usually develop early in therapy, physicians should remain alert for ulceration and bleeding in patients treated chronically with NSAIDs, even in the absence of previous GI tract symptoms. In patients observed in clinical trials for several months to 2 years, symptomatic upper GI ulcers, gross bleeding, or perforation appear to occur in approximately 1% of patients treated for 3 to 6 months, and in about 2% to 4% of patients treated for 1 year. Physicians should inform patients about the signs and/or symptoms of serious GI toxicity and what steps to take if they occur."

The relative risk of gastric ulcer complications is somewhat higher than that of duodenal ulcers (49, 51–54, 59), and less frequently, perforation and bleeding also result from ulcers in the small intestine (50) and colon (35, 52, 55). The pathogenesis of NSAID gastropathy is complex, involving both local injury due to direct contact with the gastroduodenal mucosa and systemic effects caused by inhibition of prostaglandin synthesis (41, 52, 53, 62, 65–67). Local injury develops acutely on short-term administration of NSAIDs and can be quantified endoscopically in comparative studies in normal volunteers by rating submucosal hemorrhage and erosions as well as by measuring occult GI blood loss. Unfortunately, these measures correlate poorly with the relative risk that various NSAIDs and NSAID formulations will produce GI ulceration, perforation, and hemorrhage on chronic administration to patients (62). More important in the pathogenesis of NSAID gastropathy than the acute local effects of NSAIDs are the ulcerogenic effects of longer-term administration mediated by prostaglandin inhibition. These include a decreased antisecretory effect on gastric acid production, reduced bicarbonate secretion, decreased production of protective gastric mucus, and reduction in mucosal blood flow coupled with the increased risk of bleeding associated with impaired platelet aggregation (52, 53).

No subgroup of patients that is free of the risk of developing NSAID gastropathy has been identified. There is a poor correlation between GI symptoms and ulceration; the majority of patients with these lesions have no symptoms unless bleeding or perforation occurs, and the prevalence of silent ulceration increases with age (49, 52, 54, 59). However, cohort and case-control epidemiological studies have identified a number of putative risk factors for NSAID gastropathy; some of these are fairly well substantiated and others are more controversial. Risk factors other than the individual NSAID and its dose include age above 60; female gender; history of peptic ulcer disease, GI bleeding, GI-related hospitalization, or NSAID-related GI adverse effects; concomitant treatment with corticosteroids or anticoagulants; the use of multiple NSAIDs; high level of disability; serious concomitant disease; and possibly alcohol use (35, 37, 49, 52, 54, 56, 57, 59, 62, 65, 66). Several studies suggest that *Helicobacter pylori* infection is not a risk factor for NSAID gastropathy (62, 65).

Numerous case-control and cohort studies have compared the relative risks of gastropathy reported with individual NSAIDs (58, 59, 61). Henry et al. (60) recently published meta-analyses of 12 of these studies, which revealed substantial differences in the risk of inducing gastrointestinal bleeding and ulcer perforation. Higher dose was generally a risk factor for NSAID gastropathy, a finding consistent with numerous other studies. Ibuprofen in daily doses of 1600 mg or less was associated with the lowest relative risk of severe GI toxicity; the 11 comparator drugs were associated with a 1.6-fold to 9.2-fold increase in risk compared with ibuprofen. Aspirin (1.6) and diclofenac (1.8) were among those with the lowest risk; diflunisal (2.2) and naproxen (2.2) occupied an intermediate position; and piroxicam (3.8) and ketoprofen (4.2) were near the highest.

If an NSAID is indicated for the treatment of chronic pain, give the least toxic agents at the lowest effective dose, and do not continue to prescribe an NSAID unless there is clear evidence of analgesic efficacy. If a patient is at high risk for NSAID gastropathy, consider the coadministration of misoprostol, which provides effective protection against both gastric and duodenal ulceration and is the only drug approved by the FDA for this purpose. Some histamine$_2$-antagonists and proton pump inhibitors are also used for this indication, but they appear to be more effective against duodenal than against gastric ulceration (22, 37, 52–54, 62, 63, 65).

Hepatic Adverse Effects

Aspirin and most other NSAIDs can cause small, asymptomatic, reversible elevations in serum aminotransferase levels in 1 to 15% of patients, depending on the NSAID, the dose, the duration of therapy, and the underlying disease. Rarely, NSAIDs can also cause symptomatic hepatitis and very rarely, fatal liver injury. Studies are inconsistent as to which NSAIDs are more likely to produce symptomatic liver injury, but sulindac and diclofenac have been most frequently mentioned in the U.S. literature (35, 62, 68). When NSAIDs are used for the treatment of chronic pain, serum aminotransferase levels should be assessed at baseline and periodically thereafter, and the NSAID should be discontinued if aminotransferase levels progressively increase or clinical signs or symptoms of liver disease develop (62).

Renal Adverse Effects

Prostaglandins appear to play a negligible role in renal hemodynamics in the euvolemic healthy person. However, by opposing the increased vasoconstrictive influences of norepinephrine and angiotensin II that result from activation of pressor reflexes, they play an important role in the maintenance of renal perfusion in patients with a reduction of renal blood flow or blood volume. Therefore, acute renal failure can be precipitated by NSAIDs in patients with hypovolemia, congestive heart failure, chronic renal insufficiency, cirrhosis with ascites, those taking diuretics, and the elderly. In addition, NSAIDs can affect renal tubular function, causing salt and water retention and edema as well as promoting hyperkalemia (10, 33, 35, 69, 70). If promptly recognized, these conditions can be reversed by discontinuing the NSAID.

Interstitial nephritis with or without nephrotic syndrome is a rare form of nephrotoxicity caused by a number of NSAIDs, although it has most frequently been associated with fenoprofen (10, 35, 69, 70). This syndrome also usually resolves on discontinuation of the NSAID.

NSAIDs and Hypertension

Chronic NSAID therapy can produce small elevations (3 to 5 mm Hg) in mean arterial pressure through a variety of prostaglandin-dependent mechanisms, which probably include both effects on vascular tone and effects mediated through the kidney. Of most practical importance is the realization that some NSAIDs can partially antagonize the antihypertensive effects of thiazide and loop diuretics, α- and β-adrenergic blockers, and angiotensin-converting enzyme inhibitors, and this interaction may interfere with blood pressure control in some patients (33, 71–73).

ASPIRIN AND OTHER SALICYLATES

Historically, aspirin and acetaminophen have been the mainstays and drugs of first choice in oral analgesic therapy. Until the advent of the newer NSAIDs, no single-entity oral analgesic, with the exception of large doses of oral opioids, was more effective than the usual therapeutic dose of aspirin or acetaminophen (4, 5, 11, 12, 74–78). Controlled clinical trials have shown aspirin to be effective in essentially every pain model in which it has been studied, including postoperative pain of various types, oral surgery and other types of dental pain, postpartum episiotomy and uterine cramp pain, headache, dysmenorrhea, acute musculoskeletal pain, cancer pain, rheumatoid arthritis, and osteoarthritis.

The major problem with aspirin as an analgesic is the shallow slope of its dose-response curve and/or a ceiling of analgesic effect somewhere in the 650-mg to 1300-mg dose range; however, it is unclear just where, in terms of dose, this ceiling occurs. Wallenstein (79) of the Memorial Sloan-Kettering group of Houde, Wallenstein, and Rogers found an apparent ceiling of peak analgesic effect in cancer pain at the 600-mg dose, although the 900-mg dose had a longer duration of action (Fig.33.1). On the other hand, Ventafridda et al. (80) found that aspirin 1000 mg did produce greater peak analgesia in cancer patients than a 600-mg dose.

Laska, Sunshine, and their colleagues (81) found a significant positive dose-response relation in terms of the area under the analgesic time-effect curve on administering graded doses of aspirin—325, 650, and 1300 mg—to women with postpartum pain, although the slope of this curve was relatively shallow (Fig. 33.2).

Adverse Effects of Aspirin

While the patient with chronic pain can experience any of the adverse effects associated with the use of aspirin (4, 8–10, 22, 48) certain of these present a particular problem on prolonged high-dose administration. Dyspepsia, pyrosis, nausea, vomiting, occult GI blood loss with resulting anemia, and less frequently, GI ulceration, perforation, and gross bleeding are the most frequent limiting adverse effects of chronic aspirin administration. The problem is exacerbated in patients with chronic cancer pain receiving chemotherapy, steroids, or local irradiation.

Various special aspirin formulations may somewhat reduce GI intolerance (4, 22). In particular, dependable enteric-coated aspirin is now available and has been used successfully in

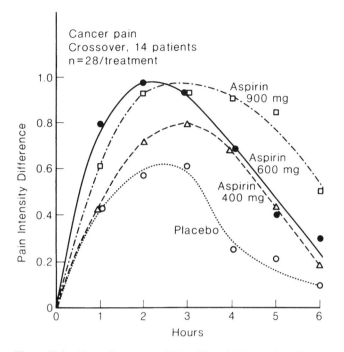

Figure 33.1.   Time-effect curves of 400, 600, and 900 mg of aspirin after crossover administration to inpatients with cancer pain. (Adapted from Wallenstein SL. Analgesic studies of aspirin in cancer patients. In: Proceedings of the Aspirin Symposium. London: Aspirin Foundation, 1975;5–10.)

reducing subjective GI intolerance in patients receiving aspirin for the therapy of rheumatic diseases (8, 9). There do not appear to be any well-controlled repeat-dose studies of plain and enteric-coated aspirin in chronic nonrheumatic pain to compare the analgesic efficacy and tolerability of these two preparations.

Another adverse effect of particular importance in cancer patients with chronic pain is aspirin's inhibition of platelet function, which in contrast to the other NSAIDs, is irreversible. In the cancer patient undergoing active treatment, depressed platelet counts due to chemotherapy and radiation seem to be more the norm than the exception, and this very much limits the use of aspirin. In patients not in active anticancer therapy, this may not be as much of a problem.

At high daily dosages, salicylism can become a problem. As the salicylate plasma level approaches and then exceeds 30 mg/dL, a progressively larger number of patients develop reversible ototoxicity characterized by tinnitus and hearing loss, headache, dizziness, confusion, nausea, vomiting, or a combination of these. While most patients can tolerate 650 mg of aspirin every 4 hours or 1000 mg every 6 hours (4 g/day) without too much difficulty, if the dose is increased beyond this to 1000 mg or 1300 mg every 4 hours (6 to 8 g/day), most patients develop salicylism and GI intolerance.

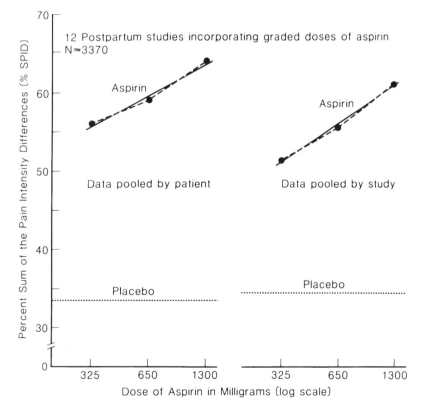

Figure 33.2.   Dose-response curves based on pooled data from 12 postpartum studies incorporating graded doses of aspirin. (Based on data from Laska EM. et al. Caffeine as an analgesic adjuvant. JAMA 1984;251:1711–1718.)

Nonacetylated Salicylates

Although sodium salicylate was the first synthetic salicylate used as an antipyretic and antirheumatic, after aspirin was introduced in 1899, the interest in nonacetylated salicylates waned. However, in recent years, renewed interest in nonacetylated salicylates has been prompted by the realization that several important adverse effects of aspirin—GI intolerance and bleeding, impairment of platelet function, and aspirin-sensitive asthma—are associated with the acetyl group (10, 48). Nonacetylated salicylates are relatively prostaglandin sparing but are still effective anti-inflammatory agents in rheumatic disease (25). Use of the nonacetylated salicylates was hampered by the lack of a suitable solid dosage form with good bioavailability, problems that seem to have been overcome with the development of choline magnesium trisalicylate. This drug appears to be equieffective to aspirin and some of the newer NSAIDs in the treatment of rheumatoid arthritis and osteoarthritis while causing substantially less gastric mucosal erosion and microbleeding and little or no effect on platelet function as compared with aspirin (82). However, there are only a few data on the analgesic efficacy of choline magnesium trisalicylate (83) and other nonacetylated salicylates in nonrheumatic pain.

ACETAMINOPHEN

Acetaminophen has proved equieffective and equipotent with aspirin in single-dose studies in pain due to cancer, postoperative pain, postpartum pain, oral surgery pain, and headache (4, 84, 85). In a study in cancer patients at the Memorial Sloan-Kettering Cancer Center, the dose-response curves for aspirin and acetaminophen were identical (79), and in another study, Houde et al. (86) showed that the time-effect curves for aspirin 600 mg and acetaminophen 600 mg were also virtually identical (Fig. 33.3).

Laska et al. (81) also explored the dose-response curve of acetaminophen 500 mg, 1000 mg, and 1500 mg in five postpartum studies (Fig. 33.4). The slope of the curve was significant; however, as in the case of aspirin, doubling of dose produced only a modest increment in analgesic effect.

Acetaminophen's mechanism of analgesic action is unknown but is clearly different from that of aspirin and the other NSAIDs. While acetaminophen has peripherally mediated analgesic effects (26), it does not inhibit peripheral COX. There is also some evidence for an analgesic effect mediated by actions in the CNS (47, 87). It is often said that acetaminophen has little or no anti-inflammatory effect; this is not true. Acetaminophen is not effective in the treatment of rheumatoid arthritis, but in some other types of inflammation it may equal or surpass the anti-inflammatory effects of aspirin.

Skjelbred, Lokken, and Skoglund (88) have done a series of studies in patients who had impacted third molars surgically removed, in which both pain relief and an objective index of inflammation (swelling) were measured. They found that acetaminophen was at least as effective if not more effective than aspirin in reducing postoperative swelling over a 3-day

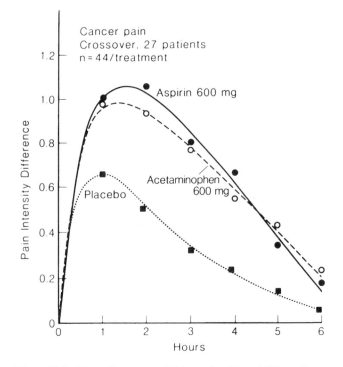

Figure 33.3.   Time-effect curves of 600 mg of aspirin and 600 mg of acetaminophen after crossover administration to inpatients with cancer pain. (Based on data from Houde RW, Wallenstein SL, Beaver WT. Clinical measurement of pain. In: de Stevens G, ed. Analgetics. New York: academic Press, 1965;75–122.)

period in this model of posttraumatic inflammation. The question then arises whether the inflammation associated with particular chronic pain states is more similar to that in rheumatoid arthritis or to that in acute tissue trauma.

When one also considers the differing pharmacokinetics of the two drugs, it is obvious that repeat-dose studies in nonrheumatic chronic pain comparing full doses of acetaminophen with aspirin and other NSAIDs are needed. This is an important issue because acetaminophen has much less in the way of adverse effects, particularly on chronic administration, than do aspirin and other NSAIDs. Acetaminophen does not produce subjective GI intolerance, GI bleeding and ulceration, an adverse effect on platelet function, or salicylism; nor does it cross-react in aspirin-sensitive asthma. If it could be shown that on repeated dosing, acetaminophen was equieffective with aspirin, acetaminophen would be very attractive as an alternative to aspirin in chronic pain.

It has been known for 30 years that acetaminophen in substantial overdose (15 to 25 g) can produce serious or fatal hepatic injury. This is due to the production of a toxic metabolite, N-acetyl-p-benzoquinoneimine, which is formed by the oxidation of acetaminophen catalyzed by the cytochrome P450 isozymes CYP2E1, 1A2, and 3A4 (85, 89). Some alcoholics and persons who are fasting are susceptible to liver injury at doses of 4 to 10 g/day and rarely from doses less than 4 g/day, apparently because of a complex interaction between acetaminophen metabolism, alcohol, and hepatic glutathione (68, 89–93). Otherwise a dosage of 4 g/day is well tolerated.

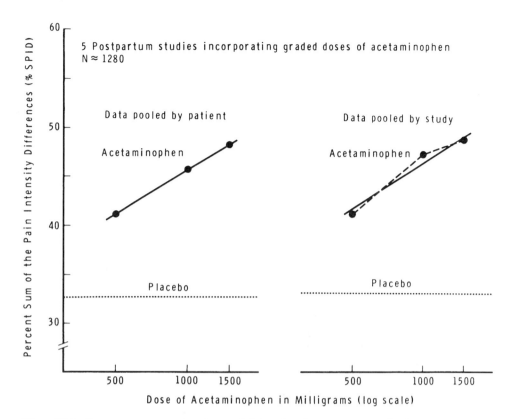

Figure 33.4.   Dose-response curves based on pooled data from five postpartum studies incorporating graded doses of acetaminophen. (Based on data from Laska EM, et al. Caffeine as an analgesic adjuvant. JAMA 1984;251:1711–1718.)

NONSTEROIDAL ANTI-INFLAMMATORY ANALGESICS

Table 33.1 lists the NSAIDs available in the United States; many others are used extensively in other parts of the world. During the past 25 years, the international pharmaceutical industry has been exceptionally prolific in the development and marketing of new NSAIDs; however, as noted earlier, only a few have been subject to well-controlled studies in non-rheumatic chronic pain. Most of what we know about their analgesic efficacy comes from studies in other pain models, such as oral surgery and postpartum and postoperative pain. The optimal daily dosage in chronic pain may well be different from that recommended on the basis of acute pain studies.

Indomethacin

Indomethacin was the first of the "newer" NSAIDs, but it is used much more extensively for the treatment of non-rheumatic pain in Europe than in the United States. In postoperative pain, Sunshine et al. (94) found that 50 mg of indomethacin was comparable but not superior to 600 mg of aspirin, while both drugs were significantly superior to placebo. This result is consistent with the results of studies comparing repeated doses of the two drugs in acute sports injury: both drugs are effective, but indomethacin is not significantly more effective than aspirin. Indomethacin produces

Table 33.1.   Nonsteroidal Anti-Inflammatory Drugs Available in the United States

Aspirin[a] (OTC)
Nonacetylated salicylates[a] (OTC)
Acetaminophen (Tylenol)[a] (OTC)
Phenylbutazone
Indomethacin (Indocin)
Mefenamic acid (Ponstel)[a]
Ibuprofen (IBU, Motrin, Advil, Nuprin)[a] (OTC)
Naproxen (Naprosyn)[a]
Naproxen sodium (Anaprox, Aleve)[a] (OTC)
Fenoprofen calcium (Nalfon)[a]
Ketoprofen (Orudis, Actron)[a] (OTC)
Flurbiprofen (Ansaid)
Tolmetin sodium (Tolectin)
Sulindac (Clinoril)
Diflunisal (Dolobid)[a]
Piroxicam (Feldene)[a]
Meclofenamate sodium (Meclomen)[a]
Diclofenac sodium (Voltaren)[a]
Diclofenac potassium (Cataflam)[a]
Bromfenac (Duract)[a]
Ketorolac tromethamine (Toradol)[a]
Etodolac (Lodine)[a]
Nabumetone (Relafen)
Oxaprozin (Daypro)

[a]Indicated as a general purpose analgesic.
OTC, available over the counter.

a higher incidence of CNS adverse effects (usually headache, dizziness, and trouble thinking) than do any of the other NSAIDs (34), and it is also more likely to cause agranulocytosis and aplastic anemia, although these adverse effects are very rare with any NSAID (35).

Mefenamic Acid

The usual 250-mg dose of mefenamic acid has been shown to be no more effective than aspirin 650 mg in cancer pain (75). Although Moore et al. (95) have shown that mefenamic acid 500 mg three times a day for 7 days was more effective than placebo in patients with long-standing chronic back pain, labeling for the drug recommends administration of a maximum total daily dose of 1000 mg for periods not to exceed 1 week.

Ibuprofen

The aromatic propionic acid derivatives, the profens, constitute the largest single class of NSAIDs and include several of the most useful general-purpose analgesics. The prototype and oldest of this class is ibuprofen, whose major analogs include naproxen, fenoprofen, ketoprofen, and flurbiprofen. The best analgesic assay sensitivity in the evaluation of ibuprofen and other NSAIDs has been obtained using the postsurgical dental pain model developed by Cooper and Beaver (96), and Cooper's series of analgesic studies (7, 97, 98) constitutes the most extensive database available for ibuprofen. Cooper et al. (78) found that 400 mg of ibuprofen was more effective than either 60 mg of codeine or 650 mg of aspirin and was comparable with the combination of these two drugs (Fig. 33.5).

Ibuprofen 400 mg was significantly more effective than 650 mg of aspirin or 600 or 1000 mg of acetaminophen in several other studies (5, 7, 97–102), and a number of studies also indicate that 400 mg of ibuprofen has a duration of action of about 6 hours, somewhat longer than the 4 hours characteristic of aspirin or acetaminophen (97–101, 103). Doses of ibuprofen above 400 mg do not provide greater peak analgesia (7, 103), but this analgesic ceiling is significantly higher than that of either aspirin or acetaminophen.

Ibuprofen has also been the subject of both single-dose (104) and repeat-dose (105, 106) controlled studies in cancer pain, and all three studies show a significant enhancement of analgesia when 400-mg or 600-mg doses of ibuprofen were added to methadone (104), an acetaminophen-oxycodone combination (105), or various oral opioids (106).

Naproxen and Naproxen Sodium

In contrast to ibuprofen, which has a plasma half-life of about 2 hours, naproxen has a half-life of 12 to 15 hours (107). In oral surgery pain, Forbes et al. (108) showed that 550 mg of naproxen sodium produced significantly higher peak analgesia and had a significantly longer duration of action than did either 650 mg of aspirin or 60 mg of codeine (Fig. 33.6). A

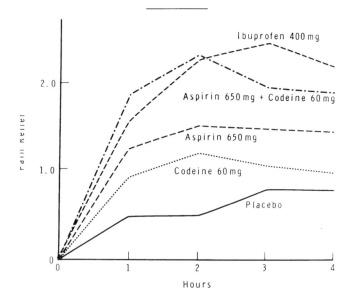

Figure 33.5. Time-effect curves from an oral surgery study of 400 mg of ibuprofen in outpatients with postoperative pain after the surgical removal of impacted third molars. (Adapted from Cooper SA, et al. Analgesic efficacy of an ibuprofen-codeine combination. Pharmacotherapy 1982;2:162–167.)

dose of 550 mg is a loading dose of naproxen sodium; the usual dosage is 275 mg every 6 to 8 hours, with a total daily dose not exceeding 1100 mg (275 mg of naproxen sodium is equivalent to 250 mg of naproxen). Although naproxen has a longer duration of analgesic action than ibuprofen, the difference is not as great as would be suggested by the difference in plasma half-life. This illustrates that the relative duration of effective analgesia produced by NSAIDs is not necessarily predictable on the basis of differences in half-life.

In patients with chronic back pain, efficacy of 14-day treatment periods with twice daily administration of naproxen sodium 550 mg or diflunisal 500 mg was significantly superior to placebo, and naproxen sodium appeared superior to diflunisal (109). In cancer patients with bone pain, naproxen sodium 550 mg every 8 hours for 3 days was more effective than 275 mg every 8 hours (110).

Ketoprofen

Ketoprofen was first marketed in France and the United Kingdom in 1973 and in the United States about 10 years later (111). Single doses of 25 to 300 mg of ketoprofen have been compared with aspirin, with codeine, and with ibuprofen in oral surgery pain (112); with acetaminophen plus codeine (113) and with acetaminophen plus oxycodone (114) in postoperative pain; with aspirin and with codeine in postpartum pain (113); and with acetaminophen plus codeine (115) and with intramuscular morphine (113) in cancer pain. In general, 25 or 50 mg of ketoprofen was significantly more effective than 650 mg of aspirin or acetaminophen and comparable in peak analgesia with the combination of 600 mg of acetaminophen with 60 mg of codeine; 100 mg of ketoprofen was superior to 400 mg of

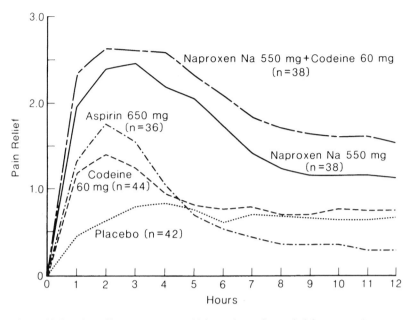

Figure 33.6. Time-effect curves over a 12-hour observation period from an oral surgery study of 550 mg of naproxen sodium in outpatients with postoperative pain after the surgical removal of impacted third molars. (Adapted from Forbes JA, et al. Analgesic effect of naproxen sodium, codeine, a naproxen-codeine combination, and aspirin on the postoperative pain of oral surgery. Pharmacotherapy 1986;6:211–218.)

ibuprofen and comparable with aspirin plus codeine and the combination of acetaminophen with 10 mg of oxycodone. The duration of action of ketoprofen was longer than most of the comparator drugs. In a single-dose study in cancer pain, Stambaugh and Drew (115) showed that the mean analgesia produced by 100 mg of ketoprofen was somewhat greater than that produced by the combination of 650 mg of aspirin with 60 mg of codeine, although the difference was not statistically significant (Fig. 33.7). This study illustrates the ceiling on analgesic effect that exists for all NSAIDs; the mean effect of the 300-mg dose of ketoprofen was less than that of the 100-mg dose.

Flurbiprofen

Flurbiprofen has been available in Europe since 1977 and is marketed in the United States for the treatment of rheumatoid arthritis and osteoarthritis. Controlled clinical studies have demonstrated the analgesic efficacy of flurbiprofen in doses ranging from 25 to 150 mg when compared with placebo and standard analgesics in postoperative oral surgery pain, postpartum pain, dysmenorrhea, postoperative pain in inpatients undergoing gynecological, orthopaedic or abdominal surgery, and musculoskeletal pain associated with trauma (116–120). The duration of analgesic action is intermediate between that of ibuprofen and diflunisal, and the analgesic dose is 50 to 100 mg (not to exceed 300 mg in 24 hours), which provides analgesia significantly superior to that of aspirin or acetaminophen (120). As with most other NSAIDs, there are few controlled studies of flurbiprofen in nonarthritic chronic pain, but the drug is useful in the treatment of cancer pain (22, 116).

Diflunisal

Diflunisal is a fluorinated salicylic acid derivative with a plasma half-life of 10 to 11 hours, but it is not biotransformed to salicylate. Forbes and his associates (121–123) have done a series of 12-hour studies comparing diflunisal with aspirin, acetaminophen, and opioid combinations in oral surgery pain. Figure 33.8 is typical of the results of these studies (122).

In addition to a peak effect that is significantly superior to that of 650 mg of aspirin, the most distinguishing characteristic of diflunisal is its exceptionally long duration of action. There is also fairly consistent evidence of a ceiling effect, in that 1000 mg is not significantly superior in peak effect to 500 mg, but the onset of analgesia after the 1000-mg dose is significantly faster than after the 500-mg dose. This is why a 1000-mg loading dose is administered followed by 500 mg two or three times a day in the treatment of acute pain.

During a 4-week treatment period in patients with chronic low-back pain, diflunisal 500 mg twice daily was significantly more effective than acetaminophen 1000 mg four times a day (124). Ventafridda (125) found that in cancer pain, single doses of 500 mg of diflunisal were significantly more effective than 800 mg of aspirin. Diflunisal produces less interference with platelet function than aspirin.

Piroxicam

Piroxicam is marketed in the United States for the treatment of rheumatoid arthritis and osteoarthritis. Well-controlled clinical trials have also demonstrated that it is effective in the man-

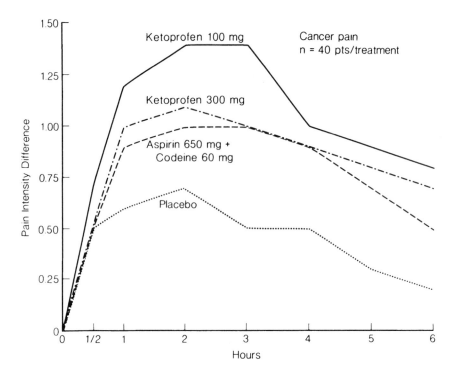

Figure 33.7. Time-effect curves of 100 and 300 mg of ketoprofen compared with 650 mg of aspirin plus 60 mg of codeine versus placebo in inpatients with cancer pain. (Adapted from Stambaugh J, Drew J. A double-blind parallel evaluation of the efficacy and safety of a single dose of ketoprofen in cancer pain. J Clin Pharmacol 1988;28[Suppl]:S34–S39.)

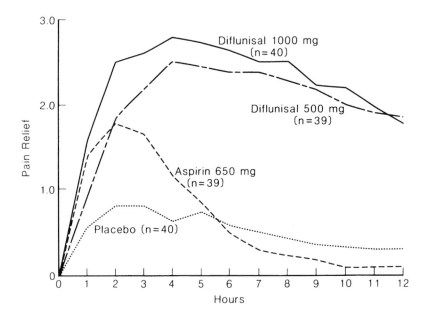

Figure 33.8. Time-effect curves from an oral surgery impaction pain study comparing 500 mg and 100 mg of diflunisal with 650 mg of aspirin and placebo over a 12-hour observation period. (Based on data from Forbes JA, et al. A 12-hour evaluation of the analgesic efficacy of diflunisal, zompirac sodium, aspirin and placebo in postoperative oral surgery pain. Pharmacotherapy 1983;3[2 Pt 2]:38S–46S.)

agement of postoperative pain secondary to general surgery, gynecological surgery, and oral surgery for the removal of impacted third molars; pain associated with acute musculoskeletal disorders and sports injuries; and dysmenorrhea (126). For the treatment of arthritis, because of its 50-hour half-life, it is effective when administered in a 20-mg single daily dose, but steady-state blood levels are not reached for 7 to 12 days. In acute pain, a 20-mg dose results in a delayed onset of analgesia with a peak effect comparable with that of 650 mg of aspirin but with a longer duration. The delayed onset of analgesia can be overcome by the use of a 40-mg loading dose. However, only one or two daily 40-mg loading doses should be administered; repeated administration of daily doses greater than 20 mg results in a substantial increase in GI toxicity.

Diclofenac

Diclofenac is available as both the sodium and the potassium salts. Diclofenac sodium is an enteric-coated formulation indicated for the treatment of rheumatoid arthritis, osteoarthritis, and ankylosing spondylitis. This formulation is not optimally suitable for analgesic use in acute pain because of delayed dissolution, although it has been used as an analgesic in other parts of the world and there are a few clinical trials demonstrating its efficacy for this purpose (127). Diclofenac potassium, which is not enteric coated, is more rapidly absorbed and is available as 50-mg tablets primarily for analgesic use. The half-life of diclofenac is 2 hours, about the same as ibuprofen's.

In studies in oral surgery pain (128) and postoperative pain (129), 50 mg of diclofenac potassium was equianalgesic to 650 mg of aspirin and had a somewhat longer duration of action, while the 100-mg dose of diclofenac had a significantly superior analgesic effect (128). The recommended maximum daily dose is 150 mg.

Etodolac

In postoperative pain after oral surgery, 100 mg of etodolac was comparable or slightly superior to aspirin 650 mg, and 200 mg of etodolac was superior; both doses of etodolac had a longer duration of action than aspirin (130). Other studies in postoperative, oral surgery, and postepisiotomy pain found 100 or 200 mg of etodolac comparable in efficacy with 650 mg of aspirin and 400 mg superior to aspirin (131). The recommended total daily dose of etodolac is 1000 mg. Initial postmarketing studies suggest that etodolac may produce less GI adverse effects than many of the older NSAIDs (52, 65), but extensive epidemiological data will be necessary to substantiate a lower risk of NSAID gastropathy.

Ketorolac Tromethamine

Ketorolac is the only injectable NSAID available for analgesic use in the United States (132–134). Injectable formulations of a few other NSAIDs are marketed in other parts of the world, but adverse reactions at the site of injection have limited their usefulness. Ketorolac has good aqueous solubility and is relatively nonirritating to tissues. Clinical trials have shown that intramuscular ketorolac is as effective and longer acting in postoperative pain than usual doses of intramuscular morphine or meperidine (135–137). A 10-mg oral dose of ketorolac is at least as effective as 400 mg of ibuprofen in oral surgery pain (100). However, the usefulness of ketorolac in chronic pain is severely limited because the drug is indicated only for short-term use, no more than 5 days. Even with parenteral administration, NSAID gastropathy can occur, and the risk is greater when the drug is used in higher doses, in older patients, or for more than 5 days (138).

SUMMARY COMMENTS ON THE NSAIDS

Adverse Effects

The adverse effects of the newer NSAIDs are qualitatively similar to those of aspirin, but there are quantitative differences. With the exception of the risk of precipitating aspirin-sensitive asthma in susceptible individuals, single or a few analgesic doses of either produce very little in the way of adverse effects.

On repeat-dose use in chronic pain, some but not all of the NSAIDs are better tolerated than equianalgesic doses of aspirin. When prescribing any NSAID, attention must be paid to the risk factors peculiar to this whole class of drugs. Patients should be made aware of the characteristic signs and symptoms of potentially serious adverse effects and should be monitored for evidence of gastropathy; hepatic or renal dysfunction; CNS dysfunction, such as problems with short-term memory and confusion; and bleeding. Do not continue a patient on an NSAID in the absence of clear evidence of analgesic efficacy.

Like aspirin and acetaminophen, the NSAIDs do not produce the CNS side effects characteristic of oral opioids. The NSAIDs have no dependence liability, and there is no evidence that tolerance to their analgesic effects develops. This represents a real advantage over the opioids when the NSAIDs are used in the treatment of chronic pain. There is also a psychological advantage in allaying physician and patient anxieties related to the use of scheduled drugs.

Efficacy

In single-dose studies, some but not all of the NSAIDs are clearly more effective analgesics than optimal doses of aspirin or acetaminophen, and some can equal or exceed the analgesic effect of full doses of opioid combination products. The extent to which this is also true on repeat-dose administration in chronic pain remains to be proved. Furthermore, there are few adequately controlled studies comparing the newer NSAIDs with each other in either acute or chronic pain.

Like aspirin and acetaminophen, there is a ceiling on the analgesic effect of all of the NSAIDs; beyond a certain dose, increasing the dose does not yield an increase in analgesic effect. However, for some NSAIDs this ceiling is substantially higher than for aspirin or acetaminophen. Anecdotal evidence suggests that as in the treatment of arthritis, individual patients may respond with more satisfactory analgesia or less adverse effects to one particular NSAID as opposed to another (8, 20). While the reason for this is unknown, it is worthwhile to switch a patient from one NSAID to another if his or her experience with a particular NSAID is unsatisfactory.

Time-Effect Considerations

A few of the NSAIDs are comparable with aspirin or acetaminophen in their time-effect curves; most have a substantially longer duration of analgesic action. This is an advantage over aspirin and acetaminophen in the treatment of chronic pain. On the other hand, while NSAIDs with longer half-lives have the convenience of less-frequent administration, these agents are also more likely to accumulate and produce toxicity in patients who are aged or have renal or hepatic dysfunction. Agents with a longer duration of action also tend to have some delay in the onset of analgesia after administration of the initial dose. Although this is of questionable relevance in the treatment of chronic pain, it can usually be remedied through the use of a loading dose.

Analgesic versus Antirheumatic Use

While all NSAIDs used in the treatment of arthritis have some analgesic activity, the relative efficacy, time-effect curves, and optimal dosage regimen of these drugs as analgesics are often not the same as their efficacy and appropriate dosage regimen as antirheumatics. One cannot just administer the usual antirheumatic dose regimen and expect to produce a predictable analgesic response. A particular antirheumatic may also be a useful analgesic, but it may require a lower dose or a loading dose for optimal analgesic effect. Some antirheumatic NSAIDs do not appear to be appropriate for use as analgesics at all. One should be guided in this respect by the labeling of the drug and the results of well-controlled analgesic studies in various types of nonrheumatic pain that define the appropriate dose and dosage regimen for analgesic use.

NSAIDs in Combination with Other Analgesics

There is evidence that the NSAIDs can be administered concomitantly with opioids to produce an additive analgesic effect (discussed later). On the other hand, there are a number of reasons to question the advisability of coadministering aspirin with other NSAIDs or these NSAIDs with each other (12, 22, 71, 139). Although rheumatologists occasionally prescribe regimens combining different NSAIDs, I do not believe this is wise when using these drugs as analgesics for the fol-

lowing reasons: Aspirin and other NSAIDs are subject to pharmacokinetic interactions of possible clinical importance; there is some evidence that combinations of NSAIDs may produce an increase in adverse reactions (59, 71, 139); and most important, there is no evidence from well-controlled clinical trials demonstrating that combinations of NSAIDs provide an analgesic effect superior to that provided by an appropriate dose of one of these agents administered alone.

Acetaminophen may constitute an exception to this caveat because its adverse-effect profile is different from that of aspirin and the other NSAIDs, as is its mechanism of analgesic action. In rheumatic disease, cancer pain, and other types of chronic pain, NSAID regimens are sometimes supplemented with acetaminophen-containing opioid combinations administered as needed or by the clock. Clinical experience suggests that this is a useful strategy, but controlled studies are lacking, and the patient must be warned not to exceed the prescribed maximum total daily dose to prevent the risk of hepatotoxicity from acetaminophen overdose.

COMBINATIONS OF NONSTEROIDAL ANTI-INFLAMMATORY ANALGESICS WITH WEAK OPIOIDS

If an optimal regimen of an NSAID alone does not provide adequate analgesia, one can *add* a weak opioid to the existing NSAID regimen. This strategy is recognized in the World Health Organization's analgesic ladder for cancer pain relief (24) and is the most appropriate use for oral opioids in view of the fact that usual doses administered alone are no more and often less effective than optimal doses of NSAIDs (5, 11, 12, 74–76).

Rationales

The first rationale for this strategy is the enhancement of efficacy achieved by combining two analgesics with different mechanisms of action. The slopes of the dose-response curves of orally administered opioids are relatively flat; the slopes for NSAIDs are even flatter, and NSAIDs have a ceiling on analgesic efficacy at some dose level. Even successive doubling of the dose of either category of analgesic produces only modest increases in analgesic effect. Opioids and NSAIDs are known to produce analgesia by different mechanisms: the former combine with specific opioid receptors in the CNS, whereas the latter exert their analgesic effect by blocking COX in the periphery at the site of tissue injury and also in the CNS. The simple additive effect of administering an opioid and an NSAID together therefore is often substantially greater than the analgesia achieved by doubling the dose of either drug administered alone.

The second rationale for combination therapy is the reduction of adverse effects. By using two drugs with different profiles of adverse effects rather than an equianalgesic dose of a single component, adequate analgesia can often be achieved while keeping the dose of each constituent below the threshold for limiting adverse effects. Specifically, one is able to reduce the dose of the opioid component, often the limiting factor, to a level that does not cause unacceptable GI and CNS side effects. On chronic administration, the development of tolerance and the risk of dependence are likewise reduced.

Evidence from clinical studies to substantiate these theories is neither optimal nor complete for any particular combination regimen. However, in the aggregate there is a reasonable body of evidence from well-controlled clinical trials in several pain models other than nonmalignant chronic pain that combination regimens of appropriately chosen doses of aspirin or acetaminophen with opioids do fulfill these objectives (12).

Opioid Combinations with Aspirin or Acetaminophen

Combinations Containing Codeine

Figure 33.9 illustrates the results of a single-dose factorial study of 600 mg of aspirin and 32 mg of codeine in cancer pain (79, 86). Each drug alone produces a significant analgesic effect, and codeine at this dose is somewhat less effective than aspirin. The combination of 600 mg of aspirin with 32 mg of codeine is clearly superior to either of the constituents alone. This has sometimes been called "potentiation" or "synergism," but on statistical analysis the effect of the combination is a *simple addition* of the effects of its two constituents.

Numerous other studies have confirmed a significant contribution of codeine, usually at a 60-mg dose, to the analgesic effect of combinations with aspirin or acetaminophen (13, 14), but the magnitude of this contribution has varied. In oral surgery pain, Cooper and his associates have consistently found 60 mg of codeine to be less effective than 650 mg of aspirin (78) or 600 mg of acetaminophen (96). Bentley and Head (140) have likewise demonstrated a significant but smaller contribution for codeine 60 mg in combination with acetaminophen 1000 mg. However, the contribution of codeine was approximately equal to the effect of 650 mg of aspirin in cancer pain (141) and to the effect of 600 mg of acetaminophen in postoperative pain (12, 142) and was greater than the effect of 600 mg of acetaminophen in one study in oral surgery pain (121).

Some types of pain may respond more dramatically to analgesics such as aspirin and acetaminophen than to centrally acting opioids such as codeine and propoxyphene (74, 143, 144). Although the full extent of this phenomenon is unclear, it most likely occurs in pain states associated with significant inflammation or mediated primarily through the release of prostaglandins. All currently used single-dose mild analgesic pain models appear sensitive to aspirin, acetaminophen, and NSAIDs. However, certain types of pain, such as rheumatoid arthritis and osteoarthritis, oral surgery pain, dysmenorrhea, and uterine cramp pain (145) appear less sensitive to codeine and other opioids than to the aspirinlike drugs. There seem to be no data relevant to this issue from studies in nonmalignant chronic pain.

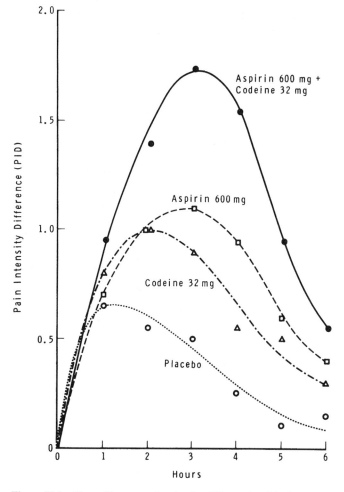

Figure 33.9. Time-effect curves for placebo, 600 mg of aspirin, 32 mg of codeine, and the combination of aspirin with codeine administered on a crossover basis to inpatients with cancer pain. (Adapted from Houde R W, Wallenstein S L, Beaver W T. Clinical measurement of pain. In: de Stevens G, ed. Analgetics. New York: Academic Press, 1965;75–122.)

On the other hand, the analgesic effect of codeine and its contribution to combinations with acetaminophen or aspirin may be greater on repeated dosing than is evidenced in single-dose studies (146), and the same may also be true for propoxyphene (74). For example, Matts (147) was able to demonstrate the contribution of 16 mg of codeine to combinations of acetaminophen or aspirin plus phenacetin when the drugs were administered on a repeat-dose basis for an 8-day period to patients with various types of chronic pain. It is very unlikely that a statistically significant analgesic effect for a 16-mg dose of codeine could be demonstrated in the usual single-dose analgesic study.

Combinations Containing Hydrocodone and Oxycodone

One of the reasons for the popularity of codeine-containing combinations is that codeine retains about two thirds of its analgesic activity when administered orally, a high oral-parenteral potency ratio relative to those of many opioids (148). The more potent codeine derivatives, hydrocodone and oxycodone, share codeine's excellent oral efficacy, and both are marketed in combination with aspirin and acetaminophen.

Hydrocodone is 6 to 8 times as potent as codeine (149). In patients with postpartum pain, 1000 mg of acetaminophen and 10 mg of hydrocodone produced comparable analgesia (Fig. 33.10), which was significantly superior to that produced by placebo (143). Both acetaminophen and hydrocodone were slightly more effective than 60 mg of codeine. As in the codeine combination studies, analgesia produced by the combination of acetaminophen with hydrocodone represented the additive effects of the two constituents. Hydrocodone combinations, like codeine combinations, are schedule III controlled substances.

Oxycodone is 9 to 10 times as potent as codeine (150, 151). In oral surgery pain, Cooper et al. (152) found that 500 mg of acetaminophen and 5 mg of oxycodone produced comparable analgesia that was significantly superior to placebo. The analgesic effect of the combination of these two drugs was at least equal to the additive effect of the two constituents, and combinations containing higher doses of one or both constituents yielded progressively greater analgesia. In chronic cancer pain, Moertel et al. (141) have likewise demonstrated the contribution of oxycodone to the analgesic effect of aspirin. Oxycodone-containing combinations, although obviously very effective analgesics, have a dependence liability greater than that of codeine combinations and have been implicated more frequently as a cause of iatrogenic opioid dependence in patients with chronic pain (153). These combinations are schedule II controlled substances.

Combinations Containing Propoxyphene

Since propoxyphene hydrochloride is pharmacologically a weak narcotic, approximately two thirds as potent as codeine (74), its analgesic effect should be additive to those of aspirin and acetaminophen, and like codeine, propoxyphene is usually prescribed in combination with these drugs. Several studies have demonstrated a significant contribution of either propoxyphene hydrochloride or napsylate to the analgesic effect of aspirin in chronic pain (154) or to the analgesic effect of acetaminophen in postpartum pain (155) and in rheumatoid arthritis (12, 74, 156).

In outpatients with cancer pain, Moertel et al. (141) compared the efficacy of crossover administration of single doses of placebo, 650 mg of aspirin, and 650 mg of aspirin combined with a variety of other analgesics and putative analgesics. Codeine 65 mg, oxycodone 9.76 mg, and pentazocine 25 mg added significantly to the analgesia produced by aspirin. The effect of 100 mg of propoxyphene napsylate was not statistically significant, but the mean analgesia produced by the propoxyphene plus aspirin fell between that provided by aspirin alone and the other combinations.

Propoxyphene has a substantially longer half-life in the blood (12 to 24 hours) than other mild analgesics. Therefore, when administered every 4 to 6 hours, as mild analgesics usu-

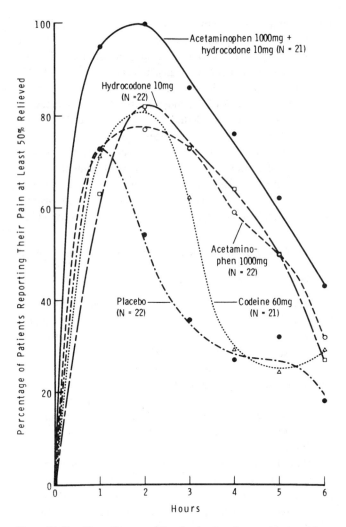

Figure 33.10.   Time-effect curves for placebo, 1 g of acetaminophen, 10 mg of hydrocodone, the combination of acetaminophen with hydrocodone, and 60 mg of codeine, administered to women with postpartum pain. (Based on data from Beaver W T, McMillan D. Methodological considerations in the evaluation of analgesic combinations: acetaminophen [Paracetamol] and hydrocodone in postpartum pain. Br J Clin Pharmacol 1980;10[Suppl]:215S–223S.)

ally are, propoxyphene accumulates to a greater extent. It is therefore possible that on the basis of blood level considerations, greater analgesia may be produced after a few repeated doses of propoxyphene (relative to alternative mild analgesics) than is seen in single-dose studies (74).

Combinations Containing Pentazocine

Pentazocine is the only mixed agonist-antagonist opioid available for oral administration, and it is marketed in combination both with aspirin and with acetaminophen. In postoperative pain, 50 mg of oral pentazocine is equianalgesic with 60 mg of codeine and 600 mg of aspirin (77). Pentazocine has been shown to make a significant analgesic contribution when combined with aspirin in cancer pain (141) and in postoperative pain (157).

It is important to note that for the patient to derive the optimal analgesia from any of these combinations, the combination should be prescribed so that the patient receives the usual full dose of aspirin or acetaminophen in combination with the desired dose of opioid. This may necessitate taking extra tablets of aspirin or acetaminophen in conjunction with the opioid combination product.

Combinations of Opioids with Other NSAIDs

As noted earlier, it would appear rational to add an oral opioid to a regimen of one of the newer NSAIDs if a full daily dose of the NSAID alone does not provide adequate analgesia. This strategy is being exploited widely for the treatment of cancer pain (3, 15, 16, 18, 22, 24) and to some extent for arthritis; however, published reports of controlled clinical trials have not kept pace with clinical practice.

Most of the studies have been done on codeine-NSAID combinations, and many have used a 30-mg dose of codeine, which almost invariably fails to produce a statistically significant increment of analgesia when given with a full dose of the NSAID. Sunshine et al. (158) have demonstrated a significant contribution of 60 mg of codeine to 400 mg of ibuprofen in mixed episiotomy and postoperative pain. Forbes et al. (108) have shown that the coadministration of 550 mg of naproxen sodium with 60 mg of codeine produces an additive analgesic effect in oral surgery pain (Fig. 33.6).

Ferrer-Brechner and Ganz (104) compared graded doses of oral methadone with and without the addition of 600 mg of ibuprofen in a single-dose study in cancer pain (Fig. 33.11).

Not only was analgesic effect significantly enhanced by the addition of ibuprofen, but one can compare the rather modest increment of effect produced by doubling the dose of methadone from 2.5 mg to 5 mg with the much larger increment of effect resulting from the addition of ibuprofen to either dose of methadone.

In the use of NSAID-opioid combinations, the physician is obviously not restricted to the analgesic combinations prepared as fixed-ratio formulations by the pharmaceutical industry. One can prescribe an optimal regimen of aspirin, acetaminophen, or another NSAID and add any of the available oral opioids to it in a dose titrated to the needs of the individual patient (12, 15, 16, 22, 159). This approach provides great flexibility in the choice of the opioid component and in the case of chronic pain, in adapting the dose of opioid to the level of narcotic tolerance present in the individual patient.

CONCLUSION

The potential contribution of appropriate dosage regimens of the NSAIDs in the management of chronic pain is often underrated; they are as effective as or more effective than either the weak opioids or modest oral doses of the strong opioids. However, attention must also be paid to the occasional serious adverse effects of NSAIDs, particularly in special-risk patients. Oral opioids are most effective when given in combination with a full regimen of an NSAID. There is obviously a need for further controlled single-dose and repeat-dose studies of both old and new NSAIDs in chronic pain.

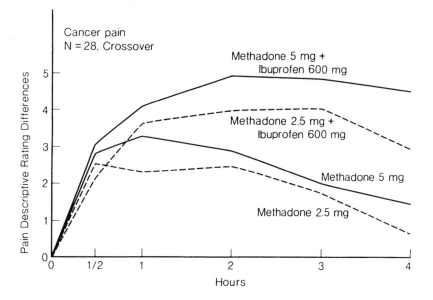

Figure 33.11. Time-effect curves of oral methadone with and without 600 mg of ibuprofen administered on a crossover basis to inpatients with cancer pain. (Adapted from Ferrer-Brechner T, Ganz P. Combination therapy with ibuprofen and methadone for chronic cancer pain. Am J Med 1984;77[Suppl 1A]:78–83.)

References

1. Eisenberg E, Berkey CS, Carr DB, et al. Efficacy and safety of nonsteroidal antiinflammatory drugs for cancer pain: a meta-analysis. J Clin Oncol 1994;12:2756–2765.

2. Acute Pain Management Guideline Panel. Acute pain management: operative or medical procedures and trauma. Clinical practice guideline. AHCPR Pub 92–0032. Rockville, MD: Agency for Health Care Policy and Research, 1992.

3. American Pain Society. Principles of analgesic use in the treatment of acute pain and cancer pain. 3rd ed. Glenview, IL: American Pain Society, 1992.

4. Beaver WT. Mild analgesics: a review of their clinical pharmacology. Am J Med Sci 1965;250:577–604.

5. Beaver WT. Impact of non-narcotic oral analgesics on pain management. Am J Med 1988;84(Suppl) 5A:3–15.

6. Brune K, Lanz R. Nonopioid analgesics. In: Kuhar M, Pasternak G, eds. Analgesics: neurochemical, behavioral, and clinical perspectives. New York: Raven Press, 1984;149–173.

7. Cooper SA. New peripherally-acting oral analgesic agents. Ann Rev Pharmacol Toxicol 1983;23:617–647.

8. Kantor TG. Peripherally-acting analgesics. In: Kuhar M, Pasternak G, eds. Analgesics: neurochemical, behavioral, and clinical perspectives. New York: Raven Press, 1984;289–312.

9. Kantor TG. New strategies for the use of anti-inflammatory agents. In: Dubner R, Gebhart FG, Bond MR, eds. Proceedings of the V World Congress on Pain. New York: Elsevier Science, 1988;80–86.

10. Sunshine A, Olson NZ. Non-narcotic analgesics. In: Wall P D, Melzack R, eds. Textbook of pain. 3rd ed. London: Churchill Livingstone, 1994;670–685.

11. Beaver WT. Mild analgesics: a review of their clinical pharmacology (Part II). Am J Med Sci 1966;251:576–599.

12. Beaver W T. Combination analgesics. Am J Med 1984;77(Suppl) 3A:38–53.

13. de Craen AJM, Di Giulio G, Lampe-Schoenmaeckers AJEM, et al. Analgesic efficacy and safety of paracetamol-codeine combinations versus paracetamol alone: a systematic review. Br Med J 1996;313:321–325.

14. Moore A, Collins S, Carroll D, McQuay H. Paracetamol with and without codeine in acute pain: a quantitative systematic review. Pain 1997;70:193–201.

15. Stambaugh JE Jr. The use of nonsteroidal anti-inflammatory drugs in chronic bone pain. Orthop Rev 1989;18(Suppl):54–60.

16. Agency for Health Care Policy and Research. Management of cancer pain. Clinical practice guideline 9. AHCPR Pub 94–0592. Rockville, MD: AHCPR, 1994.

17. Beaver WT. Nonsteroidal antiinflammatory analgesics in cancer pain. In: Foley KM, Bonica JJ, Ventafridda V, eds. Advances in pain research and therapy, vol 16. Proceedings of the II International Congress on Cancer Pain. New York: Raven Press, 109–131, 1990.

18. Foley KM, Inturrisi CE. Analgesic drug therapy in cancer pain: principles and practice. Med Clin North Am 1987;71:207–232.

19. Gerbershagen HU. Nonnarcotic analgesics. In: Bonica J J, Ventafridda V, eds. Advances in pain research and therapy, vol 2. New York: Raven Press, 1979;255–262.

20. Kantor TG. Nonsteroidal anti-inflammatory analgesic agents in management of cancer pain. In: Beaver WT, ed. Symposium on the management of cancer pain. New York: HP, 1984;30–34.

21. Levy MH. Pharmacologic treatment of cancer pain. N Engl J Med 1996;335:1124–1132.

22. Twycross RG. Pain relief in advanced cancer. London: Churchill Livingstone, 1994.

23. Ventafridda V, Fochi C, DeConno D, Sganzerla E. Use of non-steroidal anti-inflammatory drugs in the treatment of pain in cancer. Br J Clin Pharmacol 1980;10(Suppl):343S–346S.

24. World Health Organization. Cancer pain relief. Geneva: WHO, 1986.

25. Weissman G. NSAID's: aspirin and aspirin-like drugs. In: Bennett JC, Plum F, eds. Cecil textbook of medicine. 20th ed. Philadelphia: Saunders, 1996.

26. Lim RK, Guzman F, Rodgers DW, et al. Site of action of narcotic and nonnarcotic analgesics determined by blocking bradykinin-evoked visceral pain. Arch Int Pharmacodyn Ther 1964;152:25–58.

27. Ferreira SH. Prostaglandins, aspirin-like drugs and analgesia. Nature 1972;240:200–203.

28. Ferreira SH, Vane JR. New aspects of the mode of action of nonsteroid antiinflammatory drugs. Ann Rev Pharmacol Toxicol 1974;14:57–73.

29. Ferreira SH. Peripheral analgesia: mechanism of the analgesic action of aspirin like drugs and opiate-antagonists. Br J Clin Pharmacol 1980;10:237S–245S.

30. Flower RJ. Drugs which inhibit prostaglandin biosynthesis. Pharmacol Rev 1974;26:33–67.

31. Vane JR. Inhibition of prostaglandin synthesis as a mechanism of action for aspirin-like drugs. Nature 1971;231:232–236.

32. Vane JR, Botting RM. Mechanism of action of anti-inflammatory drugs. Scand J Rheumatol 1996;25(Suppl 102):9–21.

33. Brooks PM, Day RO. Nonsteroidal antiinflammatory drugs: differences and similarities. N Engl J Med 1991;324:1716–1725.

34. Fries JF, Williams CA, Bloch DA. The relative toxicity of nonsteroidal antiinflammatory drugs. Arthritis Rheum 1991;34:1353–1360.

35. Furst DE. Are there differences among nonsteroidal antiinflammatory drugs? Arthritis Rheum 1994;37:1–9.

36. Heller CA, Ingelfinger JA, Goldman P. Nonsteroidal antiinflammatory drugs and aspirin: analyzing the scores. Pharmacotherapy 1985;5:30–38.

37. Polisson R. Nonsteroidal anti-inflammatory drugs: practical and theoretical considerations in their selection. Am J Med 1996;100(Suppl 2A):31S–36S.

38. McCormack K, Brune K. Dissociation between the antinociceptive and anti-inflammatory effects of the nonsteroidal anti-inflammatory drugs: a survey of their analgesic efficacy. Drugs 1991;41:533–547.

39. Hayball P J. Chirality and nonsteroidal anti-inflammatory drugs. Drugs 1996;52(Suppl 5):47–58.

40. Cashman JN. The mechanisms of action of NSAIDs in analgesia. Drugs 1996;52(Suppl 5):13–23.

41. Jouzeau JY, Terlain B, Abid A, et al. Cyclo-oxygenase isoenzymes: how recent findings affect thinking about nonsteroidal anti-inflammatory drugs. Drugs 1997;53:563–582.

42. McCormack K. The spinal actions of nonsteroidal anti-inflammatory drugs and the dissociation between their anti-inflammatory and analgesic effects. Drugs 1994;47(Suppl 5):28–45.

43. McCormack K. Non-steroidal anti-inflammatory drugs and spinal nociceptive processing. Pain 1994;59:9–43.

44. Mehlisch DR, Hubbard RC, Isakson P, et al. Analgesic efficacy and plasma levels of a highly selective inhibitor of COX-2 (SC-58635;SC) in patients with post-surgical dental pain. Clin Pharmacol Ther 1997;61:195 (abstract).

45. Brune K. Spinal cord effects of antipyretic analgesics. Drugs 1994;47(Suppl 5):21–27.

46. Malmberg AB, Yaksh TL. Hyperalgesia mediated by spinal glutamate or substance P receptor blocked by spinal cyclooxygenase inhibition. Science 1992;257:1276–1279.

47. Urquhart E. Central analgesic activity of nonsteroidal antiinflammatory drugs in animal and human pain models. Semin Arthritis Rheum 1993;23:198–205.

48. Roth SH. Merits and liabilities of NSAID therapy. Rheum Dis Clin North Am 1989;15:479–498.

49. Agrawal N. Risk factors for gastrointestinal ulcers caused by nonsteroidal anti-inflammatory drugs (NSAIDs). J Fam Pract 1991;32:619–624.

50. Allison MC, Howatson AG, Torrance CJ, et al. Gastrointestinal damage associated with the use of nonsteroidal antiinflammatory drugs. N Engl J Med 1992;327:749–754.

51. Bateman DN. NSAIDs: time to re-evaluate gut toxicity. Lancet 1994;343:1051–1052.
52. Bjorkman DJ. Nonsteroidal anti-inflammatory drug-induced gastrointestinal injury. Am J Med 1996;101(Suppl 1A):25S–32S.
53. Blower AL. Considerations for nonsteroidal anti-inflammatory drug therapy: safety. Scand J Rheumatol 1996;25(Suppl 105):13–26.
54. Champion GD, Feng PH, Azuma T, et al. NSAID-induced gastrointestinal damage: epidemiology, risk and prevention, with an evaluation of the role of misoprostol. An Asia-Pacific perspective and consensus. Drugs 1997;53:6–19.
55. Davies NM. Toxicity of nonsteroidal anti-inflammatory drugs in the large intestine. Dis Colon Rectum 1995;38:1311–1321.
56. Fries J. Toward an understanding of NSAID-related adverse events: the contribution of longitudinal data. Scand J Rheumatol 1996;25(Suppl 102):3–8.
57. Fries JF, Williams CA, Bloch DA, Michel BA. Nonsteroidal anti-inflammatory drug-associated gastropathy: incidence and risk factor models. Am J Med 1991;91:213–222.
58. Garcia Rodriguez LA, Jick H. Risk of upper gastrointestinal bleeding and perforation associated with individual non-steroidal anti-inflammatory drugs. Lancet 1994;343:769–772.
59. Henry D, Dobson A, Turner C. Variability in the risk of major gastrointestinal complications from nonaspirin nonsteroidal anti-inflammatory drugs. Gastroenterology 1993;105:1078–1088.
60. Henry D, Lim LLY, Garcia Rodriguez LA, et al. Variability in risk of gastrointestinal complications with individual non-steroidal anti-inflammatory drugs: results of a collaborative meta-analysis. Br Med J 1996;312:1563–1566.
61. Langman MJS, Weil J, Wainwright P, et al. Risks of bleeding peptic ulcer associated with individual non-steroidal anti-inflammatory drugs. Lancet 1994;343:1075–1078.
62. Lichtenstein DR, Syngal S, Wolfe MM. Nonsteroidal antiinflammatory drugs and the gastrointestinal tract: the double-edged sword. Arthritis Rheum 1995;38:5–18.
63. Peloso PM. Strategies and practice for use of nonsteroidal anti-inflammatory drugs. Scand J Rheumatol 1996;25(Suppl 105):29–48.
64. Pincus T, Griffin M. Gastrointestinal disease associated with nonsteroidal anti-inflammatory drugs: new insights from observational studies and functional status questionnaires. Am J Med 1991;91:209–212.
65. Roth SH. NSAID gastropathy: a new understanding. Arch Intern Med 1996;156:1623–1628.
66. Silverstein F. Nonsteroidal anti-inflammatory drugs and peptic ulcer disease. Postgrad Med 1991;89:33–40.
67. Soll AH, Weinstein WM, Kurata J, McCarthy D. Nonsteroidal anti-inflammatory drugs and peptic ulcer disease. Ann Intern Med 1991;114:307–319.
68. Rabinovitz M, Van Thiel DH. Hepatotoxicity of nonsteroidal anti-inflammatory drugs. Am J Gastroenterol 1992;87:1696–1704.
69. Murray MD, Brater DC. Renal toxicity of the nonsteroidal anti-inflammatory drugs. Ann Rev Pharmacol Toxicol 1993;32:435–465.
70. Palmer BF. Renal complications associated with the use of nonsteroidal anti-inflammatory agents. J Invest Med 1995;43:516–533.
71. Johnson AG, Seidemann P, Day RO. NSAID-related adverse drug interactions with clinical relevance: an update. Int J Clin Pharmacol Ther 1994;32:509–532.
72. Houston MC. Nonsteroidal anti-inflammatory drugs and antihypertensives. Am J Med 1991;90(Suppl 5A):42S–47S.
73. de Leeuw PW. Nonsteroidal anti-inflammatory drugs and hypertension: the risks in perspective. Drugs 1996;51:179–187.
74. Beaver WT. The analgesic efficacy of dextropropoxyphene and dextropropoxyphene-containing combinations: a review. Hum Toxicol 1984;3:191S–220S.
75. Moertel CG, Ahmann DL, Taylor WF, Schwartau N.A comparative evaluation of marketed analgesic drugs. N Engl J Med 1972; 286:813–815.
76. Moertel CG. Relief of pain with oral medications. Aust N Z J Med 1976;6(Suppl):1–8.
77. Kantor TG, Sunshine A, Laska E, et al. Oral analgesic studies: pentazocine hydrochloride, codeine, aspirin, and placebo and their influence on response to placebo. Clin Pharmacol Ther 1966;7:447–454.
78. Cooper SA, Engle J, Ladove M, et al. Analgesic efficacy of an ibuprofen-codeine combination. Pharmacotherapy 1982;2:162–167.
79. Wallenstein SL. Analgesic studies of aspirin in cancer patients. In: Proceedings of the aspirin symposium. London: Aspirin Foundation, 1975;5–10.
80. Ventafridda V, Martino G, Mandelli V, Emanueli A. Indoprofen, a new analgesic and anti-inflammatory drug in cancer pain. Clin Pharmacol Ther 1975;17:284–289.
81. Laska EM, Sunshine A, Mueller F, et al. Caffeine as an analgesic adjuvant. JAMA 1984;251:1711–1718.
82. Ehrlich GE, ed. The resurgence of salicylates in arthritis therapy. Norwalk, CT: Science Media Communications, 1983.
83. Sunshine A, Marrero I, Olson NZ, et al. Analgesic efficacy of choline magnesium trisalicylate alone and in combination with controlled-release codeine for the treatment of post surgical dental pain. Phoenix: American Pain Society, 1989 (abstract 100).
84. Cooper SA. Comparative analgesic efficacies of aspirin and acetaminophen. Arch Intern Med 1981;141:282–285.
85. Prescott LF. Paracetamol (acetaminophen): a critical bibliographic review. London: Taylor & Francis, 1996.
86. Houde RW, Wallenstein SL, Beaver WT. Clinical measurement of pain. In: de Stevens G, ed. Analgetics. New York: Academic Press, 1965;75–122.
87. Björkman R, Hallman KM, Hedner J, et al. Acetaminophen blocks spinal hyperalgesia induced by NMDA and substance P. Pain 1994;57:259–264.
88. Skjelbred P, Lokken P, Skoglund LA. Postoperative administration of acetaminophen to reduce swelling and other inflammatory events. Curr Ther Res 1984;35:377–385.
89. Farrell GC. Paracetamol-induced hepatotoxicity. In: Farrell G C, ed. Drug-induced liver disease. Edinburgh: Churchill Livingstone, 1994, 205–224.
90. Whitcomb DC, Block G D. Association of acetaminophen hepatotoxicity with fasting and ethanol use. JAMA 1994;272:1845–1850.
91. Maddrey WC. Hepatic effects of acetaminophen: enhanced toxicity in alcoholics. J Clin Gastroenterol 1987;9:180–185.
92. Zimmerman H J, Maddrey WC. Acetaminophen (Paracetamol) hepatotoxicity with regular intake of alcohol: analysis of instances of therapeutic misadventure. Hepatology 1995;22:767–773.
93. Slattery JT, Nelson SD, Thummel KE. The complex interaction between alcohol and acetaminophen. Clin Pharmacol Ther 1996;60:241–246.
94. Sunshine A, Laska E, Meisner M, Morgan S. Analgesic studies of indomethacin as analyzed by computer techniques. Clin Pharmacol Ther 1964;5:699–707.
95. Moore RA, McQuay HJ, Carroll D, et al. Single and multiple dose analgesic and kinetic studies of mefenamic acid in chronic back pain. Clin J Pain 1986;2:29–36.
96. Cooper SA, Beaver WT. A model to evaluate mild analgesics in oral surgery outpatients. Clin Pharmacol Ther 1976;20:241–250.
97. Cooper SA. Five studies on ibuprofen for postsurgical dental pain. Am J Med 1984;77(Suppl 1A):70–77.
98. Cooper SA. The relative efficacy of ibuprofen in dental pain. Compend Contin Educ Dent 1986;7:578–597.
99. Forbes JA, Barkaszi BA, Ragland RN, Hankle JJ. Analgesic effect of fendosal, ibuprofen and aspirin in postoperative oral surgery pain. Pharmacotherapy 1984;4:385–391.
100. Forbes JA, Kehm CJ, Grodin CD, Beaver WT. Evaluation of ketorolac, ibuprofen, acetaminophen, and an acetaminophen-codeine combination in postoperative oral surgery pain. Pharmacotherapy 1990;10(6 Pt 2):94S–105S.
101. Forbes JA, Beaver WT, Jones KF, et al. Analgesic efficacy of bromfenac, ibuprofen, and aspirin in postoperative oral surgery pain. Clin Pharmacol Ther 1992;51:343–352.

102. Mehlisch DR, Sollecito WA, Helfrick J F, et al. Multicenter clinical trial of ibuprofen and acetaminophen in the treatment of postoperative dental pain. J Am Dent Assoc 1990;121:257–263.

103. Laska EM, Sunshine A, Marrero I, et al. The correlation between blood levels of ibuprofen and clinical analgesic response. Clin Pharmacol Ther 1986;40:1–7.

104. Ferrer-Brechner T, Ganz P. Combination therapy with ibuprofen and methadone for chronic cancer pain. Am J Med 1984;77(Suppl 1A):78–83.

105. Stambaugh JE Jr, Drew J. The combination of ibuprofen and oxycodone/acetaminophen in the management of chronic cancer pain. Clin Pharmacol Ther 1988;44:665–669.

106. Weingart WA, Sorkness CA, Earhart RH. Analgesia with oral narcotics and added ibuprofen in cancer patients. Clin Pharm 1985;4:53–58.

107. Todd PA, Clissold SP. Naproxen: a reappraisal of its pharmacology, and therapeutic use in rheumatic diseases and pain states. Drugs 1990;40:91–137.

108. Forbes JA, Keller CK, Smith JW, et al. Analgesic effect of naproxen sodium, codeine, a naproxen-codeine combination and aspirin on the postoperative pain of oral surgery. Pharmacotherapy 1986;6:211–218.

109. Berry H, Bloom B, Hamilton EBD, Swinson DR. Naproxen sodium, diflunisal, and placebo in the treatment of chronic back pain. Ann Rheum Dis 1982;41:129–132.

110. Levick S, Jacobs C, Loukas DF, et al. Naproxen sodium in treatment of bone pain due to metastatic cancer. Pain 1988;35:253–258.

111. Kantor TG. Ketoprofen: a review of its pharmacologic and clinical properties. Pharmacotherapy 1986;6:93–103.

112. Cooper SA. Ketoprofen in oral surgery pain: a review. J Clin Pharmacol 1988;28: S40–S46.

113. Sunshine A, Olson NZ. Analgesic efficacy of ketoprofen in postpartum, general surgery, and chronic cancer pain. J Clin Pharmacol 1988;28: S47–S54,

114. Sunshine A, Olson NZ, Zighelboim I, DeCastro A. Ketoprofen, acetaminophen plus oxycodone, and acetaminophen in the relief of postoperative pain. Clin Pharmacol Ther 1993;54:546–555.

115. Stambaugh J, Drew J. A double-blind parallel evaluation of the efficacy and safety of a single dose of ketoprofen in cancer pain. J Clin Pharmacol 1988;28(Suppl): S34–S39.

116. Sunshine A, ed. Control of acute and chronic pain with Ansaid (flurbiprofen). Am J Med 1986;80(Suppl 3A).

117. Sunshine A, Olson NZ, Laska EM, et al. Analgesic effect of graded doses of flurbiprofen in post-episiotomy pain. Pharmacotherapy 1983;3:177–181.

118. Cooper SA, Mardirossian G, Milles M. Analgesic relative potency assay comparing flurbiprofen 50, 100, and 150 mg, aspirin 600 mg, and placebo in postsurgical dental pain. Clin J Pain 1988;4:175–181.

119. Forbes JA, Yorio CC, Selinger LR, et al. An evaluation of flurbiprofen, aspirin, and placebo in postoperative oral surgery pain. Pharmacotherapy 1989;9:66–73.

120. Forbes JA, Butterworth GA, Burchfield WH, et al. An evaluation of flurbiprofen, acetaminophen, an acetaminophen-codeine combination and placebo in postoperative oral surgery pain. Pharmacotherapy 1989;9:322–330.

121. Forbes JA, Beaver WT, White EH, et al. Diflunisal: a new oral analgesic with an unusually long duration of action. JAMA 1982;248:2139–2142.

122. Forbes JA, Butterworth GA, Burchfield WH, et al. A 12-hour evaluation of the analgesic efficacy of diflunisal, zomepirac sodium, aspirin and placebo in postoperative oral surgery pain. Pharmacotherapy 1983; 3(2 Pt 2):38S–46S.

123. Beaver WT, Forbes JA, Shackleford RW. A method for the 12-hour evaluation of analgesic efficacy in outpatients with postoperative oral surgery pain: three studies of diflunisal. Pharmacotherapy 1983;3(2 Pt 2):23S–37S.

124. Hickey RFJ. Chronic low back pain: a comparison of diflunisal with paracetamol. N Z Med J 1982;95:312–314.

125. Ventafridda V. Diflunisal in the treatment of cancer pain. In: Huskisson E C, Caldwell A D S, eds. Diflunisal: new perspectives in analgesia. London: Royal Society of Medicine, 1979;137–139.

126. Sunshine A, ed. Use of piroxicam in the management of pain. Am J Med 1988;84(Suppl 5A)1–60.

127. Kantor TG. Use of diclofenac in analgesia. Am J Med 1986;80(Suppl 4B):64–69.

128. Mehlisch DR, Brown P. Single-dose therapy with diclofenac potassium, aspirin, or placebo following dental impaction surgery. Todays Ther Trends 1995;12:15–31.

129. Hebertson RM, Storey N. The comparative efficacy of diclofenac potassium, aspirin, and placebo in the treatment of patients with pain following gynecologic surgery. Todays Ther Trends 1995;12:33–45.

130. Gaston GW, Mallow RD, Frank JE. Comparison of etodolac, aspirin and placebo for pain after oral surgery. Pharmacotherapy 1986;6:199–205.

131. Lynch S, Brogden RN. Etodolac: a preliminary review of its pharmacodynamic activity and therapeutic use. Drugs 1986;31:288–300.

132. Beaver WT, ed. Ketorolac: a new potent analgesic for parenteral and oral administration. Pharmacotherapy 1990;10(6 Pt 2):29S–131S.

133. Buckley MT, Brogden RN. Ketorolac: a review of its pharmacodynamic and pharmacokinetic properties, and therapeutic potential. Drugs 1990;39:86–109.

134. Gillis JC, Brogden RN. Ketorolac: a reappraisal of its pharmacodynamic and pharmacokinetic properties and therapeutic use in pain management. Drugs 1997;53:139–188.

135. O'Hara DA, Fragen RJ, Kinzer M, Pemberton D. Ketorolac tromethamine as compared with morphine sulfate for treatment of postoperative pain. Clin Pharmacol Ther 1987;41:556–561.

136. Brown CR, Moodie JE, Dickie G, et al. Analgesic efficacy and safety of single-dose oral and intramuscular ketorolac tromethamine for postoperative pain. Pharmacotherapy 1990;10(6 Pt 2):59S–70S.

137. Stanski DR, Cherry C, Bradley R, et al. Efficacy and safety of single doses of intramuscular ketorolac tromethamine compared with meperidine for postoperative pain. Pharmacotherapy 1990;10(6 Pt 2):40S–44S.

138. Strom BL, Berlin JA, Kinman JL, et al. Parenteral ketorolac and risk of gastrointestinal and operative site bleeding. JAMA 1996;275:376–382.

139. Miller DR. Combination use of nonsteroidal antiinflammatory drugs. Drug Intell Clin Pharm 1981;15:3–7.

140. Bentley KC, Head T W. The additive analgesic efficacy of acetaminophen, 1000 mg, and codeine, 60 mg, in dental pain. Clin Pharmacol Ther 1987;42:634–640.

141. Moertel CG, Ahmann DL, Taylor WF, Schwartau N. Relief of pain by oral medications: a controlled evaluation of analgesic combinations. JAMA 1974;229:55–59.

142. Beaver WT, Feise GA. Comparison of the analgesic effect of acetaminophen and codeine and their combination in patients with postoperative pain. Clin Pharmacol Ther 1978;23:108 (abstract).

143. Beaver WT, McMillan D. Methodological considerations in the evaluation of analgesic combinations: acetaminophen (paracetamol) and hydrocodone in postpartum pain. Br J Clin Pharmacol 1980;10(Suppl):215S–223S.

144. Bloomfield SS, Barden TP, Mitchell J. Aspirin and codeine in two postpartum pain models. Clin Pharmacol Ther 1976;20:499–503.

145. Bloomfield SS, Mitchell J, Cissell G, Barden T P. Analgesic sensitivity of two post-partum pain models. Pain 1986;27:171–179.

146. Quiding H, Oikarinen V, Sane J, Sjoblad A M. Analgesic efficacy after single and repeated doses of codeine and acetaminophen. J Clin Pharmacol 1984;24:27–34.

147. Matts SFG. A clinical comparison of Panadeine Co, soluble codeine Co, and soluble aspirin in the relief of pain. Br J Clin Pract 1966;20:515–517.

148. Beaver WT, Wallenstein SL, Rogers A, Houde RW. Analgesic studies of codeine and oxycodone in patients with cancer: 1. Comparison of oral with intramuscular codeine and of oral with intramuscular oxycodone. J Pharmacol Exp Ther 1978;207:92–100.

149. Beaver WT. Analgesic efficacy of hydrocodone and its combinations: a review. Spring House, PA: Smith Simon, 1988.

150. Sunshine A, Laska E, Olson NZ. Analgesic effects of oral oxycodone and codeine in the treatment of patients with postoperative, post fracture or somatic pain. In: Foley KM, Inturrisi CE, eds. Advances in pain research and therapy, vol 8. Opioid analgesics in the management of clinical pain. New York: Raven Press, 1986;225–234.

151. Beaver WT, Wallenstein SL, Rogers A, Houde RW. Analgesic studies of codeine and oxycodone in patients with cancer: 2. Comparisons of intramuscular oxycodone with intramuscular morphine and codeine. J Pharmacol Exp Ther 1978;207:101–108.

152. Cooper SA, Prescheur H, Rauch D, et al. Evaluation of oxycodone and acetaminophen in treatment of postoperative dental pain. Oral Surg 1980;50:496–501.

153. Maruta T, Swanson DW. Problems with the use of oxycodone compound in patients with chronic pain. Pain 1981;11:389–396.

154. Wang RI, Sandoval RG. The analgesic activity of propoxyphene napsylate with and without aspirin. J Clin Pharmacol 1971;11:310–317.

155. Hopkinson JH, Bartlett FH Jr, Steffens AO, et al. Acetaminophen versus propoxyphene hydrochloride for relief of pain in episiotomy patients. J Clin Pharmacol 1973;13:251–263.

156. Huskisson EC. Simple analgesics for arthritis. Br Med J 1974;4:196–200.

157. Calimlim JF, Wardell WM, Davis HT, et al. Analgesic efficacy of an orally administered combination of pentazocine and aspirin: with observations on the use and statistical efficiency of GLOBAL subjective efficacy ratings. Clin Pharmacol Ther 1977;21:34–43.

158. Sunshine A, Roure C, Olson N, et al. Analgesic efficacy of two ibuprofen-codeine combinations for the treatment of postepisiotomy and postoperative pain. Clin Pharmacol Ther 1987;42:374–380.

159. McGivney WT, Crooks GM, eds. The care of patients with severe pain in terminal illness. JAMA 1984;251:1182–1188.

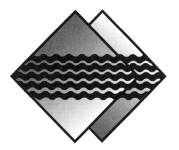

PART VII

DIAGNOSTIC AND THERAPEUTIC TECHNIQUES

CHAPTER 34

Magnetic Resonance and Radiological Imaging in the Evaluation of Back Pain

Jonathan Kleefield

TECHNICAL CONSIDERATIONS

Major advances in spine imaging have occurred during the past 25 years. For decades, plain radiography and myelography were the only methods for visualizing abnormalities involving the vertebrae, intervertebral discs, spinal cord, or nerve roots. By 1975, improvement of myelographic nerve root imaging was feasible with the substitution of nonionic water-soluble for oily contrast media, the latter having been in use since the early 1940s. Unlike oily agents, nonionic contrast carried negligible risk of arachnoiditis, was absorbable, and thus eliminated the need for its removal from the thecal sac. In 1977, the advent of whole-body computed tomography (CT) permitted direct cross-sectional imaging of both spinal and paraspinal structures. However, the spinal cord outline could be consistently demonstrated only after the intrathecal injection of water-soluble contrast, a procedure known as CT myelography (CTM). In 1982, magnetic resonance imaging (MRI) was introduced into clinical practice and has proved to be superior to CT because the spinal cord and nerve roots can be visualized without intrathecal contrast material. For the first time as well, the interior of the cord could be imaged and assessed for intrinsic pathology, such as demyelinating plaques. These may not alter the outer contour of the cord and therefore may go undetected by CTM. Second, MRI permits images in multiple planes, such as sagittal and coronal orientations, having spatial and contrast resolution equivalent to the axial plane. Last, MRI does not employ ionizing radiation and poses no known health risk.

Sagittal plane MRI is particularly advantageous for extended, expeditiously performed surveys of the entire vertebral column, the spine fortunately being oriented in the sagittal axis of the body. Recent improvements in MRI receiver coil design (phased array coil) have provided the ability to image the entire spine with high resolution in less than 10 minutes. This is especially advantageous in the search for cord compression due to metastatic spinal neoplastic disease, as these patients are often quite ill and can benefit greatly from rapid imaging. Newer pulse sequences, including half-Fourier turbo spin echo (HASTE), can yield usable images in less than 10 seconds. Additionally, this fast technique can suppress some metal-induced artifacts arising from surgical hardware, as a result producing a clearer diagnostic image. (Fig. 34.1).

Although CT is capable of producing sagittal plane spinal images, these can be obtained only by reformatting the data from prior axial plane scans. Unfortunately, the number and thickness of the axial scans limits the coverage and spatial resolution of the reformatted sagittal CT images. No such restrictions exist for sagittal plane MRI. As noted earlier, MRI is more versatile than CT because it can depict pathology not apparent on CT. Intrinsic spinal cord disease, such as syringomyelia or multiple sclerosis plaques, is uniquely delineated by MRI. MRI is performed by subjecting the patient to a sequence of radiofrequency pulses and a strong magnetic field. The use of various combinations of pulses, known as pulse sequences, allows formation of images that reflect the differing energy-releasing characteristics of a given tissue, known as the T1 and T2 relaxation constants. In general, scans emphasizing T1 characteristics clearly define the outline of an anatomical structure, such as the spinal cord, whereas so-called T2-weighted images are more sensitive in portraying a pathological process within the spinal cord, such as edema surrounding a tumor, gliosis, or demyelination.

In the past few years, helical (spiral) CT scanners have been introduced. This device, as compared with a conventional CT scanner, employs continuous x-ray tube rotation as the patient is moved by the scanning table through the aperture in the scanner gantry. This volumetric data acquisition scheme is more flexible than so-called single-slice scanning, as it permits

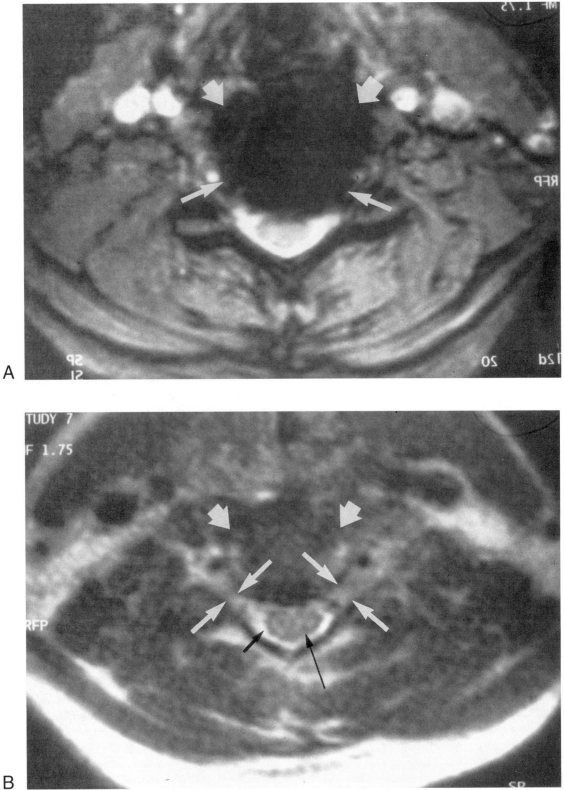

Figure 34.1. A. Conventional axial T2-weighted gradient echo image of the cervical spine. Status: post-anterior cervical fusion with metallic plates and screws. The metallic fixation devices create a large, dark artifact that totally obscures the vertebral body (thick arrows) and neural foramina (thin arrows). B. Axial HASTE image of the cervical spine, same patient and scan position as view A. Scan obtained in 10 seconds. Note clear delineation of the neural foramina (thin white arrows) and the vertebral body margins (thick white arrows). The spinal cord (long black arrow) is sharply margined by bright cerebrospinal fluid (short black arrow) within the thecal sac.

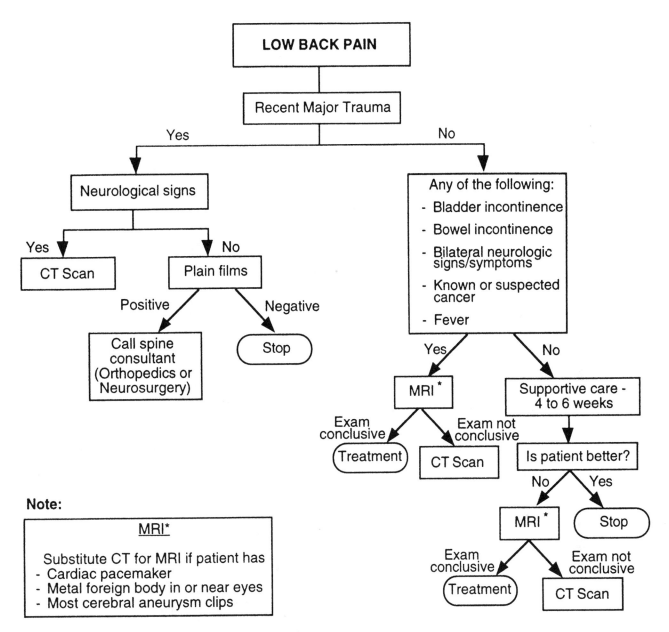

Figure 34.2.   Algorithm for radiological evaluation of low back pain.

multiplanar reconstructions of selectable *spatial* resolution. However, *contrast* resolution, critical for discerning the thecal sac and other neurological structures is, if anything, inferior to that of conventional single-slice scanning. Therefore, helical spinal CT is most helpful in imaging intrinsically high contrast bony structures and their related pathological processes, such as fractures and degenerative arthritis. Helical CT should not be viewed as a substitute for MRI.

Today, patients with neck and back pain requiring diagnostic imaging are most effectively studied by MRI. MRI should be reserved for patients who either did not respond to conservative treatment or are suspected of harboring an abnormality that may require urgent management; these include spinal cord compression from a tumor or an infection such as osteomyelitis, discitis, or epidural abscess. If an acute fracture is clinically suspected, plain films are obtained first. If they are not diagnostic, helical CT with sagittal and coronal reformatted images is used to obtain optimum bony detail. However, intrinsic spinal cord injury is best depicted by MRI. This discussion should make clear my impression that plain film radiography is overused, especially in light of its relative insensitivity in detecting disease, including neoplasm and infection. Other than as an imaging triage for acute spinal trauma, plain film usage should be curtailed in a fashion similar to the virtual disappearance of skull radiographs for evaluation of most neurological disease. These imaging recommendations have been formulated into an algorithm (Fig. 34.2).

Supplementary CT may be useful when MRI is equivocal. This situation can occur particularly in the postsurgical spine, where metallic internal fixation devices may severely degrade or even preclude MRI despite the use of the aforementioned HASTE sequences (Fig. 34.3). Additionally, CT can more reliably detect calcific or ossific lesions than MRI. For example, subtle cases of ossification of the posterior longitudinal ligament can be difficult to detect by MRI but are efficaciously depicted by CT. As such, I view CT and MRI as being complementary techniques.

In my experience it is now rarely necessary to perform CTM. CTM is reserved for patients who are unable to undergo MRI (Table 34.1) or in whom MRI and CT are nondiagnostic. In the unoperated patient conventional myelography or CTM is no longer a primary diagnostic imaging study at Boston's Beth Israel-Deaconess Hospital. These procedures carry the risks of allergic reaction to the contrast agent, introduction of infection into the thecal sac and its contents, and post-lumbar-puncture headache. I think that MRI, compared with myelography or CTM, offers superior imaging of both extradural and intradural structures with no known morbidity. Both MRI and CT directly depict the extradural compartment, which harbors the most frequent pathological processes, disc disease and facet joint arthropathy. Myelography, which fills the intradural compartment (thecal sac) with contrast medium, at best provides indirect evidence of extradural pathology by virtue of indentations on the sac or nerve root sleeves. Lesions in the extradural compartment that are not contiguous to the thecal sac or the nerve root sleeves are undetectable by myelography. No such limitation applies to MRI or CT. Recently, MRI pulse sequences have permitted the rapid acquisition of heavily T2-weighted images with high spatial resolution. These are called fast spin echo or turbo spin echo. With strong T2 weighting, the cerebrospinal fluid appears bright and essentially identical to intrathecal contrast used in CTM, (Fig. 34.4A). Thus, the CTM image equivalent is achieved *noninvasively* by MRI, which in my opinion usually obviates CTM.

As noted previously, T2 signal abnormalities in the spinal cord can signify several categories of disease, including gliosis, edema, or tumor. The differentiation among these pathological processes has been refined through the use of the MRI contrast agent gadolinium diethylene triamine pentaacetic acid (DTPA). Gadolinium, a metal in the rare earth series, is a paramagnetic element causing shortening of the T1 of tissues that accumulate it. T1 shortening translates into brightening on the MR image, which emphasizes T1 relaxation characteristics. This phenomenon is analogous to the enhancement effect of iodinated contrast. Moreover, in the human body the transport kinetics of gadolinium are identical to those of iodinated radiographic contrast agents. The gadolinium is chelated to a carrier molecule, DTPA, and is injected intravenously, usually in a volume of 10 mL. The agent carries almost no risks to the patient, with only

Table 34.1.   Contraindications to MRI

Life support equipment (e.g., ventilator)
Intracranial aneurysm clip (ferromagnetic type)
Cardiac pacemaker
Starr-Edwards Cardiac Valve-Mark 1
Metallic otological implant (e.g., stapes and cochlear)
Ocular metallic foreign body

extremely rare instances of anaphylaxis, far fewer than with iodinated contrast. Even patients with hepatic and renal compromise can tolerate gadolinium agents more readily than iodinated contrast. Nevertheless, it remains axiomatic to employ gadolinium with discretion, particularly in these debilitated patients. Gadolinium enhances most spinal tumors, postoperative granulation tissue, and many inflammatory processes.

Low-back pain is often a nonspecific symptom that may relate to paraspinal pathology involving retroperitoneal structures. Therefore, when imaging the spine with either CT or MRI, it is helpful to have at least some coverage of the paraspinal region. Pathology such as aortic aneurysms, infections, and retroperitoneal tumors can be demonstrated via either technique (1). Also, it is extremely helpful if the radiologist is provided with pertinent clinical history, particularly with regard to any localization, especially lateralization, of pain, weakness, or other neurological symptoms (Fig. 34.5). Many imaging centers have the patient note his or her perception of pain on an anatomical diagram, which I have found very useful on a number of occasions (Fig. 34.6).

DEGENERATIVE DISEASE

The most common causes of neck and back pain that can be imaged are intervertebral disc disease and facet joint degeneration. Disc disorders are more commonly found in young and middle-aged adults, whereas facet degeneration is more frequent in the elderly. Moreover, the two disease processes often coexist in older patients, in whom they can cause spinal stenosis. Although MRI depicts disc pathology with remarkable clarity, recent publications have noted the detection of disc abnormalities of varying types in asymptomatic persons (2, 3). Therefore, any *radiological* finding of disc disease must be viewed in the context of *clinical* symptoms before it should be considered significant. Furthermore, some types of disc pathology occur more frequently in the asymptomatic patient. For example, Jensen et al. (3) noted that a bulging disc, defined as a uniform, concentric expansion of disc material (Fig. 34.7), was more often asymptomatic than what was termed an extruded disc. (These authors included herniated discs in the category of extruded disc. This apparent terminological reclassification highlights the need for a more standardized nomenclature of disc abnormalities for a predictable assignment of pathological significance.) A

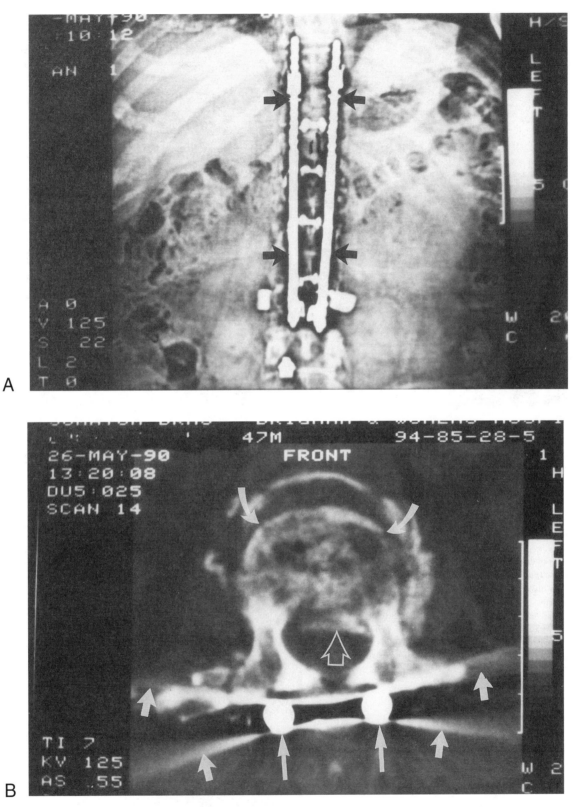

Figure 34.3.   **A.** Preliminary anteroposterior (scout) CT of the lumbar spine, used to position the axial CT scan levels, showing Harrington rods (*arrows*) overlying lumbar spine. **B.** Axial lumbar spine CT, same patient as view A. Despite linear streak artifacts (*short arrows*) generated by the rods (*long arrows*), the CT is clear enough to depict burst fracture (*curved white arrows*), including fracture fragment (*open arrow*) retropulsed into the central spinal canal. Metallic fixation devices should not necessarily preclude diagnostic CT or MRI. In most cases, myelography or CT myelography can be avoided.

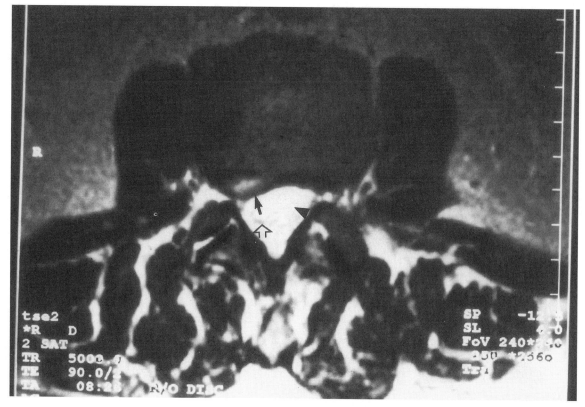

A

Figure 34.4.   A. Axial fast spin echo T2-weighted image at level of lumbar disc. Note bright area (*black arrow*) in posterior disc margin representing torn annulus with associated focal disc deformity consistent with a protrusion. Bright cerebrospinal fluid in the-cal sac provides excellent contrast against normal dark disc margin. Note speckles in spinal fluid (*open arrow*) representing the normal cauda equina in cross section. **B.** Sagittal fast spin echo T2-weighted lumbar spine image, different patient from view A. Torn annulus (*black arrow*) seen as bright area along posterior disc margin. Center of disc (*thick white arrow*) is dark, compared with other normal disc (*thin white arrow*). This is disc desiccation, thought to be an early manifestation of disc degeneration. The finding is often asymptomatic. In the normal disc is a horizontal black streak (*black arrowhead*), representing the intranuclear cleft, a normal finding as well. Note bright cerebrospinal fluid (*open arrows*) providing excellent contrast with posterior disc margins and vertebral bodies. Such high contrast imitates and therefore usually obviates CT myelography.

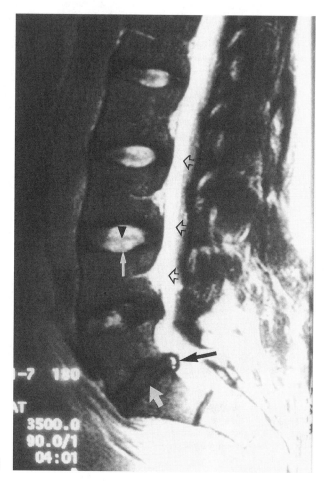

B

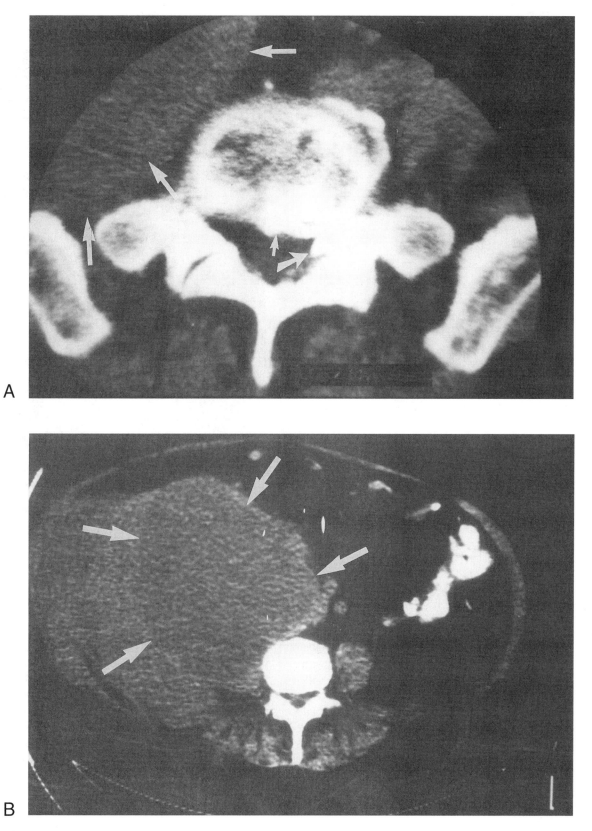

Figure 34.5.   A. Axial CT scan at L5-S1 disc level. No history supplied to radiologist other than "low back pain; rule out disc." Interpretation noted *left*-sided posterior osteophyte (*small arrow*), and *left* facet joint degeneration (*angled arrow*). *Right* paraspinal mass (*large arrows*) not described. Patient had *right*-sided back pain. **B.** Axial CT, same patient as view A, 10 days later. Huge right paraspinal mass shown (*arrows*). Diagnosis: tuberculous psoas abscess. This case emphasizes importance of communicating pertinent clinical information to consulting radiologist, particularly if findings *lateralize.*

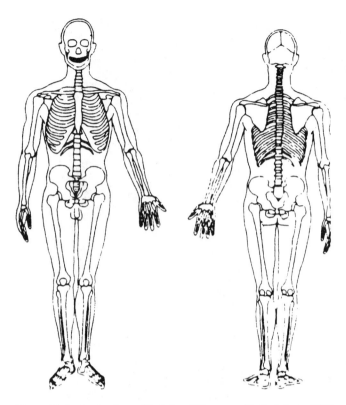

Figure 34.6. Intake sheet of Beth Israel-Deaconess Medical Center MRI department. Note drawing of body. Patient is requested to note areas of pain, paresthesias, or motor difficulties on the illustration. This information has proven its significant radiological interpretive utility on many occasions, as the information often supplements that provided on requisition.

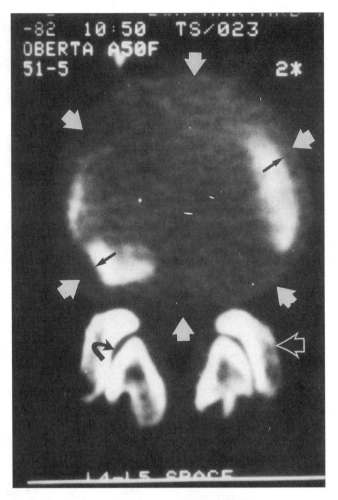

Figure 34.7. Axial CT at level of bulging disc. Note uniform, concentric expansion of disc margins *(white arrows)* beyond vertebral body margin *(black arrows)*. Normal right-sided facet joint space *(curved black arrow)* and left superior articular facet *(open arrow)* also shown.

protruding disc is a focal deformity of the outer disc margin, with a broad base relative to the anteroposterior (AP) extent of the lesion (Fig. 34.4*A*). This may also be associated with a tear of the outer disc material, the annulus, and thus is called an annular tear (Fig. 34.4*B*). The pathology of an annular tear is similar to that of a tear of a meniscal cartilage. It usually presents as an area of increased T2 signal in the annulus, highlighted from the dense collagen of the normal annulus, which is dark on T2-weighted scans. A herniated disc can be defined as a focal distortion of disc margin, in which the AP extent of the deformity approaches its width (Fig. 34.8). Extruded discs, as I define them, remain attached to the parent disc while extending cephalad, caudad, or bidirectionally relative to the plane of the disc space (Fig. 34.9). Finally, a free disc fragment is separable from the parent disc (Fig. 34.10).

In the cervical spine, midline posterior disc herniation is well demonstrated by sagittal plane MRI (Fig. 34.11). T2-weighted images can show increased signal intensity within the compressed spinal cord, suggesting cord edema or gliosis (4) (Fig. 34.12). (High T2 signal may also occur in a concurrent pathological process, such as a spinal cord tumor. The advent of intravenous gadolinium-enhanced MRI has rendered such a differentiation more reliable. In general, most spinal cord tumors enhance, whereas edema does not.) A lateral cervical disc herniation, typically causing radiculopathic symptoms, is optimally visualized by MRI in the axial plane (Fig. 34.13). The sagittal images are not as revealing in this case because of the oblique orientation of the cervical neural foramina. Similarly, in the lumbar spine, a midline disc herniation is best imaged by sagittal MRI (Fig. 34.14). However, a lateral,

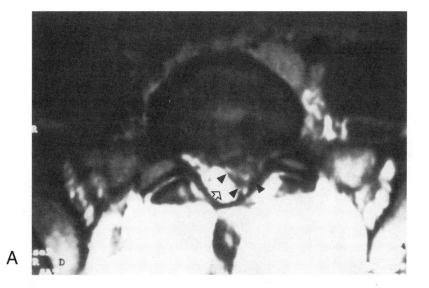

A

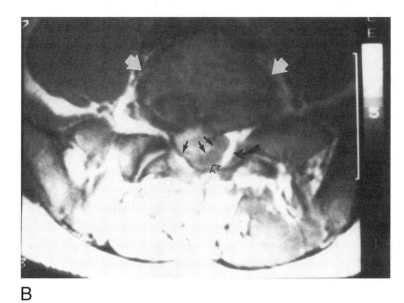

B

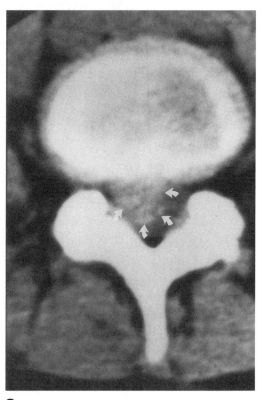

C

Figure 34.8.   **A.** Axial T2-wieghted MRI at the level of L5-S1 disc space. Large left-sided disc herniation (*arrowheads*) is shown as dark area contrasted clearly by bright spinal fluid in thecal sac (*open arrow*). **B.** Axial T1-weighted MRI at the level of L5-S1 disc space, different patient from view A. Large right-sided disc herniation (*black arrows*) shown as brighter than adjacent parent disc (*white arrows*) and distorted thecal sac (*open arrow*). Biochemical explanation for the hyperintense disc herniation is uncertain. Note very bright crescent of normal epidural fat (*curved black arrow*) providing excellent natural contrast with adjacent thecal sac and posterior disc margin. **C.** Axial CT shows huge, tongue-shaped herniated disc (*arrows*) essentially obliterating the thecal sac. Herniated discs of this size can be a surgical emergency, for example, if patient has cauda equina syndrome. However, lesions of this size are occasionally asymptomatic. Correlation of the radiological studies with clinical findings is critical for proper patient management.

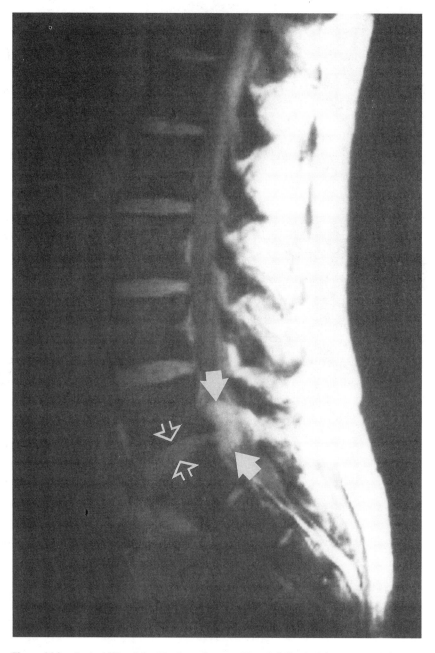

Figure 34.9.   Sagittal T2-weighted lumbar spine scan. Extruded disc (*solid arrows*) cephalad and caudad to plane of the L5-S1 parent disc (*open arrows*) creates a mushroom cap deformity.

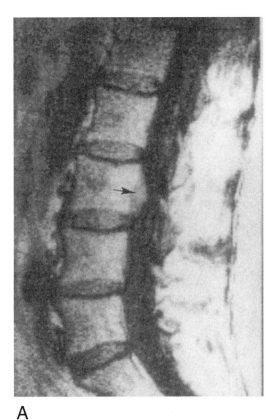

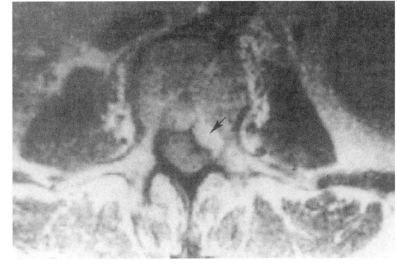

B

A

Figure 34.10.   **A.** Midline T1-weighted sagittal MRI of lumbar spine. Sequestered disc fragment (*arrow*) appears semicircular and is posterior to L3 vertebral body. **B.** Axial T1-weighted MRI at level of L3 body in same patient as in view A. Sequestered disc fragment (*arrow*), elliptical in cross-section, has high (bright) signal relative to adjacent dural sac.

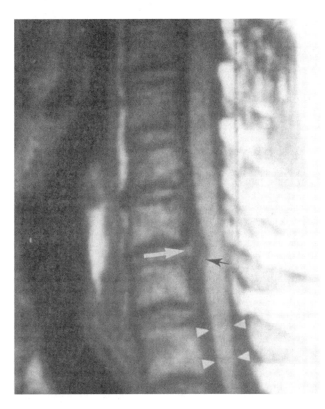

Figure 34.11.   Midline sagittal T1-weighted MRI of cervical spine. Central disc herniation (*white arrow*) displaces the epidural venous plexus posteriorly (*black arrow*), causing spinal cord compression. Note the good distinction of cord margins (*arrowheads*) provided by T1-weighted images.

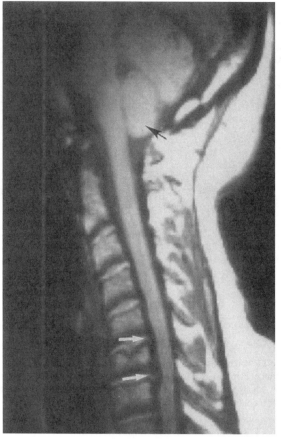
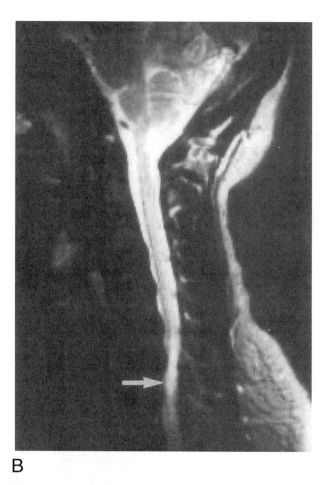

A   B

Figure 34.12.   **A.** Midline sagittal T1-weighted MRI of cervical spine. Note central disc herniations (*white arrows*) at C5-C6 and C6-C7 interspaces. The largest disc herniation is at C6-C7, causing greatest cord compression. Note good definition of normal cerebellar tonsil (*black arrow*). **B.** Midline sagittal T2-weighted MRI of cervical spine, same patient as in view A. Spinal cord outline is less clearly seen than on T1-weighted image. However, scan shows abnormally high (bright) signal in spinal cord at C5-C6 interspace (*arrow*), likely indicating edema in cord due to contiguous disc herniation. In the absence of cord compression, identical high-T2 signal in the cord can be seen in a demyelinating process.

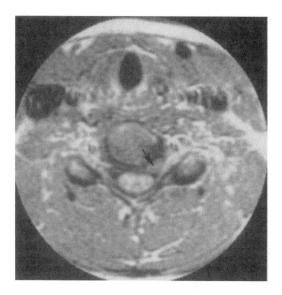

Figure 34.13.   Axial MRI of C5-C6 disc space showing large lateral disc herniation (*arrow*) within left neural foramen, compressing left sixth cervical nerve root sleeve. Compare with normal right side, where there is clear visualization of normal dorsal and ventral cervical nerve rootlets.

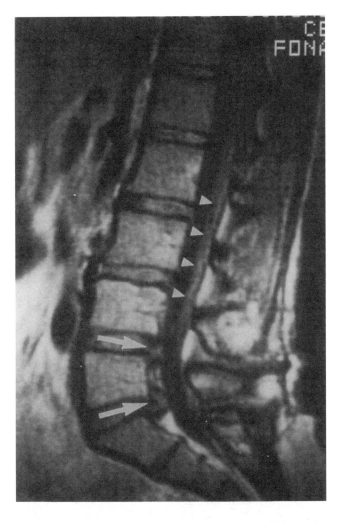

Figure 34.14. Midline sagittal T1-weighted MRI of lumbar spine. Moderate-sized central L4-L5 and large central L5-S1 disc herniations (*arrows*). Note normal cauda equina (*arrowheads*).

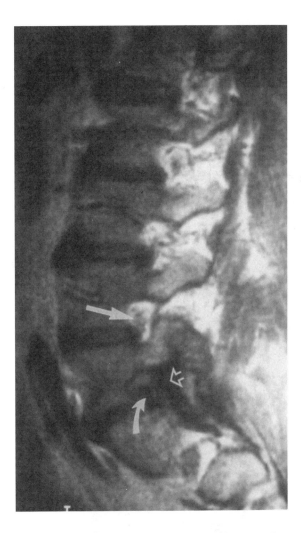

Figure 34.15. Parasagittal T1-weighted MRI of lumbar spine. Normal L4-L5 neural foramen shown exiting L4 nerve root sleeve (*large arrow*) is clearly outlined by high-signal (bright) epidural fat. At L5-S1, neural foramen is narrowed by both lateral disc herniation (*curved arrow*) and facet degeneration (*open arrow*). Both pathological processes compress nerve root sleeve, which lies superior to disc herniation.

intraforaminal lumbar disc herniation can be well shown by either axial or sagittal MRI because of the parasagittal orientation of the lumbar neural foramina (Fig. 34.15). As noted earlier, a portion of disc can separate from the parent disc, producing a free fragment (5) (Fig. 34.10). Virtually all free fragments remain in the extradural compartment. Rare cases of fragments transgressing the posterior longitudinal ligament and dura and thus lodging intradurally have been reported (6), but they are almost always diagnosed in retrospect at surgery. Lumbar MRI also can demonstrate the normal conus medullaris, thereby excluding a tumor at that site (Fig. 34.16A). On occasion a conus medullaris tumor can symptomatically mimic a disc herniation (Fig. 34.16B).

Although MRI provides excellent imaging of disc disease, axial CT is often just as effective in this regard, particularly when there are associated bone changes such as osteophytic spurs. Clinical localization is helpful in directing the CT

examination to the appropriate levels of the spine because it is impractical to scan the entire spine axially by CT.

Thoracic disc herniations were formerly thought to be infrequent. However, the incidence was likely underestimated because of limited imaging sensitivity of plain films and myelography. The ease of comprehensive thoracic spine imaging by MRI likely accounts for the more frequent imaging of disc pathology by this modality (Fig. 34.17). Nevertheless, if the herniated disc material is heavily calcified, CT may better delineate the true extent of the herniation (Fig. 34.18). This is because calcification may produce a low signal, making it difficult to distinguish from cerebrospinal fluid on T1-weighted MRI. By contrast, CT clearly delineates calcification. Calcification occurs more frequently in thoracic disc herniations than in lumbar or cervical sites.

Recently, imaging has provided some justification for conservative treatment strategies. Disc herniations, particularly

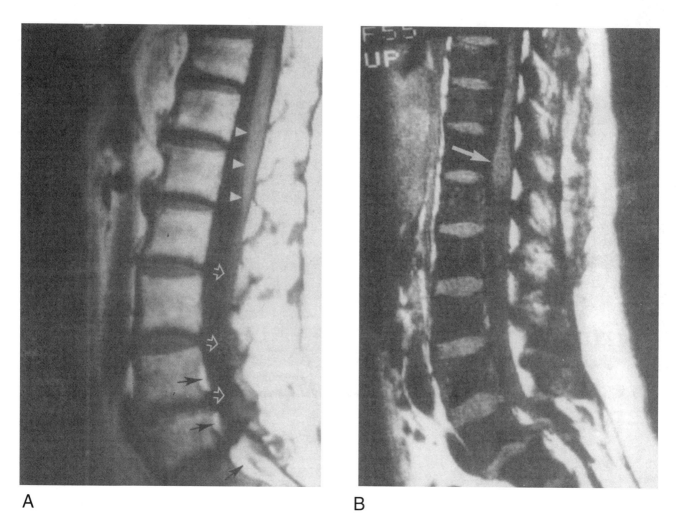

A   B

Figure 34.16. **A.** Midline sagittal T1-weighted MRI of lumbar spine. Normal conus medullaris (*arrowheads*) is conical, with its tip usually at L1-L2 interspace. Normal cauda equina rootlets are clearly distinguished (*open arrows*). Also note areas of high (bright) signal (*black arrows*), representing residual oily contrast agent (Pantopaque) from previous myelogram. **B.** Midline sagittal T1-weighted MRI of lumbar spine. Abnormal expansion of conus medullaris (*arrow*), presumably due to intramedullary breast metastasis. Note very low (dark) signal in all vertebral bodies, representing replacement of normally bright marrow fat by widely metastatic breast cancer.

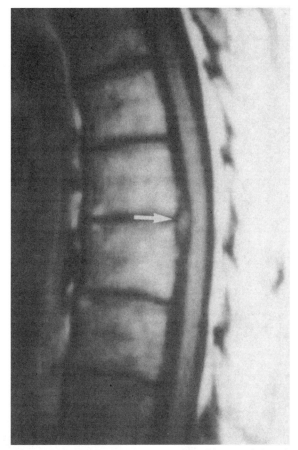

Figure 34.17.   Midline sagittal T1-weighted image of thoracic spine. T6-T7 central disc herniation (*arrow*) causes mild deformity of adjacent thoracic cord.

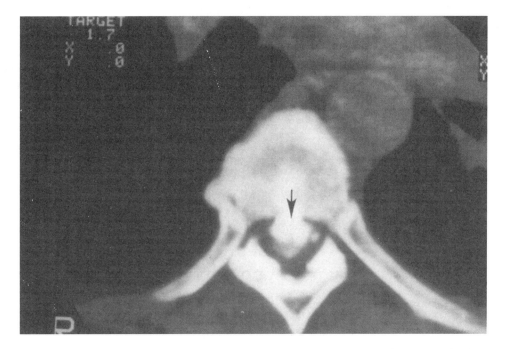

Figure 34.18.   Axial CT scan at level of T7-T8 disc. Large disc herniation shows calcification extending from nucleus pulposus (*arrow*) into central spinal canal.

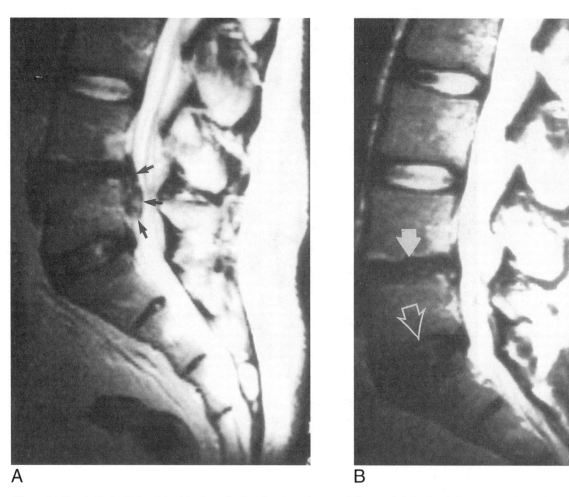

Figure 34.19. **A.** Sagittal T2-weighted lumbar spine imaging shows large caudally extruded disc herniation (*arrows*). **B.** Sagittal T2-weighted lumbar spine imaging of same patient as view A, 3 months later. This patient had no surgery but essentially complete spontaneous regression of extruded disc. Patient has recovered clinically as well. Note the residual dark (desiccated) L4-L5 disc (*arrow*). L5-S1 disc (*hollow arrow*) is also desiccated.

large ones, have been shown to regress over time without surgical intervention (Fig. 34.19). Yock (7) has noted that the herniation may have associated hemorrhagic elements, which may be resorbed over time and thus explain the apparent reduction in size.

The evaluation of the postoperative spine, particularly regarding recurrent and/or residual disc herniation, has been simplified through the use of gadolinium-enhanced MRI (8). Gadolinium enhances postoperative scar tissue to a much greater extent than disc material, usually allowing distinction between the two. We have also found that supplemental axial T2-weighted imaging can help in differentiating a disc fragment from an entrapped nerve root sleeve (Fig. 34.20).

Over the past few decades, discography has been advocated, principally by orthopaedic surgeons, as a method for delineating intrinsic disc pathology via injection of contrast material into the disc and imaging with plain radiography or CT. It has also been used as a provocative test (discomanometry) to determine whether a disc abnormality is symptomatic. Publications endorsing discography's utility have appeared, again mostly in the orthopaedic literature (9–11). However, contrary opinions are also cited (12). There has been limited acceptance of this procedure by the radiology community, particularly in view of the large accumulated experience with the noninvasive techniques of MRI and CT. Discography carries the risk of introduction of infection into the disc and adjacent bone, as well as allergic reaction to the contrast agent.

Facet joint degeneration occurs most often in the lumbar and cervical portion of the spinal column and least commonly in the thoracic spine. The regional differences reflect the greater mobility of the cervical and lumbar spine. As with any other synovial joint, degenerative arthritis can cause narrowing of the joint space with overgrowth of the bony margins of the facet joints. These bony spurs may encroach upon the spinal canal and compress the thecal sac and/or nerve root sleeves. Such spinal stenosis can be further aggravated by thickening of the ligamentum flavum posteriorly, an abnormality frequently accompanying facet joint degeneration. Moreover, facet joint

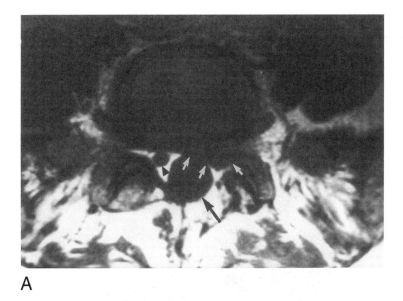

A

Figure 34.20. A. Axial T1-weighted lumbar spine MRI after laminectomy and discectomy. Patient had residual left-sided radiculopathic symptoms. Study performed to rule out recurrent disc herniation or scar tissue. Note soft tissue (*white arrows*) posterior to disc that obscures nerve root sleeve on left. Normal right-sided root sleeve (*black arrowhead*) is clearly marginated by normal epidural fat, as is the thecal sac (*black arrow*). **B.** Same axial T1-weighted section following gadolinium injection, showing enhancement (brightening) of a portion of the soft-tissue region in view A (*hollow white arrows*) except for one area (*black arrow*). The enhancement represents granulation tissue. What is the significance of the nonenhancing region? Is it a residual or recurrent disc fragment or nerve root sleeve? **C.** Axial T2-weighted section at same anatomical level shows nonenhancing region noted above to have T2 signal identical to thecal sac, making it a fluid-filled nerve root sleeve rather than a disc fragment. The *open white arrow* points at this root sleeve. Note darker dot within the sleeve, representing the actual nerve rootlet (*short black arrow*). *Long black arrow* points to black dot in thecal sac representing cauda equina rootlet.

B

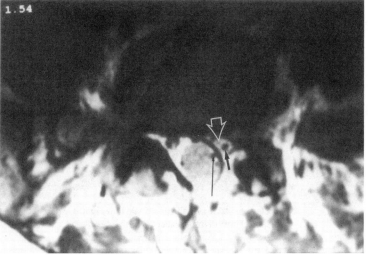

C

disease often occurs in conjunction with disc abnormalities. The two pathological processes together may cause spinal stenosis, the extent of which can be accurately demonstrated by MRI (Fig. 34.21). CT is an excellent alternative imaging study, provided the clinical examination can accurately direct the placement of the axial scans (Fig. 34.22).

If facet joint degeneration progresses, subluxation or spondylolisthesis can occur, aggravating the spinal stenosis. In nearly all cases, the vertebra that pathologically displaces does so anteriorly relative to the contiguous caudal segment. The spondylolisthesis can be visualized by plain radiographs, MRI or CT (Fig. 34.23). Degenerative spondylolisthesis should be distinguished from spondylolisthesis with an accompanying pars defect, known as spondylolysis. The defect is most readily depicted by sagittally reformatted CT and is most commonly seen at the L5 level (Fig. 34.24).

NEOPLASMS

Neoplastic disease in the spine often presents with back pain. The most common tumor is a metastasis from a breast or lung carcinoma. MRI is exquisitely sensitive in detecting bony vertebral metastatic disease (13–18) and any associated epidural tumor extension that is causing spinal cord or nerve root compression (Fig. 34.25). At Beth-Israel Deaconess

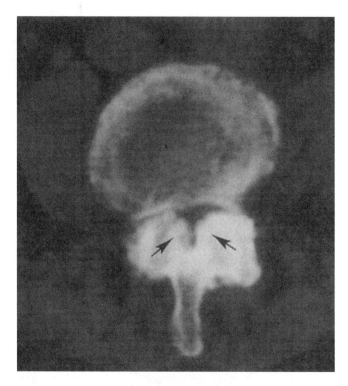

Figure 34.22.   Axial CT at level of L3-L4 disc. Note severe spinal stenosis largely due to massive degenerative facet disease (*arrows*).

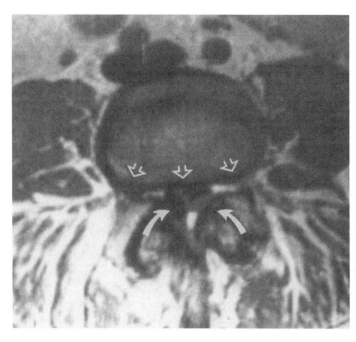

Figure 34.21.   Axial MRI at L4-L5 interspace. Bilateral facet joint degeneration accompanied by overgrowth of ligamentum flavum (*curved arrows*) and bulging disc annulus (*open arrows*), producing marked spinal stenosis with compression of dural sac.

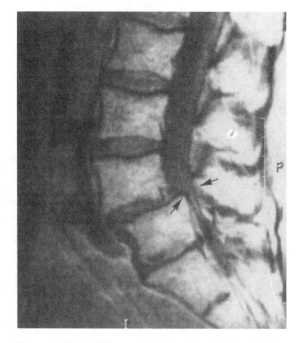

Figure 34.23.   Midline sagittal T1-weighted MRI of lumbar spine. Forward displacement of both L4 body and spinous process relative to L5, indicative of an intact neural arch (i.e., no pars defect or spondylolysis). This degenerative spondylolisthesis causes severe spinal stenosis (*arrows*).

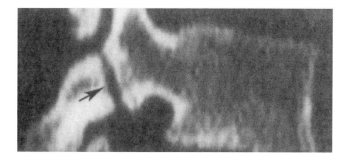

Figure 34.24.   Parasagittal reformatted CT showing pars defect (*arrow*) indicating spondylolysis. Note excellent demonstration of normal pedicle and vertebral body.

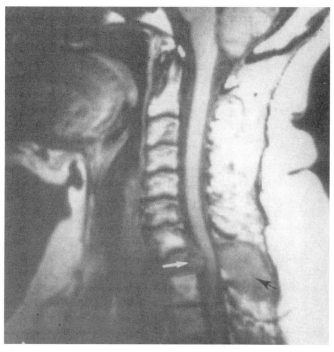

A

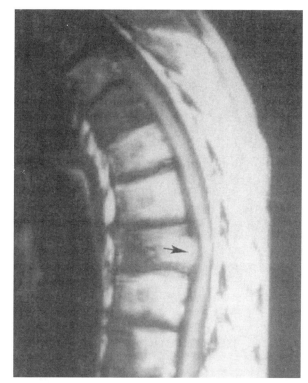

B

Figure 34.25.   A. Midline sagittal T1-weighted MRI of cervical and upper thoracic spine. Breast metastasis destroys first thoracic vertebral body (*white arrow*). Accompanying epidural tumor mass compresses and displaces the spinal cord. Large tumor also seen in the spinous process of same vertebra (*black arrow*), contacting dorsal aspect of spinal cord. **B.** Midline sagittal T1-weighted MRI of thoracic spine. Low-signal (dark) metastatic tumor foci seen in T4, T7, and T9 vertebral bodies. At T7, associated pathological fracture has retropulsed fragment compressing the spinal cord (*arrow*). Diagnosis: metastatic lung carcinoma.

Medical Center myelography is no longer performed on patients who are suffering from spinal metastases because MRI provides superior delineation of the extent of metastatic disease, which is necessary to plan radiation therapy, and also because it is completely noninvasive. Metastatic disease involving the leptomeninges can also be detected on MRI, particularly with gadolinium enhancement (Fig. 34.26). However, even with enhancement, MRI is only about a third as sensitive as serial lumbar punctures in detecting leptomeningeal spread of tumor (19).

A patient with suspected metastatic disease who is unable to undergo MRI for technical or medical reasons can be examined by CT after focusing the study on a specific region of the spine by the aid of the clinical findings, plain radiographs, and if time permits, a radionuclide bone scan. This latter study is still a very sensitive and inexpensive method of surveying the vertebral column for bony malignancy.

Intraspinal neoplasms can be classified as intramedullary or extramedullary. Intramedullary tumors are most commonly low-grade astrocytomas or ependymomas. Spinal cord gliomas can disseminate widely, up to the entire extent of the spinal cord. Again, MRI is the imaging modality of choice. These neoplasms usually expand the spinal cord and alter its signal intensity, making their visualization easy. However, it is often possible to improve discrimination of the tumor mar-

gins from accompanying cysts or edema by using gadolinium DTPA (20) (Fig. 34.27). As noted previously, this contrast agent is virtually nonallergenic and has negligible renal toxicity. Most extramedullary but intradural tumors are meningiomas or schwannomas. These neoplasms may compress both the spinal cord and the nerve roots (Fig. 34.28), findings easily demonstrable by MRI. However, distinction between meningioma and schwannoma can sometimes be accomplished with CT, which can better demonstrate calcification seen almost exclusively with meningioma. Spinal schwannomas can occur in isolation or as a manifestation of an inherited neurocutaneous syndrome, neurofibromatosis I (21).

SYRINGOMYELIA

Some intramedullary tumors may be associated with syringomyelia (22). If MRI has simplified the detection of one pathological process in the spine, that process is syringomyelia. Formerly, such invasive procedures as gas myelography and later CTM were the only methods of demonstrating cysts within the spinal cord. Chiari malformations of the hindbrain and cervical spine with tonsillar ectopia and hydromyelia are well visualized in their entirety by MRI (23) (Fig. 34.29). Often the central cavity extends the whole length of the cord. Associated cerebral and midline anomalies

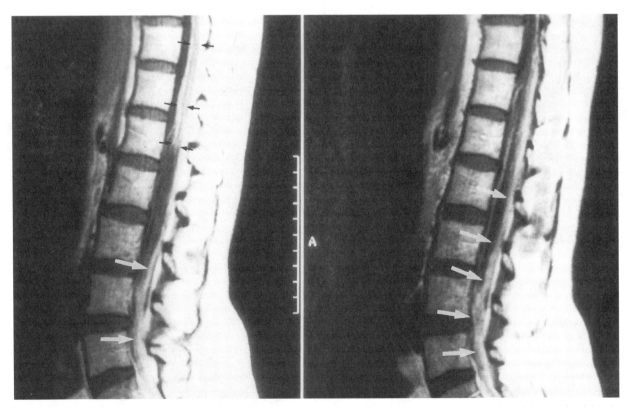

Figure 34.26. Two contiguous sagittal T1-weighted gadolinium-enhanced images of the lumbar spine. Note extensive bright areas involving the cauda equina (*white arrows*) on both images. *Left,* Note bright stripe coating distal spinal cord (*tiny black arrows*). These abnormalities represent pathological enhancement from leptomeningeal spread of metastatic tumor, in this case from breast cancer. There is no sign of bony metastases. Meningeal infection occasionally produces equivalent degrees of enhancement.

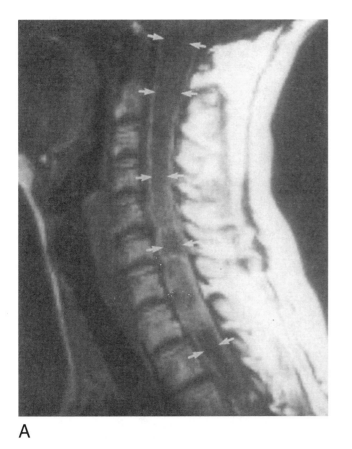

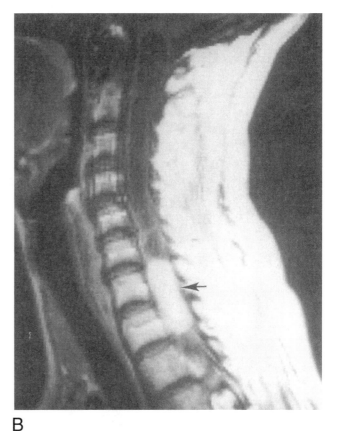

A

B

Figure 34.27.   A. Midline sagittal T1-weighted MRI of cervical and upper thoracic spine. Extensive irregularly marginated cavity (*white arrows*) of mixed signal intensity is generally lower (darker) than normal cord parenchyma. Cavity expands the spinal cord. **B.** Midline sagittal T1-weighted MRI in same patient as view A following intravenous infusion of gadolinium-DTPA. Enhancement of tumor mass (*arrow*) facilitates planning of surgical resection. Operative diagnosis: intramedullary ependymoma. Large cavity was accompanying syringomyelia.

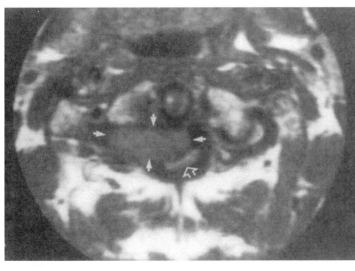

A

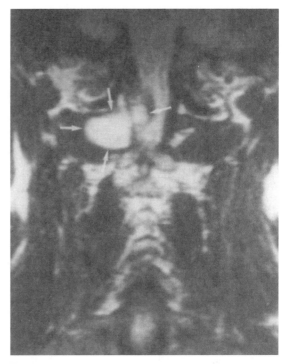

B

Figure 34.28.   A. Axial T1-weighted image of cervical spine at C1-C2 level. Tumor mass of low-signal (dark) intensity (*solid arrows*), dumbbell shaped, extends through right neural foramen into spinal canal, compressing spinal cord (*open arrow*). **B.** Coronal moderately T2-weighted image of cervical spine in same patient as view A. Tumor mass now shows high (bright) signal (*arrows*), facilitating its detection. Signal pattern is compatible with schwannoma, which was surgically proved.

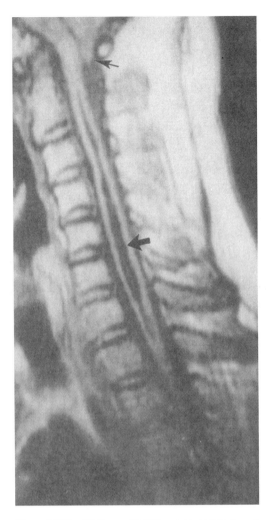

Figure 34.29. Midline sagittal T1-weighted MRI of cervical spine. Cerebellar tonsil (*small arrow*), normally above foramen magnum, extends to posterior arch of C1 vertebra. Tonsil is abnormally pointed. Low-signal (dark) cavity (*large arrow*) causes fusiform expansion of cervical cord. Findings represent Chiari I malformation with hydromyelia.

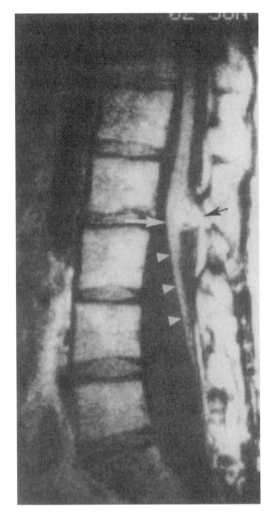

Figure 34.30. Midline sagittal T1-weighted MRI of lumbar spine. Abnormally low position of conus at L2-L3 (*white arrow*). Tumor mass (*black arrow*) with high signal (bright) intensity consistent with lipoma. Associated thickening of filum terminale (*arrowheads*). Findings represent tethered cord syndrome with associated lipoma.

may be identified when the spine is imaged. In the lumbar spine, dysraphic states such as meningoceles and tethering of the spinal cord with an associated lipoma are best imaged by MRI (24) (Fig. 34.30).

DEMYELINATING DISEASE

Demyelination in the spinal cord occasionally presents as a radiculopathy (25) clinically mimicking disc herniation, particularly in the cervical region. Before the advent of MRI, there was no method of directly imaging demyelinating plaques within the spinal cord, although frequently such lesions could be demonstrated in the brain by CT. Typically, demyelination produces one or more discrete foci of elevated T2 signal intensity within the spinal cord, at times with cord expansion if the lesion is acute. Besides the clinical features, confirmation that the signal abnormalities in the cord may be

due to a demyelinating process can be obtained by MRI of the brain, demonstrating additional areas of prolonged T2 signal in the periventricular white matter (26).

TRAUMA

Trauma to the spine has traditionally been initially imaged with plain radiographs. These studies often serve to guide subsequent CT scanning, which provides excellent imaging of the extent of most fractures (Fig. 34.31). MRI provides superior definition of soft-tissue injuries, particularly if there is an associated spinal hematoma or cord contusion (4, 27). However, particularly in the acutely traumatized patient who may be in traction or on external life-support systems, it is often physically impractical to employ MRI. The recent introduction of wide-bore, so-called open magnet systems will likely make it simpler to scan such patients.

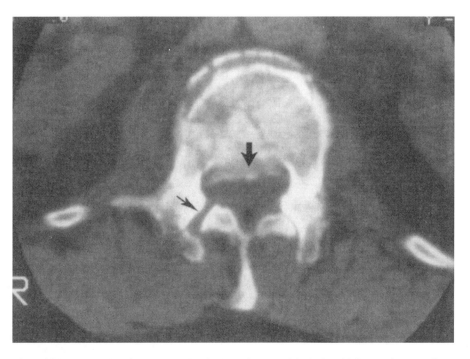

Figure 34.31.   Axial CT of L3 vertebra showing burst fracture of the body, with fracture fragment (*large arrow*) retropulsed into spinal canal. Note distraction of right L2-L3 facet joint (*small arrow*).

INFECTION

An increasingly common cause of back pain is spinal osteomyelitis and/or epidural abscess, yet their diagnosis is often fraught with difficulty. Vertebral and intervertebral disc destruction is the hallmark of discitis and osteomyelitis, yet such abnormalities occur late in the course of the disease. With epidural abscess, plain films are unrevealing and should not be relied upon to rule out an infectious process. MRI is the preferred technique for imaging osteomyelitis, discitis, and epidural abscess (28, 29) (Figs. 34.32 to 34.34) As epidural abscesses may extend discontinuously over long areas of the spine, it is recommended that the entire spine be imaged, at least in sagittal plane, with supplemental multiplanar sequences in the area of clinical symptoms. I have seen a striking increase in the incidence of spinal infections, both in intravenous drug abusers and debilitated patients. By no means is the diagnosis of spinal infection uncommon anymore.

VASCULAR MALFORMATION

Perhaps the rarest cause of back pain—one that is often associated with a myelopathy—is a vascular malformation involving the spinal cord or surrounding dura mater (30–34). In preparation for either surgical resection or therapeutic embolization of a vascular malformation, selective spinal angiography remains necessary (Fig. 34.35). However, MRI has supplanted myelography in detection of intramedullary vascular malformations (Fig. 34.36) and often dura-based arteriovenous fistulas as well (Fig. 34.37).

In conclusion, MRI is the most comprehensive imaging procedure for the evaluation of neck and back pain. Particu-

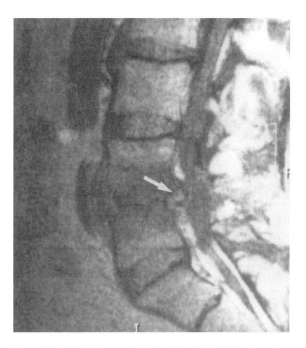

Figure 34.32.   Midline sagittal T1-weighted MRI of lumbar spine. Low (dark) signal within L4 and L5 vertebral bodies, with loss of distinction of L4-L5 disc space. Associated epidural mass (*arrow*) causes mild compression of dural sac. Diagnosis: discitis with osteomyelitis.

larly with the advent of capitated payment schemes creating ever-diminishing resources for care, an understanding by both referring clinician and radiological consultant of the appropriate indications for, capabilities, and limitations of diagnostic imaging studies has never been more relevant.

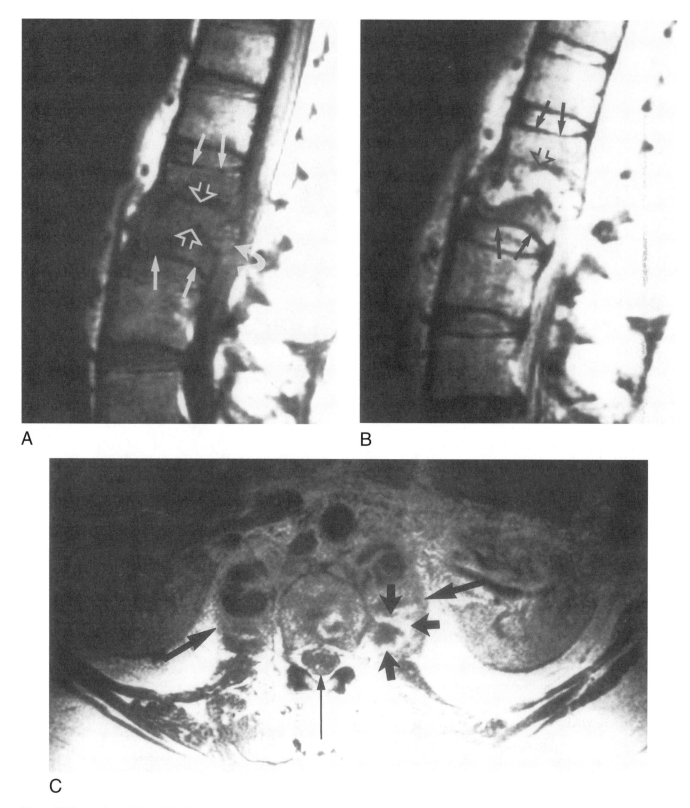

A

B

C

Figure 34.33.   A. Sagittal T1-weighted lumbar spine image. Note dark signal in contiguous vertebral bodies (*white arrows*) and marked disruption of the intervening disc (*hollow white arrows*). *Curved white arrow* points to retropulsed disc and vertebral body into central spinal canal. **B.** Sagittal T2-weighted image of lumbar spine in the same patient as view A. Formerly dark regions shown in view A now show bright signal (edema) in both the vertebral bodies (*black arrows*) and disrupted disc (*open arrow*). Diagnosis: tuberculous osteomyelitis and discitis. Retropulsed disc and bone created epidural abscess. Epidural abscesses can occur *without* accompanying osteomyelitis or discitis. **C.** Gadolinium enhanced axial T1-wieghted image through area of osteomyelitis and discitis, same patient as views A and B. Note rim enhancement of left psoas muscle abscess (*short thick arrows*). Psoas muscle margins shown by *long thick arrows*. *Thin arrow* points to normal thecal sac outlined by enhancing epidural abscess.

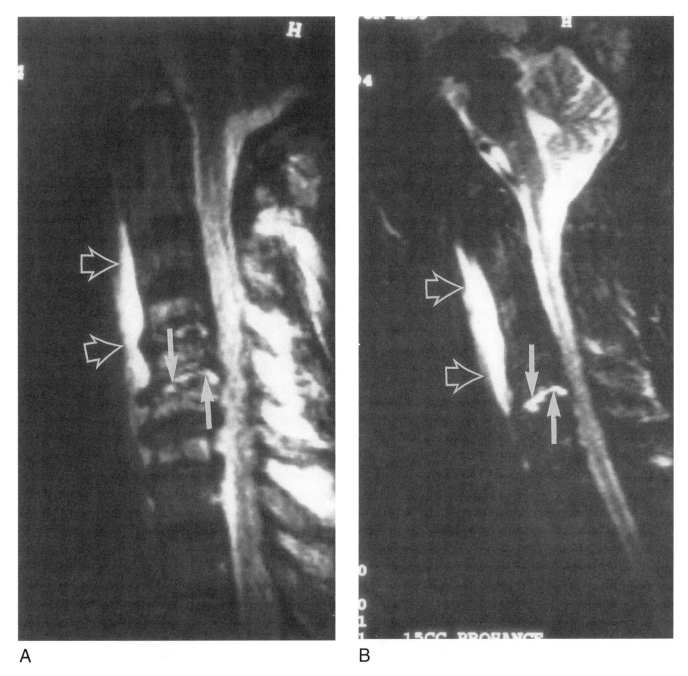

Figure 34.34. **A.** Sagittal T2-weighted cervical spine image shows prevertebral fluid collection (*open arrows*) and question of slightly elevated T2 signal in C5-C6 disc (*solid arrows*). Is there discitis? **B.** Sagittal STIR (more heavily T2-weighted image than in view A), same patient and anatomical location, unambiguously defines the high T2 signal in the C5-C6 disc (*solid arrows*), correlating this abnormality with the prevertebral fluid collection (*open arrows*). Flexible imaging strategies are often necessarily to define the extent of a pathological process, especially infectious disease.

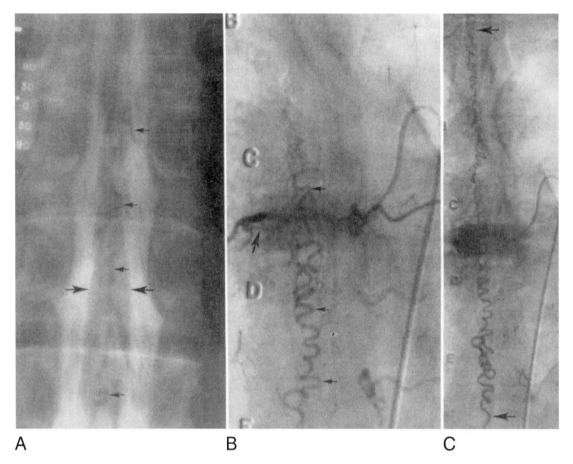

A   B   C

Figure 34.35. **A.** Myelography, anteroposterior view, shows tortuous vessel (*small arrows*) overlying spinal cord (*large arrows*).
B. Selective anteroposterior spinal arteriogram shows dural fistula (*large arrow*) and a portion of the tortuous vessel (*small arrows*)
seen on myelogram, representing an enlarged vein draining the malformation. **C.** Less magnified view of later phase of angiogram than
view B shows extent of draining vein (*arrows*).

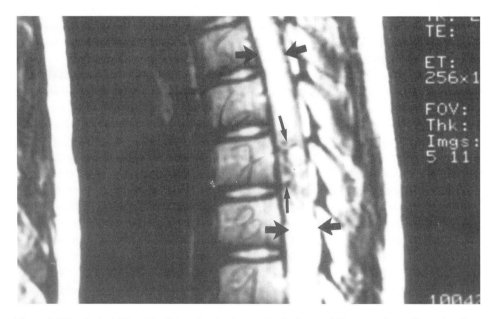

Figure 34.36.   Sagittal T2-weighted thoracic spine image showing intramedullary vascular malformation. Note
speckled appearance of the lesion (*small arrows*) representing abnormal vasculature within the cord, which would
be occult to visualization by myelography. Spinal cord (*large arrows*) shows diffuse edema, manifested as abnormally bright signal.

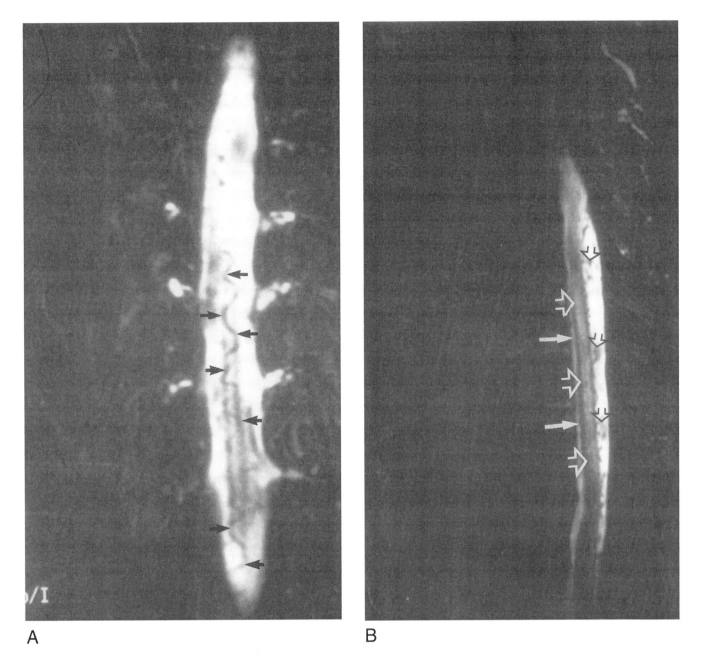

A   B

Figure 34.37.   A. Dural arteriovenous fistula. Coronal heavily T2-weighted scan of the thoracolumbar spine shows serpiginous vessel (*arrows*) along dorsal surface of the cord, representing dilated vein draining the fistula, the latter not shown on this scan. Identification of the fistula itself requires selective spinal angiography. The appearance of this scan is analogous to the myelographic image in Figure 34.35*A*. Therefore, MRI can replace myelography as the first examination searching for superficial spinal cord veins draining a dural fistula. **B.** Same patient as in view A. Sagittal heavily T2-weighted scan shows the serpiginous vessel (*black arrows*) on the dorsal cord surface, compatible with dilated vein draining the fistula. Edematous region (*open white arrows*) within the spinal cord (*solid white arrows*) likely represents venous congestion secondary to the abnormal vascular dynamics created by the fistula.

References

1. Olson P M, Wong W H M, Hesselink J R. Extraspinal abnormalities detected on MR images of the spine. AJR Am J Roentgenol 1994;162:679–684.

2. Boden S D, Davis D O, Dina T J. Abnormal magnetic resonance scans of the lumbar spine in asymptomatic subjects. J Bone Joint Surg (Am) 1990;72:403–408.

3. Jensen M C, Brant-Zawadksi M N, Obuchowski N. et al. Magnetic resonance imaging of the lumbar spine in people without back pain. N Engl J Med 1994;331:69–73.

4. Hackney D B, Asato R, Joseph P M, et al. Hemorrhage and edema in acute spinal cord compression: demonstration by MR imaging. Radiology 1986;161:387–390.

5. Masaryk T, Ross J S, Modic M T, et al. High resolution MR imaging of sequestered lumbar intervertebral disks. AJNR Am J Neuroradiol 1988;9:351–358.

6. Snow R D, Williams T P, Weber E D, et al. Enhancing transdural lumbar disc herniation. Clin Imag 1995;19:12–16.

7. Yock D. Magnetic resonance imaging of the CNS: a teaching file. ed. 3. St. Louis: Mosby, 1994;515.

8. Modic M, Masaryk T J, Ross J S. Magnetic resonance imaging of the spine. ed. 2. St. Louis: Mosby, 1994;165–175.

9. Osti O L, Fraser R D. MRI and discography in anular tears and intervertebral disc degeneration: a prospective clinical comparison. J. Bone Joint Surg Br 1992;74:431–435.

10. Linson M A, Crowe C H. Comparison of magnetic resonance imaging and lumbar discography in the diagnosis of disc degeneration. Clin Orthop 1990;250:160–163.

11. Min K, Leu H J, Perrenoud A. Discography with manometry and discographic CT: their value in patient selection for percutaneous lumbar nucleotomy. Bull Hosp Jt Dis 1996;54:153–157.

12. Gibson M J, Buckley J, Mawhinney R et al. Magnetic resonance imaging and discography in the diagnosis of disc degeneration: a comparative study of 50 discs. J Bone Joint Surg (Br) 1986;68:369–373.

13. Algra P R, Bloem J L, Tissing H, et al. Detection of vertebral metastases: comparison between MR imaging and bone scintigraphy. Radiographics 1991;11:219–232.

14. Carmody R F, Yang P J, Seeley G W, et al. Spinal cord compression due to metastatic disease: diagnosis with MR imaging versus myelography. Radiology 1989;173:225–229.

15. Smoker W R K, Godersky J C, Knutzun R K, Keyes W D. Role of MR imaging in evaluating metastatic spinal disease. AJR Am J Roentgenol 1987;8:901–908.

16. Williams M P, Cherryman G R, Husband J E. Magnetic resonance imaging in suspected metastatic spinal cord compression. Clin Radiol 1989;40:186–290.

17. Lien H H, Blomlie V, Heimdal K L. Magnetic resonance imaging of malignant extradural tumors with acute spinal cord compression. Acta Radiol 1990;31:187–190.

18. Avrahami E, Tadmor R, Dally O, et al. Early MR demonstration of spinal metastases in patients with normal radiographs and radionuclide bone scans. J Comput Assist Tomogr 1989;13:598–602.

19. Yousem D M, Patrone P M, Grossman R I. Leptomeningeal metastases: MR evaluation. J Comput Assist Tomogr 1990;14:255–261.

20. Dillon W P, Norman D, Newton T H, et al. Intradural spinal cord lesions: Gd-DTPA-enhanced MR imaging. Radiology 1989;170:229–238.

21. Elster A D. Radiologic screening in the neurocutaneous syndromes: strategies and controversies. AJNR Am J Neuroradiol 1992;13:1078–1082.

22. Poser C M. The relationship between syringomyelia and neoplasm. In American lecture series 262. American lectures in neurology. Springfield, IL: Charles C. Thomas, 1956.

23. Wolpert S M, Anderson M, Scott R M, et al. Chiari II malformation: MR imaging evaluation. AJR Am J Roentgenol 1987;8:783–792.

24. Barnes P D, Lester P D, Yamanashi W S, Prince J R. Magnetic resonance imaging in infants and children with spinal dysraphism. AJNR Am J Neuroradiol 1986;7:465–472.

25. Matthews W B. Clinical symptoms and signs. In: Matthews W B, Acheson E D, Batchelor J R, Weller R O, eds. McAlpine's multiple sclerosis. Edinburgh, Churchill-Livingstone, 1985; 104.

26. Edwards M K, Farlow M R, Stevens J C. Cranial MR in spinal cord MS: diagnosing patients with isolated spinal cord symptoms, AJNR Am J Neuroradiol 1986;7:1003–1006.

27. Schweitzer M E, Cervilla V, Resnick D. Acute cervical trauma: correlation of MR imaging findings with neurologic deficit. Radiology 1991;179:287–288.

28. Post M J D, Sze G, Quencer R M, et al. Gadolinium-enhanced MR in spinal infection. J Comput Assist Tomogr 1990:14:721–729.

29. Angtuaco E J C, McConnell J R, Chaddock W M, et al. MR imaging of spinal epidural sepsis. AJNR Am J Neuroradiol 1987;8:879–883.

30. Rosenblum B, Oldfield E H, Doppman J L et al. Spinal arteriovenous malformations: a comparison of dural arteriovenous fistulas and intradural AVM's in 81 patients. J. Neurosurg 1987;67:795–802.

31. Symon L, Kuyama H, Kendall B. Dural arteriovenous malformations of the spine: clinical features and surgical results in 55 cases. J Neurosurg 1984;60:238–247.

32. Masaryk T J, Ross J S, Modic M T, et al. Radiculomeningeal vascular malformations of the spine: MR imaging. Radiology 1987;164:845–849.

33. Terwey B, Becker H, Thron A K, Vahldiek G. Gadolinium DTPA enhanced MR imaging of spinal dural arteriovenous fistulas. J Comput Assist Tomogr 1989:13:30–37.

34. Larsson E M, Desai P, Hardin C W, et al. Venous infarction of the spinal cord resulting from dural arteriovenous fistula: MR imaging findings. AJNR Am J Neuroradiol 1991;12:739–743.

CHAPTER 35

Role of Diagnostic and Therapeutic Nerve Blocks in the Management of Pain

P. Prithvi Raj and Gabor B. Racz

The modern era of nerve blocks for pain control really began with the invention of the hollow needle by Rynd (1) in 1845 and the syringe by Pravaz (2) and Wood (3) during the 1850s. This prompted many efforts to treat painful disorders, such as trigeminal neuralgia, by injecting solutions of opioids, chloroform, bromides, tannin, alcohol, and other compounds near nerve trunks. Most of these procedures failed because all of the agents except alcohol lacked local anesthetic action. About the time that syringes and needles were being developed, in 1855, Gaedecke isolated cocaine from the juice of coca leaves; five years later Niemann (4) named it cocaine and reported its tongue-numbing effect for the first time. It was then studied extensively by many pharmacologists, including Bennett (5) and Von Anrep (6), who reported its anesthetic effects and suggested its use as a surgical anesthetic. As early as 1875 Collins, Fauvel, Saglia, and other French clinicians applied an extract of coca leaves topically to the pharynx and larynx to control the severe pain of tuberculosis and cancer (7). These were probably the first clinical applications of local anesthesia for pain control.

Unfortunately, all of these suggestions regarding its use as an anesthetic were ignored until Koller's report to the Ophthalmologic Congress in Heidelberg on September 15, 1884 (8). The report was received with enthusiasm. It prompted intensive laboratory research and the extensive clinical use of cocaine as a topical anesthetic for surgery in various parts of the body, and soon thereafter it was used widely to produce local infiltration analgesia.

Although these procedures were developed primarily for use in surgical anesthesia, it was not long before some physicians began to realize their value for the control of nonsurgical pain and other medical disorders. In 1885 Corning (9) reported the injection of cocaine into the spinal canal of dogs to produce anesthesia of the hind legs and subsequently used the method in a man who had been suffering from "spinal weakness and seminal incontinence." Corning was probably the first to produce both subarachnoid and extradural block.

DIAGNOSTIC NERVE BLOCKS

Diagnostic nerve blocks with local anesthetics are widely employed in pain management (10–20). They are performed to diagnose pain problems and predict the results of anatomical or ablative procedures (Table 35.1). Two assumptions are made if pain is relieved with local anesthetics: (*a*) the source of the pain is distal to the site infiltrated, and (*b*) pain relief predicts the long-term results of permanent ablative and/or anatomical procedures. The literature suggests that both of these assumptions may be incorrect. In fact, few studies have documented the value of performing isolated nerve blocks to help diagnose pain problems or to guide subsequent therapy (12, 21–23). While few studies assessing neural blockade have adequately demonstrated a high predictive value, these blocks continue to be performed (19, 24–26). Both the sensitivity and specificity of these blocks have been called into question by numerous studies over the past 25 years (27–30).

Differential Epidural and Nerve Blocks

Although differential nerve block resulting from the use of local anesthetics has been studied for many years, considerable controversy concerning the differential susceptibility of nerve fibers to local anesthetic conduction block remains. Some of the controversy stems from different approaches to the problem and different definitions of what constitutes differential block. Gasser and Erlanger (31) studied the effect of cocaine on the dog saphenous nerve. Although they found that

Table 35.1. Indications for Diagnostic Nerve Blocks

To diagnose pain-producing sites
To prognosticate results of ablative procedures
Caution: Sensitivity and specificity of the diagnostic nerve blocks are
undetermined

the compound action potential (CAP) of small nerve fibers disappeared before the CAP of large fibers, some of the large fibers had been blocked before all of the small fibers. This phenomenon is called a relative differential block or differential rate of block. Nathan and Sears (32) applied local anesthetics to cat spinal nerve roots. They found critical local anesthetic concentrations that would completely block small myelinated fibers without blocking large myelinated fibers. They referred to this phenomenon as an "absolute differential block" and required that equilibrium be established between the nerve and local anesthetic solution. Between small myelinated fibers and C (GR IV) fibers, they found a relative differential block; Aδ (GR III) fibers were blocked first. Franz and Perry (33) obtained single-unit recordings from the cat saphenous nerve and were able to produce an absolute differential block only when the local anesthetic was applied to less than 4 mm of nerve. When more than 4 mm of nerve was bathed in a procaine solution, a differential rate of block was obtained, with Aδ and C fibers being blocked before Aα fibers. Gissen et al. (34, 35) used desheathed rabbit vagus and sciatic nerve preparations and initially found a differential rate of block, with C fibers being blocked before Aα fibers. However, when equilibrium was established between the nerve and local anesthetic solution, the Aα fibers were blocked more extensively than were the C fibers.

While the technique of differential spinal block is not important to this discussion, it should be understood that two approaches, an anterograde and retrograde administration, are used. The latter is simpler, requiring only the use of one concentration sufficient to block all modalities, whereas the anterograde injection requires sequential use of three concentrations of local anesthetic after the saline placebo is first injected.

If the patient's pain is relieved by the first injection, the mechanism underlying the patient's pain is regarded as psychogenic. It is well established that 30 to 35% of patients who have true organic pain obtain relief from an inactive agent, so relief following the injection of normal saline may simply be a normal placebo (physiological) reaction. However, this response can usually be differentiated clinically from true psychogenic pain because the placebo reaction usually has rather short duration and is generally self-limiting. The possibility that pain is entirely psychogenic is substantiated or refuted by the findings of a psychological evaluation and when in doubt, repeated provocative tests of sympatholysis. If the patient does not obtain relief from the placebo injection and if he or she does obtain relief from the injection 0.25% procaine, a sympathetic mechanism is implicated as a basis of the patient's symptoms. This conclusion is reinforced when there are no signs of testable sensory blockade.

If the 0.25% procaine solution does not provide pain relief but the 0.5% procaine dose does, pain relief must be a factor of sensory block, that is, blockade of the Aδ (GR III) or C (GR IV) fibers, which suggests a somatic or organic basis for the patient's pain. However, if the patient does not obtain relief with either 0.25% or 0.5% procaine, 1% procaine (and some-

times when necessary 5% procaine) should be injected to produce blockade of all modalities. Should this concentration relieve the pain, the mechanism is still regarded as somatic, the presumption being that the patient has an elevated critical sensory blocking threshold. If the patient fails to obtain relief despite a complete sympathetic, sensory, and motor blockade, a central nervous system (CNS) mechanism is implicated. Central mechanisms include a lesion higher in the CNS than the level of the spinal anesthesia, psychogenic pain, the phenomenon known as encephalization, and malingering.

Although this technique of differential spinal blockade has proved to be extremely effective, it does have several drawbacks: (a) the technique is quite time-consuming because the physician must wait an adequate time after each injection to allow the various responses to become evident. When the 1% concentration of procaine does not provide a complete blockade of all modalities, an additional injection of 5% procaine is necessary; (b) each injection deposits an increasing amount of procaine in the subarachnoid space, so that considerable time is necessary for full recovery; (c) the anterograde administration requires the needle to remain in place throughout the procedure, which forces the patient to remain in the lateral position.

Because of its complexity and imposition on time, differential spinal block is now rarely used. It has been replaced by the epidural route, which can be applied at any segmental level. While an anterograde sequence of placebo solution and blocking concentrations of local anesthetics similar to the technique of differential spinal can be used, some consider the retrograde approach to have an advantage if there is a high functional or psychogenic overlay (Table 35.2). Usually normal saline followed by one of the short-acting local anesthetics, including 2-chloroprocaine, lidocaine, or mepivacaine, in a motor-blocking concentration is used. Interpretation of the results follows the same sequence as that for a spinal differential block.

Nerve Root Blocks

The study of Krempen et al. (22) is frequently quoted as support for the performance of diagnostic nerve root blocks. Krempen's study prospectively evaluated 22 patients with complicated back problems who were seen with sciatica as their major symptom. They placed needles at the site of nerve roots in an attempt to elicit the patient's typical pain. Once the pain was localized, they injected 1 mL of Pantopaque to assure needle position in the nerve root sleeve. After the characteristic radiographic pattern was obtained, they injected 1 mL of 1% xylocaine. Two patients had excellent relief of pain during the immediate postinjection period but decided against operation. Four had a negative test. Sixteen patients had excellent pain relief and proceeded to surgery; findings showed two with retained disc material, thirteen with scar tissue, and one with impingement of the articular process on the nerve root. Follow-up ranged from 8 to 24 months after surgery and showed no failures. These excellent results pro-

Table 35.2. Differential Epidural Blocks

Technique

Injection of NaCl; if there is *pain relief,* work up for psychogenic pain

If there is *no pain relief,* inject 3% 2-chloroprocaine or equivalent to cover the painful dermatome and 2 segments above

Wait for motor sensory and sympathetic block covering the painful area

Evaluate the *pain relief* when function of each nerve fiber returns (motor, sensory, sympathetic)

If pain returns with return of function of motor fiber, pain is transmitted through large A (Aβ) fibers

If pain returns with recovery of sensory fiber function, pain is transmitted through Aδ fiber

If pain does not return with return of sensory function, pain is transmitted through C fiber

vided a rationale for proceeding with diagnostic neural blockades, as individuals who responded favorably to the block had favorable outcomes with an anatomical procedure. However, the success of the operation was not assessed by an independent third party, and it is not clear what would have happened if they had operated for a negative diagnostic block. Thus, although all patients did well, it is possible that even patients with a negative response to the diagnostic blockade would have responded well to surgery; diagnostic neural blockade would simply not have been indicated.

Dooley et al. (12) also reported excellent results. They retrospectively studied 62 patients with lumbosacral radicular symptoms who had undergone nerve root infiltration, dividing them into four groups. Group 1 had typical pain reproduced by needle placement and then relieved by nerve root infiltration. Group 2 had typical pain reproduced by needle placement, but the pain was not relieved by local anesthesia and therefore indicated multiple root involvement. Patients with groups 3 and 4 did not have their typical pain reproduced by needle insertion, with or without relief of pain by local anesthesia, and were seldom relieved of radicular pain. Group 1 (44 patients) was 85% accurate in identifying a single nerve root as the sole cause of radicular symptoms; these patients had surgery. Group 2 (4 patients) showed incomplete relief and were suspected of having multiple-level root symptoms. Groups 3 and 4 (14 patients) had 6 patients defer surgery secondary to a negative response to the infiltration; only 5 patients had surgery with relief of symptoms. This study has been used to support a surgical intervention when a nerve root infiltration successfully abolishes the pain.

One should cautiously interpret Dooley and colleagues' observations. These patients could have had a positive response to the nerve block because of a placebo or systemic effects. This retrospective analysis could have been biased by the investigators' choice of cohorts. Conclusions on patient populations less than 100 (62 in this study) can be statistically flawed by an inadequate sampling number.

Onofrio and Campa (36) retrospectively studied 286 Mayo Clinic patients who had dorsal rhizotomies for intractable pain.

Of the 286, 112 had pain of unknown origin despite exhaustive investigation, and 81 had diagnostic blocks before consideration for surgery. A successful block encouraged the rhizotomy of the appropriate root. These investigators observed that the blocks were almost always unsuccessful and proved to be a very unreliable prognostic indicator of the result to be expected from section of the same roots.

Loeser (27) retrospectively studied 45 patients who had dorsal rhizotomies for relief of chronic pain. He extensively used nerve blocks in the preoperative evaluation of his patients but considered that the results of the nerve blocks did not enable the surgeon to predict the operative result. Patients with effective nerve blocks had a 20% long-term operative success rate; those with ineffective blocks had a 27% long-term success rate. Overall, 28% of the patients were successfully treated. Thus the diagnostic blocks were not helpful in guiding therapy.

Loeser's and Onofrio's results were later supported by North et al. (28), who reviewed their experience with a series of 13 patients with failed back surgery syndrome in whom dorsal root ganglionectomy was performed. Patients were selected on the basis of clinical presentation and diagnostic root blocks that suggested a monoradicular pain syndrome. The preoperative nerve block showed that nearly all patients reported 100% relief; one reported 95% relief and one, 90% relief. The block results were repeated and reproduced. Most but not all patients underwent additional blocks at other levels to confirm the specificity of their responses. Follow-up data were obtained at a mean of 5.5 years following dorsal root ganglionectomy. Treatment success (50% sustained relief of pain and patient satisfaction with the result) was recorded in two patients at 2 years after surgery and in none in 5.5 years. Equivocal success (at least 50% relief without clear-cut patient satisfaction) was recorded in one patient at 2 and 5.5 years postoperatively. Improvements in activities of daily living were recorded in a minority of patients. Loss of sensory and motor function was reported frequently by patients.

In a subsequent study North et al. (29) performed a prospective, randomized, controlled study to determine the specificity of diagnostic nerve blocks for sciatica pain; 33 consecutive patients with radicular pain of known spinal origin of at least 6 months' duration were studied. Each patient underwent a series of blocks with a total volume of 3 mL of 0.5% bupivacaine at the following sites: a single-level lumbosacral root block at L5 or S1, a medial branch posterior ramus block, a sciatic nerve block, and a lumbar subcutaneous block. Each procedure was performed under fluoroscopic guidance with a standard procedure for each patient. The results showed a specificity between 24% and 36%. Patterns of responses specific to the established diagnosis of radiculopathy had sensitivities between 9% and 42%. Statistical analysis of clinical and technical prognostic factors revealed that the only predictors of pain relief by any block were the effects of other blocks. The strongest association was between relief by sciatic nerve block and relief by medial branch posterior primary ramus (facet) block (p =.001; odds ratio, 16). There were no associations between the results of blocks and clinical findings (history, physical examination, diagnostic imaging) in these patients, chosen for their homogeneous clinical presentation and absence of functional signs. Nerve blocks do not reliably predict the results of anatomical and ablative procedures or of a successful diagnostic nerve block. The therapeutic management should consider options other than surgery.

Facet Blocks

In 1991 Goldthwait (37) demonstrated that pathology in the lumbar facet joints can result in axial pain radiating to the hips. Experimental studies on normal volunteers have shown that the lumbar and cervical zygapophyseal joints are capable of producing characteristic patterns of pain. This idea has led many to inject local anesthetics into this joint and the primary rami supplying the joints to assess for pain relief (38–45). The assumption is that if pain relief occurs with a diagnostic block, the patient will respond to a rhizolysis of the primary rami supplying that joint. However, the same problems that exist with diagnostic nerve root blocks also exist with diagnostic facet blocks; that is, a positive test with local anesthetic imperfectly predicts the outcome of permanent ablative or anatomical procedures. A range of studies have assessed the significance of diagnostic facet blocks.

Barnsley et al. (46) believed diagnostic blocks were a valid technique for the identification of painful zygapophyseal joints. They performed a randomized, double-blind, controlled comparative study of local anesthetic blocks for the diagnosis of cervical zygapophyseal joint pain, studying 47 patients with chronic neck pain following whiplash injury. Each patient was investigated with radiologically controlled blocks of the medial branches of the cervical dorsal rami to anesthetize the target cervical zygapophyseal joint. The blocks were performed with either lignocaine or bupivacaine, randomly allocated; and the patients' responses were assessed in a double-blind fashion. Any positive response was assessed by repeating the block with the complementary anesthetic. They found that 44 patients had pain relief from two blocks at a single level, of whom 31 had longer pain relief from bupivacaine (p=.0002). A subgroup had unexpectedly prolonged responses to one or both of the anesthetics. This study was valuable in its conclusion that uncontrolled diagnostic blocks could be compromised by a significant false-positive rate that seriously detracts from the specificity of the test.

Schwarzer et al. (47) questioned the existence of a facet syndrome and performed a prospective cross-sectional analytical study with 176 consecutive patients with chronic low back pain. Screening blocks were performed with lignocaine and confirmatory blocks with bupivacaine; 47% of patients had a definite or greater response to the screening injection at one or more levels, but only 15% had a 50% or greater response to a confirmatory block. They found that response to

zygapophyseal joint injection was not associated with any single clinical feature or set of clinical features.

Esses and Moro (48) wanted to ascertain the correlation between diagnostic facet blocks and treatment outcome, both surgical and nonsurgical. They reviewed 126 patients; 82 had a lumbar arthrodesis, and the rest had a variety of nonoperative therapies. Their statistical analysis failed to show any significant correlation between facet blocks and outcome for either surgical or nonsurgical patients.

North et al. (29) reviewed facet blocks' prognostic implications for radiofrequency facet denervation. Of the 82 patients studied, 42 reported at least 50% relief of pain following diagnostic medial branch posterior primary ramus blocks and proceeded to radiofrequency. Of the patients undergoing denervation, 45% reported at least 50% relief of pain at long-term follow-up. Among the 40 patients who underwent only temporary blocks, 13% reported relief (i.e., spontaneous improvement or placebo effect) by at least 50% at 1.6 years. By multivariate statistical analysis, patients undergoing bilateral blocks for bilateral or axial symptoms were significantly more likely to achieve temporary relief and to proceed to permanent denervation. There was no difference between the long-term results of bilateral denervation for bilateral or axial pain and those of unilateral denervation for unilateral pain. There was no significant difference in the rate of response between the 56 patients who had undergone lumbosacral spine surgery and the 26 who had not.

As this shows, diagnostic facet blocks have been examined by many researchers, and the interpretation of the results is in dispute. Clarity can occur when one considers this block part of the many diagnostic procedures one can offer to a patient and the results as part of the information that can be used to define an individual's pain.

Sympathetic Blocks

Recent studies indicate that the adequacy of sympathetic blockade in sympathetically maintained pain (SMP) does not consistently correlate with the degree of pain relief obtained (49). Notwithstanding the variables introduced by the widely differing technical skills, lack of uniform protocols, and as emphasized by Bonica and Buckley (11), the need for obsessive attention to detail when performing these sympatholytic regional anesthetic procedures, there are several other possible reasons for the relief of pain in the absence of successful sympathetic block. One is the previously mentioned placebo response (50, 51). A second reason is that the pain relief is due to the regional spread of local anesthetic to nearby somatic afferent nerves and their dorsal root ganglia (tracking of the solution alongside the rami communicantes, which can be avoided by the use of dynamic fluoroscopic imaging) (52). This regional spread may also occur with stellate ganglion injections and is of course inevitable when using epidural and intrathecal injections (53). A third possibility is the systemic absorption of locally injected lidocaine, which produces analgesia through an

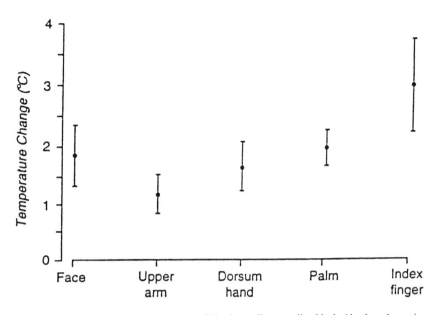

Figure 35.1.   Ipsilateral temperature change following stellate ganglion block. Absolute change in skin temperature of the ipsilateral arm increased with distance from the shoulder. Absolute temperature changes in the face were comparable with those in the palm. Error bars are plus or minus standard error of mean. (Reprinted with permission from Dellemijn HL, Fields RR, Allen WR, et al. The interpretation of pain relief and sensory changes following sympathetic blockade. Brain 1994;117:1475–1487.)

action distant from the injection site (e.g., dorsal root entry zone) (54). Fourth, in the case of pharmacological adrenoceptor blockade, drugs like phentolamine have many other effects, such as blocking ATP-regulated potassium ion channels so their site of action is not specifically on α-adrenergic receptors (55, 56). Given that none of the commonly used methods of reversible sympathetic block is truly specific, a false-positive diagnosis of SMP may be made whenever pain relief is achieved by any methods in common use. The evaluation of pain is subjective. A linear scale such as the visual analog scale (VAS), with units of 1 to 10 (or 10 to 100), with zero as no pain and 10 as excruciating (unbearable) pain, is used most commonly. As an example, a shift of 75%, for example from 10 to 3 or 7 to 0, from a patient's baseline pain on the VAS is consistent with a diagnosis of SMP. Obviously, because pain is subjective and continually variable, a smaller percentage reduction in a patient's pain symptoms, such as from 7 to 4, still represents a significant component of SMP. It also indicates some residual pain, which under the circumstances can be termed sympathetically independent pain (SIP) (57), that is, it is not affected by sympatholysis. This situation, however, presupposes that complete sympatholysis in this respect has been achieved.

In a study that compared the effects of stellate ganglion block and intravenous phentolamine in patients with a presumptive diagnosis of SMP, Dellemijn et al. (58) found that both procedures provide information that is complementary to, and may be necessary to substantiate, a clinical diagnosis (Fig. 35.1). In fact, the two procedures supply different information. For example, the change in skin temperature after sympathol-

ysis had no bearing on the relief of pain. In the case of phentolamine, usually associated with minimal skin temperature change, pain relief may correlate with the magnitude of systolic blood pressure fall. Interestingly, changes in the quantitative sensory testing (QST) over the thenar eminence following stellate ganglion block suggested that in this instance, pain relief was correlated with a partial deficit in thermal discrimination. To explain the greater relief of pain that was associated with stellate ganglion block, the authors provided at least two possibilities, neither of which is related to the degree of sympathetic blockade: systemic uptake of the local anesthetic and the potential spread to adjacent somatosensory nerves (Fig. 35.2). The foregoing aspect of this study corroborates the results of Treede et al. (49), who also found that pain relief from stellate ganglion and lumbar sympathetic conduction blocks are not related to the degree of sympathetic block. From the foregoing results, it is clear that supplemental testing of patients with a presumptive diagnosis of reflex sympathetic dystrophy or SMP requires the utmost care when monitoring the outcome of sympathetic blockade by either method. Because of its ability to document the effect of local anesthetic action on small-diameter axons, QST is useful when doubt as to the diagnosis remains. Not only should local anesthetic sympatholysis be undertaken in conjunction with the phentolamine test, but it also may be necessary to use intravenous lidocaine, when, for example, pain relief has been realized with stellate ganglion block but not phentolamine. Such an approach helps to exclude the possibility of diffusion by the local anesthetic to nearby spinal nerves.

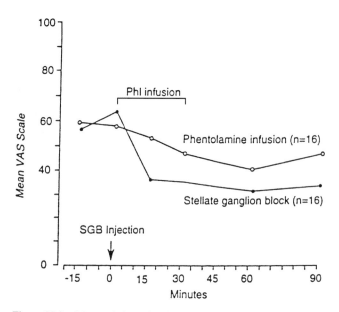

Figure 35.2. Mean pain intensity visual analog scale (VAS) scores during stellate ganglion block and phentolamine. Open circles represent phentolamine infusion, filled circles, stellate ganglion block. Phentolamine was administered at a constant rate during the 30-minute infusion period. (Reprinted with permission from Dellemijn HL, Fields RR, Allen WR, et al. The interpretation of pain relief and sensory changes following sympathetic blockade. Brain 1994;117:1475–1487.)

Lack of pain relief with effective sympathetic blockade can also occur. Obviously, if the pain is truly independent of activity within the sympathetic nervous system, no pain relief is expected. A more difficult problem is to determine whether sympatholysis in the area of interest has occurred. Obviously, only objective tests in the ipsilateral territory and not subjective observations will substantiate whether of the postganglionic sympathetic outflow has been interrupted (59, 60).

Quantitative thermal sensory testing is a useful tool for documenting blockade of small-caliber afferent axons from local anesthetic spread. With the stellate ganglion block, careful monitoring of the temperature changes on both hands may provide a better index of which patients achieve adequate blockade of sympathetic outflow than is attainable by simply measuring the temperature in the ipsilateral hand. Sympathetic block with intravenous phentolamine does not produce a sensory deficit and elicits minimal changes in skin temperature or none at all. Thus, although less potent in relieving pain at the 35-mg dose recommended by Raja et al. (61), phentolamine appears to be more specific in its action than is stellate ganglion block.

The differentiation of SMP from SIP depends on the sensitivity and specificity of the sympatholytic techniques. Unfortunately, no single technique now available is adequate to make this distinction. With this circumstance in mind, we can redefine SMP in the upper extremity as having the following characteristics: (a) pain that is relieved by both phentolamine infusion and stellate ganglion block, (b) no weakness or sensory deficit to either warm or cold stimuli

produced by sympathetic blockade by stellate ganglion injection, and (c) warmer temperature in the hand and face ipsilateral to the block following stellate ganglion block.

Problems with Diagnostic Blocks

An incorrect diagnosis with a temporary nerve block can be the result of either a false-positive or false-negative response. It is important to understand the possible sources of these experimental errors in interpreting the data.

False Positives

A false-positive result occurs when pain reduction occurs in the setting of a block but the pain relief resulted from some other factor. There are a number of possible explanations for this phenomenon: (a) the placebo response, (b) misleading reports from patients, (c) systemic uptake of local anesthetics and inadvertent spread of local anesthetics to adjacent structures, and (d) effects of needle placement.

Placebo Response

A placebo response occurs when pain reduction or abolition occurs by means other than the pharmacological conduction block by the anesthetic (62–66). Beecher (62) found that 35% of patients had a placebo response. Meleka et al. (65) noted a 50% false-positive response in patients with chronic pain undergoing diagnostic peripheral nerve blocks with normal saline solution. Accordingly, one needs to be aware of this phenomenon so that one does not perform an anatomical or ablative procedure that is not indicated.

Many psychological theories have addressed the placebo response. The psychological behaviorism theory of pain is a comprehensive new theory that can enable one to interpret placebo responses in the context of a neural blockade (67). This theory recognizes that the pain response is complex, incorporating the nociceptive input and the emotional state of the individual. It recognizes that a person who has a predominantly positive emotional state feels pain less intensely than those whose emotional state is predominantly negative. A placebo can be thought of as a stimulus that through classical (Pavlovian) conditioning, has come to elicit an emotional response in that person; this makes the placebo stimulus a conditioned stimulus. Therefore, in a placebo responder, the placebo elicits a positive emotional response, which lessens the negative emotional response elicited by the nociceptive stimulus. This functions to decrease the patient's report of pain.

If a diagnostic neural block (during which the patient experiences a large number of stimuli, some positive and some negative) is being performed and the patient reports a decrease in pain, the actual source of the decrease in pain can be confusing. If a patient has a high expectancy that a nerve block is likely to relieve the pain, the language stimuli that the practitioner uses or that a patient verbalizes may elicit a positive emotional response. Through a principle of algebraic summation, the person may have a decrease in pain from the language he or she used to describe the painful event (66) (see Fig. 35.3). One can avoid this situation by blinding the patient to one's test, performing multiple blocks at different levels and comparing the results of the block with a presumed normal (placebo) level.

Patients' Reports

Patients' reports may be misleading. Patients may feel a change in sensation in an area (e.g., warmth after a sympathetic block or numbness after a sensory block) and incorrectly state that there is decreased pain when in fact there is no change except in sensual perception. Local anesthetic blocks administered in an area of pain referral have been shown to provide temporary relief of pain, even when the source of pain is known to be remote. Some deceitful persons claim pain relief to obtain some secondary gain (i.e., further treatment, drugs).

Systemic Effects

Local anesthetics used in blocks can be systemically absorbed (68, 69). This confounds the evaluation because part of the effect witnessed may be from an unintentional central effect of one's agent. This problem can be avoided by using low volumes of local anesthetic in the block or by controlling with subcutaneous local anesthetic. Also, if one administers anxiolytic agents to individuals who have a high anxiety for pain, the simple relief of anxiety may cause a decrease in the report of pain.

Needle Placement

Myofascial pain can mimic pain from other anatomical sites. Some report a high correlation between acupuncture sites and trigger points. A treatment for deactivation of myofascial trigger points is dry needling and/or local injections of anesthetics. It is possible that trigger points can be deactivated or acupuncture sites treated in the process of performing another procedure more internal to these sites.

False Negatives

False negatives occur when a diagnostic block does not relieve pain from the site where the nidus of pain originates. This problem can arise in some of the following scenarios: (*a*) inadequate spread of local anesthetic to the involved nerve or a technically inadequate block, (*b*) referral of pain, and (*c*) misunderstanding of instructions by the patient.

Nerve fibers may not all be completely blocked, and alternative pathways may continue to provide nociceptive input from the same site or structure (70). It is possible that there are two nidi for a patient's pain. If there are multiple sources of pain and only one is anesthetized, the pain is likely to persist. With this paradigm a small number of patients may be

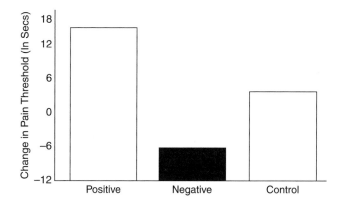

Figure 35.3. Effects of placebos on pain threshold: change in pain threshold from pretest to posttest in the positive placebo, negative placebo, and control participants.

Table 35.3.   Problems with Diagnostic Blocks

False positives
False negatives
Unreliable communications
Poor skills of the performer

missed. One may be able to overcome this problem by performing confirmatory tests with contrast to identify a structure or with a neurostimulator before performing the block.

There have been anecdotal reports of pain relief with local anesthetic blocks directed into an area of referral. Cutaneous blocks can relieve pain (71, 72). North et al. (73) documented that sciatic nerve blocks and posterior rami facet blocks may produce temporary relief in a majority of patients with known spinal pathology. Referred pain may also show a predilection for sites of previous pain (74). A nonspecific reduction in afferent input may result in temporary relief of central pain (27, 75). One must keep these possibilities in mind when performing a block.

Some patients have poor communication skills, have a difficult time rating their pain, or are unable to compare their pain before and after the procedure. Some patients may have ulterior motives and give false information; psychological evaluation usually reveals serious personality disorders (Table 35.3).

In summary, diagnostic nerve blocks lack specificity. A positive response from a single diagnostic test is difficult to interpret by itself. On the other hand, if a patient undergoes multiple blocks in a placebo-controlled manner and pain relief follows a single test, this information may help guide therapy. Negative results of diagnostic tests may also help exclude various sources of the pain. Information on the results of permanent ablative or anatomical procedures following negative test of positive results, performed in a placebo-controlled manner, are not available. Well-controlled studies addressing the role of these procedures should be carried out. Although a single positive diagnostic test result provides little information, if used in conjunction with the findings from several placebo-controlled nerve blocks or discograms, useful diagnostic information can be obtained.

THERAPEUTIC BLOCKS

In the past 30 years significant advances have been made in the understanding and management of pain. However, pain is one of the most subjective complex human experiences and one whose complete understanding is elusive. There is no general agreement among the experts in the field about the nature of the pain experience, classification of chronic pain states, underlying causes, pain mechanisms, or ways to manage pain. However, interest in the management of pain patients has increased significantly and the role of pain specialists from various disciplines has been critically evaluated.

There is a growing challenge by the other pain specialists as to the role of nerve blocks in managing chronic pain patients. Data continue to be published in the journals *Pain, Psychiatry,* and *Neurosciences,* pointing out that in management of patients with chronic benign pain, noninvasive techniques have been more successful and longer-lasting than nerve blocks. Furthermore, they argue that the nerve blocks provide only transient relief and hence not enough for chronic pain patients. Even though this concept has been held by pain specialists other than anesthesiologists generally, there is some evidence of change in these long-held views. Recently basic researches have shown that nerve blocks have prevented central sensations or diminished them over a long period. Furthermore, when chronic pain patients could not improve their functions any further, nerve blocks have provided better function by allowing the patients to comply with other facets of their program.

Generally, pain syndromes are classified as neurogenic, musculoskeletal, sympathetic, visceral, or psychogenic in origin. They can cause acute or chronic pain states. Treatment and outcome vary between acute and chronic counterparts.

In acute syndromes such as herpes zoster or early sympathetic dystrophy, prognosis is good, and aggressive therapy is recommended. In contrast, in chronic pain states such as postherpetic neuralgia, arthritis, and diabetic neuropathy, prognosis is guarded, and one expects to cope with pain and not be cured. This is best achieved by multidisciplinary modalities rather than by an individual physician's management. Cancer pain, even though it may be prolonged, is treated differently from chronic pain because of the shortened life span, and one's goal is to provide improved quality of life even if it is at the cost of function.

The techniques that are useful for pain management are (*a*) systemic analgesic administration, (*b*) intravenous (IV) local anesthetic administration, (*c*) nerve blocking with local anesthetics, opioids, or neurolytics, (*d*) surgical ablation of nociceptive pathways, (*e*) placement of electrodes for stimulation produced analgesia, and (*f*) psychotherapy. Most of the techniques of nerve blocking are described in this chapter (Table 35.4).

Intravenous Local Anesthetics

Use of intravenous local anesthetic has been beneficial in managing pain syndromes due to burns, deafferentation syndrome, Raynaud's disease, phantom limb, causalgia, diabetes, neuritis, and myofascitis.

Table 35.4.   Therapeutic Nerve Blocks: Common Procedures

Intravenous local anesthetic administration
Subcutaneous infiltration
Continuous epidural analgesia
Continuous subarachnoid infusion
Continuous peripheral analgesia
Continuous sympathetic blocks
Implantable drug delivery systems
Radiofrequency
Cryolysis
Neuromodulation

Mechanism of Action

Leriche (76) proposed that injury to tissue caused reflex vasoconstriction, resulting in anoxia, capillary dysfunction, and increased permeability. This process would lead to the accumulation of nociceptive metabolites and the irritation of peripheral nerve endings. He believed that procaine, by acting directly on the arteriolar, meta-arteriolar, and capillary endothelia, produced widespread vasodilation, thereby anesthetizing the irritated endothelial nerve endings and breaking the reflex arc.

Choice of Drug

Procaine is the classic local anesthetic agent for intravenous administration because of its potency and low toxicity; however, its short action, even at maximum dosages, is its major disadvantage. Hatangdi et al. (77) used IV lidocaine in a range of 1 to 1.5 mg/kg. They reported complete relief of lancinating pain within seconds after injection. In addition, the degree of success with intravenous lidocaine often predicted response to oral antiepileptic drugs. Boas et al. (68) used lidocaine in patients with deafferentation syndrome and noted significant pain relief within 15 to 20 minutes of starting the infusion. Recently there has been a focus on the intravenous administration of 2-chloroprocaine. Parris et al. (78) successfully used a 60-mL bolus of intravenous 3% chloroprocaine solution to control pain associated with partial splenic embolization. Schnapp (78a) used intravenous chloroprocaine to treat chronic intractable pain, and 43% of the patients reported more than 50% relief lasting longer than 30 days. Phero (78b) considered intravenous chloroprocaine to be safe and efficacious in managing certain chronic intractable pain, particularly musculoskeletal pain.

Monitoring

Monitoring of the patient during intravenous infusion of local anesthetic is essential. The patient's vital signs (electrocardiogram [ECG], blood pressure, heart rate, and mentation) are evaluated every 5 minutes.

Side Effects

The side effects of intravenous local anesthetics, which have long been documented, are associated with CNS toxicity. Early signs and symptoms include metallic taste, tinnitus, light-headedness, agitation, and drowsiness. Moderate signs of CNS toxicity include difficulty with ocular focusing, nystagmus, slurred speech, dysarthria, numbness in the lips and tongue, and tingling or a heavy feeling in the extremities.

Subcutaneous Infiltration

Subcutaneous infiltration is useful for acute herpes zoster and postherpetic neuralgia, neuroma, painful subcutaneous fibrotic nodules, and spermalgia or labial pain in the groin. For herpetic pain, a solution of 0.2% triamcinolone in 0.25% bupivacaine or dexamethasone (16 mg/50 mL) in 0.125% bupivacaine is prepared. The solution (10 to 50 mL) is injected subcutaneously throughout the area of intense pain or in the vesicular distribution. The total number of such treatments ranges from 1 to 10, with an average of 4. In acute herpes zoster, the treatments are given two to three times weekly, while in postherpetic neuralgia, it can be done weekly and may require as many as 12 treatments before pain diminishes.

For neuroma and other subcutaneous nodular or fibrotic pain, local anesthetic with steroid is injected four to six times on a weekly basis. The majority of the patients obtain tolerable pain relief with this regimen. Those with persistent pain after this may be candidates for neurolytic procedures.

Continuous Regional Blocks

Infusion techniques with catheters located in the epidural and subarachnoid spaces and on the peripheral nerves are now commonly used for acute and chronic pain patients. For patients who are suffering from acute pain, continuous infusion has been beneficial for trauma, postsurgical pain, and acute medical diseases. Similarly, for chronic pain sufferers the technique has been useful for rehabilitation of patients with chronic low-back pain, reflex sympathetic dystrophy, peripheral neuropathy, and cancer pain. If the patient needs a sensory, motor and/or sympathetic blockade that is considerably longer than that provided by long-acting local anesthetics, continuous regional anesthesia is indicated. The goal is to provide prolonged pain relief to a segregated portion of the body, using the smallest dose of the drugs infused, thus minimizing side effects. It is also indicated for facilitating early mobilization, increasing distal limb vascularity, and improving nutrition. Continuous regional anesthesia is commonly administered into epidural sites (cervical, thoracic, lumbar), subarachnoid spaces, peripheral nerves (brachial plexus, lumbar plexus, femoral, sciatic), and sympathetic nerves and plexus.

Continuous Epidural Analgesia

Continuous epidural analgesia is not a new concept (79–81). The first description of this technique, in 1949, consisted of administering intermittent boluses of a local anesthetic for 1 to 5 days postoperatively (82). Although effective analgesia was obtained, significant sympathetic blockade accompanied the pain relief with fluctuating levels of analgesia as the effect of the bolus began to regress. In addition, continuous analgesia with intermittent bolus injections is labor intensive and requires skilled personnel to reassess and treat the patient every few hours. Because of these shortcomings, continuous epidural infusion has now become commonplace.

Continuous epidural infusion offers therapeutic advantages over intermittent boluses. The primary advantage of continuous epidural infusion is that it provides continuous analgesia rather than intermittent dosing. Although single boluses of opioids such as epidural morphine may provide 12 hours of pain relief, a wide variability is reported in the duration of effective analgesia, ranging from 4 hours to 24 hours (83, 84). Because of this, it is difficult to titrate uniform levels of pain relief. Continuous infusions allow easier titration, particularly with shorter-acting opioids such as fentanyl or sufentanil. Epidurally administered fentanyl has an onset of action within 4 to 5 minutes and a peak effect within 20 minutes (85–87). This rapidity in onset facilitates adjustment in dosage because the patient quickly appreciates subjective pain relief.

For the intermittent bolus technique to be successful, longer-acting agents such as morphine and hydromorphone must be administered to provide a reasonable duration of analgesia. These opioids are associated with a higher risk of delayed-onset respiratory depression (84).

Catheter Location

Segmental limitation of epidural analgesia mandates placing an epidural catheter at sites adjacent to dermatomes covering the field of pain. This reduces dose requirements while increasing the specificity of spinal analgesia (88, 89). Suggested interspaces where catheters are usually located for epidural infusion of analgesic solutions are thoracic surgery, T2-T8; upper abdominal surgery, T4-L1; lower abdominal surgery, T10-L3; upper extremity surgery, C2-C8; and lower extremity surgery, T12-L3.

Analgesic Agents

Continuous epidural analgesia is usually provided via a local anesthetic, an opioid, or an opioid and a local anesthetic combined.

Local Anesthetic Agents   Local anesthetic agents are best used to provide analgesia and anesthesia for patients undergoing surgery and to maintain postoperative pain relief. Lidocaine and bupivacaine are both effective for achieving and maintaining adequate analgesia (87, 90). In general, lidocaine use is limited to bolus form to establish or rescue a block, whereas bupivacaine can be used as an infusion. Development of tachyphylaxis is a problem inherent in bolus administration of a local anesthetic through the epidural catheter. Tachyphylaxis does not develop when bupivacaine is administered as an infusion. Continuous infusion of dilute local anesthetic solutions has simplified maintenance and improved analgesic uniformity; however, concentrations sufficient to produce pain relief usually result in progressive sensorimotor blockade. Such deficits are undesirable, since the ability to walk is compromised.

Local anesthetic agents alone can accumulate in the systemic circulation (87, 91). This accumulation is more pronounced with the short-acting amides such as lidocaine than the longer-acting amides. The decrease in systemic effects with longer-acting agents has been attributed to more nonspecific binding of the longer-acting agents in the fat of the epidural space, compared with the shorter-acting amides.

A constant-rate infusion of 0.25% and above of bupivacaine has been associated with hypotension, muscle weakness, sensory block, and possible accumulation of toxic systemic levels of bupivacaine (87). Higher plasma levels of the agent may occur in the elderly and frail. Side effects can be attenuated by use of lower concentrations. A low-dose, constant-rate infusion of epidurally administered bupivacaine (0.03% to 0.06%) close to the dermatomal level desired for pain relief can decrease the incidence of side effects. Although a low dose of bupivacaine is effective, it provides a level of analgesia less profound than that provided by a combination of bupivacaine and low concentrations of epidurally administered morphine or the use of opioids alone (87, 92, 93).

Opioid and Local Anesthetic Combination In an effort to combine the desirable analgesic properties of local anesthetics and epidural opioids, several investigators have described the concomitant use of morphine-bupivacaine epidural infusions for pain relief (94–97). These studies demonstrate either additive or synergistic analgesic activity between a variety of opioids and dilute concentrations of bupivacaine (88, 96, 98). Such combinations provide pain relief of greater magnitude than the relief attained with either agent alone. The incidence and severity of side effects are minimized. This advantage may be explained by the different analgesic properties of each class of agents and their ability to block pain at two different sites in the spinal cord. Opioids produce analgesia by specifically binding and activating the opiate receptors in the substantia gelatinosa, whereas local anesthetics provide analgesia by blocking impulse transmission at the nerve roots and dorsal root ganglia.

Bupivacaine in concentrations of 0.03% to 0.125% has been combined most often with morphine, fentanyl, or meperidine. Morphine and bupivacaine use has resulted in effective analgesia in the management of patients after thoracic, abdominal, and general surgery (87, 93, 99, 100). However, fentanyl combined with bupivacaine had a lower incidence of side effects than the morphine-bupivacaine combination. Bupivacaine 0.03% to 0.125% mixed with fentanyl 2 to 3 µg/mL given at 8 to 10 mL/hour to a 70-kg patient usually provides excellent analgesia with minimal respiratory depression and sensory motor blockade. Bupivacaine 0.03% combined with 0.005% morphine or 2 to 3 µg/mL fentanyl and infused at 8 to 10 mL/hour achieves similar results for chronic pain patients.

Specific concentrations of drugs and rates of infusion should be tailored to individual patients. For example, it is possible to treat or prevent significant hypotension by decreasing the local anesthetic concentration, eliminating the local anesthetic, decreasing the rate of a combined local anesthetic-opioid infusion, or infusing intravenous fluids. Sedation or carbon dioxide retention can be treated by changing the specific epidurally administered opioid, decreasing the chances of respiratory depression.

Limitations of Continuous Epidural Analgesia

There are limitations to epidural infusion analgesia. One is that it cannot independently control pain from multiple sites. Epidural analgesia normally can provide analgesia for five to seven continuous dermatomal regions, such as L4-S5 or T2-T8. Patients with multiple injuries may require other forms of pain control.

In addition, the site of the epidural catheter influences the adequacy of pain relief and maintenance of normal vital function. In general, placing of the epidural catheter within the dermatomal distribution of the pain achieves the best results with the least amount of drug. For example, pain from a thoracotomy is best treated with a thoracic epidural infusion, and pain in the lower extremity requires a lumbar epidural infusion.

Patient-Controlled Epidural Analgesia

Patient-controlled epidural analgesia has been offered to patients recovering from intra-abdominal, major orthopaedic, or thoracic surgery and for chronic pain states such as those due to cancer. It has several potential advantages. Patients can titrate analgesic doses in amounts proportional to their level of pain intensity. Because of large variations of pain relief from person to person (101), this can optimize spinal opioid analgesia. Most of the published work describing patient-controlled epidural analgesia comes from Europe (101, 102). Chrubasik and Wieners (102) compared three epidural opioids using patient-controlled epidural analgesia technique. These studies showed that the self-administered morphine dosage required for effective analgesia was much smaller than the amount used with continuous epidural opioid and intravenous patient-controlled analgesia (PCA) techniques (103–105) and that the patients' serum morphine levels were very low. Table 35.5 lists various investigators, the opioids used in their studies, and the average hourly consumption.

Technique with Morphine

To apply patient-controlled epidural analgesia using morphine (106), one places catheters using standard techniques. Patients are administered a loading dose of 2 to 3 mg of preservative-free morphine, and a basal infusion of 0.4 mg/hour (0.02% solution) is started. Patients are allowed to self-administer 0.2 mg morphine every 10 to 15 minutes, with a maximum dose of 1 to 2 mg/hour. The loading dose is administered only after a local anesthetic test dose (2 to 3 mL of lidocaine 2%) has demonstrated that the catheter is not in the subarachnoid space. The optimal size of the loading dose and the timing of administration have yet to be determined; however, because of morphine's latency-to-peak effect, the loading dose must be given as early as possible. Breakthrough pain is common in these patients during the first 6 to 8 hours.

Breakthrough pain is treated with epidural morphine boluses of 0.5 to 1 mg/hour. If two doses are inadequate to provide analgesia, the catheter should be retested with local anesthetic to confirm epidural placement and to rule out dislodgment. The loading dose can be augmented with fentanyl 50 to 100 μg administered epidurally. This drug speeds the onset of the analgesia, possibly because of dual action, that is, rapid vascular uptake and epidural intense neuraxial action.

Alternative Choice of Analgesic Agents With Patient-Controlled Epidural Analgesia

Lipophilic Opioids

Fentanyl, sufentanil, and hydromorphone can be used with a patient-controlled epidural infusion technique; however, the amount of drug needed to provide effective analgesia appears to be much greater than equivalent doses of morphine. Administration of lipophilic opioids by continuous infusions and/or patient-controlled epidural analgesia has been questioned by several authors (108, 109). Estok et al. (109) showed that fentanyl administered by intravenous PCA or patient-controlled epidural analgesia provided equivalent analgesia. Epidurally administered lipophilic opioids may have special use when the drug is administered via thoracic epidural catheters, when there is a need to speed the onset of epidural opioid analgesia, and when the drug has to be given in a large volume of dilute solution or combined with local anesthetics.

Efficacy

Cohen et al. (110, 111) compared combinations of fentanyl, bupivacaine, and buprenorphine-bupivacaine for patient-controlled epidural analgesia. The average hourly doses of opioid were minimized, presumably because of the effective analgesia provided by concurrently administered bupivacaine, so that 24-hour serum concentrations were low. Lipophilic agents may be useful for breakthrough pain, especially in the first few hours postoperatively.

Local Anesthetics

Patient-controlled epidural analgesia with local anesthetics has been reported to be safe and effective during labor. The technique was first described in 1988 by Gambling et al. (112), who compared bupivacaine (0.125%) delivered epidurally via PCA with patient-controlled epidural analgesia continuous infusion. They found that bupivacaine delivered via patient-controlled epidural analgesia was better than that administered via continuous epidural infusion; patients in the patient-controlled epidural analgesia group required significantly less bupivacaine to provide similar analgesia. The technique was believed to be safe, reliable, and not associated with excessive sensory blockade (Table 35.6).

Continuous Subarachnoid Infusion

Intraspinal infusion of opioids has commonly been used for management of intractable cancer pain (117, 118). These infusions have been maintained with implanted pumps connected to intrathecal catheters. The treatment of patients with severe, chronic noncancer pain in the lower body has been difficult. Included among the possible causes of this pain are arachnoiditis, epidural scarring, vertebral body compression fracture, reflex sympathetic dystrophy, phantom limb, and/or thoracotomy. Intraspinal infusions are increasingly being used

Table 35.5.   Consumption of Opiates Based on Reports by Various Authors

Investigator	PCA Epidural Opiates (mg/hour)	Average Consumption
Sjöström (101)	Morphine sulfate	0.52
Marlowe (106)	Hydromorphone	0.10
Walmsley et al. (107)*	Morphine sulfate	0.47
Chrubasik et al. (102)*	Morphine sulfate	0.25
Sjöström (101)	Demerol	18.00

*Infusion of patient-controlled epidural analgesia

Table 35.6.   Technique of Patient-Controlled Epidural Analgesia

Author	Analgesic drug	Additional drug	Continuous infusion (mL/hr)	PCA dose (mL)	Lockout (minutes)	Comments
Gambling (113)	Bupivacaine 0.125%	1:400,000 Epinerphrine	—	4	20	Greater satisfaction with patient-controlled epidural analgesia than continuous infusion
Gambling (112)	Bupivacaine 0.125%	—	4	4	20	Patient-controlled epidural analgesia group used less local than continuous infusion group
Lysak (114)	Bupivacaine 0.125%	Fentanyl 1 μg/mL	6	4	10	Fewer top-ups needed than in continuous infusion group
Viscomi (115)	Bupivacaine 0.125%	Fentanyl 1 μg/mL	4	4	10	Fewer top-ups needed than in continuous infusion group
Naulty (116)	Bupivacaine 0.063%	Sufentanil 0.3 μg/mL	5	2	6	No advantage over continuous infusion

with minimal complications and limited instances of drug tolerance in these noncancer patients (119–123). For these infusions, programable infusion pumps have infusion rates that can be tailored to the patient's needs at any time with an external programer. These pumps have been extensively tested and found to be quite reliable and cost effective (123).

Analgesic Agents

Morphine is the usual agent for these infusions. For temporary or prolonged intraspinal infusions, in resistant cases the addition of dilute bupivacaine to the morphine infusion has improved pain relief (123, 124).

Efficacy

In a study of 15 patients with intractable pain from reflex sympathetic dystrophy and arachnoiditis with a follow-up of 2 to 44 months, pain relief was reported as excellent by 8 patients, good by 3, and fair by 4 (125); 6 patients returned to work. Few complications occurred, but most patients needed increasingly larger doses over time to maintain pain relief. Richard and Kanoff conclude that intraspinal infusion of morphine sulfate via an implanted externally programable pump is safe and effective in selected patients with intractable pain of nonmalignant origin.

They note that spinal morphine dose requirements increase over time. All patients should be started at the lowest dose possible to avoid early toxicity, overdosing, or overtreating. Each patient reaches pain relief at a different level, as evidenced by the effective therapeutic range of morphine, extending from 6.275 mg/24 hours to 57 mg/24 hours among the patients in their study group. Most patients respond fairly well with a continuous infusion at the onset of therapy. When they become active as their pain decreases, they become aware that the pain is most intense at certain times of the day. As a result, individual dose patterns must be established. Such individualization can be done efficiently only with an externally programable infusion system. The medication is well tolerated in most cases and is without significant side effects. It may allow return to a more normal lifestyle, including improved ability to perform activities of daily living and resumption of work in many cases. The best results are found among well-motivated patients with realistic goals and a clear understanding of spinal morphine therapy who have demonstrated appropriate responses during a screening trial. Meticulous attention to detail in the care and maintenance of the system and a willingness by the clinician to devote ample time to the patient maximize the effectiveness of this modality.

CONTINUOUS PERIPHERAL ANALGESIA

Peripheral continuous techniques are usually carried out exactly like a single-injection technique (126). A variety of catheter and needle systems are available for use in providing continuous blockade. Early on, catheters were inserted through needles. While providing protection of the catheter during insertion, the hole made by the needle in the sheath was often larger than the catheter, resulting in leakage of local anesthetic after removal of the needle. The use of thin-bore needles with catheters over the needle has improved the success of continuous techniques. When the sheath has been penetrated, identified by either paresthesia or with the use of a nerve stimulator, the catheter is advanced slightly as the needle is withdrawn. Sometimes it is best first to inject a test dose of local anesthetic through the needle to expand the perivascular space. If the catheter is to be used for several days or if movement is a problem, a second smaller catheter, similar to a nylon epidural catheter, can be advanced through the first catheter and further into the perivascular compartment.

Continuous Brachial Plexus Infusion

Indications

For 2 decades prolonged brachial plexus blocks have been performed perioperatively for trauma and postoperative pain (127). Prolonged sympathetic blocks have also been performed for vascularly compromised patients (128). Catheters have been placed on the brachial plexus after surgery for pain relief up to 48 hours post surgery. With the experience obtained with acute perioperative patients, prolonged brachial plexus analgesia has now been tried for intractable patients such as those with complex regional pain syndrome I and II and phantom pain (129).

Site

The brachial plexus is an ideal location for a continuous regional technique because of its well-defined perivascular compartment and the close approximation of the large number of nerves supplying the upper extremity. All techniques of brachial plexus blockade have been described as continuous, but some are easier to achieve than others. An axillary approach is easy to perform, and the technique is familiar to many. Unfortunately, movement of the upper extremity, either passive or active, can dislodge the catheter. Hair and moisture in the axilla also can make maintaining a sterile environment difficult at best. The interscalene technique can be difficult in terms of placement because the approach is 90° to the skin, making it difficult to thread the catheter. A subclavian perivascular approach allows easy threading of the catheter, and the catheter position is not affected by head or neck movements. The infraclavicular approach to the brachial plexus allows easy threading of the catheter and is not affected by patient movement (130).

All four approaches to the brachial plexus have been tried for insertion of a catheter for continuous infusion (131, 132). The most often performed technique is at the axilla, perhaps because of the familiarity of the anesthesiologist with insertion of an intra-arterial catheter. This was the impetus to try this technique initially. It has remained popular ever since. The interscalene approach has been used by some clinicians. Technically it is simple. However, the catheters do not stay at the site longer than 48 hours. The infraclavicular approach is preferred by another group of clinicians who perform this block routinely. It has the advantage of maintaining the catheter in the same position for long periods, sometimes as long as 3 weeks.

Drugs and Technique

Even though lidocaine and mepivacaine have been used for continuous infusion, the most commonly chosen local anesthetic is bupivacaine. In a typical case, after the catheter is placed on the brachial plexus, a bolus of 20 to 30 mL of 0.5% bupivacaine or a 1:1 mixture of 2% lidocaine and 0.5% bupivacaine is administered. Monitoring is mandatory for at least 45 minutes, during which time the onset of block is tested. If adequate block is present, up to 10 mL/hour of either 0.25% or 0.125% bupivacaine is administered via an infusion pump. Steady state is reached in five half-lives, that is, approximately 18 hours. The infusion should be started within 2 hours before the bolus effect wears off. Before 18 hours are reached, however, the bolus block is expected to wear off (usually after 6 hours). The infusion of 0.25% bupivacaine would not be effective to maintain analgesia for another 12 hours. If there is intolerable pain at 6 hours, it is imperative to provide another 20-mL bolus of 0.5% bupivacaine. Monitoring is required for 45 minutes, as with the initial bolus.

In the past decade adjuvant drugs have been used in brachial plexus infusions. Drugs that have been administered with bupivacaine include narcotics and clonidine. Their efficacy is still to be determined.

The plasma concentration and pharmacokinetics of brachial plexus infusion in a steady state are similar to that seen with epidural infusion. Once the steady state is reached, the drugs infused do not accumulate if infused at the same rate. The metabolites also remain at an insignificant level without causing any deleterious effect. However, brachial plexus infusion should be used with caution in patients with liver and kidney disease.

Efficacy

For periods up to 48 hours, the continuous brachial plexus analgesia is reliably efficacious. After that period, the efficacy drops precipitously, for Aδ fiber blocking. Sympathetic blocking can still be maintained for up to 2 to 3 weeks with 0.125% or 0.25% bupivacaine, quite reliably if catheters are well anchored. The best site for catheter insertion seems to be the infraclavicular region. The second best site is the axilla. The interscalene site is too superficial for reliable anchoring for prolonged periods.

Continuous Lower-Extremity Peripheral Nerve Infusion

Lumbosacral Plexus Catheterization

Placement of a lumbosacral catheter with an epidural needle has been reported by Vaghadia et al. (133). Successful blockade of the lumbar and sacral plexus was achieved for unilateral lower-extremity surgery. The catheter is placed between the quadratus lumborum and psoas muscles between the transverse processes of L4 and L5. The technique is not difficult and seems highly successful. The main disadvantage is the volume of local anesthetic needed, 40 to 70 mL.

Sciatic Nerve Catheterization

Many of the nerves innervating the lower extremity can be blocked using continuous techniques. Techniques for continually blocking the sciatic nerve have been described by Smith et al. (134). Continuous regional anesthesia can be obtained anywhere along the course of the nerve. A 16-gauge intravenous infusion needle and catheter or Tuohy needle with an epidural catheter can be used. The catheter is usually advanced 4 to 6 cm into the perivascular space. The lateral approach described by Guardini (135) can be very useful for obtaining a continuous block. The catheter is placed along the nerve just posterior to the quadratus femoris muscle in the subgluteal space.

Femoral Nerve Catheterization

Continuous techniques for the femoral nerve have been used for a variety of surgeries. Edwards and Wright (136) recently reported significantly lower postoperative pain scores and opioid requirements in patients undergoing total knee replacement with continuous infusion of 0.125% bupivacaine at 6 mL/hour within the femoral sheath than with analgesia from conventional intramuscular injections of opioids.

Drugs

The drugs administered for lower-extremity infusions follow the same principles as for brachial plexus infusions. The concentration of drug infusion depends upon the need to block Aα or Aδ fibers or C fibers, and the rate of infusion is usually 10 to 15 mL/hour. Complications include peripheral neuropathy, motor weakness, dysesthesia and decubitus ulcers secondary to sensory loss.

Efficacy

Technically lower-extremity infusions are difficult and unreliable. At best they are alternatives to lumbar epidural infusions when the latter cannot be performed (for instance because of infection or coagulation abnormality). Postoperative knee pain and complex regional pain syndrome I and II may be the best indications for these procedures.

Continuous Sympathetic Blocks

Some clinicians are routinely performing continuous sympathetic infusions (137). Continuous stellate ganglion and continuous lumbar sympathetic infusions are common. The stellate ganglion infusion is in many situations unreliable because of catheter dislodgment. Continuous celiac and lumbar sympathetic infusions are successful even in outpatients with no significant problems. These techniques are most useful in treating visceral pain secondary to cancer, complex regional pain syndrome I and II, and sympathetically maintained pain (138, 139).

Drugs

The drugs administered for sympathetic infusions follow the same principles as for brachial plexus infusion. The drug of choice is bupivacaine (0.125% to 0.25%), usually without an opioid. Morphine, fentanyl, and sufentanil have been mixed with the local anesthetic to prolong the analgesia; 6 (stellate ganglion) to 20 mL (celiac plexus, bilateral) solution is commonly infused.

Efficacy

Stellate ganglion infusion is unreliable because of catheter dislodgment. Lumbar sympathetic infusion is quite reliable, even though the lumbar plexus will eventually be blocked by diffusion of local anesthetic solution into the psoas muscle. Hypotension and nausea are rare complications of bilateral celiac plexus infusion. Not enough data are as yet available to state that continuous sympathetic infusion is a safe, reliable, and efficacious technique.

ADVANCED INTERVENTIONAL TECHNIQUES

In patients with persisting intolerable pain lasting longer than 3 months, it is necessary to find new avenues of pain management. Prolonged analgesia is one of those techniques. This can be provided by performing special procedures such as epidural analgesia with patient-controlled analgesia, implantable drug delivery system, spinal cord and peripheral nerve stimulation, radiofrequency, and cryolysis.

Implantable Drug Delivery Systems

Intraspinal opioids have dramatically influenced the way pain of malignant origin is managed; this is seen by the continued decline in the number of neurodestructive procedures performed to palliate cancer pain (140). This powerful modality has been expanded to treat selected patients suffering from chronic benign pain (141). In tandem, various implantable drug delivery systems have been developed to complement and facilitate the delivery of opioids and other drugs to the neuraxis.

Classification

Table 35.7 describes the six basic types of implantable drug delivery systems. Type 1, a simple percutaneous catheter analogous to those used for obstetric pain control, is the type most familiar to anesthesiologists. Type 2 is simply a catheter suitable for percutaneous placement and tunneling. Type 3 consists of a totally implantable injection port that is attached to a type 2 tunneled catheter. Type 4, a totally implantable mechanically activated pump attached to a type 2 tunneled catheter, in principle is a PCA device. Type 5 is a totally implantable continuous infusion pump that is connected to a type 2 tunneled catheter. Type 6 is a totally implantable programable infusion pump attached to a type 2 tunneled catheter. The programable feature of the type 6 implantable drug delivery system allows a broad spectrum of delivery rates and modes, including occasional bolus injections.

Each of these drug delivery systems has a unique profile of advantages and disadvantages (142). The pain management specialist must be familiar with the particular merits of each system if optimal selection is to be made. In this time of increasing pressure to control the costs of health care, economic factors must also play a role in the selection of an implantable drug delivery system. The cost of both the intended delivery system and the drugs to be administered through it must be considered prior to implantation. A perfectly functioning implantable drug delivery system is useless to the patient who is unable to pay for the drugs, special needles, and supplies needed to use it. Similarly, implanted systems may superimpose financial hardship upon a difficult terminal course. With planning, the financial issues can be individualized and resolved.

Issues to be Considered before Device Placement

Appropriate patient selection is crucial if optimal results in terms of pain palliation and patient satisfaction are to be achieved. Factors that must be considered prior to placement of an implantable drug delivery system are summarized in Table 35.8 (140, 142). These issues are discussed further.

Preimplantation Trial

The first responsibility to the patient being considered for an implantable drug delivery system is to make a diagnosis of the pain problem and analyze the appropriateness of the patient's current analgesic regimen. A preimplantation trial of spinal opioids is necessary to determine whether an implantable drug delivery system can adequately relieve the patient's pain. Not all pain is relieved by spinal opioids (143). A drug delivery system should never be implanted without first verifying the ability of the specific spinal drug to relieve the patient's symptoms adequately on two separate occasions. Extensive clinical experience suggests that implantation should not proceed unless the pain is reduced to less than 50%

Table 35.7.   Spinal Drug Delivery Systems

Type 1	Percutaneous epidural or subarachnoid catheter
Type 2	Percutaneous epidural or subarachnoid catheter with subcutaneous tunneling
Type 3	Totally implanted epidural or subarachnoid catheter with subcutaneous injection port
Type 4	Totally implanted epidural or subarachnoid catheter with implanted manually activated pump
Type 5	Totally implanted epidural or subarachnoid catheter with implanted infusion pump
Type 6	Totally implanted epidural or subarachnoid catheter with implanted programmable infusion pump

Table 35.8.   Preimplantation Considerations

Results of preimplantation trials of spinal drugs
Infection
Clotting disorders
Behavioral abnormalities
Physiologic abnormalities
Cost of delivery system
Cost of drugs, needles, and supplies
Evaluation of support system
Concurrent therapy

of the preinjection intensity and unless analgesia lasts at least twice the half-life of the agent; for example, 8 to 12 hours in the case of morphine (144).

Failure of a preimplantation trial may occur for several reasons: test injections made in the wrong place; psychological reasons, such as depression; advanced tolerance to opioids; incorrect dose of spinal drugs; or a principal component of the patient's symptoms being not susceptible to spinal application of opioid (e.g., some central pain syndromes (143). If a question remains about the ability of spinal drugs to provide symptom relief after two trial doses, a placebo injection may help clarify the situation.

It is widely accepted that this response to acute drug administration is highly predictive of the long-term outcome of chronic drug administration. Failure to see adequate, long-lasting analgesia under these conditions is cause to reconsider placement of an implantable opioid-delivery system.

Unless the efficacy of spinal opioids is clearly demonstrated during the preimplantation trial, the patient could be subjected to the implantation of a delivery system that will fail to achieve the desired pain relief. With the exception of electrical stimulation and spinal drugs, few invasive pain therapies allow the patient and physician to test the therapy before an irreversible result has occurred. Local anesthetic blocks are useful in educating the patient before neurodestructive procedures but cannot always predict the adequacy, extent, or complications of an irreversible destructive procedure.

Infection and Local Conditions

Infection, inflammation, or dermatitis at the proposed cutaneous site of implantation—and any generalized sepsis—are absolute contraindications to device implantation.

Anticoagulation and Hematological Abnormalities

The fully anticoagulated patient presents a special problem when considering placement of an implantable drug delivery system. Preimplantation trials of spinal drugs for the relief of pelvic and lower body pain have been performed safely in the presence of anticoagulation by administering the opioid caudally with a 25-gauge, 1.5-inch needle (145). Unfortunately,

spinal opioids administered in the lumbar or caudal region may not relieve upper body pain without a substantial increase in the dose. Carefully weigh the risk-benefit ratio of stopping anticoagulants to proceed with preimplantation trials of cervical or thoracic spinal drugs.

Coagulopathy caused by disease is also common, particularly in cancer patients. Platelet count and function and tests for procoagulant factor activity should be assessed in all cancer patients and others whose history or physical examination suggests the possibility of coagulopathy. Efforts should be made to reverse the coagulopathy if possible. If this is not possible, assess the risk-benefit ratio of proceeding with preimplantation trials.

Physiological Abnormalities

Physiological abnormalities, such as electrolyte imbalance and drug-induced organic brain syndrome, may impair the patient's ability to assess the adequacy of symptom relief (143). Many abnormalities are reversible, and an effort should be made to correct them before a trial of spinal drugs is undertaken. It should be remembered that the confusion secondary to these physiological abnormalities may be incorrectly interpreted as uncontrolled pain by the patient and pain management specialist alike.

Behavior Abnormalities

Behavioral abnormalities that are often difficult to identify may affect the patient's ability to assess the adequacy of symptom relief. These abnormalities may coexist with physiological factors, but care must be taken not to attribute inadequate symptom relief solely to behavioral factors until all possible physiological causes have been explored (146).

Support System

Use of an implantable drug delivery system requires a commitment from patients and their support systems. Someone must be available day and night to care for the system and inject the drug should the patient be unable to do so. Thus one or more persons must be designated as the patient's support system, and they must be acceptable to the patient. It should be remembered that cancer patients who inject their own implantable drug delivery systems initially may be unable to do so later in the course of disease. Inability or unwillingness by the designated support persons to care for the system has significant implications for selecting the appropriate system.

Life Expectancy

Although prediction of a cancer patient's life expectancy can be difficult, an estimate in terms of days, weeks, or months is essential to select the most appropriate implantable drug delivery system (140). Often the patient's general condition improves when adequate symptom control is provided, and this must be taken into account when estimating life expectancy.

Types of Implantable Drug Delivery Systems

Type 1: Percutaneous Catheter

The Type 1 percutaneous catheters have gained wide acceptance for the short-term administration of spinal opioids and/or local anesthetics for the palliation of acute pain, including obstetric and postoperative pain. The Type 1 system also has three applications in cancer pain management. The first is in the acute setting, where delivery of opioids into the epidural or subarachnoid space can provide temporary palliation of pain postoperatively or until other concurrent treatments, such as radiation therapy, become effective. The second is in imminently dying patients too ill for more invasive procedures (140, 143, 147). The third is in the use of a percutaneous catheter to administer test doses of spinal opioids before emplacing a more permanent system. In many centers the use of a type 1 percutaneous catheter to deliver epidural and especially subarachnoid opioids is limited. Improved catheter fixation, reduced risk of infection, and the relative ease of tunneling (140, 142, 148) has led many pain specialists to tunnel the spinal catheter to the flank, abdomen, or chest wall, even for the short-term administration of opioids. Despite several reports that the type 1 system can be used for long periods in immunocompromised patients without an increased risk of infection (149), the validity of this observation has not been established. In view of the potentially devastating and life-threatening consequences of catheter-induced spinal infection, as well as the highly favorable risk-benefit ratio of the type 2 tunneled catheter, the use of the type 1 system should be limited solely to the acute setting.

Type 2: Subcutaneous Tunneled Catheter

The subcutaneous tunneled catheter is selected for patients with life expectancies of weeks to months. The low cost, ease of implementation, and ease of catheter care and injection make the type 2 system the preferred delivery system at many centers. The type 2 system can be implanted or removed in the outpatient setting and has a lower incidence of infection than the type 1 system.

Type 3: Totally Implantable Reservoir

The totally implantable reservoir is often chosen for patients with life expectancies of months to years who have had excellent relief of symptoms with trial doses of spinal drugs (140, 149). The type 3 system has less risk of infection than with type 1 and 2 systems and a lower risk of catheter failure. Injection of the type 3 system is more difficult than with type 1 and 2 systems; this can be significant when training lay people to inject and care for this system (150). Furthermore, removal or replacement requires a surgical incision.

Type 4: Totally Implantable Mechanically Activated Pump

Poletti et al. (150a) created one of the earliest totally implantable systems for PCA. This system consisted of an implantable sterile blood bag with a hydrocephalus shunt valve in series with the bag and spinal catheter. The valve could be activated by the patient to allow self-administration of an opioid from the implanted bag. This concept has now been extended by Cordis as a totally implantable reservoir that is accessed percutaneously through a septum on the surface of the device. The device also has a mechanical valve system activated by a set of buttons on the pump surface. The patient delivers spinal drugs by depressing the buttons in the proper sequence (140). The type 4 system has less risk of infection than the types 1, 2, and 3 systems. Subarachnoid delivery is more feasible with the type 4 system than with type 1 and 2 systems. The greatest advantage of this system is that the patient can titrate the dose of the drug to symptoms and can pretreat symptoms prior to periods of increased activity.

Type 5: Totally Implantable Infusion Pump

The totally implantable infusion pump is also used in patients with life expectancies of months to years who obtained relief of symptoms after trial doses of spinal drugs (140, 151). Type 5 delivery systems may also be indicated in cancer patients with shorter life expectancies who have intermittent confusion secondary to metabolic abnormalities or systemically administered drugs. Clinical experience suggests that such patients may obtain analgesia with fewer side effects with low-dose continuous spinal opioid infusion than repeated bolus injections into a spinal catheter. Alternatively, an implanted port with an external infusion pump may suffice in this situation, although this may be more inconvenient and require more support.

Since type 5 systems require infrequent refills and run continuously, they are ideal for patients with limited medical or nonmedical family support services. The type 5 system is usually selected with an auxiliary bolus injection port to take advantage of potential drug options, such as local anesthetic injections. Advantages of the type 5 system include the minimal risk of infection after the perioperative period and the infrequent need to inject the pump relative to other implantable drug delivery systems whose pump reservoir must be refilled approximately every 7 to 20 days. The overall high cost of the type 5 system is a disadvantage that may occasionally result in selecting a less effective or more inconvenient analgesic technique.

Type 6: Totally Implantable Programable Infusion Pump

The type 6 totally implantable programable infusion pump is implanted with the same ease as the type 5 system (152). This system allows a broad spectrum of delivery rates and modes, including occasional bolus injections. Its principal application to date has been intrathecal infusion, especially in the therapy of spasticity in multiple sclerosis and spinal cord—injured patients (152, 153). There is as yet no proven advantage of programable systems over the simpler continuous infusion systems. However, there are several theoretical advantages for cancer pain patients, including the reduction of side effects that may occur with the bolus injections provided by types 1, 2, 3, and 4 implantable drug delivery systems, coupled with the added ability to pretreat symptoms associated with periods of increased activity.

Neural Stimulation: Spinal Cord and Peripheral Nerve Stimulation

Neural stimulation has been a significant part of medical history. Advances in today's technology and physiological research have helped define avenues in which this tool, when properly used, can afford society outstanding clinical and economic benefits.

The first multiprogramable electronics were introduced in 1980, and totally implantable neural stimulator systems were introduced in 1981. Eight-channel multiprogramable electronics and the first eight-electrode catheter were developed in 1986. Following this, 1988 signaled the introduction of the noninvasive programable implantable pulse generator that also had radiofrequency capabilities. In the 1990s successful adaptation of multilead electrode arrays, implantable programable pulse generators, implantable radiofrequency receivers, and more sophisticated objective patient screening methods has led to very high success rates.

Physiology

The sensitivity of neural tissue to frequency and amplitude variations significantly alters the physiological response in the living organism. High-frequency, low-amplitude stimulation silences most dorsal horn cells, including presumably noxious ones, which are active only during strong pinching or clamping. The inhibition is dramatic. Conversely, low-frequency, high-amplitude stimulation is much less effective. This may explain part of the efficacy of spinal cord stimulation or peripheral nerve stimulation for peripheral vascular disease

and reflex sympathetic dystrophy, since sympathetic fibers are normally recruited more with this type of stimulation. Inhibition of the sympathetic system is more likely by high-frequency, low-amplitude stimulation.

Stimulation recruits Aβ fibers; paresthesia is frequency dependent. If a patient is stimulated at higher frequencies, Aδ fibers are recruited and the frequency dependence is diminished. Excess Aδ stimulation causes the patient to report unpleasant paresthesia, which may feel prickling or even epicritic (sharp, well localized). However, if such a paresthesia were better able to suppress C fiber activity, pain would be less protopathic (agonal, diffuse).

Stimulating large-diameter afferents with nonnoxious stimuli may close down or inhibit messages from the ascending small diameter nociceptive fibers and interneurons. Other theories include inhibitory pathways being stimulated by spinal descending tracts. Spinal cord stimulation physiologically may be affected by a number of mechanisms. The basics include electrical contact with a cathode (negative electrode), which causes excitation of nervous tissue. The inside of living neural cells is negatively charged. Thus the exposure of an external negative charge causes depolarization to a positive potential on the inside of the cell, which therefore causes an action potential and thus a nonnoxious message.

Chronic pain sufferers have demonstrated lower levels of endorphin and serotonin in the cerebral spinal fluid than subjects who did not complain of chronic pain. Both chemicals show demonstrative increases that are subject to neural stimulation, although the analgesic effects of spinal cord stimulation have not been reversible by naloxone (154).

Indications

The general indications for spinal cord stimulation are for suppression of chronic, intractable pain of the trunk or limbs (155). Examples of specific diseases for which spinal cord stimulation may be indicated include arachnoiditis (156), spastic torticollis, intercostal neuralgia, peripheral neuropathy (157), reflex sympathetic dystrophy (158), phantom limb pain (159), radicular pain associated with intraspinal fibrosis, peripheral pain associated with ischemic vascular disease (160), and peripheral pain associated with postherpetic neuralgia. Conditions that are specifically amenable to peripheral nerve stimulation include reflex sympathetic dystrophy, causalgia, direct nerve injury, and plexus avulsion. The pathologies that respond best to peripheral stimulation are deafferentation and neuropathic conditions.

Conditions for Implantation

Guidelines have been established by the Health Care and Finance Administration (HCFA) on implantation of spinal cord and peripheral nerve simulators. Spinal cord simulators should be used only as follows:

1. As a late resort for patients with chronic, intractable pain
2. When other treatment modalities (pharmacological, surgical, physical, or psychological therapies) have been tried and do not prove satisfactory, have been judged to be unsuitable, or are contraindicated for the patient
3. When patients have undergone careful screening and diagnosis by a multidisciplinary team before implantation
4. When all of the facilities, equipment, and professional support personnel required for the proper diagnosis, treatment, training, and follow-up of the patient are available
5. When demonstration of pain relief with a temporarily implanted electrode precedes permanent implantation
6. With an objective basis for the pain
7. With documentation of no drug addiction

The screening criteria for peripheral nerve stimulation, including the previous guidelines, should also include pain confined or related to a specific nerve branch and pain that can be ablated by a peripheral nerve block. This is discussed in more detail later.

Contraindications

There are a few precautions to spinal cord stimulation as a therapeutic option:

1. Patient who fails the screening
2. Patient who is averse to electrical stimulation
3. Patient who is averse to an implant as a modality of treating his or her pain
4. An active and uncontrolled coagulopathy at the time of the planned procedure
5. Localized or disseminated pain at the time of the planned implantation
6. Physician's lack of experience or training in implanting stimulator devices
7. Patient who has a demand cardiac pacemaker
8. Patient who needs MRI in the immediate foreseeable future
9. Untreated and unresolved serious drug habituation
10. Absence of an objectively documented cause of the pain

Failed Treatment

It is extremely important to document, within the confines of the history and physical examination, what medications and therapeutic interventions have not been successful for the patient. Specifically indicate the medical, neurosurgical, orthopaedic, vascular, behavioral medicine, or other consultants who have been involved. Determine that there are no contraindications to spinal cord implantation and no better alternatives.

Implantation Procedures

Precautions

The screening stimulator lead array is implanted in a sterile operating room. Determine that adequate stimulation has been achieved on the operating table. The stimulator paresthesia must cover the area of pain if at all possible. The entire system is not implanted in a single setting. The possible exception to this is in cases of objective documentation of clinical improvement in peripheral vascular disease. Operating room screening and immediate full-system implantation is discouraged for the following reasons:

1. The patient is usually under the influence of a preoperative or intraoperative sedative administered to ease discomfort during the placement of the intraspinal lead.
2. The patient is not hearing during the time of lead implantation and is not participating in activities of daily living. Thus using a stimulator system is an unrealistic test of pain relief.
3. The transient changes in body chemistry and position may remove the pain generator. Therefore the physician may not have the opportunity to see the pain in its most exaggerated form during the brief tenure in the operating room.

Walking after temporary placement of the lead in the prone or lateral position may cause migration of a percutaneously placed lead, thus altering the area of stimulation. Be certain that the system to be implanted can withstand changing positions from recumbent to upright, and make sure that the paresthesia coverage does not vary significantly with walking.

It is recommended that the patient receive intravenous antibiotic prophylaxis approximately 30 minutes before the percutaneous implantation of the lead array. It is recommended that without exception, all leads be placed with fluoroscopic guidance. A mild sedative should be available to patients to help lessen the trauma of having a stimulating electrode placed into the spinal canal and to diminish the probability of sudden dangerous movement.

Procedure

The patient should be maintained on antibiotics as long as the percutaneous lead is present and for a brief period subsequent to total system implantation. The decision whether to place an implantable programable nerve stimulator power source or a radiofrequency receiver with external transmitter and antennae is based on a number of variables. The first and foremost is whether the capability of the electrical power generation is more in the screening system than in the implanted generator. Other factors to consider include the use of the external power source, depending somewhat on the patient being able to place the antennae if the system is guided by an audible signal. This may cause problems with patients who have impaired hearing. The problem can be overcome by teaching patients to find their radiofrequency receiver by a shrinking concentric circle motion until they reach maximal stimulation from the antennae. Once the patient is capable of properly operating the system, he or she is discharged, usually within 12 to 24 hours of the final implant.

Peripheral Nerve Stimulation

Peripheral nerve stimulation has been used since 1965. It was initially performed with cuffs containing stimulation electrodes. Technical and clinical complications were significant. Electrode migration and equipment malfunction created the need for more stable equipment design. Scar formation caused by direct contact between the nerve and the cuff led to nerve constriction. Flat electrode arrays with a thin panel of fascia between the nerve and the stimulator proved to be much more stable and clinically effective (161). Peripheral nerve stimulation has been used successfully to treat pain of neurogenic origin in upper extremities, lower extremities, and intercostal nerves. As equipment design improved, so did the clinical selection and screening procedure.

Selection Criteria for Peripheral Nerve Stimulation

Patients with single nerve pathology are the best candidates for peripheral nerve stimulation, although patients with multiple nerve lesions have been successfully screened and implanted. Clinical syndromes that have responded favorably to peripheral nerve stimulation include reflex sympathetic dystrophy, causalgia, plexus avulsion, operative trauma, entrapment neuropathies, and injection injuries. Clinical selection criteria include chronic intractable pain recalcitrant to other therapies, temporary relief from local anesthetic injection, no psychological contraindications, objective evidence of pathology (e.g., electromyography, somatosensory evoked potential, or selective tissue conductance studies), no drug habituation, and relief from temporary screen.

Complications

Complications can occur. Medical complications include infection, bleeding, adverse drug reaction, injury to the spinal cord, nerve injury, cerebrospinal fluid leak, poor pain relief, fibrosis at the tip of the stimulator, and motor stimulation. Mechanical problems include lead fracture, lead shearing and shortage, intraoperative or postoperative lead movement, extension cable fracture, battery malfunction or depletion, and transmitter malfunction and depletion.

Efficacy

Spinal cord stimulation has been reported effective in 53% to 70% of patients over 2.2 to 5 years. Reports to measure the effectiveness of spinal cord stimulation include good

to excellent pain relief, decreased consumption of opioids and other analgesias, improved tissue oxygenation, decreased incidence of amputation in peripheral vascular disease, increased activities of daily living, and return to work.

Radiofrequency Lesions

Electrical current has been used to produce neural lesions in patients for 100 years. Modern radiofrequency thermocoagulation has been used to ablate pain pathways in the trigeminal ganglion, spinal cord, dorsal root entry zone, dorsal root ganglion, sympathetic chain, and peripheral nerve. Unfortunately, the long-term effects of ablative techniques on clinical pain syndromes are incompletely known.

The radiofrequency lesion is formed when neural temperature exceeds 45° C. These temperatures are a result of frictional heat that is generated by molecular movement in a field of alternating current at radio wave frequency. Frequencies above 250 kHz produce an electromagnetic field around an active electrode. An active electrode is placed in the desired anatomical location, and an indifferent electrode is placed to minimize current passage across the myocardium. The current disperses via the second electrode, which is usually a high-area contact plate. Wattage is gradually increased and heat develops in the tissue, which conducts to the active probe. Heat is generated as current flows through a probe with a built-in thermocouple. Thus the thermocouple-needle combination allows lesioning, monitoring and injecting without movement of the appropriately positioned device. The temperature of the probe itself assumes equilibrium with the temperature of the tissue surrounding it. The heat is not emitted from the probe itself but from the current's movement, which generates the heat as it passes through the tissues. The temperature is monitored and wattage is adjusted to a target temperature, which is a primary determinant of lesion size. For low-power procedures such as facet denervation, 10 to 20 watts are used. Other factors, such as active electrode diameter and length, contribute to wattage requirements. Tissue blood flow is important because significant heat convection can occur, with significant blood flow in the area of the lesion. Homogeneous tissue is necessary for a symmetrical lesion (162).

Efficacy

Radiofrequency lesioning is a neurodestructive procedure. Therefore it has to be considered an end-of-the-line procedure for use when conservative therapeutic modalities have failed. The physician performing radiofrequency procedures must have appropriate training and experience before beginning such neurodestructive procedures. All of these procedures should be done under fluoroscopic guidance after appropriate test stimulation and verification of the tissues about to be destroyed. Different temperatures have various levels of neurodestructive capabilities. Numbness or motor paralysis occurs very rarely as a consequence of the lesioning. The tissues can be injured anywhere along the passing of the needle probe if there is a break in the insulation. Therefore supramaximal motor stimulation is always part of the procedure before lesioning is performed, in the event that the insulated portion of the needle passes near a motor nerve, such as in lumbar sympathetic lesioning. If there is a break in insulation, not only the lumbar sympathetic ganglion but also the lumbar nerve root may be destroyed, which is definitely not the desired outcome. Kline (163) described the essential information for trainees and others interested in radiofrequency techniques.

Radiofrequency lesioning can have definite advantages over alternative neurodestructive procedures, primarily because the lesion is controlled. The complications associated with neurolytic solutions, which result from intravascular injection and spread along tissue planes, can be avoided. The proximal and distal spread of the lesion beyond the uninsulated tip of the probe is only 1 mm, and the cross-sectional diameter of the lesion is 5 to 6 mm. The advantages include the following:

1. Well-controlled lesion size
2. Temperature monitored in the core of the lesion by the built-in thermal couple
3. Electrode placement verified by fluoroscopic guidance using electrical stimulation and impedance monitoring
4. Procedure that can be performed without general anesthetics
5. Procedure that can be performed on an outpatient basis and whose effectiveness can be recognized in approximately 4 weeks
6. Low morbidity and mortality associated with the lesioning itself; however, potential complications include major neurological injury, and extreme care must be taken when injecting local anesthetic and steroids, as well as during probe placement, location verification, and lesion formation
7. Procedure that can be repeated (163)

Monitor patients, because radiofrequency equipment can interact with pacemakers and spinal cord stimulators. The equipment used in the procedure must be safe, precise, and must yield reproducible results. The equipment must be able to do the following (163):

1. Measure impedance
2. Stimulate a wide range of frequencies
3. Accurately time the lesion for precise temperature measurement in the core of the lesion tissue
4. Accurately measure and indicate amperage and voltage
5. Gradually increase temperature with time

Patients should be selected according to the following criteria (163):

1. Other noninvasive conservative measures have failed.
2. Any substance abuse such as opioids, sedatives, and alcohol, has been identified and dealt with; the patient has entered a program to resolve the issues in addition to symptom control.
3. Appropriate psychological assessment and therapy for depression, anxiety, anger, and secondary gain have been performed; the patient has entered an appropriate behavioral management program.
4. The patient accepts his or her lifestyle changes, addresses psychological issues, and interacts with physicians, therapists, and psychologists in an appropriate manner.
5. Fully informed consent, including recognition of realistic expectations and procedural risks, must be obtained.

Procedural considerations must be preceded by full awareness of the anatomy, pain pathways, anticipated outcomes, and the need to have a multidisciplinary team around the person carrying out such procedures. The most commonly used procedures are performed around facet joints in the neck, thoracic, lumbar, and lumbar cervical areas. Anterior compartment pain from lumbar disease can be solved by lesioning the anterior communicating branch (164). Radiofrequency lumbar ganglionotomy, partial rhizotomy, sacral ganglionotomy, thoracic ganglionotomy, cervical ganglionotomy, cervical facets, discs, nerve roots, myofascial tissues, sphenopalatine ganglion, and radiofrequency lesioning of the stellate ganglion via the interior approach have been quite useful at C6, C7, and T1 areas.

Radiofrequency lesioning of the trigeminal ganglion, as described by Sweet (165) is an important technique in neurosurgical circles. Percutaneous cordotomy, probably the most studied and indicated procedure, especially affects the torso on the contralateral side of the lesioning. The hazards of the procedure include worse pain when the patient outlives the lesioning and the possibility of Ordine's curse (the ability to inhale but not to exhale) if bilateral lesioning is carried out. The incidence of radiofrequency cordotomies, even in patients with cancer pain, seems to have decreased since the introduction of spinal opioids, other neuroaugmentation procedures such as spinal cord stimulation, and in patients who respond favorably to more modern forms of cancer therapies. It is especially unfortunate when complications of therapy such as permanent numbness or in rare instances development of neuropathic pain persist when the cancer is no longer a problem. As a general rule, deafferentation pains do not respond to radiofrequency lesioning.

Cryolysis

Cryoanalgesia is a term for creating a nerve injury by freezing. Cryoanalgesia developments include freezing carbon dioxide and fashioning it into dry ice pencils for topical application, cooling metal rods (cryoprobes) in baths of dry ice and acetone or ether, and pressing the rods against the tissue to be frozen.

It was not until liquid air and liquid nitrogen became available, however, that another generation of more powerful cryoprobes was developed. In 1961 Cooper et al. (165a) developed the first cryoprobe. The probe employed the principle of phase change using liquid nitrogen to produce a temperature of −196° C. Later, Amoils developed a smaller, more easily controlled probe for ophthalmic surgery and introduced the enclosed gas expansion cryoprobe. This probe, which used the Joule-Thompson principle, was driven by liquid carbon dioxide and was capable of reaching temperatures of −50° C. Since that time, numerous probes have been developed using this principle and nitrous oxide as the primary refrigerant, which is capable of achieving minimal temperatures of approximately −70° C. These probes are available in many sizes and shapes and have incorporated thermocouples and nerve stimulators. Many probes can be inserted through the skin for localization and freezing of nerves percutaneously (166).

Nelson et al. (166a), Brain (166b), and Lloyd et al. (166) applied cryoprobes to various nerves, including intercostal, pharyngeal, trigeminal, sacral, and others, in the treatment of various chronic neuralgias and pain. Lloyd et al. (166), who are credited with naming the technique cryoanalgesia, have demonstrated that prolonged analgesia can be obtained after a single freeze of a peripheral nerve. They particularly stressed the safety of the procedure and reported that nerve function always returned and neuroma formation did not occur.

A cryolesion is reversible and has not been associated with neuromas. In several studies on animals, there is no evidence of neuroma formation at necropsy, and the degree of fibrosis and scarring at the site of injury is minimal. The extent of cell destruction by a cryolesion depends on several factors, but the rate of freezing and thawing and the temperature attained by the tissue in proximity to the cryoprobe are the most important (167). Evans et al. (167) showed that when a rat sciatic nerve was directly exposed to cryolesion, the time for regeneration of the nerve was independent of the duration of freezing and the application of a repeat freeze cycle. However, the temperature attained by the nerve is important. Those researchers concluded that if the temperature remained above than −20° C, the results are unpredictable. Below this temperature the interruption was prolonged and uninfluenced by greater reductions in temperature (167).

When using a percutaneous cryoprobe, the rate of cooling the tissue depends on the geometry of the cryoprobe and its capacity for heat extraction. The ice ball (probe tip to ice interface with tissue) shows a sharp temperature gradient across its radius of approximately 10°C/mL. The tissues closest to the probe attain the maximum subzero temperature, whereas the remaining tissues show a rapid rise toward 0°C. The central zone undergoes rapid cooling, while the peripheral zone is influenced by the heat generated as the surrounding tissue slowly cools. Longer freezing produces some increase in the size of the ice ball and the central zone until a plateau is reached at which heat extraction by the probe balances the heat production by the surrounding tissue. Here again, Gill et al. (167a) showed that repetitive freezing could increase the amount of tissue frozen and the rate of freezing tissue surrounding the probe. Despite debate in the literature, there is uniform agreement that temperatures below −20°C cause cellular freezing, and cells do not recover.

Specific Lesions with Percutaneous Cryoprobe

Percutaneous cryoprobe application has been used for many types of neural lesioning. In fact, any nerve that can be isolated by percutaneous or direct vision cryoprobe can undergo cryoneurolysis. The following is a review of some of the more popular uses for the cryoprobe. However, despite the lack of neuroma formation and low incidence of neuritis with a cryolesion, it is not a benign procedure, and cryoneurolysis of motor nerves should be avoided.

Facial Pain

Treatment of postherpetic and nonherpetic trigeminal neuralgia by cryoneurolysis has been described throughout the literature. Barnard et al. (168) also described the use of cryoneurolysis for posttraumatic neuralgia, malignant disease causing facial pain, and neuralgia of unknown origin. They used the cryoprobe to lyse supraorbital, supratrochlear, infraorbital, mental, and lingual nerves in 21 patients. In these patients, they compared freezing followed by sectioning with freezing alone. They found that the median time of pain relief was 116 days for cryoneurolysis alone and only 38 days for freezing and subsequent sectioning. However, sensory loss lasted 49 days for cryoneurolysis and 131 days for freezing and sectioning. They concluded that cryoanalgesia was a useful therapeutic tool for the management of intractable facial pain because it provided a reliable, prolonged, and reversible nerve block that could be achieved by a simple technique that did not appear to aggravate symptoms. Goss (169) described using cryoneurotomy for intractable temporomandibular joint pain. In his review of six consecutive patients with intractable neurogenic pain of the auricular nerves, cryoneurolysis was performed percutaneously, and all six patients had excellent pain relief for 1 year after the procedure. Four of the six had recurrent pain. He also found that repeat cryoneurolysis had decreasing effectiveness. Cryoprobes have also been described for use in oral surgery and pituitary cryoablation (170).

Thoracic Pain

Chronic and acute thoracic pain have been treated with cryoneurolysis, intraoperatively at the end of thoracotomy for acute pain and percutaneously for chronic thoracic pain.

Spinal Pain

The use of the percutaneous cryoprobe for facet rhizotomy has also been described in the literature for the treatment of low-back pain and the lumbar disk syndrome. This procedure is used to block the articular nerve of Luschka at the junction of the pedicle with the transverse process. At this site, the nerve has not yet branched into its ascending, lateral, and medial branches; therefore a single lesion can produce analgesia. However, in this technique, the nerve may be lysed at the level in question, one level above, and one level below the facet of pathology. This is due to the branching nature of the nerves innervating the facets. Schuster (171) used this technique for treating facet pain in 52 patients and found that 47 of these patients had significant relief from back pain. Of these 47, only one had recurrent pain after 9 months without pain.

Pelvic Pain

Sacral foraminal cryolesions have also been used to treat cancer, coccydynia, and sciatic pain. A bilateral S4 block is useful for treating coccydynia and perineal pain from cancer of the rectum; reportedly, this avoids bladder denervation. Also, S1 and S2 cryolesions can treat pain in sciatic distribution. However, multiple bilateral sacral block is best avoided in view of the possibility of bladder dysfunction as a complication.

Cryoneurolysis of the iliohypogastric and ilioinguinal nerves has also been described. In a study by Khiroya et al. (171a), cryoneurolysis of the ilioinguinal nerve was performed for postoperative pain relief after herniorrhaphy. These authors compared patients who had their ilioinguinal nerves frozen during surgery with those who did not, and they concluded that cryoanalgesia of the ilioinguinal nerve alone did not produce significant early postherniorrhaphy pain relief.

Peripheral Nerve Pain

Blocking peripheral nerves by cryotherapy has been used for neuroma, causalgia, flexion contractures, and nerve entrapment syndromes. The nerves to be frozen must not have a significant motor component unless motor destruction is the goal, for example in the later stages of multiple sclerosis. The reversibility of the nerve block, however, allows for return of motor function after normal regeneration. Wang reported that in patients treated for chronically painful peripheral nerve lesions, 50% of the patients treated in one study had pain relief for 1 to 12 months (172). He also reported that the pain eventually returned. However, during the period of remission, patients returned to normal activities. Wang (172) concurred with the concept that it is especially important when freezing peripheral nerves to have precise localization of the nerves to obtain adequate neurolysis.

Complications of Cryotherapy

Many of the complications reported in the literature pertain to how the use of cutaneous cryosurgery affects nerves that lie under the skin. However, some complications do exist for the use of the percutaneous cryoprobe. Cryosurgical equipment must be tested thoroughly before using to ensure that there are no leaks. A significant leakage of refrigerant can cause freezing along the shaft of the cryoprobe and consequent freezing of structures other than those intended.

The most common problem is frostbite of the skin at the entry site, which can usually be prevented by an introducer sheath. Unintended motor damage can occur, but the patient very often recovers. A frustrating aspect of cryoneurolysis is that therapeutic effectiveness cannot be predicted; pain relief can last 3 to 1000 days.

COMMON PAIN SYNDROMES IN WHICH NERVE BLOCKS HAVE BEEN USEFUL

Low-Back Pain (Table 35.9)

Epidural Steroid Injection

Epidural steroid injection is performed following failure of conservative management of discogenic pain. Even though some claim improved results with subarachnoid injection, most believe epidural steroids are safer and produce equally good results. Since the nerve root compression is extradural in discogenic disease, it is rational to introduce the steroid epidurally at the site of compression, rather than intradurally, where it will be subject to dilution, dispersion, and precipitation.

Technique

Epidural puncture should be done at the site of nerve root lesion, with the painful side down in the lateral decubitus position. When the epidural space has been identified by standard techniques, 80 mg of methylprednisolone acetate or 50 mg of triamcinolone diacetate is suspended in 10 mL of 0.25% or 0.125% bupivacaine and injected slowly in the epidural space. With previous back surgery, identification of the epidural space may be difficult. Initial local anesthetic administration will make identification of epidural space easier under these circumstances.

Following epidural steroid injection, a catheter can be introduced to inject another dose of steroid and local anesthetic, if needed, to reach the appropriate nerve root. This is determined by objectively measuring the improvement in a straight-leg-raising test and absence of radicular pain during the performance of the test. The patient is kept in the lateral position for 10 minutes to keep the injected solution on the dependent side.

The patient is reevaluated 2 weeks after the epidural steroid injection. If there is significant improvement in function and subjective pain relief, no further epidural injection is administered. However, if after the first injection the initial improvement is not maintained, another injection can be repeated up to a maximum of three. Similarly, if there is no change in the patient's condition after the first injection, alternative measures are sought.

When considering epidural steroid administration, the following points should be kept in mind: (*a*) Historical and biochemical evidence supports its use in the 30- to 50-year group with low back or cervical pain with radiculopathy. (*b*) The pain is primarily discogenic; features of this syndrome are shooting pain in brachial plexus or sciatic or femoral distribution with sensory and/or motor deficits, reflex change, and in the lower extremity a positive straight leg raising (SLR) above 30°. (*c*) Epidural versus subarachnoid injection has proponents on either side. (*d*) Meningitis or arachnoiditis after intrathecal use and no appreciable therapeutic advantage over the extradural route makes subarachnoid technique risky. (*e*) Bupivacaine 0.125% or 0.25% with either methylprednisolone acetate (Depo-Medrol) 80 mg or triamcinolone (Aristocort) 50 mg in 8 to 10 mL is commonly used.

Table 35.9.   Common Pain Syndromes for Which Nerve Blocks Have Been Useful

Low back pain
Herpes zoster pain
Complex regional pain syndrome
Cancer pain
Myofascial pain

One can ask whether the efficacy of epidural steroid injection been established. The extensive literature on this question leaves much to be desired. Most studies are purely descriptive, anecdotal, retrospective, and not randomized, controlled, or blinded. Patient populations are poorly defined and not homogeneous; treatment protocols are variable; and outcome criteria poorly defined.

The efficacy of epidural steroid injection has not been conclusively demonstrated, and it is unlikely that such a study will soon be completed. Nevertheless, many studies have confirmed good short-term success rates in selected patients. Recent reviews by Rowlingson (172a), Abram (172b), and Hammonds (172c) state the case for continued use of this therapy as part of the overall management of patients with acute radicular pain, herniated disc, or new radiculopathy superimposed on chronic back pain or cervical spondylosis. The presence of nerve root irritation is required to justify use of epidural steroid injection. Reliable patient follow-up and comprehensive management of physical, occupational, and emotional rehabilitation are necessary to avoid a too narrowly focused, block-oriented approach to these patients.

Herpes Zoster

Acute herpes zoster is reactivation of a latent viral infection (varicella zoster) of the dorsal root ganglion causing exquisite pain and vesicular rash in the dermatome subserved by the particular spinal or cranial nerve. Treatment protocols include antiviral agents, anti-inflammatory agents, and neural blockade with local anesthetics. All regimens attempt to relieve acute pain, hasten cutaneous healing, and prevent postherpetic neuralgia (PHN).

Matas (172d) first used regional anesthesia for treatment of herpetic pain with gasserian ganglion and subarachnoid injections of cocaine. In 1938, Rosenak (172e) employed paravertebral blocks of sympathetic ganglia to relieve acute herpetic pain, believing the blocks would also hasten healing of the vesicular rash. Colding (172f) later suggested that sympathetic blockade could prevent PHN when performed early in the natural history of the disease. In 1985, Tenicela et al. (172g) proved the efficacy of regional sympathetic blockade over placebo is relieving acute neuralgic pain in a randomized, double-blind study.

Justification for the treatment of herpes zoster with the invasive techniques of regional sympathetic blockade stems from the attempt to prevent the devastating pain of PHN, which in the broadest sense is pain in the distribution of a spinal or cranial nerve after resolution of the herpetic rash. The term itself is

ambiguous. The distinction between the end of acute neuralgia and the beginning of "postherpetic" neuralgia is nebulous and a function of the definition used by individual authors.

The complete lack of a randomized, double-blind, placebo-controlled study with sufficient numbers for analytical stratification by age and immunocompetence weakens the argument that sympathetic blockade prevents PHN. Furthermore, no author addresses the question whether complete resolution of pain or decrement in pain intensity signifies therapeutic success.

The definitive therapeutic modality for prevention of PHN remains elusive. Acyclovir does not prevent PHN, and the efficacy of steroids is controversial. There is the suggestion that early regional blockade may be a possible answer to this problem, though the data are far from conclusive. Without a multicenter, randomized, double-blind, placebo-controlled study of sufficient numbers to assess the effect of immunocompetence and age in therapeutic success, no definitive comment is possible regarding enhanced healing of the vesicular risk or prevention of PHN by regional sympathetic blockade.

Complex Regional Pain Syndrome

Complex regional pain syndrome (CRPS) is one of the common neuropathic syndromes. While CRPS 1, or reflex sympathetic dystrophy, is a clinical diagnosis, determining the component of the pain that is mediated or maintained by the sympathetic nervous system may play an important role in tailoring the therapeutic approach for a specific patient. Early diagnosis of SMP is important, since the painful syndrome may be progressive and debilitating. SMP is diagnosed by determining the magnitude of relief of pain with appropriate sympathetic blockade.

However, the results of local anesthetic sympathetic blocks must be interpreted with caution. It is important to know whether the sympathetic blockade is complete, especially in patients who do not have significant pain relief. The efficacy of sympathetic blockade can be objectively assessed by evaluating the effects on sympathetic sudomotor and vasoconstrictor function and by measuring changes in skin blood flow, skin temperature, and skin resistance.

When the goal is diagnosis, the sympathetic block should be specific to the sympathetic nervous system. When therapy is the goal, however, the technique need not have specificity to that system.

Once the diagnosis of SMP is made, the mainstay of treatment is sympatholysis in conjunction with appropriate psychological and physical therapy. The goal is restoration of normal function. No single therapy is effective in the rehabilitation of all patients. In general, therapy should include treatment of the precipitating injury, sympathetic blockade, and aggressive physical therapy.

What, then, is the efficacy of sympathetic blockade? Recent studies indicate that the adequacy of sympathetic blockade in SMP does not consistently correlate with the degree of pain relief obtained. Notwithstanding the variables introduced by the widely differing technical skills, lack of uniform protocols, and the need for obsessive attention to detail when performing these sympatholytic regional anesthetic procedures, there are several other possible reasons for the relief of pain in the absence of successful sympathetic block. One is that a placebo response is elicited. A second is that the pain relief is due to the regional spread of local anesthetic to nearby somatic afferent nerves and their dorsal root ganglia. This regional spread may also occur with stellate ganglion injections and is of course inevitable when using epidural and intrathecal injections. A third possibility is the systemic absorption of locally injected lidocaine, which produces analgesia through an action distant from the injection site (e.g., dorsal root entry zone).

In the final analysis it is clear that none of the methods that are directed toward interrupting the α-adrenoceptor, either pharmacologically or by conduction block, are entirely reliable, reproducible, easy to interpret, or highly specific. In fact, differential blocks by any route have the least specificity and at best can only be considered screening tests of sympathetic function. The problems of placebo, false-positive results, and the possibility that a non—adrenoceptor-dependent mechanism, albeit indirect, might indeed lower the specificity of the different methods still remain. Certainly the disparity between the relief of pain after a sympathetic block and the phentolamine test may merely reflect the failure in each case of an appropriate dose response. In support of sympatholysis by whichever method, however, are compelling data that still seem to implicate the α_1-adrenoceptor in nociception. What is clear is that interpretation of the response to sympatholysis must be taken in context with the total clinical picture. Because the diagnosis of CPRS 1 is essentially one of exclusion, any contributory tests of clinical features that are reproducibly unique to these conditions must remain a part of the standard diagnostic protocol. Sympatholysis, whether pharmacological or by conduction block, is one such test. Until new knowledge regarding a mechanism of pathophysiology suggests otherwise, regional anesthetic with the limitations already discussed in this test is a centerpiece in the diagnosis of CPRS 1 and SMP.

Cancer Pain

Various types of regional analgesic techniques have been used in patients with cancer pain (Table 35.10). Destructive solutions have been injected into nerves, ganglia, epidural, and intrathecal space for 60 years. Alcohol was first used in the early 1930s by Dogliotti (172h). It has been injected in the intrathecal and epidural spaces, celiac plexus, various sympathetic ganglia, and on pituitary in concentrations ranging from 50% to 100%.

What is the success rate, for instance, of intrathecal phenol neurolysis? Despite 60 years of use, the incidence of success has been quoted reliably at 45% to 60%. There has not been much change in technique despite decades of use. Criteria for success rates vary from one type of study to another, making comparison difficult. In addition, prospective comparisons of this technique with newer methods of pain control, that is, intrathecal morphine pump, deep brain stimulation, and dorsal root entry zone lesions, have not been done,

Table 35.10.   Types of Injected Solutions and Procedures for Regional Analgesia in Chronic Pain and Cancer Patients

Nondestructive solutions
  Local anesthetics
  Opiates
  Steroids
Destructive solutions and procedures
  Alcohol
  Phenol
  Hypertonic saline
  Chlorocresol
  Ammonium sulfate
  Radiofrequency ablation
  Cryolysis and similar procedures

making it difficult to assess its real value in pain control. Many of these techniques are intricate, and one must be cognizant of the range of therapeutic efficacy and complications when deciding upon a particular neurolytic approach.

We continue to strive for neurolytic techniques that are selective in destroying pain fibers while sparing all others. While ricin and capsaicin offer promise as selective agents, little has been reported on them. Laser, on the other hand, offers the most controlled area of neurodestruction, even though it is nonselective. However, it is limited to procedures that permit direct visualization of the target nerves. There are few reports in the literature comparing these newer agents with the more widely accepted techniques. Cryoanalgesia has the least incidence of long-term neuralgia, but studies with it have shown a short duration of relief and low efficacy. The neurolytic drugs alcohol and phenol are the premier agents still in use, and modification of their concentrations and volumes are allowing them to be used in patients even with benign causes of pain. The use of neurolytic agents in the treatment of benign pain, however, continues to remain controversial. These are drugs and techniques with infrequent but serious complications that may be more acceptable in the terminal patient with a life expectancy measured in weeks or months.

Myofascial Pain

Myofascial trigger point injection of local anesthetics are the simplest and most frequently used analgesic blocks in the treatment of pain. Simplicity and apparent innocuousness make this a method of choice among physicians treating chronic pain. Dry needling of trigger points without injecting any solution may be effective but does not equal the therapeutic effectiveness of injecting a local anesthetic. Krause (173) noted that postinjection pain follows dry needling. Sola and Kuitert (174) treated a series of 100 patients with isotonic saline in their trigger points. They found saline effective in relieving the pain. Hameroff et al. (175), on the other hand, found the long-acting local anesthetics bupivacaine, and etidocaine provide better and longer pain relief for up to 7 days post injection. We have experience with a mixture of 0.5% etidocaine and 0.375% bupivacaine and found their effect long-lasting without systemic or myotoxicity. This mixture has produced better relief than dry needling, saline, or lidocaine in my hands.

Travell and Simons (176) advocate mixing corticosteroid and a local anesthetic for trigger point injection, for two groups of patients only: those with soft-tissue inflammation (adhesive capsulitis) and those with postinjection soreness of muscles. We have experience with dexamethasone (4 mg/10 mL of local anesthetic solution), mixing it with bupivacaine and etidocaine, and found no sequelae due to its use. It is true that steroid may be responsible for a burning sensation in the area of injection 24 to 48 hours postinjection. But this subsides and patients continue to have pain relief 7 to 10 days afterward.

SUMMARY

Nerve blocks, even though questioned by pain specialists who do not perform these procedures, are useful for diagnostic, prognostic, and therapeutic purposes. They have a place in difficult and complex pain patients. They need to be performed with precision and under safe monitored conditions to obtain good outcome. Adequate training of clinicians in performing these procedures is essential. The efficacy of nerve blocks is at least as good as any other management technique available to the pain specialist. They are most useful when intolerable acute pain is to be adequately managed and when the patient's function is poor and requires tolerable pain relief to pursue aggressive physical therapy.

References

1. Rynd F. Treatment of neuralgia: introduction of fluid to the nerve. Dublin: Medical Press, 1845;13:167.
2. Pravaz CG. Sur un nouveau moyen d'operer la coagulation du sang dans les artères, applicable à la guérison des anéyrismes. CR Acad Sci (Paris) 1853;36:88.
3. Wood A. New method of treating neuralgia by the direct application of opiates to the painful points. Edinburgh Med Surg J 1855;82:265.
4. Niemann A. Über eine organische Base in der Coca. Annal Chemie 1860;114:213.
5. Bennett A. An experimental inquiry into the physiological actions of theine, caffeine, guaranine, cocaine, and theobromine. Edinburgh Med J 1873;19:323.
6. Von Anrep V. Über die physiologische Wirkung des cocaine. Arch Ges Physiol 1880;21:38.
7. Fauvel H. De l'anesthesia produite par le chlorhydrate de cocaine sur la muquese pharyngienne et laryngienne. Gas Hôp Nr 1864;134S:1067.
8. Koller C. Vorläufige Mitteilung über lokale Anästhesierung am Auge. Bericht über die 16. Versammlung der ophthalmologischen Gessellschaft. Heidelberg Beilageheft Klin Mbl Augenh 1884;60–63.
9. Corning JL. Spinal anesthesia and local medication of the cord. N Y State J Med 1885;42:483.
10. Boas RA. Nerve blocks in the diagnosis of low back pain. In: Loeser JD, ed. Low back pain. Neurosurgery Clinics of North America. Philadelphia: Saunders, 1991;807–816.
11. Bonica JJ, Buckley FP. Regional analgesia with local anesthetics. In: Bonica JJ, ed. The management of pain. Philadelphia: Lea & Febiger, 1990;1883–1966.
12. Dooley JF, McBroom RJ, Taguchi T, et al. Nerve root infiltration in the diagnosis of radicular pain. Spine 1988;13:79–83.
13. Haueisen D, Smith B, Myers S. The diagnostic accuracy of spinal injection studies: their role in the evaluation of sciatica. Clin Orthop 1985;198:179–183.
14. Herron LD. Selective nerve root blocks in patient selection for lumbar surgery: surgical results. J Spinal Disord 1989;2:75–79.
15. Krempen JF, Smith BS. Nerve root injection: a method for evaluating the etiology of sciatica. J Bone Joint Surg 1974;56A:1435–1444.
16. Macnab I. Unilateral root decompression in lumbar spinal stenosis. Orthop Trans 1988;12:77.
17. Mooney V. Injection studies: role in pain definition. In: Frymoyer JW, Ducker TB, Hadler NM, et al. The adult spine: principles and practice. New York: Raven Press, 1991;527–540.
18. Cytowic R. Nerve block for common pain. New York: Springer-Verlag, 1990;62.
19. Steindler A, Luck JV. Differential diagnosis of pain in the low back: allocation of the source of pain by procaine hydrochloride method. JAMA 1938;110:106–113.
20. Xavier AV, McDanal J, Kissin I. Relief of sciatic radicular pain by sciatic nerve block. Anesth Analg 1988;67:1177–1180.
21. Kikuchi S, MacNab I, Moreau P. Localization of the level of symptomatic cervical disc degeneration. J Bone Joint Surg 1981;63B.272–277.
22. Krempen JF, Smith BS, Defreest LJ. Selective nerve root infiltration for the evaluation of sciatica. Orthop Clin North Am 1975;6:311.
23. Lord SM, Barneley L, Wallis BJ et al. Third occipital nerve headache: a prevalence study. Neurol Neurosurg Psychiatry 1991;57:1187–1190.
24. Bogduk N, Marsland A. The cervical zygapophyseal joints as a source of neck pain. Spine 1988;13:610–617.
25. Laros GS. Differential diagnosis of low back pain. In: Mayer TT, Mooney V, Gatchel RJ, eds. Contemporary conservative care for painful spinal disorders. Philadelphia: Lea & Febiger, 1991;123–130.
26. Tile M. The role of surgery in nerve root compression. Spine 1984;9:57–64.
27. Loeser JD. Dorsal rhizotomy for the relief of chronic pain. J Neurosurg 1972;367:745–754.
28. North RB, Kidd DH, Campbell JN, et al. Dorsal root ganglionectomy for failed back surgery syndrome: A five year follow up study. J Neurosurg 1991;74:236–242.
29. North RB, Han M, Zahurak M, et al. Radiofrequency lumbar facet denervation: analysis of prognostic factors. Pain 1994;57:77–83.
30. Park W. The place of radiology in the investigation of low back pain. Clin Rheumatol Dis 1980;6:93–132.
31. Gasser HS, Erlanger J. The role of fiber size in the establishment of a nerve block by pressure or cocaine. Am J Physiol 1929;88:581–591.
32. Nathan PN, Sears TA. Some factors concerned in differential nerve block by local anesthetics. J Physiol (Lond) 1961;157:565–585.
33. Franz DN, Perry RS. Mechanisms for differential block among single myelinated and nonmyelinated axons by procaine. J Physiol (Lond) 1974;236:193–210.
34. Gissen AJ, Covino BG, Gregus J. Differential sensitivities of mammalian nerve fibers to local anesthetic agents. Anesthesiology 1980;53:467–474.
35. Gissen AJ, Covino BG, Gregus J. Differential sensitivity of fast and slow fibers in mammalian nerve: 3. Effect of etidocaine and bupivacaine in fast/slow fibers. Anesth Analg 1982;61:570–575.
36. Onofrio BM, Campa HK. Evaluation of rhizotomy: review of 12 years' experience. Neurosurg 1972;36:751–755.
37. Goldthwait JE. The lumbosacral articulation: an explanation of many cases of lumbago, sciatica, and paraplegia. Boston Med Surg J 1911: 164:365–372.
38. Dory MA. Arthrography of the cervical facet joints. Radiology 1983;148:379–382.
39. Fairbank JCT, Park WM, McCall IW, et al. Apophyseal injection of local anaesthetic as a diagnostic aid in primary low back pain syndromes. Spine 1981;6:598–605.
40. Hove B, Gyldensted C. Cervical analgesic facet joint arthrography. Neuroradiology 1990;32:456–459.
41. Jackson RP, Jacob RR, Montesaro PX. Facet joint injection on low back pain: a prospective statistical study. Spine 1988;13:966–971.
42. Mooney V, Robertson J. The facet syndrome. Clin Orthop 1976; 115:149–156.
43. Ogsbury JS, Simon RH, Lehman RW. Facet denervation in the treatment of low back pain syndrome. Pain 1977;3:257–263.

44. Raymond J, Dumas JM. Intra-articular facet diagnostic test or therapeutic procedure? Radiology 1984;15:1–11.

45. Selby DK, Paris SC. Anatomy of facet joints as connection with low back pain. Contemp Orthop 1981;11:312.

46. Barnsley L, Lord S, Bogduk N. Comparative local anaesthetic blocks in the diagnosis of cervical zygapophysial joint pain. Pain 1993; 55:99–106.

47. Schwarzer AC, Aprill CN, Derby R, et al. Clinical features of patients with pain stemming from the lumbar zygapophyseal joints: is the lumbar facet syndrome a clinical entity? Spine 1994;19:1132–1137.

48. Esses S, Moro JK. The value of facet joint blocks in patient selection for lumbar fusion. Spine 1993;18:185–190.

49. Treede RD, Davis KD, Campbell JN, et al. The plasticity of cutaneous hyperalgesia during sympathetic ganglionic blockade in patients with neuropathic pain. Brain 1992;115:607–621.

50. Roberts WJ. A hypothesis on the physiological basis for causalgia and related pains. Pain 1986;24:297–311.

51. Verdugo R, Ochoa JL. Placebo-controlled somatic and sympathetic blocks in patients with prior diagnosis of causalgia, RSD or SMP. In GF Gebhardt, DL Hammond, TS Jensen, eds. Proceedings of the VII World Congress on Pain, Progress in Pain Research and Management, vol 2. Seattle: IASP Press, 1993:560–561 (abstract).

52. Stanton-Hicks M. Blocks of the sympathetic nervous system. In: Stanton-Hicks M, ed. Pain and the sympathetic nervous system. Boston: Kluwer, 1990:153–164.

53. Löfström JB, Lloyd JW, Cousins MJ. Sympathetic neural blockade of upper and lower extremity. In: MJ Cousins, PO Bridenbaugh, eds. Neural blockage in clinical anesthesia and management of pain. Philadelphia: Lippincott, 1980:355–382.

54. Rowbotham MC, Fields HL. Topical lidocaine reduces pain in postherpetic neuralgia. Pain 1989;38:297–301.

55. McPherson GA, Angus JA. Phentolamine and structurally related compounds selectively antagonize the vascular actions of the K+ channel opener, cromakalim. Br J Pharmacol 1989;97:941–949.

56. Dunne MJ. Block of ATP-regulated potassium channels by phentolamine and other alpha-adrenoreceptor antagonists. Br J Pharmacol 1991:103:1847–1850.

57. Campbell JN, Meyer RA, Raja SN. Is nociceptor activation by alpha-1 adrenoceptors the culprit in sympathetically maintained pain? APS J 1992;1:3–11.

58. Dellemijn HL, Fields RR, Allen WR, et al. The interpretation of pain relief and sensory changes following sympathetic blockade. Brain 1994; 117:1475–1487.

59. Moore DC. Anterior (paratracheal) approach for block of the stellate ganglion. In: Regional block: a handbook for use in the clinical practice of medicine and surgery. 4th ed. Springfield, IL: Charles C. Thomas, 1975; 123–137.

60. Hardy PAJ, Wells JCD. Extent of sympathetic blockade after stellate ganglion block with bupivacaine. Pain 1989;36:193–196.

61. Raja SN, Treede RD, Davis KD, et al. Systemic alpha-adrenergic blockade with phentolamine: a diagnostic test for sympathetically maintained pain. Anesthesiology 1991;74:691–698.

62. Beecher HK. The powerful placebo. JAMA 1955;159:1602.

63. Benson H, Epstein J. The placebo effect: a neglected asset in the care of patients. JAMA 1975;232–1225.

64. Laska E, Sunshine A. Anticipation of analgesia: a placebo effect. Headache 1973;13:1.

65. Meleka S, Staats PS, Hekmat H. Evaluating the possible role of the placebo response in diagnostic peripheral neural blockade. Reg Anesth 1997 (in press).

66. Staats PS, Hekmat H, Staats A. The placebo-suggestion and pain: negative as well as positive. J Pain Symptom Mgmt 1998;15(4):235–243.

67. Staats PS, Hekmat H, Staats AW. The psychological behaviorism theory of pain. Pain Forum 1996;5:13.

68. Boas RA, Covino BG, Shahwarian A. Analgesic response to IV lignocaine. Br J Anesth 1982;54:501.

69. Woolf C, Wiesenfeld-Hallin A. The systemic administration of local anesthetics produces a selective depression of C-afferent fiber evoked activity in the spinal cord. Pain 1985;23:361.

70. Boas RA, Cousins MJ. Diagnostic neural blockade. In: Cousins MJ, ed. Regional anesthesia. Philadelphia: Lippincott-Raven, 1988:885–898.

71. Weiss S, Davis D. The significance of the afferent impulses from the skin in the mechanism of visceral pain: skin infiltration as a useful therapeutic measure. Am J Med Sci 1928;176:517.

72. Travell J, Rinzler SH. Relief of cardiac pain by local block of somatic trigger areas. Proc Soc Exper Biol Med 1946;63:480.

73. North RB, Kidd DH, Zahurak M, et al. Specificity of diagnostic nerve blocks: a prospective randomized study of sciatica due to lumbosacral spine disease. Pain 1996;65:77–85.

74. Henry JA. Cardiac pain referred to site of previously experienced somatic pain. Br Med J 1978;9:1605–1606.

75. Schechter NL. Pain and pain control in children. Curr Probl Pediatr 1985;15:1.

76. Leriche R. Simple methods of easing pain in the extremities in arterial diseases and in certain vasomotor disorders. Presse Med 1941;49:799.

77. Hatangdi VS, Boas RA, Richards EG. Postherpetic neuralgia: management with antiepileptic and tricyclic drugs. In: Bonica JJ, Liebeskind JC, Albe-Fessard D, eds. Advances in pain research and therapy. New York: Raven, 1976;1:583–587.

78. Parris WCV, Gerlock AJ, Macdonnell RC. Intraarterial chloroprocaine for the control of pain associated with partial splenic embolization. Anesth Analg 1981;60:112–115.

78a. Schnapp M, Mays KS, North WC. Intravenous chloroprocaine in the treatment of pain. Anesth Analg 1981;60:844–845.

78b. Phero JC et al. Controlled intravenous administration of chloroprocaine for intractable management. Reg Anaesth 1984;9:50–51.

79. Green R, Dawkins CJM. Postoperative analgesia: the use of continuous drip epidural block. Anaesthesia 1966;21:372.

80. Sqoerel WE, Thomas A, Gerula GR. Continuous drip analgesia: experience with mechanical devices. Can Anaesth Soc J 1970;17:37.

81. Rosenblatt RM, Raj PP. Experience with volumetric infusion pumps for continuous epidural analgesia. Reg Anaesth 1979;4:21–23.

82. Cleland JG. Continuous epidural caudal analgesia in surgery and early ambulation. Northwest Med 1949;48:266.

83. Akerman B, Arwenstrom E, Post C. Local anesthetics potentiate spinal morphine antinociception. Anesth Analg 1988;67:943–948.

84. Bromage PR, Camporesi E, Chestnut D. Epidural narcotics for postoperative analgesia. Anesth Analg 1980;59:473–480.

85. Cousins MJ, Mather LE. Intrathecal and epidural administration of opioids. Anesthesiology 1984;61:276–310.

86. Rutler DV, Skewes DG, Morgan M. Extradural opioids for postoperative analgesia. Br J Anaesth 1981;53:915–920.

87. Scott NB, Mogensen T, Bigler D, et al. Continuous thoracic extradural 0.05% bupivacaine with or without morphine: effect on quality of blockade, lung function and the surgical stress response. Br J Anaesth 1989;62:253–257.

88. Lubenow TR, Durrani Z, Ivankovich AD. Evaluation of continuous epidural fentanyl/butorphanol infusion for postoperative pain. Anesthesiology 1988;69:381.

89. Rosseel PMJ, Van Der Broeck J, Boer EC, et al. Epidural sufentanil for intraoperative and postoperative analgesia in thoracic surgery: a comparative study with intravenous sufentanil. Acta Anaesthesiol Scand 1988;32:193–198.

90. Raj PP, Denson D, Finnason R. Prolonged epidural analgesia: intermittent or continuous. In: Meyer J, Nolte H, eds. Die Kontinuerliche Peridural Anesthesia. VII International Symposium über Die Regional An-Aesthesia AM, January 7, 1982, Minden, Germany. Stultgant, Germany: George Themaverlag, 1983:26–38.

91. Tucker GT, Cooper S, Littlewood D, et al. Observed and predicted accumulation of local anesthetics during continuous extradural analgesia. Br J Anaesth 1977;49:237.

92. Gregory MA, Brock-Utne JC, Bux S, et al. Morphine concentration in brain and spinal cord after subarachnoid morphine injection in baboons. Anesth Analg 1985;64:929–932.

93. Rawal N, Sjöstrand U, Dahlström B. Postoperative pain relief by epidural morphine. Anesth Analg 1981;60:726–731.

94. Chestnut DH, Owen CL, Bates JN, et al. Continuous infusion epidural analgesia during labor: a randomized double-blind comparison of 0.0625% bupivacaine/0.0002% fentanyl versus 0.125% bupivacaine. Anesthesiology 1988;68:754–759.

95. Cullen M, Staren E, Ganzouri A, et al. Continuous thoracic epidural analgesia after major abdominal operations: a randomized prospective double-blind study. Surgery 1985;98:718–728.

96. Fisher R, Lubenow TR, Liceaga A, et al. Comparison of continuous epidural infusion of fentanyl-bupivacaine and morphine-bupivacaine in the management of postoperative pain. Anesth Analg 1988;67:559–563.

97. Logas WG, El-Baz NM, El-Ganzouri A, et al. Continuous thoracic epidural analgesia for postoperative pain relief following thoracotomy: a randomized prospective study. Anesthesiology 1987;67:787–791.

98. Hjortsø NC, Lunc C, Mogensen T, et al. Epidural morphine improves pain relief and maintains sensory analgesia during continuous epidural bupivacaine after abdominal surgery. Anesth Analg 1986;65:1033–1036.

99. Magora F, Olshwand DL, Eimei D, et al. Observation on extradural morphine analgesia in various pain conditions. Br J Anaesth 1980; 52:247–252.

100. Rutberg H, Hakannson E, Anderberg B, et al. Effects of extradural administration of morphine, or bupivacaine on the endocrine response to upper abdominal surgery. Br J Anaesth 1984;56:233–238.

101. Sjöström S, Hartvig D, Tamsen A. Patient controlled analgesia with extradural morphine or pethidine. Br J Anaesth 1988;60:358.

102. Chrubasik J, Wieners K. Continuous plus on-demand epidural infusion of morphine for postoperative pain relief by means of a small, externally worn infusion device. Anesthesiology 1985;62:263.

103. Downing JE, Stedman PM, Busch EH. Continuous low volume infusion of epidural morphine for postoperative pain. Reg Anesth 1988;13(Suppl):84.

104. Planner RS, Cowie RW, Babarczy AS, et al. Continuous epidural morphine analgesia after radical operations upon the pelvis. Surg Gynecol Obstet 1988;166:229.

105. Rauck R, Knarr D, Denson D, et al. Comparison of the efficacy of epidural morphine given by intermittent injection of continuous infusion for the management of postoperative pain. Anesthesiology 1986;65:A201.

106. Marlowe S, Engstrom R, White PF. Epidural patient-controlled analgesia (PCA): an alternative to continuous epidural infusions. Pain 1989;37:97.

107. Walmsley PNH, McDonnell FJ, Colclough GW, et al. A comparison of epidural and intravenous PCA after gynecological surgery. Anesthesiology 1989;73:A684.

108. Loper KA, Ready LB, Sandler AN. Epidural and IV fentanyl infusions are clinically equivalent following knee surgery. Anesthesiology 1989; 71:A1149.

109. Estok PM, Glass PSA, Goldberg JS, et al. Use of PCA to compare IV to epidural administration of fentanyl in the postoperative patient. Anesthesiology 1987;67:A230.

110. Cohen S, Amar D, Pantuck CB. Continuous epidural-PCA postcesarean section: buprenorphine-bupivacaine 0.03% vs. fentanyl-bupivacaine 0.03%. Anesthesiology 1990;73:A975.

111. Cohen S, Amar D, Pantuck CB. Continuous epidural-PCA cesarean section: Buprenorphine-bupivacaine 0.015 with epinephrine vs fentanyl-bupivacaine 0.015 with and without epinephrine. Anesthesiology 1990;73:A918.

112. Gambling DR, Yu P, Cole C, et al. A comparative study of patient controlled epidural analgesia (PCEA) and continuous infusion epidural analgesia (CIEA) during labour. Can J Anaesth 1988;35:249–254.

113. Gambling DR, McMorland GH, Yu P, et al. Comparison of patient controlled epidural analgesia and conventional intermittent "top-up" injections during labor. Anesth Analg 1990;70:256–261.

114. Lysak SZ, Eisenach JC, Dobson CE. Patient-controlled epidural analgesia during labor: a comparison of three solutions with a continuous infusion control. Anesthesiology 1990;72:4449.

115. Viscomi C, Eisenach JC. Patient-controlled epidural analgesia during labor. Obstet Gynecol 1989;77:A685.

116. Naulty JS, Barnes D, Becker R, et al. Patient-controlled epidural analgesia vs. continuous infusion of sufentanil-bupivacaine for analgesia during labor and delivery. Anesthesiology 1990;73:A963.

117. Coombs DW, Saunders RL, Lachance D, et al. Intrathecal morphine tolerance: use of intrathecal clonidine, DADLE, and intraventricular morphine. Anesthesiology 1985;62:358–363.

118. Auld AW, Maki-Jokela A, Murdoch DM. Intraspinal narcotic analgesia in the treatment of chronic pain. Spine 1985;10:777–781.

119. Carl P, Crawford ME, Ravlo O, et al. Long term treatment with epidural opioids: a retrospective study comprising 150 patients treated with morphine chloride and buprenorphine. Anaesthesia 1986; 41:32–38.

120. Glynn C, Dawson D, Sanders R. A double-blind comparison between epidural morphine and epidural clonidine in patients with chronic noncancer pain. Pain 1988;34:123–128.

121. Murphy TM, Hinds S, Cherry D. Intraspinal narcotics: nonmalignant pain. Acta Anaesthiol Scand Suppl 1987;85:75–76.

122. Penn RD, Paice JA. Chronic intrathecal morphine for intractable pain. J Neurosurg 1987;67:182–186.

123. Coombs DW, Pageau MG, Saunders RL, et al. Intraspinal narcotic tolerance: preliminary experience with continuous bupivacaine HCl infusion via implanted infusion device. Int J Artif Organs 1982;5:379–382.

124. Nitescu P, Appelgren L, Linder LE, et al. Epidural versus intrathecal morphine-bupivacaine: assessment of consecutive treatments in advanced cancer pain. J Pain Symptom Manag 1990;5:18–26.

125. Richard B, Kanoff DO. Intraspinal delivery of opiates by implantable, programmable pump in patients with chronic, intractable pain of nonmalignant origin. J Am Osteopath Assoc 1994;94:487–493.

126. Raj P. Continuous brachial plexus analgesia. XXII Annual Meeting, American Society of Regional Anesthesia, San Diego. Abstract Book. 1996;501–502.

127. Fisher A, Meller Y. Continuous postoperative regional analgesia by nerve sheath block for amputation surgery: a pilot study. Anesth Analg 1991;72:300–303.

128. Matsuda M, Kato N, Hosoi M. Continuous brachial plexus block for replantation in the upper extremity. Hand 1982;14:129–134.

129. Hartrick C. Pain due to trauma including sports injuries. In: Raj PP, ed. Practical management of pain. ed 2. St Louis: Mosby–Year Book, 1992;409–433.

130. Raj PP, Montgomery SJ, Nettles D, et al. Infraclavicular brachial plexus block: a new approach. Anesth Analg 1973;52:897.

131. Pham-Dang C, Meunier JF, Poirier P, et al. A new axillary approach for continuous brachial plexus block: a clinical and anatomic study. Anesth Analg 1995;81:686–693.

132. Tuominen M, Haasio J, Hekali R, et al. Continuous interscalene brachial plexus block: clinical efficacy, technical problems and bupivacaine plasma concentrations. Acta Anaesthesiol Scand 1989; 33:84–88.

133. Vaghadia H, Kapnoudhis P, Jenkins LC, et al. Continuous lumbosacral block using a Tuohy needle and catheter technique. Can J Anaesth 1992;39:75.

134. Smith BE, Fischer ABJ, Scott PU. Continuous sciatic nerve block. Anaesthesia 1984;39:155.

135. Guardini R, Waldron BA, Wallace WA. Sciatic nerve block: a new lateral approach. Acta Anaesthesiol Scand 1985;29:515.

136. Edwards ND, Wright EM. Continuous low-dose 3-in-1 nerve blockade for postoperative pain relief after total knee replacement. Anesth Analg 1992;75:265.

137. Linson MA, Leffert R, Todd DP. The treatment of upper extremity reflex sympathetic dystrophy with prolonged continuous stellate ganglion blockade. J Hand Surg 1983;8:153.

138. Raj PP. Sympathetic nerve block. In: Raj PP, ed. Practical management of pain. ed 2. St Louis: Mosby–Year Book, 1992.

139. Murray P. Continuous axillary brachial plexus blockade for reflex sympathetic dystrophy. Anaesthesia 1995;50:633–635.

140. Waldman SD, Coombs DW. Selection of implantable narcotic delivery systems. Anesth Analg 1989;68:377–384.

141. Waldman SD, Cronen MC. Thoracic epidural morphine in the palliation of chest wall pain secondary to relapsing polychondritis. J Pain Symptom Manag 1989;4:60–63.

142. Waldman SD. A simplified approach to the subcutaneous placement of epidural catheters for long-term administration of morphine sulfate. J Pain Symptom Manag 1987;3:163–166.

143. Waldman SD, Feldstein GS, Allen ML. Selection of patients for implantable spinal narcotic delivery systems. Anesth Analg 1986; 65:883–885.

144. Coombs DW, Saunders RL, Schweberger CL. Epidural narcotic infusion reservoir: implantation technique and efficacy. Anesthesiology 1982;56:469–473.

145. Waldman SD, Feldstein GS, Waldman HJ, et al. Caudal administration of morphine sulfate in anticoagulated and thrombocytopenic patients. Anesth Analg 1987;66:267–268.

146. Zenz M. Epidural opiates for the treatment of cancer pain. In: Zimmerman M, Drugs P, Wagner G, eds. Recent results in cancer research. Heidelberg: Springer-Verlag, 1989:107115.

147. Crawford ME, Anderson HB, Augustenborg G, et al. Pain treatment on outpatient basis utilizing extradural opiates: a Danish multicenter study comprising 105 patients. Pain 1983;16:41–46.

148. Peder C, Crawford M. Fixation of epidural catheters by means of subcutaneous tissue tunneling. Ugeskr Laeger 1982;144:2631–2633.

149. Downing JE, Busch EH, Stedman PM. Epidural morphine delivered by a percutaneous epidural catheter for outpatient treatment of cancer pain. Anesth Analg 1988;67:1159–1161.

150. Cousin M, Gourley G, Cherry D. A technique for the insertion of an implantable portal system for the long-term epidural administration of opioids in the treatment of cancer pain. Anesth Intens Care 1985; 13:145–152.

150a. Poletti CB et al. Cancer pain relieved by long-term epidural morphine with a permanent indwelling system for self-administration. J Neurosurg 1981;56:581–584.

151. Gestin Y. a totally implantable multi-dose pump allowing cancer patients intrathecal access for the self-administration of morphine at home: a follow-up of 30 cases. Anaesthetist 1987;36:391.

152. Waldman SD, Leak WD, Kennedy LD, et al. Intraspinal opioid therapy. In: RB Patt, ed. Cancer pain. Philadelphia: Lippincott, 1993; 285–328.

153. Waldman SD, Feldstein GS, Allen ML. A troubleshooting guide to the subcutaneous epidural implantable reservoir. J Pain Symptom Manag 1986;1:217–222.

154. Meyerson BA. Electrical stimulation of the spinal cord and brain. In: Bonica JJ, ed. The management of pain. ed 2. Philadelphia: Lea & Febiger, 1990.

155. North R, et al. Failed back surgery syndrome: five year follow-up after spinal cord stimulator implantation. Neurosurgery 1991;28:692–699.

156. Siegfried J, Lazorthes Y. Long term followup of dorsal cord stimulation for chronic pain syndromes after multiple lumbar operations. Appl Neurophysiol 1982;45:201–204.

157. Long DM, et al. Electrical stimulation of the spinal cord and peripheral nerves for pain control. Appl Neurophysiol 1981;44:207–217.

158. Racz GB, et al. Percutaneous dorsal column stimulator for chronic pain control. Spine 1989;14:1–4.

159. North RB. Spinal cord stimulation for intractable pain: indications and technique. Curr Ther Neurol Surg 1989;2:297–301.

160. Jacobs M, et al. Foot salvage and improvement of microvascular flow as the result of epidural spinal cord electrical stimulation. J Vasc Surg 1990;12:354–360.

161. Waisbrod H, Panhans CH. Direct nerve stimulation for painful peripheral neuropathies. J Bone Joint Surg 1985;67:B470–B472.

162. Cosman ER, Nashold BD, Ovelmann-Levitt J. Theoretical aspects of radiofrequency lesions in the dorsal root entry zone. Neurosurgery 1984;15:945–950.

163. Kline MT. Stereotactic radiofrequency lesions as part of the management of pain. Orlando, FL: Paul M. Deutsch, 1992.

164. Sluyter ME, Racz GB, eds. Techniques of neurolysis. Boston: Kluwer, 1989.

165. Sweet WH. The treatment of trigeminal neuralgia (tic douloureux). N Engl J Med 1986;315:174–177.

165a. Cooper IS, Grissman F, Johnson R. complete system for cryogenic surgery. St Barnab Hosp Med Bull 1962;1:11–16.

166. Lloyd JW, Barnard JDW, Glynn CJ. Cryoanalgesia, a new approach to pain relief. Lancet 1976;2:932–934.

166a. Nelson KN et al. Intraoperative intercostal nerve freezing to prevent postthoracotomy pain. Ann Thorac Surg 1974;18:280–285.

166b. Brain D. Non-neoplastic conditions of the throat and nose. In: Holden HB, ed. Practical cryosurgery. St. Louis: Mosby, 1975.

167. Evans PJD, Lloyd JW, Green CJ. Cryoanalgesia: the response to alterations in freeze cycle and temperature. Br J Anaesth 1981;53:1121–1127.

167a. Gill W, Frazier J, Carter D. Repeated freeze-thaw cycles in cryosurgery. Nature 1968;219:410–413.

168. Barnard JDW, Lloyd JW, Glynn CJ. Cryosurgery in the management of intractable facial pain. Br J Oral Surg 1978–79;16:135–141.

169. Goss AN. Cryoneurotomy for intractable temporomandibular joint pain. Br J Oral Maxillofac Surg 1988;26:26–31.

170. Duthie AM. Pituitary cryoablation. Anaesthesia 1983;38:495–497.

171. Schuster GD. The use of cryoanalgesia in the painful facet syndrome. Neural Orthop Surg 1982;3:271–274.

171a. Khiroya RC, Davenport HT, Jones JG. Cryoanalgesia for pain afer herniorrhaphy. Anasethesia 1986;41:73–76.

172. Wang JK. Cryoanalgesia for painful peripheral nerve lesions. Pain 1985;22:191–194.

172a. Rowlingson TC. Epidural steriods: do they have a place in pain management? APS J 1994;3:20–27.

172b. Abram SE. Risk versus benefit of epidural steriods: let's remain objective. APS J 1994;3:28–29.

172c. Hammonds WD. Epidural steriod injections: an unproven therapy for pain. APS J 1994;3:31–32.

172d. Matas R. Local and regional anesthesia with cocaine and other analgesic drugs, including the subarachnoid method as applied in general surgical practice. Phil Med J 1900;6:820.

172e. Rosenak S. Procaine injection treatment of herpes zoster. Lancet 1938;2:1056–1060.

172f. Colding FL. The effect of regional sympathetic blocks in the treatment of herpes zoster. Acta Anaesth Scand 1969;13:133–141.

172g. Tenicela R, Lovasik D, Eglstein W. Treatment of herpes zoster with sympathetic blocks. Clin J Pain 1985;1:63–67.

172h. Dogliotti AM. Nouvelle méthode thérapeutique pour les algies péripheriques: injection d'alcool dans l'espace sous arachnoiden. Rev Neurol 1931;11:485.

173. Krause H. Clinical treatment of back and neck pain. New York: McGraw-Hill, 1970.

174. Sola AE, Kuitert JH. Myofascial trigger point pain in the neck and shoulder girdle. Northwest Med 1955;54:980–984.

175. Hameroff SR, Crago BR, Blitt CD, et al. Comparison of bupivacaine, etidocaine, and saline for trigger-point therapy. Anesth Analg 1981; 60:752–755.

176. Travell J, Simons DG. Myofascial pain and dysfunction: the trigger point manual. Baltimore: Williams & Wilkins, 1983.

CHAPTER 36

Nonsurgical Management of Spinal Radiculopathy by the Use of Lysis of Adhesions (Neuroplasty)

Gabor B. Racz, James E. Heaver, and P. Prithvi Raj

Epidural neuroplasty (also called epidural neurolysis, lysis of epidural adhesions) is an interventional pain management technique that has emerged over the past 10 or so years. Fundamental to the development and acceptance of the procedure were (*a*) increased clarity about structural changes in the epidural and intervertebral spaces that can contribute to low-back and radicular pain; (*b*) better definition of what structures in and around the epidural space may be involved in the generation of pain; (*c*) data regarding the nature and location of pain that is perceived when different pathological structures in and adjacent to the epidural space are stimulated; (*d*) improvements in techniques for reliably and safely accessing the epidural space via the percutaneous route; (*e*) recognition of the value of epidurography as a diagnostic and therapeutic aid; (*f*) establishment of a clear rationale for the procedure and medications used to accomplish epidural neurolysis; (*g*) demonstrated patient improvement; and (*h*) acceptance of the technique by physicians qualified to judge its merits.

EPIDUROGRAPHY

Synonyms for epidurography include lumbar peridurography and canalography (1). According to these radiologists, epidurography can add a much-needed dimension to the diagnosis of difficult back problems. Their publication in 1979 in a radiology journal a report of epidurography performed on 53 patients documented the utility of this examination. They performed epidurography via the sacral approach, using a modified Seldinger technique to place a catheter for contrast injection.

TISSUE ORIGIN OF LOW-BACK PAIN AND SCIATICA

In 1991 Kuslich et al. (2) published observations they made while performing 193 operations on the lumbar spine of patients given local anesthesia for surgery. They observed that sciatica could be produced by only stimulation of a swollen, stretched, or compressed nerve root. Back pain could be produced by stimulation of several lumbar tissues, but the most common tissue of origin was the outer layer of the annulus fibrosus and posterior longitudinal ligament. Stimulation of the facet joint capsule rarely generated low-back pain, and facet synovium and cartilage surfaces of the facet were never tender.

In patients who had undergone laminectomies, there was always some degree of perineural fibrosis. While scar tissue itself was never tender, the nerve root was frequently very sensitive. Kuslich et al. (2) concluded that scar tissue compounded pain associated with the nerve root by fixing it in one position and thus increasing the susceptibility of the nerve root to tension or compression. Moreover, they concluded that "sciatica can only be produced by direct pressure or stretch on the inflamed, stretched, or compressed nerve root. No other tissues in the spine are capable of producing leg pain." Roffe (3) identified a rich nerve supply to the outer annulus as well as the posterior longitudinal ligament. This innervation is connected to the central nervous system by the sinovertebral nerve (Fig. 36.1). Literature related to the pathogenesis of sciatica was reviewed by Olmarker and Rydevik (4). Besides mechanical factors, nerve roots may also be exposed to substances from degenerated intervertebral discs or facet joints.

PRESSURE

Changes in nerves differ according to whether compression pressures are high or low (e.g., below 200 mm Hg). High pressure may induce direct mechanical effects on the nerve tissue, such as deformation of nerve fibers, displacement of nodes of Ranvier, and invaginations of the paranodal myelin sheaths. Lower pressures induce changes based on impairment of the blood supply to the nerve tissue.

Several interesting studies have been done in which pressure on the cauda equina of animals was applied by inflating

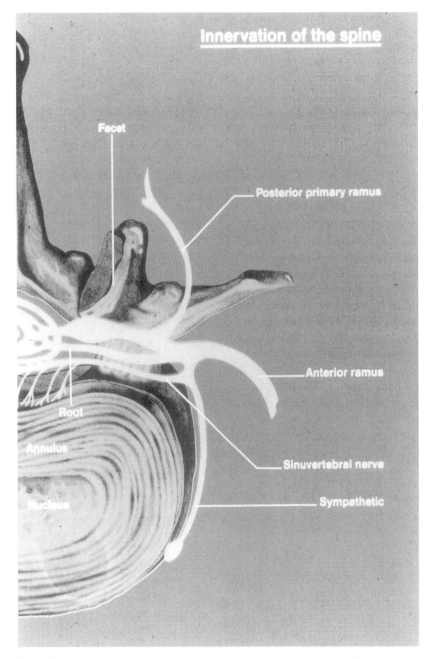

Figure 36.1. Hemi-cross-section of spine showing its innervation. The sinovertebral nerve supplies the annulus fibrosus and posterior longitudinal ligament, two structures that play an important role in back pain. (Courtesy of the Upjohn Company.)

a balloon fixed to the spine. These studies showed that when applied pressure equaled mean arterial pressure, blood flow in the cauda equina ceased. A pressure of 5 to 10 mm Hg stopped blood flow in some venules. Evidence showed that nutrient transport to nerve roots was reduced by 20 to 30% by 10 mm Hg. In addition to reducing nutrient transport, compression may induce changes in the permeability or transmural pressure of endoneural capillaries of the nerve roots producing edema. Such edema was seen after compression at 50 mm Hg for 2 minutes. Intraneural edema in chronic nerve injury is related to the formation of intraneural fibrosis. The

fibrosis may contribute to the slow recovery seen in some patients with nerve compression disorders.

When spinal nerve roots were compressed at 10 mm Hg for 2 hours with two adjacent balloons to simulate a clinical condition of multiple nerve compression, nerve conduction as reflected in recorded action potential was reduced by about 65%. One balloon compression at 50 mm Hg for 2 hours did not affect action potential amplitude. Olmarker and Rydevik concluded that a pressure of 10 mm Hg, which is known to induce incomplete venular congestion, seems to be sufficient to induce changes in nerve function when spinal nerve roots

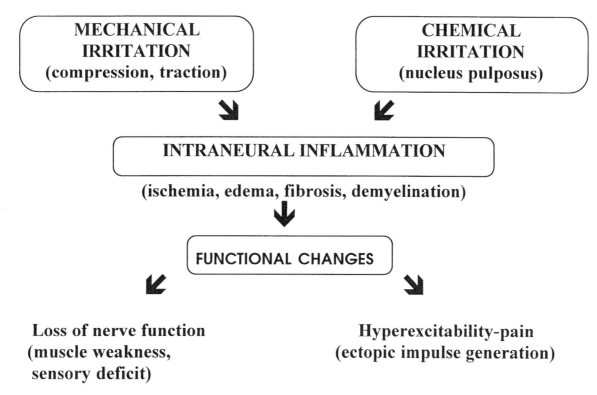

Figure 36.2.   Mechanical and/or chemical stimulation initiate as sequence of events responsible for the generation of back pain and/or radiculopathy.

are compressed at two levels. It was suggested that a herniated or protruded disc may induce higher compression pressures than does central spinal stenosis.

CHEMICAL IRRITATION

The nucleus pulposus has been identified as a source of chemicals that produce irritation when leaked into the spinal canal via a rent in the annulus fibrosis. Nerve roots compressed by disc material often show signs of inflammation. Substances that might leak from the disc and produce inflammation of nerve roots and/or meninges include lactic acid, glycoprotein, cytokines, and histamine. In addition, it has been theorized that material from the nucleus pulposus might act as a foreign protein and trigger an autoimmune reaction. Obviously, chemically induced irritation can occur in the absence of compression by the disc.

STRUCTURAL CHANGES

In a literature review, Benzon (5) pointed out that abnormalities of the intervertebral disc include degeneration, bulging, and herniation. Narrowing of the disc space as a consequence of disc pathology is frequently associated with osteophyte formation and osteoarthritis of the facet joints, which can put pressure on spinal nerves. Bulging of the intervertebral disc distends the posterior longitudinal ligament, causing localized back pain. If bulging of the disc increases, pressure may be exerted on the adjacent nerve roots, producing radicular pain.

RATIONALE FOR EPIDURAL NEUROPLASTY

The foregoing discussion indicates that one or all of the following pathological changes may be present in patients with chronic back pain and/or radiculopathy (Fig. 36.2):

- Inflammation
- Edema
- Fibrosis
- Venous congestion
- Mechanical pressure on
  Posterior longitudinal ligament
  Annulus fibrosis
  Spinal nerve

- Reduced or absent nutrient delivery to the spinal nerve or nerve root
- Central sensitization

Inflamed tissue may generate activity in nociceptors or axons that convey nociceptive information to the central nervous system. In addition, inflammation may render nociceptors or nociceptive axons more sensitive to mechanical stimuli. Sources of mechanical stimuli include pressure as described earlier or movement-induced stretch due to entrapment of a spinal nerve or root by fibrous tissue. Most experience with neuroplasty involves a chronic condition. Therefore, peripheral and central changes associated with chronic painful conditions probably are present in the patients (e.g., central sensitization).

It is therefore rational to treat back pain with or without radiculopathy with local application of (a) anti-inflammatory medication (e.g., corticosteroid); (b) agents aimed at reducing edema (e.g., hypertonic 10% saline and corticosteroid); (c) local anesthetics to block nerve axons that carry nociceptive information to the brain (hypertonic saline has local anesthetic action); and (d) fluid volume with hyaluronidase to break down scarring that prevents medication from getting to target tissue and that traps spinal nerves or roots. Our use of neuroplasty in the treatment of chronic back pain with or without radiculopathy is shown in Figure 36.3. Clearly, noninvasive conservative approaches must be tried first. A synopsis of our technique for neuroplasty is shown in Table 36.1.

EPIDURAL NEUROLYSIS VIA THE CAUDAL APPROACH (6)

Preparation

The patient's consent must be obtained prior to the procedure. The consent form should state all possible complications, including bruising, transient hypotension, transient breathing difficulty, numbness of the extremities, bowel or bladder dysfunction, paralysis, infection, sexual dysfunction, and possible catheter shearing. In selected cases, patients are shown a videotape of the procedure, which lists all of the possible complications as well as expectations in terms of treatment outcomes associated with the dilemma of the intractable progressive failed back syndrome.

Intravenous access must be established. This is necessary in the event of unintended injection of local anesthetic into the subarachnoid or subdural space or into a vascular structure. Additionally, venous access is necessary to allow the administration of sedation. It is usually necessary to administer 1 to 2 mg of midazolam and 25 to 50 μg of fentanyl. Injection of solutions in the epidural space can be quite painful for patients with epidural adhesions. This pain on injection is in all likelihood due to stretching of the affected nerve roots. The patient feels the pain in the dermatomal distribution of the nerve roots being stretched.

Although sedation is given, it is important that the patient remain awake and responsive during the procedure to ensure that the spinal cord is not compressed during the injection. The patient must be able to move the appropriate extremity and to report any weakness or loss of movement that develops during the injection.

All procedures are performed with a fluoroscope with a C-arm. It is preferable to use a fluoroscopy unit with memory capability to decrease radiation exposure. The physician should use appropriate protective measures, including leaded gloves and apron, thyroid shield, and leaded glasses. Most physicians do not routinely use radiographic guidance to place epidural catheters. To obtain maximum benefit from this procedure, however, fluoroscopy should be used to allow verification of needle placement, visualization of dye spread, and proper placement of the catheter.

Choice of Drugs

A water-soluble contrast medium is used because of the possibility of unintended subarachnoid injection. In addition, if contrast agent is injected into the epidural space, it may dissect through the adhesions into the subarachnoid space. Non-water-soluble contrast media in the subarachnoid space can cause spinal cord irritation, spinal cord seizures or clonus, arachnoiditis, and paralysis.

The steroid used for this procedure is triamcinolone. Because the particle size of triamcinolone is about 20 μm, it cannot be injected through a bacterial filter. Owing to its local anesthetic effect, hypertonic saline is used to prolong pain relief, allowing the patient to attend physical therapy twice a day.

Technical Considerations

The patient is placed prone on the fluoroscopy table with a pillow under the abdomen and with the legs abducted and the feet inverted to facilitate entry into the sacral hiatus. Monitoring equipment includes electrocardiography leads, pulse oximeter, and automated blood pressure cuff.

The sacral area is prepared and draped in a sterile manner. The sacral cornua and the sacral hiatus are palpated. The entry point through the skin is in the gluteal fold opposite the affected side, approximately 1 to 2 cm lateral and 2 cm inferior to the sacral hiatus. This site allows the needle as well as the catheter to be directed toward the affected side. Lateral needle placement tends to avoid penetration of the dural sac and subdural area by either the needle or the catheter.

The cutaneous entry point is infiltrated with a local anesthetic such as lidocaine. A 16-gauge epidural needle, preferably an R-K, is passed through the described entry point and into the sacral hiatus, with the sacral cornua used as landmarks to locate the hiatus. The needle is advanced to a level between the S2 and S3 foramina or below. Prior to injection, placement is confirmed by a lateral fluoroscopic view to confirm that the needle is within the bony canal. Radiographic confirmation of needle placement is important, because anatomical variations of the sacrum can lead to incorrect needle placement not recognized on clinical grounds alone. An anteroposterior (AP) view should verify needle tip placement toward the affected side.

After aspiration for blood and cerebrospinal fluid (CSF) is negative, 10 mL of iohexol (Omnipaque 240) or metrizamide (Amipaque) is injected under fluoroscopy. If venous runoff is noted, suggesting intravascular needle placement, the needle tip is moved during injection until contrast medium is seen spreading within the epidural space. While contrast medium is injected into the epidural space, a Christmas tree shape can be noted as the medium spreads into the perineural structures inside the bony canal and along the nerves where they exit the vertebral column. Epidural adhesions prevent the spread of contrast medium in this characteristic pattern, resulting in an absence of medium outlining the involved nerve root.

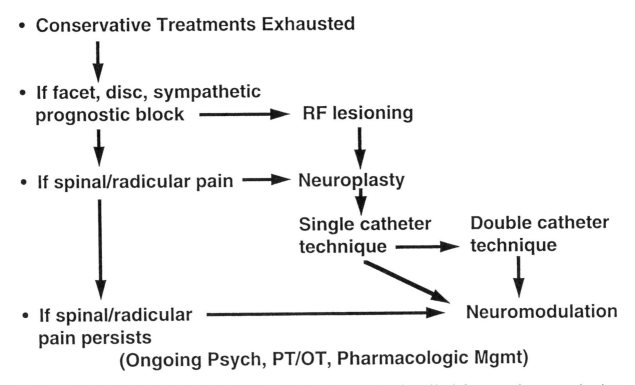

- **Conservative Treatments Exhausted**

- **If facet, disc, sympathetic prognostic block** ⟶ **RF lesioning**

- **If spinal/radicular pain** ⟶ **Neuroplasty**

Single catheter technique ⟶ **Double catheter technique**

- **If spinal/radicular pain persists** ⟶ **Neuromodulation**

(Ongoing Psych, PT/OT, Pharmacologic Mgmt)

Figure 36.3. Algorithm for the treatment of back pain and/or radiculopathy. Neuroplasty is considered after conservative treatments have been found to be ineffective and after appropriate diagnostic evaluation.

Table 36.1. Synopsis of neuroplasty

In the operating room
  Place epidural needle.
  Inject iohexol (Omnipaque-240) and visualize spread of contrast medium (epidurogram).
  If filling defect corresponding to area of pain is present, thread Racz catheter into filling defect (scar) while injecting normal saline through the catheter.
  Observe fluoroscopically to visualize washout of contrast and opening of scar.
  Inject additional iohexol to ascertain opening of scar and spread of injectate within the epidural space.
  Inject preservative-free saline with or without hyaluronidase (Wydase).
  Inject 0.25% bupivacaine and triamcinolone.
  Tape catheter in place.
In the postanesthesia care unit
  Thirty minutes after steroid and local anesthetic injection, inject 10% saline.
In the clinic area
  Once on each of the following 2 days, inject 0.25% bupivacaine; then, 30 min later, 10% saline.
  After the last treatment, remove the epidural catheter.

If the needle tip is subarachnoid, contrast medium spread is noted centrally and cephalad. If the needle tip is subdural, contrast medium spread is also central and cephalad, but not as wide as with subarachnoid injection; however, it enhances the view of the outline of the nerve roots and the dura through the circumferential spread within the less resistant subdural space. Injection of local anesthetic into the subarachnoid or subdural space results in a motor block that is notably more profound and has a more rapid onset than that seen after injection into the epidural space.

If blood is aspirated, the needle is moved until no blood can be aspirated. If CSF is aspirated, it is best to abort the procedure and repeat it the following day. If the patient is allergic to iodinated contrast media, the needle should be placed appropriately, as verified by fluoroscopy, and the procedure should be continued without contrast medium. The soft-tipped, radiographically visible Racz Tun-L-Kath catheter can be used to direct the injection of local anesthetics, steroids, and hypertonic saline as described later.

After negative aspiration, 14 mL of 0.25% bupivacaine and 40 mg (1 mL) of triamcinolone are injected in 2- to 3-mL separate small volumes through the epidural needle while the fluoroscope screen is observed. The contrast agent outlines the filling defect as the agent is displaced by bupivacaine.

A stainless steel fluoropolymer-coated spiral-tipped Racz Tun-L-Kath epidural catheter is passed through the needle into the adhesions. The bevel of the needle should face the ventrolateral aspect of the caudal canal of the affected side. This position facilitates passage of the catheter to the desired side and decreases the chance of catheter shearing. Because adhesion formation is usually uneven, multiple passes may be necessary to place the catheter into the scarred area. For this reason, it is best to use a 16-gauge R-K epidural needle or spinal cord access (SCA) catheter introducer, which is specially designed to allow the catheter to be repositioned.

After negative aspiration, another 5 to 10 mL of contrast medium is injected through the catheter. It should be seen spreading into the area of the previous filling defect. Then 9 mL of 0.25% bupivacaine and 40 mg of triamcinolone are injected through the catheter after negative aspiration. This second injection is helpful in further lysis of adhesions because the catheter tip remains in the adhesions. The area of adhesions and subsequent dissection of adhesions should be noted and recorded.

Then 30 minutes after the second injection of bupivacaine and after negative aspiration, 10 mL of 10% saline is injected in small increments or with an infusion pump over 15 to 20 minutes. The hypertonic saline has a mild, reversible local anesthetic effect and also reduces edema of scarred or inflamed nerve roots. Injection of hypertonic solutions into the normal epidural space is quite painful unless preceded by local anesthetics. If the hypertonic saline spreads beyond the level anesthetized by the local anesthetic, the patient may have severe pain and may require intravenous sedation. The pain caused by the hypertonic saline in the epidural space rarely persists more than 5 minutes.

If contrast medium is not used because of a history of allergy, the procedure is carried out in the same manner without contrast. A test dose of local anesthetic should be given to verify that the needle and subsequently the catheter are not subarachnoid or subdural. The patient notes pain with injection of bupivacaine in the dermatomal distribution of the scarred area. As the catheter is passed, resistance is felt at the level of adhesions. The catheter should be advanced carefully to avoid passage into the subdural area or subarachnoid space.

Postprocedure Considerations

When the procedure is completed, the catheter should be secured. The catheter exit site is covered with a generous amount of triple-antibiotic ointment. Two 2 × 2-inch split venous gauze dressings are used to cover the antibiotic ointment and prevent its spread. The surrounding skin is covered with tincture of benzoin. With a single curve of the catheter toward the midline, the catheter and exit site dressings are covered with a 4 × 6-inch transparent dressing (e.g., Tegaderm). Two 4 × 4-inch gauzes are placed over the course of the catheter from the exit site and the subcutaneous portion toward the sacral hiatus. Four pieces of 6-inch-long Hypafix tape are placed on top of the transparent dressing. The Hypafix tape has the unique property of being elastic yet porous, so that the patient does not sweat it off during the 3 days that the catheter is kept in place.

The catheter is connected to an injection hub adapter, which in turn is connected to a bacterial filter that is not removed during the subsequent three daily injections. The bacterial filter is capped, and the catheter is taped to the patient's flank. During the hospitalization, the patient receives cephalosporin antibiotics (Rocephin), 1 g once daily intravenously, to prevent bacterial colonization, which is especially hazardous in view of the epidurally administered steroid. Additionally, on discharge the patient is ordered oral cephalosporin type of antibiotic therapy for 5 additional days.

Technique for Subsequent Injections

The catheter is left in place for 3 days. On the second and third days, after negative aspiration of blood and CSF, the catheter is injected each day with 10 mL of 0.25% bupivacaine and 30 minutes later with 10 mL of 10% saline. On the third day, the catheter is removed 10 minutes after the last injection. While the catheter is in place, the patient should keep the insertion site dry. We also recommend that the patient keep the area dry for 48 hours after removal of the catheter to decrease the chance of infection.

Epidural neurolysis of adhesions is usually followed by significant improvement in pain and motor function. With improvement of pain, it is important to initiate aggressive physical therapy to improve muscle strength and tone, which are usually weakened from lack of use secondary to pain.

Often it is not possible to lyse existing epidural adhesions completely because of their extent. If necessary, the procedure is repeated. Because of the steroids used, a 3-month delay between procedures is necessary, during which time the patient should be encouraged to continue intensive physical therapy. A month of aquatic therapy is usually followed by aggressive graded physical therapy and work hardening.

Neuroplasty in the Cervical, Thoracic, and Lumbar Areas

The technique for epidural neuroplasty in the cervical, thoracic, and lumbar areas of the spine must be modified to ensure that initial needle placement is in the epidural space and to avoid spinal cord compression by subsequent injections.

Technical Considerations for Cervical Neuroplasty

The patient is placed in the left lateral position on the fluoroscopy table. We use a 3-D technique (direction, depth, direction) to catheterize the cervical epidural space (Fig. 36.4, Table 36.2). The paramedian approach is also used for catheterization of thoracic epidural space. The sequence of events is the same for thoracic neuroplasty as it is for lumbosacral and cervical neuroplasty. The volumes of fluids injected at the thoracic levels are 0.25% bupivacaine 7 mL; 0.9% saline 6 mL.

Catheter Placement in the Anterior Epidural Space or in an Intervertebral Foramen

Medication placed in the posterior or posterolateral epidural space may not reach the area of pathology in an intervertebral foramen or in the anterior epidural space. Therefore, it may be necessary to manipulate catheters into these areas. The direction of the catheter is controlled by (a) inserting the R-K epidural needle or SCA catheter introducer so it points to the direction the catheter is to go and (b) by placing a bend in the tip of the catheter to improve steering. To place a catheter in the anterior

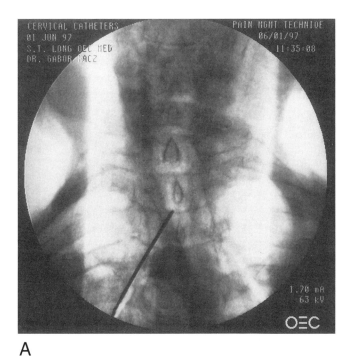

A

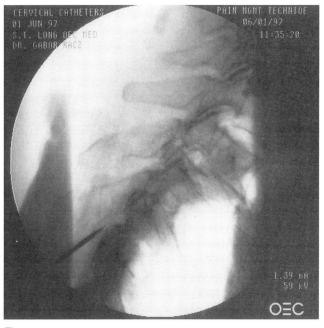

B

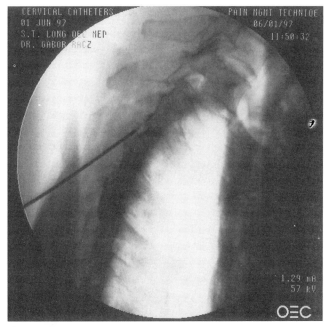

C

Figure 36.4. 3-D technique for accessing cervical epidural space. Direction, **A**; depth, **B**; direction, **C. A.** Anteroposterior (directional) view showing paramedian approach at C7-T1. **B,** Lateral (depth) view showing needle tip entering the posterior epidural space. **C,** Anteroposterior (directional) view showing needle in position and ready to receive catheter.

Table 36.2. Cervical Catheter Placement with the 3D Technique (Direction, Depth, Direction)

Before the operation
  Assess patient to determine neuropathy level and appropriate site
    for catheter placement.
  Obtain white cell count, erythrocyte sedimentation rate, bleeding time; confirm
    within normal limits prior to surgery.
During the operation
  Position patient in the left lateral decubitus position.
  Prep and drape patient.
  Enter C7-T1 or T1-T2.
  Use paramedian approach *1cm or less from midline* one interspace below the
    intended epidural access site.
  Obtain epidural access with a 16-ga R-K needle.
  Use AP fluoro to assess *direction.*
  Use lateral fluoroscopy to determine needle *depth.*
  Use AP fluoroscopy to reassess *direction* and correct if necessary.
  Advance needle to the base of the spinous process. This depth corresponds
    to the level of the lamina near the posterior aspect of the epidural space.
  Remove needle stylet.
  Attach pulsator (low-friction plastic) syringe containing 4 mL normal saline
    and 2 mL air.
  Use loss-of-bounce technique to confirm entry into the epidural space.
  Optimal needle placement is midline.
  Inject iohexol or other myelogram quality contrast 1–2 mL through the needle
    for cervical epidurogram.
  Thread catheter through the needle toward the target nerve root in the lateral
    epidural space. lateral placement is important because nociception and pain
    generators are in the lateral space. Always aspirate catheter first.
  To verify no loculation inject a small amount of dye through the catheter.
  Inject 1500 U hyaluronidase in 4–6 mL normal saline.
  Inject 6 mL 0.25% bupivacaine with 1 mL 40 mg/mL triamcinolone in
    incremental doses (2–3 mL boluses to be sure of no subarachnoid
    or subdural spread).
  Remove needle under fluoroscopy to avoid movement or displacement
    of the catheter.
  Attach connector to the catheter with bacteriostatic filter.
  Affix 3.0′ monofilament locking suture to the skin entry site
    to secure the catheter.
  Apply antibacterial or antifungal ointment to operation site. Cover catheter with
    cotton gauze, placing one loop (cephalad direction) in the catheter. Cover
    with Op-Site adhesive and affix catheter with tape to the patient's skin.
After the operation (recovery room)
  Monitor patient closely for 30 min for subdural spread of bupivacaine, which
    may have delayed onset, and motor block.
  Administer 6 mL hypertonic saline solution through the catheter via
    an infusion pump.
  Flush catheter with 2 mL preservative-free normal saline.
Each of two postoperative days (outpatient pain center)
  Aspirate the catheter
  Inject 2 mL 0.25% bupivacaine through the catheter. Wait 5 min as a
    precaution against subarachnoid or subdural spread. Inject 4 mL 0.25%
    bupivacaine. Wait 15 min as a precaution against subarachnoid
    or subdural spread.
  Infuse 6 mL hypertonic saline through the catheter via infusion pump.
  Flush catheter with 2 mL preservative-free normal saline.
  Following removal of the catheter, warn the patient of possible delayed onset of
    infection, meningitis (2–4 weeks) because of the long-lasting steroid injection.

lumbosacral epidural space via the caudal approach, the catheter should be directed there before S3. At other segmental levels, the transforaminal approach may be used.

PATIENT DATA

Data were reviewed from 1500 patients who underwent lysis of epidural adhesions between the beginning of 1989 and the end of 1992 at our institution. A hundred patients were randomly divided into two groups. Group 1 (n = 50) initially received one dose of triamcinolone plus local anesthetic followed by hypertonic saline. On the second and third days, only the local anesthetic injection was given. Group 2 (n = 50) received the same drugs as group 1 plus an injection of 1500 units of hyaluronidase prior to the injection of local anesthetic and steroid followed by 10% sodium chloride. Under fluoroscopic observation, it is apparent that the injection of hyaluronidase in saline clearly facilitated dispersal of the contrast agent.

The data were reviewed for demographics and duration of pain relief. Telephone follow-up was carried out by a neutral third party, who tabulated the patients' responses. In some instances, patients had undergone treatment 3 years before follow-up. The patients are separated according to gender, drug received, and extent and duration of pain relief.

In group 1, the nonhyaluronidase group, the failure rate was 18%, with 14% of the patients being pain free at the time of review; 68% of the patients in group 1 had various levels and duration of pain relief. In group 2, the hyaluronidase group, the complete failure rate fell by two thirds to 6.1%, and the persistent relief rate was 12.3%. The remaining 81.6% of patients had various levels and duration of pain relief.

It is recognized that an equal volume of saline without the hyaluronidase was not incorporated into this study. Therefore, the question remains whether the higher success rate is due to the effect of the hyaluronidase alone or purely the effect of the additional 10 mL of saline. A prospective double-blind study to answer this question is under way.

The Use of Steroids

At our institution, only one dose of steroid is injected, and the injection is done in the operating room under sterile conditions. The bacterial filter is kept in place for the duration of the patient's hospitalization. It has been demonstrated in the Texas Tech University Health Sciences Center laboratory that when methylprednisolone (Depo-Medrol) plus local anesthetic or triamcinolone (Aristocort) and local anesthetic are injected through a bacterial filter, the filter screens out virtually all of the steroid.

Complications

The potential side effects and complications of epidural neuroplasty include unintended subarachnoid or subdural injection of local anesthetic or hypertonic saline, paralysis, bowel and/or bladder dysfunction, and infection. Careful attention to sterile technique is necessary because steroids suppress the immune system, increasing the risk of infection. Hypertonic saline injected into the subarachnoid space has been reported to cause cardiac arrhythmias, paresis, and loss of sphincter control.

The Texas Tech University Health Sciences Center Experience

At Texas Tech, the technique described in this chapter for lysis of epidural adhesions has been performed in more than 3000 patients with very few complications. Subarachnoid or subdural injection of local anesthetic is very rare. Two of our patients undergoing epidural lysis of adhesions developed meningitis but responded to antibiotic therapy. No patients were paralyzed by this procedure, although one has transient motor weakness following a caudal procedure in which solid proximal adhesion prevented runoff of injected solution. There have been no significant long-term bowel or bladder problems following the use of this technique, although a few patients have noted mild difficulty in voiding for up to 2 weeks after the procedure. Transient perineal numbness that resolves in 1 to 2 months has been reported.

Undiagnosed Neurogenic Bowel and Bladder

The problem of undiagnosed preexisting neurogenic bladder in patients suffering from failed back surgery syndrome or spinal cord injury has resulted in a higher index of suspicion among treating physicians. The use of a consulting urologist to perform urodynamic studies and document any preexisting neurogenic bladder helps avoid incorrectly attributing voiding difficulties to the epidural lysis of adhesions rather than to a patient's underlying pathological process. Testing before the procedure is especially important in patients suffering from ongoing constrictive arachnoiditis, which can cause the development of bowel, bladder, and male sexual dysfunction. Fortunately, the typical experience of such patients who undergo epidural lysis of adhesions is an improvement rather than deterioration in both bladder function and male sexual function.

Spinal Cord Compression

As mentioned earlier, all injections should be made slowly. Rapid injections into the epidural space may cause large increases in CSF pressure, with the risk of cerebral hemorrhage, visual disturbance, headache, and compromise of spinal cord blood flow.

Infection

Patients are warned that during the first 2 to 6 weeks following the procedure, epidural infection is a distinct possibility because of the procedure as well as the immunosuppression secondary to the steroid injection. Until proven otherwise, any nausea, vomiting, neck stiffness, new pain, different pain, increased pain, weakness, numbness, or paralysis is considered to be caused by epidural infection related to the procedure and should be evaluated and treated accordingly.

The patient should be made aware of the need to contact the physician carrying out the procedure or the primary physician immediately if any of these signs and symptoms occur. Prompt intravenous antibiotic therapy that provides coverage for *Staphylococcus aureus* along with hospitalization is the appropriate treatment. As indicated previously, epidural abscess has not been a problem in the Texas Tech patient population. Because of the potentially devastating consequences of an unrecognized and untreated epidural abscess, however, a high index of suspicion coupled with careful education of the patient is mandatory.

Catheter Shearing

Catheter shearing in the Texas Tech practice occurs during the initial training of each new group of pain specialty fellows, until they can identify the sensation associated with the free and smooth movement of the catheter within the needle. Identification of this smooth, flowing movement is necessary, because the physician often has to withdraw the catheter through the specially designed R-K needle to place the catheter in an optimal location. An alternative to the R-K needle is the SCA introducer. The introducer is nonmetallic and therefore will not shear catheters. Sheared catheters usually end up in the subcutaneous tissues or at the sacral hiatus.

Part of the consent form explains that if catheter shearing occurs, surgical intervention to retrieve the sheared catheter is required. To date, there have been five such occurrences. To retrieve the sheared catheter under fluoroscopy, two needles placed from different angles help pinpoint the end of the sheared catheter. This makes removal of the catheter fragment through a half-inch incision a simple procedure. We simply do not share the view that sheared catheters are best left behind.

Sensitivity to Hyaluronidase

In a series of 1520 epidural administrations of hyaluronidase, Moore (7) indicated a 3% sensitivity reaction. Perhaps the reason this 3% sensitivity has not been seen with our technique is that steroid is placed exactly where the hyaluronidase is deposited. The steroid leaves the space more slowly than hyaluronidase and may help protect against allergic reaction. Although the two-thirds reduction of outright therapeutic failure is sufficient justification to continue the administration of hyaluronidase, one must look very carefully for any evidence of a sensitivity reaction in all patients who receive hyaluronidase.

Acceptance by Qualified Physicians

Perhaps one of the best tests of the value of a procedure is for a physician to request the treatment himself or herself.

This is so especially if the physician (*a*) is knowledgeable about the pathophysiology and treatment options for a medical condition and (*b*) has observed the treatment outcomes on numerous occasions. Physicians, including orthopaedic surgeons at our institution, have requested and received epidural neuroplasty (Fig. 36.5).

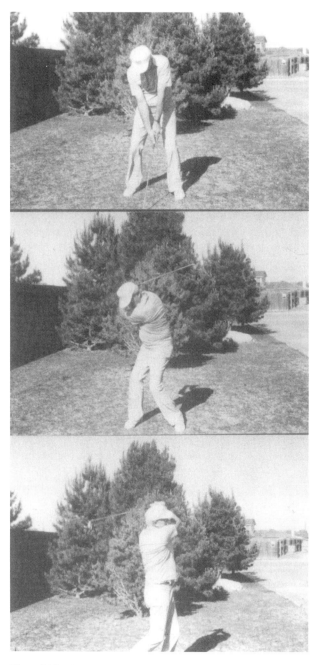

Figure 36.5 Orthopaedic surgeon golfing after having neuroplasty performed on himself. Pain relief continues 2.5 years after neuroplasty at L4-L5 level.

SUMMARY

Epidural neuroplasty is an interventional pain management technique used to treat pain originating from structures within or adjacent to the epidural space or in the intervertebral foramen at all segmental levels. The technique is based on sound scientific foundations that include substantial knowledge regarding the pathogenesis of back pain and radiculopathy. For the technique to be safe and for maximization of therapeutic benefit, strict adherence to details (technique, patient selection) as described in this presentation is recommended.

Acknowledgment

All work was performed in the Texas Tech University Health Sciences Center, Department of Anesthesiology Pain Clinic or the University Medical Center, Institute for Pain Management.

References

1. Roberson G H, Hatten H P Jr, Hesselink J H. Epidurography: selective catheter technique and review of 53 cases. Am Roentgenol R Soc 1979;132:787–793.
2. Kuslich S D, Ulstrom C L, Michael C J. The tissue origin of low back pain and sciatica. Orthop Clin North Am 1991;22:181–187.
3. Roffe P G. Innervation of the annulus fibrosus and posterior longitudinal ligament. Arch Neurol Psychiatry 1940;44:100.
4. Olmarker K, Rydevik B. Pathophysiology of sciatica. Orthop Clin North Am 1991;22:223–233.
5. Benzon H T. Epidural steroid injection for low back pain and lumbosacral radiculopathy. Pain 1986;24:277–295.
6. Racz G B, Heavner J E, Diede J H. Lysis of epidural adhesions utilizing the epidural approach. In: Waldman S D, Winnie A P, eds. Interventional pain management text. Philadelphia: Dannemiller Memorial Educational Foundation, Saunders, 1996;339–351.
7. Moore D C. The use of hyaluronidase in local and nerve block analgesia other than the spinal block: 1520 cases. Anesthesiology 1951;12:611–626.

CHAPTER 37

Intraspinal Drug Delivery Systems for Pain Treatment: When Are They Appropriate?

Serdar Erdine

INTRODUCTION

In the past 2 decades the introduction of intraspinal pain delivery systems has opened new facilities for the treatment of intractable pain. However, this development also brought several problems and questions: the appropriate selection of patients, drugs, and delivery systems; indications; contraindications; side effects; and complications. Numerous articles have appeared in many journals, most of which are uncontrolled studies and personal experiences with a wide range of results. Thus the appropriate use of intraspinal pain delivery systems is still to be discussed.

HISTORICAL PERSPECTIVES

In 1901 Katawata of Japan reported the injection of 10 mg morphine combined with 20 mg eucaine into the subarachnoid space in two patients with uncontrollable back pain. After that 70 years passed before the discovery of opioid receptors in 1971. Opioid receptors were isolated in 1973 and reported in the brain and in the spinal cord in 1974. In 1975 endorphins were identified. In 1976 analgesia mediated by a direct spinal action of opioids was demonstrated. In 1979 first reports of epidural and intrathecal analgesia in man emerged. In 1981 the era of long-term opioid delivery via epidural and intrathecal routes by delivery systems began, with further refinements of technique and instrumentation.

PREIMPLANTATION PERIOD

The overuse and wrong use of drug delivery systems may cause numerous problems. This technology is still under development, and the appropriate use is crucial for all these devices. An approach for the appropriate uses of technology has been proposed. Inappropriate uses are those likely to be unsuccessful (unlikely to benefit the patient with far advanced disease), unsafe (complications outweigh probable benefits), unkind (decrease the quality of life), unwise (divert resources from accomplishing greater good), and unnecessary (goals can be accomplished by simpler means). The best method is use of the least expensive, least invasive, yet most effective treatment possible. The success of spinal opioid delivery depends mainly on proper patient selection.

CRITERIA FOR THE APPROPRIATE USE OF SPINAL DRUG DELIVERY SYSTEMS

Spinal drug delivery systems should be used as follows:

- When the oral route and other less invasive methods are excessive and inadequate
- When the spinal drug delivery system will sustain a better pain relief and quality of life than other methods of analgesia
- When the effectiveness of analgesia is tested by preimplantation trial
- When the caregiver and the patient are trained and there is good communication among the staff, the patient, and the patient's supporters
- When the patient's general and psychological status is stable and favorable
- When the drug delivery system is cost effective

Inappropriate or contraindicated conditions for intraspinal opioid delivery are low platelet count; blood coagulation disorder; local infection; physiological abnormalities that interfere with the pain assessment, such as metabolic encephalopathy, preexisting structural abnormalities, and neurodegenerative disorders; behavioral abnormalities, such as drug dependence; psychiatric disorders; and use of pain for more medication attention seeking, or punishing caregivers.

Many factors determine the clinical efficacy of the spinal opioid delivery:

- The patient's characteristics, including life expectancy, the origin of the pain, age, weight, spinal canal assessment, and environment
- Route used, intrathecal or epidural
- Physical and chemical properties of the drugs used
- Injection technique, bolus or continuous infusion
- Characteristics of the delivery system used, internal or external
- Cost of the system used

A careful history of pain and detailed assessment of the previous therapies should be considered during the preimplantation period. It has been suggested that 90 to 95% of pain can be effectively controlled by the use of World Health Organization (WHO) guidelines for cancer pain relief. Thus first the appropriate use of oral opioids should be considered. The inappropriate use of oral analgesics should not be the first reason for implementing the spinal delivery systems for pain relief. Physician- and patient-related factors play an important role in this aspect. Poor assessment of the patient, lack of adequate information about the indications and use of opioids, and fear of addiction may cause undertreatment of pain related to the physician. Patients with drug dependence or fear of addiction and those who use pain as an attention-seeking device, do not obey the advice of the physician, or manipulate the physician are poor candidates.

CHARACTERISTICS OF THE PATIENT

Cancer Pain

The life expectancy of the patient is very important when selecting the appropriate system. For a patient with a very short life expectancy, days to weeks, a percutaneous or subcutaneously implanted catheter is appropriate. Ports or pumps should be considered for a patient with a life expectancy of months to years.

Not all pain responds to spinal opioids. The route of administration, epidural or intrathecal, differs according to opioid responsiveness. A classification of pain types responding better to intraspinal opioids has been made. Neurogenic, neuropathic, or deafferentation pain; incident pain as observed on weight bearing; bone pain; and other pain syndromes, such as pancreatic pain, rectal tenesmus, and pressure sore pain, are all relatively unlikely to respond to opioids.

However, no patient should lightly be called opioid resistant. Many patients with neuropathic pain respond to intraspinal opioids. Also, there is no correlation between specific pain source and the degree of pain relief .

A complete assessment of the spinal canal during the preimplantation period is mandatory. A space-occupying lesion in the epidural space and compression to the spinal cord may be seen. This is very important for decision making. There is a risk of passing through the tumor during epidural application, and this may cause other complications. If there is tumor compression in the epidural space, the intrathecal route may be used; however, the results are not likely to be satisfactory. The catheter should be inserted under fluoroscopic control to ensure proper place-

ment. If there are any changes of efficacy or problems of delivery during the procedure, epidurography may again be a useful tool, showing catheter tip obstruction and fibrosis sheath formation. However, epidurography cannot be used with all delivery systems. In ports with an inside filter a layer inside the port is formed enhancing the passage of the solution.

The patient's and the caregiver's ability to cope with the equipment and perform tasks associated with drug administration must be considered. An understanding of mechanics and the skill of operating the devices both internal and external are necessary for the caregiver. An appropriate home environment must provide the required conditions for medication storage and pump use as wall as access to emergency medical support.

Non-Cancer Pain

Decision making for cancer pain is somewhat easier than for non-cancer pain. Because of the limited life expectancy, follow-up of the cancer patient is easier, and the long-term complications and side effects are less significant. Opioid therapy for nonmalignant pain is still controversial. Traditionally the opioid analgesics have been used to manage acute pain. Long-term use of opioids has been discouraged because of the risk of tolerance or physical and psychological dependence. In fact there is very little evidence of drug abuse in patients who receive opioid analgesics for any type of painful chronic illness.

The incidence of opioid addiction in some 40,000 hospitalized patients was monitored in a prospective study. Among nearly 12,000 patients who received at least one strong opioid preparation, there were only four reasonably well documented cases of addiction in patients who had no history of drug abuse. These data suggest that medical use of strong opioids is rarely associated with the development of addiction.

If oral opioids can be used for nonmalignant pain syndromes, so can spinal opioid delivery systems. However, there are fewer of these patients than cancer patients. The nonmalignant pain syndromes with which spinal drug delivery systems may be considered are pain of vascular origin in the lower extremities in which surgery is contradicted or ineffective, failed back syndromes, and neuropathic pain syndromes.

In nonmalignant pain treatment, all modalities other than spinal opioid delivery, including oral opioids, should first be used for a reasonable time. Only when all other methods have failed should spinal drug delivery systems be tried, because in noncancer pain the patient will live with the system for the rest of his or her life. Thus the risk of all complications is higher. Every complication requires a new intervention. Thus the patient is likely to become a member of a drug delivery system club.

CLASSIFICATION OF SPINAL DELIVERY SYSTEMS

Several drug delivery systems are now in use. These may be categorized as follows:

- Percutaneously inserted epidural catheters
- Subcutaneously tunneled epidural and intrathecal catheters
- Implanted epidural or intrathecal catheters connected to access ports
- Implanted intrathecal manual pumps
- Implanted intrathecal or epidural infusion pumps
- External pumps

These may also be classified as internal and external systems. There should be appropriate selection criteria for all these systems. Each of them has several advantages and disadvantages. Percutaneous epidural catheters are generally used in acute intraoperative, postoperative, and obstetric pain. Percutaneously inserted epidural catheters are used during the preimplantation trial period to observe the efficacy of the method and the route of administration. It may also be used for patients with a life expectancy of days. However, prolonged use of a percutaneous catheter has been reported to be reliable and safe. If the percutaneous catheter is going to be used for a preimplantation trial, it should be inserted under fluoroscopy. It can be attached to an external infusion pump. It can easily be placed and removed, which is both an advantage and disadvantage.

The subcutaneous epidural or intrathecal catheter has the advantages of easy placement in patients with poor general status and short life expectancy, less risk of infection than the percutaneous catheters, ease of injection by nonmedical caregiver, and attachment to an external pump. The disadvantages of subcutaneously tunneled epidural or intrathecal catheters are dislodgment or migration of the catheter, kinking or obstruction, infection, irritation of the skin by bandages, and difficulty with skin cleaning.

Although it has been frequently used for the epidural route, long-term experience with patients receiving continuous opioid and bupivacaine subarachnoid infusions through an externalized subarachnoid catheter has also been reported. The choice of subarachnoid over epidural opioid treatment with subcutaneously implanted externalized catheters is still a question of a risk benefit ratio and risk of infection. We prefer the epidural route for subcutaneous catheters.

Totally implanted epidural or intrathecal catheters connected to access ports may be stable for longer periods, and the risk of infection is less. However, they have the disadvantages of multiple punctures of the skin, kinking, and obstruction of the catheter. Removal or replacement of the port system requires further surgery. Special needles are necessary for the puncture of the port, and the number of injections possible through the port is limited.

In recent years mechanical pumps, which may be activated by pushing a button, have been developed. These have several advantages over the port systems. Skin punctures are required only for filling the reservoir, and the infection risk is low. It can be used by the patient or the caregiver. However, bolus injection is not possible through these pumps, and if a dose increase is required, the reservoir capacity has to be reassessed. These pumps can be used only intrathecally, as the volume delivered is only 1 to 1.5 mL. They are confined to patients with pure opioid response. Mechanical failure with the buttons is the main cause of surgical removal.

Totally implantable infusion pumps have the advantages of lower peak cerebrospinal fluid and plasma morphine levels than the mechanical pumps, which can be used only for bolus injection. These are stable for very long periods and can be used in patients with noncancerous pain. Implanted infusion pumps also vary widely from fixed rate to programable pumps. Programable pumps are more favorable for noncancer patients, as they can be assessed easily. However, for cancer patients with limited life expectancy they may be considered too expensive, although some studies claim that these are cost effective even in cancer patients after 3 months.

There is an increasing number of externally portable infusion devices available, ranging from a relatively inexpensive syringe driver with a simple on-demand system to more expensive programable devices containing exchangeable plastic reservoirs. The patient or caregiver should successfully manage external systems at home, including changing catheter dressings, changing medication reservoirs, operating the pump, and monitoring side effects. These requirements may cause some difficulties during long-term delivery.

COST EFFECTFIVENESS

Cost effectiveness is one of the important factors for the appropriate use of spinal delivery systems. The development of delivery systems has led to multiple treatment options, the availability of which has resulted in far greater expense both in direct cost and indirect expenses. Given longer survival rates, cancer patients may live months or even years with pain and may incur significant expenses for pain treatment. Thus the life expectancy is important not only for medical reasons but should also be considered in terms of cost effectiveness. Cost-benefit analysis in pain treatment requires a different perspective of analysis. The best pain cost-benefit realization is by use of the least expensive, least invasive, yet most effective pain treatment possible. The decision to use one method of pain control over another is generally made on a case-by-case basis; no given technique has clear superiority for most procedures.

The cost of medications and methods used spinally vary widely even from country to country. For example a comparison of seven morphine products used intraspinally reveals a 21-fold range from the least to most expensive morphine preparation. The period of the use of the system also affects the cost. Savings may accrue when the patients require treatment beyond 3 months with a more expensive implanted infusion system compared with catheters and externalized pumps. The education of the performing physician about the delivery systems may also be important in the reduction of costs. The use of spinal drug delivery systems also have indirect costs to patients and the families, including wages and salaries lost and time devoted to care activities.

SUBARACHNOID VERSUS EPIDURAL DELIVERY: APPROPRIATE CHOICE

Subarachnoid drug delivery systems and tunneled epidural catheters both have distinct advantages and disadvantages. Despite the importance of appropriate selection, the crucial point is the management and follow-up of patients after implantation. Close follow-up and assessment are essential. The selection of the route and mode of administration should be individualized to the patient's circumstances.

The potential advantages of the epidural route are placement at the dermatomal level; no risk of spinal fluid leakage and related spinal headache; the ability of the dura to act as a barrier, reducing the risk of infection at the site of the tip of the catheter; and infection generally limited to the reservoir pocket. There is greater flexibility for the preference of drugs, so that drugs other than the opioids can be used either together with opioids or alone to potentiate the analgesia. The margin of safety may be increased in case of accidental overload. Side effects tend to be less intense. However, the number of catheter dysfunctions is much more in the epidural space than in the intrathecal space. In quite a number of patients fibrosis develops in the epidural space around the tip of the catheter and may occlude the catheter.

Epidural fibrosis develops generally within 2 to 3 months. In some patients a fibrotic sheath develops around the catheter from the tip through the tunneled area to the exit site. During fibrous tissue formation a resistance to the flow through the catheter develops. Dose escalation, which may be considered as pseudotolerance, can develop, the reason being that the dural thickening and fibrotic reactions in the epidural space affect the dural kinetics.

Burning pain on epidural injection is observed in a number of patients. The reasons for such pain can only be speculated upon. Fibrosis, inflammation, or infection in the epidural space may be the cause. This type of pain is sometimes so intractable that patients prefer the pain of their disease and desire removal of the system. Injection-related burning pain and fibrous tissue development are the main reasons for preferring the intrathecal route in patients whose pain responds to opioids.

The advantages of the intrathecal route are less risk of catheter obstruction, no risk of fibrosis or injection-related burning pain, less risk of catheter migration, longer and stronger analgesia, and lower dose of opioids. Generally the intrathecal dose of opioids is 10% of the epidural dose. Complications due to the spinal delivery systems seem to be less in the intrathecal route. However side effects, including nausea, vomiting, and urinary retention, are more severe with the intrathecal route. Generally pure opioids are used for the intrathecal route, but in recent years bupivacaine plus opioid infusions are also delivered intrathecally. Bupivacaine probably potentiates the morphine.

There are some disadvantages of intrathecal delivery. Cerebrospinal fluid leakage and postspinal headache are frequently seen when the catheter is inserted intrathecally, possibly because of the discrepancy between the sizes of the catheter and the needle. The incidence of postspinal headache varies from 0.2 to 24% in anesthesia. If a system inserted intrathecally has to be removed for any reason, a cerebrospinal fistula may develop. This is a very rare complication that requires careful treatment. It is mentioned in only a few studies. Meningitis may occur if the catheter is inserted intrathecally. The incidence has been shown to be higher in series with complete tunneling of the intrathecal catheter and a connection to a port than in series with a percutaneous epidural catheter.

There have been no controlled studies in patients with intractable pain comparing the epidural and intrathecal routes of administration in terms of dosage and analgesic efficiency. Guidelines for the appropriate selection of the route have still to be discussed, but the following points may be considered:

1. For cancer patients with short life expectancy the epidural route may be preferred, as the less expensive drug delivery systems, such as percutaneous, subcutaneously implanted catheters or ports can be used.
2. The use of drugs other than morphine, such as local anesthetics, may be more effectively used with the epidural route. For opioid-nonresponsive pain, combination of drugs may be used via the epidural route.
3. The epidural route should be confined to cancer patients with life expectancies of weeks to 2 to 3 months because fibrosis, occlusion of the catheter, and injection-related burning pain develop with longer durations.
4. Manually activated or infusion pumps are not feasible for the epidural route, as the volume delivered is not generally not more than 1 to 1.5 mL.
5. The intrathecal route may be more effectively used for long-term spinal delivery with more satisfactory, often complete pain relief.
6. With the intrathecal route lower doses and volume of drugs may be sufficient.
7. In nonmalignant pain intrathecal spinal opioid therapy may be continued for years with the use of infusion pumps.

APPROPRIATE SELECTION OF DRUGS

The selection of the appropriate drug for spinal administration is vitally important. The ideal opioid agent for intraspinal use should have the following characteristics:

1. Long duration of effect, up to 24 hours
2. No or minimal side effects, especially nausea, pruritus, respiratory depression, urinary retention, or mental clouding
3. No toxic effects on the spinal cord during long-term delivery
4. No pain on injection
5. Compatibility with available drug delivery systems.

Many of the pharmacokinetic and pharmacodynamic properties of intraspinal opioids can be explained by the influence of their relative solubilities on receptor binding and systemic uptake. High lipid solubility, high specific receptor affinity, low protein binding, and low ionization determine the efficacy of the drug. High molecular weight, low lipid solubility, low blood-brain barrier crossing capacity and stability of receptor binding are the properties of a long-acting drug. Thus lipophilicity and hydrophilicity are the main issues to be considered. Morphine and hydromorphone have high hydrophilic, low lipophilic properties; diamorphine, pethidine, and methadone have medium lipophilic properties; and fentanyl, alfentanil, sufentanil, lofentanil, and phenoperidine have high lipophilic properties.

The systemic reabsorption of lipophilic drugs administered intraspinally is faster and more complete. They stay in the extradural space for a shorter period, and direct transit through the dura mater is easier but slower. Diffusion along the cerebrospinal axis is increased, while concentration at the receptor level is reduced. Thus highly lipophilic drugs have a more rapid onset of peak effect, and hydrophilic drugs have a more delayed peak effect but a longer duration of action.

Opioid selection continues to be problematic. Factors such as duration of action and efficacy-safety ratio of the opioids as well as the vertebral site of injection and optimum volume of concentration of the injectate have to be addressed. A wide variety of opioid and nonopioid substances has been used, but still morphine is the gold standard. It has low lipid solubility and high receptor affinity, and the peak analgesic effect is obtained during the first hour and lasts for 6 to 24 hours. The beginning dose varies, according to several authors, from 0.5 to 10 mg. This is due to the individual characteristics of the patient at the time of the first application of the method. If the patient has been using higher doses of oral or other routes of opioids for a long time, the beginning dose is generally high.

At this point, the appropriate time of application and transferring from oral to spinal opioids should be discussed. The cancer pain relief and palliative care guidelines of WHO are somewhat contradictory. The cancer pain relief campaign of WHO insists on the oral use of opioids, while the palliative care guidelines bring the quality of life to the front. If the patient has been treated with oral opioids and many side effects have decreased the quality of life, and if this quality of life can be sustained effectively by intraspinal delivery, intraspinal analgesia is more appropriate.

Morphine is still the drug of first choice because of its long duration of action, excellent analgesia, accessibility, and relatively low cost. Because of the hydrophilic properties, rostral spread may cause delayed side effects; however, side effects such as delayed respiratory depression may be seen in opioid-naive patients but not in patients taking opioids chronically .

Sufentanil is the prototype of lipophilic agents. Analgesia begins in 10 minutes and is sustained for 2 to 5 hours. Because of its lipophilicity, analgesia is more regional and segmental, and the catheter should be near the appropriate dermatomal region. The duration of pain relief from bolus doses is relatively short. Higher doses of fentanyl and sufentanil relative to an equianalgesic dose of morphine are required for the epidural route to produce analgesia. This factor combined with venous uptake necessitates increased vigilance for early side effects, especially in the opioid-naive patient. There is a risk of respiratory depression with sufentanil.

Methadone, hydromorphone, meperidine, and diamorphine have intermediate lipophilic effects. Most of the experience with these drugs is for acute pain, not for chronic pain management.

DRUGS OTHER THAN OPIOIDS

The use of drugs other than opioids is possible. Local anesthetics in conjunction with opioids produce analgesia with a different mechanism. While the opioids interact with receptors, local anesthetics induce conducting block. A combination of opioids and local anesthetics may be used for the treatment of intractable neuropathic pain. Several other agents, including clonidine, somatostatin, calcitonin, d-ala^2-d-leu^5 enkephalin (DADL), midazolam, and droperidol, are also used for intraspinal delivery. However most of these agents are not used on daily. Thus for appropriate dose and drug selection:

- Titration and stabilization of the drug are necessary.
- Morphine is still the less cost-effective agent.
- For bolus injection, drugs with high receptor affinity, such as morphine, are most suitable.
- For infusion, a drug with low receptor affinity, such as fentanyl, may be used.
- Addition of drugs other than morphine, such as bupivacaine, may be necessary.
- Appropriate type of delivery, bolus versus infusion, must be determined.

The use of intraspinal opioids may be realized by either of two means, bolus or infusion. There are several types of drug delivery systems, and not all of them are suitable for infusion. Thus bolus and infusion types again depend on the appropriate selection of patients and devices. In the earlier periods of intraspinal drug delivery, bolus administration through externalized epidural catheters and access ports was common.

Several authors have suggested that the delivery of opioids by infusion has distinct advantages over bolus injection. There are several advantages of continuous infusion: it may sustain a more consistent level of analgesia, lower doses are required, tolerance may be delayed, and the incidence of side effects and infection is less. The handling and care of the patient are also reduced, and as a result the patient's and the family's anxiety is decreased. External devices may also be used for infusion with externalized catheters or ports, and patient-controlled anesthesia (PCA) devices may also be used for this aim. The use of bolus injection requires handling of syringes and needles. Aspiration of foreign material inside the syringe and then delivery of it through the catheter may occlude the catheter. Accidental contamination of syringes and needles may also cause infection.

However, there are also some disadvantages. These pumps are more expensive than the manual pumps or ports that deliver bolus. Trained personnel for the service and the care of the patient is required. There is always a potential for device malfunction and errors of prescribing and device refilling. In some cases there may be a potential for overtreatment and undertreatment of pain. There are limits and indications for the use of infusion over bolus injection. Thus appropriate use of bolus and infusion types should also be considered. Internal infusion pumps are not cost-effective in patients with short life expectancy because in such patients subcutaneously inserted epidural or intrathecal catheters, externalized or combined with an access ports, are generally preferred. External pumps may be used in such instances and may also be used later for other cases.

The use of fixed-rate internal infusion pumps may not be cost effective in cancer patients, because when dose increase is required, the reservoir should be refilled. Controllable pumps seem to be very expensive. If bolus injections sustain adequate pain relief, manually activated pumps may be considered in such patients. Bolus injection manually activated or external pumps are not suitable for non-cancer pain patients. In such patients controllable infusion pumps are more appropriate.

APPROPRIATE USE OF INTERNALIZED VERSUS EXTERNALIZED SYSTEMS

The spinal delivery systems may also be classified as internalized, partially externalized, or externalized systems. The internalized systems are the manually activated or infusion pumps, which are refilled regularly, depending upon the reservoir and volume of delivery. Partially externalized systems are the access ports combined with epidural or intrathecal catheter which are used either with bolus injection or with external pumps. Externalized systems are the subcutaneously implanted epidural or intrathecal catheters used either with bolus injection or external pumps. This subject has to be considered in two ways, the system inserted and the pump used. The advantages and disadvantages of the systems inserted were discussed previously.

There is an increasing number of external portable infusion devices that range from a relatively inexpensive syringe driver with a simple on-demand system to more expensive programable devices containing exchangeable plastic reservoirs. These devices vary widely in their specifications. Systems with greater accuracy should be selected when patients are sensitive to very small changes in their dosage of morphine. Cosmetic and safety considerations should also be addressed when selecting a portable infusion system. Safety considerations may sometimes preclude the use of a smaller device.

Well-designed randomized clinical trials to compare internal and external pumps are still lacking. Generally it depends on the physician's preference and experience. External pumps may be used with access ports with epidural or intrathecal

catheters. They may also be used with externalized catheters, but physicians still avoid them with externalized catheters for fear of infection.

For externalized systems the use of bolus injection requires handling of syringes and needles, while infusions require some level of mastery of ambulatory pumps. Standards of care and appropriate indications for use are needed for external pumps to be used for chronic pain. This should include both the utility of approach and the problems that may arise from its use from either the individual patient perspective or the broader health policy perspective. Externalized pumps still have a limited time of application and should be limited to cancer patients with a medium life expectancy of months. Because of the difficulty of training the patient and the caregiver, potential for device malfunction and for errors in prescribing and refilling the device, there is the risk of overtreatment and undertreatment. There are also risks of infection and mechanical catheter complications.

The use of internal infusion pumps may have several advantages if the patients are appropriately selected. In long-term delivery, especially when the intrathecal route is effective, it may be used both in cancer and noncancer pain with great comfort. Caregiver or personnel help is minimal, and the device is filled monthly with very few skin punctures. Handling and care of the internal pumps are much easier than the external pumps. Although continuous infusion alone controls pain in the majority of patients receiving intraspinal morphine with or without local anesthetic, some patients may benefit from a PCA infusion pump. The PCA enables the patient to receive either additional doses of medication within controlled physician-described limits or an intermittent bolus on demand without continuous infusion. These devices may be superior in providing constant pain control, especially for patients with breakthrough pain.

Combining continuous infusion and PCA features eliminates the need for frequent bolus administration as well as awakening to administer boluses. However, PCA should not be used unless proper supervision from a family member or visiting health professional is provided. There are still only a few controlled studies for the appropriateness of PCA in chronic pain. Clinical trials of PCA in acute pain cannot be assumed to generalize to the chronic pain setting.

SIDE EFFECTS AND COMPLICATIONS OF SPINAL DRUG DELIVERY SYSTEMS

Some authors prefer to evaluate the side effects of opioids and the complications due to the system itself together. However, most of the side effects of the opioids also develop when using other routes of delivery. Thus we believe that the complications due to the system and side effects of the opioids should be discussed separately. Side effects that develop with other routes of opioid administration may also be observed as side effects of spinal opioid delivery. They are either dose independent (these, which may occur irrespective of the opioid dose, include urinary retention, pruritus, perspiration, and sedation) or dose dependent (such as nausea, emesis, dysphoria, euphoria, and central depression, including major sedation, respiratory depression, hypotension, and tachyphylaxis).

Dose escalation does occur during long-time delivery. It is not appropriate to address every dose escalation as tolerance. True tolerance and pseudotolerance should be differentiated. In cancer pain there may be a continuous increase in nociceptive stimulus. Dose increase during long-term delivery may be due to disease progression, development of opioid-resistant pain during the time course, or changes in the epidural or subarachnoid space as dural thickening and fibrotic reactions. This is generally called pseudotolerance. In fact, various studies suggest that tolerance to the pharmacological effects of opioids other than analgesia develop; this selective tolerance is beneficial for the patient. If morphine tolerance develops, substances such as DADL, metenkephalin, β-endorphin, clonidine, labetalol, lysine acetylsalicylate, calcitonin, somatostatin, octreotide, droperidol, may be used.

There is risk of respiratory depression in opioid-naive patients when opioids are used for postoperative or posttraumatic pain, but it is nearly nonexistent in chronic spinal opioid delivery. Accidental overdose through the injection port may cause respiratory depression. Pruritus is a side effect observed only during intraspinal delivery. The incidence is between 17 and 28%. It generally subsides within days either without therapy or with the administration of antihistamine or naloxone.

The incidence of nausea and vomiting is not so high in opioid-experienced patients as it is in opioid-naive ones. Generally these symptoms subside during the delivery. Urinary retention has been observed in 20 to 40% of the patients, especially in men. It occurs within the first 2 days, and intermittent bladder catheterization may be necessary. These side effects are generally not the cause of ceasing the treatment. They generally subside within days. It has been suggested that the side effects and tolerance have been overemphasized.

COMPLICATIONS OF THE DRUG DELIVERY SYSTEMS

Complications may be due to several factors independent of the choice of the system, route, and application. However, inappropriate choice of system can cause complications. Complications of the drug delivery systems may be categorized as time related, related to the site of the catheter, related to the part of the system, and rare complications. Time-related complications are either immediate or late. Immediate complications are bleeding at the site of surgery, hematoma along the course of the subcutaneous tunneling device, epidural hematoma, early infection, cerebrospinal fluid leakage, postspinal headache, edema, pump pocket seroma, and improper placement of the system. Late complications are obstruction of the catheter, obstruction of the port or the pump, catheter kinking, catheter dislodgment, pump malfunction or failure, late infection, fibrosis, and injection-related burning pain.

Complications related to the site of the catheter are either epidural or intrathecal. Complications related to the epidural space are fibrosis in the epidural space, injection-related burning pain, epidural hematoma, epidural abscess, and fibrous sheath formation around the catheter. Complications related to the intrathecal space are leakage of the cerebrospinal fluid, fistula of the dura, cerebrospinal hygroma, spinal headache, and meningitis.

Complications related to the part of the system are either related to the catheter or to the port or the pump. Complications related to the catheter are clot formation, kinking, curling, and knotting; misplacement, displacement, occlusion, or migration of the catheter; and removal difficulties. Complications related to the port or pump are obstruction of the port, leakage from the port membrane, mechanical pump failure, pump malfunction, disconnection of the catheter; and seroma formation around the port or the pump. Rare complications are skin necrosis and skin reaction to the percutaneous or subcutaneously tunneled devices.

Some of the complications may be resolved without replacing the system. However, complications such as infection, occlusion, or displacement of the catheter and port or pump malfunction have to be taken seriously. Infections related to the drug delivery system mostly occur at the exit site of the catheter or where the port or pump is inserted. Superficial infections at the exit site occur in 6% of the patients. Epidural abscess or meningitis is related to the space of insertion. Epidural infection or abscess formation may be due to hematogenous spread or extension of the superficial infection at the port site during injection. Meningitis is mostly observed when the catheter is inserted intrathecally. It has been shown in several studies that the incidence of infection if the catheter is inserted intrathecally is 4%, while it is approximately 9% for the epidural route. Occlusion of the system may be due to the port, pump, or catheter. The catheter may be occluded by clot, fibrosis around the tip of the catheter, foreign particles in the injected solution, or kinking. Dislodgment of the catheter is also an important problem. In patients with fully inserted systems, catheter dislodgment necessitates removal of the system. Although several measures can be taken, it is still a problem in drug delivery systems. When evaluated retrospectively, the frequency of dislodgment has been shown to be approximately 8%. Valve failure in manual pumps or pump malfunction in infusion pumps may also occur. In such cases the pump has to be replaced.

FUTURE ASPECTS

Development of intraspinal delivery systems for the treatment of intractable pain is a new era in pain medicine. The appropriate use of spinal drug delivery systems should be based upon the principle of optimum benefit and minimal harm both for the patient and the health system as a whole. Technical improvement of the systems used is still necessary for a safe and effective treatment with few side effects and complications. There are still few controlled studies of long-term outcome. Pain practitioners implanting these systems create their own guidelines depending on their own empirical experience. The analgesic ladder described by WHO may be effective in 90% of the cancer pain patients, but it also means that there are still 10% of the patients needing other interventions for pain control. As the spinal delivery systems are also used for noncancer pain in recent years, the appropriate use of these systems should thoroughly be defined.

Developing algorithms and guidelines is crucially important for the appropriate use of spinal drug delivery systems.

Suggested Readings

Akerman B, Arweström E, Post C. Local anesthetics potentiate spinal morphine antinociception. Anesth Analg 1988;67:943–948.

Andersen H B, Jorgensen B C, Engquist A. Epidural metenkephalin (FK 33–824) a dose-effects study. Acta Anaesthesiol Scand 1982;26:69–71.

Arner S, Arner B. Differential effects of epidural morphine in the treatment of cancer related pain. Acta Anaesthesiol Scand 1985;29:32.

Arner S, Meyerson B. Lack of analgesic effect of opioids on neuropathic and idiopathic forms of pain. Pain 1988;33:11–23.

Arner S, Rawal N, Gustafsson L. Clinical experience of long-term treatment with epidural and intrathecal opioids: a nationwide survey. Acta Anaesthesiol Scand 1988;32:253–259.

Atanossoff P, Alon E. Accidental epidural injection of a large dose of morphine. Anaesthesia 1988;43:1056 (letter).

Ballantyne J C, Loach A B, Carr D B. Itching after epidural and spinal opiates. Pain 1988;33:149–160.

Bedder M D, Burchiel K J, Larson A. Cost analysis of two implantable narcotic delivery systems. J Pain Symptom Manag 1991;6:368–373.

Behar M, Magora F, Olswang D, Davidson J T. Epidural morphine in the treatment of pain. Lancet 1979;1(8115):527–528.

Benedetti C. Intraspinal analgesia: an historical overview. Acta Anesthesiol Scand 1987;31(Suppl 85):17–24.

Blond S, Meynadier J, Brichard D, et al. Intracerebroventricular morphinotherapy and study of the supraspinal action of morphine. Pain 1987(Suppl 4):S391.

Boersma F P, Blaak H B, Ananias T K, et al. Technical complications and sequelae of long-term epidural cancer pain control: a review of 206 cases. Pain Clin 1993;6:121–127.

Boersma F P, Meert T F, Kate A T, et al. Cancer pain control by epidural sufentanil. Eur J Pain 1990;11:76–80.

Brazenor G A. Long-term intrathecal administration of morphine: a comparison of bolus injection via reservoir with continuous infusion by implanted pump. Neurosurgery 1987;21:484–491.

Bromage P R, Camporesi E M, Durant P A C, Nielsen C H. Rostral spread of epidural morphine. Anesthesiology 1987;56:431–436.

Brown M, Rein P. Securing the epidural catheter. Anesthesiology 1985;62:373–374.

Budd K. Drug management of chronic benign pain. Int Disabil Stud 1987;9:30–33.

Bunodierer M, Colbert N, Renaud J. Sédation des douleurs cancereuses par injection péridurale quotidienne de morphine grâce à un acces sous cutane implante. Ann Fr Anesth Réanim 1984;3:129–130.

Caballero G A, Ausman R K, Himes J. Epidural morphine by continuous infusion with an external pump for pain management in oncology patients. Am Surg 1986;52:402–405.

Caute B, Monsarrat B, Gouardes C, et al. CSSF morphine levels after lumbar intrathecal administration of isobaric and hyperbaric solutions for cancer pain. Pain 1988;32:141–146.

Cherry D A. Drug delivery systems for epidural administration of opioids. Acta Anaesthesiol Scand 1987;31(Suppl 85):54–59.

Cherry D A, Gourlay G K, Cousins M J. Epidural mass associated with lack of efficacy and epidural morphine and undetectable CSF morphine concentrations. Pain 1986;25:69–73.

Cherry D A, Gourlay G K, Cousins M J, Gannon B J. A technique for the insertion of an implantable portal system for the long-term epidural administration of opioids in the treatment of cancer pain. Anaesth Intens Care 1985;13:145–152.

Cherry D A, Gourlay G K, Plummer J L, et al. Cephalad migration of pethidine and morphine following lumbar epidural administration in a patient with cancer pain. Pain 1987;(Suppl 4):69 (abstract).

Christensen V. Respiratory depression after extradural morphine. Br J Anaesth 1980;52:841 (letter).

Chrubasik J, Chrubasik S, Friedrich G, Martin E. Long-term treatment of pain by spinal opiates: an update. Pain Clin 1992;5:147–156.

Chrubasik J, Chrubasik S, Martin E. Patient-controlled spinal opiate analgesia in terminal cancer. Drugs 1992;43:799–804.

Chrubasik J, Chrubasik S, Martin E. The ideal epidural opioid: fact or fantasy? Eur J Anaesth 1993;10:79–100.

Chrubasik J, Cousins M, Martin E. Advances in pain therapy I. Berlin: Springer, 1992.

Chrubasik J, Falke K F, Zindler M, et al. Is calcitonin an analgesic agent? Pain 1986;3–276.

Chrubasik J, Meynadier J, Blond S, et al. Somatostatin a potent analgesic. Lancet 1984;2:1208–1209.

Coombs D R, Saunders R L, Gaylor M, Pageau M G. Epidural narcotic infusion reservoir implantation technique and efficacy. Anesthesiology 1982;56:469–473.

Coombs D W. Intraspinal analgesic infusion by implanted pump. Ann N Y Acad Sci 1988;531:108–122.

Coombs D W, Colburn R W, Dele J A, et al. Comparative spinal neuropathology of hydromorphone and morphine after 9 and 30 day epidural administration in sheep. Anesth Analg 1994;78:674–681.

Coombs D W, Maurer L, Saunders R, Gaylor M. Outcomes and complications of continuous intraspinal narcotic analgesia for cancer pain control. J Clin Oncol 1984;2:1414–1420.

Coombs D W, Saunders R L, Fratkin J D, et al. Continuous intrathecal hydromorphone and clonidine for intractable cancer pain. J Neurosurg 1986;64:890–894.

Coombs D W, Saunders R L, Lachance D, et al. Intrathecal morphine tolerance: use of intrathecal clonidine, DADLE, and intraventricular morphine. Anesthesiology 1985;62:358–363.

Cousins M J, Cherry D A, Gourlay G K. Acute and chronic pain: use of spinal opioids. In: Cousins M J, Bridenbaugh P O, eds. Neural blockade in clinical anesthesia and management of pain. 2nd ed. Philadelphia: Lippincott, 1988;955–1029.

Cousins M, Gourlay G, Cherry D. A technique for the insertion of an implantable portal system for the long-term epidural administration of opioids in the treatment of cancer pain. Anaesth Intens Care 1985;13:145–152.

Cousins M J, Mather L E. Intrathecal and epidural administration of opioids. Anesthesiology 1984;61:276.

Crul J B, Van Dongen R T, Snijdelaar D G. Intrathecal opioids. Pain Rev 1994;1:295–307.

De Castro J, Meynadier J, Zenz M. Regional opioid analgesia. Dordrecht: Kluwer Academic, 1991.

De Jong P C, Kansen P J. A comparison of epidural catheters with or without subcutaneous injection ports for treatment of cancer pain. Anesth Analg 1994;78:94–100.

Devoghel J C. Small intrathecal dosers of lysin-acetyl-salicylate relieve intractable pain in man. J Int Med Res 1983;11:90–91.

Du Pen S L, Ramsey D H. Diagnosis and treatment of epidural infections-a complication of long-term epidural narcotic administration. Anesthesiology 1988;69(3A):A411 (abstract).

DuPen S L, Williams A R. Management of patients receiving combined epidural morphine and bupivacaine for the treatment of cancer pain. J Pain Symptom Manag 1992;7:125–127.

Du Pen L S, Williams A R. Spinal and peripheral drug delivery systems. Pain Digest 1995;5:307–317.

Edwards W T, DeGrolami U, Burney R G, et al. Histopathologic changes in the epidural space of the guinea pig during long-term morphine infusion. Reg Anesth 1986;11:14–19.

Eisenach J C. Respiratory depression following intrathecal opioids. Anesthesiology 1991;75:712 (letter).

Erdine S, Aldemir T. Long-term results of peridural morphine in 225 patients. Pain 1991;45:155–159.

Erdine S, Özyalçýn S, Yücel A. Intrathecal morphine by implanted manual pump for cancer pain. Pain Digest 1996;6:161–165.

Erdine S, Yücel A. Long-term results of intrathecal morphine in 65 patients. Pain Clin 1994;7:27–33.

Erdine S, Yücel A. Complications of drug delivery systems. Pain Rev 1995;2:227–242.

Erstad B L, Snyder B A, Kramer T H. Epidural, intrathecal and patient-controlled analgesic use in a university medical center. J Pharm Technol 1993;9:141–143.

Feldstein G S, Waldman S D, Allen M L. Reversal of apparent tolerance to epidural morphine by epidural methylprednisolone. Anesth Analg 1987;66:264–266.

Ferrell B R, Nash C C, Warfield C. The role of patient controlled analgesia in the management of cancer pain. J Pain Symptom Manag 1992;7:149–154.

Fisher A P, Simpson D, Hanna M. A role for epidural opioid in opioid-insensitive pain. Pain Clin 1987;1:233–239.

Follet K A, Hitchon P W, Piper J, et al. Response of intractable pain to continuous intrathecal morphine: a retrospective study. Pain 1992;49:21–25.

Fraioli F, Fabbri A, Gnessi L, et al. Subarachnoid calcitonin for intolerable pain. Lancet 1982;2.

Gestin Y. A totally implantable multi-dose pump allowing cancer patients intrathecal access for the self-administration of morphine at home: a follow-up of 30 cases. Anaesthetist 1987;36:391–394.

Gestin Y, Pere N, Solassol C. Morphin thérapie isobare intrathécale au long cours. Ann F Anesth Reanim 1986;5:346–350.

Gourlay G K. Long-term use of opioids in chronic pain patients with nonterminal disease states. Pain Rev 1994;1:62–76.

Gourlay G K, Cherry B A, Cousins M J. Cephalad migration of morphine CSF following lumbar epidural administration in patients with cancer pain. Pain 1985;23:317.

Grass J A. Fentanyl: clinical use as postoperative analgesic-epidural/intrathecal route. J Pain Symptom Manag 1992;7:419–430.

Haindl H, Muller H. Eine atraumatische nadel fur die punktion von ports und pumpen. Klin Wochensschr 1988;66:1006–1009.

Hardy P A J, Wells J C D. Patient-controlled intrathecal morphine for cancer pain. Clin J Pain 1990;6:57–59.

Hassenbusch S J, Pillay P K, Maginee M, et al. Constant infusion of morphine for intractable cancer pain using an implanted pump. J Neurosurg 1990;73:405–409.

Hays R L, Palmer C M. Respiratory depression after intrathecal sufentanil during labor. Anesthesiology 1994;81:511–512.

Hoekstra A. Pain relief mediated by implantable drug delivery devices. Int J Artif Organs, 1994;17:151–154.

Hogan Q, Haddox J D, Abram S, et al. Epidural opiates and local anesthetics for the management of cancer pain. Pain 1991;46:271–279.

Hullander M, Leivers D. Spinal cutaneous fistula following continuous spinal anesthesia. Anesthesiology 1992;76:139–140.

Jennet B. High technology medicine: benefits and barriers. Oxford, UK: Oxford University Press, 1986.

Jong P C, Kansen P J. A comparison of epidural catheters with or without subcutaneous injection ports for treatment of cancer pain. Anesth Analg 1994;78:94–100.

Kaiser K G, Bainton C R. Treatment of intrathecal morphine overdose by aspiration of cerebrospinal fluid. Anesth Analg 1987;66:475–477.

Kerr I G, Sone M, De Angelis C, et al. Continuous narcotic infusion with patient-controlled analgesia for chronic cancer pain in outpatients. Ann Intern Med 1988;108:554–557.

Kitahata L M. Spinal analgesia with morphine and clonidine. Anesth Analg 1989;68:191–193.

Klepper I D, Sherrill D L, Boetger C L, et al. Analgesia and respiratory effects of extradural sufentanil in volunteers, and the influence of adrenaline as an adjuvant. Br J Anesth 1987;59:1147.

Koning G, Feith F. A new implantable drug delivery system for patient controlled analgesia. Ann N Y Acad Sci 1988;531:48–56.

Krames E S. Intrathecal infusional therapies for intractable pain: patient management guidelines. J Pain Symptom Manag 1993;8:36–46.

Krames E S, Gershow J, Glassberg A, et al. Continuous infusion of spinally administered narcotics for the relief of pain due to malignant disorders. Cancer 1985;56:696–702.

Krames E S, Schuchard M. Implantable intraspinal infusional analgesia: management guidelines. Pain Rev 1995;2:243–267.

Krames S E, Lanning M R. Intrathecal infusional analgesia for nonmalignant pain: analgesic efficacy of intrathecal opioid with or without bupivacaine. J Pain Symptom Manag 1993;8.

Kreek M J. Medical safety and side effects of methadone in tolerant individuals. JAMA 1973;223:665–668.

Kwan J W. Use of infusion devices for epidural or intrathecal administration of spinal opioids. Am J Hosp Pharm 1990;47(Suppl):1.

Lam A M, Knill R L, Thompson W R, et al. Epidural fentanyl does not cause delayed respiratory depression. Can Anaesth Soc J 1983; 30(Suppl):78.

Lazorthes Y. Intracerebroventricular administration of morphine for control of irreducible cancer pain. Ann N Y Acad Sci 1988;531:123–132.

Leavens M E, Hill C S, Cech D A, et al. Intrathecal and intraventricular morphine for pain in cancer patients: initial study, J Neurosurg 1982;56:241–245.

Linnemann M, Jonsson T. Treatment of cancer pain in outpatients with continuous infusion of local anaesthetics and opioids epidurally, employing a portable infusor. Eur J Pain 1992;13:4.

Lubenow T, Keh-Wong E, Kristof K, et al. Inadvertent subdural injection: a complication of an epidural block. Anesth Analg 1988;67:175–179.

Madrid J L, Fatela V L, Lobato R D, Gozalo A. Intrathecal therapy: rationale, technique, clinical results. Acta Anesthesiol Scand 1987;31(Suppl 85):60–67.

Malone B, Beye R, Walker J. Management of pain in the terminally ill by administration of epidural narcotics. Cancer 1985;15:438–440.

Margaria E, Gagliardi M, Palieri L, et al. Analgesic effect of peridural labetalol in the treatment of cancer pain. Int J Clin Pharmacol Ther Toxicol 1983;21:47–50.

Matber C M P, Anaes F C, Ready L B, Newman M. Inflammatory cutaneous reactions to epidural catheters. Anesthesiology 1993;78:200–203.

Maurette P, Tauzin-Fin P, Vincon G, Brachet-Lierman A. Arterial and ventricular CSF pharmacokinetics after intrathecal meperidine in humans. Anesthesiology 1989;70:961–966.

Max M B, Inturrisi C E, Kaiko R F, et al. Epidural and intrathecal opiates: cerebral spinal fluid and plasma profiles in patients with chronic cancer pain. Clin Pharmacol Ther 1985;38:631.

McQuay H J. Opioids in chronic pain. Br J Anaesth 1989;63:213–216.

Meynadier J, Chrubasik J, Dubar M, Wünsch E. Intrathecal somatostatin in two terminally ill patients. Pain 1985;23:9–12.

Millan M J. Multiple opioid systems and pain. Pain 1986;27:303–347.

Miseria S, Toressi U, Piga A, et al. Analgesia with epidural calcitonin in cancer patients. Tumori 1989;75:183–184.

Moulin D E, Inturrisi C E, Foley K M. Cerebrospinal fluid pharmacokinetics of intrathecal morphine sulfate and D-Ala-D-Leu-Enkephalin. Ann Neurol 1986;20:218–222.

Muller H, Luben V, Zierski J, Hempelman G. Long-term spinal opiate treatment. Acta Anaesthesiol Belg 1988;39(Suppl 2):83–86.

Nickels J H, Poulos J F, Chaouki K. Risks of infection from short-term epidural catheter use. Reg Anesth 1989;14:88.

Nitescu P, Appelgren L, Hultman E, et al. Long-term, open catheterization of the spinal subarachnoid space for continuous infusion narcotic and bupivacaine in patients with refractory cancer pain. Clin J Pain 1991;7:143–161.

Nitescu P, Appelgren L, Linder L E, et al. Epidural versus intrathecal morphine-bupivacaine: assessment of consecutive treatments in advanced cancer pain. J Pain and Symptom Manag 1990;5:1.

Nitescu P, Hultman E, Appelgren L, et al. Bacteriology, drug stability and exchange of percutaneous delivery systems and antibacterial filters in long-term intrathecal infusion of drugs and bupivacaine in "refractory" pain. Clin J Pain 1992;8:324–337.

Nitescu P, Sjöberg M, Appelgren L, Curelaru I. Complications of intrathecal opioids and bupivacaine in the treatment of "refractory" cancer pain. Clin J Pain 1995;11:45–62.

Nordberg G. Epidural versus intrathecal route of opioid administration. Int Anesthesiol Clin 1986;24:93–111.

Ohlsson L, Rydberg T, Eden T, et al. Cancer pain relief by continuous administration of epidural morphine in a hospital setting and at home. Pain 1992;48:349–353.

Onofrio D M, Yaksh T L, Arnold P G. Continuous low dose intrathecal morphine administration in the treatment of chronic pain of malign origin. Mayo Clin Proc 1981;56:516–520.

Oyama T, Fukushi S, Jin T. Epidural B-endorphin in treatment of pain. Can Anaesth Soc J 1982;29:24–6.

Paice J A, Magolan J M. Intraspinal drug therapy. Nurs Clin North Am 1991;26:477–498.

Patt R, Laughner J. Problems and innovations in epidural opioids. Anesthesiology 1990;72:215–216.

Pellerin M, Hardy F, Abergel A, et al. Douleur chronique rebelle des cancéreux. Press Med (Paris) 1987;65–1468.

Penn R D, Paice J A. Chronic intrathecal morphine for intractable pain. J Neurosurg 1987;67:182–186.

Penn R D, Paice J A, Gottschalk J, et al. Cancer pain relief using chronic morphine infusion. J Neurosurg 1984;61:302–306.

Penn R D, Paice J A, Kroin J S. Intrathecal octreotide for cancer pain. Lancet 1990;1:738.

Penn R D, York M M, Paice J A. Catheter systems for intrathecal drug delivery. J Neurosurg 1995;83:215–217.

Pfeifer B L, Sernaker H L, Ter Horst U M. Pain scores and ventilatory and circulatory sequelae of epidural morphine in cancer patients with and without prior narcotic therapy. Anesth Analg 1988;67:838–842.

Poletti J E, Copen A M, Todd D P, et al. Cancer pain relieved by long term epidural morphine with permanent indwelling systems for self administration. J Neurosurg 1981;55:581.

Portenoy R K. Chronic opioid therapy in non-malignant pain. J Pain Symptom Manag 1990;5:(Suppl 1S):46–62.

Portenoy R K, Foley K M, Inturrisi C E. The nature of opioid responsiveness and its implications for neuropathic pain: new hypothesis derived from studies of opioid infusions. Pain 1990;43:273–286.

Porter J, Jick H. Addiction rate in patients treated with narcotics. N Engl J Med 1980;302:123.

Racz G B, Sabonghym I. Intractable pain therapy using a new epidural catheter. JAMA 1982;248:646–647.

Rawal N, Schott U, Dahlstrom B. Influence of naloxone infusion on analgesia and respiratory depression following epidural morphine. Anesthesiology 1986;64:194–201.

Rodan B A, Cohen F L, Bean W J, Martyak S N. Fibrous mass complicating epidural morphine infusion. Neurosurgery 1985;16:68–70.

Saiah M, Borgeat A, Wilder-Smith OHG, et al. Epidural-morphine-induced pruritus: propofol versus naloxone. Anesth Analg 1994;78:1110–1113.

Samuelsson H, Hedner T. Pain characterization in epidural morphine. Pain 1991;46:3–8.

Schug S A, Merry A F, Acland R H. Treatment principles for the use of opioids in pain of non-malignant origin. Drugs 1991;42:228–232.

Scott D B, Sinclair C J. Advances in regional anaesthesia and analgesia. Clin Obstet Gynaecol 1982;9:273–289.

Shetter A G, Hadley M N, Wilkinson E. Administration of intraspinal morphine sulphate for the treatment of intractable cancer pain. Neurosurgery 1986;18:740–774.

Shir Y, Shapira S S, Shenkman Z. Continuous epidural methadone treatment for cancer pain. Clin J Pain 1991;7:339–341.

Shir Y, Yehuda D B, Polliack A, et al. Prolonged continuous epidural methadone analgesia in the treatment of back and pelvic pain due to multiple myeloma. Pain Clin 1987;1:255–258.

Sjöström S, Tamsen A, Persson P, et al. Pharmacokinetics of intrathecal morphine and meperidine in humans. Anesthesiology 1987;67:889–895.

Strong W E. Epidural abscess associated with epidural catheterization: a rare event? Report of two cases with markedly delayed presentation. Anesthesiology 1991;74:943–946.

Swanson G, Smith J, Bulich R, Shiffman R. Patient-controlled analgesia for chronic cancer pain in the ambulatory setting: a report of 117 patients. Clin Oncol 1989;7:1903–1908.

Tawfik M O. Mode of action of intraspinal opioids. Pain Rev 1994;1:275–294.

Thangathuari D, Bowles H F, Allen H W, Mikhail M S. Epidural morphine and headache secondary to dural puncture. Anaesthesia 1988;43:519 (letter).

Thi T V, Orliaguet G, Lui N, et al. A dose-range study of intrathecal meperidine combined with bupivacaine. Acta Anaesthesiol Scand 1992;36:516–518.

Tom C M L, Arias L M, Barolat G. Spinal opiate administration: a case of catheter misplacement. Clin J Pain 1990;6:60–63.

Tryba M, Zenz M, Strumpf M. Long-term epidural catheters in terminally ill patients: a prospective study of complications in 129 patients. Anesthesiology 1990;73(Suppl):784.

Vainio A, Tigerstedt I. Opioid treatment for radiating cancer pain: oral administration vs. epidural techniques. Acta Anaesthesiol Scand 1988;32:179.

Wakefield R D, Mesaros M. Reversal of pruritus secondary to epidural morphine with a narcotic agonist-antagonist nalbuphine (Nubain) Anesthesiology 1985;63(Suppl):A255 (abstract).

Weightman W M. Respiratory arrest during epidural infusion of bupivacaine and fentanyl. Anaesth Intens Care 1991;19:282–284.

Waldman S D. A simplified approach to the subcutaneous placement of epidural catheters for long-term administration of morphine. J Pain Symptom Manag 1987;2:163–166.

Waldman S D. Implantable drug delivery systems: practical considerations. J Pain Symptom Manag 1990;5:169–174.

Waldman S D, Coombs D W. Selection of implantable narcotic delivery systems. Anesth Analg 1989;68:377–384.

Waldman S D, Kennedy L D, Leak D W, Patt R B. Intraspinal opioid therapy: non-pharmacological treatment and novel approaches to management. In: Patt R B, ed. Cancer pain Philadelphia: Lippincott, 1993;285–294.

Waldman S D, Leak D W, Kennedy L D, Patt R B. Intraspinal opioid therapy. In: Patt R B, ed. Cancer pain. Philadelphia: Lippincott 1993;285–328.

Wang J K, Naus L A, Thomas J E. Pain relief by intrathecal applied morphine in man. Anesthesiology 1979;50:149–151.

Wanscher M, Rishede L, Krogh B. Fistula formation following epidural catheter: a case report. Acta Anaesthesiol Scand 1985;29:552–553.

Watson R L, Rayburn R L, Muldoon S M, et al. The mechanism of action and utility of epidurally administered morphine. In Wain H J, ed. Treatment of pain. New York: Aaronson. 1982.

Wermeling D P, Foster T S, Record K E, Chalkley J E. Drug delivery for intractable cancer pain: use of a new disposable parenteral infusion device for continuous outpatient epidural narcotic infusion. Cancer 1987;60:875–878.

Yaksh T L. The analgesic pharmacology of spinally administered mu opioid agonists. Eur J Pain 1990;11:66–71.

Yaksh T L, Onofrio B M. Retrospective consideration of the doses of morphine given intrathecally by chronic infusion in 163 patients by 19 physicians. Pain 1987;310:211–223.

Yaksh T L, Rudy T A. Analgesia mediated by a direct spinal action of narcotics. Science 1976;192:1357–1358.

Zenz M, Piepenbrock S, Glocke M. Epidural opiates: long-term experiences in cancer pain. Klin Wochenschr 1985;63:225–229.

Zenz M, Strumpf M, Tryba M. Long-term oral opioid therapy in patients with chronic non-malignant pain. J Pain Symptom Manag 1992;7:69–77.

CHAPTER 38

The Neurosurgeon's Approach to Pain

Samuel J. Hassenbusch

INTRODUCTION

Neurosurgical procedures for pain management are at a crossroad in their use for the overall management of chronic pain patients. Although many of these procedures are old, recent improvements have renewed interest in their use. While the intracranial operations traditionally have been used as later options, there is an increasing early use of them because of technical improvements and cost containment considerations. The role of spinal ablative procedures, however, appears to be stable in overall pain management. Improvements in focused radiation therapy, especially the accuracy of the gamma knife, now allow noninvasive interventional pain techniques at the intracranial level.

The relative roles of ablative and augmentative procedures are still controversial in neurosurgical pain management. Many of the ablative procedures have been available for 40 to 50 years yet in many situations have been replaced by newer augmentative procedures over the past 10 years. On the other hand, over the past 5 years techniques for intracranial ablative procedures have been improved significantly. With the use of improved stereotactic equipment and guidance by computed tomography and magnetic resonance imaging, the accuracy of intracranial procedures has been improved and the need for ventriculography largely eliminated. These procedures, which can be performed under local anesthesia, perhaps with intravenous sedation, require only a twist drill hole rather than a burr hole or a craniotomy.

While neurosurgical procedures have often been used relatively late in the overall management of patients, earlier use is now suggested by these improvements in accuracy and ease to the patient. With emphasized cost containment, one-time procedures, performed under local anesthesia with short hospital admissions and low morbidity, are now useful if not desirable.

Patients generally must have severe pain not relieved adequately by systemic medications or simple neurolytic procedures. Some of the procedures are used for chronic pain from cancer; others, such as thalamotomy and cingulotomy, have been used often for noncancer pain (1-5). As with long-term spinal infusions of morphine, it remains unclear whether delayed recurrence of pain indicates extension of the underlying tumor or other condition to involve new areas of the body or late failure of the procedure (6, 7). While the neurosurgical procedures are used for both nociceptive and neuropathic pain, it appears that with the exception of thalamotomy, pain relief is better with intracranial procedures for nociceptive pain and spinal procedures for neuropathic pain.

TECHNIQUES

The methods to place these neurosurgical lesions are relatively standard. Some of the original ablations were placed with open surgical techniques (8, 9). Now, however, closed operations using stereotaxy under ventriculogram, computed tomography, or magnetic resonance guidance have become dominant. Air or contrast ventriculography was the traditional accurate method for placing lesions at coordinates defined by the anterior commissure-posterior commissure (AC-PC) line (10, 11). This method often requires general anesthesia because of the need for ventriculography and does not adjust for variation in anatomy from patient to patient.

Computed tomography and magnetic resonance for stereotactic guidance eliminate the need for ventriculography, and there is an improved ability to correct for individual variation in anatomy (12, 13). Magnetic resonance imaging is especially useful in the identification of relevant anatomy but does offer somewhat lower accuracy as a result of magnetic field inhomogeneity (14-17).

The actual trajectory for the electrode placement, with magnetic resonance imaging, can be planned in relation to other brain structures. Special angled slices that correspond to the trajectory for the electrode placement can be performed and the target site and the actual trajectory through various brain structures found on these slices.

Radiosurgery, for example using the gamma knife, is increasingly being used to create ablative lesions for treatment of chronic pain and functional disorders. Targets in the thalamus and the anterior limb of the internal capsule have been the most widely reported (18-20). The radiosurgical technique for these pain-relieving lesions is similar to that for focused radiation (radiosurgery) for a brain tumor. Although this method is noninvasive to the brain, it is unclear to what extent the lesions become smaller and perhaps less effective at various times after the radiosurgery.

DESCRIPTION OF SPECIFIC PROCEDURES

The following procedures either are commonly used at present or according to past reports offer significant efficacy with minimal morbidity. As seen from the descriptions that follow, some of these procedures treat specific pain areas, such as the head or legs, while others treat generalized areas of pain. The order for these descriptions is based on an anatomical progression from rostral to caudal central nervous system sites.

Thalamotomy

Thalamotomy is considered usually for noncancer pain, but it can be effective for the treatment of cancer pain (21, 22). The targets have been the basal thalamus, medial thalamus, and dorsomedial thalamus affecting extralemniscal fibers, fibers terminating in the intralaminar and centromedian nuclei, and the origin of fibers projecting to the frontal lobe (23). One of the most effective sites appears to be the inferior posteromedial thalamus, containing the intralaminar, centromedian, and parafascicularis nuclei. This may affect the paleospinothalamic tract (24). Combination lesions, such as centromedian and parafasicularis lesions with dorsomedial nucleus or the thalamic pulvinar lesions, may provide greater efficacy (24). Thalamotomy is generally considered for intermittent shooting and hyperpathic or allodynic pain and not considered very effective for steady, burning, or dysesthetic components of central or deafferentation pain (22). Enthusiasm for the use of thalamotomy, however, has waned over the past few years because of concerns of pain recurrence after 6 to 12 months.

Cingulotomy

Creation of lesions in the cingulate gyrus dates to 1948, when Hugh Cairns at Oxford began to remove a portion of the anterior cingulate gyrus in an open operation (8). Use of open cingulotomy in the 1940s and 1950s produced significant improvements in psychiatric symptoms in most patients (9). The application of stereotaxy to bilateral anterior cingulotomy was described first by Foltz in 1962 for pain relief (1). Ballantine, in 1962, began to use ventriculogram-guided stereotaxy to create smaller lesions in the anterior cingulate gyrus (25).

While cingulotomy most often has been applied to patients with affective disorders, there are numerous reports of its use for severe pain control (1-3, 26-29). The mechanism for pain relief is unclear, although it presumably derives from interruption of the limbic system. According to these and more recent reports, this procedure appears most effective for diffuse, or multiply located, cancer pain that is mainly nociceptive (14, 17). Severe pain from diffuse bone metastases is a typical indication.

With the availability of these closed techniques, there appears to be no present role for open surgical techniques for cingulotomy. The specific target is the cingulate gyrus, 20 to 30 mm posterior to the anterior tip of the lateral ventricles. For ventriculogram guidance, the target is 1.5 mm lateral to midline and 15 mm superior to the roof of the lateral ventricles (25, 30). The radiofrequency method is used more commonly, with each lesion being created at 75°C for 60 to 90 seconds. The result is a cylindrical lesion approximately 10 to 20 mm long and 5 to 7 mm in diameter, centered in each cingulate gyrus.

In many historical series of patients undergoing cingulotomy, as many as 30% of patients were treated for severe chronic pain (25). Of these patients with intractable cancer pain, approximately 51% had moderate, marked, or complete pain relief 3 months after the procedure. In patients with severe pain of nonneoplastic origin, 45% had moderate, marked, or complete pain relief in evaluations more than 3 months later (2). There is some indication that the procedure is less effective in patients with noncancer pain, neuropathic pain, or longer survival times, for example longer than 8 months (14, 17).

The main complications with cingulotomy using ventriculogram guidance in the treatment of psychiatric or pain patients have been hemiplegia from intracerebral hematoma (0.3% incidence), controllable seizures (9% incidence), transient mania (6% incidence), and decreased memory (3% incidence) (25, 30, 31). In neuropsychiatric examination, the only abnormalities noted were occasional difficulties in copying complex figures, performing two tapping tests, and rarely memory on an organized serial learning test (26, 32, 33). There was a low but measurable mortality rate, 0.09%.

Hypothalamotomy

Lesions in the hypothalamus were reported first for psycho affective disorders in 1962 and for cancer pain in 1971, with 28 patients reported to have received the procedure for pain control between 1971 and 1982 (34, 35). β-Endorphin concentrations in ventricular cerebrospinal fluid have been found to be elevated by electrical stimulation of the hypothalamotomy target before actual ablation of the area and to remain elevated for at least 2 days after the hypothalamotomy ablations (36). After hypothalamotomy, degenerated axon fibers are found ipsilateral in the nucleus ventrocaudalis parvocellularis of Hassler, nucleus parafascicularis, somatosensory cortices, pallidum, and the reticular formation but not in the dorsomedial nucleus of the thalamus (37). Indications for hypothalamotomy are similar to those for cingulotomy in terms of cancer pain from rather diffuse sites, especially where there is an emotional or visceral component (38).

Although initial reports located the target 2 mm below the midpoint and 2 mm lateral to the lateral wall of the third ventricle, more recent reports suggest that more posterior lesions may be more effective (37). In one series 15 of 21 hypothalamotomy procedures were bilateral, with "good" results reported in 62% of patients; cancer pain appeared to respond better than noncancer pain (36, 38). There appear to be no significant complications, although the published reports are very limited.

Hypophysectomy

For pain relief, open operations for ablation or section of the pituitary gland include the transcranial hypophysectomy (A70) and the open microsurgical hypophysectomy (40-43). With the increasing use and improved technology of stereotactic methods, percutaneous stereotactic lesions are being accomplished more frequently by alcohol instillation, radiofrequency thermal therapy, cryotherapy, or interstitial placement of radioactive seeds. The widespread use of focused radiation therapy with the gamma knife for pituitary tumors also suggests the use of this noninvasive modality to create similar lesions.

The analgesic mechanism of action for hypophysectomy remains unclear, although it is agreed generally that it does not act on the limbic system and does not lessen psychological suffering as its primary mechanism. There is evidence both in favor of and against theories that involve hormonal, hypothalamic, and neurotransmitter release mechanisms. A postulated hormonal mechanism entails a humoral substance in the cerebrospinal fluid or hormonal changes via a direct neural mechanism (44, 42). Against this possibility it has been noted that the pain relief is almost immediate and precedes or does not correlate with tumor regression, although very small amounts of regression cannot be ruled out (45). Pain relief can occur in thalamic pain and hormonally unresponsive tumors and does not seem to correlate with the degree of pituitary ablation (41, 46-49).

In support of a hypothalamic mechanism, intrasellar instillation of alcohol has been shown to pass to the floor of the third ventricle, hypophyseal portal vessels, and the hypothalamus (45). This suggests a possible relation to the pain relief properties of the posteromedial hypothalamotomy (50), but the morphological effects of hypophysectomy, regardless of the method used to perform the ablation, appear to be in the anterior hypothalamus, specifically the supraoptic and paraventricular nuclei (51).

Projections from the paraventricular nucleus of the hypothalamus have been noted to the periaqueductal gray, rostral ventral medulla, and lamina I of dorsal horn (52-55). The effects of pituitary ablation on the paraventricular nucleus and the connections of this nucleus to important antinociceptive areas of the brain and spinal cord suggest a mechanism that entails the release of endogenous antinociceptive transmitters. It has been observed, however, that naloxone does not reverse pain relief, and no changes have been found in cerebrospinal fluid concentrations of metenkephalin or β-endorphin, although plasma concentrations of β-endorphin were elevated in one study (44, 56, 57).

Hypophysectomy generally is recommended for patients with severe cancer pain, usually from metastatic breast or prostate carcinoma with diffuse areas of pain, although it can be effective for hormonally unresponsive tumors (44, 47, 58-60). Of the various techniques for hypophysectomy, stereotactic instillation of alcohol into the pituitary gland is one of the best described and perhaps one of the most common techniques at present. The use of stereotaxy for chemical hypophysectomy using alcohol was described first in 1957 (61). Present techniques use alcohol volumes of 1 to 5 mL, with a suggestion that the results are better with volumes in the upper end of this range and clearly greater than the volume of the sella (45).

After induction of general anesthesia and placement of a stereotactic frame, the superoposterior part of the sella is chosen as the initial target. An 18-gauge, 6-inch-long spinal needle is introduced in a transnasal trajectory that passes through the floor of the sphenoid sinus. This is replaced by a 20-gauge spinal needle directed through the sella wall, with its passage monitored under lateral x-ray fluoroscopy. After the needle tip is placed at the superoposterior sellar target, absolute alcohol in a volume of 1 to 2 mL is injected in aliquots of 0.1 mL. The needle is withdrawn halfway to the floor of the sella and another 1 to 2 mL of alcohol is injected. After this second injection, the needle is withdrawn again halfway between the second injection position and the floor of the sella before a final 1 to 2 mL is injected (45). The needle is withdrawn after this last injection. During and after each injection, the eyes are monitored for evidence of compression of nerves in the cavernous sinus as evidenced by changes in pupil size or deviation of eyes from the midline.

Other techniques, such as stereotactic radiofrequency hypophysectomy, stereotactic cryohypophysectomy, and interstitial irradiation, also use standard stereotactic methods as described earlier for other intracranial targets; see appropriate references for further description (49, 62-65). The widespread use of focused radiation with the gamma knife to treat pituitary tumors suggests its use for pain control, although it appears that there are no reports of focused pituitary radiation for pain control.

In two series of more than 100 patients each, chemical hypophysectomy appeared to provide significant pain relief. Excellent pain relief was reported in 45 to 65% of all patients, and 75 to 85% of patients stopped opioid intake. With a mean postoperative survival time of 5 months, the mean length of pain relief appeared to be 3 months. Of the patients treated with alcohol injections, 50 to 75% had breast or prostate carcinoma; they appeared to have slightly better pain relief than those with other types of tumors (45). This length of pain relief was accomplished with one additional alcohol injection in 25 to 30% of patients and with two additional injections in another 3 to 9% (44, 45, 66). Approximately 25% of patients had at least one significant exacerbation of pain after the procedure, while a third of these patients had more than one exacerbation (45).

The most common complications consisted of hormonal deficiency, such as diabetes insipidus, in 5 to 20% of patients, cerebrospinal fluid leak in 1 to 10% of patients, and ocular nerve palsy or temporal field visual loss in 2 to 10% of patients (45, 67). Most of these changes, however, appear to dissipate or disappear with time (45). Less frequently reported complications included meningitis in 0.5 to 1%, hypothalamic changes, headaches, and carotid artery damage (67). While a 2 to 5% mortality rate has been reported in older reports, it seems likely that mortality is significantly lower with newer percutaneous stereotactic methods (67, 68).

Pulvinotomy

In 1966 Kudo et al. (69) first described lesions in the pulvinar of the thalamus for pain relief. By 1975, 30 patients were reported to have received this operation. Although the mechanism for pain relief remains unclear, electrophysiological studies in cats have demonstrated that the pulvinar is involved in an indirect route for afferent stimuli (70). From the pulvinar, afferent transmission connections have been traced to the temporal lobe and from there to the posterior sensory cortex (71). The oral and medial parts of the pulvinar have been shown to be involved in pain appreciation (72).

The main indication for pulvinotomy appears to be treatment of intractable cancer pain with qualities and areas of involvement similar to those indicated for cingulotomy or hypothalamotomy (73). In one series, pulvinotomy was applied to patients with phantom pain (10 patients), thalamic pain (10 patients), peripheral neuropathy (6 patients), cancer pain (5 patients), herpetic neuralgia (5 patients), and anesthesia dolorosa (5 patients) (74). Because of reports of pain relief in some patients for long periods, pulvinotomy may be indicated for cancer patients with expected survival times as long as 18 months.

Lesions have been reported in the medial or in both the medial and lateral areas of pulvinar. The lesions have been created in one hemisphere, contralateral to the site of pain, but appear to be more effective with bilateral lesions (73-75). The coordinates for pulvinar lesions have been 4 mm superior to the anteroposterior commissure line, 5 mm posterior to the anteroposterior commissure line, and lateral to the anteroposterior commissure line by either 10 to 11 mm for a medial target or 15 to 16 mm for a lateral target (73). The resultant lesions, which are 5 to 6 mm in diameter, are created with ultrasonic probes, with a setting of 75 watts and 2.5 megacycles for 30 seconds, at two to six separate sites (73). As described earlier in this chapter, stereotaxy with magnetic res-

onance guidance and radiofrequency thermal lesions has been adapted to create lesions in the pulvinar at the same target coordinates.

Preexisting pain is most affected by this operation, and there is no reported loss of somatic sensation after the procedure (75). Good to excellent pain relief has been reported in as many as 25% of patients for periods ranging from 1 to 2.5 years (71, 73). Pulvinar lesions, especially in the anterior pulvinar, have been described as more effective than centrum medianum thalamotomy (71). Better relief with thalamotomy lesions in the centrum medianum and parafascicularis have been noted when the lesions are extended backward to involve the pulvinar (76). Analysis of patients after pulvinotomy has shown no apparent changes in speech, intelligence quotient, or vision, although temporary changes in emotions have been noted (77). Other transient changes include tearfulness, childishness, and excessive excitability and euphoria (74).

Mesencephalotomy

Mesencephalic tractotomy (mesencephalotomy) has been reported to provide significant pain relief in 65 to 75% of patients on both short-term and long-term (2 to 4 years) follow-up, especially in the treatment of head and neck cancer. The target has been at the level of the superior colliculus or inferior colliculus; it appears that the inferior colliculus provides a lower incidence of ocular problems, although perhaps with lower success rates (50 to 70%). The major side effect appears to be difficulties with ocular movement and binocular vision, with mortality rates varying from 1 to 7% (79, 80).

Trigeminal Tractotomy

The clinical use of lesions in the descending trigeminal tract and the adjacent nucleus caudalis were prompted historically by the observation that such lesions affected pain and temperature but not touch sensation (81), The role of the nucleus caudalis in these lesions is based on its probable role as a relay station for pain and temperature transmission from cranial nerves V, VII, IX, and X. The nucleus lies on the surface of the medulla posterior to the dorsal spinocerebellar tract, lateral to the fasciculus cuneatus, and inferior to the restiform body (82).

This procedure appears to be indicated mainly for treatment of patients with head and neck cancer and with intractable pain in the distribution of the trigeminal nerve. Since such pain often involves more diffuse areas of the head and neck, mesencephalotomy often is more appropriate for these patients (83). Although trigeminal tractotomy has been used in the past for trigeminal neuralgia and postherpetic neuralgia, it is not indicated now for these conditions because of the availability of other percutaneous and open operations.

Both open surgical and percutaneous techniques have been described for this operation. The open operation, based on that described by Sjoqvist (81), uses a prone position with bone removal from the occiput and C1 unilaterally. After the dura is opened, the nucleus caudalis lesion is created by a transverse knife incision to a depth of 3 to 5 mm below the surface of the cervicomedullary junction. The incision, which is made 4 to 8 mm inferior to the obex, extends medially from the fasciculus cuneatus to the rootlets of the spinal accessory nerve. In an attempt to place the lesion as superior as possible but without injury to the restiform body, an oblique incision angling from superior to inferior as it is made from posterior to anterior can be used. For mouth coverage, extension of the lesion is recommended to involve part of the spinothalamic tract and part of the fasciculus cuneatus.

A percutaneous technique has been reported with needle penetration at the C1-foramen magnum area under stereotactic guidance (84, 85). An electrode with a 0.5- to 0.6-mm diameter is angled 30° cephalad and placed 6 mm lateral to the midline and 4 mm deep in the spinal cord. Electrical stimulation at 50 Hz should provide facial stimulation at low voltage. If the electrode placement is too ventral, stimulation will be felt in contralateral body areas via the spinothalamic tract, and if the placement is too dorsal, stimulation will be felt in ipsilateral areas via the fasciculus cuneatus.

Limited published reports of the results of this procedure, either with open or percutaneous techniques, suggest that about 75 to 85% of patients with head and neck cancer appear to have good pain relief, although the tractotomy often is combined with other nerve and/or root sections in the same area. Pain relief in general appears to continue for months but not years after the procedure (82). There have been patients documented, after the tractotomy, with sensory changes in the area of the pain but without pain relief.

Complications consist of changes in ipsilateral arm coordination, contralateral leg sensation, and ipsilateral arm and rarely leg proprioception. Most of these deficits are temporary; less frequent complications include Horner's syndrome, dysarthria, gait changes, and hiccoughs. Overall mortality has been estimated at 5 to 10% in patients with advanced cancer.

Combined Procedures

As these intracranial procedures become technically easier to perform, combinations of the procedures are examined. Many of these combinations are based on similar combinations in the treatment of affective disorders. One of the most reported combinations is the use of cingulotomy and anterior capsulotomy, in which lesions are created in both the cingulate gyrus and the anterior limb of the internal capsule. While this combination has been most reported in the treatment of affective disorders, it has been used for the treatment of severe cancer-related pain and appears to provide better relief for pain, including neuropathic pain, than cingulotomy alone (86). Various combinations of targets for thalamotomy also include the pulvinar as an additional target, with improved pain relief over a single site in the thalamus (76). An example

of the combination of cingulotomy and pulvinotomy is described earlier in the general techniques section of this chapter, although its use is too limited to characterize any added benefits in pain relief. As experience with these techniques and improved technology become widespread, it is hoped that there will be a research basis to provide for rational combinations of these procedures and better long-term efficacy in pain control.

Intraventricular Infusion of Opioid

For augmentative techniques at the intracranial level, the intraventricular infusion of opioid has been well described. Morphine sulfate, the usual agent, appears to provide a marked increase in potency as compared with intrathecal or epidural infusions and appears to affect supraspinal pathways for analgesia (87). Daily morphine doses for intraventricular delivery range from 50 to 700 μg/day (88, 89).

The opioid can be delivered via an implanted infusion pump placed subcutaneously in the anterior abdominal wall and connected by subcutaneous tubing to an implanted ventricular catheter. The length of action of the intraventricular injections appears to be significantly longer than with intraspinal, and some patients can be treated adequately via an implanted ventricular catheter connected to a subcutaneous Ommaya reservoir type of device with 1 to 2 injections a day (90).

This form of drug delivery appears to be indicated for head and neck cancer pain and rarely for patients with an initial good response to intraspinal infusions of opioids and subsequent development of apparent tolerance but with very limited (1 to 3 months) remaining survival time. The safety and side effects of the intraventricular injections or infusions appear to be similar to those of intraspinal infusions except that an increased risk of respiratory depression has been noted only in the first 3 days of the intraventricular delivery (88, 90).

Deep Brain Stimulation

For noncancer pain, deep brain stimulation of either the periaqueductal grey region or thalamic sensory nuclei is acutely effective in 61 to 80% of patients and has an overall success rate of 50 to 63% for noncancer pain (91-94). Transient complications include infections, hardware malfunction, implantation site pain, and mild neurological deficits. Overall permanent complications, which occur in 1 to 2% of patients, include hemiparesis, intracranial hemorrhage, and death (93).

In cancer pain, deep brain stimulation can be indicated for pain not well treated by ablative procedures, which includes pain from diffuse bone metastases; midline or bilateral pain, especially of the lower body; brachial, or lumbosacral plexopathy; and recurrent pain from head and neck cancer (95). In a series of 31 patients with cancer pain treated with deep brain stimulation, 87% had satisfactory relief, with 55% of these having relief lasting until death (95).

Cordotomy

Despite the variety of intracranial procedures, intraspinal ablative procedures have been employed more often until the past decade. Cordotomy, the best known of these procedures, is a standard option, although its use appears to be decreasing as intracranial ablative and intraspinal augmentative procedures are supported by rapidly improving technology. In the percutaneous method, x-ray fluoroscopy is used to position a radiofrequency electrode needle at the level of the C1-C2 interspace in the lateral spinothalamic tract to correlate with the area of pain (96).

In the large series of Tasker, long-term success with no pain was found in 33% of patients and partial pain relief in 12% (96). Persistent pain was noted in 6% and a dysesthetic pain in 34%, while 2.6% required a repeat cordotomy for continued pain relief. Complications included persistent paresis (2%), bladder dysfunction (2%), temporary respiratory failure (0.5%), and death (0.5%,) as well as postlesional dysesthesias and new pain either in the contralateral limb or above the level of the previous pain.

Dorsal Root Entry Zone Lesions

For noncancer pain, especially central pain from an injury or other damage to the central nervous system, creation of lesions in the dorsal root entry zone can be helpful. The goal is to disrupt the dorsal horn of the spinal cord at the level that the pain impulses are entering. The usual application of this technique is for brachial plexus avulsion pain, spinal cord injury pain, phantom limb or stump pain, or postherpetic pain (97).

The goal of the procedure is to ablate Lissauer's tract and laminae I through V in the spinal cord on the side of the pain. The central nuclear groups of the dorsal horn are affected by this ablation. The procedure was introduced by Nashold in 1976 (98). The cord lesions are directed to reduce or eliminate the cellular hyperactivity seen after deafferentation in central pain syndromes. Note that peripheral anesthetic areas are usually present in these conditions.

The technique involved a laminectomy, either unilateral or bilateral, at the dermatomal level of the area of the pain (99, 100). The dura mater is opened and an operating microscope used to visualize the area of the entry of the dorsal rootlets into the spinal cord: the dorsal root entry zone. An electrode, usually 0.25 mm in diameter with 2-mm exposed metal tip, is then inserted about 2 to 3 mm into this zone. The lesion is made using a radiofrequency thermal technique with a tip temperature of 75° C for 15 to 20 seconds. A series of such lesions are made all along the vertical line of the rootlets, spanning 2 to 3 dermatomal levels. The lesions are separated by about 1 mm, and 20 to 50 total lesions are created in a typical patient, depending on the number of dermatomes involved. There are also reported techniques using laser and ultrasound modalities to create the lesions (101, 102).

For brachial plexus avulsion pain, good pain relief in multiple reports at follow-up intervals of 12 to 48 months has ranged from 65 to 80%, although the success rate is more typically 60 to 65% in series with longer follow-up periods (97). Phantom limb or stump pain success rates appear to be lower (50 to 60%) in smaller series, although with follow-up periods to 60 or 79 months. These lesions have also been applied to pain from trauma to the conus medullaris or cauda equina; in 39 patients with a mean follow-up of 3 years, pain relief was noted in 74% of patients, although the degree of relief varied (97). Use of dorsal root entry zone lesioning for intercostal postherpetic neuralgia does not appear to be very useful.

For spinal cord injury, the dorsal root entry zone procedure is most useful for the radicular or segmental (end zone) pain that occurs at or just below the level of the injury. The success rate for good pain control has been reported at 70 to 75% for this type of pain (103, 104). The diffuse, burning pain over the lower body or phantom pain in the same areas appears to not respond as well to dorsal root entry zone lesioning.

Permanent sensory changes are found in about 10 to 13% of patients; permanent motor changes are found in about the same number of patients. Transient sensory or motor changes are seen in about 5% of patients. Infection or cerebrospinal fluid leak are seen in about 5 to 7% of patients.

Midline Myelotomy

Midline myelotomy can be performed with mechanical ablation, radiofrequency techniques, or carbon dioxide laser (105) to section midline fibers posterior to the central canal of the spinal cord. The lesions usually are created at the lower thoracic spinal cord level, although lesions at C1 also have been reported by Gildenberg (106) and others. The efficacy in moderate to marked pain relief has been approximately 70%, with only rare complications or side effects. This procedure appears to be effective for lower body pain, especially midline or bilateral for which cordotomy or other ablative lesions might not be useful. Analgesia from hyperpathia and background pain has been obtained without sensory loss but with preserved ability to localize and discriminate between sharp and dull stimuli (107).

SUMMARY

A number of neurosurgical procedures have been described in the treatment of intractable pain. Improved stereotactic technology, especially using magnetic resonance guidance, has improved greatly the accuracy and ease of application of the intracranial procedures. The technology for and use of spinal procedures has been largely unchanged in the past decade. Information about the best application of many of these procedures is still lacking. The techniques are applied, for the most part, only to patients with severe pain, since many nonsurgical options adequately manage pain that is minimal or mild in severity. Decisions for selection of a specific technique can be based on expected survival time (cancer pain patients), pain location or locations, or preference for ablative or augmentative options.

Although each of these procedures has been championed and found effective by different clinical groups, information about the best roles for specific pain syndromes is lacking. This may indicate that technology has outpaced knowledge of the most effective application for each procedure. As scientific information about the efficacy of different various pain procedures is provided over the next few years, it is hoped that the role of each of these neurosurgical procedures in the overall management of patients with severe pain will be clarified.

References

1. Foltz EL, White LE. Pain "relief" by frontal cingulumotomy. J Neurosurg 1962;19:89-100.
2. Hurt RW, Ballantine HT. Stereotactic anterior cingulate lesions for persistent pain: a report on 68 cases. Clin Neurosurg 1974;21:334-351.
3. Mempel E, Dietrich RZ. Favorable effect of cingulotomy on gastric crisis pain. Neurol Neurochir Pol 1977;11:611-613.
4. Sano K. Neurosurgical treatments of pain: a general survey. Acta Neurochir Suppl 1987;38:86-96.
5. Santo JL, Arias LM, Barolat G, et al. Bilateral cingulumotomy in the treatment of reflex sympathetic dystrophy. Pain 1990;41:55-59.
6. Coombs DW. Intraspinal analgesic infusion by implanted pump. Ann N Y Acad Sci 1988;531:108-122.
7. Yaksh TL, Onofrio BM. Retrospective consideration of the doses of morphine given intrathecally by chronic infusion in 163 patients by 19 physicians. Pain 1987;31:211-223.
8. Lewin W. Selective leucotomy: a review. In: Laitinen LV, Livingston KE, eds. Surgical approaches in psychiatry. Baltimore: University Park Press, 1972;69-73.
9. Lewin W. Observations on selective leucotomy. J Neurol Neurosurg Psychiatry 1961;24:37-44.
10. Spiegel EA. Guided brain operations. Basel: Karger, 1982.
11. Spiegel EA, Wycis HT, Marks M, et al. Stereotaxic apparatus for operations on the human brain. Science 1947;106:349-350.
12. Hadley MN, Shetter AG, Amos MR. Use of the Brown-Roberts-Wells stereotactic frame for functional neurosurgery. Appl Neurophysiol 1985;48:61-68.
13. Martinez R, Vaquero J. Image-directed functional neurosurgery with the Cosman-Roberts-Wells stereotactic instrument. Acta Neurochir (Wien) 1991;113:1769.
14. Hassenbusch SJ, Pillay PK. Cingulotomy for treatment of cancer-related pain. In: Arbit E, ed. Advances in surgical management of cancer-related pain. Mt. Kisco, NY: Futura, 1993;297-312.
15. Hassenbusch SJ, Pillay PK. Cingulotomy for intractable pain using stereotaxis guided by magnetic resonance imaging. In: Rengachary SS, Wilkins RH, eds. Neurosurgical operative atlas, vol 1. Baltimore: Williams & Wilkins, 1992;449-458.
16. Hassenbusch SJ, Pillay PK, Barnett GH. Radiofrequency cingulotomy for intractable cancer pain using stereotaxis guided by magnetic resonance imaging. Neurosurgery 1990;27:220-223.
17. Pillay PK, Hassenbusch SJ. Cingulotomy for cancer pain: two year experience. Stereotact Funct Neurosurg 1992;59:33-38.
18. Leksell L. Cerebral radiosurgery: gammathalamotomy in two cases of intractable pain. Acta Chir Scand 1968;134:585-595.
19. Lindquist C, Kihlstrom L, Hellstrand E. Functional neurosurgery: a future for the gamma knife? Stereotact Funct Neurosurg 1991;57:72-81.
20. Steiner L, Forster D, Leksell L, et al. Gammathalamotomy in intractable pain. Acta Neurochir 1980;52:173-184.
21. Sano K. Neurosurgical treatments of pain: a general survey. Acta Neurochir Suppl 1987;38:86-96.
22. Tasker RR. Thalamotomy. Neurosurg Clin North Am 1990;1:841-864.
23. Gildenberg P. Functional neurosurgery. In: Schmidek HH, Sweet WH, eds. Operative neurosurgical techniques: indications, methods, and results. New York: Grune & Stratton, 1988;1035-1068.
24. Sweet WH. Central mechanisms of chronic pain (neuralgias and certain other neurogenic pain). Res Publ Assoc Res Nerv Ment Dis 1980;58:287-303.
25. Ballantine HT, Bouckoms AJ, Thomas EK, et al. Treatment of psychiatric illness by stereotactic cingulotomy. Biol Psychiatry 1987;22:807-819.
26. Faillace LA, Allen RP, McQueen JD, Northrup B. Cognitive deficits from bilateral cingulotomy for intractable pain in man. Dis Nerv Sys 1981;32:171-175.
27. Ortiz A. The role of the limbic lobe in central pain mechanisms: an hypothesis relating to the gate control theory of pain. In: Laitinen LV, Livingston KE, eds. Surgical approaches in psychiatry. Baltimore: University Park Press, 1972;59-64.
28. Sharma T. Abolition of opiate hunger in humans following bilateral anterior cingulotomy. Tex Med 1974;70:49-52.
29. Sharma T. Absence of cognitive deficits from bilateral cingulotomy for intractable pain in humans. Tex Med 1973;69:79-82.
30. Ballantine HT. A critical assessment of psychiatric surgery: past, present, and future. In: Berger PA, Brodie HKH, eds. American handbook of psychiatry, vol. 8. New York: Basic Books, 1986;1029-1045.
31. Jenike MA, Baer L, Ballantine T, et al. Cingulotomy for refractory obsessive-compulsive disorder. Arch Gen Psychiatry 1991;48:548-555.
32. Allen RP, Faillace LA. A clinical test for detecting defects of cingulate lesions in man. J Clin Psychol 1972;28:63-65.
33. Corkin S, Twitchell TE, Sullivan EV. Safety and efficacy of cingulotomy for pain and psychiatric disorder. In: Hitchcock ER, Ballantine HT, Myerson BA, eds. Modern concepts in psychiatric surgery. New York: Elsevier North-Holland, 1979;253-272.
34. Fairman D. Hypothalamotomy as a new perspective for alleviation of intractable pain and regression of metastatic malignant tumors. In: Fusek K, ed. Present limits of neurosurgery. Prague: Avicenum Czechoslovakian Medical Press, 1971;525-528.
35. Sano K. Sedative neurosurgery with reference to posteromedial hypothalamotomy. Neurol Medicochir 1962; 4:112-142.
36. Mayanagi Y, Sano K, Suzuki I, et al. Stimulation and coagulation of the posteromedial hypothalamus for intractable pain, with reference to beta-endorphins. Appl Neurophysiol 1982;45:136-142.
37. Sano K, Sekino H, Hashimoto I, et al. Posteromedial hypothalamotomy in the treatment of intractable pain. Confinia Neurol 1975;37:285-290.
38. Amano K, Kitamura K, Sano K, et al. Relief of intractable pain from neurosurgical point of view with reference to present limits and clinical indications: a review of 100 consecutive cases. Neurol Med Chir (Tokyo) 1976;16:141-153.
39. Deleted.
40. Gros C, Frerebeau P, Privat JM, et al. Place of hypophysectomy in the neurosurgical treatment of pain. Adv Neurosurg 1975;3:264-272.
41. Silverberg GD. Hypophysectomy in the treatment of disseminated prostate carcinoma. Cancer 1977;39:1727-1731.
42. Tindall GT, Payne NS, Nixon DW. Transsphenoidal hypophysectomy for disseminated carcinoma of the prostate gland. J Neurosurg 1979;50:275-282.
43. Tindall GT, Ambrose SS, Christy JH, et al. Hypophysectomy in the treatment of disseminated carcinoma of the breast and prostate gland. South Med J 1976;69:579-583.
44. Miles J. Chemical hypophysectomy. Adv Pain Res Ther 1979;2:373-380.
45. Levin AB. Hypophysectomy in the treatment of cancer pain. In: Arbit E, ed. Management of cancer-related pain. Mt. Kisco, NY: Futura, 1993;281-295.
46. Kapur TR, Dalton GA. Trans-sphenoidal hypophysectomy for metastatic carcinoma of the breast. Br J Surg 1969;56:332-337.
47. Levin AB, Ramirez LF, Katz J. The use of stereotaxic chemical hypophysectomy in the treatment of thalamic pain syndrome. J Neurosurg 1983;59:1002-1006.
48. Maddy JA, Winternitz WW, Norrell H. Cryohypophysectomy in the management of advanced prostatic cancer. Cancer 1971;28:322-328.
49. Zervas NT. Stereotaxic radiofrequency surgery of the normal and abnormal pituitary gland. N Engl J Med 1969;280:429-437.
50. Sano K. Intralaminar thalamotomy and posteromedial hypothalamotomy in the treatment of intractable pain. Prog Neurol Surg 1977;8:50-103.

51. Daniel PM, Prichard MML. The human hypothalamus and pituitary stalk after hypophysectomy of pituitary stalk section. Brain 1972;95:813-824.

52. Nilaver G, Zimmerman EA, Wilkins J, et al. Magnocellular hypothalamic projections to the lower brain stem and spinal cord of the rat: immunocytochemical evidence for predominance of the oxytocin-neurophysin system compared to a vasopressin-neurophysin system. Neuroendocrinology 1980;30:150-158.

53. Silverman AJ, Zimmerman EA. Magnocellular neurosecretory system. Ann Rev Neurosci 1983;6:357-380.

54. Sofroniew MV. Projections from vasopressin, oxytocin, and neurophysin neurons to neural targets in the rat and human. J Histochem Cytochem 1980;28:475-478.

55. Swanson LW, Sawchenko PE. Paraventricular nucleus: a site for the integration of neuroendocrine and autonomic mechanism. Neuroendocrinology 1980;31:410-417.

56. Deshpande N, Moricca G, Saullo F, et al. Some aspects of pituitary function after neuroadenolysis in patients with metastatic cancer. Tumori 1981;67:355-359.

57. Levin AB, Katz J, Benson RC, et al. Treatment of pain of diffuse metastatic cancer by stereotactic chemical hypophysectomy: long-term results and observations on mechanism of action. Neurosurgery 1980;6:258-262.

58. Katz S, Levin AB. Treatment of diffuse metastatic pain by instillation of alcohol into the sella turcica. Anesthesiology 1977;46:115-121.

59. Perrault M, LeBeau J, Klotz B, et al. L'hypophysectomie totale dans le traitment du cancer sein: premier cas français: avenir de la méthode. Therapie 1952;7:290-300.

60. Williams NE, Miles JB, Lipton S, et al. Pain relief and pituitary function following injection of alcohol into the pituitary fossa. Ann R Coll Surg Engl 1980;62:203-207.

61. Greco T, Sbaragli F, Cammilli L, et al: L'alcolizzazione della ipofisi per via transfenoidale nella terapia di particoloari tumori maligni. Settim Med 45:355-356, 1957.

62. Benabid AL, Schaerer R, De Rougemont J, et al. Clinical evaluation of stereotactic isotope hypophysectomy in advanced breast cancer. Rev Endocrine Rel Cancers 1978; (Suppl): 111-117.

63. Rand RW. Stereotactic transsphenoidal cryohypophysectomy. Bull L A Neurol Soc 1964;29:40-48.

64. Talairach J, Aboulker J, Tournoux P, et al. Technique stéréotaxique de la chirurgie hypophysaire par voie nasale: suites opératoires: indications thérapeutiques. Neurochirurgie 1956;2:3-20.

65. West CR, Avellanosa AM, Bremer AM, et al. Hypophysectomy for relief of pain in disseminated carcinoma of the prostate. Adv Pain Res Ther 1979;2:393-400.

66. Madrid JL. Chemical hypophysectomy. Adv Pain Res Ther 1979;2:381-391.

67. Tasker R. Neurosurgical and neuroaugmentative intervention. In: Patt RB, ed. Cancer pain. Philadelphia: Lippincott, 1993;471-500.

68. Lipton S. Percutaneous cervical cordotomy and pituitary injection of alcohol. In: Swerdlow M, ed. Relief of intractable pain. Amsterdam: Elsevier, 1983;269-304.

69. Kudo T, Yoshii N, Shimizu S, et al. Effects of stereotactic thalamotomy to intractable pain and numbness. Keio J Med 1966;15:191-194.

70. Kudo T, Toshii N, Shimizu S, et al. Stereotactic thalamotomy for pain relief. Tohoku J Exp Med 1968;96:219-230.

71. Laitinen LV. Anterior pulvinotomy in the treatment of intractable pain. In: Sweet WH, Obrador S, Martin-Rodriguez JG, eds. Neurosurgical treatment in psychiatry, pain, and epilepsy. Baltimore: University Park Press, 1977;669-672.

72. Strenge H. The functional significance of the pulvinar thalami. Fortschr Neurol Psychiat 1978;46:491-507.

73. Yoshii N, Mizokami T, Ushikubo Y, et al. Comparative study between size of lesioned area and operative effects after pulvinotomy. Appl Neurophysiol 1982;45:492-497.

74. Yoshii N, Fukuda S. Effects of unilateral and bilateral invasion of thalamic pulvinar for pain relief. Tohoku J Exp Med 1979;127:81-84.

75. Sweet WH. Central mechanisms of chronic pain (neuralgias and certain other neurogenic pain). Res Publ Assoc Res Nerv Ment Dis 1980;58:287-303.

76. Mayanagi Y, Bouchard G. Evaluation of stereotactic thalamotomies for pain relief with reference to pulvinar intervention. Appl Neurophysiol 1976;39:154-157.

77. Yoshii N, Fukuda S. Several clinical aspects of thalamic pulvinotomy. Appl Neurophysiol 1977;39:162-164.

78. Reference deleted.

79. Frank F, Fabrizi AP, Gaist G. Stereotactic mesencephalic tractotomy in the treatment of chronic cancer pain. Acta Neurochir (Wien) 1989;99:38-40.

80. Shieff C, Nashold BS. Stereotactic mesencephalic tractotomy for thalamic pain. Neuro Res 1987;9:101-104.

81. Sjoqvist O. Studies on pain conduction in trigeminal nerve: a contribution to the surgical treatment of facial pain. Acta Psychiatr Neurol 1938;17 (Suppl):1-139.

82. White JC, Sweet WH, eds. Pain and the neurosurgeon: a forty-year experience. Springfield, IL: Charles C. Thomas, 1969;232-251, 314-320.

83. Spiegel EA, Wycis HT. Mesencephalotomy in the treatment of "intractable" facial pain. Arch Neurol 1953;69:1.

84. Nashold BS Jr, Crue BL Jr. Stereotaxic mesencephalotomy and trigeminal tractotomy. In: Youmans JR, ed. Neurological surgery. 2nd ed.. Philadelphia: Saunders, 1982;3702-3716.

85. Schvarcz JR. Spinal cord stereotactic techniques re trigeminal nucleotomy and extralemniscal myelotomy. Appl Neurophysiol 1978;41:99-112.

86. Hassenbusch SJ, Pillay PK. Ablative intracranial neurosurgery for cancer pain: three-year experience and modification of techniques. J Neurosurg 1992;76:396A (abstract).

87. Tseng LF, Fujimoto JM. Differential actions of intrathecal naloxone on blocking the tail flick inhibition induced by intraventricular beta-endorphin and morphine in rats. J Pharmacol Exp Ther 1985;232:74-79.

88. Dennis GC, DeWitty RL. Long-term intraventricular infusion of morphine for intractable pain in cancer of the head and neck. Neurosurgery 1990;26:404-408.

89. Lazorthes Y. Intracerebroventricular administration of morphine for control of irreducible cancer pain. Ann N Y Acad Sci 1988;531:123-132.

90. Brazenor GA. Long term intrathecal administration of morphine: a comparison of bolus injection via reservoir with continuous infusion by implanted pump. Neurosurgery 1987;21:484-491.

91. Gybels J, Kupers R. Deep brain stimulation in the treatment of chronic pain in man: where and why? Neurophysiol Clin 1990;20:389-398.

92. Kumar K, Wyant GM, Nath R. Deep brain stimulation for control of intractable pain in humans, present and future: A ten-year follow-up. Neurosurgery 1990;26:774-782.

93. Young RF. Brain stimulation. Neurosurg Clin North Am 1990;1:865-879.

94. Young RF, Tronnier V, Rinaldi PC. Chronic stimulation of the Kolliker-Fuse nucleus region for relief of intractable pain in humans. J Neurosurg 1992;76:979-985.

95. Young RF. Electrical stimulation of the brain for the treatment of intractable cancer pain. In: Arbit E, ed. Management of cancer-related pain. Mt. Kisco, NY: Futura, 1993;257-269.

96. Tasker RR. Percutaneous cordotomy: the lateral high cervical technique. In: Schmidek HH, Sweet WH, eds. Operative neurosurgical techniques: indications, methods, and results. New York: Grune & Stratton, 1988;1191-1205.

97. Iskandar BJ, Nashold BS. Spinal and trigeminal DREZ lesions. In: Gildenberg PL, Tasker RR, eds. Textbook of stereotactic and functional neurosurgery. New York: McGraw-Hill, 1998;1573-1583.

98. Nashold BS Jr. Introduction to second international symposium on dorsal root entry zone (DREZ) lesions. Appl Neurophysiol 1988;51:76-77.

99. Cosman ER, Rittman WJ, Nashold BS Jr, et al. Radiofrequency lesion generation and its effect on tissue impedance. Appl Neurophysiol 1988;51:230-242.

100. Cosman ER, Nashold BS Jr, Ovelmen-Levitt J. Theoretical aspects of radiofrequency lesions in the dorsal root entry zone. Neurosurgery 1984;15:945-950.

101. Young RF. Clinical experience with radiofrequency and laser DREZ lesions. J Neurosurg 1990;72:715-720.

102. Dreval ON. Ultrasonic DREZ-operations for treatment of pain due to brachial plexus avulsion. Acta Neurochir (Wien) 1992;122:76-81.

103. Edgar RE, Best LG, Quail PA, et al. Computer-assisted DREZ microcoagulation: posttraumatic spinal deafferentation pain. J Spinal Disord 1993;6:48-56.

104. Friedman AH, Nashold BS Jr. DREZ lesions for the relief of pain related to spinal cord injury. J Neurosurg 1986;65:465-469.

105. Fink RA. Neurosurgical treatment of nonmalignant intractable rectal pain: microsurgical commissural myelotomy with the carbon dioxide laser. Neurosurgery 1984;14:64-65.

106. Gildenberg PL, Hirshberg RM. Limited myelotomy for the treatment of intractable cancer pain. J Neurol Neurosurg Psychiatry 1984;47:94-96.

107. Schvarcz JR. Stereotactic extralemniscal myelotomy. J Neurol Neurosurg Psychiatry 1976;39:53-57.

CHAPTER 39

Physical Therapy: Evaluation and Treatment of Chronic Pain Patients

Harriet Wittink and Theresa Hoskins Michel

INTRODUCTION

Many of the patients we see in our daily practice complain of chronic pain, and their management remains a difficult challenge. Patients often relate to their physicians that at best past physical therapy had no effect on their pain. It is all too common for chronic pain patients to complain that physical therapy always makes them worse. Why, then, should a physician refer to physical therapy again? Merely asking if a patient has had physical therapy without asking what that consisted of, is like asking if a patient is taking medications without asking which ones. Physical therapy consists of a broad array of techniques and approaches, some of which are not helpful to patients with chronic pain. At the heart of past treatment failures may be a number of factors: persistent failure of physical therapists to recognize and treat the differences between acute and chronic pain states, past treatment that was uni-disciplinary and did not address the emotional and cognitive aspects of chronic pain, and the patient's inability to recognize anything less than total pain relief as success. A dynamic exercise approach may have been tried with the result that the patient had muscle soreness that was misinterpreted as a new injury. The patient, then complaining vociferously about this "new pain," may have caused the physician to stop physical therapy. Indeed, any or all of these factors may have played a part in a patient's history of treatment failure. Mutual trust and communication between the physician and the physical therapist are extremely important in the treatment of these patients. We must operate as a team and share common goals and objectives for the patient. Any disagreement in this team may result in treatment failure.

To place the importance of physical therapy into a wider framework of caring for pain, a disablement model is suggested. There are three major schemes, discussed by Jette (1). These all help describe restrictions in the patient's performance by identifying the relationship among pathology, impairments, functional limitations, and disability. Physical therapy treatment is directed at the prevention of disability and the restoration of functional ability. In acute pain there are clear relations among nociception, perceived pain, and impairments. Therefore, treatment focuses on the elimination of pain. As a result, impairments improve, functional ability is restored, and disability is prevented. In chronic pain patients, however, the relations among pain, impairments, and disability is unclear. Chronic pain patients may never return to work even when the only impairment identified is pain. Treatments that address chronic pain as an acute phenomenon, a warning of tissue damage, have no ability to alter the illness and disability behavior of the chronic pain patient. More appropriate physical therapy treatment addresses behavioral changes and is ideally a component of a multidisciplinary approach. Apart from a strong behavioral management focus, treatment of chronic pain patients should include education of the patient on the nature of their problem, resolution of treatable impairments, instruction in independent management of pain, and instruction in methods to prevent future problems, such as ergonomics and pacing techniques.

Referral to physical therapy is appropriate when pain impairs a patient's optimal functional ability or inhibits a patient's independence in activities of daily living. The physical therapist's evaluation entails the identification of cardiopulmonary, musculoskeletal, and neuromuscular impairments that may cause functional limitations. A diagnosis, the orders "evaluate and treat," and any precautions should be provided to allow the physical therapist to use clinical judgment in designing an appropriate treatment program. It is also helpful to the physical therapist to know that the physician intends to wean a patient off pain medications, as patients may complain of increased pain and seek medications elsewhere. Frequent communication between the physician and the physical therapist helps the team stay focused on the goals set for the patient and solve any problems encountered that would interfere with attaining these goals.

PHYSICAL THERAPY EVALUATION

The following purposes of evaluation are identified:

1. To establish a baseline from which to plan and begin interventions
2. To assist in the selection of appropriate interventions
3. To evaluate the efficacy of interventions

Physical therapists are comfortable with the assessment of physical impairments, such as flexibility, strength, and endurance. Most of the information needed to develop an appropriate treatment plan should be obtained during an interview and the physical examination (2).

Interview of the Patient

The process of collecting information from a pain patient begins with the patient interview of the patient, which guides all future examination procedures. The physical therapist asks the patient about the pain: intensity, pattern, location, duration, onset, what makes it better, what makes it worse, what does the patient think is causing the pain. The answers to each of these questions guide the next series of questions. Red flags that make the therapist suspicious that there is a more serious medical problem are identified immediately, and the therapist may refer the patient back for further medical workup. Examples of this are severe flank pain in a man who has a history of kidney stones and neck pain with jaw ache in an obese man with hypertension who smokes. Pain location is a very important clue to direct further questions and the physical examination. Abdominal pain that worsens with eating suggests a gastrointestinal cause rather than a musculoskeletal or neuromuscular one. Pains that are mechanical in nature may be worst in the morning, then less by evening after a day of general activity, as in osteoarthritis, or may be worse on weight bearing but eased by non-weight bearing positions. The physical examination can then begin to differentiate some of the mechanisms of the pain. The interview should also provide clues to the classification of pains: neuropathic, somatic, visceral, sympathetically maintained, or some combination. The medications that help control pain the most will assist in this classification. Positions of comfort versus discomfort also help to classify mechanical causes of joint pain. For more definitive differentiation of back and neck pain, see Quebec Task Force on Spinal Disorders (3).

Physical Examination

The physical examination should consist of the following elements:

1. Observations of movement, posture, and affect are done even before the patient is aware that the assessment has begun. Transitional movements are observed when the patient sits, stands, walks, or climbs onto a plinth.
2. Muscle testing, with observed active motions at joints, and resisted motions may be done. Objective performance measures using dynamometers are sometimes obtained for future comparison.
3. Joint motion in a voluntary range should be observed, and should be measured in particularly impaired areas so that improvement or loss of joint range will be detected. Quality of motion can be very distorted, and jerky, dysfunctional movement patterns should be noted. Muscle guarding and pain behaviors are often displayed during the physical examination and should be noted.
4. Posture in standing and sitting should be evaluated for asymmetries and altered spinal curvatures.
5. Palpation is used to determine the presence of muscle spasm, trigger points (the jump sign), edema, skin turgor, and subcutaneous nodules. Areas of tenderness should be determined, which may represent pain from viscera or deeper structures, should be determined.
6. Sensory testing for light touch, temperature, pressure, proprioception, and sharp pinprick should be done to assess nerve root involvement. Deep tendon reflexes are tested with a reflex hammer if sensory disturbances in a dermatomal distribution appear. Patients' reports of dysesthesias, burning, and sharp stabbing pain are clues to neuropathic pain and suggest further neurologic testing.
7. Pain measurement is essential to the evaluation of the patient in pain. Both the sensory and the emotional aspects of pain must be assessed. Although limited to the dimension of pain intensity, a visual analog scale or a numeric rating scale is useful, especially in acute pain situations. The Present Pain Intensity Scale found on the McGill Pain Questionnaire (4) assigns a numeric score for the affective reaction to pain. For the more complex pain states, such as mixed acute and chronic pain or chronic pain syndrome, measurement of pain should be taken over time, and along several dimensions, including behavioral, psychosocial, and functional. The McGill Pain Questionnaire combined with a disability questionnaire, such as the Roland-Morris Disability Questionnaire (5), that is specific for back pain provides the functional picture and many of the pain dimensions of a complex chronic pain patient. These instruments have been tested for reliability and are much more sensitive than intensity scales to the

types of complex issues surrounding chronic pain. Physical therapists are frequently called upon to evaluate and treat patients with neuralgias, causalgias, diabetic polyneuropathies, sympathetically maintained pain, and pain resulting from damage to central somatosensory pathways. These are most likely chronic conditions and are associated with hyperalgesia, allodynia, lancinating pain, and severe disability. For these conditions it may be important to add to the evaluation process sensory mapping, temperature mapping of involved parts, volumetric or girth measurements for edematous body parts, nerve conduction studies, muscle performance measures including isokinetic testing, and even electromyography.

8. Function testing should always be done with direct observation of the patients' performance rather than taking the patient's word for it. Some functional tests that have been applied to a chronic pain population include the 6-minute walk test (meters walked in 6 minutes), and the "get up and go" test (6). Aerobic fitness can be estimated from submaximal bicycle ergometer tests (7), and from a 6-minute walk test. The therapist should note inconsistencies in performance, such as giveaway weakness, voluntary muscle guarding, complaint of radicular pain with straight leg raising in supine but not in sit position, as this may reflect the patient's behavioral response to pain or secondary gain issues.

The chronic pain patient commonly has secondary impairments, such as muscle strain patterns, muscle weakness and tightness, and trigger points, that are a direct result of the chronic pain state. The avoidance of activities, the patterns of protection of painful parts, and the distortion of movement can lead to secondary impairments and new pain. A common secondary impairment of chronic pain states is that of deconditioning. A precise measure of physical work capacity can be very helpful as a part of the physical capacity assessment, involving indirect calorimetry using the analysis of expired air during steady-state exercise. This, however, is a time-consuming and costly test and not available to all physical therapists. The 6-minute walk test offers a reasonable alternative as an indicator of physical capacity (6).

Additional very common secondary impairments in chronic pain are depression and anxiety, which should be factored in to the plan of care by the physical therapist, even if another member of the multidisciplinary team performs the evaluation of mood.

Disability evaluation is another multidisciplinary area of concern. The physical therapist's role includes but is not limited to job task analyses, evaluation of risks to the individual patient returning to a job, impairment assessment, and deciding how a job may be modified to assist the individual's safe return to the job. A functional capacity evaluation (FCE) (see Appendix to Chapter 4) is usually performed to determine patients' physical capacity to perform work. Assessment includes the patient's ability to lift weights from the floor to waist and from the waist to overhead, to carry, crawl, squat, sit, stand, walk, climb stairs, and push and pull weights. Aerobic fitness may be determined from a (submaximal) bicycle or treadmill test. Additional specific tests may be performed such as fine motor skills for the hands and hand grip strength may be performed. An FCE is always somewhat subjective, as it can only document how much a patient is willing to do on a given day. Therefore, inconsistencies in effort and pain behaviors should be noted and documented. Although the use of isokinetic machines has been advocated, there is little scientific evidence to support their use for medicolegal purposes (8).

PHYSICAL THERAPY TREATMENT OF CHRONIC PAIN AND CHRONIC PAIN SYNDROME PATIENTS

To determine a treatment plan, it is helpful to differentiate between chronic pain patients and chronic pain syndrome patients. For the purposes of this chapter, chronic pain patients, or patients with persistent pain, are defined as patients with little or no disability associated with their pain. Their pain, impairments, and associated functional limitation are in direct proportion to objective findings. Often their main complaint is diminished quality of life. They have few dysfunctional beliefs and require little cognitive restructuring. These patients require less intensive treatment and respond well to passive treatment modalities in combination with active treatment and education on independent pain management.

Chronic pain syndrome patients, on the other hand, present with considerable abnormal illness behaviors and complain of disability and pain out of proportion to objective findings. Waddell et al. (9) showed that the relation of pain to physical impairments (r =.27) and disability (r =.31) in chronic back pain patients is poor. These patients believe they are "sick," and it is this belief that renders them incapable of functioning. Unfortunately, this belief is often reinforced by health care providers who tell patients to stop when it hurts, reinforcing the sick role. Illness behaviors include fear of pain (10), fear-avoidance behaviors (9, 11) and fear of movement and injury or reinjury (10), which independently lead to functional limitations and secondary impairments. These patients are passive, dependent, helpless, and hopeless, and they require intensive treatment. As the pain is chronic, the focus of physical therapy treatment should not be on passive treatment techniques that deny patients control over their own physical health. Treatment of pain in these patients will not decrease their disability perception, nor will it improve their quality of life. The focus of physical therapy treatment should be on helping patients to regain control over their lives by active participation in their pain therapy program and independent management of their pain. To achieve this, an active partnership must be established between the patient and the physical therapist. The physical therapist becomes a guide, leading the patient to the desired goals of independent pain management and improved functioning by way of appropriate physical therapy treatment in an environment sufficiently secure to reduce fear and promote self-confidence. Included in physical therapy treatment are behavioral methods, such as quota-based progressive exercise programs, to decrease fear of injury and physical activity, education on hurt versus harm, and performance-contingent rewards, and of functional goals.

The role of the physical therapist is that of a motivator, a challenger, and educator. The patient does the work by following through with the home program, taking responsibility for his or her own pain management and achievement of functional goals.

Physical therapy should be time limited and have an observable end point associated with the following:

1. Reduction of the influence impact of pain on the patient's life, that is, reduced disability
2. Improvement of the patient's knowledge of independent pain management
3. Resolution of treatable impairments that interfere with normal function (12)
4. Attainment of measurable functional goals within a limited time frame

Central to all treatment of chronic pain patients are the following:

1. Education
2. Self-management techniques
3. Functional goal setting
4. Behavioral modification techniques
5. Active modalities: exercise
6. Passive modalities: massage, joint mobilization, electrotherapy, heat and cold
7. Ergonomics

Education

Perhaps most important is education about pain treatment itself and the expectations of the patient and the health care providers involved. The patient and the team must agree on the goals of treatment to prevent confusion and disappointment on both sides and to increase patient compliance. Shutty et al. (13) showed that common treatment goals are strongly related to increased treatment satisfaction and to a lesser extent decreased disability ratings a month after treatment. Patients must understand that usually after a functional restoration program, a medical end point will be declared and that it may have legal implications. For instance, a declaration of medical end point allows them to settle their worker's compensation claim. Their work capacity will be assessed at the end of treatment, and they should know that their current disability status will not be supported if they are physically capable of work.

Common misperceptions by patients include the notion that their pain could be cured if only someone would diagnose them correctly and that increasing their function may result in potentially fatal injury leading to life in a wheelchair or even death. Education on the difference between acute and chronic pain, on the anatomy of the affected body part, the pathophysiology of their diagnosis, and the difference between "hurt" (soreness) and "harm" (injury) should help dispel these notions.

Patients also need to understand that the focus of treatment is return to function, rather than return to a pain-free state. Education on the fluctuating course of pain, and knowledge that pain perception is influenced by a host of circumstances, including psychosocial factors, is important. Continuous education takes place during treatment on body mechanics, proper execution of movement patterns, and on the importance of correct posture. When treating patients in a group, education comes from other patients as well. They may share solutions to functional problems, ways to better pace their activities, or independent pain management techniques they have found helpful.

Self-Management Techniques

Chronic pain patients must learn to relinquish their dependence on health care providers for their pain management and learn techniques that enable them to take control and manage their pain independently. Self-management techniques include the use of pain-control modalities (e.g., ice, heat, and self-massage) and a structured home exercise program. Getting patients to invest in their use can be difficult, as many patients have a history of treatment failures and may feel that these relatively simple techniques will be insufficient in helping them manage their pain. Chronic pain patients have a tendency to do more on days they feel good and less on days when they feel more pain and fatigue. This "pain-contingent" behavior results in a cycle of the patient doing too much one day and nothing at all the next. The home exercise program is progressive quota based, beginning at a submaximal level to ensure early success with an appropriate rate of increase built in. This structure allows for achievement of functional goals and the disconnection of activities from pain.

Functional Goal Setting

Focusing on function allows the entire treatment team and the patient to avoid issues that may disrupt a successful rehabilitation approach (14). Therefore treatment starts with patients setting their own goals. Common goals include being able to walk for an hour, sit through a meal or a movie, carry and lift a certain amount, and perform essential job components. Return to work or vocational rehabilitation should be part of the treatment plan. A directive return-to-work approach has been shown to be successful in chronic pain patients (15). The goals must be realistic and attainable within a reasonable time frame. It is helpful to set the number of treatments per week and the number of weeks of treatment before initiating treatment. Having a definite end point increases patient compliance and gives a framework to the treatment team and the patient in which to achieve goals and a behavioral change.

Behavior Modification Techniques

Illness beliefs, such as fear of pain and fear of movement and injury or reinjury (10), and illness behaviors such as fear-avoidance (9, 11), limping, and using ambulatory devices etc. lead to functional limitations and secondary impairments independent of the amount of pain the patient has. Avoidance behavior (16) is postulated to be one of the mechanisms in sustaining chronic pain disability. Patients receiving disability compensation report more pain of movement and injury or reinjury than those who do not receive any compensation (10). It is the physical therapist's task to help patients overcome their fear of movement and injury or reinjury and to achieve a cognitive change in the patients' perception of what they think they are able to do versus what they actually can do.

The operant behavioral approach to pain management (16) involves having patients set their own goals and rewarding the accomplishment of each goal (positive feedback). It also includes ignoring pain behaviors such as sighing, rubbing, and complaining about pain (no feedback). Because pain patients are not being rewarded for expressing their pain, their pain behaviors gradually disappear.

The cognitive-behavioral approach challenges dysfunctional beliefs by pointing out to patients that they are performing a task they previously stated they were unable to accomplish. Repeated exposure to avoided activities has been shown to decrease anxiety and fear about them (17). In fact, it has been shown that **chronic pain levels stay the same or decrease despite significant increases in activity levels** (11, 17–20). During baseline trials of prescribed exercises the patient works to tolerance without interruption at each exercise, and then carefully records how many times the exercise can be repeated before the need to stop is felt. The numbers of repetitions for each exercise can be averaged. The average baseline number of repetitions for each exercise is set. Quotas are then set for each exercise. Each quota should be less than the average number of baseline repetitions (16). The key element is that the patient is certain the first quota can be met. This will set the patient up for success and thus positive reinforcement. The quota is determined by the physical therapist's judgement of how well the patient will be able to perform. Quotas are then increased at a predetermined rate. Upper limits are set to the number of repetitions for each exercise. This allows the patient to overcome his or her fear and learn that increased activity does not equal an increase in pain. It allows the physical therapist to know that the patient is exercising safely, that is, within the boundaries of his or her physical ability, without damage to any tissues through overuse.

Active Modalities: Exercise

The hypothesis that pain control systems become more active with long-lasting muscle exercise is supported by the finding that immobilized and inactive patients suffer more from pain than active ones do. It is important to keep the patient mentally and physically stimulated, and muscle-training programs should be included in the rehabilitation of pain patients (21). Encouraging patients to take greater responsibility for their care can strengthen the sense of personal control over a person's pain and function. Physical exercise is perceived by many as something that healthy people do and thus has the potential to detach patients from their sick role. The physical therapist should encourage patients to rehearse functional activities while addressing impairments that interfere with their ability to function. Chronic pain patients are deconditioned from lack of activity and present with loss of strength, endurance, flexibility, and aerobic capacity. Many patients present with muscle imbalance, which is a specific pattern of muscle tightness and weakness (22, 23) that presents itself as abnormal posture. The physical therapist develops a specific program for each patient, addressing that patient's specific impairments and functional needs. Exercise can be subdivided into three categories: strengthening, and endurance, exercise and stretching.

The purpose of stretching is to regain normal flexibility around joints to allow them to function in their optimal position. As tight muscles are thought to inhibit their antagonists (22, 23), stretching muscle indirectly helps to restore muscle strength.

Directly increasing muscle strength is achieved by high-intensity, short-duration exercise. Neuronal adaptation occurs first by increased efficiency to recruit motor neurons, followed by an increase in myofibrillar protein after about 6 weeks of exercise. Increased muscle strength helps patients perform functional tasks such as lifting and carrying. It may also be helpful in decreasing pain perception. Increasing strength has been shown to decrease neck pain in patients with neck pain (24, 25). Lack of trunk muscle endurance plays an important role in chronic back pain (26–28).

Endurance exercise is the term used for two types of exercise:

1. Exercise targeted to increase maximal aerobic power or cardiovascular functioning by exercising patients at 65 to 80% of their maximal heart rate, usually by treadmill walking, biking, or any form of dynamic exercise of large muscle groups. Work and functional tasks such as walking, climbing stairs, repetitive lifting, fighting fires, carrying loads, scaling walls, and running, as necessary for police work, have a significant aerobic endurance component. Many tasks are defined by their energy cost as expressed in oxygen consumption or metabolic equivalents (METS). Patients need a maximum aerobic power high enough to perform functional tasks (work) without excessive fatigue (7).

2. Exercise (low intensity, long duration) targeted to increase the aerobic capacity of a specific muscle so that the muscle can sustain contraction for long periods without fatiguing. This improves neuromotor control and coordination and thus prevents injury to passive structures during prolonged activities. Physical forces provide important stimuli to tissues for the development and maintenance of homeostasis. Endurance exercise of specific muscles is not only associated with increased capillary density of that muscle, but also with increased strength of muscle, bone, and tendons. It results in thicker, stronger ligaments that maintain their compliance and flexibility and that are stronger at the bone-ligament-bone complex (29). Synovial fluid lubricates the ligamentous structures of the joint and provides nourishment to cartilage, menisci, and ligaments. Repetitious motion enhances this transsynovial nutrient flow (30). Endurance exercise thus improves the body's ability to withstand repetitive physical forces and muscle fatigue. As most functional tasks are repetitive in nature, most patients have a greater need of increased endurance than of increased strength. For instance, many back pain patients have significant lack of leg and gluteal endurance, which does not manifest with strength testing, but is apparent with repetitive squatting. Lack of leg endurance results in patients lifting with their back and arm muscles instead of with their leg muscles. Improving the endurance of the muscle groups that are important for proper lifting prevents reinjury.

Aerobic exercise is thought to have beneficial effects on pain perception and mood. It appears that pain inhibition through exercise can be mediated through the opiate and the non-opiate systems. Analgesic effects of exercise have been found at submaximal workloads of around 63% of $VO_{2\,max}$ (31). Droste et al. (32) found that pain threshold elevations were most pronounced during maximal exertion, at which time the subjects reported the greatest fatigue. The elevations in pain threshold were correlated with rating of perceived exertion (RPE). This exercise-induced elevation in pain threshold did not appear to be directly related to plasma endorphin levels. Rhythmic exercise stimulates the $A\delta$ or group III afferents arising from muscle. Histologically, $A\delta$ or group III afferents are a prominent group of fine myelinated fibers located in skeletal muscle nerves. More recent investigations indicate that these afferents respond to muscle stretch and contraction with low-frequency discharge (33). For this reason, Kniffki et al. (34) called the endings of these afferents **ergoreceptors.** Thoren et al. (33) and Lundeberg (21) hypothesize that rhythmic exercise activates the ergoreceptors, which then activates the descending pain modulating systems.

Moderate aerobic exercise has been shown to be effective in the treatment of mild to moderate forms of depression and anxiety (35, 36). The data from the meta-analysis by North et al. (35) suggest that exercise is as effective an antidepressant as psychotherapy and that anaerobic exercise is as effective as aerobic exercise. Exercise was not as effective an anti-depressant as exercise and psychotherapy together, suggesting that an additive effect of treatments may exist.

Passive Modalities

The use of passive modalities, unless self-administered, can be detrimental to chronic pain syndrome patients, as it tends to increase these patients' dependence on others and confirm disability beliefs. The application of modalities such as ice and heat is easy for patients to learn and can play a role in effective treatment, but should be linked to function. For instance, heat or ice can be used after treatment as a reward for meeting quotas, or performing a functional activity. Ice can be used before an activity to numb the painful area, so that the patient is able to perform the activity. In chronic pain patients, passive modalities can play an integral role in treatment, but should not be the only treatment the patient receives. Active exercise should always be a part of treatment of all chronic pain patients. Passive modalities include joint mobilization, soft tissue mobilization, electrotherapeutic modalities, ice, and heat.

Joint Mobilization

Joint mobilization is a technique used to improve joint mobility when the ligamentous and capsular structures limit passive range of motion. It can restore normal capsular extensibility by applying carefully directed forces across the articular surfaces. All collagenous tissues rely heavily on movement to ensure adequate nutrition and respond to loading much as bone does, according to Wolff's law. When not stretching the tissues, joint mobilization can be used to decrease pain by stimulation of the type I and II mechanoreceptors. Joint mobilization is usually combined with ultrasound or heat, as this is thought to make the tissue more extensible and treatment thus more effective. Findings to support the efficacy of use of mobilization or manipulation in chronic low-back pain are yet inconclusive, although there are indications that manipulation may be beneficial for certain (subgroups) of patients (37).

Soft-Tissue Mobilization

Soft-tissue mobilization includes massage, passive stretching, and myofascial techniques such as myofascial release and craniosacral therapy. Massage can provide symptomatic relief by reducing pain through increasing local circulation and by stimulating $A\beta$ fibers. Trigger point massage in combination with passive stretching is thought to inhibit trigger points in muscle (38), thus reducing muscle pain. It is helpful to instruct the patient in self-massage as an active pain control modality by use of using a cane, umbrella handle, or tennis balls. The patient can use these devices to press against a trigger point and apply ischemic pressure or slowly rotate the ball around a painful area.

Myofascial and somatoemotional release and craniosacral therapy are techniques that are founded on the notion that the fascia spans the entire body. A scar in the fascia can thus provoke pain elsewhere in the body. Craniosacral therapy is based on the idea that the cranial sutures are capable of movement and that spinal fluid has a rhythm of its own that can be felt by the experienced therapist when palpating the cranial sutures. Somatoemotional release is a technique that regresses patients to what is thought to be their initial trauma. Having the patient relive the trauma is considered therapeutic. We found only one study (39) in the peer-reviewed literature on these techniques. This study compared a myofascial technique with a conventional technique and found the conventional technique to be superior. At best these techniques can be considered quackery that may provide a relaxation response; at worst they make the patient more dependent and disabled. Somatoemotional techniques in chronic pain patients should be avoided. Tinkering by a physical therapist with a patient's emotional past is dangerous unless the physical therapist is also a licensed psychologist or psychiatrist.

Electrotherapy, Ice, and Heat

Physical therapy with electrotherapy, ice, and heat is summarized Table 39.1.

Ergonomics

A job description, as detailed as possible, should be obtained if return to work is a goal. Components of the job description can be practiced with the physical therapist and at home. Ergonomics is concerned with ensuring that the work place is so designed that work-induced injuries and aggravation of existing impairments are prevented and safety is ensured (61). Nonneutral postures, forceful exertions, constrained or static postures, repetitive work, use of pinch grip, work over shoulder height, prolonged periods of time with the trunk inclined forward, heavy lifting, twisting while lifting, and whole-body and segmentally applied vibration are risk factors for work-related musculoskeletal disorders (62). Common ergonomic instruction during physical therapy concerns itself with education of the patient on manual handling and lifting, optimal seated postures and activities, and the relationship of the seat to the work bench or desk. The patient is

Table 39.1. Modalities' Mechanism of Action in Treatment of Pain

Type of Modality	Acute Pain	Chronic Pain
Heat (self-apply)		
Hot packs	↑ Neuronal activity of spindle secondary endings (40)	Large A fiber input to dorsal horn
Electric heating pads	↓ Muscle spasm (41)	as pain gating mechanism (42)
Paraffin baths		
Infrared lamp		
Heat (P.T. apply)		
Ultrasound	↑ Vasodilation (ischemic pain) (43)	↑ Sedation, relaxation (44)
	Restores tissue regeneration (45)	↑ Edema (46)
Microwave diathermy	↑ Pain threshold (47)	
Shortwave diathermy	↑ Collagen distensability (48)	
Hydrotherapy	Debridement (49)	Sedation (44)
	Tissue regeneration (49)	
Cold (self-apply)		
Ice massage	↑ Large A fiber input (42)	↑ Coping with pain (50)
Brief intense icing	↓ Swelling (51)	
Prolonged ice pack	↓ C fiber conduction velocity (52)	
Prolonged cold pack		
Cold (P.T. apply)		
Vapocoolant spray	Counterirritation (53)	
	↓ C fiber conduction velocity (52)	
	↑ Anxiety for some (54)	
Electrical stimulation		
TENS (self-apply)	↑ Large A fiber input; restores inhibitory input to dorsal horn (55)	Same as for acute pain
P.T. apply		
Interferential stimulation	Deeper heating of tissues (56)	Same as for acute pain
	Tissue regeneration (57)	
High-volt galvanic current	↑ Large A-fiber input for gating pain (57)	
Electroacuscope	Tissue regeneration (58)	
Functional Electrical Stimulation	Stimulation of muscle contraction (59)	Same as for acute pain
Biofeedback (self and P.T. apply)	Muscle relaxation (60)	Same as for acute pain

P.T., Physical therapist.

taught about taking "stretch breaks" during work or alternating job components.

At the end of treatment a functional capacity evaluation should be performed and matched with the job description. Recommendations for return to work are based on this evaluation. Changes in the job that would enable the patient to return to work may be suggested. If possible, a work site analysis should be performed to help identify risks to the patient, and to suggest changes into the work environment to accommodate the patient. Three major classes of risk factors can be identified: (*a*) the force exerted on the job, (b) the postures of the arms and trunk, and (*c*) the time elements of the job (frequency and duration of activities) (62). For return to work, a light-duty job is usually recommended and/or gradual increase in the hours worked per day. In work hardening and some pain programs patients participate 8 hours per day. After discharge from these programs a full-time return to work is appropriate. For more detailed descriptions of job evaluations see Rodgers (63, 64).

SUMMARY

Evaluation and treatment of the chronic pain patient is a difficult task that is best performed in an interdisciplinary team. In the absence of such a team close cooperation between the referring physician and the physical therapist as well as the psychologist can be helpful in guiding patients to a more functional life with significantly reduced disability.

References

1. Jette A. Physical disablement concepts for physical therapy research and practice. Phys Ther 1994;74:380–386.
2. Michel T H. Evaluation of chronic pain patients. In: Wittink H, Michel T H, eds. Chronic pain management for physical therapists. Boston: Butterworth-Heinemann, 1997;57–93.
3. Quebec Task Force on Spinal Disorders. Scientific approach to the assessment and management of activity related spinal disorders: a monograph for clinicians. Spine 1987;12 (Suppl):S8–S39.
4. Melzack R. The McGill Pain Questionnaire: major properties and scoring methods. Pain 1975;9:275–277.
5. Roland M, Morris R. A study of the natural history of back pain: 1. The development of a reliable and sensitive measure of disability in low back pain. Spine 1983;8:141.
6. Harding V R, Williams A C, Richardson P H, et al. The development of a battery of measures for assessing physical functioning of chronic pain patients. Pain 1994;25:367–375.
7. Astrand P O, Rodahl K. Textbook of work physiology, physiological bases of exercise. 3rd ed. New York: McGraw-Hill, 1986.
8. Newton M, Waddell G. Trunk strength testing with iso-machines: 1. Review of a decade of scientific evidence. Spine 1993;13: 801–811
9. Waddell G, Newton M, Henderson I, et al. A fear avoidance beliefs questionnaire and the role of fear avoidance beliefs in chronic low back pain and disability. Pain 1993;52:157.
10. Vlayen J W S, Kole-Snijders A M J, Boeren R G B, et al. Fear of movement/(re)injury in chronic low back pain and its relation to behavioral performance. Pain 1995; 62:363.
11. Fordyce W, McMahon R, Rainwater G, et al. Pain complaint-exercise performance relationship in chronic pain. Pain 1981;10:311–321.
12. Wittink H, Michel T H, Cohen L J, Fishman S. Physical therapy treatment. In: Wittink H, Michel T H, eds. Chronic pain management for physical therapists. Boston: Butterworth-Heinemann 1997;119–157.
13. Shutty M S, DeGood D E, Tuttle D H. Chronic pain patient's beliefs about their pain and treatment outcomes. Arch Phys Med Rehabil 1990;71:128.
14. Gatchel R J. Occupational low back disability: why function needs to "drive" the rehabilitation process. Am Pain Soc J 1994;3:107–110.
15. Catchlove R, Cohen K. Effects of a directive return to work approach in the treatment of worker's compensation patients with chronic pain. Pain 1982;14:181.
16. Fordyce W E. Operant conditioning: an approach to chronic pain. In: Jacox A, ed. Pain source book for nurses and other health professionals. Boston: Little Brown, 1977;275–284.
17. Dolce J J, Crocker M F, Moletteire C, Doleys D M. Exercise quotas and anticipatory concern and self efficacy expectancies in chronic pain: a preliminary report. Pain 1986;24:365.
18. Geiger G, Todd D D, Clark H B, et al. The effects of feedback and contingent reinforcement on the exercise behavior of chronic pain patients. Pain 1992;49:179–185.
19. Linton S. The relationship between activity and chronic pain. Pain 1985;21:289–294.
20. Rainville J, Ahern D, Phalen L, et al. The association of pain with physical activities in chronic low back pain. Spine 1992;17:1060–64.
21. Lundeberg T. Pain physiology and principles of treatment. Scand J Rehab Med 1995;32(Suppl):13–41.
22. Janda V. Muscle weakness and inhibition (pseudoparesis) in back syndromes. In: Grieve G, ed. Modern manual therapy of the vertebral column. Edinburgh: Churchill-Livingstone, 1986.
23. Janda V. Muscles and cervicogenic pain syndromes. In: Grant R, ed. Clinics in physical therapy of the cervical and thoracic spine. New York: Churchill-Livingstone, 1988;152.
24. Berg H, Berggren G, Tesch P. Dynamic neck strengthening effect on pain and function. Arch Phys Med Rehabil 1994;75:661
25. Highland T R, Dreisinger T E, Vie L L, Russell G S. Changes in isometric strength and ROM of the isolated cervical spine after eight weeks of clinical rehabilitation. Spine 1992;17:S77.
26. Jorgensen K, Nicolaisen T. Trunk extensor endurance: determination and realtion to low back trouble. Ergonomics 1987;30:259.
27. Roy S H, DeLuca C J, Casavant D A. Lumbar muscle fatigue and chronic lower back pain. Spine 1989;14:992.
28. Andersson G, Bogduk N, DeLuca C, et al. Muscle. In: Frymoyer J W, Gordon S L, eds. New perspectives on low back pain. Park Ridge, IL:American Academy of Orthopaedic Surgeons 1989;14.
29. Frank C, Akesow W H, Woo S L Y, et al. Physiology and therapeutic value of passive joint motion. Clin Orthop 1984;185:113–125.
30. Twomey L. A rationale for the treatment of back pain and joint pain by manual therapy. Phys Ther 1992;72:12.
31. Gurevich M, Kohn P, Davis C. Exercise induced analgesia and the role of reactivity in pain sensitivity. J Sports Med 1994;12:549–559.
32. Droste C, Greenlee M, Schreck M, Roskamm H. Experimental pain thresholds and plasma beta endorphin levels during exercise. Med Sci Sports Exerc 1991;23:334–342.
33. Thoren P, Floras J, Hoffman P, Seals D. Endorphins and exercise: physiological mechanisms and clinical implications. Med Sci Sports Exerc 1990;22:417–428.
34. Kniffki K, Mense S, Schmidt R. Muscle receptors with fine afferent fibers which may evoke circulatory reflexes. Circ Res 1981;48(Suppl 1):125–131.
35. North T C, McCullagh P, Tran Z V. Effect of exercise on depression. Exerc Sports Sci Rev 1990;18:379–415.
36. Crews D J Landers D M. A meta-analytic review of aerobic fitness and reactivity to psychosocial stressors. Med Sci Sports Exerc 1987;19;S114–S120.
37. Koes B W, Assendelft W J J, van der Heijden G J M G, Bouter L M. Spinal mobilization and manipulation for low-back pain: an updated systematic review of randomized clinical trials. In: Tulder M W, Koes B W, Bouter L M, eds. Low back pain in primary care. Amsterdam: Faculteit der Geneeskunde VU, EMGO Instituut, 1996;149–171.

38. Travell J G, Simons D G. Myofascial pain and dysfunction: the trigger point manual, vol 1. Baltimore: Williams & Wilkins, 1983.

39. Hanten W P, Chandler S D. Effects of myofascial release leg pull and sagittal plane isometric contact-relax techniques on passive straight leg raise angle. J Orthop Sports Phys Ther 1994;20:138–144.

40. Mense S. Effects of temperature on the discharges of muscle spindles and tendon organs. Pflugers Arch 1987; 374;159.

41. Low J, Reed M. Electrotherapy explained: principles and practice. Oxford, UK: Butterworth-Heinemann, 1990.

42. Melzack R, Wall P. The challenge of pain. New York: Penguin Books, 1982.

43. Lehmann J F, DeLateur B J. Therapeutic heat. In: Lehmann J F, ed. Therapeutic heat and cold. 4th ed. Baltimore: Williams & Wilkins, 1990;429–432.

44. Warren C G, Lehmann J F, Koblanski J N. Heat and stretch responses: an evaluation using rat tail tendon. Arch Phys Med Rehab 1971;52:465.

45. Dyson M, Suckling J. Stimulation of tissue repair by ultrasound: a survey of mechanisms involved. Physiotherapy 1978;64:105.

46. Lota M J, Darling R C. Change in permeability of the red blood cell membrane in a homogenous ultrasonic field. Arch Phys Med Rehab 1955;36:282.

47. Lehmann J F, Brunner G D, Stow R W. Pain threshold measurements after therapeutic application of ultrasound, microwaves and infrared. Arch Phys Med Rehab 1958:39:560.

48. Gersten J W. Effect of ultrasound on tendon extensibility. Am J Phys Med 1955;34:662.

49. Abraham E. Whirlpool therapy for treatment of soft tissue wounds complicated by extremity fractures. J Trauma 1974;4:222.

50. Kvien T K, Nilson H, Vik P. Education and self-care of patients with low back pain. Scand J Rheum 1981;10:318–320.

51. Matsen F A, Questad, K, Matsen A L. The effect of local cooling on post fracture swelling. Clin Orthop 1975;109:201.

52. Lee J M, Warren M P, Mason S M. Effects of ice on nerve conduction velocity. Physiotherapy 1978;64:2.

53. Gammon G D, Staff I. Studies on the relief of pain by counterirritation. J Clin Invest 1940;20:13.

54. Day M J. Hypersensitive response to ice massage: report of a case. Phys Ther 1974;54:592.

55. Frampton V M. Pain control with the aid of transcutaneous nerve stimulation. Physiotherapy 1982;68:77–81.

56. Savage B. Interferential therapy. London: Faber & Faber, 1984.

57. Low J. Electrotherapeutic modalities. In: Wells P E, Frampton V, Bowsher D, eds. Pain management by physical therapy. 2nd ed. Oxford, UK: Butterworth-Heinemann, 1994;144.

58. Hanen D T, Howson D C. Bibliography on electroanalgesia. Phys Ther 1978;58:1484–1492.

59. Delitto A, Snyder-Mackler L. Two theories of muscle strength augmentation using percutaneous electrical stimulation. Phys Ther 1990;70:158–164.

60. Roberts A H. Biofeedback techniques: their potential for the control of pain. Minn Med 1974;57:167–171.

61. Bullock M I, Bullock-Saxton J E. Low back pain in the work place: an ergonomic approach to control. In: Twomey L E, Taylor J R, eds. Physical therapy of the low back. Clinics in Physical therapy. 2nd ed. New York: Churchill Livingstone, 1994;305–329.

62. Wells R. Task analysis. In: Ranney D, ed. Chronic musculoskeletal injuries in the work place. Philadelphia: Saunders, 1997;41–65.

63. Rodgers S H. Job evaluation in worker fitness determination. Occup Med 1988;3:219–239.

64. Rodgers S H. A functional job analysis technique. Occup Med 1992;7:679–711.

Pain Management Program at New England Medical Center
MODIFIED FUNCTIONAL CAPACITY EVALUATION

Patient name: John Doe
age/gender: 36 year old male
NEMC #:
Diagnosis: neck and back pain
Date of injury: 06/18/95
Insurance Carrier:
Employer: Computerboss
Job title: engineer
Date: 12.16.96 with f/u 02.21.97

AEROBIC CAPACITY; ESTIMATED VO2 MAX PER ASTRAND BICYCLE TEST:
low 12/16/96 /somewhat low/average/**somewhat high 02/21/97** /high for age range and gender.
Norm for age range and gender: 2.8-3.4 L/MIN

PHYSICAL ACTIVITY	PATIENT ABILITY before	after	COMMENTS
sitting	30 min	1.5 hours	patient report
standing	30 min	2 hours	patient report
walking	30 min	2 hours	patient report
stair climbing	able		observed
pushing	6 kg	10 kg	repetitive, observed
pulling	6 kg	16 kg	repetitive, observed
repetitive squatting	able		observed
lifting			
floor to waist	30#	50#	repetitive, observed
waist to overhead			
carry 25 meters	30#	50#	repetitive, observed

PATIENT SELF REPORT MEASURES:

SF-36 scores (scale 0-100, optimal score = 100)

	before	after		before	after
physical functioning	70	83.3	vitality	25	45
role physical	25	50	social functioning	50	75
bodily pain	40	41	role emotional	100	100
general health	62	72	mental health	72	80

Items complete: 97.2%
consistency of responses: 100%

**Pain Management Program at New England Medical Center
page 2: modified functional capacity evaluation**.

Krause-Weber tests: N=normal   G=Good   F=Fair   P=Poor

1. Double straight leg raise. (Lower abdominal strength)
N.............Able to keep back flat while raising the legs for 10 seconds 2/21/97
G.............Able to raise the legs for several seconds, but back curves part way through test 12/96.
F.............Able to raise legs but back curves as soon as legs are raised.
P.............Unable to raise both legs.

2. Partial sit-up. (Upper abominal strength)
N...............Able to raise shoulder blades with knees bent, hands behind neck 2/21, 12/96
G.............. Able to raise shoulder blades with knees bent, hands across chest.
F.............. Able to raise shoulder blades with knees bent, arms out straight.
P.............. Not able to raise shoulder blades with knees bent and feet flat.

3. Upper Back strength.
N...............Able to lift head and trunk with hands behind head for 10 seconds 2/21, 12/96
G...............Able to lift head and trunk with hands behind head momentarily.
F...............Able to lift head and trunk with arms at the sides for 10 seconds.
P...............Unable to lift trunk.

4. Lower Back strength.
N................Able to lift both legs and hold for 10 seconds 2/21
G................Able to lift both legs and hold momentarily 12/96
F................Able to lift one leg at the time and hold for 10 seconds.
P................Unable to lift either leg.

5. Lateral Trunk strength
N................Able to raise upper body completely and hold for 10 seconds.
G................Able to raise upper body with difficulty momentarily.
F................Able to raise upper body only minimally.
P................Unable to raise body off floor.

FUNCTIONAL TESTS:
1. ONE MINUTE STAND UP FROM CHAIR....from 16 to 19.....SIT-STANDS
2.. 30 SECONDS SQUATS......from 11 to 24 ....SQUATS
3. PILE TEST.........50.............POUNDS.........26.........TIME........128............HR
comments:
Full effort

PAIN AND PAIN BEHAVIOR:
None

ASSESSMENT:
Patient is a 36 year old male with the following work capacity:

**Pain Management Program at New England Medical Center
page 3: modified functional capacity evaluation.**

PHYSICAL DEMAND CHARACTERISTICS OF WORK

LEVEL	WEIGHT LIFTED	FREQUENCY OF LIFT	WALKING/ CARRYING	ENERGY	patient ability
SEDENTARY	10# or less	infrequently	none	1.5 mets	YES
SED/LIGHT	15# 10# or less	infrequently frequently	intermitted self pace, no load	2.0 mets	YES
LIGHT	20# 10# or less	infrequently frequently	2.5 mph or slower speed with 10# or less	2.5 mets	YES
LIGHT/ MEDIUM	35# 20# or less	infrequently frequently	3.0 mph or slower speed with 20# or less	3.0 mets	YES
MEDIUM	50# 25# or less	infrequently frequently	3.5 mph or slower speed with 25# or less	3.5 mets	YES
MEDIUM/ HEAVY	75# 35# or less	infrequently frequently	3.5 mph, no load or 115# wheelbarrow 2.5 mph no grade	4.5 mets	MAYBE
HEAVY	100# 50# or less	infrequently frequently	3.5 mph with 50# or less	6.0 mets	NO
VERY HEAVY	>100# 50-100#	infrequently frequently	3.5 mph with 50# or more load	7.5-12.0 mets	NO

RECOMMENDATIONS:

RETURN TO WORK FULL-TIME WITHOUT RESTRICTIONS.

Sincerely,

Harriet Wittink MS PT OCS.

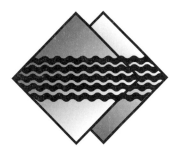

PART VIII

Special Topics

CHAPTER 40

Nonpharmacological Approaches to Pain Relief: Hypnosis, Self-Hypnosis, Placebo Effects[1]

Martin T. Orne and Wayne G. Whitehouse

INTRODUCTION

Recognition of the contribution of distress and suffering in the experience of pain can be traced to ancient times. Over the centuries and across cultures, efforts to relieve disease-related pain, as opposed to that provoked by acute injury, often involved spiritual/psychological interventions, such as the exorcism of evil spirits, letting of presumably virulent bodily fluids, prayer, and attempts to appease the gods, in accordance with extant beliefs (1). The modern scientific zeitgeist that developed in the mid-19th century heralded a shift toward discovering the anatomical structures that give rise to pain as a pure sensory phenomenon, which in turn promised to point the way for developing effective pharmacological and surgical treatments. While the emotional and motivational aspects of pain continued to be appreciated clinically, it took approximately another 100 years before science was prepared to conceptualize and to develop techniques to address the essential multidimensionality of the problem (2–4). Modern day nonpharmacological approaches to pain treatment seek to apply psychological and/or biobehavioral procedures optimally to modify a patient's perceptual, emotional, and evaluative responses to pain. Although these techniques are in many ways derivative of centuries-old antecedents, they have also benefited from significant scientific advances in understanding their mechanisms, specificity, and efficacy. In this chapter, we examine such issues as they pertain to the application of hypnotic and self-hypnotic procedures for pain management.

Consider for a moment being stung by a bee, stubbing a toe, touching a hot utensil, waking up with a toothache, or having stomach cramps after the ingestion of unripe apples. None of these experiences generally tends to be particularly

frightening and all are known to cause pain of relatively brief duration. Since our commonsense view of pain is largely based on experiences such as these, one tends to focus on the sensation aspect of the pain experience, considering it as a simple and direct consequence of a noxious stimulus, closely analogous to other sensory experiences.

The sensory experience of pain, however, is greatly modulated by the circumstances under which it occurs. A bee sting to someone with many allergies can be terrifying, as can a toothache to an individual with an unfortunate dental history. Similarly, pain of no greater intensity than a stomach cramp occurring in a cancer patient may involve a vastly greater amount of suffering. Conversely, as Beecher (5, 6) dramatically demonstrated during World War II, soldiers who had lived through the continuous bombardment of the Anzio beachhead and had received serious shrapnel injuries involving compound fractures required little or no opioid medication when they were brought to the medical aid stations. Instead of showing concern, they tended to be euphoric, since their wound meant that they would soon be evacuated and would no longer have to endure the intense stress of combat. Thus, Beecher distinguished between the suffering and the sensation components of the pain experience and documented the profound effects of the psychological significance attached to the wound and to the degree of suffering associated with it.

In addition to the immediate context, many aspects of the individual's history affect his or her responses to pain. Who has not observed a child fall, look doubtfully at his or her mother, and being met with a reassuring smile, return happily to play, while a friend, having the same kind of fall and seeing the mother's horrified expression, promptly begins to cry and apparently experiences considerable pain. To a large extent a child's definition of what constitutes pain is learned and inevitably influences future pain experiences, leading to

1Adapted from Ng L K Y, Bonica J J, eds. Pain, discomfort, and humanitarian care. New York: Elsevier North Holland, 1980;253–292.

relatively stable differences among various cultural groups and their pain responses.

We have thus far considered acute pain for which the nature of the noxious stimulus is clearly understood. While it is commonly recognized that factors associated with anxiety, motivation, and perception of the meaning of pain affect an individual's experience of pain, most of us are nevertheless astonished when we see a clear-cut example of such psychological factors overriding the neural events that would normally be experienced as severe pain. For instance, it is not uncommon for athletes to suffer injuries during a game without becoming aware of any discomfort; however, once the game is over, they quickly succumb to the exquisite pain of the injury.

HYPNOTICALLY INDUCED ANESTHESIA

The use of hypnosis as the sole anesthetic for major surgery was employed sporadically during the first half of the 19th century but was generally abandoned with the clinical demonstration of the efficacy of ether and chloroform for surgical anesthesia. There continue to be, however, well-authenticated cases in which hypnosis served as the sole anesthetic (7). These range from appendectomies to thyroidectomies, from cesarean sections to open heart surgery (8, 9). Although with today's broad range of safe chemical anesthesias hypnosis is rarely indicated as a surgical anesthetic, the fact that it is possible to carry out major surgery with hypnosis as the only form of anesthesia is perhaps the most dramatic and clear-cut example of the profound effects that psychological factors can exert on the sensation of pain.

The work of Hilgard and Hilgard (9) and their associates, using normal college students and experimental pain of a kind that mimics important aspects of clinical pain, has gone a long way toward addressing some of the questions concerning the factors that affect hypnotic analgesia. Using immersion in ice water, as well as ischemic muscle pain, they have shown the remarkable lawfulness of the effect of hypnotically induced analgesia on subjects' reports of their pain experience. The single most important factor has turned out to be the individual's ability to respond to hypnosis.

Whereas at one time the basis of the hypnotic phenomenon was sought in the special skill of the hypnotist, modern studies have amply documented that it is the skill of individuals to respond that determines whether they are hypnotized. There are wide individual differences in this ability. Thus, following a standardized hypnotic induction procedure, some persons (5% to 10%) respond to very difficult suggestions, including positive and negative hallucinations, whereas those at the other end of the normal distribution (5% to 10%) cannot respond at all, with most falling between the two extremes (10).

The importance of the subject's skill in being hypnotized is illustrated in a study by Hilgard and Morgan (11), who assessed the response to hypnosis using standardized typical hypnotic suggestions other than analgesia and on this basis subdivided subjects into three groups of high, average, and low hynotizability. They then tested the response of subjects in each group to suggestions of hypnotic analgesia during a cold-pressor test. Using subjects' pain ratings as a criterion, they showed that of 15 highly hypnotizable subjects, only 7% failed to reduce pain by less than 10%, while 67% reduced pain by 33% or more. Conversely, with 16 subjects who had little ability to experience hypnosis, 56% showed less than a 10% pain reduction, and only 13% reduced pain by 33% or more (Figure 40.1). The group with medium hypnotic responsiveness fell between these two extremes. Similar findings were reported by Karlin et al. (12), who simultaneously monitored electroencephalographic (EEG) activation and subjective pain reports during hypnotically induced analgesia for cold-pressor stimulation. These investigators observed that following induction of hypnosis, pain ratings and degree of contralateral hemispheric EEG activation during 1-minute periods of immersion of the hand in ice water were significantly less for highly hypnotizable subjects than they were for those of moderate hypnotic talent, although both groups reported decreased pain during hypnosis. However, findings from an investigation of the cold-pressor paradigm with children 6–12 years of age suggest that there may be developmental limitations on the extent to which hypnotizability is a factor in hypnotic analgesia; younger children appear to derive less benefit from analgesia suggestions administered during hypnosis than older children (13). Nevertheless, the ability of the subject to benefit from hypnotic suggestions of analgesia in a laboratory setting seems generally to be related to the ability to respond to other kinds of hypnotic suggestions.

There have been a great many reports about the effective use of hypnosis to suppress clinical pain. An excellent example is its use with burns in children and adults, in whom the repeated trauma associated with the changing of burn dressings and the debridement of wounds could in many instances be greatly negated (14, 15). Similar reports have been made in the control of pain associated with a wide range of other noxious medical procedures (9). In the few studies that formally assessed hypnotizability, the findings parallel those of laboratory investigations; that is, the amount of benefit derived from the use of hypnotic procedures for pain reduction covaried with the patients' ability to experience hypnosis (15–18). Unfortunately, in the vast majority of clinical studies, relatively little systematic information about the patients' hypnotizability is available. Despite this oversight, it is instructive to note that hypnotic techniques appear to enjoy a remarkably high degree of success in suppressing pain in a dental context (19). Clearly, given what is known about the distribution of hypnotizability in the general population, factors other than hypnosis must also be playing a role in these situations. Next we consider some of the mechanisms that may be involved.

PAIN REDUCERS

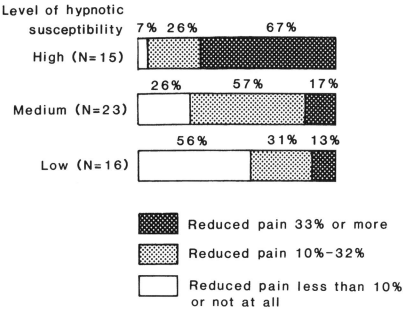

Figure 40.1. Reduction of pain through hypnotically suggested analgesia as related to susceptibility to hypnosis. (Reprinted with permission from Hilgard E R, Morgan A H. Heart rate and blood pressure in the study of laboratory pain in man under normal conditions and as influenced by hypnosis. Acta Neurobiol Exp 1975;35:741–759.)

HYPNOTIZABILITY, THE PLACEBO RESPONSE, AND PAIN RELIEF THROUGH SUGGESTION

One tends to think of the placebo response as a manifestation of the same psychological processes that account for hypnosis. Elsewhere we have reported in-depth findings that challenge this assumption (20, 21). We outline the relevant aspects of this rather complex study here because it addresses some basic questions about the nature of hypnotic analgesia.

The response to suggestions of anesthesia following an induction procedure was compared between two groups of subjects, 12 highly hypnotizable persons and 12 subjects who had repeatedly failed to respond to hypnosis. One of the problems with such a comparison, however, is that the unhypnotizable group not only fail to enter hypnosis but also do not expect hypnosis to help them, whereas those who are able to enter deep hypnosis have every reason to believe that the technique should help them tolerate pain. Since our interest was to compare the effect of hypnosis, we wanted both groups to have the expectation that this method would help them. For this reason the unhypnotizable subjects participated in yet another hypnotic induction session with a different investigator, which was carefully designed to use elaborate relaxation procedures over a long period without any hypnotic suggestions being given, since these subjects would almost certainly have failed to respond to any of these.

After a procedure lasting some 50 minutes, which induced profound relaxation—a phenomenon that is often associated with but is not identical to hypnosis—another lengthy tech-

nique was used to induce glove anesthesia of the right hand. Without asking the subject to comment on the anesthesia, he or she was asked to tolerate a mild electric shock, which was administered to both the right and left hands. The subject was subsequently awakened with instructions to have lost track of time but otherwise to recall everything that had happened. (Again, even unhypnotizable individuals become unaware of the passage of time during a lengthy procedure of this kind.)

When asked, all of the subjects indicated that much to their surprise, this time the hypnotic procedure had been effective and that there was indeed a modest but striking difference in the electric shock between the right and left hand. They typically expressed considerable satisfaction that they had finally been able to achieve a hypnotic experience and eagerly looked forward to participating in further studies. The manner in which this result was achieved, however, had little to do with hypnosis. When the experimenter tested the right hand, he simply decreased the amount of current applied to the hand without, of course, informing the subject. The manner in which the testing was presented to subjects conveyed that the experimenter merely wanted to assess their response, and the investigator indicated that he too was pleased that the subject had been able to have the experience. Carefully carried out, the manipulation was extremely plausible and resulted in a group of subjects still unable to respond to hypnosis but sharing the conviction of the hypnotized group that they would benefit from hypnosis when attempting to control pain.

All subjects subsequently came to the laboratory and participated in an ischemic pain procedure, which involved applying a blood pressure cuff at 200 mm Hg to their arm and then asking that they pump water from one flask to another by repeatedly squeezing a rubber bulb. This task becomes exceedingly painful as the amount of ischemia mounts. Subjects are asked to indicate pain threshold but also to continue pumping as long as possible. Both the time blood flow is occluded and the amount of work performed have been shown by Dorpat and Holmes (22) and Lasagna et al. (23) to be systematically related to pain threshold.

The experimenter was not told which subjects were able to enter hypnosis. After an initial baseline session, subjects were asked to return for a second session that would involve hypnosis. During that session, hypnosis was induced by the same relaxation procedure mentioned earlier, and the experimenter was careful to avoid any test of hypnotic responsiveness that would indicate whether the subject was in fact hypnotizable. He then suggested analgesia of the hand and arm and repeated the same test. Again, pain threshold and tolerance were assessed.

Finally, the subjects were asked to come for yet a third session in which it was explained to them that a powerful analgesic would be employed to assess how long and how much water they could pump if the pain was effectively controlled and the only limiting factor was the amount of anaerobic energy in the muscle. Subjects were given a pill, and about 20 minutes later the ischemic muscle test was repeated. (Although all subjects received placebo, all members of the laboratory other than the director believed that a double-blind comparison was being carried out between propoxyphene hydrochloride (Darvon) and a placebo. Thus the placebo was given with conviction by the investigator, while we had the benefit of having all subjects in the placebo treatment.)

Figure 40.2 summarizes the basic findings for pain thresholds and pain tolerance across all three sessions. It should be noted first that the level of response to placebo in session 3 was virtually the same for the highly hypnotizable group as for the unhypnotizable group. There is no meaningful difference in the level of placebo response between these two groups. Certainly this speaks against the notion that hypnotizability is related to the placebo response.

Looking at the placebo response of the unhypnotizable group, it is interesting that the magnitude of response overall is virtually the same as that to hypnosis. Indeed, there is a correlation of .76 between the amount of pain relief that the unhypnotizable subject obtains from hypnosis and from placebo. However, if one examines the hypnotizable group, it is obvious that the amount of benefit they derive from hypnosis is vastly greater than the amount of benefit they derive from placebo. Of course, it might be possible for hypnosis to be more effective, and still a high correlation between the response to hypnosis and placebo in highly hypnotizable subjects could exist. This is not the case, however; within this group the relation of pain relief from hypnosis and that from placebo is .06.

Figure 40.2 shows that the hypnotizable group derived significantly more benefit from hypnosis than did the unhypnotizable group, but their response to placebo was no different from that of the unhypnotizable group. Thus, the dramatic effect of hypnosis on pain cannot be explained solely in terms of subjects' expectations but rather again turns out to be directly related to hypnotizability. Nonetheless, the unhypnotizable subject also derives considerable benefit from hypnosis. Although it is less than the amount of benefit seen in the hypnotizable person, the effect is still significant. Since this effect is highly correlated with the amount of relief obtained by placebo, we have conceptualized it as a placebo effect of the hypnotic procedure. For some purposes it is useful to think of it in this fashion; however, in the context of the present discussion it points up important effects of the hypnotic induction procedure that occur even if the subject fails to be hypnotized. It appears to us that these effects are worth studying in their own right and may in many instances be extremely important clinically.

THE PLACEBO RESPONSE

In many ways the placebo has the properties of an active drug. More than 40 years ago, Gruber (24) not only showed that placebo was effective in the treatment of headaches but demonstrated that the "dosage" was important and that two placebo pills were almost twice as effective as one. Similarly, Rickels et al. (25) showed that when patients suffering from anxiety consulted a medical practitioner, they obtained considerable relief from placebo, and again the administration of four placebos a day was considerably more effective than one per day.

These and other studies emphasize that the effectiveness of placebo depends on the conviction with which it is administered, the kind of expectations that the therapist conveys when placebo is administered, and the congruence of such expectations with the patient's own attitudes and beliefs. For example, in the study by Rickels et al. (25), patients who were seeking relief in the form of medicine tended to be helped greatly by placebo, whereas those who had sought psychiatric help did not show any improvement with placebo.

The expectancies that the therapist communicates when administering the placebo may actually override a potent drug effect. For example, Fisher (26) administered 10 mg of the stimulant D-amphetamine (Dexedrine) to volunteers who were to help him assess the effectiveness of a new sleeping pill. Under such circumstances, d-amphetamine did not interfere with sleep. Again, Lyerly et al. (27) showed that sleeping medication administered as a new form of stimulant did not cause drowsiness nor, as Fisher had already shown, did amphetamines administered as sedatives cause subjective arousal.

A review (28) of six double-blind studies determined that the index of efficiency of placebo compared with a standard dose of a potent analgesic such as morphine was .56, indicating that placebo is 56% as effective as morphine. Surprisingly, when the index of placebo efficiency was compared

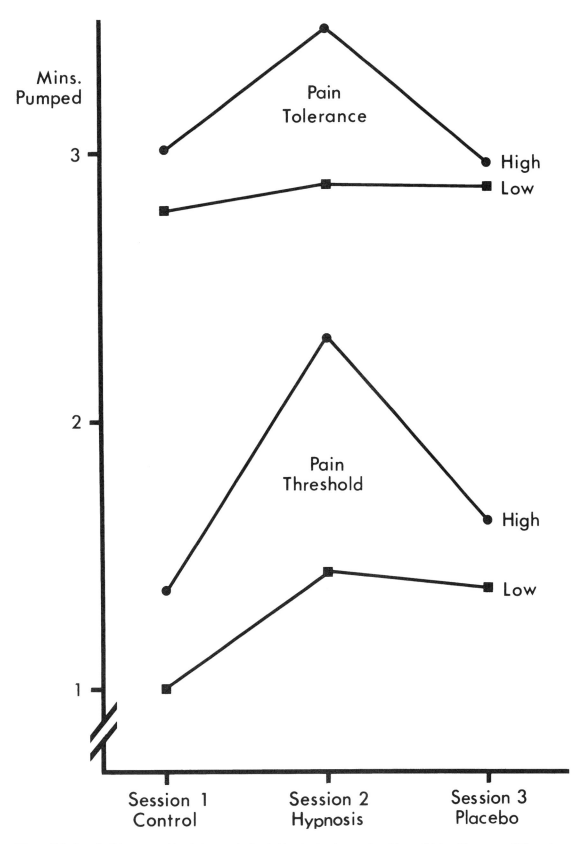

Figure 40.2. Length of time pumped in relation to pain threshold and pain tolerance for subjects of high and low susceptibility to hypnosis during control, hypnotic analgesia, and placebo ischemic muscle pain performance. (Reprinted with permission from McGlashan T H, Evans F J, Orne M T. The nature of hypnotic analgesia and placebo response to experimental pain. Psychosomat Med 1969;31:227–246.)

with aspirin in nine studies, it proved to be .54. Again, the efficiency of placebo when compared with an intermediate-strength analgesic such as propoxyphene hydrochloride or codeine was found to be .56.

The effectiveness of placebo compared with a standard dose of a specific analgesic drug administered in a double-blind study seems to be constant, indicating that placebo is powerful indeed when it is given with morphine but it is pro-portionately less powerful when it is given with aspirin. Thus, it appears that the doctor's belief about the effectiveness of the active drug determines the effectiveness of the placebo.

Although much has been written about placebo effects and their many fascinating puzzles, such as why red placebos are more effective than blue ones, a limited amount of research has been carried out to understand the mechanisms that determine how a placebo works. As we have seen, the belief of the inves-tigator or doctor about the effectiveness of the drug is a criti-cal determinant of the level of placebo response. In addition, however, early work by Beecher (5) demonstrated that placebo is vastly more effective on the battlefield than in a civilian con-text. Apparently, the higher the patient's level of anxiety, the more effective the placebo. Similarly, in another study, Beecher (29) showed that when postoperative wound pain was at its greatest, morphine relieved 52% of the patients, whereas placebo relieved the pain of 40% of the same patients. Later, when the pain was much less with these patients, the same standard dose of morphine relieved the pain of 89% of the patients, whereas placebo was effective with only 26%.

Although the concept of placebo was designed as a control for nonspecific factors in treatment, an important area of research involves the elucidation of specific mechanisms, such as the level of state anxiety, that are responsible for what have heretofore been considered general nonspecific effects. As such mechanisms become recognized and better understood, it will be possible to use this information to design more power-ful ways of modifying pain in specific treatment programs.

THE EFFECT OF HYPNOSIS VERSUS THE EFFECT OF HYPNOTIC INDUCTION

As was pointed out earlier, people vary in hypnotizability. This ability is a generally stable trait of the individual, and while motivational factors may impede a person's ability to enter hypnosis, for the most part, provided he or she is rea-sonably cooperative and has a moderately good relationship with the hypnotist, motivation is not particularly important.

Clinically, the use of hypnosis is not limited to those who are profoundly responsive but may be employed with the vast majority of persons, even those who have a minimal skill for entering hypnosis and respond only by relaxation. As long as suggestions that are too difficult for the patient to carry out are avoided, he or she may feel adequately responsive to hyp-nosis. It is useful, however, to distinguish between the benefit the subject derives from actual hypnosis and benefits that accrue from other nonspecific effects of hypnosis. Again, like

the study of placebo effects, it is important to begin to isolate some of the components that can be specified and that will cause a hypnotic induction procedure to help even patients who are not actually hypnotizable.

SOME EXAMPLES OF THE EFFECT OF THE HYPNOTIC INDUCTION IN THE CLINICAL CONTEXT

The use of a hypnotic procedure alters many aspects of the doctor-patient relationship. Furthermore, by asking the patient to attend to some ideas and to ignore others, important cogni-tive changes may be brought about. Not only can the hypnotic induction procedure affect the patient directly, but it may also radically change the way the doctor behaves, which in turn can have profound effects on what the patient experiences.

Consider the effect of hypnosis during a dental procedure with an anxious patient. Instead of minimizing the patient's fears and treating him or her with annoyance, the dentist who elects to use hypnosis will show concern about the patient's comfort, establish rapport, and then carefully induce hypno-sis, even though this may not be his or her normal chairside behavior. Throughout the hypnotic session, the dentist main-tains an almost continuous stream of suggestions and remains very sensitive to the patient's reactions. While he or she may have given suggestions of analgesia, the dentist schooled in the use of hypnosis will promptly terminate any activity that brings about even minor evidence of discomfort, renewing suggestions of relaxation and proceeding subsequently only with great caution, often augmenting hypnotic analgesia with a suitable amount of local anesthetic.

From the patient's point of view, even if he or she is rela-tively unhypnotizable, the hypnotic situation is radically dif-ferent from the typical dental encounter. Instead of feeling that the dentist wants urgently to get on with the technical aspects of the procedure, the patient perceives a heightened sense of concern for his or her own level of comfort. Instead of being largely ignored, with the dentist either quietly work-ing or maintaining a conversation with the assistant, there is a continuous show of interest on the part of the dentist and an obvious sensitivity to even slight evidence of discomfort. It is hardly surprising that under such circumstances patients become more relaxed and trusting, and exhibit an increased ability to tolerate discomfort. These effects have little to do with the state of hypnosis; rather, they may be a function of the patient's increased feeling of control and safety.

Several studies have shown that giving subjects control over the timing of painful stimuli (30), instilling the belief that they can control noxious events (31–33), or even instill-ing only the belief that they can terminate aversive stimuli (34) increases their tolerance for discomfort and decreases their physiological reactivity. Analogously, it is well known that procedures that give patients the feeling of control in a dental context can in and of themselves bring about a marked rise in pain threshold. Similarly, the patient comes to believe that the dentist will not inflict serious pain, another factor that increases pain tolerance, since a small amount of pain no longer serves to signal the inevitable advent of more severe pain. The reduction of anxiety associated with the total procedure also decreases the sensitivity to pain. Simply being talked through a dental procedure is infinitely more reassuring than being left to one's own devices, which permits fears and fantasies to multiply. Both the direct and indirect effects discussed here that follow from the use of hypnotic procedures have little to do with the patient's entering hypnosis. Nonetheless, they profoundly alter the patient's experience. This may well account for the high success rate reported for hypnosis in dentistry, although only 15% to 20% of patients are able to achieve a moderately profound hypnotic response that would lead to dental analgesia in the sense of a hypnotically suggested negative hallucination for pain.

HYPNOSIS IN THE TREATMENT OF CANCER PAIN

Although it is estimated that 38 to 70% of patients with advanced cancer have severe pain (35, 36), the profound and progressive sense of isolation, helplessness, and despair as family, friends, and caretakers gradually withdraw, all focus the patient on his or her body and accentuate the severity of pain. In turn, the pain prevents the patient from enjoying some of the few pleasures that remain, and at times the pain itself and behavior related to pain become the principal means of communication with others.

Orne has had the opportunity to treat a number of patients with terminal cancer, and certainly those who are fortunate enough to have the skill of experiencing deep hypnosis can derive a remarkable degree of relief. However, we have become increasingly aware of the complex and important role that hypnotic induction and its consequences—not related to the presence of hypnosis—can sometimes play in reversing what had appeared to be a progressive worsening of the patient's overall condition. Thus, the induction of hypnosis and/or training in self-hypnosis provide the opportunity to offer relief in a manner that entails the patient's active participation.

In the context of a structured treatment program, those around the patient can be assigned responsibility to help him or her to better achieve the skill of pain control. For the first time in a long while, it may become possible for the patient to accomplish something of personal importance and to focus on one or another aspect of improvement, be it increased pain tolerance, the decrease of nausea, a modest weight gain, or the ability to read a newspaper. The specifics of the accomplishment matter little; the fact that progress can be perceived matters a great deal. Some sign of progress, however slight, is important, not only for the patient but at times even more so to help his or her caregivers maintain their ability to interact meaningfully and to focus on the positive things that can be shared rather than solely the pain and suffering, which may be equally unbearable to all concerned.

Much has been written about the importance of factors such as these in making what remains of life livable and meaningful, but it has rarely been emphasized how the use of the hypnotic situation can provide the context that for many patients permits the kind of changes we have tried to sketch in this chapter. While the patient who is able to experience hypnosis can reap the benefits of suggested analgesia as well as the benefits that follow from the induction procedure, many of the changes that hypnotic techniques, particularly the use of self-hypnosis, can bring about in the patient's perception of the situation and interaction with others have little or nothing to do with the ability to enter hypnosis. On the contrary, they reflect the response on the part of the doctor, who suddenly feels there is something that can be offered to the patient to bring about relief; on the part of the family, who suddenly may be encouraged to share positive experiences with the patient and find the interaction less enervating; and on the part of the patient, who begins again to feel able to control some aspects of his or her experience.

In discussing the effect of hypnosis on cancer pain, we have touched on a kind of pain that involves chronicity as well as the other psychobiological effects of cancer, which others have discussed in more detail elsewhere (35, 37). The treatment of chronic pain inevitably involves dealing with complex psychosocial aspects, partly caused by the pain and partly maximizing the pain and making it difficult for the patient to obtain relief except through drugs that numb consciousness. When one considers the treatment of chronic pain, it becomes particularly useful to consider a variety of approaches to pain.

HYPNOSIS IN THE TREATMENT OF PAIN ASSOCIATED WITH SICKLE CELL DISEASE

Issues quite similar to those in the management of chronic malignant pain also apply to progressive diseases in which pain is a salient, unpredictable, and recurrent symptom. An example of a disorder with these features is sickle cell disease, which is genetically transmitted and affects primarily individuals of African heritage. Persons with this disease have red blood cells that are susceptible to periodic deformation called sickling. When this occurs, the sickle cells occlude blood vessels and capillaries, promoting sudden episodes of ischemic pain, organ failure, and other serious health problems (38, 39). In many patients symptoms develop in early childhood and tend to increase in severity and frequency with age (40). Mild to moderate pain episodes are typically managed at home with nonopioid analgesics; more severe crises may require emergency room treatment, often consisting of hydration and opioids, with occasional blood transfusions for cases involving other serious medical complications (41, 42).

Work by our laboratory suggests that children and adolescents with frequent sickle cell pain may be behaviorally disadvantaged in that they restrict their activities and are absent from school on 30% of the days they have pain (43). We have also found that the pain disturbs their sleep, which can exacerbate problems with daytime functioning and school attendance (44). Because there is no way to anticipate the painful episodes, persons with sickle cell disease must learn to cope with and control their pain in such a way that the pain itself, as well as the methods for its control, interfere as little as possible with their everyday activities and quality of life.

Training in self-hypnosis appears to be a particularly useful adjunct to standard medical treatments for the management of sickle cell-related pain (45). Our laboratory's experience with this approach has attempted to exploit both the specific (i.e., related to the ability to enter hypnosis) and nonspecific components (i.e., placebo effects of hypnotic induction, regular group training sessions, supportive involvement of family and friends) of a programmatic cognitive-behavioral intervention centered on self-hypnosis. The principal objective was to teach child, adolescent, and adult patients the requisite skills to induce a condition of self-hypnosis that would enable them to reduce their pain experiences when they occurred. A secondary yet critical aspect of the program was to provide a legitimizing, conducive, and motivating context to ensure that patients would practice these skills and use them as needed. By sharing their concerns and experiences with self-hypnosis in regular group training sessions, patients were able to allay any fears, develop effective therapeutic metaphors for their self-hypnosis exercises, forge a group identity with which to confront their common medical problem, and reinforce the desire to take personal control over their pain.

Compared with a 4-month baseline period during which patients relied only on conventional medical management of sickle cell pain, the subsequent 18 months, during which the cognitive-behavioral and self-hypnosis program was in effect, were associated with a significant reduction in pain days (Fig. 40.3). Both the proportion of bad sleep nights and use of opioid medications also decreased significantly during the self-hypnosis treatment phase. However, patients continued to report disturbed sleep and to require medications on days during which they did have pain. That is, although there was less pain overall during the self-hypnosis treatment phase, that which did occur tended to be the more severe episodes, both in intensity and duration. Such a finding is consistent with expectations that a cognitive-behavioral intervention should be better suited to alleviating less severe rather than severe bouts of pain.

Just as with the design of interventions for the relief of chronic pain, the use of hypnotic procedures for the treatment of recurrent episodic pain requires a great deal of attention, not only to training of the appropriate hypnotic, imaginal, and relaxation skills, but most important, to contextual factors that ultimately determine the extent to which patients can integrate these skills into their daily lives. The ability to derive benefit from self-hypnosis for pain management is not the exclusive province of a handful of patients who happen to possess considerable hypnotic talent. Rather, the very multidimensionality of the pain experience virtually assures that given an appropriately supportive context, even minimally hypnotizable patients who have an earnest desire to improve their quality of life can be expected to realize tangible benefits from regularly carrying out their self-hypnosis treatment exercises. While the basis for improvement in many patients may reside in nonspecific—including placebo—aspects of treatment, the doctor should be concerned foremost with developing the most effective care delivery program available for each patient, regardless of the specific mechanisms that contribute to treatment outcome.

EFFECTIVE TREATMENT OF CHRONIC PAIN: A MANDATE FOR FURTHER RESEARCH

Perhaps because most of us are fortunate enough that our personal experiences have included only acute pain, we tend to have little understanding of the nature of chronic pain. Severe chronic pain is not so common as severe acute pain and is very different from a continuing acute pain. Behavior modification and cognitive-behavioral interventions, for example, have little role in the treatment of acute pain but are effective in the treatment of chronic pain, particularly to alter pain-related behavior that prevents the patient from undertaking activities that would in themselves help ameliorate suffering (46, 47).

It is useful to distinguish between the treatment of pain associated with end-stage malignant disease and other forms of chronic pain. The cancer patient suffers not only from physical pain but also from a debilitating illness that progressively diminishes the ability to function, making him or her acutely aware of the inevitable outcome. Although severe pain as such is a problem in many patients, it can generally be controlled by analgesic drugs, which should not be withheld because of an undue fear of addicting a dying patient. By the same token, psychological factors play a major role in the patient's ability to tolerate growing incapacity, to withstand the side effects of cancer treatment, and to be able to live his or her remaining days with a sense of dignity and a modicum of satisfaction.

The treatment of chronic pain associated with non-life-threatening illnesses is complicated by the fact that many pain-killing drugs are addictive. For example, the doctor treating a condition such as shingles, which may involve extreme pain over long periods, knows the patient is suffering and yet must be rightfully concerned about the addictive potential of opioid drugs that would provide true relief. The very considerable number of persons who suffer from severe chronic pain find their lives profoundly affected by the fact that they are unable to obtain safe and enduring relief. These patients suffer all the more because they know that there are drugs that can provide virtually instant relief but that must be withheld as soon as it becomes clear that the problem is chronic. By that time, the patient's course is likely to be already complicated by varying degrees of addiction, making it even more difficult for the doctor to assess the nature of the chronic pain. Too often the doctor, concerned with addiction, further complicates the patient's treatment by a judgmental attitude, in effect blaming the patient for seeking relief from suffering.

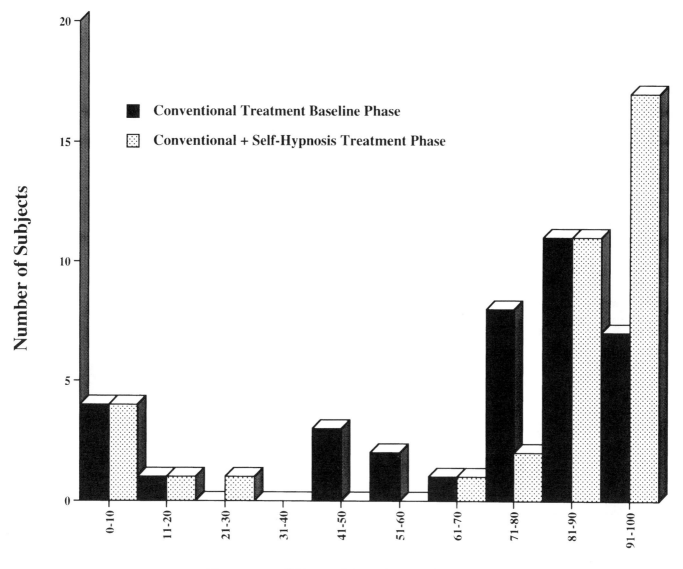

Percent of Days Free from SCD Pain

Figure 40.3   Relative frequency distributions of median percent of sickle cell-related pain-free days during 4-month baseline and 18-month self-hypnosis treatment phases of the investigation. (Reprinted with permission from Dinges D F, Whitehouse W G, Orne E C, et al. Self-hypnosis training as an adjunctive treatment in the management of pain associated with sickle cell disease. Int J Clin Exp Hypn 1997;45:417–432.

While more basic information about the nature of the pain experience and how it may be modified is ultimately relevant to the treatment of all pain, the treatment of chronic pain in particular is an area demanding innovative approaches that must, in the final analysis, be evaluated with the patient population. During the past several years, there has been an increasing amount of research on the neurobiology of pain. However, there has been less scientific progress in understanding the psychological factors that affect pain. Thanks to the evolution of multidisciplinary pain clinics, the importance of psychological factors has been more generally recognized; however, their systematic study has continued to lag. Although it will always be appropriate to support isolated studies to document

the effect of some particularly important aspect of motivation or the examination of some relevant cognitive factors on the pain experience, we need to begin to go about the study of psychological factors affecting the pain experience in a more programmatic and multidisciplinary fashion.

The development of multidisciplinary pain clinics that seek to apply our current knowledge must be matched with the development of multidisciplinary pain research groups, as proposed by Bonica (37), which will seek to increase our understanding of the pain experience. Fortunately, effective laboratory models can be used for systematic exploration of the effect of psychological factors in modifying the pain experience under tightly controlled conditions. Such research groups of course, must have an appreciation of clinical pain and blend a wide variety of skills and techniques—ranging from psychophysical scaling to the use of signal detection techniques and from the assessment of behavior to the study of the experience by means of interviews and psychophysiological measures—in a concerted effort to objectify the pain experience.

Of necessity, much of the research will focus on acute pain. Nonetheless, as has already been pointed out, we must be equally concerned with chronic pain and the psychological concomitants of such pain. Chronic pain cannot be studied entirely in the laboratory context because only a few animal models exist. It must be studied with chronic pain patient volunteers. It is essential for pain research centers to maintain close contact with clinical pain services and doctors who treat chronic pain on a day-to-day basis.

It is difficult to convey the plight of the chronic pain patient. Not surprisingly, a person who is exposed to continual severe pain becomes difficult to be with; the doctor who has been unable to provide relief often seeks to avoid the patient, and those around him or her (made equally uncomfortable by the suffering) may shun the person in pain. Such circumstances, combined with the patient's inability to obtain relief, often lead to suspiciousness and hostility well above the norm, as well as definite signs of depression. This patient group, who have sought and failed to obtain relief from conventional medicine, may prevail upon alternative or complementary medical interventions that have yet to be scientifically accepted (48); worse, they may be victimized by charlatans and quacks.

It is not only possible but essential that the effectiveness of procedures developed for the treatment of chronic pain be scientifically evaluated. Because of the nature of the problems, chronic pain patients given the opportunity of participating in a research study are almost always eager to do so. In providing an opportunity to take part in research on chronic pain, the investigator not only may help assess procedures that could provide enduring relief in an acceptable fashion but also helps the patient, who can identify with the project and feel he or she is working toward a solution, to gain renewed hope of ultimate relief.

SUMMARY

The fact that major surgery can be carried out in suitable patients, with hypnosis as the sole anesthetic, serves to illustrate the power of psychological factors to modify the pain experience. An effort has been made to show that it is possible to identify a number of different psychological mechanisms that alter the experience of pain. Furthermore, it has been suggested that a concerted effort should be made to develop pain research centers to study the psychological factors affecting pain experience. Such centers should concern themselves with the difficult but essential task of developing appropriate measures for pain so that this essentially private experience can be objectified more effectively. Such techniques will facilitate the study of both clinical and laboratory pain. In addition, the programmatic study of chronic pain, recognizing its special features, is particularly important.

As our understanding of pain grows, the links between research focusing on neurobiological mechanisms and research seeking to clarify psychological processes that affect the pain experience are bound to become increasingly strong. While this discussion is at the level of psychological and psychosocial factors, the experience of pain ultimately has a physiological basis. The links that must be formed to understand psychological and neurobiological aspects of pain should lead to important scientific insights as we seek to provide more effective tools to alleviate the suffering of our fellow man.

Acknowledgments

The substantive research on which this chapter is based was supported in part by the following agencies: Grants M H 19156 and M H 44193 from the National Institute of Mental Health, the van Amerigen Foundation, Hasbro Foundation, MBNA America Bank, N.A., Stratford Foundation, Arcadia Foundation, Curry Foundation, The Auxiliary of Pennsylvania Hospital, the Commonwealth of Pennsylvania, and the Institute for Experimental Psychiatry Research Foundation. We are grateful to our colleagues, Emily Carota Orne and David F. Dinges, for their valuable suggestions and thoughtful review of this paper.

References

1. Bonica J J. Pain. New York: Raven Press, 1980.
2. Melzack R. The McGill Pain Questionnaire: major properties and scoring methods. Pain 1965;1:277–299.
3. Melzack R, Wall P D. Pain mechanisms: a new theory. Science 1965;150:971–975.
4. Price D D, Barrell J, Gracely R. A psychophysical analysis of experiential factors that selectively influence the affective dimension of pain. Pain 1980;8:137–149.
5. Beecher H K. Relationship of significance of wound to pain experienced. JAMA 1956;161:1609–1613.
6. Beecher H K. Pain: one mystery solved. Science 1966;151:840–841.
7. Orne M T, Dinges D F. Hypnosis. In: Wall P D, Melzack R, eds. Textbook of pain. 2nd ed. London: Churchill Livingstone, 1989;1021–1031.
8. Finer B. Hypnosis and anesthesia. In: Burrows G D, Dennerstein L, eds. Handbook of hypnosis and psychosomatic medicine. Amsterdam: Elsevier North Holland, 1980.
9. Hilgard E R, Hilgard J R. Hypnosis in the relief of pain. Los Altos, CA: William Kaufmann, 1975.
10. Hilgard E R. Hypnotic Susceptibility. New York: Harcourt Brace & World, 1965.
11. Hilgard E R, Morgan A H. Heart rate and blood pressure in the study of laboratory pain in man under normal conditions and as influenced by hypnosis. Acta Neurobiol Exp 1975;35:741–759.
12. Karlin R A, Morgan D, Goldstein L. Hypnotic analgesia: A preliminary investigation of quantitated hemispheric electroencephalographic and attentional correlates. J Abnorm Psychol 1980;89:591–594.
13. Zeltzer L K, Fanurik D, LeBaron S. The cold pressor pain paradigm in children: Feasibility of an intervention model: 2. Pain 1989;37:305–313.

14. Bernstein N R. Observations on the use of hypnosis with burned children on a pediatric ward. Int J Clin Exp Hypn 1965;13:1–10.
15. Schafer D W. Hypnosis use on a burn unit. Int J Clin Exp Hypn 1975;23:1–14.
16. Hilgard J R, LeBaron S. Relief of anxiety and pain in children and adolescents with cancer: quantitative measures and clinical observations. Int J Clin Exp Hypn 1982;30:417–442.
17. Hilgard J R, LeBaron S. Hypnotherapy of pain in children with cancer. Los Altos, CA: William Kaufman, 1984.
18. VanDyck R, Zitman F G, Linssen A C, Spinhoven P. Autogenic training and future oriented hypnotic imagery in the treatment of tension headache: Outcome and process. Int J Clin Exp Hypn 1991;39:6–23.
19. Barber J. Rapid induction analgesia: a clinical report. Am J Clin Hypnosis 1977;19:138–147.
20. McGlashan T H, Evans F J, Orne M T. The nature of hypnotic analgesia and placebo response to experimental pain. Psychosom Med 1969;31:227–246.
21. Orne M T. Mechanisms of hypnotic pain control. In: Bonica J J, Albe-Fessard D, eds. Advances in pain research and therapy, vol 1. New York: Raven Press, 1976;717–726.
22. Dorpat T L, Holmes T H. Mechanisms of skeletal muscle pain and fatigue. Arch Neurol Psychiatr 1955;74:628–640.
23. Lasagna L, Tetreault L, Fallis N E. Analgesic drugs and experimental ischemic pain. Fed Proc 1962;21:326.
24. Gruber C M. Interpreting medical data. Arch Intern Med 1956;98:767–773.
25. Rickels K, Hesbacher P T, Weise C C, et al. Pills and improvement: a study of placebo response in psychoneurotic outpatients. Psychopharmacologia 1970;16:318–328.
26. Fisher S. Nonspecific factors as determinants of behavioral response to drugs. In: DiMascio A, Shader R I, eds. Clinical handbook of psychopharmacology. New York: Science House, 1970;17–39.
27. Lyerly S B, Ross S, Krugman A D, Clyde D J. Drugs and placebos: the effects of instructions upon performance and mood under amphetamine sulfate and chloral hydrate. J Abnorm Soc Psychol 1964;68:321–327.
28. Evans F J. The placebo control of pain: a paradigm for investigating non-specific effects in psychotherapy. In: Brady J P, Mendels J, Orne M T, Rieger W, eds. Psychiatry: areas of promise and advancement. New York: Spectrum, 1977;129–136.
29. Beecher H K. Evidence for increased effectiveness of placebos with increased stress. Am J Physiol 1956;187:163–169.
30. Averill J R. Personal control over aversive stimuli and its relationship to stress. Psychol Bull 1973;80:286–303.
31. Bowers K. Pain, anxiety and perceived control, J Consult Clin Psychol 1968;32:596–602.
32. Staub E, Tursky B, Schwartz G E. Self-control and predictability: their effects on reactions to aversive stimulation. J Pers Soc Psychol 1971;18:157–162.
33. Glass D C, Singer J E, Leonard H S, et al. Perceived control of aversive stimulation and the reduction of stress responses. J Pers 1973;41:577–595.
34. Lanzetta J, Cartwright-Smith J, Kleck R E. Effects of nonverbal dissimulation on emotional experiencing and autonomic arousal. J Pers Soc Psychol 1976;33:354–370.
35. Bonica J J. Treatment of cancer pain: current status and future needs. In: Fields H L et al., eds. Advances in pain research and therapy, vol 9. New York: Raven Press,,1985;589–616.
36. Foley K M. Pain syndromes in patients with cancer. In: Bonica J J, Ventafridda V, eds. Advances in pain research and therapy, vol 2. New York: Raven Press, 1979.
37. Bonica J J. Pain research and therapy: past and current status and future needs. In: Ng L K, Bonica J J, eds. Pain, discomfort, and humanitarian care. New York: Elsevier North Holland, 1980;1–46.
38. Gil K M. Coping with sickle cell disease. Ann Behav Med 1989;11:49–57.
39. Nagel R L, Fabry M E, Billett H H, Kaul D K. Sickle cell painful crisis: a multifactorial event. Prog Clin Biol Res 1987;240:361–380.
40. Platt O S, Thorington B D, Brambilla D J, et al. Pain in sickle cell disease: rates and risk factors. N Engl J Med 1991;325:11–16.
41. Shapiro B S. The management of pain in sickle cell disease. Pediatr Clin North Am 1989;36:1029–1045.
42. Shapiro B S. Management of painful episodes in sickle cell disease. In: Schechter N L, Berde C B, Yaster M Y, eds. Pain in infants, children, and adolescents. Baltimore: Williams & Wilkins, 1993;385–410.
43. Shapiro B S, Dinges D F, Orne E C, et al. Home management of sickle cell related pain in children and adolescents: natural history and impact on school attendance. Pain 1995;61:139–144.
44. Dinges D F, Shapiro B S, Reilly L B, et al. Sleep/wake dysfunction in children with sickle cell crisis pain. Sleep Res 1990;19:323.
45. Dinges D F, Whitehouse W G, Orne E C, et al. Self-hypnosis training as an adjunctive treatment in the management of pain associated with sickle cell disease. Int J Clin Exp Hypn 1997;45:417–432.
46. Fordyce W E. Learning processes in pain. In: Sternbach R A, ed. The psychology of pain. 2nd ed. New York: Raven Press, 1986;49–65.
47. Turk D C, Meichenbaum D H. A cognitive-behavioural approach to pain management. In: Wall PD, Melzack R, eds. Textbook of pain. 2nd ed. London: Churchill Livingstone, 1989;1001–1009.
48. Eisenberg D M, Kessler R C, Foster C, et al. Unconventional medicine in the United States: prevalence, costs, and patterns of use. N Engl J Med 1993;328:246–252.

CHAPTER 41

Pain Centers: Treatment for Intractable Suffering and Disability Resulting from Chronic Pain

Gerald M. Aronoff

INTRODUCTION

Relief of suffering has been the medical profession's primary objective throughout time. In the past 2 decades, we have seen the proliferation of theoretical concepts designed to help patients suffering from chronic pain and clinicians faced with the treatment of this difficult problem. This discussion concerns chronic nonmalignant pain. When this type of pain is intractable, its causative factors can remain obscure, the time course may be variable, and the symptoms often evade most conventional medical treatment.

Despite therapeutic advances, chronic pain often remains a medical enigma. Most treatment approaches have been based on a dichotomy between physiological and psychological causes. This dualism greatly reduces the treatment available to the patient. It reinforces the tendency to isolate the symptoms from the person in pain and to focus treatment on target organs. Although this dichotomy has not been universally rejected, medical science has made significant contributions to the theory of pain as a multidimensional phenomenon (1).

Increasingly, chronic pain is recognized as a major public health problem afflicting 30% of the U.S. population at an estimated $70 billion a year in medical costs, lost workdays, and compensation payments. The frequency and impact of chronic pain are expected to increase over the next decade as the average age of the work force increases (2).

DEFINING PAIN

For the purpose of this chapter, pain is defined as a complex, personal, subjective, unpleasant sensory and perceptual experience that may or may not be related in any way to an injury, illness, or other bodily trauma. Psychosocial, ethnocultural, motivational, as well as biological, physiological, chemical, and other factors influence it. In managing a patient with intractable chronic pain and the inevitable accompanying suffering, which often leads to chronic debilitation, the pain should be viewed as a form of learned goal-directed behavior and the process itself as a conditioned psychosocioeconomic disorder.

This does not imply that the pain is not real, severe, or debilitating, that the patient need not be treated, or that the patient does not require thorough diagnostic evaluation. However, we often overevaluate and overtreat these patients, who are prime candidates for iatrogenic complications (1).

Pain patients, in their desperate search for the elusive cure, often chase windmills and persuade their doctors to perform a myriad of invasive tests and procedures. Those involved in their treatment must find improved ways to detect this highly susceptible population, establish a therapeutic alliance, and short-circuit their pain careers. Our health care system of finite resources cannot rely solely on the traditional methods of medical and surgical approaches so often used with this population (3).

It is unfortunate that most of the medical educational process deals with chronic pain as if it were simply an extension of acute pain. To superimpose the acute pain model onto the chronic pain patient is a mistake, since they may bear little resemblance to each other. It is inappropriate to apply the same parameters used in evaluating a patient with acute pain to someone who has a complicated chronic pain syndrome (4). Whereas acute pain may be a biologically useful indicator to warn the patient of an underlying problem requiring treatment, chronic pain generally serves no such function. Bonica (5) describes chronic pain as a "malefic force that imposes severe emotional, physical, economic, and social stresses on the patient, on the family and on the society." However, in accordance with the traditional medical model, most treatments are directed at the patient alone and seek to discover and alleviate the source of the presumed nociceptive stimulation. Little or no attention is directed to the overall effect of the condition on the patient's life. Within the constraints of the acute model, patients are initially evaluated conservatively. If the problem is refractory, more aggressive diagnostic evaluations and therapeutic maneuvers are suggested, often including opioids, nerve blocks, implanted stimulators or opioid pumps, and conventional and stereotactic surgery (4).

Unlike acute pain, treatment aimed at the relief of a specific nociceptive stimulus is unlikely to be successful with a chronic pain syndrome (CPS). The current use of this term refers to nonmalignant pain in which the subjective pain complaints, resultant suffering, and pain behaviors are excessive and disproportionate to the actual pathophysiology. In addition, there generally is accompanying life disruption and dysfunctional, maladaptive behavior demonstrated by impairments in physical and psychosocial functioning. The following characteristics are common in this patient population: "preoccupation with pain, strong and ambivalent dependency needs, feelings of isolation and loneliness, characterological masochism (meeting other people's needs at their own expense), inability to take care of self needs, passivity, lack of insight into self-defeating behavior patterns, difficulty dealing appropriately with anger and hostility, and the use of pain as a symbolic means of communication" (6, 7). The multidisciplinary team approach to management of intractable CPS has been shown to be an effective treatment option.

THE MULTIDISCIPLINARY APPROACH TO TREATMENT

A multidisciplinary pain center (MPC) is one that offers multidisciplinary and interdisciplinary evaluation, treatment, and a cohesive pain team approach directed toward understanding and treatment of pain and suffering. For residual pain the goal is to eliminate maladaptive pain and drug-seeking behaviors and replace these with more adaptive coping skills. All comprehensive pain programs should have a rehabilitation philosophy with a goal of functional restoration and whenever possible, interrupting the disability process (4, 7a). In addition, "a comprehensive pain center must address the medical, psychological, and social contributions to the pain problem, be involved in teaching and research, and be staffed by a dedicated staff with appropriate training and experience in managing pain" (8, 8a).

A multidisciplinary pain treatment team is one in which physicians work in an interdisciplinary and collaborative role with other health professionals (e.g., dentists, nurses, psychologists, social workers, physical and occupational therapists, and vocational and rehabilitation counselors). The team functions as an interactive, cohesive unit, with concurrent assessments using a behavioral medicine biopsychosocial approach. The physician reviews medical records, symptoms, and signs to assess whether further diagnostic evaluation is warranted. *Diagnostic evaluation and invasive procedures are not recommended simply because we have the technology or because we work in a fee-for-service health care delivery system. It is my belief that one of the problems facing pain centers is a direct result of having done too much to too many for too long without demonstration of significant benefit. This has appropriately sensitized insurance carriers, who often feel that they have in the past been abused.* The traditional behavioral model has been modified to a more cognitive-behavioral model, as described in detail by Turk (Chapter 24). Psychological evaluation assesses for dysfunctional pain behaviors, comorbid psychopathology, and cognitive distortions. Pain patients frequently have faulty cognitions regarding the implications of their pain, its effects in the present and for the future, and their ability to resume a productive life. These are all targets for evaluation and intervention. The team's cohesiveness is also important in addressing the manipulative behavior of some patients, which can be an attempt to split the efforts of the team (6, 7).

The medical director may have a subspecialty in any of a number of areas—neurology, neurosurgery, orthopaedics, physiatry, anesthesiology, or psychiatry—depending on the type of pain treatment focus. However, the expertise, interest in, and philosophy of pain management are often more important than the area of specialization. Table 41.1 lists the common goals of MPCs. The following services are the responsibility of the treatment team (6):

1. A thorough medical assessment of the pain complaints, including detailed review of previous evaluations and treatments to ensure that pertinent workups and treatment options have been addressed. If further evaluation is needed, it is obtained. However, an MPC should not be viewed primarily as a diagnostic center, since most patients have already been extensively evaluated. These diagnostic services should be used for testing deemed necessary if the pain evaluation is incomplete, if results need further clarification, or for necessary management of ongoing medical problems.
2. Medical history, physical examination, and monitoring of other medical problems.
3. Psychosocial evaluation (including psychological testing) to determine pertinent underlying (prepain) and resultant (postpain) psychological problems and coping styles that have an impact on the patient's CPS. Individual and group psychotherapy and education address problem areas.
4. Family assessment and intervention based on the view that pain is a systems problem and recognizing that although the patient is defined as the one having the problem, the family is also affected and either covertly or overtly may complicate the patient's recovery. The family can also be an ally in implementing the treatment plan.
5. Physical therapy evaluation to assess structural limitations and restrictions (objective findings versus pain complaints), body mechanics and postural deviations, range of motion, strength, and flexibility and to teach pain control modalities (i.e.,

Table 41.1.   MPC Goals

Clarify the diagnosis. Review medical records and the need for further diagnostic studies or invasive procedures.
Improve pain control (eliminate pain if possible) through physical therapies:
  Help the patient to be more comfortably active, with a return to a functional and productive lifestyle.
  Promote the use of alternative, noninvasive pain control modalities other than potent medications.
  With individually structured exercise programs, reduce the patient's fear of reinjury.
  Teach proper body mechanics and postural awareness.
  Evaluate limitations and restrictions.
Improve psychological functioning.
  Define and address psychosocial issues influencing the CPS.
  Relieve drug dependency.
  Treat depression and its frequently associated insomnia.
  Address primary and secondary gains from pain.
  Assess family system.
  Strengthen support network (e.g., personal, family, and community).
Provide access to occupational and vocational rehabilitation and any other significant health care personnel, and resolve disability when possible.
Communicate with the patient's referring physician via discharge summary, phone, or personal meetings to obtain any information that will assist in the continued management of the patient.
Reduce inappropriate use of the health care system.
Decrease the cost of medical care associated with the CPS.

transcutaneous electrical nerve stimulation [TENS] and ice massage) and maximize function.

6. Systematic relaxation training with biofeedback as indicated.
7. Primary nursing coordination of the entire patient care plan (work in the previously mentioned areas, development of more productive coping strategies, overall health behaviors, and medication management).
8. Vocational assessment to determine whether a patient can return to a former job or requires retraining; appropriate testing and intervention to assist in return to the work force.
9. When indicated, determination of residual functional capacity, followed by a systematic program of gradually progressive occupational and vocational activities in simulated work and home environments.

Not every chronic pain sufferer requires an MPC. Many respond to single-modality treatment (e.g., use of TENS, ice massage, or other physical therapy techniques; nerve blocks; or relaxation techniques, often with biofeedback training), with resolution of their pain or at least adequate pain control and diminished suffering. However, patients who have not benefited from conventional pain treatments, whose lives continue to be severely disrupted by their pain, and who often have complicating psychosocial problems are best treated at a comprehensive MPC. Others may require primarily psychotherapy or work with social services if psychosocial issues are paramount (6, 7).

Credit must be given to Bonica (5) for both conceptualizing the form, function, and structure of the multidiscipli-

nary pain center and persevering in its growth and development, beginning in the 1940s. During the 1950s, there emerged a number of pain centers using an anesthesiology model. However, not all of the early pioneers in the pain center movement subscribed to Bonica's model (9). In 1960, the neurosurgeon Crue (10) established the City of Hope Pain Center in Duarte, California, based on the concept that most CPS patients and their referring physicians were incorrect in viewing the problem as if there were something abnormal in the periphery that must be located and fixed by the physician, either by cutting or blocking a sensory nerve or pathway. He emphasized placing the responsibility for the treatment outcome on the patient as quickly as possible, while understanding that patients themselves are fixed in the organic medical model and are sometimes incapable of accepting the responsibility for their own pain treatment. It is his opinion that by the time a clinician has enough experience to evaluate the results of diagnostic nerve blocks, the blocks are usually a waste of time for both the patient and the physician. Indeed, a study quoted in *Pain* (11) suggests that whereas nerve blocks are widely used in pain programs directed by anesthesiologists, they are infrequently used in pain centers directed by nonanesthesiologists.

Although MPCs initially were viewed with enthusiasm by payors, it did not take long before "the new growth industry" (as Medical World News called pain clinics of the early 1980s) was viewed with skepticism. By the early 1990s the pain clinic movement was in trouble, with image problems, such that some programs closed and others changed their names to "functional restoration" or "work conditioning programs" to avoid using the word "pain" as a descriptor. What happened, and was it preventable? Was it simply our capitalist free enterprise system and some of the inherent problems of the fee-for-service procedure-driven American health care system, in which the greater the number of procedures, the greater the reimbursement? As I rethink the many lessons I learned from Crue, Loeser, Hollister, Rosomoff, Seres, Addison, Brena, and others who shaped the field of pain medicine, the most important had to do with listening to our patients, hearing their suffering, and recognizing that most of it does not come from the periphery but from central generators as products of learned goal-directed pain and illness behaviors. Consequently, early in my career I viewed the anesthesia-based interventionalist model as inappropriate. I have since modified my position. Chronic pain conditions at times respond best to an interventionist approach, at other times to a cognitive-behavioral and rehabilitation approach, and sometimes to a combination of the two. Our knowledge about clinical uses of analgesics and adjuvant analgesics continues to improve, and interventional approaches are being used with greater specificity and with better-defined selection criteria. It is to be hoped that this will assist in improving our outcomes and redeem our raison d'être in the eyes of health care payors, colleagues, and patients.

MPC TREATMENT OUTCOMES

A review of MPC follow-up studies of patient outcomes during the past 20 years indicates consistently positive post-treatment results (i.e., reduced medication use, decreased use of the health care system, and improved mood and quality of life). Although many follow-up studies in this area have methodological flaws and further research is necessary, the overall ability of an MPC to help reduce the suffering and pain behavior components of CPS is clear (12).

Painter et al. (13) mailed 500 questionnaires to patients who had attended the Northwest Pain Center in 1977 and found that 77% of the patients felt improved as a result of their pain center experience, with an average pain reduction of 35%. Further improvement followed discharge, with an average reduction in pain of 21%. Deterioration was reported by 27% of the patients sampled. On admission, approximately 90% of patients were unemployed, whereas on follow-up, 48% were employed. Also, 61% of the patients reported that they had no further medical care for their pain, and 17% stated that they were seeking other medical solutions; 20% reported having returned to the use of opioid medications, which had been eliminated by the pain unit program. They found that the failure group demonstrated fewer incentives for maintaining their gains, with most continuing to receive financial compensation for their pain. Also, the failure group was more likely to assume a passive-dependent stance, with depression the mood most characteristic of the group. Finally, the failure group had done little to change their environment and continued to find reinforcement for pain behavior.

Wang et al. (14) studied 406 patients for 1 to 3 years following treatment. (These patients responded to the questionnaire that was mailed to 725 patients.) Pain intensity, medication used, daily activity, ability to work, and patient's belief in the benefit of treatment were assessed. Of those answering, approximately 50% had no pain or mild pain or were merely uncomfortable from their pain; 60% reported decreased or no use of medications for the pain; and 56% noted that their activity was increased even if occasionally somewhat difficult. The number of patients able to work increased by 50%, and 45% of the patients believed that their treatment had been beneficial.

Similar variables were assessed by Crue and Pinsky (10) in their study of 151 patients who responded out of a total of 299 mailed questionnaires. Length of time from discharge from the program for these patients varied from 3 months to 5 years. The variables of interest reported were medication use, medicosurgical treatment of pain, pain rating, results of an open-ended questionnaire about chronic pain, general life outlook, and attitude. The drugs about which the patients were queried were opioids, barbiturates, major and minor tranquilizers, and muscle relaxants. As compared with their condition at the time of admission, after 4 years 38% were using none of these drugs, 31% were using less than they had prior to admission, and 31% used more drugs. The data showed that 2 years after treatment, 89% had no invasive or medical treatment (e.g., surgery or nerve blocks) for their pain. By 4 years, 85% had no invasive treatment for their pain. In rating overall pain intensity at 1 year, approximately 50% said their pain was the same as or worse than it had been before admission, whereas 50% said that it had improved. By 4 years, their percentages had not changed. The authors also stated that 75% of their patients seemed to have positive attitudes, both in regard to their pain and their general lifestyle.

Turk (15), in his review of the efficacy of MPCs in the treatment of chronic pain not only found them to be effective, but in reviewing the criteria for success found the consensus of research had demonstrated the following:

1. Pain reduction
2. Reduction or elimination of opioid medication
3. Increase in activity
4. Return to work (an average of 67% in the treated group based on 11 studies)
5. Decreased use of the health care system
6. Closure of disability claims
7. Cost effectiveness

Turk states, "Interestingly, third-party payors who review these statistics are often reluctant to pay for rehabilitation at MPCs. Yet they seem to have few reservations about paying for invasive medical and surgical interventions that achieve less impressive results" (15). His review of studies on intractable chronic back pain comparing surgical treatment (including neurostimulation) with MPC data indicated that on all criteria of success MPC programs appeared to be superior to surgery. Turk noted, "When considering the success rates of MPCs we must acknowledge that the population served have the most recalcitrant problems and have failed many other treatment efforts including surgery. As such, the population of pain patients referred to and treated at MPCs is at higher risk to fail any treatment. It is against this backdrop that MPC outcome studies must be assessed."

Cutler et al. (16) in a review and meta–analysis of the literature found that nonsurgical pain center treatment of chronic pain was successful in returning patients to work. The proportion of patients working increased from 20% to 54% post chronic nonsurgical treatment. The results indicated that (a) chronic nonsurgical treatment returned patients to work; (b) increased rates of return to work were due to treatment; and (c) benefits of treatment were not temporary. In another study, Fishbain et al. (17) found that chronic pain patients' perceptions about their preinjury jobs often determined their intent to return to the same type of job post pain facility treatment. In a review of their outcome data from 1989 through 1996, 1 year post discharge statistics indicate a 71% reduction in pain, 75% improvement in functional status, and 77% improvement in quality of life; 72% were employed or work ready, 81% were not using opioid medications, and 79% were satisfied with treatment.

One of the criticisms of pain center treatment has been that patients' gains are not lasting. While there is some recidivism, our findings at the Boston Pain Center and Presbyterian

Rehabilitation Center for Pain Medicine are consistent with an earlier study by Painter et al. (13) indicating that the patients who regress often had little incentive to maintain their gains (e.g., continued reinforcement for maintenance of their disabled status through ongoing workers compensation, other litigation, or environmental reinforcement), had ongoing depression, and did not follow through with the recommendations of the treatment team. In addition, we have found that job dissatisfaction and ongoing pain-prone characteristics contribute to poor prognosis in patients who at a given point in life may use pain as a way of satisfying previously unmet dependency needs so that finally it is they who are taken care of. In these patients, pain may be an indirect and symbolic means of communication.

An updated review of the literature on MPC treatment outcome studies through 1996 supports the contention that this model of treatment continues to improve functional ability and quality of life for many chronic pain sufferers and their families. However, many of the same methodological flaws and research limitations noted in Aronoff et al.'s (12) survey of the literature are still problematic (i.e., lack of operational definitions of successful outcome; lack of comparison and control groups; use of subjective self-report measures; and low sample size, to name a few).

PATIENT SELECTION

At the Presbyterian Rehabilitation Center for Pain Medicine (chronic pain rehabilitation and functional restoration section), treatment is limited to nonmalignant CPS. Low-back pain, myofascial pain, fibromyalgia, neuropathic pain, and head and neck pain syndromes are by far the most common. More than half of our patients have had industrial accidents, and the remainder have non–work-related personal injuries or pain secondary to a disease process or medical condition (e.g., chronic headaches, fibromyalgia and other rheumatological pain syndromes, postherpetic neuralgia, complex regional pain syndrome 1 (CRPS 1, or reflex sympathetic dystrophy), chronic abdominal and pelvic pain, peripheral neuropathy, and phantom limb pain). Of this latter group, pain is often disproportionate to the degree of organic pathology or uncharacteristic of the disease process (e.g., persistent postthoracotomy chest wall pain, in which intercostal neuritis, neuroma, and other organic causes have been excluded; or nonischemic chest pain in an anxious patient with known stable cardiac disease who has become a cardiac cripple, inappropriately using nitroglycerine for noncardiac pain).

Pain centers are sometimes regarded as the treatment of last resort. This erroneous impression is beginning to change as more health care providers recognize that early referrals may help eliminate needless or multiple surgeries, reduce health care costs, and promote the patient's return to productivity. Insurance carriers and employers may ultimately benefit from chronic pain programs. Failed surgical procedures, multiple physician visits, medication dependency, repetitive evaluations, unsuccessful treatments, iatrogenic complica-

tions, and lost workdays may be reduced (18). The way the patient views referral to a pain center often depends on the referring physician's presentation of the suggestion. The following should be incorporated in the presentation:

1. A pain center embodies a specialized, comprehensive approach to exploring and treating multiple aspects of a pain problem that has become the disease and is not resolving.
2. Although patients with CPS often have a complex interaction between physiological and psychological factors, their pain is rarely all psychological.
3. At the time of discharge from a pain center, patients may have some residual pain, but for most there is substantially diminished suffering and pain behavior; the majority of patients at discharge do not find their pain to be disabling.
4. The vast majority of patients with CPS can be taught effective pain control techniques. By the time of discharge, most have less suffering without analgesic therapy than they did on admission while using analgesics (18).

Multiple factors play a part in the prognosis and must be explored and understood. These include ethnocultural, family, value system, character, personality, support system, and motivational factors (18). Just as the anesthesiologist, orthopaedist, or neurosurgeon is selective in choosing patients likely to benefit from a given nerve block or operative procedure, pain centers also must be selective in their admission process. As part of the pain center program, behavior modification to reinforce adaptive behaviors and extinguish self-defeating maladaptive behaviors also requires the patient's capacity for insight and self-change. Some patients are incapable of this process and if detected initially, are recognized as being inappropriate candidates for a pain center treatment program. Patients with major cognitive deficits from cerebral vascular accidents or dementing illnesses and those with severe hearing deficits not improved by hearing aids generally do not do well in this type of pain program. Those who have limited comprehension in the primary language used at the pain center also have difficulty in grasping the concepts of the program and interacting in any meaningful way with the other patients in the therapeutic community. As do other clinicians, pain center personnel must be aware of factors that may place the treatment of many pain patients beyond their grasp (4).

The screening process is extremely important, especially when the issue of disability compensation is involved. If, on the basis of the initial evaluation, it is thought that the patient's motivation for behavioral change is marginal or that he or she is content to collect compensation and be taken care of, thus assuming a passive dependent role, treatment at the pain center should be deferred. This must be clearly expressed to the patient in a nonjudgmental way, and it also should be the patient's right and privilege to continue with the pain and suffering if he or she so chooses. An interpretation and clarification should address the issues very candidly. The primary concern should not be with the patient's reaction but rather with assisting the patient to recognize motivational and attitudinal deficits, psychological factors complicating the disability, and issues of primary and secondary gain.

One should attempt to clarify life stressors, traumatic life events, past patterns of disability in the patient or other family members, a history of family member illness or chronic pain, unmet dependency needs, childhood deprivations, and substance abuse. All of these are important in understanding how the patient became the person now seeking treatment. This information is essential in formulating an individual treatment program and understanding prognosis, as well as in making statements about vocational matters and disability (4).

Our goal must be to determine more carefully patients for whom impairment (physical or psychological) warrants receiving disability compensation and to assist those patients in any way we can to receive the assistance they deserve. However, clinicians should not encourage anyone to remain disabled when there are more appropriate alternatives.

If I were to subdivide the chronic pain population I have worked with, initially at the Boston Pain Center (1976–1994) and subsequently at the Presbyterian Rehabilitation Center for Pain Medicine (since 1994), approximately one third of the patients truly desire to be actively involved in their health care, with the goal of suffering less with pain, using less medication, and returning to a more active, productive life than was the case at the time of their admission. This group generally is reasonably self-motivated and eagerly awaits training in new techniques to help them better live with pain and suffer less. Another third of this population is composed of those who have learned how to be pain patients; that is, they have developed goal-directed conditioned pain behaviors (learned helplessness), often maintaining these unconsciously. Nonetheless, these patients are "stuck," and investigation has revealed patterns of self-defeating behaviors. These patients, although somewhat more defensive than those in the first group, are at least receptive to participating in a structured program designed to maximize function and minimize dysfunction and to replace maladaptive coping with more adaptive techniques, so that they can learn to not be disabled by pain. Generally, these two segments of the chronic pain population do quite well in MPCs. We can have a major influence on the quality of their lives and also serve society by returning to it more functional members.

It is the remaining third of this population that is of greatest concern, because, although this last group tends to be the most abused by the health care system, it is also the group that abuses the health care system and society.

Increasingly, it appears that there are some patients who cannot be helped, who at a given point in time may not want to be helped, and whose agenda of being enmeshed in the health care system has nothing to do with receiving health care, but more with receiving benefits. We must more efficiently identify this segment of the population and not treat them. Regardless of a patient's complaints, once we have established that the tools at our disposal are unlikely to ameliorate his or her symptoms, we should establish a series of recommendations. If the patient is unable or unwilling to consider these, it may be that the system has adequately fulfilled its responsibility to that person and should no longer attempt treatment (19).

A WELLNESS MODEL

Based on experience in evaluating and treating chronic pain patients, both in our inpatient and outpatient facilities, I conclude that the majority of these patients can be effectively treated in an outpatient setting. This avoids costly hospitalization.

Inpatient versus outpatient costs were compared by Cicala and Wright (20) of the University of Tennessee Center for Pain Management on 25 patients treated in 1985 on an inpatient basis versus 25 patients treated in 1987 on an outpatient basis. They found that "total hospital costs paid through third-party reimbursement for all 25 patients treated in 1985 was $321,500 in 1987 reduced to $61,000. When office visits, procedures, and other charges were considered, the total expenses to third-party payers were $571,200 in 1985 and $191,000 in 1987. The average cost for each patient treated had decreased from $22,848 to $7,640 when the two periods were compared."

The outpatient setting more realistically simulates typical activities of daily living. Follow-up of these day patients indicates that for the majority of them, there was a much less difficult transition from the treatment program to their usual lifestyle. Unfortunately, this has been one of the major problems with the hospital model since its inception. Many patients find that after being confined in a sheltered and artificial environment, they ultimately have a difficult transition returning to the workplace or normal daily activities. Many insurance carriers also have great difficulty with the high cost of inpatient programs. Table 41.2 highlights some of the advantages and disadvantages of MPC treatment in each setting.

I believe that treatment for those with difficult chronic pain problems should be based on a wellness model, recognizing that their pain does not make them sick in the acute medical sense of the word but rather that it interferes with their optimal functioning in various areas of their lives. These patients generally do not require around-the-clock medical or nursing care.

After the primary goal of alleviating pain and suffering, treatment should be directed toward helping patients to overcome the disabling effects of chronic pain and return them to productivity rather than continued dependency on the health care system. Although the presence of active or unstable medical problems or major medication dependency may require an inpatient setting, even patients with a difficult home situation or those who must travel a considerable distance to the center often can be housed in groups at a local hotel, attending the program during the day and continuing the therapeutic milieu dur-

Table 41.2.   Inpatient versus Outpatient MPC Treatment

Inpatient	Outpatient
Indications	
Global life disruption	Global life disruption
Depression, high suicide risk	Depression, not overtly suicidal
Major medication dependency (especially with substance abuse disorder)	May be taking medication but without significant dependence
Unstable medical problems requiring inpatient monitoring	No trial of outpatient pain center treatment
Nonambulatory	
Previous unsuccessful outpatient pain center treatment	Home responsibilities (e.g., child care) preclude inpatient admission
Advantages	
Ability to confront noncompliance (e.g., nonparticipation due to "pain")	Wellness model
	Reduced cost
Patient removed from disruptive home situation and treated in therapeutic milieu	Permits incorporation or simulation of normal daily routine and activities (e.g., driving to and from MPC)
	Easier transition from treatment program back to workplace or other activities of daily living
Disadvantages	
Illness model	Behavior modification more difficult (home environment may reinforce pain behavior)
Greater cost	
More difficult to simulate normal daily activities during program	May call in sick secondary to pain; more difficult medication management in substance-dependent patient (especially in marginally motivated patient)
Fosters dependency	

ing the evening. Our MPC treatment program focuses on several major patient problem areas, including the following:

1. The pain-depression-insomnia cycle
2. Pharmacological reevaluation, eliminating nonessential medication and treating substance dependencies
3. Pain-related physical dysfunction and deconditioning
4. Psychosocial factors affecting the pain syndrome
5. The distinction between impairment and disability
6. Early return to work, school, or other productive activity
7. Resolving cognitive distortions

DISABILITY INTERVENTION

It is important to distinguish between the pain patient who is difficult by virtue of a medical problem, psychiatric problem, or both and the unmotivated, manipulative, hostile, and negative patient, who may be exploiting the health care system for personal gain. The behavioral aspects of multidisciplinary pain programs are often based on some traditional American values, which include maturity and the work ethic. If we assume that assisting patients to return to productive, functional lifestyles is desirable for them and for society and that these patients' support systems can be sources of distraction from the pain problem itself, the more meaningful a person's support system is, the less that person is to suffer from the pain (21).

There is no linear relationship between the degree of medical or psychiatric impairment and the resulting disability rating. The findings of a multidisciplinary medical panel from Boston University Medical Center emphasize this. In this study, 111 consecutive chronic low-back pain patients referred by the Office of Workers Compensation Programs (OWCP) were assessed. Of these, only 13 (11.7%) were found to have evidence of significant objective impairment that by itself warranted total disability. Of the 13, roughly half were physically impaired and half were psychiatrically impaired. In none of the 6 patients granted psychiatric disability was the psychiatric impairment found to be work related. In other words, the insurance carrier for the employee was paying for a claim that was not its responsibility. Strang (22) discusses the chronic disability syndrome in which individuals who are capable of working choose to remain disabled. He writes, "They lack motivation to recover and return to productivity. The disability is often the result of a fairly minor injury but actually represents an inability to cope with other life problems."

Brena and Chapman (23) describe the five D's, a cluster of symptoms often seen in chronic pain patients: *d*ramatization (of vague, diffuse, nonanatomical pain complaints); *d*rug abuse (misuse of habit-forming pain medications); *d*ysfunction (bodily impairments related to various physical and emotional factors); *d*ependency (passivity, depression, and helplessness); and *d*isability (pain contingent on financial compensation and pending litigation claims).

Several authors have contributed to our understanding of why pain-related disability and litigation are such major problems. Brena and Chapman (24) reviewed several studies of the disability process, indicating that certain characteristics make patients prone to have a disabling injury. In one study, Weinstein (25) noted these factors: (*a*) low self–esteem in a dependent person, (*b*) inability to deal competently with stress, (*c*) a demanding job, and (*d*) tension at home. The injury is viewed as a socially acceptable way out of a stressful situation.

Ellard (26) enumerates some significant characteristics of patients who have psychological reactions to injury. (*a*) They lack the usual objective signs of suffering (a disparity between verbal pain complaints and untroubled manner). (*b*) Objective clinical findings do not correlate with the complaint (e.g., no atrophy of a paralyzed limb). (*c*) Poor motivation is exhibited (the patient remains a passive sufferer, vehemently asserting his or her problem and desire to get well yet failing to participate effectively in treatment). (*d*) The patient exhibits unusual responses to treatment. Initially, these patients may not actively seek treatment; once treated, they fail to benefit from it, although they continue to pursue it. Ellard notes that many of these patients show no evidence of a stated psychopathological condition preceding the accident. He summarizes the diagnostic and treatment dilemma these patients create, stating that the symptoms may represent a conscious or unconscious desire for the person to establish that he or she is sick, "not so much because of his personal pathological condition, but because of the social consequences of the sick role." He notes that when financial gain is involved, legal rather than medical processes most often remedy the complaints. Brena and Chapman (24) noted the demoralized behavior of many patients in chronic pain management programs when consistently confronted with situations in which they could not control the outcome. They demonstrated elements of depression, passivity, and lack of initiative in attempting to affect situation outcomes. They point to the common features between these behaviors and those previously noted in workers prone to chronic disability following a work-related injury.

Bigos et al. (27) and Fordyce et al. (28) in the frequently quoted Boeing studies found that mood or psychological state, personality characteristics, and job happiness may have greater predictive value than biomechanical or ergonomic factors as predictors or risk factors of workers filing back injury complaints.

Waddell et al. (29) found that the best predictor of return to work after a reported back injury was the worker's fear-avoidance beliefs about what would happen to symptoms and to his or her body upon return to work. The degree of anticipation of reinjury was more predictive of return to work than the presence or severity of symptoms. Disability is more difficult to treat once it has continued for 6 months or longer. Thus early recognition of features predicting poor prognosis and prompt intervention is important. Seres and Newman (30) note that 80 to 90% of workers with back injuries return to work within days or weeks of the injury. Of the remaining injured, 5 to 15% have prolonged or permanent disability.

McGill (31) noted in his study of industrial back problems that a lengthy period of disability predicted a low chance of ever returning to work. Those out of work longer than 6 months had a 50% probability of return; those out of work for more than 1 year had a 25% chance of return, and those out of work longer than 2 years were extremely unlikely to return. Waddell's (32) more current study confirms these statistics.

Brena et al. (33) recommend using some of the funds now paid to maintain workers in the sick role to provide economic incentives for injured workers. They point out that such a practice would encourage a return to work when the acute phase of the injury is over and when the attending physician has released the worker for productive activities. He also recommends employer economic incentives for rehiring employees as soon as they have recovered, at different duties when necessary.

I have written on the disability epidemic (34, 34a), which is most prominent in the United States and other countries where entitlement programs are viewed as appealing alternatives to gainful employment. If this epidemic is to be reversed, the compensation and disability systems must be changed so that they encourage early intervention, prevention of chronicity with incentives toward rehabilitation, and early return to work.

The Social Security disability system, for example, discourages potentially disabled workers from even attempting rehabilitation. To be eligible for disability benefits, a claimant must prove that he or she is unable to engage in any substantial gainful employment because of a medical impairment that is anticipated to continue for at least 12 months. On the other hand, to be eligible for rehabilitation, the claimant must demonstrate both the potential for work and that rehabilitation would be beneficial. As the Pain Commission (U.S. Department of Health and Human Services) (35) stated in 1987, the need to vigorously prove and reprove one's disability under the current system works against the rehabilitation provisions. The beneficiaries themselves may have little incentive to try to be rehabilitated after being found disabled. Often the patient's attitude and motivation, coupled with his or her support system, is likely to determine whether a given patient allows pain to be totally disabling. It especially is a reflection of underlying personality style and goals in life. We should encourage rehabilitation, not disability, and we should help patients retain a sense of purpose and self-worth. However, certification of disability because of chronic pain sometimes occurs as a result of collusion between health care providers and patients (21).

It is important to distinguish between disability (a legal term) and impairment (a medical term), since they are sometimes erroneously used interchangeably. Medically, impairment can be defined as reduction of body or organ function (36) or as "an anatomic or functional abnormality, nonprogressive and fully rehabilitated" (33). Disability can be defined as a task-specific limitation of performance (37). Therefore, the presence of a disease does not necessarily mean impairment. There may be disability from certain tasks but not necessarily from the skills necessary for the patient's job. The American Medical Association (AMA) *Guide to the Evaluation of Permanent Impairment* (38) emphasizes the difference between impairment and disability. Impairment is determined medically as any anatomic or functional abnormality or loss; disability is judged administratively, based on the patient's actual or presumed ability to engage in gainful activity (35). In addition to consideration of (permanent) impairment in determining disability, Ziporyn (39) notes other factors that must be taken into account, such as the patient's age, sex, education, economic, and social environment. Richman (36) believes that disability definitions should further distinguish between occupational disability (total or partial), which "inherently involves a decline in earning power, and non-occupational disability (never total), which involves customary vocational and recreational activities, but without adverse effect on earning power."

Research indicates that decreased function depends not only on pathophysiology but also on illness behaviors or pain behaviors (e.g., inactivity, drug misuse, learned helplessness) (33). Patients with lengthy disabilities are special in several respects. Snook (40) found that patients receiving workers compensation for back injuries were less likely to have objective findings or a definitive diagnosis than those with back injuries who were not receiving compensation.

In discussing patients with chronic low-back pain claims, Carron (41) indicated that the three most striking factors were as follows: (*a*) 78.7% of the subjective complaints were not supported by physical findings; (*b*) 60% were taking dependence-inducing drugs, and (*c*) 49.3% had a previous back injury. In those injuries (occult), which were neither witnessed nor reliably documented and with pain as the major manifestation of injury, he noted a high incidence of previous compensable injury, drug dependency, obesity, low income, and nonsupervisory work. In one study by Leavitt et al. (42), 70% of workers receiving compensation for back injuries reported a specific work activity or event triggering the pain or injury, but only 35% of workers not receiving compensation for low-back pain reported such a clear-cut work-related event.

Brena and Turk (43) note the importance of return to work as a goal of MPCs:

If the goal of a health care provider is to restore the patient's physical, emotional, and social wellness, return to work functioning whenever feasible should be a major goal of any pain treatment program, equal in importance with the subjective pain reduction and the correction of physical and emotional disorders a clear understanding of the chronic pain patient's problems, of the third party payor's specific needs and of the structure of the present day disability programs, is imperative.

Catchlove and Cohen's (44) 1982 retrospective review of two groups of chronic pain patients receiving workers compensation support this. When a directive return-to-work approach was incorporated into their treatment, 60% of patients returned to work, and 90% of them continued to work an average of 9.6 months later. They were also receiving fewer compensation benefits and less additional pain treatment than a group of patients similarly treated but for whom a return-to-work directive was not included. Only 25% of the latter group returned to work. Although the improvements may have been related both to selection factors (a treatment contract that patients had to affirm) and to treatment efficacy, the results were quite promising.

Of back pain patients treated at MPCs, many have undergone multiple pain-related surgeries. In Waddell's (44a) 1979 study of failed lumbar disc surgery in compensation patients following industrial injuries, 97% had some persistent pain complaints. Another finding was that 77% continued with impaired functioning, and of those who had third or fourth operations, outcomes were progressively worse, with increased psychological dysfunction. I have cited recommended criteria for patients who should have a second opinion prior to elective surgery (Table 41.3).

As low-back operations are being performed more selectively and less frequently, pain centers should be viewed as a positive alternative for treatment, not only by concerned physicians and health care providers but also by cost-conscious insurance carriers and employers.

Assessment of primary or secondary gain from pain and disability is crucial in evaluating the prognosis for return to work. Financial gain from litigation or disability compensa-

Table 41.3.   Second Opinion Prior to Elective Surgery

Two or more pain-related surgeries without beneficial results
One or more pain-related surgeries with negative findings
Attorney-referred patients involved in pain-related litigation
Known or highly suspected major psychopathology
History of unjustified overuse of health care system

tion may reinforce the decision to remain out of work. Attorneys receiving contingency fees, who stand to gain more when the client remains outwardly disabled by pain, sometimes foster the view of illness as a means of economic gain.

Seres and Newman (30) indicate that low-back injuries are the most frequently litigated claims and the most common type of cumulative trauma injury. Many studies (31, 40, 42, 44b) indicate that pain treatment is less successful for those receiving workers compensation or with pending litigation than for those without. Some pain centers actually decline admission to patients with pending litigation. However, another more recent study has reported contradictory results. Dworkin et al. (45) found that in 454 chronic pain patients, only employment status at initial evaluation predicted treatment response (employed patients had better outcomes than those not employed). Neither litigation nor compensation was a significant predictor of treatment outcome. Similarly, Peck et al. (46) found no significant effects of either litigation or representation by attorneys on the pain behavior of patients with pending workers compensation claims.

Review of the literature regarding pain center success in returning patients to the workplace indicates results ranging from 20 to 81% (47, 48; McAlary PW, unpublished doctoral dissertation, May 1989).

In a review of outcomes from a number of chronic pain center programs, Brena and Chapman (23) and Chapman and Bradford (48) noted that 20 to 50% of patients had returned to work within 1 year or less following treatment. In one study, for example, 86% of a sample of 40 patients treated at an inpatient pain management program were unemployed on admission (the other 14% were running a household). Follow-up questionnaires 6 months to 3 years after treatment indicated that 47% were employed, 28% running a household, and only 25% unemployed (49). At the Northwest Pain Center (13), approximately 90% of patients were unemployed on admission and only 52% remained so at follow-up; 70% of patients were receiving compensation at admission and only 45% at follow-up. Vasudevan et al. (50) contacted 149 patients 1 year after discharge from a pain center and found that employment levels rose from a pretreatment rate of 19% to 45%.

In a retrospective review of work placement records, Addison (47) noted that in 1978 the return to work rate was 51%; in 1979, 70.8%; and during the first 6 months of 1980, 81%. Most placements (72%) involved a former employer (previous job or modified one); 28% were in new jobs. Informal analysis of this population 3 years after discharge indicated that many had been promoted or achieved upward mobility in their employment area. Unfortunately, the author's data gathering methods and prior patient work records were not reported.

A report from the Ohio Pain and Stress Treatment Center (51) noted a 100% return to work rate among 19 private utility company employees who were referred by the company. These patients had been disabled by pain and had been unemployed for 9 months to 21 years (an average of 8 years). At 6-month follow-up, all 19 patients had returned to full employment. The treatment cost of the pain center amounted to only 2% of the projected disability cost, theoretically saving the company about $1.8 million. The small sample size and relatively short follow-up period (6 months) must be considered when evaluating the results.

Newman et al. (37) reported on 36 patients with low-back pain who were followed up 18 months after treatment at the Northwest Pain Center. At that time, most patients reported improved ability to cope with pain, higher activity level, and less analgesic use; 30% of them were employed.

Meilman et al. (52) conducted personal interviews of 56 chronic pain patients (31 with back and leg pain), 18 months to 10 years following pain center treatment. Significantly, more patients were employed at follow-up than prior to treatment. Of these patients, 19 were working 30 hours or more per week, 3 were working 20 hours per week, and 1 worked 10 hours per week. An additional 12 patients were housewives, and three had retired for non–pain-related reasons. As with most of these studies, a limitation was the lack of comparison groups (treated versus untreated patients) and the use of different treatment modalities.

In an outcome study by Guck et al. (53), treatment and no treatment groups were used to compare follow-up results 1 to 5 years after pain center discharge. They compared 20 treated patients with a control group of 20 untreated patients who met admission criteria but lacked financial coverage to participate in the program. They found that 60% (or 12 of the treated patients) met a stringent set of criteria for success, whereas none of the untreated patients did. These criteria, compiled by Roberts and Reinhardt (54), included the following:

1. Employment (or unemployed for non–pain-related reasons), housewife by profession, attending school or training, or doing volunteer work by profession, all requiring being up and active at least 8 hours per day.
2. Not being compensated for pain problems.
3. No pain-related hospitalizations or surgeries since evaluation or treatment.
4. Not using prescription opioid or psychotropic medications.

Among 57 treated patients not used for the study, significantly more were employed at follow-up and met these criteria than on initial evaluation. Treated patients also reported that pain interfered less with daily activities, including work, chores, outdoor activities, shopping, sexual activity, physical and recreational activity, and sleep than did the untreated group. The patients noted less depression and pain and were out of bed more of the time than the untreated group. Records also noted fewer hospitalizations and pain-related operations (none in the treated group) and less overall use of the health care system among treated patients.

Unpublished follow-up data on 14 of the first 20 patients who completed the South Shore Pain Center program, an outpatient MPC that I directed, noted a 64% return to work rate (full time, part time, or light duty) within 1 to 4 months post discharge. These patients were all out of work because of pain prior to admission.

In this time of cost containment in the U.S. health care system, the necessity for and effectiveness of all treatments and therapies is weighed and scrutinized. Payors are asking rehabilitation providers to demonstrate empirically both clinical and cost effectiveness in their programs. These data will be used to compare providers and will likely contribute to more preferred-provider relationships. Among the trends in medical rehabilitation, the following are noted:

1. An increase in rehabilitation services for persons with traumatic brain injury, back injuries, and chronic pain.
2. A proliferation of cost-effective outpatient and day treatment programs.
3. Enhanced vocational services, including work hardening, work site modifications, and direct return-to-work services.
4. An emphasis on timely reports and communication and collaboration with referral sources and payors (2).

The measure of successful pain center treatment has increasingly become the return of the worker to the workplace. In some cases especially insurance carriers responsible for the injured worker now see this as virtually the sole measure of treatment success. With the proliferation of pain management services over the past decade, the need to address this issue by developing a valid profile of which patients are most likely to return to work has arisen. Although we understand and support the insurance carrier's focus on closing claims and work returns, we still must be concerned with helping patients with CPS achieve a better overall quality of life.

CONCLUSION

Assisting individuals to return to productivity can provide patients with a positive distraction from pain. This may account in part for the phenomenon whereby individuals so often perceive pain as worse during the night than at other times. Interaction with the therapeutic community of fellow patients within the MPC helps many to focus less on their pain and in general, somatize less than prior to admission. One of the goals of the pain program is to help patients incorporate these values and techniques into activities of daily living during the program and after discharge.

A person's support system, that is, what he or she will return home to and whether the home itself is a source of stress and anxiety or of comfort, is extremely important. The sounder the support system, the less the suffering component of his or her pain may be. I have found that many of the patients treated in the inpatient pain program did well while hospitalized in a structured program, insulated from the life stressors of home or work, and often denied the existence of these problems. Many of these conflicts become somatized, and it can be anticipated that individuals who do not deal with these life stressors may manifest increased physical and psychological symptoms upon return to their stressful environments at home or work. Those who adequately address these life stressors as part of the pain program find alternative coping mechanisms. Some actually resolve various life stressors and continue to do well following discharge. Recidivism is then significantly less, as manifested by various measures, such as reliance on the health care delivery system, use of analgesic and sedative-hypnotic medications, and self-reports of functioning. Treating these patients in a structured outpatient setting has encouraged patients to incorporate the necessary problem solving into their treatment programs and lifestyles on an ongoing basis.

Certainly, some persons, for medical or psychiatric reasons, cannot return to any type of employment; however, they are in the minority. I have treated a number of persons who upon admission presented letters claiming total and permanent disability or who had been told by physicians that they would be unable to engage in specific physical or work activities. At the conclusion of their pain program, they were able to resume many of their formerly abandoned activities. All too often, the traditional health care system fosters disability or creates it iatrogenically.

Many studies suggest that chronic pain continues to be a major cause of patients seeking disability status, with disability for low-back pain said to be increasing at approximately 14 times the population growth in the U.S. It is apparent that we have far to go in our understanding of pain and suffering as it affects our patients' social roles. Although the biomedical model for chronic pain assessment has been appropriately changing to a biomedical-psychosocial model, many of our colleagues still refuse to accept that pain medicine is as much an art as a science.

Although physicians and other health care providers cannot unilaterally change social prejudices against hiring handicapped or elderly persons, our reports can more clearly reflect not only the factors that emphasize the amount of physical impairment, but also the residual capacities and capabilities of the individual and any other factors that will help create a fair disability hearing. In so doing, we are benefiting the patient by helping him to retain a sense of purpose and self-worth and to decrease pain–related suffering and disability (3).

References

1. Aronoff G M, Evans W A. Evaluation and treatment of chronic pain at the Boston Pain Center. J Clin Psychiatr 1982;43:47.
2. Schwartz G E, Watson S D, Galvin D E, Lipoff E. The disability management sourcebook, vol. 6. Washington Business Group on Health and Institute for Rehabilitation and Disability Management, fall 1989.
3. Aronoff G M. Clin J Pain 1985;1:13 (editorial).
4. Aronoff G M. The role of the pain center in the treatment of intractable suffering and disability from chronic pain. Semin Neurol 1983;3:377–381.
5. Bonica J J. Report of the panel on pain to the national advisory neurological and communicative disorders and strobe council. Pub 811912. Washington: National Institutes of Health, 1980;4.
6. Aronoff G M, McAlary P W. Organization and function of the multidisciplinary pain center. In: Aronoff, G M, ed. Pain centers: a revolution in health care. New York: Raven Press, 1988;55.
7. Aronoff G M, McAlary P W. Organization and personnel functions in the pain clinic. In: Ghia J N, Raj P P, eds. Organization, personnel functions and pain management in the multidisciplinary pain center clinic. Current management of pain. Boston: Martinus Nijoff, 1988.
7a. Aronoff G M. The role of the pain center. In: Aronoff G M, ed. Evaluation and treatment of chronic pain. 1st ed. Baltimore: Urban & Scharzenberg, 1985; 507–509.
8. Aronoff G M, Wagner J M. The pain center: development, structure and dynamics. In: Burrows, Elton, Stanley, eds. Handbook of chronic pain management. New York: Elsevier, 1987;407, 424.
8a. Aronoff G M, Wagner J M. Pain centers: a community resource. In: Mediguide to pain, vol 7. New York: Delacorte Press, 1986;12.
9. Bonica J J. Evolution of multidisciplinary and interdisciplinary pain programs in pain centers. In: Aronoff, G M, ed. Pain centers: a revolution in health care. New York: Raven Press, 1988;55.
10. Crue B L, Pinsky J J. Chronic pain syndrome: four aspects of the problem. New Hope Pain Center and Pain Research Foundation. In: Lorenz and Ng KY, eds. NIDA research monograph series. Rockville, MD: NIDA, 1981;37.
11. Khoury G, Varga C A. Does frequency of utilization of nerve blocks in pain clinic vary with the specialty of the director? Pain 1988;33:265.
12. Aronoff G M, Evans W O, Enders P L. A review of follow up studies of multidisciplinary pain units. Pain 1983;16:1.
13. Painter J R, Seres J L, Newman R I. Assessing benefits of the pain center: why some patients regress. Pain 1980;8:101.
14. Wang J K, Ilstrup D M, Nauss L A, et al. Outpatient pain clinic: a longterm followup study. Minn Med 1980;63(9):663–666.
15. Turk D C. Efficacy of multidisciplinary pain centers in the treatment of chronic pain. In: Cohen M J M, Campbell J N, eds. Pain treatment centers at a crossroads: a practical and conceptual reappraisal. Progress in pain research and management, vol 7. Seattle: IASP Press, 1996; 257–274.
16. Cutler R B, Fishbain D A, Rosomoff H L, et al. Does nonsurgical pain center treatment of chronic pain return patients to work? Spine 1994;19:643–652.
17. Fishbain D A, Rosomoff H L, Cutler R B, Rosomoff R S. Do pain patients' perceptions about their preinjury jobs determine their intent to return to the same type of job post–pain facility treatment? Clin J Pain 1995;11:267–278.
18. Aronoff G M, McAlary P W, Witkower A, Berdell M S. Pain treatment programs: do they return workers to the workplace? Spine State Art Rev 1987;2:123–136.
19. Aronoff G M. What is happening to medicine? Clin J Pain 1988; 4:65–66 (editorial).
20. Cicala R S, Wright H. Outpatient treatment of patients with chronic pain: an analysis of cost savings. Clin J Pain 1989.
21. Aronoff G M. Pain treatment: is it a right or a privilege? Clin J Pain 1986;1:18788 (editorial).

22. Strang J P. The chronic disability syndrome. In: Aronoff G M, ed. The evaluation and treatment of chronic pain. 1st ed. Baltimore: Urban & Schwartzenberg, 1985.

23. Brena S F, Chapman S L. The learned pain syndrome. Postgrad Med 1981;69:5362.

24. Brena S F, Chapman S L. Pain and litigation. In: Wall P D, and Melzack R, eds. Textbook of pain. New York: Churchill Livingstone, 1984;832–839.

25. Weinstein M R. The concept of the disability process. Psychosomatics 1978;19:94–97.

26. Ellard J. Psychological reactions to compensable injury. Med J Aust 1970;349–355.

27. Bigos S J, Battie M C, Spengler D M, et al. A Longitudinal prospective study of industrial back injury reporting. Clin Orthop 1992;279:21–34.

28. Fordyce W, Bigos S, Battie M, Fisher L. MMPI Scale 3 as a predictor of back injury report: what does it tell us? Clin J Pain 1992;8:222–226.

29. Waddell G, Newton M, Henderson I, et al. A fear–avoidance beliefs questionnaire (FABQ) and the role of fear–avoidance in chronic low back pain and disability. Pain, 1993;52:157–168.

30. Seres J S, Newman R I. Negative influences of the disability compensation system: perspectives for the clinician. Semin Neurol 1983;3:4.

31. McGill C M. Industrial back problems: a control program. J Occup Med 1968;10:174–178.

32. Waddell G. The epidemiology of back pain. In: Clinical Standards Advisory Group. The epidemiology and cost of back pain. Annex to the clinical standards advisory group's report on back pain. London: HMSO, 1994;1–64.

33. Brena S F, Chapman S L. Chronic pain states: their relationship to impairment and disability. Arch Phys Med Rehab 1979;60:387–389.

34. Aronoff G M, McAlary P W. Multidisciplinary treatment of intractable chronic pain syndromes. Adv Pain Res Ther 1990;13:270.

34a. Aronoff G M. The disability epidemic. Clin J Pain 1989;5:203–204 (editorial).

35. United States Department of Health and Human Services. Report of the Commission on the evaluation of pain. In: Osterweis M, Kleinman A, Mechanic D, eds. Pain and disability. Washington: National Academy Press, 1987.

35a. Institute of Medicine. Conflicts and contraindications in the disability program. In: Pain and disability. Washington: National Academy Press, 1987;7071.

36. Richman S I. The conflicting social objectives underlying the confusion. Chest 1980;78(Suppl):367–369.

37. Newman R I, Seres J L, Yospe L P, Garlington B. Multidisciplinary treatment of chronic pain: long term follow up of low back patients. Pain 1978;4:283.

38. American Medical Association. Guides to the evaluation of permanent impairment. 4th ed. Chicago: AMA.1993.

39. Ziporyn T L. Disability evaluation: a fledgling science? JAMA 1983; 250(7):873–880.

40. Snook S H et al. A. Study of three preventative approaches to low back injury. J Occup Med 1978;20:478–481.

41. Carron H. Compensation aspects of low back claims. In: Carron H, McLaughlin R E, eds. Management of low back pain. Boston: PSG, 1982.

42. Leavitt S S, Beyer R D, Johnston T L. Monitoring the recovery process: pilot results of a systematic approach to case management. Med Surg 1972;41:25–30.

43. Brena S F, Turk D C. Vocational disability: a challenge to pain rehabilitation programs. In: Aronoff G M, ed. Pain centers: a revolution in health care. New York: Raven Press, 1988.

44. Catchlove R, Cohen K. Effects of a directive return to work approach in the treatment of workers compensation patients with chronic pain. Pain 1982;14:181191.

44a. Waddell G et al. Failed lumbar disc surgery following industrial injuries. J Bone Joint Surg 1979;61:201–207.

44b. Leavitt F, Garron D C, McNeill T W, Whisler W W. Organic status, psychological disturbance and pain report characteristics in low back patients on compensation. Spine 1982;7(4):398–402.

45. Dworkin R H, Handlin D S, Richlin D M, et al. Unraveling the effects of compensation, litigation, and employment on treatment response in chronic pain. Pain 1985;23:4959.

46. Peck J C, Fordyce W E, Black. The effect of pendency of claims for compensation upon behavior indicative of pain. Wash Law Rev 1978;53:257–278.

47. Addison R G. Treatment of chronic pain: The Center for Pain Studies Rehabilitation Institute of Chicago. In: Ng L K, ed. New approaches to treatment of chronic pain: a review of multidisciplinary pain clinics and pain centers. pp. NIDA Research Monograph. Rockville, MD: NIDA, 1981;1232.

48. Chapman S L, Bradford L A. Treatment outcome of a chronic pain rehabilitation program. Pain 1981;11:255.

49. Malec J, Cayner J J, Harvey R F. Pain management: long term follow up of an inpatient program. Arch Phys Med Rehab 1981;62:369.

50. Vasudevan S V, Lynch N T, Abram S. Effectiveness of an ambulatory chronic pain management program. Pain 1981;1(Suppl):S272.

51. Podobnakar I G, MacIntosh S. Pain center: a cost–effective approach to the treatment of chronic pain due to industrial injury. Pain 1981;1:S195.

52. Meilman P W, Skultety F M, Guck T P, Sullivan K. Benign chronic pain: 18 month to ten year follow up of a multidisciplinary pain unit treatment program, Clin J Pain 1985;1:131.

53. Guck T P, Skultety F M, Meilman P W, Dowdy E T. Multidisciplinary follow up study: evaluation with a no treatment control group. Pain 1985;21:295.

54. Roberts A H, Reinhardt L. The behavioral management of chronic pain: long term follow up with comparison groups. Pain 1980;8:151.

CHAPTER 42

Functional Performance Evaluation in Patients with Chronic Pain

Karen S. Rucker and Michael D. West

Thousands of persons' lives are disrupted every day because of functional limitations caused by chronic pain. According to a poll of Americans, one quarter of adults report having pain strong enough to interfere with their daily activities every month (1). While pain can be debilitating, it can also be costly, causing more than $55 billion a year in lost work days (2).

Across the country, the functional performance evaluation (FPE) has become big business with rehabilitation programs and physical therapy groups. They are used for a number of purposes, including (*a*) to predict ability to return to a former job, (*b*) for preemployment testing for potential jobs, and (*c*) for determination of functional limitations for compensation purposes.

Functional performance evaluations are intended to measure a person's performance of specific tasks and from this viewed performance to predict ability to perform those specific tasks and related tasks, usually in a work environment. There is great variation in the tasks measured, the names of the evaluations, the length of time over which performance is evaluated, the qualifications of the evaluator, and the use of the data produced. There is no nationally accepted standardized functional capacity evaluation. A large number of published tests evaluate a wide and diverse range of abilities, from psychosocial, cognitive, and sensory skills (vision, hearing, smelling) to physical tests of strength, mobility, flexibility, and ability to perform specific physical tasks. There is considerable variability in the ways function is assessed and reported: self-report, observed performance, predicted performance based on examination and evaluation and so on.

A worldwide literature search funded by the Social Security Administration (SSA) and conducted by Virginia Commonwealth University/Medical College of Virginia's Department of Physical Medicine and Rehabilitation in 1996 identified more than 600 function-related evaluations from 20 countries (3). While many of the functional assessment rating scales, such as the Functional Independence Measure (FIM) and the Patient Evaluation Conference System (PECS) included a broad array of functional indicators, none could adequately assess function as it relates to all types of physical, cognitive, and psychiatric impairments. It is significant that the majority of functional assessment instruments relied upon self-report of symptoms. As will be discussed later in this chapter, self-report assessments frequently do not agree with more objective measures, such as observing the patient and results of physical examinations.

While a number of the instruments reviewed effectively correlate clinical measures with a person's ability to perform various activities and tasks, efforts to assess functional capacity are hampered by various methodological shortcomings. For example, validation strategies rely extensively upon concurrent validity approaches, correlating the outcomes of a particular measure with those of related measures. Instruments that have undergone extensive examinations of their content or predictive validity generally correlated clinical measures with "rehabilitation outcomes," typically improved activities of daily living or improvement in the person's health status at discharge. The relation of these criterion variables to the process of determining whether a person can engage in substantial gainful activity has not been sufficiently documented across the spectrum of functional assessment instruments and should be a focus of further research.

Outside of academia, where the tough questions must be answered or at least an educated guess given regarding a person's ability to perform certain tasks, a bevy of function-related performance evaluations are done every day in an effort to answer the questions of employers, insurance companies, doctors, and disability companies. There is no gold standard because measuring and predicting ability to perform specific tasks are limited and influenced by many factors that are very difficult to control. Pope (4) identified many of these factors that can lead to significant variability in the outcome of functional testing (Table 42.1).

Complicating the issue further is the many inconsistent terms used for functional evaluations. What is done for an FPE in one city may be very different from what is done in another city or even from another provider of services in the same area. It is imperative to determine as specifically as possible what information is needed from the testing. Does one need to know whether a person can perform a specific job safely, specific tasks once, or specific tasks consistently and repetitively over time? Or is more general information on what a person can do needed to assist in making recommendations about job types? The focus of this chapter is on FPEs, which are used to assess and predict the performance of a person with chronic pain and chronic pain syndrome.

Chronic pain has had its greatest effect on the working age population, ages 18 to 60, costing billions of dollars in medical care, lost work days, and disability pay. Yet despite its increasing medical and economic cost, many aspects of pain assessment and treatment remain unclear (5).

The sensation of pain is subjective and therefore not directly measurable. Thus the inability to identify specific organic pathology in many patients with persistent pain, continued reports of pain following the correction of pathological conditions, and continued complaints of pain following the expected period of resolution of an injury have led to a lack of consensus about basic definitions and inconsistencies in measurement and assessment techniques (5, 6). Musculoskeletal pain, particularly in the back and neck, is one of the most common, most expensive, and most functionally limiting of all chronic pain problems.

Studies have shown that there is no way to prove or disprove the presence of pain in a particular person (7) and that pain is inferred by way of both verbal and nonverbal expressions or actions, called pain behaviors. Fordyce (8) lists these behaviors as verbal complaints of pain and suffering; nonlanguage sounds such as moans and sighs; body posturing and gesturing, including limping, rubbing painful body part or area; and displays of functional limitations or disability, such as reclining for excessive periods. Other pain behaviors, such as the frequent reliance upon the health care system by those seeking medical consultation, excessive use of nonessential medications, multiple surgeries, therapy, and work disability have also been noted (7, 9). These pain behaviors are influenced not by the pathological process identified but often by the effects of naturally occurring learning processes and social reinforcement (10).

Because chronic pain patients demonstrate large individual differences in response to injury, many believe that these pain behaviors should be the focus of assessment and treatment, rather than the subjective pain reports that are often used (5). Pain behaviors, it is suggested, may offer a more objective assessment of responses referring to pain than patients' self-reports, which may be purposely distorted or at a minimum, inaccurate. One measure of functional limitations from pain

Table 42.1.   Possible Sources of Variability in Functional Testing

Discomfort
Pain
Medications
Drugs, alcohol
Other health conditions
Malingering
Gender
Body weight
Learning effect
Motivation
Height
Fatigue
Obesity
Strength
Range of motion
Fitness
Fear of injury
Psychosocial issues

Adapted from Pope MH. Clinical efficacy and outcome in the diagnosis and treatment of low back pain. New York: Raven Press, 1982.

are measures of the patient's concentration and cognitive processes, activities of living, emotional status, and functional abilities as perceived by the patient and physicians (6).

With the disclaimer that the same titles of evaluations may not reflect the same evaluations, there follow some general guidelines of what should be expected from FPEs in general. It is the responsibility of the person ordering the evaluation to determine whether the test will measure what is desired, taking into account that there is a lack of standardized, reliable, and valid tests.

For the purposes of this chapter, the term functional performance evaluation (FPE) will be used, and it is recommended as a permanent change in the nomenclature of functional performance testing. In the early 1990s at a National Institutes of Health (NIH) conference on chronic pain in persons with physical disabilities, it was emphasized that the appropriate term should be functional performance evaluation. The stated reason for this is that as clinicians, we can only *evaluate* what a person is *willing* and *able* to do at *a single point in time* as opposed to what a person is *capable* of doing.

UNDERSTANDING THE TERMINOLOGY

Since the introduction of functional performance testing, various terms have been used interchangeably to identify the same test, including functional capacity assessments, functional abilities assessments, functional capacity evaluation, etc. Because of this confusion in terminology, these individual tests do not always reflect the areas being assessed (10). This is often due to the labels being applied inappropriately, such as screening versus assessment versus evaluation; capacities versus abilities; and functional versus physical versus work-related (11). It is important then, that the distinction among these terms be made when ordering, performing, and interpreting assessments.

Screening versus Assessment versus Evaluation

A *screening* evaluation can be an assessment to identify general status and assist the physician in referring persons to the appropriate treatment or rehabilitation program. It is based on interviews or tests that are designed according to skills. An *assessment* is an investigation of the abilities, or strengths, and limitations, or weaknesses of a particular body function and comparison to expected levels, that is, the norm. An *evaluation* is simply a measurement appraisal process designed to find values or amounts that describe performance levels (11).

Capacity versus Ability

The distinction between capacity and ability also is important. *Capacity* is the limits of the anatomical, physiological, and psychological systems of the person. These capacities depend on gender, age, body type, and so on. *Ability,* on the other hand, reflects human capacities as modified by individual behavioral attitudes, in addition to external factors such as injury, pain, and environmental and social stressors (11).

Physical versus Functional versus Work-Related Factors

Understanding the differences among physical, functional, and work-related attributes is also very important to the complete comprehension of functional performance testing. For these purposes, *physical* attributes include static and dynamic muscular strength, flexibility, mobility, alertness, steadiness, gait, balance, posture, coordination, and muscular and cardiovascular endurance. *Functional* measures include sitting, standing, walking, kneeling squatting, lifting, carrying, pushing, pulling, and manual dexterity. *Work-related* factors are demands that are specific to the job or occupation in question, such as frequently lifting 50 lb (11).

TYPES OF FUNCTIONAL PERFORMANCE EVALUATIONS

Functional performance evaluations are viewed as a means of testing such parameters as lifting and carrying capability, positional tolerance, general endurance level, and ability to lift to certain heights. Work capacity testing tends to be more job specific and requires more assessment in actual job task simulation to be truly appropriate. The primary distinctions are cost and time spent in testing (12).

A typical functional performance test is performed over 2 days for a total of 4 to 6 hours. By breaking the test into 2 days, the evaluator allows for follow-up response from the patient regarding the demands of the previous day's testing. Work capacity requires more time, approximately 1 week. Several types of evaluations have been described in the area of human performance testing (11).

Physical Capacity Evaluation

The physical capacity evaluation measures the maximum levels of physical performance of the person, such as maximum weight that can be lifted, number of stairs climbed, and number of times reaching overhead. These measurements in turn assess fundamental parameters such as strength, flexibility, and endurance.

Functional Abilities Assessment

The functional abilities assessment addresses the acceptable level of performance at a certain point in time and usually produces data regarding parameters such as lifting, carrying, walking, and standing. The patient is not pushed to a maximum performance level.

Work-Related Assessments

Work-related assessments test the person's ability to meet or exceed the physical demands of the work with specific reference to a job and the tasks involved (duration, load, repetition, and so on). These assessments measure the level at which a worker must perform to safely meet job demands. Among these demands are standing, walking, sitting, lifting, carrying, pushing, pulling, climbing, balancing, stooping, kneeling, crouching, crawling, reaching, handling, fingering, feeling, talking, hearing, and seeing. These factors are the elements of this type of assessment. Various work-related assessments are described below and the more commonly used ones are summarized in Table 42.2.

Work Capacity Evaluation

The work capacity evaluation is a series of tests that can vary from several consecutive days to daily over 2 weeks. It is geared to measure the worker's ability to handle material, such as lifting, carrying, pushing, and pulling; to tolerate sustained postures such as sitting, standing, walking, crouching, and climbing; and to do repetitive activities such as bending, reaching, and squatting. It should combine measurements of strength, endurance, and flexibility with knowledge of proper posture and body mechanics and give some indication of the worker's effort, cooperation, and receptiveness to instruction. These tests are typically strenuous and expensive evaluations (13). Brief, limited work capacity evaluations can be used to assess a worker's functional ability prior to initiation of a rehabilitation or work-hardening program. This gives a baseline from which to compare and help identify areas at risk for reinjury.

Work Tolerance Screening

The work tolerance screen is geared to reflect specific critical job requirements. It requires performance of simulated activities in the same sequence and frequency that they would

Table 42.2.   Components of Commonly Used Work-Related Evaluations

Work tolerance screening
  Performance of simulated activities reflecting critical job requirements
  Requires performance in same sequence and frequency as job
  Typically a 4-day assessment
  Requires detailed job description
  Difficult to duplicate extrinsic factors such heat, glare, stress
Fitness for duty
  Assesses ability to perform critical job requirements
  For worker off only short time
  Useful for workers in hazardous jobs
Work hardening
  Progressively increases worker's physical ability to accomplish job
    requirements or maximize ability
  Rehabilitation of entire body as well as specific injury
  Includes instruction in posture and body mechanics
  Daily progression in hours, i.e. from 3–4 hours to 6–8 hours
  Length of time usually 3 weeks
  Can use in conjunction with light duty or part-time work
Work Conditioning
  1 to 2 hr/day, 3 to 5 days/week
  General conditioning exercises
  Some specific return to work activities
  May precede work hardening
On-site Job Analysis
  To determine whether job description accurately reflects job responsibilities
  Assessment of equipment and supplies
  Measurement of number and height of lifts, bends, and reaches
  Assess other factors such as uneven ground, work area congestion,
    awkward equipment

be performed on the job. Several days are required for an adequate evaluation. The work tolerance screening is thought to be the best test to assess whether a worker can return to the specific job because the actual number of repetitions and postures are performed over several consecutive days (13). If the worker is deemed unable to return to his previous employment, a work tolerance screening can be used to assess a person's ability to do other work. A specific job description is critical to maximize the usefulness of these evaluations. However, it is difficult to duplicate all the factors of a job, such as environmental factors of temperature, noise, distractions, and stress (13).

Fitness for Duty

This is usually a 2- to 4-hour evaluation during which the worker performs only the critical job requirements. It is used for the worker who has been out of work only for a short time and is thought by the physician to be ready to return to work (13).

Work Hardening

Work hardening is a treatment program, not an evaluation, designed to increase the worker's physical ability until he or she reaches critical job requirements or maximum physical ability. Through the use of functional activities, this program requires rehabilitation of the entire body. This also allows for instruction and reinforcement in proper lifting techniques and use of proper body mechanics to prevent reinjury (13).

Initially the worker performs the motions required by the job but at a reduced weight. As strength and technique improve, the weight is increased. The program typically is daily, starting at 3 to 4 hours a day and progressing to 6 to 8 hours a day. It should be an individualized program that reflects the critical job requirements. Work hardening usually lasts 3 weeks; however, the duration is determined by the initial physical condition of the worker and the critical job requirements that must be met. Communication to the therapist doing the work hardening regarding the specific performance goals is critical to prevent the patient from being required to perform activities not needed in his or her job.

Pain should not prevent a worker from participating in work hardening. The emphasis should shift from measurement of pain to measurement of function. The question should be whether the worker can perform critical job requirements without significant increase in pain rather than whether the worker is pain free. It should be noted from clinical experience that almost every patient reports increased pain when beginning work hardening and then decreasing pain levels after the first 2 weeks (13).

Work hardening is often combined with light duty and part-time work. A typical course of action is for the worker to participate in work hardening for half a day to increase his or her lifting capacity and then work half a day with the employer in an effort to increase tolerance for activity. It is very important, however, to be aware of the duties being required and performed at the job site so as to avoid both reinjury and hampering the worker's ability to continue in work hardening (13).

The physician should be provided with a report on the work hardening program outlining attendance, cooperation of the worker, the program, and the person's status in terms of reaching the critical job requirements. Ideally, this is a one- to two-page letter that lists in table form the percentage of job requirements met. It should also include recommendations for further treatment or return to work (13).

On-Site Job Analysis

Typically physicians receive a job description and are asked to make a decision as to whether or not the employee can return to that work. Frequently, these job descriptions are provided via telephone interviews or a meeting with the employer set up by the insurance company or a case manager who is not even at the actual work site. It is very important that the job description reflect the critical job requirements. A good job analysis requires a work site visit during which equipment and supplies are actually weighed and measured. The numbers of times and the distance a person must lift, bend, and reach should be identified and recorded, in addition to any other factors that might affect the worker, such as uneven ground, congested work area, or awkward equipment (13). Here, the ideal person for the on-site job analysis is one who has been specifically trained in ergonomics and job analyses.

Job site analyses allow the evaluator to see firsthand the worker's job requirements, enabling more practical and specific instructions on how to perform the job safely. Key to establishing a comprehensive job site analysis is having a detailed, quantifiable job description (13). This should include specifics regarding the rate of work, lifting requirements, and lifting frequency. Using broad terms such as occasionally or frequently and wide ranges such as 100 to 200 times does not help the evaluator to determine proper work requirements. An effective job description should also specify the level at which items are lifted and placed, for example, from waist level to the floor, from floor level to overhead. These levels are significant differences and left too vague, can result in jobs that may be dangerous.

FUNCTIONAL PERFORMANCE EVALUATIONS IN GENERAL

The FPE involves various parties, including the physician, the evaluator, and the patient. Each plays a vital role in the outcome of the FPE and consequently the selection of the treatment and rehabilitation protocol. Abdel-Moty et al (11). offer a schematic presentation of the interaction between the various entities involved in a given case referral to a functional test (Fig. 42.1).

The Physician

The physician is usually the first to examine the patient to formulate a medical diagnosis and develop an appropriate medical treatment plan. This treatment plan can include the use of exercises, physical therapy, medications, surgery, or referrals for specialty consultations, education, or counseling (14).

The physician is often asked to determine the ability of the patient to perform tasks and return to work or other daily activities. However, because this can rarely be determined via a typical medical examination, the physician may refer the patient to a functional performance evaluator. After assessing the measurements obtained through the FPE, the physician looks for any discrepancies between those findings and the medical diagnosis (14). This includes consideration of present and future pathological or biomechanical concerns of the patient that should be taken into account when the rehabilitation plan is developed.

The Functional Performance Evaluator

It is the role of the functional performance evaluator to determine the ergonomically safe level of function of the patient through objective testing (15). Objective information regarding functional performance enables the physician and rehabilitation team to design an appropriate rehabilitation protocol. The evaluator is responsible for preparing written and oral reports on the physical abilities and limitations of the

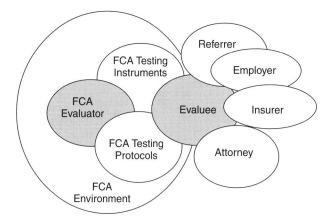

Figure 42.1. Interactions among the various entities involved in a given case referral. The evaluee and the evaluator interact through the FPE test instruments and protocols in a facility (test environment). Though slightly involved in the testing itself, the referrer may be involved with other entities, all of whom are to some some degree committed to one or more aspects of the case. FCA, functional capacity assessment. (Reprinted with permission from Abdel-Moty E, Compton R, Steele-Rosomoff R, et al. Process analysis of functional capacity assessment. J Back Musculoskeletal Rehab 1996;6:223–236.)

evaluee. This information is used in the interpretation of (*a*) true physical impairment, (*b*) functional abilities and deficits, (*c*) symptom magnification, (*d*) physical abilities versus physical demands of a potential job, (*e*) need for further treatment, and (*f*) options for continued rehabilitation (14).

It is essential that the evaluator thoroughly understand the neuromusculoskeletal system. This includes muscle, nerve, soft tissue, and bone physiology, along with normal and dysfunctional characteristics of each. Kinesiology, pathokinesiology, and cardiopulmonary implications are necessary in the evaluation of dynamic movements. The physical therapist and orthopaedically trained occupational therapist most often have this professional preparation (14).

The Occupational and Physical Therapist

Occupational and physical therapists specializing in the prevention and management of chronic diseases do possess the perspective and expertise to evaluate and make recommendations to the physician regarding the patient's functional capabilities and where applicable, return-to-work potential (16). With this expertise, combined with comprehensive training in anatomy, kinesiology, biomechanics, ergonomics, and task analysis, physical and occupational therapists can (*a*) understand the existing pathology; (*b*) analyze the worker's job and identify biomechanically unsound tasks that may have contributed to the pathology; (*c*) provide conservative treatment in conjunction with a primary treating physician; (*d*) facilitate on a gradual basis return to function (restoration of range of motion, coordination, strength, and endurance) after surgery; (*e*) identify the level of work capacity at any point during or after medical rehabilitation and factors interfering with achievement of optimal work capacity; (*f*) offer solutions to improve function and work capacity through 7 task and tool modifications; (*g*) expediently but not prematurely plan with the worker, physician, and employer the return of the worker to biomechanically sound work; and (*h*) monitor the worker's condition after he or she has returned to work (17).

The Patient

The primary role of the patient (evaluee) in the FPE is voluntary and active participation in his or her own rehabilitation (14). To do this, the patient must understand in layman's terms why the FPE is being performed, including perceived benefits and outcomes. The patient is to be informed of all treatments recommended and delivered to him or her prior to initiation of the treatment (18). With this knowledge the patient will be able to make an informed decision concerning compliance with the rehabilitation plan. The patient has the right to refuse any treatment; however, if compensation benefits are an issue, they may be terminated or suspended as determined by law.

FACTORS AFFECTING FUNCTIONAL PERFORMANCE EVALUATIONS

FPEs are primarily conducted as the result of a person's report that he or she is disabled or impaired and unable to return to work. The patients among whom this issue is most common are those who report that their chronic pain is restricting them from returning to their previous employment or to any employment at all (5). Chronic pain and chronic pain syndrome complicate the assessment of functional performance immensely because of the variability of ways pain affects persons, the inability to measure pain, the many psychosocial factors that accompany pain, fear of increasing pain, fear of injury or reinjury, the effects of single efforts versus repetitive efforts on pain, and the effect of effort exerted over time on pain. Because of the chronicity of their condition, these patients present for an FPE with considerable environmental, psychosocial, and behavioral factors that can influence their conduct during the evaluation (5).

Environmental Factors

Because rehabilitation involves such a wide array of parties, including physicians, the functional performance examiner, third-party payors, employers, attorneys, case managers, and family members, this multitude of outside influences can play a significant role in the success or failure of the rehabilitation effort. These same parties can also affect the outcome of the FPE, as outlined below.

The Physician

Physicians often look to the results of an FPE to assist them in making a decision regarding a patient's treatment,

rehabilitation, and ultimately, his or her functional capacity. Thus, the expressed or implied expectations of use of the results of the FPE may directly influence the examiner's selection of tests as well as the presentation and interpretation of the results (5). Further, advice and/or restrictions placed on the patient by the physician may affect the amount of effort expended during the FPE and the patient's willingness to attempt certain functional tasks. The physician should communicate to the evaluator the purpose of the assessment and any specific questions to which they are seeking answers.

The Third-Party Payor

Another significant influence, and one that continues to grow, is the insurance company and other third-party payors. It is this group that is responsible for payment of the medical care, including the FPE, while also pushing for cost containment and case closure (5). In addition, the rehabilitation consultant, who is often hired by the insurance company, is commonly responsible for managing the evaluation process in chronic pain cases and determining the person's ability to return to work. With this goal in mind, the rehabilitation consultant may already have formed impressions of the patient's functional abilities or limitations well before the FPE referral and may seek to obtain information needed to test his or her own hypotheses (5).

The Employer

Employers can also have a significant influence on the outcome of FPEs. Depending upon the relationship between employee and employer and the employee's belief about the future health of the company (e.g., pending layoffs, restructuring), these factors can significantly influence the patient's performance on the FPE (5). This relationship can influence the employee's desire or lack of desire to return to work. It is helpful for the physician and evaluator to be aware of the employer-employee relationship.

The Attorney

When the employee-employer relation is questioned because of mistrust of the employer, observations of previous cases at the company, or a question of liability related to the injury, complex litigation and other legal issues are an important factor that may affect the outcome of FPEs (5). Unfortunately, attorneys often coach their clients on how to behave and what to say during the FPE because they believe there is opportunity for financial restitution. This in turn can affect the patient's performance indirectly and directly. Again, it is important for the evaluator to be aware of these issues, which can influence performance and interpretation of the assessment.

Test-Specific Factors

Subjective versus Objective Measurements

Clinical research suggests that self-report assessments of status frequently do not agree with more objective measures, such as observations or physical examinations of the patient (19). Many persons either underreport or exaggerate their symptoms for a number of reasons. For example, underreporting may occur because patients believe they are actually getting better when they are simply accepting or adjusting to their new, diminished status. Or they may underreport symptoms in acquiescence to the examiner, as a defense mechanism, or simply because they have unrealistic beliefs about their condition. As will be discussed later, exaggeration of symptoms may result from a desire to receive assistance or rehabilitative services that might otherwise be unavailable. Although self-report instruments have a number of advantages, including economy of time and expense (3), the potential for misrepresentation cannot be disregarded.

The Functional Performance Evaluator

The evaluator's determination of his or her role in the FPE is often guided by the environmental factors discussed earlier. For example, referral sources, including insurance companies and attorneys, can exert considerable influence on the examiner regarding preconceived opinions of the patient's capabilities or legitimacy of his or her symptoms (5). In addition, an examiner who has had previous contact with the patient and is aware of his or her functional abilities may deviate from the testing protocol to confirm an impression. Thus the attitudes and behaviors of the evaluator can have a significant influence on the evaluation, including test selection, test administration, interpretation of the data, and reporting of the results (5).

The amount of experience the evaluator has with a specific type of assessment (standardization or lack thereof, use of normative data, and so on) affects the conduct of the test and the interpretation of the results. After considerable use, some examiners begin to personalize and adapt the test to their own preferences and expertise, often invalidating the results and eliminating the opportunity to collect standardized data (5).

Most important, the evaluator's own beliefs about pain and how it is expressed determine how observed behaviors are interpreted. Likewise, if the examiner believes that a patient is providing his or her best effort, pain complaints during the testing may be taken more seriously; but if the patient is viewed as deliberately faking or exaggerating the pain, the examiner's attitudes and the how the FPE is conducted also change (5).

The Testing Protocol

Testing procedures can be significantly influenced by examiner bias. This can involve a rephrasing of instructions by the examiner based on his or her familiarity with the patient. Likewise, patients look to the evaluator to decide when they

Table 42.3.   Task-Specific End points and General End points

Task-specific end points: Technique
  Shortness of breath
  Dizziness
  Pause between repetitions> 7 seconds
  Decreasing weight
General end points
  Psychophysical: voluntary test termination
  Aerobic: achievement of 85% of age-determined maximum heart rate
  Safety: anthropometric safe limit or 55–60% of body weight
  Completion of maximum repetitions

Adapted from Mayer TG, Gatchel RJ. Functional restoration for spinal disorders: the sports medicine approach. Philadelphia: Lea & Febiger, 1988.

should stop the testing with comments such as my back is hurting; do you want me to keep going? If the examiner is being cautious, possibly for medicolegal reasons, he or she may indicate to the patient that it is okay to stop the task. Conversely, if the examiner is suspicious of the patient's effort, he or she may push the patient to do more. It is important for the evaluator to recognize that subtle but very influential cues by the examiner, including simple changes in voice tone or facial expressions, can significantly alter the verbal message being given to patients (5). Evaluators should use consistent task-specific end points and general end points to avoid deviating from the test protocol. Examples of these end points are found in Table 42.3.

Rating the intensity of pain is a common component in the evaluation of persons reporting pain (5). However, the relevance of these reports become less significant when dealing with chronic pain patients because other factors enter the picture, including emotional distress and depression, which may influence the level of pain perceived (20). Since many chronic pain patients tend to focus heavily on their pain, continual questions about pain during testing may negatively influence patients' performance by directing their attention to the pain (5). Standardized cheerleading responses should be used: "Let's keep trying," "Do the best you can," and "Can you continue?" The evaluator should use each statement once per task.

Psychosocial and Behavioral Factors

It should be recognized that many characteristics specific to the individual patient can influence the results of the functional capacity test. Many of these characteristics involve the role of behavioral and/or psychosocial factors, including self-efficacy expectations, fear-induced avoidance of activity, interpretation of meaning of pain (supposed to live with it versus creating more injury), and litigation.

A self-efficacy expectation is a personal conviction that one can successfully perform certain behaviors in a given situation (21). A negative perception of physical capabilities leads to failure to perform the activities because of these perceptions of incapacity, creating a vicious circle (22).

Furthermore, the fear of pain is strong enough to make many chronic pain patients avoid situations or behaviors that they believe will cause them further harm. These already formed expectations of what activities will cause harm guide their choice of what activities will be attempted and with how much effort and what activities will be avoided (5). Avoidance learning therefore reduces the opportunity to disprove these expectations, creating a vicious circle. Thus, the motor impairment seen in many chronic pain patients is due in part to the patient's avoidance of certain types of motor activity because of expectations of pain (5).

These factors, and other psychosocial factors, are thought to have a substantial influence on patients' performance on functional capacity tests. This presents a challenge to the evaluator, who often, as a physical or occupational therapist, is not trained in or even comfortable with evaluating psychosocial factors. Nevertheless, Rudy et al. (5) suggest that these factors should be addressed, because failure to do so limits the therapist's ability to understand the scope of the problems contributing to the patient's disability as well as the ability to achieve maximal outcomes. However, to address psychosocial factors appropriately, psychometrically sound instruments must be used. This is not to suggest the use of comprehensive and costly psychological assessments; rather, the examiner should use brief, cost-effective psychosocial screening instruments and be trained in interpretation of data obtained from the instrument (5). Then, if significant psychosocial factors are found during the screening, referral to a psychologist may be warranted.

The functional performance evaluator must recognize the importance of psychosocial and/or behavioral factors that can influence the results of the testing being performed. This includes understanding that people respond to stimuli, observe the results of their behavior, and then present, transform, and categorize these stimuli in idiosyncratic fashion, thus determining some of the stimuli they experience and playing a vital role in guiding patients' responses to their overall condition and to the evaluation process in particular (5).

Sincerity of Effort

It is difficult in general to predict a patient's performance at work or on a functional evaluation. It is even more complicated when a patient reacts inappropriately or magnifies his or her symptoms. In a pain study at Virginia Commonwealth University's Medical College of Virginia in Richmond, funded by the Social Security Administration (23), a very broad sample of patients (18%) were thought by the physician to have an exaggerated response or magnified symptoms. These same physicians were asked to predict what type of effort the patient would give if a functional capacity evaluation was performed. It was interesting to find that physicians predicted that of these patients, 40% would give a maximum effort, 33% would give a moderate effort, 10% would give minimum effort, and 2.6% would give no effort at all.

Sincerity of effort is critical to the FPE (24). The main goal of functional performance testing is to identify what a patient can and cannot do from a functional perspective. The testing is based on the assumption that the evaluee will cooperate and will do his or her best when performing the various tasks involved in the test. If this cooperation does not exist, the abilities of the evaluee will be inaccurately assessed and the conclusions drawn from the evaluation will be erroneous (24).

When discussing the issue of sincerity of effort, a differentiation must be made between malingering and magnification or exaggeration of symptoms. There are many reasons chronic pain patients may magnify or exaggerate their symptoms besides the feigning of an illness or disability (19). For example, patients may magnify symptoms in an effort to gain recognition of their pain, which otherwise may not produce objective findings. They may feel a need to magnify their symptoms to be believed and to get the attention which they feel is appropriate for their suffering. In addition, patients may have a fear of pain in the area being tested and consequently avoid tasks that they perceive will bring on that pain. The recognition by the physician that a patient is magnifying or exaggerating his or her symptoms should not invalidate that patient's complaint. Instead, magnification of symptoms should provide the physician with additional information about the patient's perception of his or her problems and psychological state. In fact, magnification of symptoms may be pain behaviors in many patients, and therefore must be treated in addition to the physical findings (23).

Malingering, on the other hand, is the conscious and deliberate feigning of an illness or disability (23). It involves the fabrication of symptoms and complaints to achieve a specific goal. Many algologists, as well as representatives from the Commission on the Evaluation of Pain, believe that malingering is readily detected with appropriate medical and psychological tests.

Many behaviors can be associated with both malingering and magnification or exaggeration of symptoms, including grimacing, groaning, use of a cane, and so on. Many clinicians tend to label these behaviors as chronic pain behaviors, which is misleading because patients with either chronic or acute pain can and do use the same behaviors, sometimes on purpose to call attention to themselves or to manipulate people and situations for secondary gain (25).

Nevertheless, these behaviors can be judged as appropriate or magnified, acute or chronic, only when a complete understanding of the pathological process in a given patient is known. With this knowledge, the evaluator can make behavioral observations. Then, if a determination of malingering or magnification of symptoms is made, the evaluator can constructively confront the patient with the inconsistencies found, thus diminishing or eliminating the problem (25).

Often confirming sincerity of effort is not as simple as making behavioral observations. For various reasons, including secondary gain or fear of pain, some patients do not put forth maximum effort during functional performance testing.

To address this propensity to expend less than maximum effort, the degree of effort expended should be evaluated using grip tests, isometric strength tests, and so on. These methods are based on the assumption that people who are performing to their maximum capability give a consistent performance, while patients who perform submaximally will not (26). Specific tests using the Jamar dynamometer have proven effective in determining sincerity of effort. They are discussed later in this chapter. Other factors affecting the level of participation include the patient's perception of the effort being expended, the difficulty of the task, and the importance of the task to his or her work situation. These factors also must be taken into account by the examiner to understand the patient's performance and behavior (26).

CHARACTERISTICS OF AN EFFECTIVE FUNCTIONAL PERFORMANCE EVALUATION

What makes an effective FPE? Unfortunately, there is insufficient reliability and validity of existing FPEs, which make their application somewhat questionable and very confusing to physician and evaluator alike. Because of this lack of standardization, however, it is up to the physician and evaluator to determine which evaluation can provide the information needed to make the best decision for the patient. Various factors, including (a) safety, (b) reliability, (c) validity, (d) practicality, and (e) utility, ideally are addressed in the selection and use of any functional test (27).

Safety

No testing performed on the patient should lead to reinjury or new injury. This can be ensured by complete understanding of the patient's injury, including pathology, ergonomics of injury, and patient's understanding and use of correct techniques. In addition, FPEs should be administered only by trained personnel and under the supervision of the attending physician.

Reliability

Test scores should be dependable across evaluators, patients, and the time of day the test is administered (27). Various qualified professionals should be able to administer the FPE. The two most important methods of establishing reliability are interrater reliability and test-retest reliability (reliability of the rater) (26).

Interrater Reliability

Interrater reliability refers to the ability of a test to produce similar scores when administered by a different similarly trained evaluator (28). This is important because sometimes one therapist administers the FPE prior to the work-hardening program but a different therapist administers the test after the program is complete. Consistency must be maintained to ensure that significant differences in scores are not a result of the use of different examiners.

Test-Retest Reliability: Reliability of the Rater

This method of reliability ensures that consistency of measurements is maintained by the same examiner across time (28). This is done by determining an appropriate interval that is long enough to minimize a learning effect from the first test for both the subject and examiner but short enough that the patient's medical condition will not have changed significantly between tests (26).

Ensuring reliability also entails a system of checks and balances to detect inconsistencies and sincerity of effort, as described earlier. Instruments should not need calibration, and if they do, must be easily calibrated (27).

Validity

A measurement is considered valid if it measures the attribute it claims to measure (28). The FPE should do what it says it is going to do and should account for factors that may cause variability in a person's performance, including height, weight, gender, age, fear of injury, depression, and learning effect. The interpretation of a test score should predict or reflect the patient's performance in a target work setting, and the test must focus on primary physical job demands (27).

Different types of validity are different ways to support the attributes measured. Most important is criterion-related validity. This method compares scores from the test in question with other independent measures of the same attribute (26). There are two types of criterion-related validity.

Predictive validity measures the ability to predict future occurrences, that is, to predict return to work and at what level. For example, if FPE scores predict that a subject will be able to engage in heavy manual labor and the subject is successful in returning to a heavy manual job, the FPE demonstrates good predictive validity (26). *Concurrent validity* identifies those who are performing in a certain way in an independent setting. An example of this is FPE scores that distinguish between those who are unable to perform heavy manual labor and those who are performing heavy manual labor successfully; the FPE demonstrates good concurrent validity (26).

Practicality

Functional performance evaluations must be cost effective. We can't rely on expensive equipment and lengthy periods of administration by highly trained professionals or we are going to price ourselves right out of the market. Matheson et al. (27) define cost in terms of the direct expense of the test procedure plus the amount of time required of the patient plus the delay in providing the information derived from the procedure to the referral source. Furthermore, the equipment used should be widely available and inexpensive.

Utility

Because the need for and use of FPE results involve various parties, including physicians, payors, referral sources, and employers, the usefulness of the FPE should meet the needs of all of these parties. Therefore, the FPE should help the treating physician to determine the patient's ability to return to work; when the patient has reached his or her functional plateau; and at what functional level the patient is likely to return to work (27).

In addition to the aforementioned factors, the domains of the variables used in FPEs should be covered as comprehensively as possible. One method of determining comprehensiveness is to review how many of the U.S. Department of Labor's 20 physical demands of work (29) are addressed. However, it is not enough to use various domains. Rather, each domain should be evaluated thoroughly and produce an objective, specific, and quantifiable score, not just a pass or fail score (26). Another example of the need for a comprehensive FPE involves work tolerance screenings. If only 99% of the patient's former work activities were tested, the evaluation cannot state that the worker can perform all aspects of the job (13). Even minor requirements of the job, if not tested, should be addressed in the report as such.

In addition to meeting the aforementioned requirements of an effective FPE, the testing should be spread out over time. The FPE should take place over at least 4 days to assess the cumulative effect of increased activity to the worker's pain. This allows the examiner to identify activities that may aggravate the injury and whether the pain level decreases after completing the aggravating activity or remains consistent. It is expected that the worker's pain will increase gradually because of the nature of testing throughout the day; whether this pain continues into the next morning is the important finding (13). If the worker reports severe or incapacitating pain over the several days following testing, this suggests a poor response to activity, perhaps poor technique used, or fibromyalgia. Conversely, if the worker reports having no muscle soreness at all on the second or third day of testing, this should raise the question as to whether the patient gave a maximal effort.

THE FUNCTIONAL PERFORMANCE EVALUATION

The goal of the FPE is to measure a person's current physical abilities. To meet this goal, the objectives of an FPE are (a) to determine whether a person can safely meet the physical demands of a general category of job; (b) to quantify the physical impairment and functional performance of the injured worker; and (c) to assist in determining guidelines for the development of a vocational rehabilitation plan (14).

Choosing the Appropriate Test

When assessments are ordered, the therapist should know the goals of the evaluation so an appropriate test can be designed. The therapist should be creative, adapting the evaluation to the realistic ability of the worker and the practical resolution of the case (13). The physical therapist should have the clinical knowledge to design programs that minimize strain on the injured area.

Many evaluations are requested for persons who have been out of work 6 or more months and who will not likely return to their previous employment (13). The therapist should maintain an appropriate level of communication with the physician and/or rehabilitation counselor to determine any limitations placed upon the patient and to identify employment options available. The therapist can then design an evaluation that is useful and practical and does not require tasks outside of the critical job requirements.

Performing the wrong test at the wrong time can lead to underestimation of a worker's potential for employment or to injury of the worker, prolonging time out of work. The order of testing should be flexible to obtain maximal performance. For example, if a patient has a knee disorder, floor-to-waist lifting should be postponed until the end of the evaluation to avoid increase in pain due to aggravation of the injury (13). This may not be indicated in the report but should be told to the physician.

The safest plan would be for all injured workers whose jobs require strenuous activity to have a fitness-for-duty evaluation prior to return to work. If the worker does not pass this evaluation, a work-hardening program should be initiated to improve the areas in which the worker was unable to perform. When the worker is able to perform critical job requirements, a work tolerance screening should be performed prior to returning to the physician. If the worker has been deemed unable to return to previous employment, a vocational evaluation may be done to identify more appropriate job types. The work-hardening program could then focus on alternatives for employment and again, discharge of the patient when critical job requirements can be performed (13). If a worker complains of reinjury or a new injury, the physical therapist should be able to recognize the problem and refer him or her in a timely manner to the physician for evaluation and further treatment, preventing delays in treatment or increased injury (13).

Test Components

Although there is great variation in the realm of functional performance testing, as has been demonstrated in this chapter, several essential components are shown to be effective methods of assessing a patient's functional limitations.

Medical History

Information with regard to the specific injury is obtained from medical records and interviews with the patient. Initial questions should include how the injury occurred and what residual deficits were sustained as a result of the incident. The therapist should become familiar with the treatment course thus far that pertains to this particular injury, including the level of relief, if any, provided by this treatment. Assessment of cardiovascular risk factors should also be performed at this stage.

Following these questions, the therapist should attempt to identify how the patient views his or her own injury and subsequent limitations or deficits as a result of that injury. Also important to the medical history is the patient's history of previous injuries. This may signal additional problems that should be observed (17).

Neuromusculoskeletal Examination

The purpose of the neuromusculoskeletal examination is to quantify true physical impairment and rate symptom magnification, to determine the injured worker's perception of his or her own disability, and to list the specific quantifiable patient problems. The performance of this examination will provide the evaluator an opportunity to identify and evaluate any risks of or possible contraindications to the functional portion of the FPE. Therefore, the purposes of the neuromusculoskeletal examination are to (a) determine whether the patient is medically stable and does not have any contraindications for testing and (b) quantify physical impairment for possible permanent impairment rating, for any posttesting comparisons, and for any comparisons with functional limitations if necessary.

Activities of Daily Living

The patient should be asked about the level of independence with activities of daily living. Any difficulties with self-care should be noted and considered when determining residual function. Also important is whether the worker is using the injured extremity (17).

Work History

The patient's work history is taken in an effort to identify how the worker has been at his or her place of employment and to understand the type of work the patient has done in the past. Patients should also be questioned as to their willingness to return to their previous position in the same capacity. Responses should be provided in the report.

A full job description is also obtained during the work history. This can be found in the *Dictionary of Occupational Titles* (29) which provides narrative descriptions of jobs as well as their physical demands. A more accurate analysis of the person's job is discussed earlier in the chapter, where specific types of functional performance testing are reviewed. SSA is also studying the development of a new occupational classification system as part of the SSA disability redesign process now under way.

Pain Assessment

Because pain can interfere with function, the therapist should assess the worker's experience of pain and the degree to which the worker perceives that pain interferes with func-

tion (16). The use of pain diaries is the most common method of assessing activity (30). Usually they consist of forms that are completed by the patient every day and that track the levels of pain and activity in the person. Pain drawings have also shown to be helpful in assessing a person's level of pain.

Physical Examination

During the physical examination, the focus is on the patient's functional capabilities. Specific goniometric measurements are not as critical in and of themselves as they are in relation to the job's physical demands and the worker's ability to perform those job demands (17).

The physical examination should include observation and documentation of the overall appearance of the injury. Following this, evaluation of active range of motion should be made by instructing the patient to perform active range of motion movement patterns and noting any gross deficits. Often further evaluation is recommended via a goniometer, and the evaluation of passive range of motion is also performed. Discrepancies in active and passion motion should signal a need for further exploration (17).

Lifting Tasks

The assessment of lifting is a vital component of any FPE. Prior to initiation of the lifting portion of the evaluation, the therapist should be familiar with the maximum lifting requirements demanded of the worker in the actual work setting. This should include the frequency of this lifting, the size and weight of the material being lifted, and the manner in which the material will be lifted (e.g., waist to floor, floor to overhead). Before lifting tasks begin, the therapist should review with the patient proper body mechanics for the tasks. This should be done both verbally and with a demonstration (17). During the performance of the lifting tasks, the patient should be instructed to stop if there is any discomfort. Upon completion of the evaluation, the therapist should reevaluate the worker's physical status with regard to pain and discuss with the patient his or her current pain level, possibly using the pain drawing sheet again (17).

Functional Working Postures

A general FPE should include a variety of tests in each of the functional working postures. This includes sustained postures and repetitive motions as well as the handling of materials. Some evaluations only estimate the worker's tolerance for sitting, standing, and walking instead of observing and measuring them during other tests. The report should reflect how the data were collected. For example, while observing for signs of symptom magnification, the worker's tolerance for sitting or standing can also be documented. Likewise, by having the worker perform various activities in different locations, his or her tolerance for walking can be observed and measured (13).

Grip Tests

Except for research on the use of a hand dynamometer to measure grip strength, which has been shown to be a reliable indicator of effort, there has been no significant research on measurement of effort.

Five-Position Testing

It has been demonstrated that when the five positions of the hand dynamometer are graphed, maximal effort produces a bell curve across the five positions, with the greatest grip force occurring between two and four. Conversely, true weakness produces the same type of curve but with a reduced force at each position (31). Therefore, an abnormal curve probably demonstrates submaximal effort (24).

Rapid Exchange Test

Another test used to identify submaximal effort was developed by Hildreth et al (32). The rapid exchange test requires patients to perform the five-position hand grip test with the dynamometer set at the position at which the greatest force occurred. The subjects are then instructed to switch hands rapidly on the dynamometer, maximally gripping each time.

Electromyogram

Some researchers have recommended the electromyography (EMG) to measure sincerity of effort (24). The theory is that because EMGs measure overall neural drive, sincere maximal hand grip tests can be distinguished from faked maximal tests by the detection of differences in amplitude and frequency data of the EMG. According to the research on these tests, a positive rapid exchange test and a flat curve for the five-position grip test, all with low-amplitude EMG data in someone with low-back pain would provide good (some would say conclusive) evidence of malingering (24). However, according to Hoffmaster et al. (33), clinicians who suspect malingering should not simply use one test to confirm or deny it. Instead, the evaluator should have the patient participate in the five-position grip test and the rapid exchange grip test. If further confirmation is warranted, EMG measurements can, according to some (24), "provide additional data that even a skilled malingerer should find difficult to circumvent."

Environment

Every effort should be made to conduct the test in an area specifically designated as the testing area and should allow for minimal distraction. In addition, no one except facility personnel should be permitted to attend the FPE. The test can be compromised and produce inaccurate results if attorneys, rehabilitation specialists, or social workers are allowed to attend the testing (11). This should also apply to third-party requests to videotape the evaluation. Videotaping should be performed only if the evaluator finds it useful for an objective evaluation. Even in that case, permission to videotape is required and the video should be destroyed immediately after the completion of the report (11).

THE REPORT

Many physicians, employers, third-party payors, and so on look to the evaluation report to determine the injured worker's ability to safely return to work. Findings also enable the worker to make clear work restrictions rather than vague ones such as no repetitive motion or light work only (17).

The report should clearly and succinctly provide information on the pertinent data obtained during the evaluation. Tests should be clearly defined or described in the report. The report should give a clear picture of what the worker did, such as number of lifts and distance carried or walked. Most of the tests should be replicable from the information provided in the report. The actual work performance should be given in a format that is understandable, and the report should not consist solely of the examiner's opinion. Furthermore, the report should detail inconsistencies noted by the therapist during the worker's performance on the tests and should provide specific examples of these inconsistencies. Any tests that were administered but not completed should also be included in the report.

The effect of each activity on the estimated pain level should be documented. This should include clinical observations on the ease of movement and inability to maintain proper form and balance. From this report the physician should easily be able to identify activities that are particularly aggravating to the worker's pain as well as those that can be done easily. This information will be helpful in determining employment options.

All data or scores must be explained or interpreted. Norms and their source must be provided or indicated for all items. If norms are not available for a particular test, the report must provide a reasonable and justifiable interpretation. If a job description was used, specific reference to the demands of the specific job or to jobs in that work category should be made (11).

The summary section of the report should address the original questions or reasons that led to the referral. Narratives should be individualized and specific to the evaluee. If the report includes recommendations, these should be problem and goal oriented and provide details for implementation (11). Recommendations should include specific information regarding appropriate timing of return to work and at what capacity (full time or part time).

SUMMARY AND FUTURE DIRECTIONS

In chronic pain patients, physical examinations and x-ray and laboratory findings have not correlated with pain complaint, disability, or functional abilities. This, combined with the wide variability in how physicians assess impairments that cause disability, makes the FPE a critical factor in determining function, disability, and return to work. However, to date we have no valid scientific data from controlled studies to determine the accuracy of these testing programs. The Commission on the Evaluation of Pain and the Institute of Medicine have placed significant emphasis on the need for FPEs.

In 1992, after a review of functional muscle testing protocols, Malcolm Pope (4) wrote, "Science has not kept up with the marketing of this industry." There is no uniformly acceptable series of activities, no standardization of the evaluations. As can be seen from the scope of this chapter, the focus of assessments can vary from analysis of a single job and specific task to a more comprehensive assessment designed to be applicable across multiple job settings. There are no valid scientific data from controlled studies to be used to determine the accuracy of these tests. Women, the elderly, members of minorities, and persons with disabilities have been particularly underrepresented in the few studies that have been done. Yet despite the limitations, FPEs are being used clinically, and they provide a snapshot of a person's capabilities (10).

From the review of functional testing instruments discussed earlier, it appears that the direction of development in functional assessment instruments is to incorporate not only somatic complaints and symptoms but also the effect of symptoms on the fulfillment of social roles and expectations, including home management, self-care, engagement in social and leisure activities, financial self-support, well being, and employment.

As we continue to be asked the tough questions by insurance companies, employers, and even the patient—*When can the patient return to work? What are the restrictions? Can I get disability?*—the vital need for standardized, valid, and reliable FPEs will continue to be evident.

References

1. Mellman Lazarus Lake. Presentation of Findings, Mayday Fund 1993. Washington, DC: Mellman Lazarus Lake, 1993.
2. Naisbitt's trend letter. New York: Morrow, 1993.
3. Rucker K S, Wehman P, Kregel J. Analysis of functional assessment instruments for disability/rehabilitation programs. Report submitted on completion of SSA contract 600-95-21914, 1996.
4. Pope M H. Clinical efficacy and outcome in the diaagnosis and treatment of low back pain. New York: Raven Press, 1982.
5. Rudy T E, Lieber S J, Boston J R. Functional capacity assessment: influence of behavioral and environmental factors. J Back Musculoskel Rehab 1996;6:277–288.
6. Rucker K S. Standardization of chronic pain assessment: a multiperspective approach. Clin J Pain 1996;12:94–110.
7. Osterweis M, Kleinman A, Mechanic D, eds. Pain and disability: clinical, behavioral, and public policy perspective. Washington: National Academy Press, 1987.
8. Fordyce W E. Behavioral methods for chronic pain and illness. St. Louis: Mosby, 1976.
9. Vasudevan S V, Monsein M. Evaluation of function and disability in the patient with chronic pain. In: Raj PP, ed. Practical management of pain. 2nd ed. St. Louis: Mosby-Year Book, 1992.
10. Vasudevan S V. Role of functional capacity assessment in disability evaluation. J Back Musculoskel Rehab 1996;6:237–248.
11. Abdel-Moty E, Compton R, Steele-Rosomoff R, et al. Process analysis of functional capacity assessment. J Back Musculoskel Rehab 1996;6:223–236.
12. Keane G P, White A H. Back rehabilitation programs: sorting through the options. J Back Musculoskel Rehab 1991;1:29–36.
13. Carruth M K. Commentary: ???FCE-WTS-WH-WCE-FFD-WC??? J 1993;3:86–94.
14. Trinkle K L, Hart D L, Bunger S D. Roles and responsibilities of team members in the functional capacity evaluation and rehabilitation of the injured worker. J Back Musculoskel Rehab 1993;3:61–67.
15. Hart D L, Isernhagen S J, Matheson L N. Guidelines for functional capacity evaluation of people with medical conditions. J Orthop Sports Phys Ther 1993;18:682–686.
16. Schultz-Johnson K. Assessment of upper extremity-injured persons' return to work potential. J Hand Surg 1987;5:950–957.
17. Williams K. Functional capacity evaluation of the upper extremity. Work 1991;1:48–64.
18. Coy J A. Autonomy based informed consent: ethical implications for patient noncompliance. Phys Ther 1989;69:826–833.
19. Bech P. Rating scales for psychopathology, health status and quality of life: a compendium of documentation in accordance with the DSM-III-R and WHO systems. Berlin: Springer-Verlag, 1993.
20. Waddell G, Frymoyer J W. Acute and chronic pain. In: Pope M H, Andersson G B, Frymoyer J W, Chaffin D B, eds. Occupational low back pain: Assessment, treatment, and prevention. St. Louis: Mosby-Year Book, 1991.
21. Bandura A. Self-efficacy: toward a unifying theory of behavioral change. Psychol Rev 1977;84:191–215.
22. Schmidt A J M. Cognitive factors in the performance level of chronic low back patients. J Psychosom Res 1985;29:183–189.
23. Pain assessment instruments development project. Final report on completion of SSA contract 600-90-0263.
24. Simonsen J C. Validation of sincerity of effort. J Back Musculoskel Rehab 1996;6:289–295.
25. Decker M J. A response to redefining chronic pain programs for the injured worker population. J Back Musculoskel Rehab 1993;3:88–90.
26. Lechner D, Roth D, Straaton K. Functional capacity evaluation in work disability. Work 1991;1:37–47.
27. Matheson L N, Mooney V, Grant J E, et al. Standardized evaluation of work capacity. J Back Musculoskel Rehab 1996;6:249–264.
28. Feinstein A L, Josephy B R, Wells C K. Scientific and clinical problems in indexes of functional disability. Ann Intern Med 1986;105:413–420.
29. US Dept of Labor, Employment and Training Administration. Dictionary of occupational titles. 4th ed revised. Washington: US Government Printing Office, 1991.
30. Follick M J, Ahern D K, Laser-Wolston N. Evaluation of a daily activity diary for chronic pain patients. Pain 1984;19:373–382.
31. Stokes H M. The seriously uninjured hand: weakness of grip. J Occup Med 1983;25:683–694.
32. Hildreth D H, Breidenbach W C, Lister G D, Hodges A D. Detection of submaximal effort by use of the rapid exchange grip. J Hand Surg 1989;14A:742–745.
33. Hoffmaster E, Lech R, Niebuhr B R. Consistency of sincere and feigned grip exertions with repeated testing. J Occup Med 1993;35:788–794.

CHAPTER 43

The Befallen Community: Ethical and Spiritual Considerations in the Treatment of Chronic Pain

Laurie Zoloth-Dorfman

INTRODUCTION

Chronic pain represents, in the view of the medical team, in the view of the patient, and in the popular imagination, the worst that a secular crisis can possibly offer. It is a failure of the essential premise of American medical science: to fix that which has been broken. It is a physical reminder of the limits of our clinical knowledge and our power, the dark borders of our country of language and etiology. More deeply it represents a failure of rationality and order itself in the face of the mystery and messy complexity of the creaturely, embodied life.

For a religious apprehension of the world, however, physical pain and attendant suffering are a simple constancy of human life itself. Chronic pain, the agonistic persistence of pain, is itself a reminder of the fragility and contingency that frames human existence, the tragic necessity that make faith a correspondent necessity for the millions of Americans who look to religious traditions as the organizing authority for existence.

What are we to make of the place of faith in the narrative of pain? For both the physician and the patient beset by pain, faith has a critical place in both how we recount and how we address the issue. For physicians in particular new questions emerge: Will we experience the loss of control as the end or as the beginning of our work with patients? How can we mobilize the power of faith in our efforts to bring healing and compassion to the patients we treat?

THE PLACE OF FAITH: SOME NOTES TOWARD A GENERAL RESPONSE

This chapter reminds the reader that when treating chronic pain, the religious dimension is centrally important to many patients and that the problem of faith and spirituality also critically important in the ethics, values, and sense of an ordered moral life for the physician. This chapter is not a definitive account of all that is available to the practitioner who treats pain. In part, this is because of the wide variety of faith and because of a sense of humility in the face of the importance of each tradition to any one particular patient. Rather, I want to speak of the similarities between the varieties of the religious experience itself and of how a clear apprehension of the nature of the religious experience raises important questions in a variety of clinical venues.

Human persons, confronted with the event of befallenness, loss, and illness, react with a multiplicity of languages, images, rituals, sacraments, and action. But what is striking is the commonalties of the religious choice as a narrative frame and explanatory narrative for such gestures. It is not obvious that this should be the case. After all, the popular imagination is surrounded by seductive and persuasive alternatives to religion. Amid a world dominated by the secular concern, the moral and spiritual endeavor stands as radically opposed to the secular choice. Yet when confronted by illness, pain, and befallenness, it is the religious response, even for the heretofore not faithful, that often dominates the clinical encounter.

Responding to pain and illness as a believer in a religion sense is to make a choice, quite apart from the intellectual quest for understanding, that meaning is critical. Once the event is understood rationally, the intellectual and emotional work of the person in pain is to make meaning of his or her life and of this pivotal problem in that life. How will the illness or injury be understood; how can one go on? In the story of the illness the believer seeks, when cure is elusive, a return, a denouement, a closure of the crisis of acuity and sense made of the new life that the chronic illness will demand. Returning to the path of a sensible, meaningful, and hence organizable life becomes an attempt to create meaning out of the problem of befallenness in human life itself. To ask the question of faith is to face head on the most difficult questions of justice, desert, and desire. Pain and suffering are always mediated by the making of meaning. Thus all faith traditions speak of the inherent tension between the experience of eudemonia—of pleasure and the good life—and the simple human constancy of loss and death.

MAKING OUR DEAL

The modern American health care system can be understood as the physically embodied working out of a vast social bargain. Patients enter the system and are willing to put down money on the hope that we can keep them from dying. They are willing to endure a great deal of painful intervention based on this premise: that by so doing they will be rescued from death. In the hospice context, however, the bet has been called: they have come to understand that we cannot offer them a path away from death. It is often at this moment that pain control becomes a different matter.

Chronic pain is like the case of death: whether or not the underlying condition of illness is physically life threatening, the pain itself and its essentially uncontrolled nature lead us to the insight that medicine is a limited, rather modest proposal after all. It is at this moment that one turns to other strategies. What turns pain into travail is the failure of any strategy to alter suffering.

In Peter Berger's book *Death and the Sacred Canopy* (1) the deep structure of a religious turn is revealed. Berger contends that all of religion is involved in the creation of a sacred canopy, a spiritual protection against our own foreknowledge of death, which is what makes us unique in our creatureliness.

THE MIND-BODY SPLIT: DESCARTES AND THE LIMITS OF FAITH

Given the centrality of pain in the human condition, what is striking is the paucity of medical philosophy in response. In far too many contexts, the notion that the human person has no resources other than opioids is common. In the face of chronic pain, we quickly run through most of our medical and social responses. How feeble we can seem in understanding and alleviating chronic pain; how isolated individual patients feel when the traditional armamentarium fails them.

In large measure, as Eric Cassell points out in his book *The Nature of Suffering* (2), this was due to the emergence of science from the range of clerical and canonical critique in the 18th century, a strategy of René Descartes to allow for an epistemics of the physical world. Descartes cedes the mind and hence the soul to the arena of faith and the domain of the church, leaving the consideration of the body to the realm of physical science. It is this realm that enlarges, pushed by the explosion of the scientific gaze, the development of the new technology of medicine, the constantly expanding and cheerily optimistic positivism of the next two centuries of medicine and science. Progress is a promise of redemption and of an escape from death and befallenness itself.

In a terrain that had been firmly in the domain of faith the medical enterprise began to define nearly the whole of the territory, offering cause and effect, germ theory, or genetics to explain suffering and circumstance. Where moral agency, the concept of sin, choice, and ineffability had once explained events, medical explanations triumphed. For example, note how the nature, causation, and solution to drug abuse and addiction or infertility or tuberculosis changes over time. What was once understood as a set of sinful and avoidable moral dilemmas became framed by the medical narrative as having a physical origin with a physical solution in the hands of the physician.

Cassell notes that the enlargement of the physical self as the person has two effects: "an enlarged belief in a self as legitimate entity entirely apart from God and a decline in the power of belief" (2). Belief in God becomes, for many who have chosen to be entirely driven by the medical enterprise, an oddity, a near pathology, and certainly not "true" in the sense that laboratory values and x-ray films are "true" and rational belief patterns. Thus split from an ensouled meaning and no longer subject to individual or collective spiritual effort, the suffering becomes reduced to the pain of the physical body, rather a thin account of the dimension of chronic pain.

But how different the cultural response to pain can be is illustrated by close attention to nearly any alternative culture. The postenlightenment problem with pain and suffering suggests that pain and the response to pain are framed and defined by the strongest, oldest, and perhaps most deeply felt cultural narratives. Pain is a reminder of contingency and death, and for that there is a robust response and a thick community.

DYING AND DIVERSITY

How diverse and how thickly described can be illustrated by an act of attention to the questions raised by suffering. In researching cultural response to the problem of suffering, my colleagues and I conducted a series of interviews in depth at one hospital in West Los Angeles (research was done within the Kaiser Permanente system at a series of workshops on ethics and cultural diversity in 1994 and 1995). We asked how the participants reacted to death and pain in their cultures. Here are some brief representative examples:

• A Korean doctor told us that to die in a hospital was considered a mark of dishonor. This came as a surprise to the medical staff, to whom he had never mentioned it. He explained that dying in a hospital in his tradition meant that your family had abandoned you to the care of strangers.
• A nurse manager from Senegal told us how as the eldest daughter, she had sewn her parents' death shrouds, special linen garments that are to be made ceremoniously in their last illness. She did this prior to her immigration to America. She had told no one of this in the 23 years she had lived in this country.
• An Orthodox Jew shared her experiences on the Chevra Kadisha, the volunteer Jewish funeral society that receives the bodies of the Jewish dead from the hospital and washes them and ritually prepares them for burial before they place them in specially constructed caskets. Despite years of close

association, she had never detailed to her coworkers the special rituals or the meaning of the social gestures that surround death in her culture.

• An African-American nurse remembered how she had witnessed the effect of cultural influences on pain control very graphically: she reported that women from different cultures asked for pain medication so differently in labor that the babies were narcotized in varying levels dependent on their ethnicity.

• In reporting on cultural influences on her experience of pain, one Filipina recovery room nurse reflected on her training in a Roman Catholic program in which she was urged to "offer her pain up to God" rather than ask for medication when she herself was ill or injured.

There is nothing new, of course, in understanding that culture influences the perception and experience of pain. Post et al. (3) have pointed out the critical role of culture and gender in pain management.

> "Women [in a study by Karen Calderone] were . . . given analgesia less frequently and sedatives more frequently than men. . . . Both men and women under 61 years of age received more frequent pain medication. . . . A 1993 study by Knox Todd et al. of patients treated for long-bone fractures at the UCLA Emergency Medical Center found that Hispanics were twice as likely as non-whites to receive no medication for pain. Todd et al. explain the distinction as (1) culturally influenced expressions of pain, and (2) the failure of health care professionals to recognize the presence of pain in patients whose cultures differ from their own . . . [and explain that] the estimates of pain in both groups were consistently lower than the patients themselves."(3)

We know from other research that the construction of language, the linguistic strategies, and the expressive parameters themselves permit or do not permit the apprehension of events as meaningful or meaningless, expected or unexpected, welcome or dreaded. What was surprising to these participants was the extent to which the protocols of the normative institutional experience of death and illness matched no one's cultural ideal. It became clear to our participants and ourselves that what changed physical pain into the existential experience of suffering and what enabled the patient to make meaning of the experience was the cultural and largely the religious meaning ascribed to the pain.

RESOURCES OF THE FAITH TRADITIONS

While medicine as a whole took a turn from religious understanding, the faith traditions continued to respond to emerging clinical realities. Issues of power and meaning that surround surgery, complex diagnostic techniques, and high-tech intervention such as organ transplants and renal dialysis became questions for every tradition. Unlike the modern sci-

entific and secular reality, which interpreted pain in a world focused on production, seeing pain as a distraction and a profoundly personal problem, most religious traditions understood the suffering person as a person facing a range of moral as well as physical choices that could influence his or her experience of suffering, and as dwelling in a moral location of particularity within a larger, responding community.

The apprehension of religion by medical practitioners is a challenge: to the ordering of the cognitive operational world, to the surety of the medical epistemic stance, and finally to the verities of one's own belief system. But it is information that is critical to understanding how to best address human suffering, the goal and purpose of the physician who is dedicated to the practice of the treatment of chronic pain.

What follows is not an exhaustive account of the complex religious responses to pain. Such a study is best accomplished by the rigorous approach of the Park Ridge Center in Chicago, which in conjunction with the Martin Marty at the University of Chicago publishes an excellent series on the specific responses of the religious of both the Western industrialized world and the Eastern and indigenous spiritual traditions. Called the Project X series (after the original intent to focus on 10 faith traditions) this project now includes nearly twice that number (4). Providers who want to study seriously a particular religion's approach to healing or who are confronted with a religious tradition in the clinical encounter that they seek to understand better are urged to consult this invaluable reference.

BUDDHISM: PRESENTNESS IN THE ACTUAL MOMENT

Expression of the Buddhist tradition varies among the disparate cultures and countries in which it has flourished. What follows is a general description of the response of Buddhist normative tradition. Buddhism offers a distinctive view of life as a series of journeys. This physical body has certain tasks and yet is merely one in a series of lives that will be experienced in a larger journey of the larger self. In such a life, suffering (*duhkha*) is to be expected. Wisdom consists of

> [R]ecognizing the fact of suffering means understanding the truth of impermanence: everything is in a constant state of changing, disappearing, and dissolving from moment to moment. The path of the Buddha is of one who alone discovered the way of emancipation from the universal predicament of suffering. *Karma* plays a role in the etiology of some pain (5).

Buddhism assumes that suffering is a fundamental characteristic of all human existence (6). All of life as perceived by the person is actually a fleeting, temporally shifting and mutable collection of transitory perceptions, illusions without enduring actuality. The goal of a satisfactory spiritual journey is transcendence, understanding that clinging to the illusion of permanence, to the material world, or to any particular phenomenon is the root cause of suffering. In other words, it is the inability of the unenlightened person to transcend the self that leads to the suffering. Nirvana, or true liberation from suffering, can be achieved only in slow steps, with discipline and patience, as human cravings are supplanted by a steady and conscious practice. Pain, suffering, and unmet desire are the ground for human physical residence itself; it is the constancy of suffering and illusion that creates the necessity for inner reflection and practice.

Each particular life is constantly recycled through reincarnation. Caring for the ill person is a meritorious act that accelerates one's own progress in the next life. The ill are not to be seen as weak but as those who of course need our help and support in what is essentially a spiritual piece of work, a task of freeing oneself from the cycles of death, pain, illness, and ordained (*karmic*) misery. It is a paradox: your practice is enhanced by your compassionate care of the sufferer, yet in some existential way, their suffering too is an illusion, an impermanence (7).

As a young man, the prince who was to become the Buddha is described as being raised in a kingdom carefully kept free of illness and death, aging, and prayer. Confronted by these images as an adult, the Buddha flees into solitude, transfigured by the pain of human existence. As such, pain is the problem at the heart of the philosophy. Buddhist thought is developed as a Middle Path between the extremes of hedonism that marked the Buddha's earliest life and the starkness of asceticism practiced by the monks of the period.

The Middle Path is defined by the Four Noble Truths, which the Buddha preached to the villages and eventually spread throughout Asia. "They are the Truth about Suffering (illness), the Truth about the Origin of Suffering (its cause), the Truth about the Surcease of Suffering (its annihilation), and the Truth about the way to end Suffering (the Noble Eightfold Path)" (7).

What is meant by this, and how does it influence the understanding of pain? The path out of suffering is ultimately the practice of "mindfulness," the understanding that destructively chosen patterns can be altered and that the energy required to heal the body can be harnessed. It is clear that if pain and illness are not seen as an unexpected, random, and essentially unfair burden in a life that is meant to be cheerful and pain free, the sufferer is seen as the person in the fullness of his or her existential journey. Understanding suffering as the principal journey of a human life makes the narrative of the patient normative. Traditional Buddhist teachings argue that a completed life cycle is marked by four inevitable sufferings: birth, sickness, old age, and death. Hence: "For humans with a full span of life, sickness is inevitable. This particular form of suffering constitutes one of the common meeting ground in the intensely shared reality of suffering that links all humans in and experiential fellowship (8)."

Anyone who is unenlightened is considered ill—that is, their full capacities and energies are impaired—and it is the

enlightenment process itself that is equated with the healing process (8). Hence, there is no separation between the spiritual practice of the tradition—meditation, breathing exercises, visualization, prayer, confession, repentance—and the cultivation of insight. It is the mind that fundamentally is the seat of illness, hence it is the process of focusing and calming the mind that is key to healing. In fact, disease can be seen as an opportunity to be reawakened into the dramatic realization that suffering is immediate, constant, and that it is necessary to overcome it without procrastination. The physical manifestation of illness can reveal unsuspected karmic currents that once revealed, can be transformed (8).

For Buddhists, the goal of medicine is to us the proper technical means to remove the object whereby the patient is afflicted (7). Folk medicine has for generations been used by Buddhists to address the symptoms of illness: a series of potions, medicinal herbs, and heat and cold treatments are described in the earliest texts. By the same token, modern Western medicine is to be used, but it is seen as limited in the face of the enormous existential challenge presented by illness. Mindfulness and not obliteration of the experience is the aim of coherent response.

CHRISTIANITY: WITNESS AND REDEMPTION

There is a vast range of Christian faith, and several Christian traditions, notably Christian Scientists, Seventh Day Adventists, many evangelical faiths, and Jehovah's Witnesses, have made health and healing central to their observance. For the purpose of this general account I look at only two of many leading Christian theologians.

For Christians, the central story of Jesus and the metaphor of the suffering servant of God on the cross is the organizing metaphor for understanding illness and pain. Here is a paradox: the one in pain, near death, degraded and crucified, is at once the Messiah, whose pain is sent as atonement and expiation for the collective sins of humankind. Suffering is figured as redemption, the only means of overcoming sin, death, and constraint. Hence, only through a suffering journey can one be truly born into the release of knowing faith. As with Buddhism, suffering, illness, and death are the essential ground of existence, sin the original position. But escape from the ravages of sin and pain is available to those who "radically surrender" their previous egocentrism to the grace of God through Christ (9).

Paul avers: "As we share abundantly in Christ's suffering so through Christ we share abundantly in comfort, too." . . . At present, he who is one with—or in the body of—Christ will indeed continue to suffer. He has the promise, however, that he will not be left to suffer continually, but will eventually overcome that suffering through his faith in Christ. Christ himself is the evidence that, as he overcame suffering and death, so may the worshipper (9).

The faithful one is intended to follow the path of Jesus and can relay the story of Jesus, inhabiting the body of a man, to lead the faithful to the same release. We are to understand that the incarnation of God in the embodied form of Jesus is proof of the reality that the pain of ordinary life, the suffering of illness, and the apparent chaos of chronicity are meant to be transcended, will be transcended, certainly, by the redemption and resurrection into the grace of afterlife, the life of the spirit.

For a Christian, the task of the healer is to be a witness, an unfailing presence in the midst of the world of sin and pain. Stanley Hauerwas (10), a leading Protestant theologian, in what is perhaps the most careful account of the critical nature of Christian witness as response to suffering, describes this act as one of establishing a community into which the sufferer-worshipper was welcomed and supported:

> For the early Christians, suffering and evil . . . do not have to be "explained." Rather, what was required was the means to go on even if the evil could not be "explained." . . . Indeed, it was important not to provide a theoretical account . . . since such an explanation would undercut the necessity of a community capable of absorbing the suffering.

For Hauerwas, the problem of suffering is addressed by finding a common narrative, one that we are born into, that we do not have to invent by ourselves, that we are given by a merciful God to makes meaningful the plot of our lives in common. We cannot offer a solution to pain but only a witness to it. In commenting on the painful death of leukemic children, one of the most difficult examples of innocent suffering, Hauerwas reminds us that Christians believe thus:

> [We] have no theodicy that can soften the pain of our death and the death of our children, but we believe that we share a common story which makes it possible for us to be with one another especially as we die. There can be no way to remove the loneliness of the death of leukemic children unless they see witnessed in the lives of those who care for them a confidence rooted in friendship with God and with each other. That, finally, is the only response we have to "the problem" of the death of our children (10).

The larger metaphor of the cross encompasses many Christian faiths. In the clinical world, Roman Catholic tradition is a distinctive perspective for many. In reflecting on the resources that Christian faith brings to both patients and healers, Richard McCormick, noted Roman Catholic theologian, draws our attention to the *Ethical Guidelines for Catholic Health Care Institutions,* a document that was developed over 2 years by a group of Roman Catholic theologians, ethicists, and health care personnel. While this is not a papal document, it has been widely accepted by a broad cross-section of Roman Catholics. I quote in full guideline 21, which addresses pain control:

> Though suffering and death are realities that cannot be eliminated, appropriate means should be taken to reduce suffering and preserve life. What means are appropriate is determined by a due proportion between the burden and the benefit of the treatment to the patient. If the treatment would only secure a precarious and burdensome prolongation of life, it may be refused by the patient or the family on behalf of the patient. Medications and other therapies whose purpose is to alleviate pain may be given as needed, with the consent of the patient or his or her agent, even if a side effect is the shortening of life. A person who is dying presents the health care team with one of its greatest challenges and opportunities. It is the challenge and opportunity to be with the dying and the family in a way which reproduces and mediates the fullest and final sense of Christ's healing love. Any medical treatment at this critical point must aim not at simply prolonging life, but at reducing the human diminishments of the dying process, maximizing the values the patient treasured in life, and bringing comfort (11).

The Catholic tradition clearly understands the occasion of illness as an opportunity for grace, of the "gradual shedding of the sinful self" (11). The appropriate response involves the ritual of the sacrament of anointing the sick, which is the sacrament not only for the dying but for anyone who is seriously confronts the possibility of death. From a Christian point of view, then, grave illness must be seen as an intensifying conformity to Christ. In this sense, as the body weakens and is devastated, the strength of Christ is shared by those baptized into his death and resurrection (11).

McCormick adds that the critical act of witness is part of the redemptive act of love that is the practice demanded of Christians in the daily world. To count on loving and honest encounters creates the possibility of transforming the medical encounter, the patient's experience of illness, and finally, the physician as well. It is not only the passion of Christ that animates that response to suffering, it is the "as I have loved you" aspect of the actions of Jesus (11). A Christian response to illness creates the possibility to "nourish, protect and support the medical encounter as a truly human (not merely technological) one: compassion, honesty, self-denial and generosity" (11). And a profession that is "deeply penetrated" by these virtues and by persons aspiring to achieve them will be a different, a transformed profession.

In the clinical world, argues McCormick, the values of biological life, or freedom from pain, can distort the relationship, allowing for a mesmerizing fixation on technology, ego, or cost. Death is seen as a defeat for these goals. But for a Christian, death is not an unmediated evil. Other virtues and other values also have their place as a corrective to the "idolization of life and the profession's ability to preserve it" (11). Christian practice requires us to remember that a moral life is both girded by and redeemed by the meaning made possible by liberation of resurrection.

JUDAISM: A COMMUNITY OF RESPONSE

Jewish tradition is an amalgamation of many disparate texts, histories, and reflections, so the perspective on any given problem is essentially multivocal: many voices converse and disagree in the classic tradition about how a problem is to be addressed. In the modern period, the four branches of Judaism vary in their reliance on the Talmudic texts and on how much one is obligated to follow the commandments inscribed in those texts.

In Jewish thought, the crucial text is the Torah. It was here in the scriptural source that analysis of contemporary problems such as issues in medical ethics begins. (When confronted with a contemporary problem, a question of how to behave in the face of the AIDS crisis, for example, *halakhists* go first to the text and commentary to seek solutions.) Since the Torah text itself is laconic, elliptical, and contradictory, with much unsaid, the commentaries on the text are numerous, spanning the 2000 years of the Oral Law. (The Oral Law or the Oral Tradition is, of course, predominantly written. In the Talmud, "technical discussions dealing with complex legal issues are often juxtaposed with ethical teachings or sayings; the legal and ethical are often confused, as in the tractate Baba Batra where charity and compassion for the poor are defined as religious obligations (12).) The *Talmud,* the written compilation of Jewish Oral Law, is divided into two areas, the *Mishnah,* which contains aphoristic delineation and exposition on the Torah text, and the *Gemara,* which contains recorded historic comments and debates on virtually every phrase of the *Mishnah* by rabbinic scholars (*Hazal,* or the Sages, the rabbinic commentators).

The Talmud is not arranged systematically. It is the complex, multitemporal record of a long and often rambling discourse. Scattered throughout are ethical considerations, stories, and legal discourses. Talmudic disputes are often left unresolved. At times the section of the debate ends with the phrase *tayku,* which means, in effect, the question stands (until the Messiah comes to resolve it; such disputes are one of the things that will be resolved once the Messiah comes).

There are tensions as well within the Talmudic text between the weight of the old and the importance of the new, between the pull of the majority and the rights of the minority. If even a minority position can be found among the Talmudic debates, or if a later commentator has furthered a minor point, these data can be considered relevant proof text for an ethical argument. An ethical argument cannot be made, however, within the horizontal and vertical community of Judaism without a commentary or proof text that is based on Scripture or the Talmud.

Hence Jewish thought offers a range of responses to the nature and meaning of suffering and to the most appropriate stance of patient and practitioner in the face of chronic pain. Like the other religions, Jewish thought sees suffering as part of the essential character of human life—embodied, vulnerable, and a subject of a far larger universe that while essentially good (*ki tov*), is not perfected and not in the ownership or control of human persons. There is a persistent suggestion that right conduct, true awareness, and the acceptance of the covenantal relationship lead to a life that if not free of pain, is best equipped to handle pain. Some rabbinic texts suggest that suffering is more directly related to misconceptions, hubris, or wrongdoing (9). Others suggest that suffering is attendant on spiritual progress, that insight, prophecy, and compassion emerge from lives deepened by the encounter with pain (9).

Medical intervention, knowledge of the most sophisticated techniques of any particular culture in which Jews found themselves, has traditionally been a part of Jewish life (13). Jews are seen as partners in the act of creation and flourishing of the universe. It is a religious duty to visit the sick, "not [to] stand idly by the blood of your fellow" (Lev. 25:35), and to violate even the Sabbath laws to ensure the life and health of your fellow (Orah Hayyim 329:3). The Talmud and the subsequent Responsa literature stress the necessity for public health, for careful epidemiological rules to prevent infectious disease, and for the avoidance of hazardous pregnancy (13).

The normative Jewish view is that there is no concrete and personal afterlife but that when the messianic age eventually comes, dead ones will be restored to life, a meaning left undelineated and understood differently by different branches of Judaism. Jews therefore turn for support to the idea that the community bears the burden of pain with the one who is afflicted. Healing is a stance that is required of each Jew. Those who can ought to acquire the best skills to administer medicine, but even lay persons in the community are obligated to visit, feed, nurture, and provide for the physical and emotional needs of the other, the stranger, and the vulnerable, impoverished and ill. This spirit animates the aggressive approach to pain control. Chronic pain in particular is the responsibility of an entire community that understands that the sufferer is to be attended to with constancy.

Can pain make a life impossible? At least some authoritative sources argue that this is the case. Philosopher Baruch Brody has written of the importance of 14th century thinker Rabbi Nissim of Gerundi (14). Gerundi follows a Talmudic tradition that regards prayer for a swift death an appropriate stance in the face of unrelenting pain:

> It seems to me that this is what the [Talmudic passage under review] was saying: there are times that one [must] pray about the sick person that he should die since he is in a great deal of pain because of his illness and he cannot live. As it says in *Ketubot,* "When she saw how . . . much he was in pain, she prayed that it should be God's will that the immortal [God's will] should win over the mortal [the desire of men]. The rabbis would not stop praying for his survival. She took a jar and threw it on the ground. They stopped praying. Reby died." (Ketubot 104a) (14)

What are we to make of this? The passage concerns a classic and well-known story of the death of the great compiler of the Talmud, Rabbi Judah haNasi, whose students gathered at his bed to pray for his recovery. Seeing his unrelenting pain, his maidservant startled them into stopping their prayers and he died swiftly. The later rabbinic authority cites this as a proof text for his ruling that such action in the face of severe pain is permitted. This text is used by 20th century Orthodox Jewish authorities to permit the withdrawal of advanced life support and aggressive pain control measures even if such would shorten life. Since the rabbinic understanding was that prayer was a serious matter and carried significant efficacy, the injunction was to stop prayer for cure and move to prayer for the end of life.

What the Jewish commentators have in mind is that in the face of pain, the sufferer is neither abandoned nor deceived, is paradoxically aggressively cared for and alertly attended to. When the life is beyond cure, the physician is still obligated to be present, to stand by as comrade, not as healer. The skills of presence mean that the separate world of illness needs to be seen, to be included in our world. Yet in a society focused on production, it is difficult to allow for this focus without faith and a valuing community. Jewish thought, like Christianity and Islam, struggles to make meaning of pain. In the reflections on pain there is textual tension between the necessity of vulnerability and weakness and the retributive aspects of pain:

> The Lord tries the righteous (Ps XI.5). The potter does not test crack vessels; it is not worthwhile to tap them even once because they would break; but he taps the good ones because, however many times he taps them, they do not break. Even so God tries not the wicked, but the righteous." (Rabbi Yonaton, in Genesis Rabbah 32.3) (9).

It is the vulnerable, the broken, the weak, and the lost in exile that like God's chosen ones Israel, are the special responsibility of God and by extension, of the people of God. This view is at the heart of a paradox shared by several religious traditions. Judaism, for obvious historical reasons made most especially acute in the post-Holocaust era struggles actively with the problem of befallenness and pain. And it is the acknowledgment of the essentially unredeemed quality of the world—the messiah not yet come, ourselves not yet completed, our tasks not yet finished—that at times allows suffering to envelop us.

The individual is yet not an individual; he or she is seen as in the center of the responsible and responding community. The rabbinic world is one in which pain is a presence and prayer a necessity. The role of the rabbinic healer—the teacher–moral actor who serves as the later model for the physician—is to care in an embodied way for the vulnerable. To be ceaselessly present to the one in pain, to be utterly responsible for a response, is to be chosen. In rabbinic literature the messiah is not an avenging warrior but a wounded beggar, found among those "wrapping and unwrapping his bandages at the gates of the city."

ISLAM: SUBMISSION AND RESISTANCE

One of the fastest-growing religions in the world is Islam, and its discrete and particular views of illness, suffering, and pain are becoming a feature in the practice of many physicians. Islam, like Buddhism, begins in the sacred texts and specific journey of a man, given to wealth and power, who rejected this path to reflect on the problems of Meccan society (15). Muhammad came to believe that a new religion was called for, one that recognized monotheism and that confronted the inequities in the economic and social order. Driven from Mecca by conflicts with the wealthy, he established a sovereignty in Medina, where as both secular and religious leader, he was able to establish a religious state, governed by allegiance to the laws of the Qur'an. Hence the whole fabric of life, intimate and public, family, person, and state, are governed by the code of the Qur'an and the derivative, later remembered oral commentary of the Prophet. But also important are the records of the performative acts, or deeds of Muhammad. Both major contemporary branches of Muslims, the Shi'a and the Sunni, also use the report of these deeds as collected by scholars to create, with the Qur'an, a binding canon for daily behavior.

The stance toward pain emerges from the view of illness itself: "Health is the most excellent of God's blessings upon man after the faith Islam, for without it man can neither carry on his life business well nor can he obey God's commands" (15).

Paradoxically, both death in good health and death by illness are considered martyrdom; both types of statements are made, and once part of the canon, are resolved by the understanding that both have their own meanings; both reflect the possibility that it is the response of the worshipper that is key. Hence, the one in pain must bear his or her burden with understanding: "But how about the person who is ill, who has not deliberately brought on his illness, bears his illness and pain with patience, tries treatments created by God and discovered by humans, provides others the opportunity to give of tier mercy—is he or she any less a martyr?" (15) In this description of illness, it is important that the ill one has a key religious and social role to play for his or her society. It is that pain that gives others a chance to serve; it is that nobility in the face of suffering that allows for prayer and mercy. Note here as well that God sends both cure and physicians who understand the techniques of cure.

Suffering in Islamic tradition is both test and trial on the one hand and an enactment of punishment on the other (9). God is the ultimate judge of all actions and the arbitrator of divine justice; hence the Qur'an stresses that sinners will be ultimately punished. Such suffering can bring about insight into the ways the sinner has erred in observance, or it may be a result of unfairness to another, or it may be that the sufferer has faltered in belief. Evil is a part of the essential human condition, but God is perfectly just; if suffering exists, then, it is deserved or needed (9).

But directly opposite views exist: suffering is also a test, a way to sort out the true believer from the false one. Pain comes to both the good and the evil one and serves different functions for each. The response to suffering that Islam advises is a complex one and is essentially different from either the Jewish or the Christian viewpoint. In Islam, suffering is not a welcome way of proving one's faith; neither is it something to be avoided. Rather, Islam sees suffering as a necessary though unfortunate component of life that should be alleviated where possible and endured otherwise (9). Islam's paradoxical response to suffering understands that the alleviation of pain is a religious responsibility, part of the task to rid the world of suffering in a larger sense, for the relief of pain, both the physical responses to pain and the spiritual ones, are considered critical.

IN CONCLUSION: ATTENTION TO THE WORLD OF COMPLEXITY

Neither faith nor pain is simple: both are opaque to the outsider and particular in their expression; both are among the most essential of human responses and the most widely divergent. Yet in the clinical world we, from the gaze of the scientific, the rational, objective, "see" a body in pain, the outside of the self, which offers us perhaps the least of the information that we need to address the pain itself. For the physician who treats the chronic pain patient, the mystery at the heart of therapeutic response is even more opaque. Here the patient will need to find ongoing meaning in the narrative of pain. We may assist with our interventions, or we may not; part of the task of the good physician is to hear the voice of the patient as clearly as he or she hears the powerful guiding voices of science and rationality.

Another central task is to understand one's own journey, both the culture that shapes one and the way that the role-specific duties of the physician are shaken by the depths of the power of pain and by the power to deal with pain that we see in the clinical world.

Finally, seeing the patient and the self clearly means seeing the limits of the embodied and broken human world. Try as we may, pray as we may, the grief that shapes us as surely as the joy is inexorable. We can be sensitive, we can be culturally aware, but we still err and we still feel defeated by pain. However, this chapter recalls for us that what may be a great failure in the clinical world will be a moment of truth, compassion, and deep victory in the world of faith, if we allow for the full human flourishing and honoring of that faith.

Richard Niebuhr, speaking of the importance of faith in the modern world reminds us:

The faith we speak of is not an intellectual assent to the truth of certain propositions, but a personal practical trusting in, reliance on, counting on, something. Faith in other words, always refers primarily to character and power rather than to existence. . . . Now is it evident that without such active faith or such reliance and confidence on power we do not and cannot live."

Religion is in one sense an attempt to create meaning of the problem of befallenness in human life. Medicine is another. Both are discourses of power, passion, risk and daring, faith and goodness, and perhaps centrally, both are about a lifetime of learning.

When medicine as a whole took a turn from religious understanding, it created a breach in the self. It separated what is embodied, ours to reach and change, ours to name as real: the body, seen as a fixable set of parts; and what is holy, perhaps unreal, inner, disruptive: the soul. Pain and suffering teach us of the interconnection between that which can be borne and that which cannot. Any physician who overlooks the serious contribution that the faith community can make and is bidden to make, in all the cases that we discussed in Buddhist, Christian, Jewish, and Islamic communities, overlooks a critical set of allies in the work of healing and ultimately addresses an incomplete self.

For we see at last that the ability to address pain is ultimately not a personal problem, not a problem of lost work time, but a failure of a community to find the resources to respond fully to the one in pain.

Not all who are in pain, lost and alienated, retreating into a personal story of despair can be reached. But for many, far more than we suspect, calling carefully on the full resources of the culture, the faith tradition and the believing community, can offer reembrace into another narrative altogether. For it is to the ineffable that women and men have turned for generations for help. In the times of the oldest of losses, we see that record in every religious tradition: in Psalms and Upanishads, prayers and chants. We see that image repeated: of the one in pain, and the one who is answered, by this turn to the sacred.

It is the task of the physician both to seek and to honor that source of strength: the possibility for the miraculous and for the enduring and for the transcendence that can be found in the rich and complex variety of the religious traditions.

REFERENCES

1. Berger PL. The sacred canopy. New York: Anchor Press, 1969.
2. Cassell EJ. The nature of suffering. New York: Oxford University Press, 1991;33–34.
3. Post, Blustein, Gorden, Dubler. Pain: ethics cultures and informed consent to relief. J Law, Med Ethics 1996;24:348–360.
4. Marty ME, Vaux K, eds. Health and Medicine and the Faith Traditions. Philadelphia: Fortress Press, 1982.
5. Juergensmeyer M, Carmen M, eds. Bibliographic guide to the comparative study of ethics. Cambridge: Cambridge Press, 1991.
6. Smith JZ, ed. The Harper-Collins dictionary of religion. San Francisco: Harper-Collins, 1995;1029.
7. Buddhist philosophy. In: Eliade M, ed. The encyclopedia of religion, vol. 2. New York: Collier Macmillan, 1987;541–543.
8. Birnbaum R. Chinese Buddhist tradition of healing and the life cycle. In: Sullivan L, ed. Healing and restoring. New York: Macmillan, 1989.
9. Suffering. In: Eliade M, ed. The encyclopedia of religion, vol. 14. New York: Collier-Macmillan, 1987;100–105.
10. Hauerwas S. Naming the silences: God, medicine and the problem of suffering. Grand Rapids, MI: William B. Erdmans, 1990.
11. McCormick R. Health and medicine in the Catholic tradition. New York: Crossroad, 1987.
12. Wineburg S, Dorfman LZ. Jewish ethics. In: Juergensmeyer M, Carmen J, eds. A bibliographic guide to the comparative study of ethics. Cambridge, UK: Cambridge University Press, 1991;309–337.

13. Feldman D. Health and medicine in the Jewish tradition. New York: Crossroad, 1986.

14. Brody B. Jewish casuistry on suicide and euthanasia. In: Brody B, ed. Suicide and euthanasia. Boston: Kluwer, 1989.

15. Rahman F. Health and medicine in the Islamic tradition. New York: Crossroad, 1987.

Suggested Reading

Brody BA, ed. Suicide and euthanasia: history and contemporary themes. Dordrecht: Kluwer, 1989.

Brody H. The healer's power. New Haven: Yale University Press, 1992.

Cassell EJ. The nature of suffering and the goals of medicine. New York: Oxford University Press, 1991.

Droge AJ, Tabor JD. A noble death: suicide and martyrdom among Christians and Jews in antiquity. San Francisco: Harper-Collins, 1992.

Foucault M. The birth of the clinic: an archaeology of medical perception. New York: Vintage Books, 1975.

Hauerwas S. Dispatches from the front: theological engagements with the secular. Durham, NC: Duke University Press, 1994.

Hauerwas S. Suffering presence: theological reflections on medicine, the mentally handicapped, and the church. Notre Dame, IN: University of Notre Dame Press, 1986.

Numbers RL, Amundsen DW. Caring and curing: health and medicine in the western religious traditions. New York: Macmillan, 1986.

Statman D, ed. Moral luck. Albany: State University of New York Press, 1993.

Sullivan LE. Healing and restoring: health and medicine in the world's religious traditions. New York: Macmillan, 1989.

Verhey A, Lammers SE, eds. Theological voices in medical ethics. Grand Rapids, MI: William B. Eerdmans, 1993.

CHAPTER 44

Alternative Medicine for Chronic Pain: A Critical Review

Wen-Hsien Wu and Adewunmi A. Akande

INTRODUCTION

Throughout human history maintaining wellness or health has been emphasized. The philosophy has been keeping the person well, in balance; restoring balance. This approach is a holistic one. The philosophy of health care is intertwined in the cultural and historical heritage of human society. Culture includes nonmaterial attributes, such as attitudes, assumptions, beliefs, myths, concepts, approaches, and traditions, and material attributes, such as habits and clothing customs, the design of institutions, and delivery systems for goods and services such as health care. Culture characterizes the human species, and each human group possesses its own culture. A culture is dynamic and responsive to the material and the nonmaterial attributes that rise from within or without.

Human societies are constantly changing. In the mid-17th century, reason began to prevail. Syndenham suggested bedside teaching and separation of symptoms from the underlying diseases. Descartes asserted the separation of mind and body. Morgagni advocated the association of symptoms with the malformation of specific organs. In 1850, Virchow's demonstration of the cellular basis of diseases indeed solidified the reductionist approach to science. Reductionism strengthened the separation of psyche and body. Consequently, the accepted "science" in medicine is largely based on physical reality. Contemporary reductionists' biomedical paradigm consists of four elements: objectivism (observer is separate from the observed); reductionism (complex phenomena are explainable in terms of simpler component phenomena); positivism (all information can be derived from physically measurable data); and determinism (a phenomenon can be predicted from knowledge of scientific law and the initial conditions). In this paradigm, it is assumed that all beings are uniformly created. Thus, a unified input leads to a predictable outcome. This paradigm is used to create a biochemical

model of the health delivery system that is acceptable to our society. Eventually this leads to the development and expectation of high-tech medicine. However, in the process, the aspect of a unique individual interacting with the members of society and the environment is lost. Complementary alternative medicine (CAM) embraces the mind, spirit, and body aspects in the healing process. The contemporary biomedical paradigm is based on newtonian physics and predarwinian biology. Newtonian physics can be used to explain and produce many observations of everyday experience and explain the mechanics of them. Quantum physics carries the concept beyond newtonian mechanics, for example, matter-energy duality, unified field of the energy in the matter, and in the wave functions. All matter is a manifestation of energy. Einstein's equation, $E = mc^2$, means that the energy contained within a particle is equivalent to its mass multiplied by the speed of light squared. This tremendous energy storage is yet to be tapped in the healing art. This einsteinian conceptual approach may be necessary to establish new paradigms for research and investigation in the field of CAM.

CAM systems are rooted in the human history. When the reality of the therapeutic effectiveness is observed, it is up to the medical scientist to explain the mechanism. If the current technology and methodology cannot explain the phenomenon, one should not deny its existence. For instance, myasthenia gravis existed long before the pathophysiology was discovered. In this context CAM will be reviewed with the newtonian scientist paradigm and with comments from the einsteinian scientist's vintage points.

CAM includes a wide variety of disciplines. They include acupuncture, subtle energy (e.g., *qi gong*), low-level laser therapy (LLLT), mind-body (e.g. meditation), aroma therapy, ayurveda, bioenergetics, Chinese medicine, color therapy, dance therapy, detoxification, dietetics, electromagnetism, environment medicine, enzyme therapy, ethnomedicine, gem therapy, herbalism, immunostimulation, iridology, kinesiology, manual medicine, massage, music therapy, naturopathy, nutrition, organotherapy, osteopathy, oxygen therapy, polarity therapy, prayer, radionics, reflexology, shamanism, shiatsu therapeutic touch, thermal medicine, Tibetan medicine, vibrational therapy, wet cupping, yoga, and so on. Due to the space limitation, this review will include only acupuncture, *qi gong,* LLLT, and meditation.

ACUPUNCTURE

The earliest detailed Chinese description of acupuncture is in the Yellow Emperor's Classic of Internal Medicine (2nd to 3rd century B.C.). Acupuncture continued to be developed until its official banning during the Ching Dynasty (1644 to 1911 A.D.). However, its use was continued. In the 1960s, Mao Tse Tung of the People's Republic of China advocated the integration of the traditional Chinese medicine with Western science and established acupuncture and moxibustion (herb burning) research institutes. Since then the scientific basis of Chinese traditional medicine continues to be expanded.

Acupuncture is one of the Chinese traditional therapies for relieving pain and treating diseases. In ancient China, 12 important internal organs were designated in the body, six solid yin organs (heart, liver, kidney, lung, spleen, and pericardium) and six hollow yan organs (small intestine, gallbladder, urinary bladder, large intestine, stomach, and triple burners). The triple burners do not exist in Western anatomical concepts. Some of these internal organs indicate functions of several organ systems in an anatomical sense. These 12 internal organs are believed to be connected to specific distal parts of the body by an imaginary channel called *jing,* translated as meridian in French.

The vital energy *qi* was believed to circulate among the 12 internal organs through their meridians. In good health, the flow of *qi* is smooth and full. Whenever the flow is unbalanced (deficient, obstructed, or in excess) disease results, and the acupuncture points along the corresponding meridian may become tender. Inserting needles into these acupuncture points reestablishes the balance. This is accomplished by manipulations, namely tonification (for deficiency or emptiness) or sedation (for excess or fullness).

In addition to the 12 meridians, there are 2 (of 8) important extra meridians, namely the governing and conception meridians, which run along the midline of the dorsal and ventral body surface, respectively. Each main meridian possesses one collateral branch, *lo* vessel, connected transversely to the corresponding meridian. there are a total of 15 *lo* vessels. When *lo* vessels are full, the *qi* overflows into a smaller vessel system of the skin. The condition causes changes in the color and consistency of the skin. This is the basis for traditional acupuncturist's diagnosis of the fullness of *qi.*

Acupuncture points are located on meridians and designated by specific series of numbers in Western literature. The *qi* flows from the point with lower numbers to those higher num-

bers within the same meridian. The skin resistance of acupuncture points is lower (higher conductance) than in the surrounding areas. In unhealthy states this resistance is further reduced.

Acupuncture points are found to have more nerve endings than the surrounding skin areas. Gunn et al. grouped the acupuncture points into four types. Type 1 points generally correspond to motor points (47 of 70 commonly used acupuncture points). In many instances, these points also correspond to trigger points or tender points in myofacial pain syndrome. Type 2 points are found in the sagittal plane, where the superficial nerves from both sides of the body meet. Type 3 points generally lie over the superficial cutaneous nerves or nerve plexus. Type 4 points correspond to the muscle-tendon junctions. There are approximately 1000 acupuncture points in the body, of which approximately 100 are used commonly for therapy.

Auricular acupuncture was described in ancient China. It was not commonly recognized in the West until 1956, when Dr. P. Nogier presented the concept that different organs and parts of the body are represented in specific parts of the ear in an arrangement resembling an upside-down fetus. He further mapped the detailed projections of various organs in the auricle and developed physical techniques for auricular diagnosis and auriculotherapy. Recently, the effectiveness of auriculotherapy for relief of chronic pain has been disputed.

The exact mechanism of the action in acupuncture is still not completely understood. Many remain skeptical about the effectiveness of acupuncture and believe that acupuncture is a hoax involving perhaps hypnosis or placebo effect. However, the acupuncture phenomenon can be explained by a biomedical or biophysical model. The biomedical model is supported by recent neurophysiological research data. The analgesic effect of acupuncture and electroacupuncture demonstrate local and systemic physiological changes in both humans and animal experiments.

To understand the neurobiological effect of acupuncture a brief review of neurobiology is in order. In 1965, Melzack and Wall postulated that a gate control mechanism is present in the dorsal horn of the spinal cord. They explained that the segmental activation of large afferent fibers would close the gate to the pain afferent pathway transmitted by the small myelinated Aδ fibers and nonmyelinated C fibers. The large and small fibers project to the substantia gelatinosa and central transmission and via the lateral spinothalamic tract to the thalamus and cerebral cortex. The impulses synapse in the dorsal horn and are modulated by various neurochemical receptors and transmitted via the wide dynamic range neurons. Modulation of the spinal cord level depends on the antinociceptive and nociceptive receptors, which include opioid receptors, substance P receptors, and noradrenergic, serotonin, GABA, adenosine, acetylcholine and peptide receptors (enkephalin, dynorphins and β-endorphins).

The anatomical substrate of the body self is a widespread network of nervous system consisting of loops between the thalamus and cortex as well as between the cortex and the limbic system. The entire network (initially determined genetically and modified by sensory input) can be labeled a neuro-matrix. The reported cyclical processing and synthesis of nerve impulses through the neuromatrix imposes a character-istic pattern called the neurosignature. All inputs from the body undergo cyclical processing and synthesis so that char-acteristic patterns are impressed on them in the neuromatrix. The neurosignature, which is a continuous outflow from the neuromatrix, is projected to areas in the brain called the sen-tinel neural hub (SNH). The four components of the new con-ceptual nervous system then are (a) body self-neuromatrix; (b) cyclical processing and synthesis in which the neurosignature is produced; (c) SNH, which converts the neurosignature into the flow of awareness; and (d) activation of an action neuro-matrix to provide the pattern of movement to bring about the desired goal. Needle acupuncture is known to activate multi-ple afferent fibers and receptors, which send signals to the spinal cord via large myelinated Aβ fibers, small Aδ, and C fibers. The primary afferent fibers can synapse in substantia gelatinosa (SG) of the dorsal horn of the spinal cord before projecting to higher levels of the central nervous system. Stimulation of these primary afferent fibers produces segmen-tal analgesia at the level of SG by closing the gate and/or releasing enkephalins locally through the short-axon enkepha-linergic interneurons to suppress the release of substance P and thus inhibit the transmission of nociceptive stimuli.

The first evidence of neurohumoral-mediated analgesia in acupuncture was that the cerebrospinal fluid (CSF) from a donor rabbit undergoing acupuncture produced analgesia in a recipient rabbit. The time hysteresis of the analgesia (delayed onset with prolonged effect) resembled that seen after periaqueductal gray stimulation. Endorphin is implicated in acupuncture analgesia. Recently results from the cross-circulation experiment recon-firmed the transferability of endorphin through the bloodstream and showed that the effect could be reversed by naloxone. Fur-thermore, the observed acupuncture-induced increase of endor-phin in the CSF was absent in hypophysectomized animals, sug-gesting the origin of endorphin.

The second line of evidence deals with the central sero-toninergic inhibitory system in the brainstem (periaqueductal gray nuclei and raphe magnus nuclei). Two distinct pathways, one descending and one ascending, originate here. The descending pathway originates from raphe magnus nucleus, inhibiting nociceptive transmission at the spinal cord level, while the ascending pathway sends fibers to the forebrain struc-tures. The role of this ascending pathway is not yet fully under-stood. This system is preferentially activated by small C fibers, such as electrical or needle stimulation on acupuncture points.

The third neurohormone related to acupuncture analgesia is norepinephrine (NE). Early in 1964 Zhao et al. first observed a decrease of NE content in the rat brain after elec-troacupuncture. Further studies suggested that intraventricular administration of NE antagonized the effect of acupuncture-induced analgesia. In most situations, acupuncture inhibits both central and peripheral sympathetic activities, increases the pain threshold, and changes certain physiological indices (increased palm temperature, increased blood flow in finger plethysmogram, and galvanic skin response). This inhibitory effect on the adrenergic system (i.e., vasodilation and improve-ment of microcirculation) is useful in acupuncture treatment. Other therapeutic effects of acupuncture that may be related to pain relief or improving disease conditions are relaxing mus-cle spasm, normalizing T and B cell immune response, increasing circulating ACTH and cortisol, and decreasing serum triglyceride, phospholipid, and cholesterol levels.

The biophysical model is an important conceptual under-standing of bioenergetics of which acupuncture is a part. Three aspects will be discussed: concept, conductance of acupuncture point, and interaction between points.

1. Concept: It is known that every atom, ion (inorganic, organic or macromolecule), cell, organ, and organism carries a characteristic energy (electromagnetic, EM) pattern. When any of these ions are accelerated, EM radiation is emitted. At each of these levels, there is a summation of the EM waves from its component (e.g., atom, ion, cell). This phenomenon has been used for diagnostic procedures, including electroencephalography (EEG), electrocardiography (ECG), and electromyography (EMG). However, for therapy, its use has not been accepted into the mainstream medicine. In the course of travel, these EM waves can be absorbed, reflected, or refracted at interfaces (e.g., bones or soft tissues), producing interference patterns. This interference produces standing waves (Zhang CL, Popp A, unpublished work) that are unique to a given organ or person. These wave patterns from internal EM fields are relatively stable but interact dynamically with the environmental EM field.

2. Conductance of acupuncture: As stated above, superposition of all of the EM waves forms standing waves. The junction points of the standing waves coincide with the traditional acupuncture points (Zhang CL, Popp A, unpublished work), which carry the highest skin conductance.

3. Interaction between acupuncture points: It is the contention of Zhang and Popp that acupuncture points are not separate entities. They are the distribution of standing wave superposition. The net wave form at one anatomical site represents that of the entire body at a specific boundary condition. Thus, certain changes at these sites represent conditions of the entire body. Morphology of the standing wave is expected to shift from time to time, leading to movement over the body. This may be the phenomenon of *qi*. This hypothesis is attractive in its holistic approach in explanation of acupuncture. However, its value and predictive power have yet to be verified by measurable parameters.

In addition to treating chronic pain syndromes, acupunc-ture has been used to treat various diseases and symptoms. Before initiating any acupuncture treatment, proper diagnosis of the disease must always be made using modern methods. The chronic pain states shown in controlled studies to have a good responses to acupuncture are migraine, tension headaches, cervical cephalgia, trigeminal neuralgia, facial or dental pain, cervical or lumbar spondylosis, intercostal neuralgia, postherpetic neuralgia, mild sciatica of herniated nucleus pulposus, osteoarthritis, and low-back pain. Acupuncture has also been shown to be beneficial in gastrointestinal dysfunctions, bronchial asthma, hiccups, hypertension, sprain of extremities, tenosynovitis, deafness, rhinitis, and sinusitis, alcoholism and drug addiction, insomnia, smoking, and psychophysiological disorders. Numerous studies have shown that 30 to 50% of patients with migraine headaches and 22 to 68% of those with chronic low-back pain had relief lasting longer than 6 months. The patients with nociceptive pain have been shown to have the best long-term pain relief (longer than 6 months). However, these studies were not randomized, double-blinded, or controlled. The overall results of acupuncture treatment of patients with chronic pain are at best moderate.

The principles of selecting acupuncture points are primary points around the sites of lesions of the nerve distribution in the affected area and secondary points determined by identifying the meridians associated with the diseased organ. For example, large intestine 4 (L14) is used for orifacial, head, and neck problems, stomach 36 (ST36) for abdominal disorders, spleen 6 (SP6) for genitourinary disorders, urinary bladder 40, 60 (BL 40, 60) for low-back problems, and corresponding points in the auricle.

Insertion of needles is performed as quickly and painlessly as possible. A needle guide can be used to facilitate rapid insertion through the skin. When the needles are placed successfully, the patient is likely to experience a sensation known as *de qi,* which is described as a feeling of fullness, numbness, tingling, warmth, and/or soreness. Stimulation, either manual or electric, can be applied through the needles.

Electroacupuncture uses an electric, sometimes battery-operated, unit to stimulate the acupuncture point through the inserted needle. It offers several advantages over the traditional manual manipulation of needles, including (*a*) delivery of a continuous, uniform, and lengthy stimulation, (*b*) control of the intensity and frequency of the stimulation, and (*c*) simultaneous stimulation of multiple acupuncture points. For these reasons, electroacupuncture has grained popularity recently in the West as well as the East.

Acupuncture is a relatively simple and easy technique to learn. However, successful acupuncture requires that the practitioner be experienced and have a thorough understanding of the patient's physical and mental conditions. Acupuncture therapy should be preceded by a complete diagnostic workup and physical examination. Careful analysis of the treatment indication is a prerequisite for correct selection of primary and secondary acupuncture points. The effectiveness of the treatment should be evaluated continually to modify the treatment program if indicated.

Summary

The biochemical basis of acupuncture has been well established in animal studies. It seems to fit well into current understanding of neurobiology. However, its mechanism in the domain of biophysics and bioenergetics remained to be elucidated. An interesting hypothesis by Zhang and Popp may serve as a unified explanation of many phenomena observed in acupuncture (Zhang CL, Popp A, unpublished work). In its clinical application acupuncture research faces the problem of subjectivity (nonacupuncture point is not an adequate control). Its acceptance awaits results from biophysical studies.

LOW-LEVEL LASER THERAPY

Background

The properties of the laser include parallel, synchronized, and monochromatic light with a specific wavelength. Master's work on LLLT promoting healing sparked wide interest in the field. The earlier term, laser biostimulation, has been replaced by LLLT because of its bidirectional biological effects. The types of lasers commonly used are the helium neon (HeNe), ruby argon, and krypton lasers and more recently, gallium-arsenide (GaAs) and gallium-aluminum-arsenide (GaAlAs) infrared (IR) semiconductor laser diodes.

The parameters of useful lasers in LLLT are wavelengths of 632.8, 820, 830, or 904 nm, powers of 1 to 90 mW, waveforms of continuous or pulsed (1 to 4000 Hz) dosage, and site of 1 to 4 J/cm², spot size less than 1 mm², focused, defocused, and scanning, and duration several seconds to 30 seconds, daily or every other day. Other important parameters are duty cycle, subtotal energy, beam divergence (3 to 8° or more for IR laser diodes), delivery (fiberoptic, direct) and polarity. Karu and Basford published comprehensive reviews of laboratory research. Tissue absorption governs depth of penetration and refraction. The red light (632.8 nm) of a HeNe laser penetrates 0.5 to 1 mm before losing 1/e (37%) of its intensity, while IR light (820 to 940 nm) penetrates at least 2 mm before losing 37% of its energy. The effects of LLLT are nonthermal, and temperature elevations less than 0.5 to 7.5° C are wavelength dependent. The laser under discussion is LLLT, which is usually imperceptible and is capable of producing physiological effects. The mechanism is not well understood. However, it influences mitochondrial respiratory activities in a frequency-dependent manner, and many consider that this may be the basis for LLLT.

Validation of its clinical application is difficult because of the multifactional nature of pain syndromes and highly individualized responses to external stimuli. In the past decade better-designed, better-controlled, and more carefully blinded studies became available. This discussion is divided into biological and cellular studies and clinical studies (LLLT) sections.

Biological and Cellular Studies

LLLT increases or decreases protein synthesis and cell growth and differentiation, and it increases cell motility, membrane potential and binding affinities, neurotransmitter release, ATP synthesis, and prostaglandin synthesis. Tendons of tenotomized rabbits irradiated in vivo with HeNe laser (1 or 5 mJ/cm^2, pulsed for 20 days) show no collagen fibril production. Rochkind et al. showed that no more than 17 mW HeNe irradiation improves neurological viability and healing in rats and rabbits with both peripheral nerve and central nervous system injuries. Recently de Breakt found that 1 J/cm^2 830 nm IR irradiation for 10 treatments did not alter wound healing or maxillary arch dimensions in beagles following surgery. Basford found that visible and IR irradiation stimulates capillary growth and granulation and alters cytokine production. Noble et al. showed altered keratinocyte motility and fibroblast movement following laser irradiation. In additional studies laser irradiation was found to enhance, inhibit, or have no effect on the function of a variety of microorganisms and cells.

Master reported alterations of bacterial growth following HeNe laser irradiation. McGuff and Bell found that a 0.5-mW HeNe laser irradiation had no effect on bacteria, such as *Staphylococcus aureus* and *Pseudomonas aeruginosa.* Others found that some bacteria were sensitive to 6 to 40 mW, and dye-mediated laser sensibility has been shown also.

LLLT produces hypoalgesia as measured by tail flick test; LLLT of 4 Hz produces hypoalgesia of rapid onset and short duration, while the response to 60 Hz was delayed and long lasting. This analgesia or hypoalgesia is partially but significantly reversed by high dose of naloxone when measured by hotplate but not by tail flick method. This suggests that mechanisms other than endogenous opioids may be involved in LLLT-induced hypoalgesia. Laser biostimulation—induced hypoalgesia in rats is not naloxone reversible. Animal studies offer some positive findings, particularly in the earliest phases of wound healing in rabbit and rodent. Thus, the applicability of these findings to humans is undetermined. Similar experiments with pigs, which have skin more similar to that of humans, showed no benefit.

Clinical Studies

LLLT at acupuncture point (Ho Ko) in blindfolded subjects in a soundproof chamber did not alter somatosensory evoked potential (SEP) latency between 0 and 50 ms but did inhibit the late-phase (150 to 350 ms) SEP potentials. This latter change was due to anticipation and habituation. LLLT has been applied to numerous clinical conditions. However, the diversity of parameters make a cross-study comparison extremely difficult. Nonetheless, some important controlled clinical trials for the most intensively investigated LLLT will be reviewed.

For rotator cuff tendinitis conventional therapy (heat, ice, rest, exercise, massage, nonsteroidal anti-inflammatories, and corticosteroid injections) does not produce rapid or predictable outcome. Recently England et al. investigated 30 patients with supraspinatus or bicipital tendinitis. The subjects were divided into three groups: active treatment (3 mW, 904 nm, 5 minutes and six treatments), dummy treatment, and a group treated with nonsteroidal anti-inflammatory drugs only. The laser group had significantly better range of motion and analgesia than the other two groups. In this study, the patients and investigators were blinded, but the treating therapists were not. Vecchio et al. divided 30 patients with shoulder tendinitis randomly into LLLT (30 mW, 830 nm, 3 J/cm^2 maximum of 5 points) and sham LLLT groups. Improvement in movement, strength, and pain reduction occurred similarly in both groups.

In rheumatoid arthritis many IR and visible lasers are shown to decrease pain, swelling, morning stiffness, and medication use. The improvement is not accompanied by any consistent laboratory changes (immune complexes, C-reactive protein, and sedimentation rates). Ankylosing spondylitis treated with HeNe and IR lasers yielded similar clinical improvement. Despite the positive findings in some studies of rheumatic disease, others showed negative results. A large-scale study did not show enough positive evidence to persuade the U.S. Food and Drug Administration (FDA) panel in the mid-1980s to recommend approval for clinical use.

The effect of laser irradiation on nerve tissue is studied widely. Clinical studies in neurological conditions showed that LLLT did not alter nerve conduction. Rochkind's group showed that HeNe laser irradiation of the operative site of tethered spinal cords improves recovery. Bork and Snyder-Mackler find that irradiation using HeNe (1 mW) laser prolongs superficial radial nerve latencies. Wu et al. in a multicenter study and Basford et al. found that 1-mW HeNe laser irradiation reproduced neither prolongation of the superficial radial nerve latencies nor inhibition of the action potentials.

Higher power (30 to 60 mW) IR laser diodes (820 to 830 nm, 10 to 12 J/mm^2) LLLT alters superficial radial and median nerve latencies by several percent. The mild change could be produced by conventional modalities.

LLLT is advocated for carpal tunnel syndrome. A large, well-designed, double-blinded, randomized, controlled multicenter study of 160 automobile workers with electrodiagnostically confirmed and clinically symptomatic carpal tunnel syndrome has recently completed its treatment phase. The workers were divided into two groups, each of which took part in an exercise and ergonomic modification program. One group was treated with a 90-mW array of three 830-nm laser diodes; the other received sham irradiation. Final results are not yet available, but it appears that both groups improved in such measures as grip strength. In addition, the laser group reportedly had a better return-to-work rate and demonstrated a statistically significant symptom reduction relative to the sham group. Other factors, such as nerve conduction velocities, distal latencies, and blood flow are being evaluated. If the final results are strongly positive, this study may serve as the basis of an FDA review.

The FDA has approved LLLT for dental surgery. In a double-blind study of chronic orofacial pain Hansen and Thoroe found placebo more effective than pulsed 904-nm IR irradiation. In another double-blind study Ferando et al. and Masse et al. found that mixed laser (30 mW, 4 J/cm^2 830 nm, 2.5 minutes), HeNe (0.27 mW), and IR (80 mW) irradiation neither lessens pain, reduces swelling, nor improves healing following tooth extraction.

LLLT's effects on wound healing were studied by Master and associates in the late 1960s and early 1970s. They reported that HeNe laser irradiation (1 to 4 J/cm^2) promoted healing of chronic nonhealing soft tissue ulcer, with a cure rate above 70%. This observation stimulated use of laser therapy. In a well-controlled and blinded human wound healing study Lundeberg and Malm divided 46 patients with venous ulcers into two groups. All were treated with a program of paste-impregnated bandages and compressive wraps. Half received HeNe laser irradiation (6 mW, 4 J/cm^2, twice a week for 12 weeks), the other half sham irradiation. No significant differences in healing were found, supporting their earlier findings.

In chronic low-back pain many treatments evoke slow responses, and they are not always more effective than rest and a gradual return to normal activity. Despite many difficulties for objective evaluation, Klein and Eek studied 40 subjects; all received a standard exercise program. Half received 904 nm IR diode irradiation (1.3 J/cm^2, pulsed, 3 times a week for 4 weeks); the others were "treated" with a sham device. No statistical differences were found between the two groups in pain, disability, or range of motion parameters.

Patellofemoral pain was studied in 40 persons with arthroscopically documented chondromalacia patellae in a double-blinded fashion by Rogvi-Hansen et al. Subjects received either an active or a sham GaAs laser (17 mW, pulsed, 1000 Hz, 10 minutes, 8 times); there was no statistically significant difference between the groups at the end of 5 weeks. However, a trend showed 50% and 30% improvement in the treated and the sham group, respectively.

Tennis elbow (lateral epicondylitis) is another painful condition from repetitive injury. Local LLLT as well as laser acupuncture treatment protocols have been examined in double-blinded studies. For example, two acupuncture studies by Hacker and Lundeberg showed no benefit following a single HeNe laser treatment or 1 or 10 treatments from 0.07-mW and 12-mW pulsed GaAs IR devices. In a double-blinded controlled study of 30 subjects Vasseljen et al. found that eight local treatments with a 904 nm, 18 mW, 3.5 J/cm^2, array of pulsed IR diodes produced statistically significantly improvements in visual analog scale (VAS) scores and wrist extension as compared with the control group. However, even with these results, the investigators found that the benefits were limited if irradiation was performed in isolation from other therapy (splints, heat, ice, epicondylar straps, massage, injection, and activity modification).

Laser therapy for trigger point (tender points with a well-described pattern of referred pain) has been examined also. Responsiveness to LLLT HeNe CW laser 0.95 mW was studied by Snyder-Mackler in a double-blind controlled study of 24 patients. They found both a statistically significant reduction of pain and increased skin resistance at the trigger points in the group that was irradiated. Another study of 18 subjects by Olavi et al. was performed with a higher-power 904-nm IR laser. They also found that the irradiation significantly increased pain thresholds.

Acupuncture or auriculotherapy using lasers in many uncontrolled studies typically shows 80% or more improvement or cure after treatment. Unfortunately, in the controlled study of lateral epicondylitis Hacker and Lundeberg reported less impressive results. Another double-blinded and controlled study Brockhaus and Elger found that needle acupuncture altered thermal pain thresholds, whereas similar treatment with an HeNe laser (10 mW, repetitive, pulsed) did not. In contrast, King et al. used a 1-mW HeNe laser to evaluate 80 subjects using auriculotherapy in a controlled manner. Although it is not clear how well the evaluators were blinded, they found a statistically significant elevation of the pain threshold, 18%, in the treated group.

Meta-analysis on LLLT is available. Although meta-analysis requires the grouping of dissimilar LLLT regimens and conditions, some researchers think this approach would provide a more objective overview of LLLT than a review. This is arguable, but attempts have been made. In 1992 Beckerman et al. published an overview in which they evaluated 36 randomized LLLT studies of musculoskeletal pain and skin disorders, such as chronic ulcers. Despite the fact that more than 1700 subjects were included, variation of study design and quality limited the analysis. In fact, pooling was not possible. No conclusion about skin conditions was possible; and in the "better" musculoskeletal studies there was a tendency for LLLT to be more effective than placebo.

Gam et al. presented another meta-analysis, which was more strenuously restricted than that of Beckerman et al.; it was limited to 23 musculoskeletal pain trials. No differences were found between active and placebo treatment in the studies deemed "adequately blinded"; only a 9.5% difference occurred in the "insufficiently blinded" subset. As the confidence interval of both groups included no effect, it is not unexpected that these authors concluded that LLLT has no proven musculoskeletal effectiveness.

Summary

The value of LLLT has not been established, but some progress has been made. Better designed studies become more common. The relative standardization of the LLLT parameters (IR diodes or HeNe, 1 to 4 J/cm^2) become widely accepted. Several conclusions can be drawn from this review:

(*a*) Laboratory studies support the concept that laser irradiation can modify cellular processes in a wavelength-dependent, nonthermal manner. (*b*) Laser intensities sufficient to produce these cellular effects can be delivered to superficial tissues for LLLT. (*c*) Whether by a category-by-category analysis or by meta-analysis, high-quality trials still show marginal clinical effectiveness. LLLT may be particularly effective for neurological disorders. (*d*) Further clinical studies are needed.

MEDITATION

Meditation is a term applied to a diverse group of practices with the common goal of producing desired mental states and promoting personal well-being. Meditation is most often taught within the context of a religious discipline, so that the expected benefits have often been described in terms of spiritual progress. Recently in the Western societies, there has been an explosive increase of interest in meditation, such as transcendental meditation (TM), meditating yoga, and *ch'an*. Kanellakos and Lukas reviewed the lasting effects of TM on psychological variables and proposed that the practice of TM leads to the experience of a fourth major state of consciousness (the first three being waking, dreaming, and nondreaming sleep states) explained in Hinduism. Perhaps because the International Meditation Society is headed by a Hindu guru, Maharishi Mahesh Yogi, the TM movement has placed a great emphasis on physiological responses and scientific research.

Many patients with chronic pain require a comprehensive, multidisciplinary treatment including somatic, behavioral, and psychological therapies. Meditation can be conceptualized as a behavioral modality and a relaxation technique (Choi). Choi's approach to understanding meditation will be highlighted later. Buddhist practitioners study the function of the human mind, including sensations, behaviors, and various conscious experiences. To grasp the essence of meditation, one must believe that the intellect permits us to reach the limits of our mental capacity, at which words and thoughts cease and intuition replaces reason. It is reason that separates us from the completeness and universality of our true nature.

Many in the modern world are impressed with *ch'an* Buddhism because it does not accept any preconceived ideas, opinions, dogmas, or rituals of faith. *Ch'an* keeps aloof from all that popularly goes under the name of religion. *Ch'an* meditation will be discussed in more detail. It emphasizes irrationality and a lack of objectivity. Under the apparent irrationality of *ch'an* there is a solid basis of rationality because *ch'an* does not depend on any belief in dogma, ritual, or traditional thought, but relies on direct experience and unprejudiced observation. Experience gives rise to both science and mysticism. The only difference between these two realms of experience is that the truth of science is objectively verifiable, while mystic experience can be verified only subjectively. For the past decades, the very principle of objectivity in science has been challenged by development of the theories of relativity and quantum physics. This stimulated considerable interest in intellectual approaches to the mystical realm. In this respect, pain becomes a point where modern medicine meets Buddhism. There has been a growing interest among researchers in exploring the relation between behavior therapy and Buddhist psychology. In this chapter the relations among pain and religion, psychology of meditation, Buddhism and behavior modification, and various meditations independent of the religious beliefs will be discussed.

Pain and Religion

Relaxation training, biofeedback, operant conditioning, hypnosis, and cognitive-behavioral therapies as useful psychological interventions in chronic pain have recently been reviewed. Eastern Buddhist meditation can be defined as a form of cognitive-behavioral therapy. Buddhist mindfulness meditation aims at restructuring subjective experience and increasing insight by identifying distortions in mental processing. As with any other meditative technique, concentration of attention is necessary for eliciting the state of awareness. The initial concentration on the breath leads to relaxation, which allows the attention to scan in an open focus, shifting freely from one perception to the next. No sensation is considered an intrusion. The practitioner should be able to discern any association in thoughts, images, or emotions arising from internal and external stimuli. No branching of thought is allowed. Should any pain arise, the sensations should be turned into the focus of concentrated attention. By continuing this confronting observation of the pain, one gradually recognizes the sequence of events in the mind as they arise, culminate, and vanish. This technique is widely accepted in the West. Sternbach emphasized psychological and behavioral strategies for pain control. Melzack and Wall stressed motivational and cognitive aspects of chronic pain. The gate control theory provided a psychophysiological model for conceptualizing that the modulating effects of attention, distraction, suggestion, anxiety, and other emotional states can modulate the perception and interpretation of pain. There is anatomical and physiological evidence for three interacting dimensions of the pain experience: sensory-discriminative, motivational-affective, and cognitive-interpretive. As discussed earlier, the activity in the cognitive and/or motivational domains can modulate sensory transmission at the spinal cord entry level via the descending pathways, thereby influencing the sensory dimension of the pain experience. The potential benefit of using meditation for self-regulation of chronic pain depends on one's ability to separate the sensation from the self. Through practice one can obtain an attitude of detached observation in the field of awareness when a sensation becomes prominent and to uncouple the sensation and its painful meaning. This uncoupling of "sensation" and of "meaning pain" reduces power of the pain experience—the hurt, the suffering. This uncoupling, once learned, goes beyond the period of meditation. It becomes accessible in everyday life via the conscious use of the learned attentional and attitudinal shift. The practice of mindfulness meditation was used by Kabat-Zinn in a 10-week stress reduction and relaxation program to train 51 chronic pain patients in self-regulation. At 10 weeks, 65% of the patients showed a reduction of more than 33% in the mean total pain rating index of Melzack, and 50% showed a reduction of more than 50%. Kabat-Zinn concluded that this form of meditation can be useful for chronic pain patients by reducing the experience of suffering via cognitive reappraisal.

The Psychology of Meditation

There is some resemblance between the meditation and various relaxation therapies, such as self-hypnosis and progressive relaxation, autogenic therapy, and perhaps biofeedback training, particularly with electroencephalographic (EEG) α- or θ-rhythm training. Proponents of meditation throughout history have aimed to induce certain peak experiences. The attainability and importance of these experiences (samadhi, satori, nirvana, *kkaech'im,* cosmic consciousness, and so on) are attested to in the literature. Much of mystical experience is expressed in literary, poetic, and/or religious terms. The philosopher Stace showed the lists of mystical consciousness derived from a careful analysis from the mystic literature: (*a*) deep feeling of positive mood, described as bliss, peace, love, and so on; (*b*) experience of unity, or the oneness of all things; (*c*) a sense of ineffability; (*d*) an enhanced sense of reality, authenticity, meaning; (*e*) alteration of time and space perception; (*f*) paradoxic acceptance of a proposition that in normal consciousness seems contradictory. There is also a sense of sacredness. Meditation is a process that when viewed as merely relaxation has been reported to have some negative consequences, such as the subject being threatened by the idea of relaxing and paradoxically becoming more anxious. These experiences are similar to the boundless "big I" (versus ego-oriented "small I") in Buddhist meditation. The big I allows one to exercise the perfect freedom at will. The practice of detached observation is to open the gate to the realm of big I. Some psychologists consider the motivation to practice meditation a positive one. Weil contends that the desire to alter our state of consciousness is normal and universal. Maslow has written much about the positive effects of such peak experiences.

Using a reductionist paradigm, one faces a major difficulty in meditation research because of the lack of acceptable objective validation criteria for the person's presumed meditative state. At present, however, the only way to validate "successful meditation" is by the subjective statement of clear recognition of the desired change in consciousness. Eastern thought, as opposed to Western thought, is not interested in approximate or relative knowledge. It is concerned with absolute knowledge involving the understanding of the totality of life, namely a holistic viewpoint.

The Eastern sages are generally not interested in explaining things but rather in obtaining a direct nonintellectual, intuitive experience of the unity of all things. To free the human mind from words and explanations is one of the main aims of Eastern religion. Therefore, it seems to be easier for Eastern religion to deal with mind research than it is for Western reductionist intellects. There is no agreement on an accepted core of psychological features in various meditative practices. However, a prominent feature of most meditations is profound sensory detachment from the external environment. This sensory detachment is an inward direction of attention. Yet a vital characteristic of successful meditation (particularly where concentration practices are employed) is the active or, more often, passive suppression of thinking. This refers particularly to verbal thinking ("internal dialogue") but also to a certain extent to various nonverbal thinking processes.

Buddhism and Behavior Modification

For about 2500 years many Buddhist practitioners have been studying the functioning of the human mind, including sensations, convert behavior and processes, and the related subjective conscious experiences. A vast Buddhist literature contains a wealth of psychological information. Recently there has been increasing interest on the interrelationship between Buddhism and behavior modification. There are many commonalities of approach between the two. Both encourage increased awareness of the body and mind. Both emphasize the importance of learning self-control. The combination of the two covers several domains of behavior and experience, including behavioral, personal, and transpersonal domains. The behavioral domain includes all behavior, overt and covert, such as motor, verbal, psychological, and thinking. This domain is emphasized in behavior modification. Buddhism also stresses this domain as the foundation for changes in the other domains. Buddhism's main goal is to achieve fuller living in the present realm, leading to a more direct perception of the eternal present. Both encourage perceiving reality as it is. The personal domain includes one's subjective experience of the behavioral domain. Behavior modification produces changes in the personal domain through changes in the behavior domain. Buddhism encourages objective study of the phenomena of the personal domain and points out problems related to identifying with a particular sense of self. The transpersonal domain deals with a conscious space embracing all objects of consciousness. It arises prior to the experience of the personal domain. The knowledge of this domain arises only when one goes beyond the limitations of the personal domain. Western psychology, and particularly behavior modification, have had little to say of this domain; Buddhism, in contrast, has much to contribute here. Mikulas claims that this integration would be not just a combination but the development of more principles of psychology that apply in various domains.

Types of Meditation

There are many types of meditation. All great religions embrace some measure of meditation, since religion needs prayer and prayer needs concentration of mind. Tsung-mi, one of the early Chinese *ch'an* masters, classified the five main types of *ch'an*. Although they have some variations in leg crossing, hand folding, or breath control, there are three common basic elements: an erect sitting posture, correct control of breathing, and concentration. In these types, they do present differences in the substance and purpose. The first of these types, the "ordinary" *ch'an*, is purely for improving physical and mental health without any philosophic or religious content. Through practice one learns to concentrate, control and free one's mind, and indeed to restrain one's thoughts. An enrichment of personality and strengthening of character inevitably follow, because the three basic elements of mind—intellect, feeling, and will—develop harmoniously. The quiet sitting practiced in Confucianism seems to have stressed mainly these effects of mind concentration. Most medical applications of meditation shown in recent publications fall into this category. The second kind of *ch'an* is the Outside Way, which is used in teachings other than Buddhism. This is a meditation related to religion and philosophy yet not to Buddhism. Hindu yoga, the quiet sitting of Confucianism, and contemplative practices in Christianity all belong to this category. The third type is the Small Vehicle, which takes one from one state of mind (delusion) to another (enlightenment). It is designed to accommodate only one's self but not to reach the Buddha's enlightenment, in that unity with the cosmos in its totality is achieved. The fourth type is called Great Vehicle (Mahayana), and this is a truly Buddhist *ch'an*, for it allows one to see into one's essential nature and realize the Way in one's daily life. For those able to comprehend the Buddha's own enlightenment and with a desire to break through their own illusory view of the universe and experience absolute and undifferentiated reality, the Buddha taught this kind of *ch'an*. The fifth type is the Highest Vehicle, the crown of Buddhist *ch'an*. This *ch'an* was practiced by all of the Buddhas of the past and is the expression of absolute life, life in its purest form. It involves no struggle for enlightenment or any other object. When correctly practicing it, one has the firm conviction that *ch'an* is the actualization of one's true nature and that the day will come, feeling, "Ah, this is it!" The Lin-chi Buddhist sect places a Great Vehicle *ch'an* uppermost and the Highest Vehicle beneath it, whereas the Tsao-t'ung sect does the reverse. There are three aims of *ch'an*: (*a*) development of the power of concentration, (*b*) awakening, and (*c*) actualization of the Supreme Way in daily life. These three form an inseparable unity: mindfulness meditation, or insight meditation in Mahayana Buddhism, Tsao-t'ung *ch'an* practice, and yoga traditions as described by Krishnamurti. This approach emphasizes the detached observation from one moment to the next of a constantly changing field of objects.

Having achieved stability of attention, the field of objects expands ultimately to include all physical and mental experiences (body sensations, thoughts, memories, emotions, perceptions, intuitions, and fantasies) as they occur.

Summary

Meditation can be viewed as a cognitive-behavior therapy. Its backgrounds, pain and Buddhism, psychology and usefulness in pain therapy, lead to the recent growing trend toward the combination of Buddhism and behavior modification. Exploration of this approach has led to further understanding the role of Buddhism in modern medicine. *Ch'an* Buddhism rejects any religious dogma, including its own. It also rejects formulated beliefs. These concepts impressed the scientific and antireligious attitudes of modern Western intellectuals. Unfortunately, there is no way to validate the meditative state objectively. The objectivity criterion used by Western reductionism finds a great deal of difficulty in dealing with meditation research. Further research with an expanded paradigm is needed in mind research.

"Pain" in human existence was such a primary concern to Buddha that it prompted him to abandon his luxurious life and set out to discover the cause of human suffering. The Buddha's teaching is about self-development. Its basic aspects were introduced along with the varieties of meditation. Meditation is not only a form of behavior modification but also a way to understand the fundamental values of human inner experience of reality. With the ability of uncoupling of pain and its meaning meditation, practitioners can reduce the pain experience.

A CRITICAL EVALUATION OF COMPLEMENTARY ALTERNATIVE MEDICINE

Qi Gong

Qi gong was first described by Chu Yuan (342–278 B.C.), who discussed the principles of *qi gong* induction, introspective awareness, proper behavior, elimination of interfering thoughts, quietness, concentration, and breathing techniques to "cultivate the proper *qi*." In *The Yellow Emperor's Classic Internal Medicine*, *qi* was described as a part of the dynamic energy system of the universe. The universe includes the sun, moon, earth, and every other matter. This subtle energetic phenomenon can be recorded using technology, literature, and mathematics. This unified natural system has been used as a health maintenance system ever since. The practice of *qi gong* is popular in China, Japan, and Hong Kong and has recently gained popularity in the United States as part of CAM.

Contemporary medicine is based on a biochemical model, while much CAM is based on an integrated biophysical and biochemical model. *Qi gong* is an electromagnetic phenomenon and a part of CAM. Our analysis will be divided into chemical, physical, and biological studies and human studies.

Chemical, Physical, and Biological Studies

Chemical and physical evidence of the *qi gong* effect is quite rich. Using LiF (Mg, Ti) thermal γ-detector to measure the activities at eight sites in an auditorium before and after a 3-hour gathering conducted by a *qi gong* master showed progressively stronger activities toward the master, which was higher than the stable baseline in the control (sham master).

Qi emission by a master appears to have chemical and physical effects on various molecules. Infrared imaging and fluorescence spectrometry were used to measure activities of the test tubes containing 12 substances (l-arginine, bovine serum albumin, vitamin B_1, rhodium, Cd^+, Ni^+, and Cu^{++} solutions, and so on). *Qi* emission caused the temperature to rise by 1.5 to 5.2° C, with that of the control unchanged. The optical absorption (at wavelengths 239 and 256 nm) of fish DNA solution (10 mm/mL) increased by 4.8 to 45%, with control of 0 to 4.8%. Similarly, the absorption spectrum at 241 and 270 mm of thymidine solution (10 μg/mL) increased significantly after *qi* emission. *Qi* emission released free radicals from a sample of silver bromine sealed in black paper wrapping and produced an effect similar to that of light as measured by electron magnetic resonance apparatus.

Muehsami et al. demonstrated that *qi* emission significantly reduced phosphorylation (approximately 10%; p < .05) of a cell-face myosin preparation. This effect is similar to those observed in applied magnetic fields. *Qi* emission for 20 minutes produced a significant cytotoxic effect on the cultured cells (human cervical carcinoma SGC-7901 and gastric carcinoma cell lines) with a kill rate of 30.7 and 25.2%, respectively, with control of 0%. In C 56 BL mice after intraperitoneal injection of 5% sheep red blood cells (SRBC) (0.2 mL per mouse) the experimental groups received *qi* emission 20 minutes a day for 5 days. At the end of the fifth day, the peritoneal giant macrophages were examined for phagocytosis, intracellular acid phosphatase activity, mice splenic cell count, and induced anti-SRBC immunoglobulin-μ. All parameters were significantly higher than those of the control. Cytotoxicity to the harvested tumor (EAC) cells from the ascites was studied. The tumor cell survival rate after *qi* emission for an hour was 20% versus 3% in the control (p < .01) at 12 hours. The cytotoxicity power varies with different *qi gong* masters. When *qi* was applied to tumor-transplanted mice, the tumor was smaller than that of the control (p < .05). *Qi* emission promotes maturation of lymphoblast as well as Roset formation against SRBC as compared with control (p < .05). In NIH mice with immunosuppression induced by cyclophosphamide, *qi* emission for 10 to 15 minutes a day for 7 days) showed a higher thymus index (p < .005), indicating reduction of the thymus injury; thicker glandular cortex (p < .001), and thinner medullary substance (p < .05) than the control. In the New Zealand rabbit, a reperfusion myocardial injury model was established by ligating a branch of the left descending coronary artery for 60 minutes, then releasing the obstruction for 20 minutes. The *qi gong* group (n = 10) received *qi* emission

30 minutes a day for 20 days prior to surgery and throughout the surgery. The control group (n = 7) received no *qi*. The *qi gong* group showed lactate dehydrogenase (LDH) of 66.62 U/dL versus the control 106.31 U/dL (p < .05). Myocardial adenosine triphosphate (ATP) concentrations were not different. However, the myocardial adenosine diphosphate (ADP) concentration in the *qi gong* group was 42.75 μmol/mg, lower than the control group's 97.98 μmol/mg (p < .05). Thus, the ATP-ADP ratio is higher in the *qi gong* group (8.81×10^{-2} than in the control group (5.56×10^{-2}; p < .05). The postperfusion microscopic findings, including myofibril swelling, necrosis, loss of staining, contraction, and focal eosinophil infiltration, were less in the *qi gong* group. With microelectrodes to record the spontaneous electrical activity of rat brain cells in anesthetized rats, after *qi* emission for 1 to 2 minutes, the *qi gong* master left the laboratory. The recording was compared with that of the sham group. Of 25 brain cells, 23 were recorded long enough for data analysis, and 8 cells increased the spontaneous activity (average interval in milliseconds, a reduction of 16 ms; p < .05), representing excitatory cells. Another 8 cells showed reduction of the spontaneous activity (average interval from 12.6 to 211.6 ms; p < .05), representing inhibitory cells. The other 9 cells responded to the wish of the *qi gong* master's idea. The excitatory idea led to an increase in activity (the average interval from 83.1 to 32.6 ms; p < .05). In the same cells the master's inhibitory idea led to reduced activity (the interval of 24.5 to 491.2 ms; p < .05). The sham master had no effect on the recordings. Two cells did not respond to the *qi* emission. In rats pain threshold was measured by the K^+ iontophoresis method. The challenge was delivered three times with an interval of 30 seconds. *Qi* emission was delivered by a master to the rats for 15 minutes. Then the pain threshold was measured immediately and every 10 minutes for 4.5 hours. Group 1 was the control. Group 2 was divided into two subgroups, each of which received the *qi* emission from a different *qi gong* master. Group 3 received *qi* from a sham master. Group 1 showed no change. The threshold in both subgroups of group 2 (n = 15 and 16) increased (p≤ .01). The threshold peaked 30 or 40 minutes after cessation of the *qi* emission. The maximum duration of effect was 4.5 hours. Group 3 (n = 6) and group 1 showed no threshold difference. These studies were repeated with additional groups in which the rat periaqueductal gray matter (PAG) was lesioned stereotactically under general anesthesia with sham operation as control. After lesioning, the observed change from *qi gong* disappeared, suggesting a PAG mechanism involved in *qi gong*—induced analgesia.

Human Studies

In humans *qi gong* has also been found beneficial. Some of the studies are summarized here. Physiological parameters of 111 *qi gong* practitioners were measured 10 minutes before and 15 minutes after *qi gong* practice and 40 minutes after completion of *qi gong;* and recording continued 10 minutes thereafter. The changes included respiratory rate 70.8 plus or minus 4.5 to 13.6 plus or minus 7.7/minute (p < .05); pulse rate 71.4 plus or minus 11.8 to 76.2 plus or minus 14.7/minute (p < .01); skin temperature 31.5 plus or minus 2.3 to 33.4 plus or minus 1.7°C (p < .05) . During *qi gong* practice, the EEG showed a reduction of δ-waves and an increase of αθ-waves (p < .05). During the practice, the urinary epinephrine and the norepiniphrine (NE) excretion increased (p < .05) in subjects (n = 10), with significant EEG changes.

In another clinical study, after *qi gong* practice, 68 patients with chronic illnesses (hypertension, coronary heart disease, peptic ulcer, gastritis, emphysema, chronic bronchitis, arthritis, depression) showed mean changes in blood serotonin from 0.42 plus or minus 0.21 to 0.21 plus or minus 0.13 μg/mL (normal range 0.15 plus or minus 0.04 μg/mL) (P < .001); epinephrine from 0.27 plus or minus 0.13 to 0.35 plus or minus 0.27 μg/ml (p .01); dopamine from 0.86 plus or minus 0.69 to 1.19 plus or minus 0.81 μg/ml (p < .02) .

In 58 male hypertensive patients after a year of *qi gong* practice (n = 34) there was an increase of plasma estrogen (E) concentration and decrease of E_2/testosterone ratio, with no change in the control (n = 24). Sun studied 123 terminal cancer patients, all of whom received same pharmacotherapy. They were divided into the *qi gong* (n = 93) and non—*qi gong* groups (n = 30). Cancer types included gastric, 42.23%; intestinal, 31.7%; breast, 11.29%; and esophageal and pyloric, 8.12%. The *qi gong* regimen was 2 hours daily for 3 months per course. Improvements of fatigue was seen in 81.7% of patients; appetite, 63%; bowel irregularity and diarrhea, 33.3%; the control group showed improvement in 10, 10, and 6% of patients, respectively (p < .01). Body weight increased by 3 kg or more in 5.4% and reduction by 3 kg or more in 5.4%, while in the control group weight gain or weight loss occurred in 13.33 and 30%, respectively (p < .01). In a study of 345 cancer patients 6 to 9 months of *qi gong* practice was associated with the following observations: (*a*) There was constitutional improvement in factors such as appetite, sleep, strength, mood, and secondary infection. (*b*) Hematological changes (mean) included the average white blood cell count increasing from 1700 to 7800 and platelet count from 5.1×10^4 to 15.7×10^4/mL and hemoglobin from 5.2 to 14.3 g/dL. (*c*) There was improvement in malaise, pain, hemoptysis, and swallowing disturbance. In the 93 cases of breast cancer in this series, symptomatic relief occurred in 83.6%. In the 115 cases of lung cancer, improvement occurred in 75.1%. In the 72 cases of intestinal cancer, 68.2% improved. In the 65 cases of nasal pharyngeal cancer, 64.4%. (*d*) There was increased tolerance to chemotherapy with reduced side effects, such as vomiting, dizziness, headache, fatigue, insomnia, and dyspepsia. Regrowth of hair and eyebrows was more rapid. (*e*) Tumor mass appeared to be softening, reducing in size, and occasionally disappearing. (*f*) There was coincidental improvement of other coexisting diseases .

In 10 human subjects suffering from various chronic diseases, with white blood cells and platelet and at the lower normal limits, the subjects received 16 sessions of *qi* emission from a master, with the parameters measured before and after each session. In all 10 subjects, the average results were as follows: the platelets went from 6.7×9^4/mL to 8.2×10^4 /mL (p < .01); white cells, from 4493/mL to 5187./mm³ (p < .05). Serum red albumin showed bidirectional changes (in 10 cases 9.98 to 10.44 mg/100 mL ; p < .01) in seven patients; after 14 sessions red and white blood cell counts, hematocrit, hemoglobin, mean corpuscular volume (MCV), mean corpuscular hemoglobin concentration (MCHC), mean corpuscular hemoglobin (MCH), and platelets except MCHC all increased. These changes continued to rise an hour after cessation of *qi* emission, then returned to baseline

Wu et al. studied 24 refractory patients in late stage complex regional pain syndrome 1 (reflex sympathetic dystrophy) diagnosed under the uniform criteria. In a quasi-randomized fashion they were divided into two age-, disease stage-, pain intensity-matched groups. All were treated similarly except that the control group got visual and music stimulation and were exposed to a sham master. The *qi gong* regimen included visual and music stimulation, *qi gong* exercise, and *qi* adjustment, one session a week for 6 weeks. Psychological instruments used to monitor all patients included symptoms checklist 90, Carleton University Responsiveness to Suggestion Scale, and patients' expectations. Outcome measures included thermography, range of motion, visual signs (swelling, mottling, dystrophy, muscle wasting, and dystonia) VAS, medication, and pain awakening. In the *qi gong* and control groups, respectively, 11 and 9 patients completed the program. Both groups felt their *qi gong* masters to be real masters. The *qi gong* group had postsession short-term analgesia but not long lasting (p < .05), and prolonged reduction of anxiety (p < .01) at 6 weeks over the control. All other parameters showed no significant differences between the two groups. However, 3 patients in the *qi gong* group showed dramatic reduction in swelling, pain, and medication and increase in range of motion, and one patient showed an increase in weight-bearing limits and activity levels, not all of which could be explained by long-standing (longer than 12 months) prestudy stabilized condition. During this study, (conducted in a room with constant temperature) we also observed that the Laogun acupuncture point of the *qi gong* master warmed up 4°C during *qi* emission. This temperature increase is in agreement with some of the Chinese studies using similar methodology.

Qi gong practice (54 minutes twice a day for 30 days) was taught to 60 healthy workers average 40.5 years old, with a control group of 20 minerotherapy workers average age 36.4 years old who received no treatment; exercise reserve was measured. The post—*qi gong* value increased from the baseline by 574.94 kilogram-meters (kgm)/minute; the control group increased by 83.75 kgm/minute (p < .05).VO_{2max} increased by 0.97l/minute in the *qi gong* group and in the control group by 0.14l/minute (p < .05). The baseline mean heart rate was 73.4/minute. During the 54-minute practice, it increased to a mean of 94.3/minutes with a maximum of 124.4 beats/minute, and returned to 82.7/minute 10 minutes post *qi gong*. This suggested the *qi gong* practice is a low load and does not exceed the VO_{2max} by 50%, hence is suitable for cardiac patients.

In a study of 120 patients with hypertensive coronary heart disease with similar blood pressure, eye ground changes, abnormality of electrocardiogram, and types of medication, they were randomly assigned to two groups. One group (n = 60) received *qi gong,* and the control group (n = 60) did not. The courses of disease after entry into the study were different. After a year of practice, the *qi gong* group had normalized blood pressure in 86.7%, symptomatic improvement in 62.6%, and electrocardiography (ECG) improvement in 52.9%. Values for the control group were 65, 34.8, and 22.2%, respectively (p < .052 to .001). In 30 cases of hypertensive coronary heart disease, after a year of the practice the cardiac output increased and ejection fraction increased significantly. In 20 cases of hypertensive patients, serum hydroxybutyric dehydrogenase (DBH) activity decreased from 19.67 plus or minus 1.54 IU to 18.23 plus or minus 1.51 IU after 6 months of *qi gong* practice. In another 30 hypertensive patients a 6-month practice led to significant improvement of the platelet adhesiveness. In another 30 hypertensive patients a 6-month practice led to significant decline in triglyceride and total cholesterol coupled with an increase of high-density lipoprotein (HDL) .

Summary

The laboratory data on *qi gong* effects are grouped into chemical, physical, biological, and clinical studies. The laboratory studies are easier to accept from a newtonian mechanical perspective. The clinical studies can be viewed as preliminary investigations. However, the observations open up many interesting aspects to potential research areas because none has tried to explain the findings. It may need a new concept to integrate biochemical and biophysical (subtle energetics) information and accept new concepts of matter and energy duality and new technology for basic research in this area.

CONCLUSION

Noxious stimuli are transmitted through the paleospinothalamic and neospinothalamic tracts in a slow and fast manner. When the signals reach the brainstem, midbrain, and hypothalamus through the slow tract, they are transmitted to the modulating circuit at multiple levels, including the powerful descending inhibitory pathway at their spinal cord level. These signals in the central nervous system participate in the sensory-discriminatory, emotional-interpretive, and cognitive-behavioral domains and thus are processed and interpreted. This recent understanding of neurobiology has created emphasis on the concept of holism, which is the centerpiece of CAM. The four subjects reviewed in this chapter share several characteristics in the perspective of science:

1. Subjectivity is a unique experience in all four practices: chemical, biochemical, physical, cellular, and biological data support their effects. However, an expanded paradigm (einsteinian conceptual of duality) is needed to conduct mind research.
2. Mind, spirit, and body interact and finally express one's behavior in unity. Holism is needed to remove mainstream science's barriers to the study of chronic diseases and wellness maintenance.
3. Research in subtle energy in maintenance of proper biological functions may gain recognition in the 21st century.

Suggested Reading

Abergel RP, Dwyer RM, Meeker CA, et al. Laser treatment of keloids: a clinical trial and an in vitro study with Nd: YAG laser. Lasers Surg Med 1984;4:291.

Anderson RR, Parrish JA. The optics of human skin. J Invest Dermatol 1981; 77:13–19.

Anderson W. Open secrets: a western guide to Tibetan Buddhism. New York: Viking, 1979.

Bal HS. The skin. In: Senson MJ, ed. Dukes' physiology of domestic animals. 9th ed. Ithaca, NY: Cornell University Press, 1977;493–503.

Basford JR. Low-energy laser treatment of pain and wounds: hype, hope, or hokum? Mayo Clin Proc 1986;61:671.

Basford JR, Daube JR, Hallman HO, et al. Does low-intensity helium-neon laser irradiation alter sensory nerve action potentials or distal latencies? Lasers Surg Med 1990;10:35–39.

Basford JR, Hallman HO, Matsumoto JY, et al. Effects of 830 nm continuous wave laser diode irradiation on median nerve function in normal subjects. Lasers Surg Med 2993;13:597–604.

Basford JR, Hallman HO, Sheffield CG, Mackey GL. Comparison of the effects of cold quartz ultraviolet, low energy laser, and occlusion on wound healing in a swine model. Arch Phys Med Rehab 1986;67:151–154.

Baxter GD, Allen JM, Bell AJ, et al. Effect of laser (830 nm) upon conduction in the median nerve. American Society for Laser Medicine and Surgery Abstracts. Laser Surg Med Suppl 1991;3:79.

Beckerman H, deBie RA, Bouter LM, et al. The efficacy of laser therapy for musculoskeletal and skin disorders: a criteria-based meta-analysis of randomized clinical trials. Phys Ther 1992;72:483–491.

Bliddal H, Hellesen C, Ditleven P, et al. Soft-laser therapy of rheumatoid arthritis. Scand J Rheumatol 1987;16:225.

Bork CE, Snyder-Mackler L. Effect of helium-neon laser irradiation on peripheral sensory nerve latency. Phys Ther 1988;68:223–225.

Brackhaus A, Elger CE. Hypalgesic efficacy of acupuncture on experimental pain in man: comparison of laser acupuncture and needle acupuncture. Pain 1990;43:181–185.

Brown BB. new mind, new body: biofeedback, new directions for the mind. New York: Harper & Row, 1974.

Brucke RM. Cosmic consciousness. Secaucus, NJ: Citadel, 1961.

Brunner R, Haina D, Landthaler M, et al. Application of laser light of low-power density: experimental and clinical investigations. Curr Probl Dermatol 1986;15:111.

Cao XD, Xu SF, Lu WX. Inhibition of sympathetic nervous system by acupuncture. Acupunct Electrother Res Int J 1983;8:25–35.

Chang HT. Neurophysiological basis of acupuncture analgesia. Sci Sin 1978;21:829–846.

Chang L, et al. *Qi gong* effects on the immunosuppressed mice. Proceedings of I World Congress on medical *qi gong.* Beijing, 1988:13.

Chao S, et al. The inhibitory effect of *qi gong* on transplanted tumor cells in mice, preliminary study. Proceedings of I World Congress on medical *qi gong.* Beijing, 1988:20.

Chen CH. The neurophysiological mechanism of acupuncture treatment in psychiatric illness: an autonomic-humoral theory. Am J Clin Med 1979;7:188–1187.

Choy DSJ, Purnell F, Jaffee R. Auricular acupuncture for the cessation of smoking. In Schwartz JL, ed. Progress in smoking cessation. Proceedings of international conference on smoking cessation. New York: June 21–23, 1978. New York: American Cancer Society, 1979;329–334.

Conze E. The perfection of wisdom in eight thousand lines and its verse summary. Bolinas, CA: Four Seasons Foundation, 1973.

Davidson JM. The physiology of meditation and mystical states of consciousness. Perspect Biol Med 1976;19:345–378.

England S, Farrell AJ, Coppock JS, et al. Low power laser therapy of shoulder tendonitis. Scand J Rheumatol 1989;18:427–431.

Fernando S, Hill CM, Walker R. A randomised double blind comparative study of low level laser therapy following surgical extraction of lower third molar teeth. Br J Oral Maxillofac Surg 1993;31:170–172.

Fork RL. Laser stimulation of nerve cells in aplasia. Science 1971;171:907–908.

Fox EJ, Melzack R. Transcutaneous electrical stimulation and acupuncture: comparison of treatment for low back pain. Pain 1976;2:141–148.

Franz DN, Iggo A. Dorsal root puncture hypalgesia is mediated by afferent nerve impulses: an electrophysiological study in mice. Exp Neurol 1979;66:398–402.

Fung LD, et al. The effect of external *qi gong* on human tumor cells. Proceedings of I World Congress on medical *qi gong.* Beijing, 1988:1.

Fung LD, et al. The effect of external *qi gong* on mucous immune function. Proceedings of I World Congress on medical *qi gong.* Beijing, 1988:3.

Gam AN, Thorsen H, Lonnberg F. The effect of low-level laser therapy on musculoskeletal pain: a meta-analysis. Pain 1993;52:63–66.

Gartner C. Low reactive level laser therapy (LLLT) in rheumatology: a review of the clinical experience in the author's laboratory. Laser Ther 1992;4:107–115.

Goldman JA, Chiapella J, Casey H, et al. Laser therapy in rheumatoid arthritis. Lasers Surg Med 1980;1:93.

Goleman D. The Varieties of meditative experience. New York: Dutton, 1977.

Greathouse DG, Currier DP, Gilmore RL. Effects of clinical infrared laser on superficial radial nerve conduction. Phys Ther 1985;65:1184.

Guenther HV. Buddhist philosophy in theory and practice. Berkeley: Shambhala, 1976.

Guenther HV, Kawamura LS. Mind in Buddhist psychology. Emeryville, CA: Dharma, 1975.

Gunn CC. Type IV acupuncture points. Am J Acupunct 1977;5:51–52.

Gunn CC, Ditchburn FG, King MH, et al. Acupuncture loci: a proposal for their classification according to their relationship to known neural structure. Am J Chin Med 1976;4:183–195.

Haker E, Lundeberg T. Laser treatment applied to acupuncture points in lateral epicondylalgia. Pain 1990;43:243–247.

Hans JS, Terenius L. Neurochemical basis of acupuncture analgesia. Annu Rev Pharmacol Toxicol 1982;22:193–220.

Hansen HJ, Thoroe U. Low power laser biostimulation of chronic oro-facial pain: a double-blind placebo controlled cross-over study in 40 patients. Pain 1990;43:169–179.

Hokfeldt T, Ljungdahl A, Terenius L, et al. Immunohistochemical analysis of peptide pathway possibly related to pain and analgesia: enkephalin and substance P. Proc Natl Acad Sci U S A 1977;74:3081–3085.

Hosobuchi Y, Adams JE, Linchitz R. Pain relief by electrical stimulation of central gray matter in humans and its reversal by naloxone. Science 1977;197:183–186.

Huang GS. Beneficial effects of *qi gong* on cancer treatment. Proceedings of I World Congress on medical *qi gong.* Beijing, 1988:69.

Hunter J, Leonard L, Wilson R, et al. Effects of low energy laser on wound healing in a porcine model. Lasers Surg Med 1984;3:285–290.

In de Braekt MMH, Van Alphen FAM, Kuijpers-Jagtman AM, Maltha JC. The effect of low-level laser treatment on maxillary arch dimensions after palatal surgery on beagle dogs. J Dent Res 1991;70:1467–1470.

Jacobson E. Progressive relaxation. Chicago: Chicago University Press, 1938.

James W. The varieties of religious experience. New York: Modern Library, 1929.

Jessell TM, Iversen LL. Opiate analgesics inhibit substance p release from rat spinal trigeminal nucleus. Nature 1977;268:549–551.

Kaada B, Jorum E, Sagvolden T, et al. Analgesia induced by trigeminal nerve stimulation (electro-acupuncture) abolished by nuclei raphe lesions in rats. Acupunct Electrother Res Int J 1979;4:221–234.

Kabat-Zinn J. An outpatient program in behavioral medicine for chronic pain patients based on the practice of mindfulness meditation. Gen Hosp Psychiatry 2982;4:33–47.

Kan JS, Hutschenreiter G, Haina D, Waidelich W. Effect of low-power density laser radiation on healing of open skin wounds in rats. Arch Surg 1981;116:293.

Kanellakos DP, Lukas JS. The psychobiology of transcendental meditation. Menlo Park, CA: Benjamin, 1974.

Kao FF. China, Chinese medicine and the Chinese medical system. Am J Chin Med 1973;1:59.

Kao FF, Baker RH Jr, Leung SJ, et al. Efficacy of acupuncture for the treatment of sensorineural deafness. Am J Chin Med 1973;1:283–304.

Karu TI. Photobiological fundamentals of low-power laser therapy. IEEE J Quant Elect 1987;23:1703.

Karu TI. Molecular mechanism of the therapeutic effect of low-intensity laser radiation. Lasers Life Sci 1988;2:53–74.

King CE, Clelland JA, Knowles CJ, Jackson JR. Effect of helium-neon laser auriculotherapy on experimental pain threshold. Phys Ther 1990;70:24–30.

Klein RG, Eek BC. Low-energy laser treatment and exercise for chronic low back pain: double-blind controlled trial. Arch Phys Med Rehabil 1990;71:34–37.

Kolari PJ. Penetration of unfocused laser light into the skin. Arch Dermatol Res 1985;277:342–344.

Krishnamurti J. Freedom from the known. New York: Harper & Row, 1969.

Krishnamurti J. The wholeness of life. New York: Harper & Row, 1979.

Kutz I, Caudll M, Benson H. The role of relaxation in behavioral therapies for chronic pain. In: Stein JM, Warfield CA, eds. International anesthesiology clinics. Pain management, vol. 21. Boston: Little, Brown, 1983;193–199.

Lam TS, Abergel RP, Meeker CA, et al. Laser stimulation of collagen synthesis in human skin fibroblast cultures. Lasers Life Sci 1986;1:61–77.

Lau B, Wang D, Slater J. Effect of acupuncture on allergic rhinitis: clinical and laboratory evaluations. Am J Chin Med 1975;3:263–270.

Lazarus AA. Psychiatric problems precipitated by transcendental meditation. Psychol Rep 1976;39:601–602.

Lee Peng CH, Yang MP, Kok SH, Woo YK. Endorphine release: a possible mechanism of acupuncture analgesia. Comp Med East West 1978;6:57–60.

Li SP, et al. The effect of *qi gong* on the electron magnetic resonance spectrum of Ag Br. Proceedings of I World Congress on medical *qi gong*. Beijing, 1988:82.

Liu BH, et al. *qi gong* effects on plasma monoamines in man. Proceedings of I World Congress on medical *qi gong*. Beijing, 1988:34.

Lu CY, Wong YL. A method in measuring the *qi* activity. Proceedings of I World Congress on Medical *qi gong*. Beijing, 1988;75.

Lundeberg T, Haker E, Thomas M. Effects of laser versus placebo in tennis elbow. Scand J Rehabil Med 1987;19:135–138.

Lundeberg T, Malm M. Low-power HeNe laser treatment of venous leg ulcers. Ann Plastic Surg 1991;27:537–539.

Lyns RF, Abergel RP, White RA, et al. Biostimulation of wound healing in vivo by a helium-neon laser. Ann Plast Surg 1987;18:47.

Macmillan JD, Maxwell WA, Chichester CO. Lethal photosensitization of microorganisms with light from a continuous-wave gas laser. Photochem Photobiol 1966;5:555–565.

Mahesh Yogi M. The science of being and art of living. London: Unwin, 1963.

Marcarian HQ, Calhoun ML. Microscopic anatomy of the integument of adult swine. Am J Vet Res 1966;27:765–772.

Marcus P. Treatment of migraine by acupuncture. Acupunct Electrother Res In J 1979;4:137–147.

Martin AR. The fear of relaxation and leisure. Am J Psychoanal 1951;11:42–50.

Maslow AH. Religions: Values and Peak Experiences, revised edition. New York: Viking, 1970.

Masse JF, Landry RG, Rochette C, et al. Effectiveness of soft laser treatment in periodontal surgery. Int Dent J 1993;43:121–127.

Mayer DJ, Price DD, Rafii A. Antagonism of acupuncture analgesia in man by the narcotic antagonist naloxone. Brain Res 1977;121:368–392.

McGuff PE, Bell EJ. The effect of laser energy radiation on bacteria. Med Biol III 1966;16:191–194.

Melzack R. The McGill Pain Questionnaire: major properties and scoring methods. Pain 1975;1:277–299.

Melzack R. Acupuncture and musculoskeletal pain. J Rheumatol 5:1978;2:119–120 (editorial).

Melzack R, Casey KC. Sensory, motivational and central control determinants of pain: a new conceptual model. In: Kenshalo D, ed. The skin senses. Springfield, IL: Charles C. Thomas, 1968;423–439.

Melzack R, Katz J. Auriculotherapy fails to relieve chronic pain. JAMA 1984;251:1041–1043.

Melzack R, Wall DP. Pain mechanism: a new theory. Science 1965;150:971–979.

Melzack R, Wall PD. Psychophysiology of pain. Int Anesthesiol Clin 1970;8:3–34.

Merton T. Mystics and zen master. New York: Dell, 1961.

Mester E, Mester AF, Mester A. The biomedical effects of laser application. Laser Surg Med 1985;5:31.

Mester E, Spiry T, Szende B, Tota JG. Effect of laser rays on wound healing. Am J Surg 1971;122:532.

Mester E, Toth N, Mester A. The biostimulative effect of laser beam. Laser Basic Biomed Res 1982;22:4.

Mikulas WL. Four noble truths of Buddhism related to behavior therapy. Psychol Rec 1978;28:59–67.

Mikulas WL. Buddhism and behavior modification. Psychol Rec 1981; 31:331–342.

Muehsami DJ, Markow MS, Muehsami PA, et al. Effects of *qi gong* on cellface myosin phosphorylation: preliminary experiments. Subtle Energies 1994;5:93–104.

Noble PB, Shields ED, Blecher PDM, Bentley KC. Locomotory characteristics of fibroblasts within a three-dimensional collagen lattice: Modulation by a helium/neon soft laser. Lasers Surg Med 1992;12:669–674.

Nogier P. Face to face with auriculotherapy. Acupunct Electro ther Res Int J 1983;8:99–100 (letter).

Nyanaponika T. The heart of Buddhist meditations. New York: Weiser, 1962.

Olavi A, Pekka R, Pertti K. Effects of the infrared laser therapy at treated and non-treated trigger points. Acupunct Electrother Res Int J 1989;14:9–14.

Omura Y. Patho-physiology of acupuncture treatment: effects of acupuncture on cardiovascular and nervous systems. Acupunct Electrother Res Int J 1975;1:51–140.

Oyamada Y. Biostimulation effect for rheumatoid arthritis by low power He-Ne laser surgery. In: Joffe SN, Goldblatt NR, Atsumi K, eds. Laser surgery: advanced characterization, therapeutics and systems. Bellingham, WA: International Society for Optical Engineering, 1989;1066.

Parwatikar SD, Brown SD, Stern JA, et al. Acupuncture, hypnosis and experimental pain: study with volunteers. Acupunct Electrother Res Int J 1978;3:161–190.

Passarella S, Casamassima E, Molinari S, et al. Increase of proton electrochemical potential and ATP synthesis in rat liver mitochondria irradiated in vitro by helium-neon laser. FEBS Lett 1984;175:95.

Peng A. Acupuncture treatment for deafness. Am J Chin Med 1973;1:155:158.

Pomeranz B. Brain's opiates at work in acupuncture. New Scientist 1977;6:12–13.

Pomeranz B, Chang R, Law P. Acupuncture reduces electrophysiological and behavioral responses to noxious stimuli: pituitary is implicated. Exp Neurol 1977;54:172–178.

Pomeranz BH, Chiu D. Naloxone blockade of acupuncture analgesia: endorphin implicated. Life Sci 1976;19:1757–1762.

Ponnudurai RN, Zbuzek VK, Niu HL, Wu W. Laser photobiostimulation—induced hypoalgesia in rats is not naloxone reversible. Acupunct Electrother Res Int J, 1988;13:109–117.

Ponnudurai RN, Zbuzek VK, Wu W. Hypoalgesic effect of laser photobiostimulation shown by rat tail flick. Acupunct Electrother Res Int J 1987;12:93–100.

Popp FA. Erfahrungsheikunde. Acta Medical Empirica 1990;4:240.

Qi gong Research Center, Beijing Chinese Medical School. *Qi gong* effects on myocardial reperfusion injury. Proceedings of I World Congress on medical *qi gong*. Beijing, 1988:17.

Quickenden TI, Daniels LL. Attempted biostimulation of division in *Saccharomyces cerevisiae* using red coherent light. Photochem Photobiol 1993; 57:272–278.

Reichmanis M, Becker RO. Physiological effects of stimulation at acupuncture loci: a review. Comp Med East West 1978;6:67–73.

Reichmanis M, Marino AA, Becker RO. DG skin conductance variation at acupuncture loci. Am J Chin Med 1976;4:69–72.

Research Group of Acupuncture Anesthesia, Peking Medical College: The role of some neurotransmitters of brain in finger acupuncture analgesia. Sci Sin 1974;17:112–130.

Rhys Davids TW. The Questions of King Melinda (part 2). New York: Dover, 1963.

Ribari O. The stimulating effect of low power laser rays: experimental examinations in otorhinolaryngology. Rev Laryngol Otol Rhinol (Bord) 1981;102:531–533.

Rochkind S, Alon M, Ouakin GE, et al. Intraoperative clinical use of LLLT follow up surgical treatment of the tethered spinal cord. Laser Ther 1991;3:113–118.

Rochkind S, Barrnea L, Razon N, et al. Stimulatory effect of He-Ne low dose laser on injured sciatic nerves of rats. Neurosurgery 1987;20:843.

Rogvi-Hanser B, Ellitsgaard N, Funch M, et al. Low level laser treatment of chondromalacia patellae. Int Orthop (SICOT) 1991;15:359–361.

Sabolovic DMV, Michon C. Effect of acupuncture on human peripheral T and B lymphocyte. Acupunct Electrother Res Int J 1978;3:97–107.

Santoianni P, Monfrecla G, Martellotta D, Ayala F. Inadequate effect of helium-neon laser on venous leg ulcers. Photodermatology 1984;1:245–249.

Schultz W, Luthe W. Autogenic training. New York: Grune & Stratton, 1969.

Schwartz M, Doron A, Erich M, et al. Effects of low-energy He-Ne laser irradiation of posttraumatic degeneration of adult rabbit optic nerve. Lasers Surg Med 1987;7:51.

Shapiro DH, Zifferblatt SM. Zen meditation and behavioral self control: similarities, differences, and clinical applications. Am Psychol 1976;31:519–532.

Sjölund BH, Erikson MBE. The influence of naloxone on analgesia produced by peripheral conditioning stimulation. Brain Res 1979;173:295–302.

Snyder-Mackler L, Barry AJ, Perkins AI, Soucek MD. Effects of helium-neon laser irradiation on skin resistance and pain in patients with trigger points in the neck or back. Phys Ther 1989;69:336–341.

Soto JJM, Moller I. La lasertherapia como coadyuvante en el tratemiento de la AR (artritis reumatoidea). Bol Central Document Laser 1987;14:4.

Stace WT. Mysticism and philosophy. Philadelphia: Lippincott, 1960.

Sternbach RA. Clinical aspects of pain. In: Sternback RA, ed. The psychology of pain. New York: Raven Press, 1978;241–264.

Surinchak JS, Alago ML, Bellamy RF, et al. Effects on low-level energy lasers on the healing of full-thickness skin defects. Lasers Surg Med 1983; 2:267–274.

Suzuki S. Zen mind, beginner's mind. New York: Weatherall, 1970.

Tong TM, et al. Physiological effect of *qi gong* preliminary study. Proceedings of I World Congress on medical *qi gong*. Beijing, 1988:10.

Tsui YH, et al. *qi gong* effects on the absorption spectrum of the fish DNA. Proceedings of I World Congress on medical *qi gong*. Beijing, 1988:81.

Turner JA, Chapman CR. Psychological interventions for chronic pain: a critical review. 1. Relaxation training and biofeedback. Pain 1982;12:1–21.

Turner JA, Chapman CR. Psychological interventions for chronic pain: 2. Operant conditioning, hypnosis and cognitive behavioral therapy. Pain 1982;12:23–46.

Van Breugel HHFI, Bar PR. HeNe laser irradiation affects proliferation of cultural rat Schwann cells in a dose dependent manner. J Neurocytol 1993;22:185–190.

Vasseljen O Jr, Hoeg N, Kjeldstad B, et al. Low level laser versus placebo in the treatment of tennis elbow. Scand J Rehab Med 1992;24:37–42.

Vecchio P, Cave M, King V, et al. A double-blind study of the effectiveness of low level laser treatment of rotator cuff tendinitis. Br J Rheumatol 1993;32:740–742.

Veith I. The yellow emperor's classic of internal medicine (translated). Berkeley: University of California Press, 1970.

Vizi ES, Mester E, Tizza S, Mester A. Acetylcholine releasing effect of laser irradiation on Auerbach's plexus in guinea pig ileum. J Neural Transm Park Dis Dement Sect 1977;40:305.

Walker JB, Akhanjee LJ, Cooney MM, et al. Laser therapy for pain of rheumatoid arthritis. Clin J Pain 1987;3:54–59.

Wei LY. Scientific advance in acupuncture. Am J Chin Med 1977;7:53–75.

Weil A. The natural mind. Boston: Houghton Mifflin, 1972.

Whitehead PC. Acupuncture in the treatment of addiction: a review and analysis. Int J Addict 1978;13:1–16.

Wong TS et al. *qi gong* improves cardiac functions and reduces the risk factors. Proceedings of I World Congress on medical *qi gong*. Beijing, 1988:42.

Wu W, Ponnudurai R, Katz J, et al. Failure to confirm report of light-evoked response of peripheral nerve to low power helium-neon laser light stimulus. Brain Res 1987;401:407.

Wu W, Wei XB, Karmel B, Koos S. Somatosensory evoked potential laser acupuncture. The IV Congress of the International Society for Laser Surgery. Tokyo, Nov. 23–27, 1981.

Wu WH, et al. Effects of *qi gong* on late-stage reflex sympathetic dystropy: a preliminary report. Project Summary Report, OAM, NIH, Bethesda, MD, 1995.

Yang KY, et al. The effect of periaqueductal lesion on *qi gong*-induced analgesia in rats. Proceedings of I World Congress on medical *qi gong*. Beijing, 1988:28.

Yang KY, et al. Analgesic effect of *qi gong* in rats. Proceedings of I World Congress on medical *qi gong*. Beijing, 1988:29.

Yang KY, et al. *Qi gong* effects on the pain threshold in rats. Proceedings of I World Congress on medical *qi gong*. Beijing, 1988:29.

Yao YC, et al. Effects of *qi gong* on spontaneous electrical activities of rat cerebellar neurons recorded by microelectrode. Proceedings of I World Congress on medical *qi gong*. Beijing, 1988:26.

Ye M, et al. *Qi gong* effects on peripheral lymphocytes in vitro. Proceedings of I World Congress on medical *qi gong*. Beijing, 1988:21.

Young S, Bolton P, Dyson M, et al. Macrophage responsiveness to light therapy. Lasers Surg Med 1989;9:497–505.

Zhao JC, Yen YL, Zhang QZ, Li ZL. The effect of electroacupuncture on norepinephrine content in the rat brain. Proceedings of the Annual Meeting of the Clinical Society of the Physiological Sciences. Dalian, Peoples Republic of China, 1964:169 (Chinese).

Zimmermann M. Dorsal root potentials after c-fiber stimulation. Science 1965;150:971–979.

CHAPTER 45

The Application of Ethical Principles in the Management of Cancer Pain

Nathan Cherny and Nessa Coyle

Surveys indicate that pain is experienced by 30 to 60% of cancer patients during active therapy and more than two-thirds of those with advanced disease (1). Unrelieved pain is incapacitating and undermines quality of life; it interferes with physical functioning and social interaction and is strongly associated with heightened psychological distress. Persistent pain interferes with the ability to eat (2), sleep (3), think, and interact with others (4). The relation between pain and psychological well-being is complex and reciprocal; mood disturbance and beliefs about the meaning of pain in relation to illness can exacerbate perceived pain intensity (5, 6), and the presence of pain is a major determinant of function and mood (7). The presence of pain can disturb normal processes of coping and adjustment (8–10) and augment a sense of vulnerability, contributing to a preoccupation with the potential for catastrophic outcomes (8). This relation is further evidenced by the observations that uncontrolled pain is a major risk factor in cancer-related suicide (11–14) and that psychiatric symptoms have commonly been observed to disappear with adequate pain relief (15).

The alleviation of suffering is universally acknowledged as a cardinal goal of medical care (16–21), and the World Health Organization asserts that the relief of pain and other symptoms is a right of the patient with advanced and incurable cancer (22).

The management of pain of pain in cancer patients, particularly those at the end of life, requires a working knowledge of ethical principles. The four cardinal principles of all ethic constructs are respect for the person and their autonomy, justice, beneficence, and nonmaleficence.

RESPECT FOR PERSON AND AUTONOMY

Respect for person recognizes the individual as an autonomous agent and protects the rights of the person with diminished autonomy to decide for himself or herself according to beliefs, values, and a life plan. It requires the clinician to enter into a dialog with the patient: listening to the patient's priorities, transmitting information to enable informed decision making, respecting the choice to limit exposure to potentially harmful information, exploring the patient's decision making to ensure that it is not based on misconceptions.

BENEFICENCE

Beneficence is an activist principle that dictates that one ought to prevent or remove evil or harm and to promote good. This principle invokes a duty to act and includes all of the strategies that health care professionals employ to support patients and families and reduce suffering. This duty to care clearly includes the effective treatment of pain and other symptoms. Both proposed treatments and in some instances, the active withdrawal of other treatments can be evaluated in terms of their potential to relieve suffering and thereby promote good. Treatment plans that are concordant with the goals of care that a patient sees for himself or herself convey beneficence.

NONMALEFICENCE

The principle of nonmaleficence is embodied in the concept that one ought not to inflict evil or harm. In the setting of a patient with far advanced cancer and severe pain this principle implies recognition of the patient's extreme vulnerability and mandates a commitment to minimize harm through care. Potential sources of maleficence in this setting are manifold; they include continued aggressive life-prolonging or cure-oriented treatment that is not suited to the person's needs or wishes; unnecessary and unwanted oversedation; unrequested or uninformed withdrawal of treatment; physical or psychological pain caused by performing unnecessary tests or procedures; and insensitive history taking, physical examination, or conveying of information. Thus this ethical principle requires of the clinician a high level of vigilance and awareness of the needs, desires, and sensitivity of the specific patient under care.

JUSTICE

Justice deals with the concept of a fair distribution of resources. Justice in this setting is related primarily to the appropriate allocation of medical resources between patients with competing needs. In some instances this principle requires a balancing of the needs of the individual with the needs of the community. This is a complex ethical concept that often requires the weighing of competing claims. Decisions and actions that may seem morally compelling and appropriate for a particular person may not be allowable because of the wider risk they present to other members of society. Thus justice may limit autonomy in the context of the greater good. This sort of decision making integrally involves the values upon which the society is based.

THE RELIEF OF PAIN AS AN ISSUE OF RIGHTS

It has been argued and asserted that to leave a person in avoidable pain is a fundamental breach of human rights (23). This right is derived from the universal concepts of respect for all persons and is inextricably linked to the concept of human ethics. The corollary of the right of patients to have adequate relief of avoidable pain is the duty of care incumbent on the heath care system and the individual participating members to provide adequate relief.

This duty of care has widespread implications in terms of medical systems and individual clinicians. That this right is so commonly breached is partly a reflection of the very complex interaction between the various systems and persons whose cooperation is required for the effective and efficient relief of avoidable suffering due to uncontrolled pain. This complex interaction involves government, medical and nursing schools, licensing authorities, hospitals and health care maintenance organizations, physicians and nurses (Table 45.1).

On the basis of this model one can audit a health care system. With regard to government responsibility, data are available for only few of these tasks. In many countries analgesics for strong pain are not readily available and restrictive regulations interfere with the prescription, dispensation, and administration of analgesic care. We lack global data on the assumed role of government in setting standards relating pain relief in the accreditation of medical schools, licensing of clinicians, and accreditation of health care institutions. Anecdotally, few notable steps have been taken: as an outcome of an inquiry into the care of the dying in 1989 the government of Victoria, Australia, declared that the provision of palliative care education be an accreditation criterion for medical schools, and policy statements regarding the relief of pain have been endorsed by

Table 45.1.   A Model of the Hierarchy of Responsibilities in the Relief of Avoidable Pain

Government
  Ensure availability of analgesic medications
  Provide license for physicians to prescribe, pharmacists to dispense, clinicians to administer analgesics
  Ensure accredited health care vocational schools provide adequate education in the relief of pain
  Ensure that licensed clinicians are adequately skilled in pain relief
  Ensure that health care institutions meet standards in the assessment and treatment of pain relief
Health care vocational schools
  Emphasize the ethical responsibility to relieve avoidable pain
  Teach skills of pain assessment and management
  Audit the effectiveness of ethics and skills education
Hospitals and health care maintenance organizations
  Set standards of institutional care
  Provide medication
  Provide skilled staff
  Provide infrastructure for assessment and documenting of pain as part of routine standard of care
  Monitor system efficiency and outcomes to identify institutional deficiencies for remedial action
Senior clinicians
  Emphasize relief of avoidable pain as a central aspect of clinical care
  Lead junior staff by example
  Maintain high clinical standard in assessment, prophylaxis, treatment
  Monitor treatment outcomes
  Judicious use of expert clinicians
  Monitor outcomes to identify institutional deficiencies for remedial action
Junior clinicians
  Maintain high clinical standard in assessment, prophylaxis, treatment
  Monitor treatment outcomes
  Judicious use of expert clinicians
  Monitor outcomes to identify institutional deficiencies for remedial action

Presidential Commission (21) and consensus statements from major professional organizations in medicine and ethics (19, 22, 24–29). Similar evaluation can be applied to health care vocational schools, hospitals, health care maintenance organizations, and senior and junior clinicians.

Neglect of responsibility for the relief of pain is commonplace at all levels of the hierarchy. Neglect can be naive or informed; that is to say, in some situations the neglectful party may not even appreciate that his or her behavior is neglectful. For instance, the nurse who administers a placebo treatment for pain at the behest of a physician may be absolutely unaware of the inappropriateness of the order. Fulfillment of that order may be a result of lack of appreciation of that placebo injection is not an acceptable standard of practice. Alternatively, neglect can be culturally syntonic or dystonic. In some cultures activities involved in pain relief are routinely ignored. The nurse may have known that the order was inappropriate but in his or her cultural context nurses don't overtly question medical directives. Indeed, in some cultures only low priority has been ascribed to the control of avoidable pain.

The moral significance of negligence is influenced by these factors. The informed clinician who is practicing in a context in which pain is expected to be adequately relieved and who chooses to ignore a patient's request for relief or who willfully prescribes an inappropriately weak medication may be criminally negligent (23). Clinicians who work in the context of negligent systems with a chain of ignored responsibility may be individually negligent but because of the context of their practice they may plead diminished responsibility. More often than not, the negligent practice emerges in the context of a negligent system. Since the problem is systemic and diffuse, often no one has a sense of personal responsibility, let alone moral responsibility.

The degree to which one can label a neglectful health care system as morally deficient is unclear. What is clear, however, is that nonneglectful systems can facilitate the moral sensitivity of the participants within the system and that this effect is to the betterment of the participating clinicians, patients, and community at large. This is an example of a positive cascade of care. In the culture of such a system, no one wants to be a bad guy. However, where the system does not enforce the relief of pain as a high medical and moral priority, the "bad guys" are endemic and no one seems to care. This is clearly not a desirable state of affairs, and it is therefore incumbent upon persons sensitive to the issue of human suffering to try to address deficiencies in our own health care environment. As Eldridge Cleaver said, "You're either part of the solution or part of the problem."

NEGLIGENCE IN THE MANAGEMENT OF CANCER PAIN

There is substantial evidence that the management of cancer pain by medical, radiation, and surgical oncologists often falls short of accepted standards of practice and that remedial action is urgently needed (30). Despite valid and widely reproduced data to indicate that with vigilant application of sound practice guidelines, 70 to 90% of cancer pain can be relieved (31–36), the undertreatment of cancer pain remains routine in many settings.

Bonica reviewed data from 13 published surveys conducted between 1959 and 1987 and found that pain was relieved in only 30% of patients (1). Recent data indicate that the pain outcomes of patients under the care of cancer specialists are commonly suboptimal. In a survey of 1308 oncology outpatients being treated by Eastern Cooperative Oncology Group (ECOG) physicians, Cleeland et al. (37) found that 67% had pain during the week preceding the study and that the pain was severe enough to impair function in 36%. In this latter group, 42% were not given appropriate analgesics for the severity of their pain according to the criteria of the analgesic ladder (37). In a similar study performed by Larue et al. (38) in France, 57% of 601 patients reported pain due to their disease, and more than two thirds of them rated their worst pain at a level that impaired their ability to function. Among 151 patients being treated for ovarian cancer, Portenoy et al. (39) found that 42% reported persistent or frequent pain during the preceding 2 weeks and that pain usually was severe enough to

affect activity, mood, work, and overall enjoyment of life. Among 145 patients with lung and colon cancer receiving outpatient treatment by medical oncologists, 90% of patients were in pain more than 25% of the time and the pain interfered at least moderately with general activity and work in approximately 50% of patients (40). Finally, in the validation study of the Memorial Symptom Assessment Scale, also by Portenoy et al. (41), pain was present in 63% of 246 randomly selected inpatients and outpatients undergoing active treatment for prostate, colon, breast, or ovarian cancers, and pain was rated as moderate to severe by 43% of respondents. An indirect indicator of the status of pain control achieved by cancer specialists can be derived from pain data derived at the time of intake into palliative medicine and hospice services: three recent surveys of this kind have indicated that pain was inadequately relieved in 64 to 80% of patients at time of intake (42–44).

Discrepancies between results achieved among selected patients in phase 2 studies and those in routine care are well recognized in medical oncology. Such discrepancies are generally due to irreproducibility of the initial data (which brings into question the validity of the initial data), selection bias in the initial study, or failure to adhere to the established methodology. With regard to the treatment of cancer pain, the data relating to the effectiveness of the analgesic ladder approach has been replicated in no fewer than six studies (31–36). The problem of pain control appears to be due to a lack of application of established strategies.

The relief of cancer pain is a multistep process that entails (a) reports from the patient, (b) physician's assessment and evaluation of the pain syndrome, (c) development of a therapeutic plan, (d) provision of medications, (e) monitoring of outcomes with regard to analgesia and adverse effects, and (f) therapeutic adjustments in response to outcome or with longitudinal changes in the patient's condition. Recent research indicates that barriers to the effective relief of pain can occur at any of these steps.

Medical, surgical, and radiation oncologists and oncology nurses provide the bulk of care for cancer patients and are more exposed to the problem of cancer pain than virtually any other medical practitioners. Patients therefore have a reasonable right to expect that their treating cancer specialist will be vigilant and expert in the management of cancer-related pain. Data indicate that many cancer patients receive inadequate pain treatment by their oncologist (37–40, 42–44), that oncologists commonly underestimate the prevalence and severity of pain in their patients (37, 38, 45, 46), that many oncologists have substantial knowledge deficits regarding the pharmacotherapy of cancer pain (37, 45, 47, 48), and that in many cases these knowledge deficits are not appreciated by the clinicians involved (47, 48).

That so much suffering could be controlled but is not is at best unfortunate and at worst an indictment of professional standards. Professor Margaret Sommerville of the McGill Center for Medicine, Ethics and Law argues that inadequately controlled pain that is due to the delivery of substandard treatment constitutes medical negligence (23).

These findings highlight the need for a practical and visible restatement of clinical priorities that reflects a serious intent to remedy the inadequate manner in which cancer pain has been routinely treated by the oncology community thus far (30). Tangible steps to improve this situation have been described (Table 45.2). Recent years have seen many communities and institutions take active steps to identify systematic shortcomings in the delivery of adequate pain relief with concerted and ongoing remedial and quality improvement programs. The American Pain Society has described quality assurance standards for the relief of acute pain and cancer pain (49) and has issued quality improvement guidelines for the treatment of acute and cancer pain (26). The National Cancer Institute of Canada requires documentation of cancer pain, its treatment, and its outcome as a criterion for the accreditation of facilities (50, 51). Steps such as these emphasize centrality of the relief of pain to the clinical endeavor of cancer medicine and help ensure the maintenance of appropriate professional standards in the care of pain by cancer specialists.

ADVERSE EFFECTS OF ANALGESIC THERAPIES: COUNSELING THE PATIENT

Unfortunately, all contemporary analgesic tools have potential for adverse effects (Table 45.3). The ethical doctrines of beneficence and nonmaleficence require the treating physician to offer the treatment options likely to have the most favorable balance between optimal relief, minimal adverse effects, and maximal convenience. Convenience includes to convenience of administration, cost, and availability. Since all of the available options have some adverse effects, the doctrine of autonomy requires that the clinician offer a reasonable explanation of the potential benefit and risks of the proposed treatment to enable the patient to make as well-informed a decision as possible about their treatment.

Often several treatment options differ in their potential for benefit, risk, and convenience. The doctrine of autonomy suggests that the clinician should explain the available options and their benefits and risks to facilitate an informed choice by the patient. This is a process that is demanding of the clinician's resources, especially time, and it requires a patient who wishes to participate in treatment selection.

In general, the process of decision making is predicated on an understanding of the goals of care for the individual patient (52). These goals can generally be grouped into three broad categories: (*a*) prolonging survival, (*b*) optimizing comfort (physical, psychological, and existential), and (*c*) optimizing function. With the hope and knowledge that it may be possible to achieve adequate relief without compromising interactional function, the patient who equally desires comfort and function may elect to pursue only approaches with modest morbidity despite a relatively low or indeterminate likelihood of success. As the goals of prolonging survival and

Table 45.2.　Recommendations for Improvements in Pain Management by Oncologists

Individual oncologists
　Routinely focus attention on evaluation and management of pain among their own patients
　Document that any pain has been evaluated and its severity, cause, treatment, and outcome
　Remind themselves, their colleagues, and students to think about pain and need for adequate relief at all stages of illness
　Routinely include pain evaluation and management strategies in case presentations at rounds and postclinic conferences
　Know practice guidelines and contemporary cancer pain literature
Oncology professional groups
　Raise priority of clinical outcome and ensure development and maintenance of appropriate professional standards
　Ensure trainees be trained in evaluation and treatment of pain; reinforce through formal and informal clinical audit
　Examinations for medical, surgical, and radiation oncologists to include a defined number of questions on assessment and management of pain
National Cancer Bodies
　Routine documentation of cancer pain, treatment, and outcome should be incorporated into standard of care and be subject to formal audit in hospital accreditation
　Title "comprehensive cancer center" should be contingent on fulfillment of standards and provisions of expert-run programs for management of pain
Oncology researchers
　Must be encouraged to participate in cancer pain research
　Evaluation of pain using validated assessment tools should be incorporated into phase II, III, and IV studies of conditions which a high prevalence of pain is anticipated
　Methodology systematically applied to palliative surgical, radiotherapeutic, and cytotoxic interventions

optimizing function become increasingly unachievable, priorities often shift. When comfort is the overriding goal of care and the principal goal of any intervention is lasting relief, there may be no tolerable time frame for exploring other therapeutic options. In this situation interventions of low or indeterminate likelihood of success are often rejected in favor of more certain approaches, even if they may impair cognitive function or shorten survival. These processes of setting priorities for goals and informed decision making require candid discussion that clarifies the prevailing clinical predicament and presents the alternative therapeutic options. Other relevant considerations, including existential, ethical, religious, and familial concerns, may benefit from the participation of a religious counselor, social worker, or clinical ethics specialist.

Not all patients want to be involved in decision making, and they should not be compelled to do so; patients have the right to delegate decision making to a family member or health care proxy or to choose uninformed consent based upon trust in a clinician.

Benevolent paternalism describes the relationship in which the physician, based on consideration of the patient's best interest, makes a treatment decision for a consenting patient without consulting the patient. Some patients, and indeed some cultures, prefer and expect physicians to present

Table 45.3.   Potential Adverse Effects of Analgesic Therapies

	Common	Uncommon
Nonopioid analgesics	Peptic ulceration	Confusion
	Bleeding	Blood dyscrasias
	Renal failure	
Systemic opioids analgesics	Constipation	Respiratory arrest
	Itch	Seizure
	Sweating	Psychological dependence
	Nausea, vomiting	
	Drowsiness	
	Confusion	
	Myoclonus	
	Physical dependence	
	Respiratory depression	
Adjuvant analgesics	Dry mouth	Cardiac arrest
	Drowsiness	
	Constipation	
	Confusion	
Spinal opioid analgesics	Itch	Life-threatening infection
	Urinary retention	Paraplegia
	Confusion	
	Drowsiness	
	Infection	
Neuroablative procedures	Motor dysfunction	
	Bladder, bowel dysfunction	
	Neuropathic pain	

a singular recommendation for treatment rather than a range of options for complex deliberation. Since frequently one does not know a priori to what degree the patient wishes or expects to participate in decision making, it is sound practice to ask patients if they would prefer an explanation of the available options or a simple recommendation.

In the world of busy clinics and wards, the doctrine of distributional justice is often an intruding factor. On occasion there is simply insufficient time to counsel all patients on all of their treatment options. Whenever possible, it may be preferable to reschedule complex patient counseling to allow adequate time for the process or to delegate part of this responsibility to other members of the care team, such as a specialist pain nurse. When this is not possible, benevolent paternalism maybe an appropriate, though less desirable, fallback option.

THE ETHICAL SIGNIFICANCE OF THE DISTINCTION BETWEEN "REFRACTORY" AND "DIFFICULT" PAIN

The relief of intolerable pain in patients with far advanced cancer and other terminal diseases is a moral imperative. In that situation, the principles of nonmaleficence and beneficence require that the clinician determine whether the pain is refractory or merely difficult. The term refractory can be applied when pain cannot be adequately controlled despite aggressive efforts to identify a tolerable therapy that does not

compromise consciousness (53). This designation has profound implications, suggesting that suffering will not be relieved with routine measures, thus possibly justifying or even requiring nonroutine treatments such as controlled sedation. In deciding that a pain problem is refractory, the clinician must perceive that further invasive and noninvasive interventions are either (*a*) incapable of providing adequate relief, (*b*) associated with excessive and intolerable acute or chronic morbidity, or (*c*) unlikely to provide relief within a tolerable time frame. Refractory pain must be distinguished from difficult pain, which may respond within a tolerable time frame to noninvasive or invasive interventions and yield adequate relief and preserved consciousness without excessive adverse effects. Since clinicians want neither to subject severely distressed patients to therapies that provide inadequate relief or excessive morbidity nor to sacrifice conscious function when viable alternatives remain unexplored, this is an important and ethically significant distinction.

A stepwise strategy for the management of patients with cancer pain offers a model for a clinical approach that aims to identify patients with truly refractory pain. An opioid is titrated to a maximal tolerated dose. Side effects are treated, and appropriate adjuvant analgesics are considered. If dose-limiting toxicity precludes adequate relief, alternative opioids and various anesthetic and neuroablative therapies are considered. Patients must be evaluated repeatedly to determine therapeutic failure and weigh the risks and benefits of the next approach. The clinician must address the same set of questions as each new intervention is considered (Fig. 45.1). Since subjective patient variables influence the evaluation of these questions, the patient must collaborate in this decision process.

Clinician evaluation of the patient, the pain syndrome, and therapeutic options is critical. Since knowledge in the assessment and management of cancer pain is frequently deficient among physicians who lack specific training in this field (30), expert evaluation or consultation should be considered. At Memorial Sloan-Kettering Cancer Center, a survey observed that a pain service consultation identified a previously undiagnosed cause for the pain in 64% of 376 referred patients, including new neurological diagnoses in 36% of patients and an unsuspected infection in 4%; a substantial proportion of these patients received radiation therapy, surgery, or chemotherapy based on the findings of the pain consultant (54). Similarly Coyle et al. (55) reported a series of cases of crescendo pain in which evaluation of the patient identified an unsuspected delirium, treatment of which restored adequate pain control. As part of the evaluation, previous analgesic approaches must be assessed in a systematic manner by a clinician who is expert in the management of cancer pain. Specific questions include the following:

1. Are primary therapies (chemotherapy, radiation therapy, surgery, or antibiotic therapy) feasible, and if so, are they likely to improve outcome?
2. Has the opioid dose been titrated up to maximal tolerated doses?
3. Have side effects been addressed through appropriate drug therapy or by trials of alternative opioids?
4. Have appropriate adjuvant analgesics been considered or tried?
5. Have spinal opioids been considered?
6. Have other anesthetic or neurosurgical options been considered?

The principles of beneficence and nonmaleficence should guide the decision making process. Since individual clinician bias can influence decision making, a case conference approach is prudent when assessing a challenging case (nonmaleficence). This conference may include oncologists, palliative care physicians, anesthesiologists, neurosurgeons, psychiatrists, nurses, social workers, and others. The discussion attempts to clarify the remaining therapeutic options and the goals of care. When local expertise is limited, telephone consultation with physicians who are expert in the management of cancer pain is encouraged (beneficence and nonmaleficence).

If the clinician perceives no treatment is capable of providing adequate relief of intolerable symptoms without compromising interactional function, or that the patient would be unable to tolerate specific therapeutic interventions, refractoriness to standard approaches should be acknowledged. In this situation, the clinician should explain that by virtue of the severity of the problem and the limitations of the available techniques, the goal of providing the needed relief without the use of drugs that may impair consciousness is probably not achievable.

The offer of sedation is often received as an empathic acknowledgment of the severity of the degree of the patient's suffering. The enhancement of the patient's trust in the commitment of the clinician to the relief of suffering may in itself influence decision making, particularly if there are other tasks or life issues that must be completed before a state of diminished function develops. The patient can decline sedating therapies, acknowledging that the pain will be incompletely relieved but secure in the knowledge that if the situation becomes intolerable, this decision can be rescinded. Alternatively, the patient can assert comfort as the predominating consideration and accept potentially sedating therapies.

This situation becomes more complicated when the clinician is less certain that the standard approaches will fail. Therapeutic decisions are strongly influenced by the patient's readiness to accept the risk of morbidity and enduring discomfort until adequate relief is achieved. As always, evaluation of therapeutic options by the patient requires a candid disclosure of the options, including information regarding the likelihood of benefit, the procedural morbidity, the risks of side effects, and the likely time to achieve relief. If these are acceptable to the patient, further trials of standard therapies should be pursued. If the patient requires relief and the procedural morbidity, the risks of adverse effects or the likely time to achieve relief is unacceptable, refractoriness should be acknowledged and sedation should be offered.

ADVERSE EFFECTS OF ANALGESIC THERAPIES: THE PRINCIPLE OF DOUBLE EFFECT

As described in the previous section, in some instances pain can be relieved only by treatments that may have unavoidable adverse effects or a high risk thereof. High-dose opioids or induced sedation may compromise the ability of a suffering patient to interact and may shorten life. Neurolytic techniques may provide relief only at a cost of impaired neurological function that may have major consequences, such as paraplegia or incontinence.

According to Roy (56), there exists an emancipation principle of palliative care: "[One should] spare no scientific or clinical effort to free dying persons from twisting and racking pain that invades, dominates and shrivels their consciousness, that leaves them no psychic or mental space for the things they want to think and say and do before they die." From this perspective, the provision of adequate relief of symptoms is an overriding goal that must be pursued even in the setting of a narrow therapeutic index for the necessary palliative treatments (16, 57–60). This conclusion has been endorsed by a presidential commission (21) and consensus statements from major professional organizations in medicine and ethics (19, 22, 24–29).

The ethical validity of treatments that relieve pain at a high cost of unavoidable adverse effects is commonly justified on the basis of the principle of double effect, which distinguishes between the compelling primary therapeutic intent

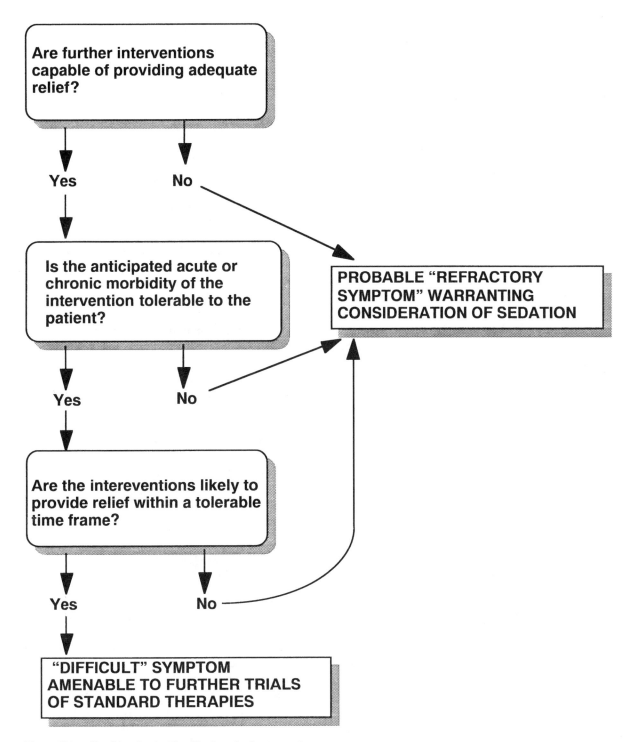

Figure 45.1.   Algorithm for the identification of refractory pain.

(to relieve suffering) and unavoidable untoward consequences (such as the likely diminution of interactional function and the potential for accelerating death) (61). The use of analgesic therapies with potentially unavoidable adverse effects meets all four of the conditions for this principle:

1.   The treatment is at least neutral (if not beneficial) but may have untoward as well as beneficial consequences.

2.   The clinician intends the beneficial outcome (relief of pain), but the foreseen untoward outcome may be unavoidable.
3.   The untoward outcome is necessary to achieve the beneficial outcome.
4.   The beneficial outcome (adequate relief of unendurable pain) is an appropriately compelling reason to place the patient at risk for the untoward outcome.

The principle of double effect is most commonly invoked in the use of high-dose opioid analgesics or induced sedation in the management of otherwise refractory pain (62). The principle of double effect is predicated on the axioms that (*a*) intent is a critical ethical concern and (*b*) the distinction between foreseeing and intending an unavoidable maleficent outcome is ethically significant.

The principle of double effect has been the subject of philosophical and ethical criticism. Some contend that one is equally responsible for outcomes that are intended and those that are foreseen as unavoidable. This can be countered by the argument that the principle is contingent upon proportionality, that the significance of the primary outcome must justify the risks that are being taken. More recently, Quill (63), the advocate of assisted suicide, has argued that clinical intentions are sometimes much more complex and ambiguous than those classically presented and that clinicians are sometimes self-deceptive such that the so-called unavoidable untoward outcomes are indeed desired and intended; thus the use of an opioid infusion may in some instances constitute slow euthanasia (64). This critique emphasizes that the ethical invocation of the principle requires introspective analysis of intent by those participating in the decision to prevent abuse of the principle by those who misrepresent their true intentions.

These criticisms do not diminish the fact that the invocation of this principle in good faith allows the patient and treating clinician to maintain an ethical equilibrium in an ethically and clinically difficult situation. In the absence of this ethical equilibrium, the moral reservations of clinicians or family members may result in either the undertreatment of catastrophic symptoms or a feeling of guilt and its morbid psychological sequelae.

COMMON CONFLICTS AND THEIR RESOLUTION: BENEFICENCE AND MALEFICENCE

Beneficence and maleficence are related concepts, and clearly some treatments are beneficent in one situation and maleficent in another. At the heart of the issue is the goal of care. As described, the goals of care can generally be expressed in terms of optimization of comfort, function, and duration of survival. The relative priority of these three goals is dynamic, and it commonly changes as clinical circumstances evolve. Thus, whereas the prolongation of survival may take priority over comfort and function for the patient with curable sarcoma that requires the amputation of a limb, in the situation of terminal dyspnea from advanced pulmonary metastases, the priorities may be reversed. This change in goals can have a profound effect on the evaluation of the relative beneficence or maleficence of many treatment options.

Decisions about the management of pain often provoke conflicts for family and staff members regarding their relative beneficence or maleficence. Common questions that arise include these: What is the optimal level of sedation? One that

maintains the ability of the patient to interact but also to suffer or a level of sedation in which the ability to interact is lost, as are visible signs of suffering? Will someone die of starvation if he or she cannot eat because of the level of sedation required to control pain? Does sedation in the management of otherwise intractable pain hasten death, and if so is this a form of euthanasia? How does one reach a balance between the risk of hastening death and increasing opioids, sedatives, and sedation to control intractable pain and distress?

These issues and conflicts are best addressed through regularly scheduled family and staff meetings. Evaluating these issues is often assisted by the participation of a clinical expert in pain or palliative care. Family members should be encouraged to vent and express their concerns or grievances. Further discussion is best predicated on a joint understanding of the condition, therapeutic options, goals of care, and expressed wishes of the patient and goals of the treating staff. This dialog is often facilitated when the patient has a living will explicitly addressing preferences for care at the end of life. Indeed, involvement of the family in counseling and decision making before the initiation of treatment often prevents confusion regarding the patient's preferences when he or she is no longer able to participate in the dialog. The tone of such meetings should reflect the beneficent intent of the treating staff, the primacy of the patient's autonomy, and sensitivity to the concerns and well-being of the family members. Among staff members, regular interdisciplinary staff meetings provide an opportunity for staff to present different viewpoints and to explore the decision-making process, focusing on goals of care, patient's wishes, and the family advocacy role. The principle of double effect is an important tool in ethical dialog with both the family and staff.

THE LIMITS OF AUTONOMY IN THE MANAGEMENT OF PAIN

In the management of cancer patients with pain there are several common conflicts related to the patient's autonomy. Patients may refuse treatment of pain for reasons founded on accurate or inaccurate assessment of risk of untoward consequences. When patients refuse treatment to relieve pain, beneficence dictates that the clinician should explore the reasons for refusal to ensure that it is based on valid reasoning and accurate information. Some patients choose to put up with suboptimal relief because they fear excessive drowsiness or nausea, and in some cases this precludes readiness to try further therapy. In such cases, fears should be recognized and discussed and options to avoid the feared side effects should be explained. Beneficence requires that the clinician express the desire to help the patient achieve the goal of relief without excessive adverse effects and that suboptimal outcomes of either persistent pain or excessive side effects require a reevaluation of the treatment plan. Expression of availability and commitment to follow-up help to foster the trust that enables the patient to take risks that are often needed to achieve the desired outcome.

A patient's refusal based on misinformation represents an illusion of autonomy rather than an expression of true autonomy. Respect for autonomy requires that the clinician explore the patient's reasoning to identify and correct misinformation, such as exaggerated estimations of the risk of addiction or tolerance, which are commonplace.

Some patients request treatment for pain that is considered disproportionate or inconsistent with the ethical framework of the treating clinician. Common examples are requests for assisted suicide and euthanasia in the treatment of pain.

EUTHANASIA AND ASSISTED SUICIDE IN THE TREATMENT OF PAIN

Hippocratic medicine has traditionally defined the purview of medical practice in normative situations. According to the Hippocratic paradigm, medicine is seen as a vocation of compassion in which the quality and quantity of human life are critical concerns and the imperative to alleviate suffering precludes killing the sufferer. The Hippocratic Charter may be summarized as follows:

1. To abhor suffering and preventable premature death
2. To strive to prevent or to cure illness that generates suffering and shortens survival
3. When cure is not possible, to find the optimal balance between relief of suffering and prolongation of survival
4. The relief of suffering to be achieved by means other than the termination of the life of the sufferer

The Hippocratic purview of medicine, in summary, requires that suffering be acknowledged, that its causes be identified, and that steps be taken to provide adequate relief with haste and effect until adequate relief is achieved.

For some practitioners and ethicists the data indicating that the treatment of pain and suffering are frequently ineffectual are sufficient to justify elective death by euthanasia or assisted suicide as beneficent options (16, 65–67). Besides absolutist reservations about the deliberate termination of human life, standard objections to this approach include the so-called slippery slope argument (of progressive precedent) and the argument from potential for abuse (61). Data from the Netherlands indicate that an institution policy permissive of euthanasia is difficult to regulate and that abuses are commonplace (68). More recently several other objections to the legalization of euthanasia or assisted suicide have taken increasing prominence.

1. The not yet argument: Several clinicians have argued that the legalization of either euthanasia or assisted suicide without first ensuring universal availability of expert care in symptom management or at very least the requirement of expert assessment of candidates, may result in the maleficent shortening of the lives of some patients when other appropriate options were untested and unexplored (17, 69–78). They assert that

the focus of public discussion on these life-curtailing options is inappropriate when so little has yet been done to ease suffering without having to kill patients or assist them to kill themselves.

2. The nature of rights objection: Arguing from the nature of rights, some have challenged the contention that the ethical principle of autonomy can be extrapolated to claim a right to choose one's time and mode of death. Given that a valid right implies a duty to respond that cannot be *reasonably*—refused (79, 80) and that reasonable moral compunction about either killing patients or assisting in their suicide is acknowledged, it is argued that there is no right to die by euthanasia or physician-assisted suicide (58). By this logic, euthanasia or physician-assisted suicide in the relief of suffering may be described as justifiable in certain circumstances but not as a right. In contrast, the right of dying patients to relief of intractable pain is undisputed, and it demands an appropriate and effective response (16, 57, 58, 61, 81).

3. The coercive element in choice: It is argued that choice is not a neutral experience and that choices themselves have implicit coercive capacity that may cause harm (82). Patients with terminal illness are a vulnerable population who frequently see themselves as a burden to their families and society (83). For some vulnerable patients, the very option of euthanasia or assisted suicide may exert coercive influence by implication that elective termination of life may be easier for the family or society than continued management of pain to facilitate living until death (82).

4. The argument from nonnecessity: Proponents of this view argue that sedation for patients with refractory suffering provides adequate relief without necessitating the death of the patient (53, 84, 85). In contrast to euthanasia or assisted suicide, in which the death of the patient is the intended outcome, deep sedation obliterates the perception of distress, and the death of the patient, when it occurs, is a foreseen contingency but not an intended or essential outcome.

Controlled sedation is a widely accepted strategy in the management of otherwise unendurable suffering. It is routinely used to manage the severe pain and anxiety associated with noxious procedures, such as major surgery, that would otherwise be intolerable (86). The loss of interactional function associated with sedation precludes its application in the routine management of chronic physical, psychological, or existential distress, since the therapeutic goal is to achieve adequate relief with preserved function. At the end of life, however, the goals of care may change such that the relief of suffering predominates over all other considerations, and induced sedation is an option of last resort to provide relief with certainty and speed.

The offer of sedation is often received as an empathic acknowledgment of the severity of the degree of the patient's suffering. The enhancement of the patient's trust arising from the commitment of the clinician to the relief of suffering may in itself influence decision making, particularly if there are other tasks or life issues to be completed before function diminishes. Some patients decline sedation, acknowledging that symptoms will be unrelieved but secure in the knowledge that if the pain becomes intolerable, this decision can be rescinded. Other patients reaffirm comfort as the predominating consideration and request the initiation of sedation.

Sedating pharmacotherapy for refractory symptoms at the end of life should not be initiated until a discussion about cardiopulmonary resuscitation (CPR) has taken place with the patient or if appropriate, with the patient's proxy, and there is agreement that CPR will not be initiated. CPR at the time of death is almost always futile in this situation (87, 88), and furthermore is inconsistent with the agreed goals of care (87).

The literature describing the use of sedation in the management of refractory pain is anecdotal and refers to the use of opioid, neuroleptic, benzodiazepine, and barbiturate drugs. In the absence of controlled relative efficacy data, guidelines for drug selection are empirical. The details of sedating pharmacotherapy are reviewed elsewhere (53). Irrespective of the agent or agents selected, administration initially requires dose titration to achieve adequate relief, followed by ongoing therapy to maintain the effect. The depth of sedation necessary to control symptoms varies greatly. For some patients, a state of conscious sedation, in which they retain the ability to respond to verbal stimuli, may provide adequate relief without total loss of interactive function (84, 89). Some authors suggest that doses can be titrated down to reestablish lucidity after an agreed interval or for planned family interactions (84, 85). This, of course, is a potentially unstable situation, and the possibility that lucidity may not be promptly restored or that death may ensue as doses are again escalated should be explained to both the patient and family.

Once adequate relief is achieved, the parameters for monitoring and the role of further dose titration is determined by the goal of care. If the goal of care is to ensure comfort until death to an imminently dying patient, the only salient parameters for ongoing observation are those pertaining to comfort. Since downward titration of drug doses places the patient at risk for recurrent distress and does not serve the goal of care, it is not recommended even as the patient approaches death.

EXCEPTIONAL SITUATIONS THAT JUSTIFY EUTHANASIA OR ASSISTED SUICIDE

Although euthanasia and assisted suicide are not necessary for the adequate relief of even refractory suffering in routine care, occasionally extreme situations justify actions that are beyond the realm of normative Hippocratic practice. For example:

A medic and a soldier are alone on an isolated battlefield. They are without communication or medicines. The soldier is mortally wounded. His bleeding viscera spill from his abdomen; his impending death is certain. He is conscious and screams in agony. In desperation, he turns to the medic to plead for a bullet to end his suffering. "I will not let you die in pain," responds the medic. In tears, he gently strokes the soldiers hair as he places his rifle at the nape of the soldier's neck and dispenses the bullet of mercy.

This anecdote presents an extreme situation: the soldier was either to die in agony or in the absence of other options, obtain relief by death at his own hands or by the assistance of his comrade. For the medic this was not a choice between right and wrong but a choice between right and also right that demanded an urgent prioritization. Given the imperative of the relief of suffering, the option to refuse collaboration and to offer only soothing words of solace seemed pitifully inadequate. Given the imperative of the sanctity of human life, the option of killing his ward was unbearably difficult. Even though his behaviors transgressed Hippocratic norms, few people would condemn the acquiescence of the medic to the pleas of his dying friend. The behavior of the medic in the anecdote of the soldier seems justifiable because the situation was not normative. The absence of other means is the defining quality of the nonnormative state in which the purview of compassionate care can be expanded to incorporate killing the sufferer.

In the routine clinical setting, does the situation of dying patients with severe suffering constitute such a nonnormative situation? The answer to that question depends on the availability of effective palliative resources. In a time of widespread drug availability and ready access to expert resources, it is extremely rare that the necessary means to provide adequate relief are unavailable.

However, the provision of the necessary relief requires a mobilization of personal, medical, and community resources to this purpose. Indeed, to maintain the moral fabric of society in general and especially the health care profession, this is an ethical and social imperative.

SUMMARY

For treatment of the cancer patient with pain, the global aim of care is to provide adequate relief of distress to both the patient and family while maintaining the moral integrity of the patient, family, and staff. Ethical dilemmas are frequent in the care of such patients, and successful care requires the clinical skills to identify, manage, and if possible, prevent such conflicts. Goal setting, family and staff meetings, and a clear understanding of the concepts of autonomy, beneficence, nonmaleficence, justice, and the principle of double effect contribute to achieving these goals.

References

1. Bonica JJ, Ventafridda V, Twycross RG. Cancer pain. In: Bonica JJ, ed. The management of pain. 2nd ed. Philadelphia: Lea & Febiger, 1990;400–460.
2. Feuz A, Rapin CH. An observational study of the role of pain control and food adaptation of elderly patients with terminal cancer. J Am Diet Assoc 1994;94:767–70.

3. Thorpe DM. The incidence of sleep disturbance in cancer patients with pain. In: VII World Congress on Pain: Abstracts. Seattle: IASP, 1993;abstract 451.
4. Massie MJ, Holland JC. The cancer patient with pain: psychiatric complications and their management. Med Clin North Am 1987;71:243–258.
5. Bond MR, Pearson IB. Psychosocial aspects of pain in women with advanced cancer of the cervix. J Psychosom Res 1969;13:13–21.
6. Barkwell DP. Ascribed meaning: a critical factor in coping and pain attenuation in patients with cancer-related pain. J Palliat Care 1991;7:5–14.
7. Daut RL, Cleeland CS. The prevalence and severity of pain in cancer. Cancer 1982;50:1913–1918.
8. Fishman B. The treatment of suffering in patients with cancer pain: cognitive behavioral approaches. In: Foley KM, Bonica JJ, Ventafridda V, eds. II international congress on cancer pain. Advances in pain research and therapy, vol 16. New York: Raven Press, 1990;301–316.
9. Lazarus RS, Folkman C. Stress, appraisal and coping. New York: Springer, 1984.
10. Syrjala KL. Integrating medical and psychological treatments for cancer pain. In: Chapman CR, Foley KM, eds. Current and emerging issues in cancer pain: research and practice. New York: Raven Press, 1993;393–409.
11. Bolund C. Medical and care factors in suicides by cancer patients in Sweden. J Psychosoc Oncol 1985;3:31–52.
12. Breitbart W. Suicide in the cancer patient. Oncology 1987;1:49–54.
13. Cleeland CS. The impact of pain on the patient with cancer. Cancer 1984;54:2635–2641.
14. Baile WF, Di Maggio JR, Schapira DV, et al. The request for assistance in dying: the need for psychiatric consultation. Cancer 1993;72:2786–2791.
15. Breitbart W. Cancer pain and suicide. In: Foley KM, Bonica JJ, Ventafridda V, ed. II International Congress on Cancer Pain. Advances in pain research and therapy, vol 16. New York: Raven Press, 1990;399–412.
16. Wanzer SH, Federman DD, Adelstein SJ, et al. The physicians responsibility toward hopelessly ill patients: a second look. N Engl J Med 1989;120:844–849.
17. Roy DJ. Relief of suffering: the doctor's mandate. J Palliat Care 1991;7:3–4 (editorial).
18. Angell M. The quality of mercy. N Engl J Med 1982;306:98–99.
19. American Medical Association Council on Ethical and Judicial Affairs. Decisions near the end of life. JAMA 1992;267:2229–2233.
20. American Nursing Association. Position statement on promotion of comfort and relief of pain in dying patients. Kansas City: ANA, 1991.
21. President's Commission for the Study of Ethical Problems in Medical and Biomedical and Behavioral Research. Deciding to forgo life sustaining treatment: ethical and legal issues in treatment decisions. Washington: U.S. Government Printing Office, 1983.
22. World Health Organization. Cancer pain relief and palliative care. Geneva: WHO, 1990.
23. Somerville MA. Death of pain: pain, suffering and ethics. In: Gebhart GF, Hammond DL, Jensen TS, eds. Proceedings of the VII World Congress on Pain: Congress Abstracts: progress in pain research and management. Seattle: IASP, 1994;41–58.
24. American College of Physicians Health and Public Policy Committee. Drug therapy for severe chronic pain in terminal illness. Ann Intern Med 1983;99:870–880.
25. American Pain Society. Principles of analgesic use in the treatment acute pain and chronic cancer pain: a concise guide to medical practice. 3rd ed. Skokie, IL: APS, 1992.
26. American Pain Society Committee of Quality Assurance Standards. American Pain Society quality assurance standards for the relief of acute pain and cancer pain. In: Bond MR, Charlton JE, Woolf CJ, ed. Proceedings of the VI World Congress on Pain. Pain research and clinical management, vol 4. Amsterdam: Elsevier, 1991;185–190.
27. Spross JA, McGuire DB, Schmitt RM. Oncology nursing society position paper on cancer pain: 2. Oncol Nurs Forum 1990;17:751–760.
28. Spross JA, McGuire DB, Schmitt RM. Oncology Nursing Society position paper on cancer pain. Oncol Nurs Forum 1990;17:595–614.
29. American College of Physicians Ethics Committee. American College of Physicians ethics manual. 3rd ed. Ann Intern Med 1992;117:947–960.
30. Cherny NI, Catane R. Professional negligence in the management of cancer pain: a case for urgent reforms. Cancer 1995;76:2181–2185.
31. Walker VA, Hoskin PJ, Hanks GW, et al. Evaluation of WHO analgesic guidelines for cancer pain in a hospital-based palliative care unit. J Pain Symptom Manag 1988;3:145–150.
32. Ventafridda V, Tamburini M, Caraceni A, et al. A validation study of the WHO method for cancer pain relief. Cancer 1987;59:851–856.
33. Takeda F. Results of field-testing in Japan of W. H. O. draft interim guidelines on relief of cancer pain. Pain Clin 1986;1:83–89.
34. Schug SA, Zech D, Dorr U. Cancer pain management according to WHO analgesic guidelines. J Pain Symptom Manag 1990;5:27–32.
35. Grond S, Zech D, Schug SA, et al. Validation of World Health Organization guidelines for cancer pain relief during the last days and hours of life. J Pain Symptom Manag 1991;6:411–422.
36. Grond S, Zech D, Lynch J, et al. Validation of World Health Organization guidelines for pain relief in head and neck cancer: a prospective study. Ann Otol Rhinol Laryngol 1993;102:342–348.
37. Cleeland CS, Gonin R, Hatfield A, et al. Pain and its treatment in outpatients with metastatic cancer. N Eng J Med 1994;330:592–596.
38. Larue F, Colleau SM, Brasseur L, et al. Multicentre study of cancer pain and its treatment in France. BMJ 1995;310:1034–1037.
39. Portenoy RK, Kornblith AB, Wong G, et al. Pain in ovarian cancer patients: prevalence, characteristics, and associated symptoms. Cancer 1994;74:907–915.
40. Portenoy RK, Miransky J, Thaler HT, et al. Pain in ambulatory patients with lung or colon cancer: prevalence, characteristics and impact. Cancer 1992;70:1616–1624.
41. Portenoy R, Thaler HT, Kornblith AB, et al. The Memorial Symptom Assessment Scale: an instrument for the evaluation of symptom prevalence, characteristics and distress. Eur J Clin Oncol 1994;30:1326–1336.
42. Tay WK, Shaw RJ, Goh CR. A survey of symptoms in hospice patients in Singapore. Ann Acad Med Singapore 1994;23:191–6.
43. Brescia FJ, Portenoy RK, Ryan M, et al. Pain, opioid use, and survival in hospitalized patients with advanced cancer. J Clin Oncol 1992;10:149–155.
44. Donnelly S, Walsh D. The symptoms of advanced cancer. Semin Oncol 1995;22(Suppl 2):67–72.
45. Von Roenn JH, Cleeland CS, Gonin R, et al. Physician's attitudes and practice in cancer pain management: a survey from the Eastern Cooperative Oncology Group. Ann Intern Med 1993;119:121–126.
46. Grossman SA, Sheidler VR, Swedeen K, et al. Correlation of patient and caregiver ratings of cancer pain. J Pain Symptom Manag 1991;6:53–57.
47. Larue F, Colleau SM, Fontaine A, et al. Oncologists and primary care physicians' attitudes towards pain control and morphine prescribing in France. Cancer 1995;76:2375–2382.
48. Cherny NI, Ho MN, Bookbinder M, et al. Cancer pain: knowledge and attitudes of physicians at a cancer center. Proc Am Soc Clin Oncol 1994;12:1490 (abstract).
49. American Pain Society Quality of Care Committee. Quality improvement guidelines for the treatment of acute pain and cancer pain. JAMA 1995;274:1874–1880.
50. Colton MC. Pain management now part of standards for care in cancer centres. Can Med Assoc J 1995;153:741–742 (letter).
51. Hagen N, Young J, MacDonald N. Diffusion of standards of care for cancer pain. Can Med Assoc J 1995;152:1205–9.
52. Cherny NI, Portenoy RK. Practical issues in the management of cancer pain. In: Wall PD, Melzack R, ed. Textbook of pain. 3rd ed. Edinburgh: Churchill Livingstone, 1994;1437–1467.
53. Cherny NI, Portenoy RK. Sedation in the treatment of refractory symptoms: guidelines for evaluation and treatment. J Palliat Care 1994;10:31–38.

54. Gonzales GR, Elliot KJ, Portenoy RK, et al. The impact of a comprehensive evaluation in the management of cancer pain. Pain 1991;47:141–144.
55. Coyle N, Breitbart W, Weaver S, et al. Delirium as a contributing factor to "crescendo" pain: three case reports. J Pain Symptom Manag 1994;9:44–47.
56. Roy DJ. Need they sleep before they die? J Palliat Care 1991;6:3–4.
57. Latimer EJ. Ethical challenges in cancer care. J Palliat Care 1992;8:65–70.
58. Pollard BJ. Dying: rights and responsibilities. Med J Aust 1988;149:147–149.
59. Scanlon C, Fleming C. Ethical issues in caring for the patient with advanced cancer. Nurs Clin North Am 1989;24:977–986.
60. Smith RS. Ethical issues in cancer pain. In: Chapman CR, Foley KM, ed. Current and emerging issues in cancer pain: research and practice. New York: Raven Press, 1993;385–392.
61. Latimer EJ. Ethical decision-making in the care of the dying and its applications to clinical practice. J Pain Symptom Manag 1991;6:329–336.
62. Cavanaugh TA. The ethics of death-hastening or death-causing palliative analgesic administration to the terminally ill. J Pain Symptom Manag 1996;12:248–54.
63. Quill TE. The ambiguity of clinical intentions. N Engl J Med 1993;329:1039–1040.
64. Billings JA, Block SD. Slow euthanasia. J Palliat Care 1996;12:21–30 (see comments).
65. Quill TE, Cassel CK, Meier DE. Care of the hopelessly ill: proposed criteria for physician assisted suicide. N Engl J Med 1992;327:1380–1383.
66. Smith G. Recognizing personhood and the right to die with dignity. J Palliat Care 1990;6:24–32.
67. Brody H. Assisted death: compassionate response to medical failure. N Engl J Med 1992;327:1384–1388.
68. van Delden JJ, Pijnenborg L, van der Maas PJ. The Remmelink study: two years later. Hastings Cent Rep 1993;23:24–27.
69. Brescia FJ. Killing the known dying: notes of a death watcher. J Pain Symptom Manag 1991;6:336–339 (editorial).
70. Foley KM. The relationship of pain and symptom management to patient requests for physician-assisted suicide. J Pain Symptom Manag 1991;6:289–297.
71. Latimer EJ. Euthanasia: a physician's reflections. J Pain Symptom Manag 1991;6:487–91.
72. Cundiff D. Euthanasia is not the answer: a hospice physician's view of the "death with dignity" debate. Totowa: Humana Press, 1992.
73. Twycross RG. Assisted death: a reply. Lancet 1990;336:796–798.
74. Saunders C, ed. Hospice and palliative care: an interdisciplinary approach. London: Edward Arnold, 1990.
75. Foley KM. Pain, physician-assisted suicide and euthanasia. APS J 1994.
76. Pollard BJ, Winton R. Why doctors and nurses must not kill patients. Med J Aust 1993;158:426–429.
77. Conolly ME. Alternative to euthanasia: pain management. Issues Law Med 1989;4:497–507.
78. Wilkinson J. The ethics of euthanasia. Palliat Med 1990;4:81–86.
79. Feinberg J. Rights: 1. Systematic analysis. In: Reich WT, ed. Encyclopedia of bioethics. New York: Macmillan, 1978;1507–1511.
80. Macklin R. Rights: 2. Rights in bioethics. In: Reich WT, ed. Encyclopedia of bioethics. New York: Macmillan, 1978;1511–1516.
81. Latimer EJ. Caring for seriously ill and dying patients: the philosophy and ethics. Can Med Assoc J 1991;144:859–64.
82. Velleman JD. Against the right to die. J Med Philos 1992;17:665–81.
83. Cherny NI, Coyle N, Foley KM. Suffering in the advanced cancer patient: a definition and taxonomy. J Palliat Care 1994;10:57–70.
84. Greene WR, Davis WH. Titrated intravenous barbiturates in the control of symptoms in patients with terminal cancer. South Med J 1991;84:332–337.
85. Truog RD, Berde CB, Mitchell C, et al. Barbiturates in the care of the terminally ill. N Engl J Med 1992;327:1678–1682.
86. Agency for Health Care Policy and Research Acute Pain Management Panel. Acute pain management: operative or medical procedures and trauma. Clinical Practice Guideline. Washington: U.S. Department of Health and Human Services, 1992.
87. Haines IE, Zalcberg J, Buchanan JD. Not-for-resuscitation orders in cancer patients: principles of decision making. Med J Aust 1990;153:225–229.
88. Rosner F, Kark PR, Bennett AJ, et al. Medical futility. Committee on Bioethical Issues of the Medical Society of the State of New York. N Y State J Med 1992;92:485–488.
89. Burke AL, Diamond PL, Hulbert J, et al. Terminal restlessness: its management and the role of midazolam. Med J Aust 1991;155:485–487.

Status of Chronic Pain Treatment Outcome Research

David A. Fishbain, R. Brian Cutler, Hubert L. Rosomoff, and Renee Steele Rosomoff

OUTCOME RESEARCH

The purpose of this chapter is to acquaint the reader with outcome research and the concept of outcomes and to review the current status of chronic pain treatment outcome research. The end result of medical care and the effects of the health care process on individual patients and patient populations are the concerns of outcome research. Outcome research has recently become extremely important. The results of outcome research, specifically which medical treatments work best and for whom, are now used by insurance companies, employers, state and federal governments, and consumers to make decisions about appropriate care (1). For example, the U.S. Agency for Health Care Policy and Research has stated that the objective of health care is to achieve good and improved patient outcomes (2). It follows that outcome research should determine whether the process of care provides good outcomes and/or the process of that medical care is one that is thought or known to be associated with good outcomes (process measurement).

One way to think about outcome research is to contrast it with traditional randomized controlled studies. These clinical efficacy studies test the success of treatments in controlled environments. In contrast, outcome research, or effectiveness research, evaluates the results of the health care process in real life (doctor's office, hospital, health clinics, home) (1). Thus, it is a misconception that treatment outcome research requires large or small randomized controlled studies. On the contrary, this type of research often involves the following types of studies: nonrandomized contemporaneous controls, nonrandomized historical controls, cohort studies, case-control studies, cross-sectional studies, surveillance (database, registers) studies, consecutive case studies and even single case reports (1). The key to performing outcome research is to understand what treatment outcomes are and how they are measured. A number of books and papers addressing this issue have recently been published (3–5).

The emphasis on outcome research has resulted in three major paradigm shifts in clinical practice. The first shift is a change in the diagnostic evaluation to an emphasis on how the disease process has affected life functioning. The second shift, to treatment focused on symptoms rather than generic disease treatment, resulted from studies indicating that focused symptom treatments are more efficacious, efficient, and cost effective. The third shift relates to measurement of treatment outcome. Here it was determined that two measurements, one before beginning treatment and one at completion of treatment, although economical, cannot specify in what way a positive outcome was positive and did not provide specific information on how treatments could be modified or tailored to a specific case. This has initiated the concurrent measurement approach, which is multiple intermediate time-patient measurements plus measurements before and after treatment. This approach can indicate which treatments produce gains more quickly and provides specific indicators of change during course of treatment. As a result, one can modify interventions during the course of treatment more quickly (6).

TREATMENT OUTCOMES

Treatment outcomes are the final health status measurements after the passage of time and the application of treatment. From another standpoint, treatment outcomes and outcome systems can be thought of as accountability methods. Thus, treatment outcomes can be used not only for determining treatment effectiveness and treatment benefit but also for cost of care, cost of complications, performance, and satisfaction with process of medical care and outcome of medical care (6). Typical outcomes are mortality, morbidity, functional status, health status, and quality of life (to be discussed in detail later). These lead to benefits, costs of complications, and satisfaction or dissatisfaction with outcome. It is interesting that these outcomes closely approximate the rank order of outcomes that surveys have determined to be important to patients: (*a*) to live as long as possible; (*b*) to be free of pain and other physical and psychological symptoms; (*c*) to function normally; (*d*) to be free of iatrogenic problems; and (*e*) to remain solvent (1). The sequence of this hierarchy is important to pain treatment outcome for two reasons: first, because people in general appear to put a very high value on living a pain-free life and second, because in pain treatment, treatment of functional deficits is often stressed over the actual treatment of pain. This dilemma often leads to disappointment and dissatisfaction on the part of the patient.

Thus, the process of care can also dissatisfy the patient. As presented earlier, the process of care in attempting to generate a positive outcome can also be measured in various ways. These measurements can include preventive measures, diagnostic testing, procedures, treatments, and other care activities. These process variables lead to cost of care and most important, patient and payor satisfaction with the process (5).

PATIENT SATISFACTION

Patient satisfaction is an often used and quoted treatment outcome. This variable relates to perceived satisfaction with any and all aspects of medical care. The relations among patient satisfaction, quality of life (QOL) (discussed later), and other outcomes is shown in Figure 46.1. Satisfaction is demonstrated to be the end result of a number of outcome measurement domains and is therefore difficult to relate to actual medical outcome. Thus, although patient satisfaction is important, it has not been shown to be an accurate measure of treatment outcome and is actually a poor measure of clinical improvement (6). For example, Atkisson and Zwick (8) showed that symptom improvement explained only 10% of the variance in patient satisfaction. Similarly, it appears that there is very little relation between pain reduction and satisfaction of chronic pain patients (CCPs) (9). This is surprising. It suggests that satisfaction with the process of care may color the view of the health care system. This last point should be kept in mind when interpreting patient satisfaction results. A number of instruments have been developed to measure patient satisfaction (10) and specifically for CPPs (11).

QUALITY OF LIFE

QOL as a treatment outcome variable has recently drawn much attention (12), and much has been written about it (13–16). However, there is no universally accepted definition for this concept. In general, QOL can be thought of as the functional effect of an illness and its therapy on a patient as perceived by the patient (13).

QOL can be divided into dimensions, domains, and indicators. There are 5 to 10 dimensions. Some of these are opportunity, health perceptions, function, morbidity, and mortality. For each dimension there may be a number of domains. For example, for the functional dimension there are four domains: social, psychological, cognitive, and physical. In turn, for each domain there are a number of indicators subject to measurement by indices and scales. For the physical domain, the indicators are activity restrictions and fitness.

Usually tools, inventories, and scales measure different combinations of dimensions and/or domains (13). This concept is demonstrated in Table 46.1. Here it can be seen that these widely used general health surveys encompass a number of domains and dimensions, hence are not disease specific. However, many disease-specific QOL measures are available. These are usually specific to a diagnosis or patient groups, such as pain (17-19), or to an impairment dimension or domain. Some researchers have recommended the use of these measures over general QOL measures and suggest choosing measures according to the specific purpose of the research (16). A number of scales have been specifically developed for pain and have been demonstrated to be reliable and valid (19).

As pointed out earlier, QOL is defined from the patient's perspective. Thus, it is not surprising to note that when QOL inventories are administered to providers and patients, there is little correlation between the answers. For example, a recent study (20) investigating this problem found moderate agreement on symptoms and function, less agreement on physical health, and little or no agreement on social relations and occupational aspects of QOL. This last point indicates that clinicians should be very careful in making judgments about patients' QOL status and that these judgments should be checked against patient perceptions.

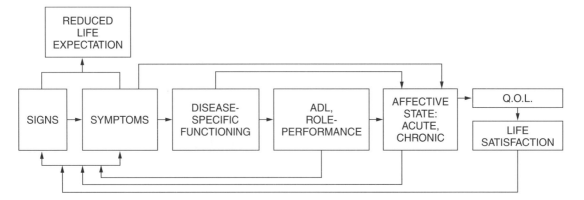

Figure 46.1. Relations among measures of patients' signs, symptoms, outcomes, and satisfaction. (Adapted from Kopec J A, Esdaile J M. Spine update functional disability scales for back pain. Spine 1995;20:1943–1949.)

Table 46.1.   Summary of Information about Widely Used General Health Surveys

	QWB	SIP	HIE	NHP	QLI	COOP	EURO-QOL	DUKE	MOS FWBP	MOS SF–36
CONCEPTS										
Physical functioning	•	•	•	•	•	•	•	•	•	•
Social functioning	•	•	•	•	•	•	•	•	•	•
Role functioning	•	•	•	•	•	•	•	•	•	•
Psychological distress		•	•	•	•	•	•	•	•	•
Health perceptions (general)			•	•	•	•	•	•	•	•
Pain (bodily)		•	•	•		•		•	•	•
Energy/fatigue	•		•	•				•	•	•
Psychological well-being			•					•	•	
Sleep		•		•				•	•	
Cognitive functioning		•						•	•	
Quality of life			•			•			•	
Reported health transition						•			•	•

QWB, Quality of Well-Being Scale; SIP, Sickness Impact Profile; HIE, Health Insurance Experiment surveys; NHP, Nottingham Health Profile; QLI, Quality of Life Index; COOP, Dartmouth Function Charts; EUROQUOL, European Quality of Life Index; DUKE, Duke Health Profile; MOS FWBP, MOS Functioning and Well-Being Profile; MOS SF-EY, MOS 36-item Short-Form Health Survey;

Rows are ordered in terms of how frequently concepts are represented; only concepts represented in two or more survey are listed.

Adapted from Ware J E. The status of health assessment 1994. Anne Rev Public Health 1995;16:327–349.

PAIN TREATMENT FACILITIES

Pain treatment facilities were developed specifically to treat chronic, intractable pain. They evolved out of the concept of pain relief clinics developed to control the continuous severe pain of battle injured World War II soldiers. In this situation, a coordinated team was required to manage the different types of pain (21). Multidisciplinary pain clinics or centers may have evolved from this concept in the early 1970s. Here it was observed that a significant percentage of low-back pain and neck pain patients did not improve with traditional medical treatment; they remained disabled (21). These patients demonstrated a host of behavioral and psychosocial problems in relation to their chronic pain. These problems required the intervention of disciplines besides those of the neurosurgeon, orthopaedic surgeon, and anesthesiologist (22). In addition, these patients required a "concurrent highly integrated multidisciplinary treatment approach" (21) that would deal with all the patient's problems simultaneously.

There are approximately 1500 to 2000 pain treatment facilities in the United States (21). They differ in their staff makeup, size, philosophy, and most important, treatment approach. The training or specialty of the medical director determines the philosophy and treatment approach of the facility. The professional specialty of the medical director of pain facilities varies (23). This variation in staff makeup and treatment approach has blurred the distinction among the different types of pain treatment facilities in the minds of physicians and the public. Because of this problem, the International Association for the Study of Pain (IASP) developed definitions for four types of pain treatment facilities (Table 46.2).

Table 46.2 indicates a clear distinction between modality-oriented clinics and pain clinics versus each other. There are

Table 46.2.   IASP Classification of Pain Facilities

Modality-oriented clinic
  Provides specific type of treatment, e.g. nerve blocks, transcutaneous nerve stimulation, acupuncture, biofeedback
  May have one or more health care disciplines
  Does not provide an integrated, comprehensive approach
Pain clinic
  Focuses on the diagnosis and management of patients with chronic pain or may specialize in specific diagnoses or pain related to a specific region of the body
  Does not provide comprehensive assessment or treatment. Institution offering appropriate consultative and therapeutic services would qualify but never an isolated solo practitioner.
Multidisciplinary pain clinic
  Specializes in the multidisciplinary diagnosis and management of patients with chronic pain or may specialize in specific diagnoses or pain related to a specific region of the body
  Staffed by physicians of different specialties and other health care providers
  Differs from a multidisciplinary pain center only because it does not include research and teaching
Multidisciplinary pain center
  Organization of health care professionals and basic scientists that includes research, teaching, and patient care in acute and chronic pain
  Typically a component of a medical school or a teaching hospital
  Clinical programs supervised by an appropriately trained and licensed director
  Staffed by a minimum of physician, psychologist, occupational therapist, physical therapist and registered nurse
  Services provided integrated and based on interdisciplinary assessment and management
  Offers both inpatient and outpatient program

Adapted from Loser J D. Desirable characteristics for pain treatment facilities: report of the IASP taskforce. In: Bond M R, Charleon. J E, Woof C J, eds. Proceedings of the VI World Congress on Pain. 1991;411–415.

also clear differences between these two types of pain facilities and multidisciplinary clinics and multidisciplinary pain centers (MPCs). The only difference, however, between multidisciplinary pain clinics and multidisciplinary pain centers appears to be the research and teaching in MPCs. These definitions also indicate that MPCs may be more likely to have both inpatient and outpatient treatment and to have larger and more diversified multidisciplinary staffs, including more than one physician specialty. As a consequence, MPCs are likely to offer a wider range of treatments than multidisciplinary pain clinics. This last statement is important to the discussion that follows. Finally, most of the outcome pain facility treatment studies relate to MPCs.

Outcome Research in Pain Facilities

Pain facilities have been around since the 1970s, and because early in their development they had to demonstrate outcome results (25), there is a large body of literature on the subject. In a recent review, Fishbain et al. (26) found 164 studies in which the effect on chronic pain of nonsurgical pain facility treatment was evaluated with some kind of outcome variable. Since that 1993 publication, the number of treatment outcome studies of chronic pain facilities stands at more than 200. In these studies, the types of outcome variables that have been used according to domains are the following (26–28):

- Demographics: numbers of CPPs in retraining or in school
- Medical history: decreased analgesic use, decreased medical system use, decreased use of opioid medications, improved sleep, decreased hospitalizations for pain
- Physical examination: improved all ranges of motion of spine, improved hip flexion, improved straight leg raising, decreased weight, increased lumbar strength
- Biomechanical testing: improved sitting tolerance, improved endurance, improved lower extremity strength, improved ability to lift, improved walking tolerance, improved climbing ability, improved aerobic capability, increased ability to do activities of daily living
- Compensation litigation: number of patients on compensation status, return to work, increased ability to do activities of daily living, number of patients completing or settling litigation
- Pain: decreased pain, increased ability to control pain, decreased frequency of pain, decreased pain on McGill pain questionnaire, decreased pain behavior
- Psychological testing: decreased scores on Minnesota Multiphasic Personality and Millon Behavior Health Inventories
- Other behavioral variables: decreased depression as measured by the Beck Depression Scale, Center for Epidemiological Studies Depression Scale, Symptom checklist 90-R, or other depression inventories; decreased anxiety scores; decreased alcohol and/or illicit drug use; decreased perception of disability

- Functional status: improvement in scores on Health Assessment questionnaire; improvement in Arthritis Impact Measurement Scale; improvement in Fibromyalgia Impact Questionnaire and Self-Efficacy Scale; improvement in ability to do activities of daily living; decreased scores on the Sickness Impact Profile inventory
- Work variables: return to work

This extensive literature has been reviewed by numerous authors (26–42). Unfortunately, these reviewers have not arrived at consistent conclusions about the efficacy of pain facility treatment on chronic pain or the efficacy of specific pain treatments (26–42).

The basic reasons for this problem have to do with the nature of chronic pain and its effect on function. Chronic pain patients are not all the same. Chronic pain is not static but is characterized by good periods punctuated by exacerbations, and CPPs may improve over time without treatment. This last point is demonstrated by two recent follow-up studies (43, 44) on unoperated discogenic back pain. Here it was shown that the vast majority of patients improved over time. Therefore, with these groups of patients, outcome variables would spontaneously improve without treatment, making the evaluation of the effect of treatment difficult to evaluate without an untreated control group. A recent study by Fishbain et al. (45) has identified another possible cofounder of this type of outcome research. Here, CPPs were followed up postpain facility treatment as part of a study on the prediction of return to work. It was found that approximately 36% of the CPPs changed or "moved" the outcome variable work status over time. Fishbain et al. (45) pointed out that such movement can confound outcome results and must be taken into account.

CPPs also differ according to the nature of their organic pathology; they may be more or less difficult to treat according to the nature of their physical problem. Although some pain facility treatment outcome studies have demonstrated positive outcomes with specific populations, such as those with failed back syndrome (46), patients suffering from disc herniation (47, 48), and geriatric CPPs (49, 50), most studies lump CPPs into one group. This has also been a source of error. These reasons and the difficulties in using good control groups are the likely reasons for inconsistent findings in outcome studies of CPP treatment in pain facilities.

A new approach was needed to solve this problem. Because of the sheer number of studies in the pain treatment outcome literature, researchers have been able to approach pain treatment outcome via a recently developed statistical tool: meta-analysis. Meta-analyses provided a new perspective by which these inconsistencies could be researched.

Meta-Analysis

Meta-analysis is a statistical analysis of a collection of results from individual studies for the purpose of result integration (51, 52). In meta-analysis the researcher integrates and synthesizes the data of each study into an effect size. Individual effect sizes are averaged across studies to provide a global portrait of the relation. Thus, meta-analyses do not rely on statistical significance tests, as do individual studies, but on effect sizes to draw general conclusions (53).

Meta-analysis has become necessary because of sampling errors, measurement errors, and other artifacts that affect the statistical power of individual studies (53). These errors have led to conclusions of no effect when there is an effect (type II error) in many individual studies (53). These type II errors within individual studies lead to erroneous conclusions within narrative reviews, which are usually based on traditional interpretations of statistical significance tests (53). Meta-analysis is useful when different studies display conflicting results that make it difficult to arrive at a conclusion in a traditional review. Finally, meta-analysis is also useful when the effect sizes of the interventions are small or the event rates are low (54). Thus, because of these advantages over a traditional review, the meta-analysis review has become the "supreme court" in determining whether an effect exists. Some authors claim that meta-analysis will end many arguments about treatment effectiveness (55).

Pain Treatment Meta-Analyses

Interestingly, large numbers of pain treatment meta-analyses have been performed on the outcome literature. Our group has reviewed (56) these meta-analyses to derive some conclusions about the quality of this literature and to answer questions about the efficacy of the used treatments. For this study we located 11 meta-analyses, described and broken down into groups in Table 46.3. We abstracted the following data: (a) types of pain problems, (b) treatments used, (c) outcome variables analyzed, (d) calculated effect size, (e) and numbers of studies examined in each category. Next we calculated the standard error for each category when not provided and where possible, a p value. The results of these abstractions and calculations are presented in Tables 46.4, 46.5, and 46.6.

From a review of these tables, we arrived at the following observations and conclusions. Close to 46% of the meta-analyses examined pain facility treatment outcome. Overall, they were remarkably *consistent* in demonstrating that pain facility treatment is effective for most outcome variables, especially for return to work. Pain facility treatment also appears to be effective for most types of chronic pain. Biofeedback, cognitive therapy, and operant conditioning as individual treatments were demonstrated to be efficacious, while the package of treatments also showed that distinction. Within the headache treatment grouping, relaxation or biofeedback and propranolol were shown to be efficacious for tension headache and migraine headaches. Antidepressant treatment showed efficacy for tension headaches and chronic low back pain, while psychoeducation was efficacious for pain, depression, and disability. These observations led to a number of general conclusions. First, the reviewed meta-analyses were consistent in demonstrating the efficacy of pain

Table 46.3.   Meta-Analyses of Pain Treatment Outcome

Study	Comments
Pain Facility Treatments	
Cutler et al. (141)	Does nonsurgical pain center treatment of chronic pain return patients to work?
Malone and Strube (137)	Meta-analysis of nonmedical treatments for chronic pain.
Fernandez and Turk (138)	Utility of cognitive coping strategies for altering pain perception.
Curtis (140)	Efficacy of multidisciplinary treatment programs for chronic low back pain.
Flor et al. (139)	Efficacy of multidisciplinary pain treatment centers.
Headache Treatments	
Holroyd and Penzien (142)	Client variables and the behavioral treatment of recurrent tension headache.
Holroyd and Penzien (143)	Pharmacological versus nonpharmacological prophylaxis of recurrent migraine headache.
Specific Treatments	
Mullen et al. (144)	Efficacy of psychoeducational interventions on pain; disability in people with arthritis.
Onghena and Van Houdenhove (145)	Antidepressant-induced analgesia in chronic nonmalignant pain.
Gam et al. (146)	Effect of low-level laser therapy on musculoskeletal pain.
Patel et al. (147)	Meta-analysis of acupuncture for chronic pain.

Adapted from Fishbain D A, Cutler R B, Rosomoff H L, Steele-Rosomoff R. Pain facilities: a review of their effectiveness and referral selection criteria. Cur Rev Pain 1997;1:107–115.

facility treatment for a wide range of outcome variables. However, it was not clear for what outcome variable or type of pain that this treatment was most successful. Second, some specific treatments appeared to be efficacious (56).

Results of meta-analyses depend on the quality of the data within the selected studies. Pain treatment studies have often been criticized for the following methodological problems: poor definition of outcome variables; time sampling differences between studies; different treatment populations within studies; different outcome variables making comparisons difficult between studies; different selection criteria making comparisons between studies problematic; different patient adherence patterns, again making comparisons difficult; different and poorly described methods of treatment; and poor control for nontreatment factors that affect outcome variables such as return to work (26, 40–42, 57, 58). These methodological problems could have affected the results of the reviewed meta-analyses (56). There are also technical factors, not reviewed here, that can be sources of error in performing a meta-analysis (56). Therefore, we concluded that the result of our review of reviews at this time should be interpreted with caution (56). However, the meta-analysis evidence is consistent in indicating that pain facilities are effective for the treatment of pain as measured by some outcome variables.

Table 46.4.　Details of Meta-Analyses of Pain Facility Treatment

Study	Variables	Effect Size	Number of Studies	95% Confidence Interval	P Value
Malone and Strube (137)	Type of pain				
	Back or neck	0.97	6	0.23–1.71	<0.05
	Cancer	0.41	1	—[a]	—[a]
	Dental or facial	1.21	10	0.12–2.30	<0.05
	Joint	1.05	8	0.11–1.99	<0.05
	Headache				
	Migraine	0.54	13	0.31–0.77	<0.001
	Mixed	0.41	2	3.53–4.35	NS
	Tension	0.96	12	0.00–1.92	NS
	Mixed group	1.16	11	0.42–1.91	<0.01
	Other	0.83	1	—[a]	—[a]
	Treatments				
	Autogenic	2.74	2	−2204–27.52	NS
	Biofeedback	0.95	24	0.45–1.45	<0.001
	Cognitive	0.76	4	0.26–1.26	<0.05
	Hypnosis	2.67	1	—[a]	—[a]
	Operant	0.55	3	0.28–0.82	<0.05
	Package	1.33	11	0.91–1.75	<0.001
	Placebo	2.23	3	−4.25–8.75	NS
	Relaxation	0.67	7	0.15–1.49	NS
	TENS	0.46	2	0.43–1.35	NS
	Outcome variables				
	Activity level	1.48	6	−0.66–3.62	NS
	Pain duration	1.42	7	−1.00–3.84	NS
	EMG or temperature	0.67	5	0.11–1.23	<0.05
	Pain frequency	0.75	18	0.35–1.15	<0.01
	Improvement	0.81	1	—[a]	—[a]
	Index	1.18	21	0.57–1.79	<0.0001
	Pain intensity	0.75	25	0.31–1.19	<0.0001
	Medication	1.21	6	−0.95–3.37	NS
	Mood	1.91	9	1.16–2.66	<0.001
	Other	3.80	2	−35.72–43.32	NS
	Subjective symptoms	1.12	7	0.72	<0.001
Fernandez and Turk (138)	Specific cognitive treatments				
	Neutral imaginings	0.74	7	0.05–1.43	<0.05
	Pleasant imaginings	0.64	20	0.41–0.87	<0.001
	External focus of attention	0.49	14	0.25–0.74	<0.001
	Rhythmic cognitive activity	0.44	5	0.08–0.80	<0.05
	Pain acknowledging	0.34	15	−0.03–0.71	NS
	Cognitive strategies vs expectancy	0.35	12	−0.01–0.71	NS
	Expectancy vs no treatment	0.03	9	−13.81–13.87	NS
Flor et al. (139)	Outcome variables				
	Somatic	0.94	37	0.77–1.11	<0.01
	Psychophysiologic	2.04	5	0.29–3.79	<0.05
	Behavioral	1.19	158	1.03–1.35	<0.001
	Pain	1.59	97	1.20–1.98	<0.001
	Interference	0.50	20	0.29–0.71	<0.001
	Mood	1.91	10	−0.43–4.25	<0.001
	Other	0.76	104	0.60–0.92	<0.001
	Outcome time				
	Short term	1.51	34	0.98–2.04	<0.001
	Long term	1.31	24	0.85–1.77	<0.001
Curtis (140)	Outcome variables				
	Physical fitness	0.5+	—	—[a]	—[a]
	Subjective distress	0.5+	—	—[a]	—[a]
	Daily activity	0.5+	—	—[a]	—[a]
	Medication	0.5+	—	—[a]	—[a]
Cutler et al. (141)	Work	40%	40	0.24–0.56	<0.001

[a]Cannot be calculated for n-1 or lack sufficient information to calculate.

EMG, electromyelography; NS, not significant; TENS, transcutaneous electrical nerve stimulation.

Adapted from Fishbain D A, Cutler R B, Rosomoff H L, Steele-Rosomoff P. Pain facilities: a review of their effectiveness and referral selection criteria. Curr Rev Pain 1997;1:107–115.

Table 46.5.   Details of Meta-Analyses of Headache Treatment

Study	Variables	Effect Size	Number of Studies	95% Confidence Interval	P Value
Holroyd and Penzien (142)	Treatments				
	EMG biofeedback	46	26	0.26–0.66	<0.001
	Relaxation	45	15	0.17–0.72	<0.01
	Relaxation, biofeedback	57	9	0.19–0.95	<0.05
	Noncontrolled biofeedback	15	6	−0.22–0.53	NS
	Headache monitor	5	10	0.10–0.18	NS
Holroyd and Penzien (143)	Treatments				
	Relaxation/biofeedback	47	22	0.25–0.69	<0.001
	Propranolol	44	12	0.12–0.75	<0.05
	Placebo	12	15	0.06–0.30	NS
	Untreated	0	15	0.02–0.03	NS

EMG, electromyelography; NS, not significant.
Adapted from Fishbain D A, Cutler R B, Rosomoff H L, Steele-Rosomoff R. Pain facilities: a review of their effectiveness and referral selection criteria. Curr Rev Pain 1997;1:107–115.

Table 46.6.   Details of Meta-Analyses of Specific Treatments for Chronic Pain

Study	Antidepressants	Variables	Effect Size	Number of Studies	95% Confidence Interval	P Value
Mullen et al. (144)	Psychoeducational	Outcome variable				
		Pain	0.21	14	0.08–0.34	<0.01
		Depression	0.28	11	0.12–0.44	<0.01
		Disability	0.09	14	0.04–0.22	NS
Onghena and Van Houdenhove (145)	Antidepressants	Type of pain				
		Rheumatologic	0.37	10	−0.06–0.80	NS
		Not specified or mixed	0.23	7	−0.01–0.47	NS
		Tension headache	1.11	6	72–1.50	<0.01
		Chronic back pain	0.64	5	28–1.00	<0.05
		Migraine	0.82	4	10–1.54	NS
		Atypical facial pain	0.81	3	−0.27–1.89	NS
		Postherpetic neuralgia	1.44	2	−4.91–7.79	NS
		Diabetic neuropathy	1.17	1	—[a]	—[a]
		Central pain	0.70	1	—[a]	—[a]
		Dysesthetic pain	−0.60	1	—[a]	—[a]
		Treatments				
		Antidepressants	0.64	40	0.42–0.82	—[a]
		Analgesics	0.48	10	0.07–0.89	<0.01
		Outcome variables				
		Physician	0.82	15	50–1.14	<0.001
		Patient	0.51	11	0.26–0.74	<0.001
		Global assessment				
		VAS (intensity)	0.47	16	0.19–0.75	<0.05
		X-point verbal scale	0.42	24	0.90–0.75	<0.01
		McGill Pain Questionnaire	0.17	3	−0.95–1.29	<0.05
		Other	0.41	30	0.08–0.74	NS
Gam et al. (146)	Low-level laser	Outcome variables				
		Double-blind pain	0.00	9	−0.10–0.11	<0.05
		Controlled pain	0.09	4	−0.03–0.22	NS
Patel et al. (147)	Acupuncture	Outcome variable				
		Pain	Weighted average of the risk difference used, calculated at 0.184	14	—[ab]	NS

[a]Cannot be calculated for n-1 or lack sufficient information to calculate.
[b]No significant effect found in placebo-controlled studies.
NS, not significant; VAS, visual analog scale.
Adapted from Fishbain D A, Cutler R B, Rosomoff H L, Steele-Rosomoff R. Pain facilities: a review of their effectiveness and referral selection criteria. Curr Rev Pain 1997;1:107–115.

Which Treatments Make Pain Facility Treatment Effective?

If pain facility treatment is effective for a number of outcome variables, which treatments or combination of treatments are responsible for this effect? Pain facilities generally use multiple treatment regimens integrated into a treatment package (56). For details of these treatment packages, see Fishbain et al. (56). This review of reviews demonstrated that the package treatment has been reported to be consistently effective. Yet we do not as yet know which aspects of that package make it effective.

For a partial answer we have to review non–meta-analysis evidence. Here the evidence indicates that treatments under one category, such as behavior, may have equal efficacy. For example, operant conditioning has been found to be as effective as cognitive-behavior (61). In addition, different treatments within one category appear not to be additive. For example, outpatient group cognitive therapy, relaxation training, and cognitive therapy combined with relaxation training have all been demonstrated to be equally efficacious (59). On the other hand, treatments from different groups may have an additive effect. For example, cognitive-behavioral methods may provide additive benefit to physical therapy. The combined package of cognitive-behavioral group pain treatment with physical therapy has been found to be superior to physical therapy alone (60). Thus, it may be advantageous for pain facilities to offer as many groups of treatments as possible. This may improve overall efficacy.

At this time, it is unclear what combinations delivered by pain facilities in a treatment package are effective. It is therefore unclear what combination of treatments is necessary for an effective package. It is also possible that the effectiveness of pain facilities rests in their ability to deliver this treatment package and an ability to integrate treatments into a package. This last issue may influence overall effectiveness but has not been explored in the literature.

Part of the managed care onslaught on medical care has been the concept of bundled charges. Here the payor negotiates for a set program fee for the patient rather than pay for individual treatments. Under these circumstances, treatment program incentive is to minimize rather than maximize the number of different treatments the patient will receive in order to maximize program profits. However, as we do not yet know which specific treatments in a package are effective or what combination is effective, there is the possibility that the minimization of different treatments decreases overall efficacy. Consequently, it is likely that bundled charges will obstruct pain facility outcomes and will therefore impair patient care.

OUTCOME OF TREATMENTS OTHER THAN SURGERY AND PAIN FACILITY TREATMENT

Other types of nonsurgical and non-pain facility treatments are epidurals, intraspinal opioids delivered via implantable drug and administration devices, spinal cord stimulators, various types of blocks, oral opioid maintenance, physical therapy, back schools, work hardening, and transcutaneous electrical nerve stimulation (TENS). There are few if any studies or efficacy reviews of these treatments and no meta-analyses except for TENS, back schools, and spinal manipulation. The treatment efficacy review that follows, where possible, presents conclusions of reviewers and where not possible, presents some recent topic outcome studies.

Physiotherapy Exercises

In pain facilities physical therapy exercises and activation are usually the cornerstone of treatment. However, in a 1991 review based on randomized controlled trials published from 1966 to 1990, Koes et al. (62) concluded that "the quality of intervention research on physiotherapy exercises is disappointingly low. Exercise therapy has not been shown to be more efficacious than other treatment modalities nor has it been shown to be ineffective. There is little evidence in favor of a specific exercise regimen." Faas (63) updated Koes's review and reviewed randomized studies published between 1991 and 1995. He found 11 randomized trials. Of them 4 dealt with acute pain, 1 with subacute pain, and the rest (6) with chronic pain. Studies dealing with acute pain showed strong evidence for lack of efficacy for either type of exercise in acute pain. The trial of subacute pain reported substantial positive results concerning return to work and sick leave. Concerning chronic back pain, all trials comparing exercise therapy with placebo or waiting list reported positive results with exercise therapy. Faas (63) concluded that "in patients with acute back pain exercise therapy is not effective. Graded activity programs with exercises in sub-acute pain and intensive extension exercises or fitness exercises in patients with chronic pain should be further investigated." Difficulties in demonstrating the efficacy of exercise physiotherapy probably relate to some of the factors discussed earlier.

Back Schools

Back schools originated in Sweden in the late 1970s. These are essentially teaching programs that include small group education sessions on anatomy and back function, correct techniques of carrying and lifting, and usually a simple back exercise program (64). The objective of back schools was to assist coping with back problems and to prevent relapse (64). With one exception, uncontrolled observational studies reported impressive benefits from this type of treatment. Yet, randomized studies produced conflicting efficacy results (64). This literature was first reviewed by Koes et al. (65) in 1994. They reviewed 21 papers reporting on 16 randomized clinical trials. Only two studies scored more than 50 points of 100 for quality. Seven studies indicated that the back school program was more effective than the reference treatment, and seven reported it to be no better or worse than the reference treatment. The best studies indicated that back schools may be effective in an occupational setting in acute recurrent or chronic conditions. The most promising back school programs were those that were modified to an intensive treatment setting (3- to 5-week stay in a specialized center) that was much like pain facility treatment (65). This review was followed by a meta-analysis (66). The results were interesting because DiFabio (66) divided the back school outcome studies into those that originated from a modified comprehensive program and those that were like the original primary back schools. He also analyzed the data according to whether the studies originated from an inpatient or outpatient program. The results indicated that the average effect size was greater for comprehensive back schools over primary back schools, with primary back schools not generating a significant efficacy effect. Similarly, inpatient back schools generated a significant efficacy effect, while outpatient back schools did not (66). It was concluded that back schools in their original format were not effective. Modified back schools were found to be effective.

Work Hardening

The Commission on Accreditation for Rehabilitation Facilities (CARF) Standards Manual for Organizations Serving People with Disabilities describes work hardening as "a comprehensive approach that addresses biomedical and psychosocial problems, uses graded work simulation and requires a coordinated interdisciplinary team. The team should include an occupational therapist, physical therapist, psychologist, and a vocational specialist." These programs focus on getting the client physically ready for return to work. Their emphasis is on "simulating that client's job and returning him to that job."

Work-hardening outcome literature can be described as meager at best. Niemeyer (67) in a recent review was able to find only five studies (68–72) that could be construed to originate from a work-hardening program. All outcome studies were retrospective case reports, with two studies (69, 70) neglecting to report the numbers of involved patients. Claims for return to work in these studies ranged from 55 to 100%. As part of this review, Niemeyer (67) reported on a study she performed to determine the outcome for return to work via a survey study of 36 work-hardening programs for consecutive client admissions. For 351 survey forms returned, 21 clients were still in the programs. Of the remaining 330 clients, 38 (11.5%) were not accepted into work hardening, the most common reason being medical instability. Of the 292 clients accepted, 72 (24.6%) did not complete the program, the most frequent reason (40%) being medical instability necessitating further treatment. Consequently, of 330 referrals, 220 (66.6%) actually completed the programs. Of the 220, 167 (75.9%) returned to work. Thus, of all referrals, 50.6% returned to work.

Contrary to pain facilities, work-hardening interdisciplinary teams do not include physicians but are usually led by a physical or occupational therapist. This type of interdiscipli-

nary team therefore cannot deal with medically complex patients, as is usually the case with CPPs. Thus, work-hardening programs have to select patients without medical problems and with little pain behavior. Niemeyer's study (67) demonstrates this problem well. At this point, work-hardening outcome studies require some improvement, and pending that improvement, it is not possible to gauge the value of work-hardening in the rehabilitation of the CPP.

Spinal Manipulation

Spinal manipulation involves a high-velocity thrust to a joint beyond its restricted range of motion. Spinal mobilization involves low-velocity passive movements within or at the limits of joint range. It is difficult to separate these two procedures in the literature, and therefore spinal manipulation will be used here to cover spinal manipulation and mobilization. There have been a significant number of studies on the outcome of spinal manipulation, but the results are in conflict. Consequently, there have been two meta-analyses (73, 74) performed on this literature. In both, the effect sizes were positive but small. The authors interpreted these effect sizes as indicating that there is very limited empirical support for the efficacy of spinal manipulation. This literature was also recently reviewed by Koes et al. (34). They also concluded that the efficacy of spinal manipulation for acute and chronic low back pain has not been demonstrated but that it may be effective for some subgroups of patients.

Transcutaneous Electrical Nerve Stimulation

TENS is a method of applying low-voltage electrical current through the skin at various sites using surface electrodes for the purpose of pain relief. It was developed in the early 1970s as a screening technique for predicting which CPPs would respond to implantable stimulators with good pain relief (75). Since that early era, the efficacy of TENS for the treatment of pain has been widely studied in more than 600 publications (76).

The issue of TENS' efficacy has been discussed in a number of review articles, most recently by Gersh and Wolf (77) and by Long (78). Gersh and Wolf (77) concluded that the literature indicates that TENS is efficacious for the treatment of acute pain; however, in reference to chronic pain, they noted that the weakest part of the TENS research literature was its sole reliance on the CPPs' reports of pain to establish TENS efficacy rather than using other measures of treatment outcome, such as functional activities or socialization. They suggested that researchers concentrate on the long-term effectiveness of TENS in CPPs (77). Long (78) reviewed the TENS literature and concluded the following: (*a*) nearly all studies indicate that TENS has a beneficial effect on patients suffering from pain of diverse origins; (*b*) in chronic pain intractable to other treatments, TENS has a short-term benefit in about 50% of patients, and for about 25% TENS is the only therapy necessary for years after treatment begins; (*c*) the effect of stimulation is beyond that which can be explained by placebo; and (*d*) there are few long-term follow-up studies available (78).

To date only seven studies (79–85) address the effect of long-term TENS use on outcome variables besides pain reduction. Here five studies (79–82, 84) reported that long-term TENS use helped the CPP reduce medication intake. One study reported an associated increase in socialization (79) with TENS use, and one study reported an associated increase in sleep (81). One study (83) in this group used a non-TENS treatment control group. This study demonstrated a significant increase in activity level in the group of CPPs using TENS versus those not using TENS; however, there was no difference in analgesic intake between the two groups at 1-year follow-up. A recent study (85) reported on the isolation of a TENS long-term user group who had used and benefited from TENS for more than 6 months. In this group changes in ratings for a number of outcome variables from the pre-TENS period to the treatment period improved and were statistically significant. These outcome variables were the following: pain interference with work, home, and social activities; activity level; pain management; use of other therapies (e.g., physical therapy, occupational therapy, chiropractic); and use of all classes of drugs.

Because of the large numbers of studies on TENS efficacy, this research is open to meta-analytic review. Recently there have been two meta-analyses performed on this literature but published in abstract form only (86, 87). The first (86) compared TENS, sham TENS, and no TENS for postoperative acute pain. In the 22 studies included in the meta-analysis no difference was found between TENS and sham TENS, but both were superior to no treatments, and both treatments were associated with less postoperative medication use than was no treatment. The second meta-analysis (87) included 117 studies and demonstrated a robust effect size for TENS use that was statistically significant compared with the placebo and control groups. However, effect sizes were smaller for chronic pain treatment than for acute pain treatment.

These data indicate that TENS has a place in the treatment of acute and chronic pain. They also demonstrate that meta-analyses may not be consistent in their results and that their results often depend on the studies chosen for inclusion.

Epidurals

Koes et al. (88) reviewed 12 randomized clinical trials evaluating epidural steroid injections. Of the four best studies (method score at least 60 of best possible 100), two reported positive outcomes and two reported negative results. Koes concluded that the efficacy of epidural steroids has not yet been established and benefit, if any, is short-lived (88). He also indicated that epidural research methodology should be improved. These same conclusions had been previously reached by Hammonds (89). Interestingly, Hammonds pointed out that for steroids most case report information supported the efficacy of epidurals.

Intraspinal Opioids

Infusion of intraspinal opioids by implantable devices has been reported to be efficacious for the treatment of intractable cancer pain (90, 91). In addition, there are a number of studies (92–94) on the use of this type of pain treatment for chronic nonmalignant pain. In two studies (93, 94) subjective pain levels decreased by 59 and 67.4% respectively. Function levels improved 50% in one study, (93) and QOL improved 81% in another study (94). Current practice and clinical guidelines for this type of treatment approach have also been developed (95). Due to the limited number of studies for this type of treatment, no firm conclusions can be drawn on its efficacy.

Spinal Cord Stimulations

De la Porte and Velft (96) recently reviewed the use of spinal cord stimulation for CPPs whose back surgery had failed. They found a success rate for improvement in pain to be 15 to 88%. Turner et al. (97) were the next to review this procedure for CPPs whose back surgery had failed. They found 39 studies, all case studies. They observed that an average of 59% of the CPPs had pain relief of 50% or more. However, they concluded that the lack of randomized trials precluded any conclusions concerning the effectiveness of this procedure relative to other treatments, placebo, or no treatment.

In addition to being used for the pain of failed back syndrome, a number of studies have used spinal cord stimulation for other types of pains. Thus, this procedure has been used for severe intractable angina (98), peripheral neuropathy of various types (99) and diabetic peripheral neuropathy (100). In the angina study, 80% of the patients reported reduced frequency of anginal attacks. The peripheral neuropathy outcome study (99) reported that 47% of the patients achieved long-term success in control of the pain. The diabetic peripheral neuropathy outcome study (100) reported at 3 months' follow-up 80% of the patients had statistically significant pain relief and that their exercise tolerance had significantly improved.

Three other studies have investigated the effect of this procedure on actual function. In a Belgium study, 147 patients with different kinds of pains, 61.4% being post failed back surgery CPPs, received spinal cord stimulators (101). Of these, at 1- to 3-year follow-up, only 3 to 4% had returned to work. Yet of another group of 70 CPPs receiving spinal cord stimulation, 52% were judged to have a very good or good effect (101). In the second study (102) of 40 CPPs treated for intractable leg pain with a spinal and stimulation procedure, various outcome variables besides overall pain relief were evaluated. It was found that this procedure decreased medication use, significantly decreased sickness impact profile scores, and significantly improved leg isometric performance strength scores (102). In the final study (103), 70 CPPs who had received a stimulator were followed for a year. All pain and QOL measures showed statistically significant improvement. For the success criteria, 50% pain relief and CPP assessment of procedure as fully or partially beneficial or worthwhile, 55% of the CPPs were judged a treatment success. Yet medication usage and work status were not significantly changed. These data indicate that in the case of spinal cord stimulation, improvement in pain may not necessarily translate into functional improvement and that this device requires further outcome research in order to determine its effect on function.

Therapeutic Blocks

Stalker et al. (104) recently reviewed the management of spinal pain by blockade. They reported the following summary of outcome results studies for various therapeutic blocks as the percentage of success (at least 50% pain relief): percutaneous facet denervation, 35 to 94% short-term and 27 to 93% long-term pain relief; percutaneous partial rhizotomy, 50 to 91% short-term and 22 to 85% long-term pain relief; radiofrequency lesion of the communicating ramus, 63% long-term pain relief; epidural steroids, 15 to 100% short-term and 19 to 72% long-term pain relief; epidural adhesiolysis, 13 to 64% long-term pain relief; and radiofrequency lesion of lumbar sympathetic trunk, no information. No other types of outcome results are yet available. Only two of the Stalker-reviewed studies (104) dealing with percutaneous facet denervation had a controlled design. All in all, this line of outcome research is extremely limited. Little can be concluded except that in uncontrolled studies, some patients appear to respond to therapeutic blocks. Whether this translates into functional improvement has not yet been determined.

Chronic Oral Opioid Therapy for Chronic Nonmalignant Pain

There is much controversy over the chronic use of opioids for chronic nonmalignant pain. This controversy relates to concerns about efficacy, adverse effects, tolerance, and addiction to opioids. Also, from their early inception one of the cornerstones of pain facility treatment was the weaning of the CPP off opioids. The rationale was the belief that opioid use contributed to psychological distress, poor treatment outcome, impaired cognitions, and reliance on the health care system (105). Recently some pain physicians, notably Portenoy and Foley (106) have tried to demonstrate that some CPPs are good candidates for chronic opioid analgesic therapy. This issue remains mired in controversy, as neither side has until recently produced convincing evidence for its position.

Although there has been a significant amount of research in this area, there are few randomized studies. Brown et al. (107) reviewed this literature and found case series reports on a total of 566 patients but no controlled studies. They concluded that chronic opioid analgesic therapy is safe and effective for many patients with recalcitrant chronic low-back pain. In another recent review Jamieson (105) reviewed 5 studies on this issue. Most CPPs, as expected, perceived pain relief

with these drugs. Pain relief was often associated with an increase in functional ability. In one of these studies of 16 patients, 12 increased their level of activity and returned to work (108). Jamieson (105) concluded that because of lack of randomized studies no conclusions could be drawn to endorse specified treatment guidelines on opioid therapy for chronic nonmalignant pain. Since these reviews, Fishbain is aware of one randomized study that has addressed this research area. Maulen et al. (109) performed a randomized double-blind crossover study in 46 patients with chronic nonmalignant pain. Oral morphine treatment resulted in statistically significant pain relief over placebo but no functional benefit (109). It was concluded that oral opioid therapy confers analgesic benefit with low risk of addiction but is unlikely to yield psychological or functional benefit (109).

As a final information point, the American Pain Society and the American Academy of Pain Medicine have recently published a consensus statement on the use of oral opioid maintenance for the treatment of chronic nonmalignant pain (110). Any physician contemplating maintaining CPPs on oral opioids should be aware of the positions of these national organizations, and standard legal procedures should be followed (111).

WHAT PAIN TREATMENTS ARE COST EFFECTIVE?

Although cost effectiveness appears to be a simple concept, it is difficult to measure accurately. This is because the cost of health care is made up of not only direct medical costs but also direct nonmedical costs, indirect morbidity costs, and indirect mortality costs (112). Direct medical costs include the materials and labor productivity consumed in preventing or treating a condition. Direct nonmedical costs reflect activity variances resulting from the care of the patient, as when a spouse misses a day of work to take the patient to a clinic. Indirect morbidity costs are incurred from lost contributions to larger systems resulting from limited activity by the person with the medical condition, such as economic value of time lost from work because of the condition or treatment consequences. Indirect mortality costs are the economic value of early death from poor health. The last two categories are the most difficult to measure (112). Each of these categories breaks down into a number of specific types of costs; costs associated with medications are one type of direct medical costs. In reference to pain there have been attempts to identify specific types of costs that are typically related to pain treatment. These have been published (113).

There are a number of different ways of comparing or looking at costs. The first of these is cost minimization. Two or more therapeutic alternatives with the same intended outcome are compared, for example, comparing costs of oral and intramuscular opioid treatment for pain. The second method is cost-benefit analysis, in which it is asked by how much in terms of monetary equivalents do the benefits of a particular treatment exceed its costs. Cost-benefit analysis requires placing a monetary value on both the costs and benefits of a given treatment, including health outcomes and human life. Cost-benefit analysis is advanced as the gold standard, as it forces decision makers to set explicit values on both the cost and the health consequences of alternative clinical actions (114). One can compare different interventions with cost benefit analyses. The third method is cost effectiveness analysis, in which the unit outcome is a reflection of treatment effect, for example cost per pound of weight loss. The fourth method is cost-utility analysis. This is similar to cost effectiveness except that in using effectiveness (e.g., pounds lost), one uses a QOL measure. This is usually a quality-adjusted life year or well year. The final measure, cost of illness, allows a calculation of costs that can be avoided by disease prevention. Either disease prevalence rates or disease incidence rates are used.

There are numerous cost-of-illness studies for low back pain, but few are outcome assessments of treatment costs. There have been some attempts to measure treatment costs, and these are reviewed later in the chapter.

In reference to pain facility treatment, Simmons et al. (115) demonstrate that when CPPs are exposed to a multidisciplinary treatment program, cost saving occurred. A year after the program medical costs of care were 58% lower than they were a year before it. Similar cost savings were also found with behavioral medicine intervention programs for chronic pain (116, 117). For example, in the first year posttreatment a 36% reduction in clinic visits was observed. This translated into a $12,000 cost saving for the year. In addition, the issue of referral to a pain facility has been examined in reference to long-term cost saving. Gallagher and Myers (118) examined the cost of delayed referral to a pain facility for 23 CPPs. Delayed referral has been shown to be a significant problem that affects the quality of pain treatment. In a recent study (119) from England, medical records of 703 CPPs were reviewed for treatment received before referral to a pain facility. Most of the CPPs (79%) had had their chronic pain condition for more than a year, and the vast majority had not received any simple treatments for their pain, such as antidepressants, anticonvulsants, or nerve stimulation. In addition, Engel et al. (120) demonstrated that a minority of patients with pain in primary care account for the majority of health care costs. They suggested that this group of patients should be targeted for behavioral interventions aimed at dysfunction, pain persistence, and depression to prevent accumulation of high health care costs. Such care is usually available only at pain facilities.

Cost effectiveness has also been demonstrated in a controlled study for back schools (121). A back school program in industry reduced absenteeism by at least 5 days per year per employee compared with the control group. There has also been one case report attempting to demonstrate the cost

effectiveness of work hardening (122). There have been a limited number of reports on cost effectiveness of individual treatments. These include the cost effectiveness of oral methadone over other opioid analgesics (123); opioid delivery systems (124, 125); cost analysis of opioid route of administration (126); and use of TENS to decrease medication and physical therapy use (127).

Patient satisfaction influences cost effectiveness. This was demonstrated in a recent study by Carey et al. (128). These researchers, in comparing medical costs for the treatment of low back pain, found orthopaedic and chiropractic treatment to be more expensive than that of primary care practitioners. However, the treated patients were most satisfied with chiropractic care. Such studies indicate that it may be difficult to decrease costs if the patient is not satisfied with the cheaper treatments.

A final issue in cost effectiveness is that of inpatient versus outpatient pain facility treatment. It is obvious that outpatient treatment should be less costly (129). However, the issue of which type of treatment is more efficacious is still being researched. The current status of this area of research is as follows. Cairns et al. (130) were the first to compare inpatient and outpatient outcomes. They found that for most outcome variables, including return to work, outpatients did better. This, however, was not a controlled study, and CPPs were not assigned randomly to these treatments. Tait et al. (131) compared QOL scores for inpatient and outpatient CPPs and found superior scores in the outpatient group. There was also no random treatment assignment in this study. Cicala and Wright (129) compared treatment costs for inpatients and outpatients when they developed an outpatient program. They found that costs decreased but that their success rate as measured by return to work did not change. Peters and Large (132) were the first to report on a randomized controlled trial comparing inpatient and outpatient pain facility treatment with a control group. Both treatment groups demonstrated significant differences in all outcome variables in reference to the control group but not to each other. Mellin et al. (133) and Harkapaa et al. (134) were the next to compare inpatient and outpatient treatments, using random assignment and a control group. On follow-up, the inpatient group showed more improvement in physical functioning. Peters et al. (135) reported a follow-up study of their original (132) inpatient and outpatient comparison. A greater percentage of inpatients met criteria for success than outpatients, although the inpatients had higher inpatient scores at pretreatment. Williams et al. (136) were the most recent to report on this issue, performing a randomized controlled trial. Both the inpatient and outpatient groups were significantly improved on all outcome variables versus controls, but the inpatient group made significantly greater gains than the controls.

There is enough evidence in this series of studies to conclude that inpatient pain facility treatment is superior to outpatient treatment, while both are superior to no treatment. The issue of inpatient versus outpatient treatment presents a dilemma: the more expensive treatment is clearly better. The focus of the research in this area should therefore not be on cost effectiveness but on trying to identify CPPs who can be treated effectively in the less expensive setting. As can be seen, pain treatment cost research, except for the inpatient versus outpatient controversy, has been limited in scope. Much work must be done to delineate which treatments are cost effective.

Table 46.7.   Levels of Evidence as Applied by the Agency for Health Care Policy and Research for Guideline Development

Type of evidence
  I. Meta-analysis of multiple, well-designed controlled studies
  II. At least one well-designed experimental study
  III. Well-designed, quasi-experimental studies, such as nonrandomized controlled, single group before and after, cohort, time series, or matched case-controlled studies
  IV. Well-designed nonexperimental studies, e.g., comparative, correlational, descriptive, case studies
  V. Case reports and clinical examples
Strength and consistency of evidence
  Evidence of type I or consistent findings from multiple studies of types II, III or IV
  Evidence of types II, III or IV and findings generally consistent
  Evidence of types II, III or IV but findings inconsistent
  Little or no evidence or type V evidence only
  Panel consensus: practice recommended on the basis of opinion of experts in pain management

Institute of Medicine Committee to Advise the Public Health Service on Clinical Practice. Clinical practice guidelines: directions for a new program. Washington: National Academy Press, 1990.

SUMMARY AND CONCLUSIONS

In 1990, the Agency for Health Care Policy and Research published some criteria by which it suggested that study evidence should be weighed. These criteria are presented in Table 46.7. As can be seen, these criteria are divided into type of evidence and strength and consistency of the evidence. We have used these criteria to weight the outcome evidence for each of the discussed pain treatments (Table 46.8). Table 46.8 also includes one other important criterion: are there studies indicating that the pain treatment improves function?

As can be seen from Table 46.8, the strongest consistent evidence for efficacy relates to pain facility, antidepressant, modified back schools, and TENS treatments. This evidence is backed up by meta-analysis. The evidence for the efficacy of spinal cord stimulation and chronic oral opioid therapy is weaker, and there is no evidence for improved functional status. The evidence for the efficacy of physical therapy, spinal manipulation, epidurals, intraspinal opioids, and therapeutic blocks is even weaker. The evidence for work hardening is the weakest of all. This is the current status of this aspect of pain outcome research. As can be seen, much work must be done.

Acknowledgment

We wish to thank Donna Hillman for her help in typing the manuscript. Our research was partially supported by grant H133A00032 from the National Institute of Disability and Disability Research.

Table 46.8.   Types of Pain Treatments and the Strength and Consistency of the Evidence for Their Efficacy and Effect on Functional Status

Type of Pain Treatment	Strength and Consistency of the Evidence for Efficacy					Some Studies Demonstrating Functional Improvement with Treatment
	A	B	C	D		
Pain facility	X					X
Antidepressants	X					X
Physical therapy exercises for chronic pain			X			X
Modified back schools	X					X
Work hardening				X		
Spinal manipulation			X			X
TENS for acute pain	X					NA
TENS for chronic pain	X					X
Epidurals			X			
Intraspinal opioids			X			X
Spinal cord stimulators		X		?		
Therapeutic blocks			X			
Chronic oral opioid therapy		X				

NA, not applicable.

References

1. Andersson G B J, Weinstein, J N. Introduction health outcomes related to low back pain. Spine 1994;19:20265–20275.

2. Using clinical practice guidelines to evaluate quality of care, vol. 1. Issues. Washington: US Department of Health and Human Services. AHCPR pub 95-0045, 1995.

3. Sederer L, Dickey B. Outcomes assessment in clinical practice. Baltimore: Williams & Wilkins, 1995.

4. A journal focusing on outcome research: focus on outcome analysis. London: Armstrong Information (in press).

5. Fuhrer M I. Conference report: an agenda for medical rehabilitation outcomes research. J Pros Orthop 1995;7:35–39.

6. Sperry L. Treatment outcomes: an overview: Psych Ann 1997;27:95–99.

7. Deleted.

8. Atkisson C, Zwick R. The clients' satisfaction questionnaire: psychometric properties and correlations with service utilization. Eval Prog Plan 1982;5:233–237.

9. Ward S E, Gordon D B. Patient satisfaction and pain severity as outcomes in pain management: a longitudinal view of one setting's experience. J Pain Symptom Manag 1996;11:242–251.

10. Stump T E, Dexter P R, Tierney W M, Wolinsky F D. Measuring patient satisfaction with physicians among older and diseased adults in a primary care municipal outpatient setting. Med Care 1995;33:958–972.

11. Chapman S L, Jamison R N, Sanders, S H. Treatment helpfulness questionnaire: a measure of patient satisfaction with treatment modalities provided in chronic pain management programs. Pain 1966;68:349–361.

12. deLateur B J. Quality of life: a patient-centered outcome. Arch Phys Med Rehabil 1997;78:237–239.

13. Spieker B. Quality of life assessments in clinical trials. New York: Raven Press, 1990.

14. Wilson I B, Clearly P D. Linking clinical variables with health related quality of life: a conceptual model of patient outcomes. JAMA 1995;273:59–65.

15. Testa M A, Nackley J F. Methods for quality of life studies. Ann Rev Public Health 1994;15:535–59.

16. Spector W D. Functional disability scales in quality of life and pharmacoeconomics. In: Spilker B, ed. Clinical trials. 2nd ed. Philadelphia: Lippincott-Raven, 1996;133–143.

17. Fairbank J C T, Couper J, Davies J B, O'Brien J P. The Oswestry low back pain disability questionnaire. Physiotherapy 1980;66:271–273.

18. Roland M, Morris R. A study of the natural history of back pain: 1. Development of a reliable and sensitive measure of disability in low-back pain. Spine 1983;8:141–142.

19. Kopec J A, Esdaile J M. Spine update functional disability scales for back pain. Spine 1995;20:1943–1949.

20. Sainfort F, Becker M, Diamond R. Judgments of quality of life of individuals with severe mental disorders: patient self-report versus provider perspectives. Am J Psychiatry 1996;53:497–502.

21. Steele-Rosomoff R. The pain patient. Spine 5:417–427.

22. Bonica J. A review of multidisciplinary pain clinics and pain centers. NIDA Res Monogr 1981;36:VII–X.

23. Rosomoff H L, Steele-Rosomoff R. Comprehensive multidisciplinary pain center approach to the treatment of low back pain. Neurosurg Clin North Am 1991;2:877–890.

24. Deleted.

25. Sanders S H, Brena S F. Pain management program in the United States: a problem of image and credibility. Focus Pain 1993;1:3.

26. Fishbain D A, Rosomoff H L, Goldberg M, et al. The prediction of return to the workplace after multidisciplinary pain center treatment. Clin J Pain 1993;9:3–15.

27. Williams R C. Toward a set of reliable and valid measures for chronic pain assessment and outcome research. Pain 1988;35:239–251.

28. White K P, Harth M. An analytical review of 24 controlled clinical trials for fibromyalgia syndrome (FMS). Pain 1996;64:211–219.

29. Large R, Peters J. A critical appraisal of outcome of multidisciplinary pain clinic treatments. In: Bond M R, Charlton J E, Woolf C J, eds. Proceedings of the VI World Congress on Pain, 1991;417–425.

30. Gross A R, Aker P D, Quartly C. Manual therapy in the treatment of neck pain. Rheumatol Dis Clin North Am 1996;22:579–98.

31. Bendix T, Bendix A F, Busch E, Jordan A. Functional restoration in chronic low back pain. Scand J Med Sci Sports 1996;6:88–97.

32. Manniche C. Clinical benefit of intensive dynamic exercises for low back pain. Scand J Med Sci Sports 1996;6:82–7.

33. Campello M, Nordin M, Weisers K M. Physical exercise and low back pain. Scand J Med Sci Sports 1966;6:63–72.

34. Koes B W, Assendelft W J J, Geert J M G, et al. Spinal manipulation for low back pain: an updated systematic review of randomized clinical trials. Spine 1996;21:2860–2873.

35. Manniche C. Assessment and exercise in low back pain: with special reference to the management of pain and disability following first time lumbar disc surgery. Danish Med Bul 1995;42:301–313.

36. Aronoff G M, Evans W O, Enders P L. A review of follow-up studies of multidisciplinary pain units. Pain 1982;16:1–11.

37. Aronoff G M, McAlary P W, Witkower A, Berdell M S. Pain treatment programs: do they return workers to the workplace? Occup Med 1988;3:123–136.

38. Wells J C D, Miles J B. Pain clinics and pain clinic treatment. Br Med Bul 1991;47:762–785.

39. Bonica J. A review of multidisciplinary pain clinics and pain centers. NIDA Res Monogr 1981;36:VII–X.

40. Turk D C, Rudy T E. Neglected factors in chronic pain treatment outcome studies referral patterns, failure to enter treatment, and attrition. Pain 1990;43:7–25.

41. Turk D C, Rudy T E. Neglected topics in the treatment of chronic pain patients: relapse, noncompliance, and adherence enhancement. Pain 1991;44:5–28.

42. Turk D S, Rudy T E, Sorkin B A. Neglected topics in chronic pain treatment outcome studies: determination of success. Pain 1993;53:3–16.

43. McCoy, C E, Selby D, Henderson R, et al. Patients avoiding surgery: pathology and one-year life status follow-up. Spine 1991;16(6 Suppl):S198–S200.

44. Smith S E, Darden B V, Rhyne A L, Wood, K E. Outcome of unoperated discogram-positive low back pain. Spine 1995;20:1997–2000.

45. Fishbain D A, Cutler R B, Rosomoff H, et al. "Movement" in work status after pain facility treatment. Spine 1996;21:2662–2669.

46. Steele-Rosomoff R, Rosomoff H L, Fishbain D A, et al. Pain center treatment: outcome for the "failed back syndrome." IASP VII World Congress on Pain. 1993;A1627, 604.

47. Saal J A, Saal J S. Nonoperative treatment of herniated lumbar intervertebral disc with radiculopathy an outcome study. Spine 1989;14:431–437.

48. Ellenberg R R, Ross M, Honet J C. Prospective evaluation of the course of disc herniation in patients with proven radiculopathy. Arch Phys Med Rehabil 1993;74:3–8.

49. Cutler R B, Fishbain D A, Lu Y, et al. Prediction of pain center treatment outcome for geriatric chronic pain patients. Clin J Pain 1994;10:10–17.

50. Cutler R B, Fishbain D A, Rosomoff R S, Rosomoff H L. Outcomes of treatment of pain in geriatric and younger age groups. Arch Phys Med Rehab 1994;75:457–64.

51. Glass G V. Primary, secondary, and meta-analysis of research. Educat Res 1976;5:3–8.

52. Glass G V, McGaw B, Smith M L. Meta analysis in social research. Beverly Hills; Sage, 1981;21–34.

53. Schmidt F L. What do data really mean? research findings, meta-analysis, and cumulative knowledge in psychology. Am Pychol 1992;47:1173–1181.

54. Haselkorn J K, Turner J A, Diehr P K, et al. Meta-Analysis, and cumulative knowledge in psychology. Am Psychol 1992;47:1173–1181.

55. Mann C. Meta-analysis in the breech. Science 1990;249:476–80.

56. Fishbain D A, Cutler R B, Rosomoff H L, Steele-Rosomoff R. Pain facilities: a review of their effectiveness and referral selection criteria. Curr Rev Pain 1997;1:107–115.

57. Roberts A H. All cats are not gray; all pain programs are not alike. Pain 1989;39:368–369.

58. Gallon R L. Reply to Dr. Roberts. Pain 1989;39:370–371.

59. Turner V A, Jensen M P. Efficacy of cognitive therapy for chronic low back pain. Pain 1993;52:169–177.

60. Nicholas M K, Wilson P H, Goyen J. Comparison of cognitive-behavioral group treatment and an alternative nonpsychological treatment for chronic low back pain. Pain 1992;48:339–347.

61. Turner J A, Clancy S. Comparison of operant behavioral and cognitive-behavioral group treatment for chronic low back pain. Clin Psychol 1988;56:261–266.

62. Koes B W, Bouter L M, Beckerman H, et al. Physiotherapy exercises and back pain, a blinded review. BMJ 1991;302:1572–1576.

63. Faas A. Exercises: which ones are worth trying, for which patients, and when? Spine 1996;21:2874–2879.

64. Leclaire R, Esdaile J M, Suissa S, et al. Back school in a first episode of compensated acute low back pain: a clinical trial to assess efficacy and prevent relapse. Arch Phys Med Rehabil 1996;77:673–679.

65. Koes B W, van Tulder M W, van der Windt W M, Bouter L M. The efficacy of back schools: a review of randomized clinical trials. J Clin Epidemiol 1994;47:851–62.

66. DeFabio R P. Efficacy of comprehensive rehabilitation programs and back school for patients with low back pain: a meta-analysis. Phys Ther 1995;75:865–78.

67. Niemeyer L, Jacobs K, Lynch K, et al. Work hardening: past, present, and future: the work programs special interest section national workhardening outcome study. Am J Occup Ther 1994;28:327–335.

68. McElligott J, Miscovich S J, Fielding L P. Low back injury in industry: the value of a recovery program. Conn Med 1989;53:711–715.

69. Gow L, Ryder W. The return to work program at New England Memorial Hospital, Stoneham, Massachusetts. In: Ogden-Niemeyer L, Jacobs K, eds. Work hardening: state of the art. Thorofare, NJ:Slack, Inc. 1989.

70. Anzai D, Wright M. Workers' evaluation and rehabilitation center, Loma Linda University Medical Center, Loma Linda, California. In: Ogden-Niemeyer L, Jacobs K, eds. Work hardening: state of the art. Thorofare, NJ:Slack, Inc. 1989.

71. Flinn-Wagner S M, Madonicky A, Goodman G. Characteristics of workers with upper extremity injuries who make a successful transition to work. J Hand Ther 1990;3:51–55.

72. Bettencourt, C M, Carlstrom P, Brown S H, et al. Using work simulation to treat adults with back injuries. Am J Occup Ther 1986;40:12–18.

73. Ottenbacher K, Difabio R. Efficacy of spinal manipulation/mobilization therapy: a meta-analysis. Spine 1985;10:833–837.

74. Anderson R, Meeker W C, Wirick B E, et al. A meta-analysis of clinical trials of spinal manipulation. J Manip Physiol Ther 1992;15:181–194.

75. Shealy C N. Transcutaneous electrical stimulation for control of pain. Clin Neurosurg 1974;21:269–77.

76. Shealy C N, Mauldin C C Jr. Modern medical electricity in the management of pain. Clin Podiatr Med Surg 1994;11:161–75.

77. Gersh M R, Wolf S L. Applications of transcutaneous electrical nerve stimulation in the management of patients with pain: state-of-the-art update. Phys Ther 1985;65:314–36.

78. Long D M. Fifteen years of transcutaneous electrical stimulation for pain control. Stereotact Funct Neurosurg 1991;56:2–19.

79. Eriksson M B E, Sjölund B H, Neilzen S. Long term results of peripheral conditioning stimulation as an analgesic measure in chronic pain. Pain 1979;6:335–47.

80. Vielvoye-Kerkmeer A P E, Ruigrok N J F, van der Kaaden M N. Transcutaneous electrical nerve stimulation (TENS): retrospective study of its effect on pain and analgesics consumption. Pain 1987;S4:S369.

81. Fried T, Johnson R, McCracken W. Transcutaneous electrical nerve stimulation: its role in the control of pain. Arch Phys Med Rehabil 1984;65:228–231.

82. Bremerich A, Wiegel W, Thein T, Dietze T. Transcutaneous electric nerve stimulation (TENS) in the therapy of chronic facial pain. J Craniofac Surg 1988;16:379–81.

83. Sternbach R A, Ignelzi R J, Deems L M, Timmermans G. Transcutaneous electrical analgesia: a follow-up analysis. Pain 1976;2:35–41.

84. Nathan P W, Wall P D. Treatment of post-herpetic neuralgia by prolonged electrical stimulation. Br Med J 1974;3:645–647.

85. Fishbain D A, Chabal C, Abbott A, et al. Transcutaneous electrical nerve stimulation (TENS) treatment outcome in long-term users. Clin J Pain 1996;12:201–214.

86. Ballantyne J, Deark L J, Chalmers T, et al. Transcutaneous nerve stimulation (TENS) and sham TENS are equally effective for post-operative pain: preliminary results of a meta-analysis. IASP VIII World Congress, Vancouver, Canada. 1996;86 (A286).

87. Delisle D. Relief of power of transcutaneous electrical nerve stimulation (TENS) on clinical pain: a meta analyses. IASP VIII World Congress, Vancouver, Canada. 1996;86 (A287).

88. Koes B W, Scholten R J P M, Mens J M A, Bouter L M. Efficacy of epidural steroid injections for low back pain and sciatica: a systematic review of randomized clinical trials. Pain 1995;63:279–288.

89. Hammonds W D. Epidural steroid injections: an unproven therapy for pain. APS J 1994;3:31–32.

90. Karavelis A, Foroglou G, Selviaridis P, Fountzilas G. Intraventricular administration of morphine for control of intractable cancer pain in 90 patients. Neurosurg 1996;39:57–61.

91. Anderson J S, Markers P I, Valentin N. Treatment of severe cancer pain via spinal catheters. Ugeskr Laeger 1966;158:6613–6616.

92. Paice J A, Penn R D, Shott S. Intraspinal morphine for chronic pain: a retrospective, multicenter study. J Pain Symptom Manag 1966;11:71–80.

93. Tutak U, Doleys D M. Intrathecal infusion systems for treatment of chronic low back and leg pain of noncancer origin. South Med J 1966;89:295–300.

94. Winkelmuller M, Winkelmuller W. Long-term effects of continuous intrathecal opioid treatment in chronic pain of nonmalignant etiology. J Neurosurg 1966;85:458–467.

95. Krames E S. Intraspinal opioid therapy for chronic nonmalignant pain: current practice and clinical guidelines. J Pain Symptom Manag 1966;11:333–352.

96. de la Porte C, Velft E. Spinal cord stimulation in failed back surgery syndrome. Pain 1993;52:55–61.

97. Turner J A, Loeser J D, Bell K G. Spinal cord stimulation for chronic low back pain: a systematic literature synthesis. Neurosurg 1995;37:1088–1095.

98. Eliasson T, Augustinsson L E, Mannheimer C. Spinal cord stimulation in severe angina pectoris: presentation of current studies, indications and clinical experience. Pain 1996;65:169–179.

99. Kumar K, Toth C, Nath R K. Spinal cord stimulation for chronic pain in peripheral neuropathy. Surg Neurol 1996;46:363–369.

100. Tesfaye S, Watt J, Benbow S J, et al. Electrical spinal-cord stimulation for painful diabetic peripheral neuropathy. Lancet 1996;348:1698–701.

101. Kupers R C, Van den Oever R, Ban Houdenhove B, et al. Spinal cord stimulation in Belgium: a nation-wide survey on the incidence, indications and therapeutic efficacy by the health insurer. Pain 1994;56:11–216.

102. Ohnmeiss D D, Rashbaum R F, Bogdanffy G M. Prospective outcome evaluation of spinal cord stimulation in patients with intractable leg pain. Spine 1996;21:1344–1351.

103. Burchiel K J, Anderson V C, Brown F D, et al. Prospective, multicenter study of spinal cord stimulation for relief of chronic back and extremity pain. Spine 1996;21:2786–2794.

104. Stalker R J, Vervest A C M, Groen G J. The management of chronic spinal pain by blockades: a review. Pain 1994;58:1–20.

105. Jamieson R N. Comprehensive pretreatment and outcome assessment for chronic opioid therapy in nonmalignant pain. J Pain Symptom Manag 1996;11(4):231–241.

106. Portenoy R K, Foley K M. Chronic use of opioid analgesics in nonmalignant pain: report of 38 cases. Pain 1986;25:171–186.

107. Brown R L, Fleming M F, Patterson J J. Chronic opioid analgesic therapy for chronic low back pain. J Am Board Fam Prac 1966;9:191–204.

108. France R D, Urban B J, Keefe F J. Long-term use of narcotic analgesics in chronic pain. Soc Sci Med 1984;19:1379–1382.

109. Maulen D E, Iezzi A, Amireh R, et al. Randomised trial of oral morphine for chronic noncancer pain. Lancet 1996;347:132–137.

110. Haddox J D, Joranson D, Angarola R T, et al. The use of opioids for the treatment of chronic pain: a consensus statement from the american academy of pain medicine and the american pain society. Clin J Pain 1997;13:6–8.

111. Wilson P R. Opioids and chronic pain. Clin J Pain 1997;13:1–2.

112. Zbrozek A S. Cost-effectiveness issues to consider in designing and interpreting pain studies. APS Bull 5–6, October/November 1994.

113. Ferrell B R, Griffith H. Cost issues related to pain management: report from the cancer pain panel of the agency for health care policy and research. J Pain Symptom Manag 1994;9:221–233.

114. Conrad D A, Deyo R A. Economic decision analysis in the diagnosis and treatment of low back pain: a methodologic primer. Spine 1994;19:2101S–2106S.

115. Simmons J W, Avant W S, Demski J, Parisher D. Determining successful pain clinic treatment through validation of cost effectiveness. Spine 1988;13:342–344.

116. Caudill M, Schnable R, Zuttermeister P, et al. Decreased clinic utilization by chronic pain patients after behavioral medicine intervention. Pain 1991;45:334–335 (letter).

117. Caudill M, Schnable R, Zuttermeister P, et al. Decreased clinic use by chronic pain patients: response to behavioral medicine intervention. Clin J Pain 1991;7:305–310.

118. Gallagher R M, Myers P. Referral delay in back pain patients on worker's compensation costs and policy implications. Psychosomatics 1996;37:270–284.

119. Davies H T, Crombie I K, Macrae W A. Why use a pain clinic: management of neurogenic pain before and after referral. J R Soc Med 1994;87:382–385.

120. Engel C C, Von Korff M, Katon W J. Back pain in primary care: predictors of high health-care costs. Pain 1996;65:197–204.

121. Versloot J M, Rozeman A, van Son K L, van Akkerveeken P F. The cost-effectiveness of a back school program in industry: a longitudinal controlled field study. Spine 1992;17:22–27.

122. Greenberg S N, Bello R P. The work hardening program and subsequent return to work of a client with low back pain. J Orthop Sports Phys Ther 1996;24:37–45.

123. Gardner-Nix S. Oral methadone for managing chronic nonmalignant pain. J Pain Symptom Manag 1996;11:321–328.

124. Bedder M D, Burchiel K, Larson A. Cost analysis of two implantable narcotic delivery systems. J Pain Symptom Manag 1991; 6:368–373.

125. Johnson M S, Pesko L J, Wood C F, Reinders T P. Cost and acceptability of three synringe-pump infusion systems. Am J Hosp Pharm 1990;47:1794–1798.

126. Goughnour B. Cost considerations of analgesic therapy: an analysis of the effects of dosing frequency and route of administration. Postgrad Med J 1991;6(Suppl 5):S87–S91.

127. Chabal C, Fishbain D A, Weaver M, Wipperman-Heine L. Long-term transcutaneous electrical nerve stimulation (TENS) use: impact on medication utilization and physical therapy costs. Clin J Pain 1998;14:66–73.

128. Carey T S, Garrett J, Jackman A. Researchers examine outcomes of back pain treatments provided by chiropractors, surgeons, and general physicians. N Engl J Med 1995;333:913–917.

129. Cicala R S, Wright H. Outpatient treatment of patients with chronic pain: an analysis of cost savings. Clin J Pain 1989;5:23–226.

130. Cairns D, Mooney V, Crane P. Spinal pain rehabilitation: inpatient and outpatient treatment results and development of predictors for outcome. Spine 1984;9:93–95.

131. Tait R C, Duckro P N, Margolis R B. Quality of life following treatment: a preliminary study of in- and outpatients with chronic pain. In J Psych Med 1988;18:271–283.

132. Peters J L, Large R G. A randomised control trial evaluating in- and outpatient pain management programmes. Pain 1990;41:283–293.

133. Mellin G, Harkapaa K, Hurri H, Jarvikoski A. A controlled study on the outcome of inpatient and outpatient treatment of low back pain. Scand J Rehab Med 1990;22:189–194.

134. Harkapaa K, Jarvikoski A, Mellin G, Murri H. A controlled study of the outcome of inpatient and outpatient treatment of low back pain. Pain 1990(Suppl 5):A746, S386.

135. Peters J, Large R G, Elkind G. Follow-up results from a randomised controlled trial evaluating in- and outpatient pain management programmes. Pain 1992;50:1–50.

136. Williams A CdeC, Richardson P H, Nicholas M K, et al. Inpatient vs. outpatient pain management: results of a randomised controlled trial. Pain 1996;54:13–22.

137. Malone M D, Strube M J. Meta-analysis of non-medical treatments for chronic pain. Pain 1988;34:231–244.

138. Fernandez E, Turk D C. The utility of cognitive coping strategies for altering pain perception: a meta-analysis. Pain 1989;38:123–135.

139. Flor H, Fydrich T, Turk D C. Efficacy of multidisciplinary pain treatment centers: a meta-analytic review. Pain 1992;49:221–230.

140. Curtis J E. The efficacy of multidisciplinary treatment programs for chronic low back pain: a meta-analysis. Dissert Abstr Int 1992;53:4948.

141. Cutler R B, Fishbain D A, Rosomoff H L. Does nonsurgical pain center treatment of chronic pain return patients to work? A review and meta-analysis of the literature. Spine 1994;19:643–652.

142. Holroyd K A, Penzien D B. Client variables and the behavioral treatment of recurrent tension headache: a meta-analytic review. J Behav Med 1986;9:515–536.

143. Holroyd K A, Penzien D B. Pharmacological versus nonpharmacological prophylaxis of recurrent migraine headache: a meta-analytic review of clinical trials. Pain 1990;42:1–13.

144. Mullen P D, Laville E A, Biddle A K, Lorig K. Efficacy of psychoeducational interventions on pain, depression, and disability in people with arthritis: a metaanalysis. J Rheumatol 1987;14:33–39.

145. Onghena P, Van Houdenhove B. Antidepressant-induced analgesia in chronic nonmalignant pain: a meta-analysis of 39 placebo-controlled studies. Pain 1992;49:205–219.

146. Gam A N, Thorsen H, Linnberg F. The effect of low-level laser therapy on musculoskeletal pain: a meta-analysis. Pain 1993;52:63–66.

147. Patel M, Gutzwiller F, Paccaud F, Marazzi A. A meta-analysis of acupuncture for chronic pain. Int J Epidemiol 1989;18:900–906.

148. Institute of Medicine Committee to Advise the Public Health Service on Clinical Practice. Clinical practice guidelines: directions for a new program. Washington: National Academy Press, 1990.

CHAPTER 47

Managed Care: Predator or Rescuer?
Implications and Recommendations for Pain Care

Joel R. Saper

Our most highly skilled, seasoned, and accredited medical specialists and clinical researchers have become the enemy. Physicians are gagged in their discussions with patients. Offsite personnel veto the treatment recommendations of experienced treating physicians. Patients are denied admission or forced out of hospitals against physicians' judgments. Appropriate tests and treatment are denied. Emergency department visits for severe or frightening symptoms are rejected. Physicians are given incentives for withholding interventions and treatments and offered partnerships in hospitals and buyout proposals to give them a stake in the methods and in the profits. Glaring conflicts of interest, so compelling that they would not be tolerated in our judges or elected officials, are overlooked, if not encouraged, and allowed to influence the decisions that affect people's lives.

Is this truly managed care? Or is it *managed profits* through *mismanaged care?* Are the gatekeepers now the jailers? Is capitation now no more than decapitation? What was intended to be a responsible initiative to hold down medical costs has turned the culture and tradition of medicine and medical care over to business and profit-driven interests, whose methods and strategies are prostituting U.S. medicine and waging a savage though not necessarily intended assault on the pursuit of excellence in medical care. In search of reduced medical costs, managed care strategies and policies have placed at risk the welfare of our patients, the ethical foundations of medicine, the training of our medical students and residents, and our ability to sustain excellence in medicine. The physician's historical authority in determining the course and nature of care and the core morality of medicine are suffocating under the weight of this 800-lb gorilla.

Does society understand the effects of putting cost containment above all else and with reckless disregard for the methods used, selling out our finest medical traditions and culture just to save a buck? What price are we as a society willing to pay to dismantle that which has taken so long to develop and mature and which will take so long to reassemble once destroyed? Does society really wish to place at risk its outstanding physician training programs and innovative centers of excellence?

AN EXAMPLE OF THE NONSCIENCE NONSENSE: A CASE HISTORY

Recently I assessed a 28-year-old man with an 8-year history of typical cluster headaches. For 6 of these 8 years the patient had made the rounds in a health maintenance organization (HMO), being evaluated by several primary care physicians and neurologists. His symptoms were severe and persistent despite treatment. Formal requests by his primary care physician for referral to a tertiary center for head pain were denied. Desperation and suicidal thoughts emerged.

(Ironically, while denied referral to a comprehensive center for headache care, he was referred, at his own travel expense, to a university-based surgical program several states away. The neurosurgeon proposed intracranial surgery that carried significant morbidity and a less than one in five chance of helping. The patient declined the offer.)

Treatment for his headaches included daily steroids, which he took for several years with periodic interruption. And during the past 3 years, in addition to the steroids, he took sumatriptan (Imitrex) daily by self-injection, reaching a maximum dose of 4 to 6 injections each day. (Sumatriptan is generally not recommended for use more than 2 days a week.) On this regimen the patient received modest benefit but still suffered multiple severe daily attacks. Increasingly desperate, the patient was finally referred to a tertiary center for head pain.

The patient was severely cushingoid and had many of the sequelae of chronic steroid use, including hyperlipidemia. He was depressed and suicidal and more than once had considered approaching Kevorkian for assisted suicide. The patient had increased intraocular pressure, presumably related to steroid use. He had four to six severe headaches each day. The patient was hospitalized. Discontinuance of sumatriptan, gradual reduction of steroids, and the implementation of a more appropriate medication program for cluster headaches resulted in dramatic reduction in his headaches during the first week of care. Periodic follow-up and regular medication adjustments, now a year and a half since hospitalization, maintain treatment success.

By the time of referral to the comprehensive center, the patient had received thousands of doses of sumatriptan. Based upon usage patterns and general prescription prices, his monthly bills for medicine alone during the previous 2 years were estimated to average approximately $4,000 to $6,000 a month.

The expenditure and risks imparted to this young man were the result of inexperience, arrogance, and mismanagement by his HMO. This example illustrates the difficulty many managed care systems have when confronting pain. While this behavior is easily blamed on the managed care concept, we must look to ourselves as well. We have not effectively made the case for comprehensive pain care nor dispelled the myths and biases against pain patients and pain doctors. We have not effectively articulated the separate and distinct body of knowledge and science of pain nor demonstrated that most physicians and general specialists have little or no exposure to it. Nor have we convincingly shown that added training, accreditation, and experience are necessary to maximize the outcome benefits to our patients. In short, we have not effectively argued on behalf of our own existence; nor have we confronted the utilization abuses, block shops, and pill mills that are assumed by many to be representative of pain medicine. Because we have not done our work, we cannot expect others to accept our declarations. So where are we going? The following concepts and history are relevant.

THE BACKGROUND

History

King and Moore (1) have traced the history of health care reimbursement. A brief review is relevant. The history of negotiated health care contracts between payors and physicians began early in this century. Publicly and privately administered inoculation and quarantine programs were begun in municipal hospitals in the British colonies in the 17th and 18th centuries. In the 19th century the Veteran's Health Care System evolved, and by the 1920s workers compensation and welfare programs emerged. Despite these significant changes and programs, the physicians' dominance over patient care decisions was assumed and honored.

Direct fee for service was the norm until the 1900s, but early in this century health insurance as an industry emerged with indemnity plans and later, after World War I, prepaid plans. In 1929 a physician-directed prepaid plan, Blue Cross, and Blue Shield were introduced. Subsequently a surgeon, Sidney Garfield, promoted a prepaid plan for workers who

were building the aqueduct from the Arizona desert to Los Angeles. Later these workers went on to build the Grand Cooley Dam. Henry Kaiser, a subcontractor at the Grand Cooley Dam project, introduced a similar program at the San Francisco shipyards during World War II. The first health maintenance organization was conceived.

On July 30, 1965, President Johnson introduced legislation establishing Medicare and Medicaid. The physician's role in decision making remained paramount and fundamental.

Is Traditional Medical Care Reimbursement to Blame or to Revere?

In part, the momentum toward managed care is driven by the notion that fee-for-service medicine is the dinosaur primarily responsible for massive health care costs. This theory has never been confirmed and is frankly not likely. But even if it were, the products of this system have been ignored as we assail its proposed villainy. The fee-for-service health care system, with its flaws and costs, has nonetheless nurtured the maturation of the best medical care in the world and made available superb specialty training programs and advanced care systems. To those in need, this "dinosaur" has assured the availability of superior and advanced systems of care and a corps of highly trained physicians and other health professionals. It has made possible a health care delivery system that almost daily generates breakthrough clinical research and technology.

It is true that this fee-for-service system has been burdened by its own potential conflict of interest: the more service given, the more money the provider makes. However, managed care imposes a more troubling *conflict of interest:* the less care provided, the more money is made by both the provider and the managed care group. Left unregulated and to its own self-interest, this concept places patients at risk and diverts funds from the support of medical services, innovation, and research into the hands of corporate investors and compromised providers.

CAN MANAGED CARE HOLD DOWN COSTS WITHOUT COMPROMISING QUALITY OF CARE?

Existing data are not sufficient for the question to be answered with certainty. An outcome report from Health Care Financing Administration (HCFA) (2) comparing health care outcomes under capitated and fee-for-service programs demonstrated better outcomes for fee-for-service patients than for those under managed care. In another study by HCFA (3) the authors concluded that managed care and capitation do not save money for Medicare. In a study supported by the Rand Corporation (4) it was concluded that patients receiving care in prepaid programs were significantly less likely to have their depression detected or treated during their visits than were patients receiving fee-for-service care. A 1995 report by the Robert Wood Johnson Foundation (5) concluded that managed care was more likely to cause difficulty for the patient in gaining access to a specialist, that examinations were not as thorough, that the time spent with the physician was often not adequate for the condition, and that the physician did not explain or teach to the same extent as in a fee-for-service system.

But the literature does not universally condemn managed care. According to Berwick (6) and others (7-9), managed care systems can reduce costs and maintain quality of care to an extent equal to or better than the fee-for-service system. In a study by Carlisle (10), HMO enrollees with acute myocardial infarction received better in-hospital care than fee-for-service patients. These findings also appeared to apply to newly diagnosed colorectal cancer, diabetes, urinary tract infection, pelvic inflammatory disease, vaginitis, pregnancy outcomes, blood pressure control, and care for patients with chronic mental illness (6).

Reassuring as this may be, these studies are seriously flawed. Such research rarely evaluates capitation as a free-standing variable (6). Moreover, the majority of these studies are already several years old, and in the current environment of growing competition and rapid organizational change, the data may not apply. Also, most of these studies evaluated relatively short-term outcomes and assessed results only after a year or two, even for chronic illnesses such as diabetes and hypertension. According to Ginzberg (11), there are no reliable data supporting the view that health care costs are significantly lower in areas where managed care in entrenched. Perhaps equally important, managed care systems have for the most part not yet absorbed the high-cost chronically ill patient, including the intractable pain patient. Thus, economic and outcome data do not yet reflect these populations. Some believe that *reality* for managed care systems has not yet struck.

THE BACKLASH AGAINST MANAGED CARE

The Legislative Backlash

A backlash against the subtle and not so subtle practices and strategies of managed care has begun. By 1996, thousands of pieces of legislation attempting to regulate or weaken HMOs had been introduced in state legislatures (12). Some 56 laws have been passed in 35 states. Patient complaints about managed care services and the media's coverage of horror stories are increasing. Physicians losing their autonomy and right to speak out on behalf of patients has gained national attention, as has federal and local concern for oppressive managed care practices.

In Michigan and elsewhere, the debate over assisted suicide (the Kevorkian phenomenon) and quality of life issues have merged with consumer rights issues, gaining the attention of legislators. Whether patients have access to quality care—pain care and otherwise—is being questioned. The *Detroit Free Press* (13), in a week-long front-page series, recently profiled the lives and medical care of Kevorkian's approximately 50 "patients." In at least 17 of them, and probably many more, pain problems appeared important, if not a primary motivation to assisted suicide.

Several HMO practices have generated the greatest concern from legislators. These are the so-called gag rules and length-of-stay limitations. Gag rules are contract clauses imposed by HMOs that forbid physicians from advocating treatments or services that the HMO will not approve or that are costly. Physicians are also prevented from offering an opinion about various HMO policies that might be considered adverse to its public image. Proposed legislation in several states and at the federal level addresses these policies.

Federal attention has also focused on the length of hospital stay for labor and delivery and mastectomy, as well as for terminating physician contracts without cause and denial of payment for emergency department visits.

At the time of this writing, additional legislation being readied in both houses of Congress and in several states collectively addresses the rights of patients in a managed care system. Access to care provisions and other safeguards thought to be critical to the protection of patients and physicians are being developed. Recently, President Clinton appointed a special commission to propose national consumer protection standards for persons in HMOs.

These actions reflect increasing concern and are a predictable reaction to the strategies and practices of many managed care systems. Targeted issues include full and timely access to appropriate care, unfettered communication between health care professionals and enrollees, choice of and accessibility to health care professionals, and the arbitrary definitions of experimental care. Several of the bills attempt to preserve the physician's right to make clinical decisions and require that outcome data and information about managed care plans be open to the public. Also targeted is the need for expeditious and fair resolution of enrollees' complaints. Thirteen states have passed bills that in principle require HMOs to pay for visits to the emergency department for medical conditions that if not addressed immediately would, *in the mind of a prudent lay person,* be likely to have resulted in serious injury to the mental or physical function of that patient.

Other areas are addressed by proposed legislation. One requires point-of-service options. Another addresses coverage for any device or drug approved by the FDA, whether or not the drug or device has been approved for the enrollee's specific condition or illness, *as long as the treating professional determines that the drug or device is medically necessary and appropriate for that enrollee's condition.*

Patients with chronic illnesses, such as AIDS, and the professionals who treat chronic illnesses have begun to unite, forming coalitions that are lobbying on both national and state levels against denial of access to care for patients with these disorders. In at least three states (Florida, Massachusetts, and Michigan) comprehensive pain care bills have been introduced.

Passage of any of the pending federal bills will be difficult. Nonetheless, Congress and state legislators, as well as the White House, have begun to acknowledge publicly that managed care, despite its arguable potential value for cost control, imposes risks and hardships to patients and physicians who participate in it.

The Litigation Backlash

Lawsuits naming HMOs as defendants are increasing, and a nonprofit legal center has been established to attract patients who require protections or redress from HMOs. Jury decisions worth millions of dollars have been awarded to patients and families who have suffered as a result of denied access or treatment (14, 15).

Moreover, the profit incentives related to denied access are being confronted by malpractice lawyers, legislators, and the general public, who have become increasingly disturbed by the monetary incentives created by HMOs for their executives and "cost-conscious" physicians. Increasingly attractive to HMOs and managed care groups is the capitation plus bonus method of reimbursing providers (16, 17). This concept allows increasing percentages (up to 50%) of a physician's income to be given in the form of bonuses, exerting significant influence upon physician prescribing and treating patterns. In principle, this influence can quickly catalyze the conversion from gatekeeper to jailer, and potentially places at risk the very core of medical morality, objectivity, and common sense. Gate keeping is in some ways a positive concept, but gate shutting, (12), the withholding of specialty, ancillary, or hospital services in pursuit of augmenting personal income, must not be tolerated.

In 1996 the federal government attempted to require HMOs to disclose certain incentive payment systems, but this effort was put on hold after a wave of protest by HMO interests (18).

The salaries of chief executives of HMOs, who on average earn 62% more than chief executive officers of other corporations of similar size, are also gaining attention (19-21). How defensible can it be for these high rewards to accrue to those responsible for policies and practices that some authorities claim are denying necessary care to those who need it and undermining our training programs and foundations of medical service?

Other Forms of Backlash

The backlash is also seen in other arenas. Provider-sponsor organizations, in which providers and businesses contract directly and thereby eliminate the HMO middleman, have gained interest in a majority of state medical societies. Moreover, recently passed federal legislation (Health Insurance Portability and Accountability Act of 1996) includes a pilot project that offers tax-exempt medical savings accounts (MSA) to 750,000 people.

Championed by organized medicine and indemnity insurance companies, the MSA is potentially one of the most significant challenges to the managed care system. Each employer can set aside a certain number of dollars per year in a tax-exempt account for patients to use for their medical care. A catastrophic insurance policy to cover hospitalization and other high-cost events can be purchased by the employer. The employee can use the money in the MSA to pay for

health care. The amount that is not used can be distributed to the employee, without taxation, much like an individual retirement account. Health care expenses and physician fees would be paid directly by patients from the MSA and (it is believed) prompt more prudent medical care shopping by the public. This establishes a market-driven method of controlling costs. MSAs are likely to be particularly appealing to healthy, young employees who will not generally require much medical care and who could be protected against unexpected, catastrophic events by supplemental coverage policies. MSAs would severely threaten HMOs because they would attract healthy people. Groups remaining in HMOs will contain a higher percentage of high-cost, high-risk individuals. This is likely to force managed care or HMO systems to raise their premiums to levels that are less competitive and thus less desirable to business.

OTHER RELEVANT OBSERVATIONS

In Minneapolis, where there were once 40 HMOs, there are now 3, each a powerful near-monopoly. With even greater control, it is feared that HMOs will be more inclined to divert corporate dollars intended for employee health care to profit and administrative expense. To circumvent this, direct business-to-provider networking has begun, working around the HMOs in a way that may set a model for the rest of the country.

In the minds of an increasing number of people (1), managed care will not be capable of controlling the rising cost of health care without compromising the quality of patient care, access to it, and the choice of providers. Left unregulated, it will continue to subvert much of the research and medical education infrastructure which sustains our traditional health care system as it introduces layer upon layer of expensive bureaucracy into the system. Providers have been forced to seek redress through labor unions, professional organizations, legislative initiatives, and legal action.

The following anecdote may be interesting in this regard. Not long ago I was asked to address a focus group of HMO directors on the issues of pain and its economic cost to business and managed care industries. As a group, these health care "leaders" did not appear knowledgeable about the effects of chronic illness on their costs nor current in their knowledge of treatment. Instead, they were clearly focused on immediate cost control. One stated that he was concerned only with next year's contract negotiations, since he must bring to the bargaining table the lowest monthly rates. Another claimed that patients would not travel to a center of excellence more than 40 miles away, even if he or she suffered a complex illness that could not be cared for in the existing system of care. Another director admitted that when comparing one treatment with another, he would choose the less costly treatment, independent of clinical efficacy. Another director rejected data from a recent *New England Journal of Medicine* study on the basis that the study's conclusion did not match his *perceptions* regarding a clinical matter. I recall only one director convincingly asserting that patients' welfare should be placed above profitability or who viewed cost effectiveness in the long-term perspective rather than a short-term one.

THE BATTLEGROUND

Medicare will be the major battleground. The outcome is uncertain. It is to be hoped that excess compensation for chief executives, high administrative costs, capitation-plus-bonus payments, and other hurtful practices of managed care will be challenged (12). Moreover, it is likely that a bipartisan coalition of legislators will attack barriers to specialty care and insist that Medicare enrollees have access to accredited specialists and specialty care systems (centers of excellence). Point-of-service options may be used (12).

THE IMPLICATIONS FOR QUALITY PAIN CARE

In the managed care environment patients with chronic and complex illnesses ("special needs" patients) are in particular jeopardy. These persons often require advanced comprehensive care services, well beyond what the primary care physician can generally provide. Such illnesses often require referral to well trained (and disciplined) subspecialists or to advanced comprehensive systems of care. The cost of such services is often beyond the customary and usual fees that have been arbitrarily established by managed care organizations for the treatment of day-to-day, routine illness. In a capitated environment, without special rules that apply to these special needs patients, negative incentives for referral are likely.

In my view, our challenge here is at least twofold. First, we must recognize and respond to the abuses within our own provider system. One size fits all pain care, block shops, pill mills, and interventional assembly lines must be confronted and modified. Even responsible insurance executives (and there are some) characterize all pain care practitioners and systems like these examples.

Second, we must restructure our thinking away from treatment algorithms to a strategy based upon levels of care. The overall complexity and treatment difficulty of a case must be determined, and according to this finding, the patient should be assigned to the appropriate level of care. This must begin with an accurate identification of key clinical variables that influence the treatment and prognosis of each patient. Then we must define the various levels of care and the interventions and responsibilities most appropriate to that level. This must be followed by guidelines for timely triage to the appropriate level of care, consistent with the severity of illness of the individual case. At each level, evidence-based decision making must be influential, and the *severity of illness and case complexity* must be responsibly matched with the appropriate *intensity of service.*

It is essential that the concept be implemented in the early phases of a chronic illness, such as pain, at a time when cost-effective and preventive measures can be applied with maxi-

mum benefit. Failure to do so will predispose at-risk, complex, and multiple-diagnosis patients to prolonged overuse of services, sequelae, irreversible disability, and avoidable iatrogenic consequences.

The key elements to cost-effective treatment of complex pain patients include the following:

- Accurate and effective diagnosis
- Delineation of comorbid, confounding clinical factors and variables
- Early identification of at-risk (special needs) patients
- Timely and efficient triage to the appropriate level of care for each case
- Appropriate interventions for key clinical variables at each level of care
- Avoidance of excessive treatments or procedures (overuse) that contribute to the complexity of that case
- The implementation of secondary preventive measures early in the course of the illness

I propose the following:

We must develop an integrated diagnostic and treatment approach that addresses not only the specific pain diagnosis but the overall *severity* of the case and the *complexity* of the patient. *We must focus on treating the patient with pain, not the pain of the patient.* We must develop severity and complexity ratings and measures that reflect comorbid diseases, previous treatment interventions and sequelae, confounding clinical variables, duration of symptoms, disability factors, psychological profiles, and overall case difficulty.

The following illustrates the point. Two patients each have the diagnosis of migraine. One, a healthy 24-year-old woman, has intermittent menstrual migraine that is easily treated with symptomatic medication each month. The other, a 37-year-old single parent, suffers from five severe migraine attacks a week. The patient is severely depressed and suicidal, has a history of chemical dependency, and seeks emergency department treatment for meperidine (Demerol) injections 5 to 6 times per week. She is an insulin-dependent diabetic, has cocaine in her urine, and has recently been told that her cardiogram is abnormal.

Clearly, both patients have migraine. However, their clinical needs are strikingly different. The first patient should be expected to respond well to primary care. The second patient requires a comprehensive system of care at which a different intensity of service and experience must be available.

Triage guidelines to direct patients to the appropriate level of care *at the appropriate time and according to case severity and complexity* must be developed. (Because pain care, unlike established medical specialties, is profoundly interdisciplinary in its composition, it is unlikely in the near future that a universally accepted treatment algorithm can gain national consensus.) To aid in the triage I suggest the use of two clinical tools. One is a *pain staging system* similar to that being developed for headache, which I and members of my staff first proposed to the American Association for the Study of Headache in 1992 and again in 1995 (22, 23). I also suggest the use of an updated version of the International Pain Society's axis diagnostic system, which would complement the staging tool and would be based upon the same clinical variables. It can be argued that the Diagnostic and Statistical Manual (DSM) and its axis diagnostic system brought order and universality to the diagnosis and treatment of mental illness, and I suggest that the staging tool and an axis-based diagnostic system would do the same for pain care.

If order and cost effectiveness in the treatment of patients in pain require appropriate and timely triage within the health care system, recognition and definition of various levels of care available for the treatment of pain is essential. We must clearly define and profile at least three levels of care: the primary level, the secondary level, and an advanced, comprehensive, fully accredited level. At each level a set of services appropriate to that level of care can be identified, as well as the level of severity and complexity of patients best served by that level. Assignment to levels of care would be determined by case staging and triage guidelines. Triage up and down would be prompted by staging and restaging scores and outcome data. Progress and cost effectiveness would be reflected by sustained reduction of staging score and other cost- and outcome-sensitive variables. Treatment guidelines could be created to apply to different levels of care but may become somewhat less critical because cost and outcome measures will justify or challenge the care being provided, thus lessening the need to delineate formal algorithms within a given system. Managed care organizations, together with accredited advance care systems, would be partners in contractually determined relationships. Risk-sharing incentives are possible. Fee schedules could be based upon complexity of each case and level of care required.

Thus, in my view, cost-effective and clinically effective treatment of pain requires the identification of global complexity of each case, the timely triage of patients to the appropriate level of care, and the prompt implementation of evidence-based treatments. The use of preventive strategies and avoidance of iatrogenic sequelae from mismanagement and overuse of services will be required for meaningful long-term cost savings.

A set of strategic criteria must be developed for triage to each level of care at the appropriate time in the clinical course of the patient. Each partnership (managed care organization and advanced center) could determine such guidelines or use nationally developed ones. Various clinical tools, such as the staging system and the multiaxial diagnosis system, will be helpful.

FINAL THOUGHTS AND RECOMMENDATIONS

Many consider the current influence of managed care to be destructive and compromising. In large measure, this is so. However, in the longer view and anticipating that through reg-

ulation and experience the managed care concept (if it survives) will mature and be forced to modify its hurtful and destructive tendencies, it is possible that the more subtle benefits of managed care might emerge. This is true particularly if managed care organizations direct their energies at long-term outcome rather than short-term cost control. Here are some suggestions:

- *Appropriate* care must be more highly valued than discounted care. Managed care organizations must learn to distinguish populations with customary, standard illness from chronically ill, complex, multiple diagnoses populations. (In the former, there are standard pathways of appropriate care. In the latter, including the chronically and acutely painful population, the same well-delineated pathways of treatment and measurements for outcome success do not exist.)
- Complex illness must be treated through an integrated, multilevel system of care based upon severity ratings (staging), triage guidelines, and outcome-based decision making at each level.
- The advanced trained and accredited specialist should be viewed not as a villain but as a resource for patient care, education of primary care physicians, clinical research, and new concepts and ideas, to work with managed care representatives to promote innovative strategies and advanced care services.
- Civil discourse between knowledgeable and authoritative health professionals and managed care organizations will be required.

Innovative concepts of triage and access determination, principles regarding maintenance of care, educational programing to enhance the quality of care that can be provided at primary and secondary levels, and partnerships between managed care organizations and accredited advanced care systems for the treatment of the multiple diagnoses populations are all possible. Ultimately, this will further the goals of *all* those concerned about the treatment of chronic illness, particularly and most importantly those who suffer from it.

In short, managed care, despite its current misguided policies and strategies, as well as its battle cry "profit now," can become the lightening rod for an integration of evidence-based treatment networks, bringing together worthwhile but diverse systems that are now operating independently and inefficiently.

Thus, managed care organizations may well have an important contribution to make, but they must first prove that they are not, by their own nature and structure, either dangerous to the interests of patients or the *predator* of innovation and advanced quality of medical service. Managed care organizations can become partners in the direction of care, encouraging and sponsoring the development of responsible, innovative clinical partnership concepts. New ideas and cost-effective approaches to treatment and services are welcome and worthwhile.

Innovative and protective solutions are likely if an atmosphere of cooperation and creative development can be achieved. However, to date efforts to ask tough questions and challenges of managed care are often met with defensive threats that suggest that any tampering or even questioning of the managed care concept as it is currently practiced will undermine all efforts at cost containment.

Surely, if the concept of managed care is sound, controls to protect patients, the infrastructure of medical excellence, and the viability of advanced care services in this country should not impose an undue burden. Only if the managed care concept is so fundamentally flawed that its survival depends on short-term oppressive, dictatorial solutions rather than responsible, creative, and innovative ones, should discourse and reasonable protection of patient rights and the survival of excellence in medical care be threatening propositions.

References

1. King RB, Moore B. Managed care: past, present, and future. Arch Neurol 1996;53:851–855.
2. Shaughnessy PW, Schlenker RE, Hittle DF. Home health care outcomes under capitation and fee-for-service payment. Health Care Financ Rev 1994;16:187–222.
3. Brown RS, Clement DG, Hill JW, et al. Do health maintenance organizations work for Medicare? Health Care Financ Rev 1993;15:7–23.
4. Wells KB, Hays RD, Burnam MA, et al. Detection of depressive disorder for patients receiving prepaid or fee-for-service care. JAMA 1989;262:3298–302.
5. Robert Wood Johnson Foundation, Princeton, NJ. June 28 1995.
6. Berwick DM. Payment by capitation and the quality of care, part 5. N Engl J Med 1996;335:1227–1231.
7. Freund DA, Rossiter LF, Fox PD, et al. Evaluation of the Medicaid competition demonstrations. Health Care Financ Rev 1989;11:81–97.
8. Retchin SM, Clement DG, Rossiter LF, et al. How the elderly fare in HMOs: outcomes from the Medicare competition demonstrations. Health Services Res 1992;27:651–659.
9. Lurie N, Christianson J, Finch M, et al. The effects of capitation on health and functional status of the Medicaid elderly: a randomized trial. Ann Intern Med 1994;120:506–511.
10. Carlisle DM, Siu AL, Keeler EB, et al. HMO vs. fee-for-service care of older patients with acute myocardial infarction. Am J Public Health 1992;82:1626–30.
11. Ginzberg E. A cautionary note on market reforms in health care. JAMA 1995;274:1633–1634.
12. Bodenheimer T. The HMO backlash: righteous or reactionary? N Engl J Med 1996;335:1601–1604.
13. The suicide machine. Detroit Free Press March 3, 1997.
14. Larson E. The soul of an HMO. Time January 22, 1996:44–52.
15. Felsenthal E. When HMOs say no to health coverage, more patients are taking them to court. Wall Street Journal May 17, 1996:B1.
16. Woolhandler S, Himmelstein DU. Extreme risk: the new corporate proposition for physicians. N Engl J Med 1995;333:1706–1708.
17. Swartz K, Brennan TA. Integrated health care, capitated payment, and quality: the role of regulation. Ann Intern Med 1996;124:442–448.
18. Pear R. U.S. health plan to limit rewards to HMO doctors. New York Times July 8, 1996:1.
19. Mitka M. HMO executives claim back paychecks. Am Med News Feb 5, 1996:3–23.
20. HMO chief execs highest paid. Washington Post Jan 2, 1996:E3.
21. U.S. health care chief will get $1 billion. New York Times June 15, 1996:14.
22. Saper JR, Hamel RL, Sell L, Winters M. A staging system for primary headache disorders. Headache 1992;32:257–258 (abstract).
23. Saper JR, Lake AE III, Hamel RL, et al. The Michigan headache staging system: defining the severity/complexity of a headache case. Award lecture at the American Association for the Study of Headache meeting. Boston, 1996.

CHAPTER 48

Listen to Your Patients

Gerald M. Aronoff and pain center alumni: Vanessa Allen, Marianne Cordillo, Karen Gallagher, Cooper Gilman, Patricia Giunta, Maureen Miller, Valerie Pearl, Katherine Pratt, and Ray Wilson

Earlier in this book, I indicated that patients with chronic pain syndromes are an enigma to the health care delivery system, which is often unresponsive to their total management needs. Most commonly, the problem does not arise with diagnostic evaluation but rather with the health care provider's failure to recognize the patient's gradual deteriorating spiral in spite of the treatment process. Much of this evolves because of the physician's preoccupation with making an accurate diagnosis and achieving resolution of the symptoms. This attempt to superimpose the acute medical model on a patient's chronic pain syndrome often results in dismal failure for the patient and physician. I am not suggesting that chronic pain patients do not deserve a thorough evaluation. I am, however, urging that when patient progress is monitored, the emphasis not merely be on pain-related complaints and examinations primarily geared to physical findings. It should also include such areas as depression, marital discord, vocational disruption, sexual problems, escalating use of both prescribed and nonprescribed substances and the fear so common for many patients with chronic pain syndromes that they are losing control of their lives.

Most of us have had a patient who because of personality factors or the duration of our professional contact with them, leads us astray. In such cases we miss certain cues indicating that we should bring in other consultants or refer the patient to colleagues who may try a different approach.

These comments are not meant to be harsh. Pain centers are often the last resort for patients with intractable pain syndromes. There is no question that it is easier to be critical retrospectively than it is to be prophetic. At the pain center, my patients almost always represent treatment failures of the health care delivery system. I rarely see the surgical successes, nor do I see those who responded to conservative medical treatment. In an attempt to be helpful to clinicians, I have asked nine alumni of the pain center to comment on their experiences with their own chronic pain problem; their stories follow this discussion. They present an overview of their problems, including what they found helpful at the pain center. They summarize with comments directed toward helping physicians to better understand patients with chronic pain.

Because more than 70% of the patients at our pain center have chronic low-back syndromes, four of the patients selected have with this problem. Each emphasizes a different and important clinical issue. Two of the patients are nurses; as they indicate, that sometimes worked against them. One of the nurses is married to a physician, a factor that certainly has complicated her pain experience. All three patients did exceptionally well during their treatment course at the pain center. There is no question that this influences the comments of some, who state that pain centers should not necessarily be considered only as a last resort for patients who suffer for many years while nothing else is working effectively. Each patient, in retrospect, would have preferred an earlier referral and perhaps a more conservative treatment approach. The third patient articulates the difficulties that previously active and energetic individuals have in accepting and coping with the inactivity and changes in lifestyle that so often accompany chronic pain. Her story also emphasizes that many of our older patients can have the aging process and overall deterioration accelerated by depression; this at times is reversible within the context of pain centers, with their strong emphasis on a therapeutic milieu.

Chronic abdominal pain, pelvic pain, and headaches are frequently seen in pain centers, and they present an interesting contrast. Few physicians would doubt the urgency of treating the abdominal pain of pancreatitis, and most would readily accept the patient's subjective complaint of pain as factual. Opioid medication usage is frequent; often chronic opioid use is the rule for pancreatitis. What we hear from a registered nurse with chronic abdominal pain secondary to pancreatitis is more than a pain problem with medical and surgical complications. We learn of her associated depression, physical and psychological drug dependency, secondary psychosocial problems, and her ultimate recognition that living with the pain of pancreatitis is greatly influenced by one's attitude, motivation, and overall life outlook.

Another physician's wife discusses her frustration at seeing several physicians, initially not getting a diagnosis, then getting a diagnosis but not relief with pharmacological and surgical treatment for severe endometriosis. Her struggle to maintain her social role as wife and mother and the importance of getting adequate analgesics to function is emphasized.

We hear from a patient with severe and incapacitating headaches of mixed type. His symptoms remained intractable despite pharmacological and conventional outpatient treatment approaches, including psychotherapy. Diagnostic evaluations had been unrevealing, and his symptoms were incapacitating to the point that they interfered with his professional and personal life. His pain and disability were every bit as real as that of the other pain patients discussed, yet because of the paucity of objective findings, there is often a tendency to minimize the complaint of headache. Let me remind you that headache pain at times does reach suicidal intensity. For this patient, as of this writing, the trend has been reversed, and he has resumed a functional and productive lifestyle, as well as being personally more content. This is not to say that many headache patients cannot be treated outside a comprehensive multidisciplinary pain center. It is, however, a plea to consider as candidates for pain centers those whose symptoms remain intractable despite thorough evaluation and treatment.

In conclusion, I suggest that when patients have chronic pain syndromes unresponsive to all therapies offered to them and when they and you are becoming increasingly frustrated with the course of their illness, it is essential that the advantages and disadvantages, risks and potential benefits of each should be discussed in an attempt to assist them in making the best educated choice about issues important to their health and well-being.

CASE 1

This is the history of a 35-year-old nurse with chronic low back and right leg pain, multiple operative procedures, and secondary depression.

My name is Pat. My part in this chapter addresses chronic pain associated with multiple surgeries and intractable lumbar radiculitis with nerve damage. As a student nurse, I fell, rupturing the disk between L4 and L5. After 2 months of conservative treatment, my orthopaedist decided that a laminectomy with fusion was necessary. The procedure was not discussed with me, nor were other possible options. Not knowing what to expect, I found my immediate postoperative period extremely difficult.

As it turned out, the ensuing year of healing was my longest period of pain-free existence. I did well until the fall of 1968. At that time, backaches and sciatica in both legs started slowly and increased in intensity and frequency. I was not coping well and spent a lot of time crying because of pain and frustration. Only medication enabled me to tolerate the pain.

My fusion had dissolved, and in 1969 a refusion was performed. Some 8 months later I was eager to start work, and with clearance from my doctor, started as charge nurse in geriatrics on a full-time basis. It was not long before sciatica and backaches began creeping back into my life, disrupting work attendance. I knew I was in trouble. Frequently, I would take a leave of absence for bed rest, then return to work part time.

The pain was so severe by 1973 that I consulted a neurosurgeon, who after a myelogram, operated for removal of scar tissue and nerve root decompressions. Again, surgery was presented without alternatives and without measurable pain relief. I tried to work wearing a special corset, driven to prove to myself that I could function as well as any nurse without a back problem. I decided to stop working when it took three oxycodone (Percodan) to survive an 8-hour shift. This was devastating to my self-esteem and hard to accept. Although I was determined to tough it out and live with the pain, I eventually gave in to it and pleaded with my doctor to do something. Pain was subtly becoming my master physically and emotionally.

The last operation, in 1974, resulted in life-threatening complications of septicemia, thrombophlebitis, and pulmonary emboli. During this time I felt at various times humiliation, frustration, anger, helplessness, and apathy. Any euphoria over being alive soon turned to self-pity because the surgery did nothing to relieve the pain. In the months that followed I often thought that I and my family would have been better off had I not lived.

My husband is very supportive and has always accepted my physical limitations without complaint. It has been extremely difficult for me to accept my condition. Guilt was a big factor when he took over what I considered my share of responsibilities, such as cleaning, washing, and grocery shopping. My self-esteem was beginning to falter badly.

After going to doctor after doctor, who offered much sympathy but little else, I sought relief through acupuncture, hypnosis, and faith healing. Then followed 3 years of epidural, caudal, and facet blocks. The blocks gave me relief for 3 months at best; more often it was 3 weeks to none. I willingly subjected myself to these blocks even though, to my horror, I went through drug withdrawal at home. Why? Because I was desperate, and there was always the chance that the next series would work.

Fortunately, my neurosurgeon understood far better than I the physical and emotional hell I was going through. He knew the importance of providing pain relief, no matter for how long, to try to build up my supply of endorphins, long before depleted. His suggestion to think about a pain clinic went ignored for more than a year. My attitude was completely negative. Pain clinics were to help people live with their pain, and I wanted to be pain free. People who went to pain clinics were losers with no hope.

Friends and family were painfully aware of my progression from an optimistic outgoing person to someone deeply depressed, under great stress, and withdrawing from life. I couldn't see these changes as clearly as they. It was a frustrating time for them, and I could not accept anything they had to say. Pain is a very private experience understood only by another sufferer. Communicating the seriousness of my problems to those in the medical profession was difficult. I have always been able to hide my pain from all but those closest to me and did not look like someone in pain. No doubt this was a form of denial. My days were spent in bed, and hypersomnia became a way of life. I was mentally and physically exhausted. Suicidal thoughts became increasingly frequent, and I was frightened. Ultimately, it was my depression more than the pain that led me to the pain center.

Finally I asked my doctor to give me a referral to the pain center. My biggest fear was that I wouldn't be accepted into the program. It turned out to be the best thing I have ever done. With a combination of strenuous physical exercises, relaxation techniques, and ice massage, my pain is under control for the first time in 17 years. I actually have occasional pain-free days and lead a full and more active life. I have conquered my depression through psychotherapy. My positive attitude enables me to risk finding my limitations without fear.

It may be true that I had to hit bottom before trying a pain control program. However, the reverse may also be true. Had I known about alternatives to surgery that were available over the past 17 years, it is distinctly possible that some surgery, with resulting disabilities, could have been avoided. I cannot stress too strongly the importance of informing patients about all of the treatment options. The many physical, psychological, and psychosocial problems that affect persons with acute, and especially chronic, pain must be dealt with as a whole for best results.

I believe that treating and dealing with people with chronic pain is difficult and frustrating for both patients and physicians. A physician who understands the problems involved and who is aware of all treatments available is surely better equipped to deal with and offer the patient a chance for a better life.

CASE 2

This is the history of a 34-year-old nurse and physician's wife with chronic low-back and right leg pain, multiple operative procedures, complicated hospital courses, and much residual displaced anger at the health care delivery system.

I am registered nurse, and nearly 2 years ago I injured my back while lifting a patient. In the following 17 months, I had six hospital admissions and spent a total of more than 4 months in four hospitals. I had many procedures: three myelograms, four computed tomography (CT) scans, two bone scans, numerous other spinal radiographs, a urology workup, and three electromyographies (EMGs), culminating in surgery, an S1 nerve root decompression, and laminectomy. This was followed by two series of facet injections and three lumbar sympathetic nerve blocks. The last block resulted in a right pneumothorax requiring chest tube placement and an additional hospitalization. Many minor complications, such as urinary tract infection, phlebitis, drug reactions, paralytic ileus, transient right leg paralysis, and drug dependence, also occurred in association with the procedures. Yet I still had low-back pain with right sciatic radiation into my right foot, muscle wasting, weakness, foot drop, and areas of decreased sensation. In addition, following surgery I began experiencing a raw sensation down the back of my right leg, along with waves of chills, frequent hypothermia of my leg and foot, and skin changes. This was diagnosed as sympathetic nerve disruption secondary to surgery.

Prior to admission to the pain center, my activity level was minimal and I was quite depressed despite use of antidepressant drugs. I was being thoroughly destroyed by the pain and felt that I had become useless both physically and emotionally. The pain obliterated any illusions I had about my ability to cope, and I was no longer the person I had been. When I was finally told that I would have to learn to live with the pain, I felt absolutely helpless and hopeless. I had frequent thoughts of suicide, not as an end to life but as an escape from constant pain. I had slowly isolated myself both physically and emotionally.

This was all very threatening to my relationship with my husband, a surgical house officer in a very competitive residency, and to my ability to care for my four children (two by each previous marriage). We had recently moved across country and had few friends and no family to turn to for assistance.

Because my husband is a doctor and I am a nurse, I think we had some unique problems, thoughts, and feelings. I felt guilty about the possible adverse effect on his career of absences from work when he took time to be with me during the hospitalizations or when he had to care for our children and assume routine household and business responsibilities to compensate for my inability to function properly. I wanted to be a help; instead I thought I was a hindrance, and I felt it was an unbearable workload for him.

I wanted so much from my husband. He could not be my doctor, and yet I would ask him questions about my problems and wanted definitive answers. When he came home from a 60-hour stretch of call duty, I would want empathy. Yet I thought, how could I expect it when all of his patients were much sicker than I, and he was frequently dealing with life-threatening situations. Mine certainly paled in comparison. When I was really desperate, I asked him to obtain prescriptions for pain medications from his colleagues and yet feared the repercussions this would have on him.

Doctors are taught to look at their patient's overall appearance as one of the first steps in physical assessment. I have always had a strong need to try to be as attractive as I can be. This need became exaggerated during this time. I tried very hard not to appear ill. I was frequently told, in essence, that I looked too good to be in much pain.

There were many frustrations for my husband, including his desire but inability to "fix" his wife when he could do so much for so many others. He attempted to remove himself from the role of doctor and yet could not withhold his opinion of other doctors' diagnoses, management, and results. He thought I should take a more active personal responsibility for my medical care and urged me to be decisive and "do something." He obtained several consultations for me with highly reputable and well-known doctors, but none would take me as a regular patient. We were told I was the worst possible combination of factors for a patient; I was a nurse and a doctor's wife, and I had back pain. The tendency in such cases is for undertreatment or overtreatment.

We both frequently felt caught in the middle of a no-win situation. As a nurse and a doctor, it seemed we were prejudged, and more was expected of us by medical personnel as well as everyone else. Yet we had the same or more fears and anxieties as anyone else in our situation. An overheard conversation in the hall during one hospitalization ("Just because her husband is a doctor and she's a nurse, she thinks she's a princess and should get anything she wants; she should know better") left me very hurt and angry. I was trying very hard to be a good patient and not be any trouble. After all, I knew these people and worked in the same hospital. When I tried relaxation techniques and tapes, I was ridiculed by nursing personnel for believing in "that mumbo-jumbo." These were my peers! I began trying to hide my identity and become invisible.

There were times when I felt trapped, with no good treatment options available. For instance, when surgery was proposed, it seemed as though the decision had already been made for me, and I would be foolish not to comply. In defense of the doctor, I must say he was kind and had a reputation for being conservative.

I believe that even if my pain was not diagnosed or accepted as chronic pain prior to admission to the pain center, the treatment and counseling offered and the skills learned there (ice massage, exercise, psychological and relaxation techniques) would have been very beneficial to me in coping with my pain. I also believe that if I can reduce other stressors in my life, I can better manage my pain. Conversely, as I become less pain-centered and require less emotional energy to cope with my pain, I can channel that energy into dealing with the stress in my life without exceeding my stress threshold. This experience has been invaluably educational for me and my husband.

I think I am developing a more positive approach to my pain and to life in general. Instead of thinking, "I can't do this because of the pain," I now ask myself, "What adaptation has to be made so that I can do this?"

Recently, while walking alone at the water's edge on a deserted strip of beach, I was sensing the sun's heat on my back, the feel of the cool wet sand on my feet, the sight and sound of the gentle blue waves, and the fresh smell of the sea. I hugged myself with sheer joy and thought, "Dear God, it is so fantastic to be alive! It is so good to be able to feel, think, love, nurture and function!"

CASE 3

This is the history of a 73-year-old writer with chronic low back and left leg pain, diffuse osteoarthritis, degenerative disk disease, and peripheral neuropathy. Because of the associated inactivity, she became increasingly depressed and disabled.

The unpredictable on-and-off Vermont winter of 1983 was a downer, even for the skiers and especially for retired senior citizens. I speak from experience. Last January I was in bad shape physically and mentally. Pain was dominating my life. The chronic pain was from a 12-year battle with osteoporosis of the lower lumbar region and from arterial dysfunction and some nerve damage in both legs. On top of that, although I didn't realize it at the time, I was suffering from the crippling pain that some misguided people make for themselves when they bottle up anger, frustration, and depression. I felt completely discouraged and didn't know what to do about it. The medication I was taking didn't seem to be doing much of anything to relieve my symptoms.

Even in a small country town like the one I now live in, community affairs can keep you very busy, but when the springtime we never had this year rolled around, I had become increasingly housebound, saying a painful "Sorry, I can't do it" to far too many outside activities. Something had to give.

A book titled *There's a Dance in the Old Dame Yet,* by Harriet Robey (1), was brought to my attention. I had never heard of a pain center as such but was impressed by the apparently successful results of Robey's experiences during the weeks she was a patient in this setting. This delightful autobiography, short and to the point, spoke to my condition so directly that I made an impulsive phone call. The charming 83-year-old author turned out to be most friendly and helpful when I finally reached her.

Because of a previous evaluation appointment with Dr. Aronoff, I had a general idea of what to expect after signing in, although I was in no way prepared for the many surprises in store. After the first few utterly confusing days, pieces of the puzzle began to fall in place. Fellow patients, women and men of all ages, became identified. Members of the staff were all warmly welcoming. The results of thorough physical examinations by several doctors went on record. Appointments with the medical physician, psychiatrist, psychologist, and nurse case manager were scheduled, and the physical therapist assigned to my case started daily treatments right away. So much attention all of a sudden was bewildering and extremely comforting at the same time. Everyone seemed genuinely to care. I had been living alone with my pain for too many years.

Due to the constant combined therapies plus new medications, my chronic pain became less severe. The alarmingly high blood pressure I brought with me, carefully monitored every day, gradually went down and stayed down. I was able to overcome my initial fear of exposing embarrassing inner feelings during group sessions, even to the point of sharing an unexpected and rather frightening incident that took place during the end of the second week, when I was still getting adjusted to the demanding schedule.

There are so many things to be said for this integrated field of medicine. Endless details and incidents are at the tip of my pen, but this is not the place to write many of them down. I can only say that I'm sorry not to have had this healing experience a long time ago.

Constant activity made the weeks go by quickly. I had to stay with it for an extra week after the usual 4-week program was completed. Apparently I was a tough old nut to crack. It had been very hard for me to express the repressed feelings that can cause depression, even on a one-to-one basis. I had enjoyed an adventurous life until my early 60s, working, traveling, playing lots of golf, and writing feature articles for newspapers all over the country after raising a family and adjusting to middle-aged divorce.

When arthritis began to take over, I did not accept being somewhat physically handicapped at all gracefully. Outdoor sports became too painful. Traveling began to be too much of a hassle. I could still drive and was not grounded, and until last winter I was keeping my spirits up and earning a little money by writing for a local weekly newspaper. Life indeed became bleak when I couldn't get around to interview likely prospects.

When finally dismissed from the pain unit with love and blessings heaped upon me, I came happily home with a brand new outlook on life in general and my aging body in particular. The neurotic hang-ups that had bedeviled me for such a long time were drowned in the river. I know I'll never be entirely free from pain, but because of the techniques learned from all those wonderful people, I also know how I can keep on top of the pain. Daily exercises. Relaxation exercises. Take deep breaths . . . as long as I stick with my good resolutions I'll be just fine.

CASE 4

This is the history of a nurse with intractable abdominal pain, chronic pancreatitis, and multiple medical and surgical procedures with many complications. Her illness was complicated by alcoholism, chronic depression, marital strain, and inability to be self-sufficient.

I am a 33-year-old married registered nurse with chronic abdominal pain as the result of chronic pancreatitis with multiple acute exacerbations since 1975. In the fall of 1974 I developed cholecystitis and subsequently underwent a cholecystectomy. My first episode of pancreatitis occurred in February 1975 and I was told at this time the cause was biliary obstruction, probably a result of adhesions or scar tissue from the prior surgery. During 1975 I had many acute attacks of pancreatitis requiring lengthy hospitalizations. My symptoms almost always included nausea and vomiting, elevated white blood count and amylase, fever, dehydration, bacteremia, and severe upper left quadrant abdominal pain radiating to the left scapula. In December 1975, following a relentless episode that left me severely malnourished, I was transferred to a hospital for hyperalimentation and surgical evaluation. After being built up with hyperalimentation, I underwent an exploratory laparo-

tomy with insertion of a draining gastrostomy tube and a feeding jejunostomy tube. Hyperalimentation was tapered, tube feedings were started, and the symptoms decreased. I was discharged home with the gastrostomy tube clamped and continued the tube feedings at home. In February 1976, when the tubes were pulled and a diet was started, I again became symptomatic. At this time a decision was made to perform further surgery, which consisted of a 50% pancreatectomy with a Roux-en-Y resection and incidental splenectomy. Following this, I enjoyed good health with very few mild exacerbations over the next 3 years. In January of 1979 I developed acute symptoms requiring hospitalization. This episode, complicated by bacteremia and malnutrition, lasted until April 1979. From that point until a Bilroth II procedure in the spring of 1981, I was treated in and out of the hospital for symptoms, especially pain, which had always been controlled with hydromorphone (Dilaudid). Needless to say, I had become extremely dependent on the opioid even when I was not in severe pain.

Gradually depression overcame me; I started to feel useless. Because of the almost constant pain, my nursing career was put on hold and my marriage deteriorated, which reinforced my feelings of uselessness. During this period, I started to abuse alcohol. This only increased the frequency and severity of my episodes of pancreatitis. From the fall of 1981 until the time I came to the pain center, I literally lived in either acute care hospitals for the treatment of the pancreatitis or alcohol rehabilitation centers. Between the pain, which vacillates from a severe acute type to a chronic nagging ache in my upper left quadrant, and the severe emotional problems that had developed, I was desperate for help and realized that I needed a program that could address the entire scope of my medical and psychological problems. Finally, a nurse where I was being treated for pancreatitis showed me a pamphlet from the pain center. We talked about it and I decided to follow through.

During my first few days at the pain center, I was doubtful that the treatments I was witnessing could help me at all. It was not long before I was able to see how the various components of the program fit together. I began to talk about how my pain, illness, and substance abuse had devastated all areas of my life. For the first time I was able to see the emotional effect as well as the physical problems; I believe this was the key for me. Because I had been inactive for so long, physical therapy helped with general conditioning and muscle strengthening and helped teach me I could be active in spite of pain. Group psychotherapy was probably the most important aspect of my care plan. Like so many other patients with chronic pain, I was depressed and beginning to question my sanity. During my stay, I was weaned, without discomfort, from hydromorphone. This was an area I was fearful of, and I feel it is important to let patients on opioids or tranquilizers know that the deceleration process is not anything to fear.

After I understood how stress was affecting me physically, I began to grasp the relaxation techniques being taught. Not only did I find relaxation therapy helpful with my pain, but also with the nausea and dumping syndrome I have periodically.

At the end of my 5-week stay at the pain center, I was able to put the various areas of the program together. I had control over most of my pain and was able to begin taking care of myself, something I had not done in a very long time. Before leaving I put together the all-important support system needed after discharge. This, for me, consisted of dietary reinforcement, weekly outpatient group therapy, and weekly individual psychotherapy. After discharge, I began to live again; I was able to work and continue to deal with my psychological problems honestly.

In closing, I would like to address general surgeons, internists, and gastroenterologists. You probably have many patients with chronic pancreatitis; when they progress to the point I had reached, if not before, you may consider referring them to a pain program. I firmly believe it will help them regain their interest in living a productive life and aid in controlling this overwhelming disease.

CASE 5

This is the history of a 55-year-old executive with intractable headaches, chronic depression, and a history of peptic ulcer disease, all complicated by his perfectionist hard-driving type A personality.

I am a 55-year-old financial executive. During the past 20 years, I have continuously been in a troubleshooting role, with a large number of assignments. Recognition has been quick, with rapid advancement and significant financial rewards. However, the stress has been continual and intense and the geographical moves frequent, with far too great a toll on my physical and emotional health.

For the past 16 years, I have been plagued with chronic headaches that when severe were incapacitating. The pain started as a dull ache at the base of my skull but at its worst would radiate around my head. It then felt as if a medieval torture cap were clamped around my skull and tightened beyond reason. My comparison of the worst headache pain level is with kidney stones, of which I have had two resembling a very spiny cocklebur the size of a pea. Believe me, the pain comparison is no exaggeration.

Although I've suffered through many episodes of intense pain, by far the worst problem was its constancy. Any chronic pain sufferer can easily understand why the ancient Chinese water torture of regularly timed drops of water on the forehead was so effective. It may not be so bad most of the time, but it just doesn't stop.

During this period, I consulted with at least 23 doctors all over the country and endured countless tests with invariably the same result. Everything checked out okay except that the headaches continued unabated. Because my charge to the doctors was always "Get me over the next 6 months and things will level out" (of course, things didn't happen that way), ever-increasing dosages of a wide variety of medications were prescribed, with steadily decreasing effectiveness.

Although I continued to wonder if the headaches weren't caused by some physical damage due to a concussion I'd suffered in Korea, I had to admit that they were probably stress-related. Unhappily, I perceived the causes of the stress to be short-lived. In a way they were, but I continued to accept positions with a whole new set of problems, so I put myself back into the same box over and over again. As a result, my headaches and the resulting depression worsened. A number of times over the last 6 years I've remarked, "If I were to kick off tomorrow, I can say I've had a very full life. I'm really lucky." Baloney. I was so deeply depressed I didn't care if I lived or not.

Having a major seizure in July 1983 was a blessing in disguise. I finally realized that I had to do something radically different or the rest of my life would be of little value to me. When outpatient treatment for chronic pain at a major clinic was not effective, I was referred to the chronic pain center. Two months earlier, I didn't know that such a place existed. Now I was going to have the treatment that would change my life. I soon learned that to be successful in the program, we had to conquer the stress cycle of pain, anxiety, stress, and more pain. Although this was true with all of us, it was true particularly for me. My problem was primarily stress, so almost every major pain treatment in the pain center was helpful to me.

Obviously, the measure of any program is the results. In my case, it may be too soon to tell, because I've been back to work for just 3 months. The box score at this point reads no days lost and no headaches that I haven't been able to control without medication. It isn't easy to change my work habits, but I'm doing it. I may not continue to do heroic things, but I will make a contribution and be more relaxed doing it. My new approach has delighted my wife and family. Instead of suffering in my own private hell, it is now fun to be alive.

In retrospect, I have to wonder why nobody told me about the chronic pain center earlier. Hadn't I shown that I was in enough chronic pain? I wonder why nobody told me that I was suffering from severe depression; I was being given antidepressants as a tension reliever. I wonder why nobody stressed the strong possibility of side effects from all the medications. I wonder why nobody suggested physiotherapy; I'd certainly indicated that I was physically tense and had been for years. Finally, I wonder why I, a fairly intelligent guy, didn't stop playing the busy executive long enough to do a little problem solving on my own, and, with professional help, start straightening out my own life long before now.

CASE 6

This is the history of a 35 year old physician's wife with chronic pelvic pain and increasing frustration and disappointment with the health care system.

My name is Karen, and I am a 35-year-old homemaker. My occupation is in medical management; I am taking several years off to raise my two small sons. My husband is a gastroenterologist. Without him, dealing with this pain would be nearly impossible. He has been in a very difficult situation, however, as he would like to remain my husband and not be my at-home physician. He is constantly caught as an intermediary between me and my physicians. It has been very straining being a physician's wife and suffering from chronic pain as well as having had several complicated acute and emergent illnesses in the past several years.

My chronic pain is caused by endometriosis. It affects nearly 3 million women in our country. Before being diagnosed, I had suffered for years and had numerous consultations with both gynecologic and urologic physicians because of bladder symptoms as well as severe cyclic pelvic and lower abdominal pain. I was very frustrated for nearly two years seeing physicians, who as well were frustrated having normal test results, but a patient with pain symptoms and no diagnosis to pinpoint and treat. I was treated with antibiotics and even at one point thought to probably have a STD; however, I was livid at this suggestion having been monogamous. I was so depressed to learn that a diagnosis was not found; however, I knew my pain was real and I was determined to find the cause and get better.

I was referred to a physician who performed a laparoscopic examination and confirmed widespread endometriosis. I was prescribed suppressive medications to decrease the amount of the disease. These medications had harsh side effects. After exhausting the medications and the length of time they could safely be taken, I was referred for laparotomy, ablation of the disease, and a presacral neurectomy. The endometriosis had widely spread throughout the abdominal cavity, bowel, and bladder. The posterior bladder wall had to be reconstructed because of the penetration of the disease. This was a 5-hour surgery, again followed by suppressive medications in an attempt to put the disease into remission. Then 2 years later, a right-sided oophorectomy was performed for regrowth of the disease severely affecting the right ovary and fallopian tube, as well as an orange-sized endometrioma that caused significant distress.

My depression escalated, as my chances of having children were now extremely slim. I sought counseling on my own. I was functioning at work but had trouble concentrating, as I was preoccupied with my illness and my inability to conceive. I was taking 8 to 12 opioid pain tablets a day when needed, and I was practicing healing visualization, which I think was beneficial if only for the relaxation. I did whatever I could on my own, as I was not aware any other treatment modalities were available. I felt I needed antidepressant therapy; however, the counselor I saw thought I was "too young" for this therapy.

After removal of my affected ovary, I realized my complete obsession and exhaustion with this illness. I stopped all medications except for a multivitamin. My pain was greatly decreased at this time, and I was able to discontinue the pain medications. I tried to focus on hobbies my husband and I enjoyed.

Then, 6 months later, without the aid of medications or fertility drugs, we conceived our first child, and we delivered a healthy boy in August 1993. What an incredible miracle. Another pregnancy followed in 1994; however, I had a complete small-bowel obstruction at 16 weeks' gestation; 18 inches of small bowel were resected with many postoperative complications, including another partial small-bowel obstruction 2 months later. Our baby was prematurely stillborn.

Recent knowledge obtained through an article I perused reveals that postoperative abdominal adhesions occur in 60 to 90% of patients who have undergone major or repeated gynecological surgery, and the adhesions are the most common cause of intestinal obstruction. Other adhesion- and endometriosis-related complications include chronic pelvic pain, urethral obstruction, and voiding dysfunction.

My recovery from these operations was slow. I was nutritionally depleted and suffering with severe pain and bowel dysfunction. I was placed on total parenteral nutrition for nearly 4 months. I also had fat malabsorption and a rapid gut syndrome (my oral to cecal transit was under 15 minutes). My only relief came from a combination therapy of Lomotil and Percocet.

I became pregnant again in 1995, and all medications were discontinued at that time. I did well during the pregnancy. We delivered a full-term boy in May 1996, but 2 months after delivery and while still nursing, I developed pain in the pelvic region that slowly over the next 6 months progressed to become incapacitating. I discontinued nursing and was back on Percocet, increasing the dosage rapidly.

My physicians studied my bowel, but there were no significant findings other than what was previously revealed. Laparoscopy in December 1996 resulted in lysis of adhesions but with very little benefit. The pain continued, and I asked my physician about acupuncture or a pain clinic. At the time, both were considered experimental and were not covered by our insurance carrier. When my pain medication increased to nearly a dozen tablets daily, my discomfort of using this amount while caring for my boys superseded any monetary situation. (After my initial consultation, my physician was able to get authorization for me to begin the pain management program.)

My first thought was that I was finally going to be pain free, and when it was explained to me that this was not the case but that I would learn how better to cope, I felt somewhat sad. I wanted so much to be rid of the pain; I finally was blessed with two wonderful boys, and I wanted to function fully and enjoy them.

I was nervous that I would be unable to fulfill the program requirements, but I was willing to try anything. I learned how to cope, and I began to strengthen my body with physical therapy and functional restoration. I worked daily with the stretches and corrected my poor posture, which can exacerbate any painful condition. It was at times difficult to meet the requirements with two small children, pain, and fatigue, but I pushed myself most days and felt a sense of accomplishment and overall better body mechanics. I am very much aware now of errors in lifting, exercising, and overall posturing.

My referring physicians were still without a confirmed diagnosis for my pain, and I dreaded any thoughts that they may have believed that it was due to past marital conflicts or the death of our second baby, as I felt certain that I had worked through these well from a psychological standpoint. I understood their frustration that there were no objective findings on my tests, but I also knew how I felt and that this pain was both real and worsening and I needed help. My physician at the pain center stepped out on a limb at this point; there was no clinical evidence to support his continued treatment. I could not return to my clinicians, who felt they had exhausted tests, radiographs, and so on and were uncomfortable treating a patient, albeit the wife of a colleague, with opioids.

I previously had no knowledge or experience with the long-acting opioids. I felt terrible taking high amounts of the short-term medications, only to repeat this regimen again in 3 to 4 hours. I've done very well on my pain management therapy, and in the beginning I was very upset with the program, as I was still wanting someone to give me an answer. Surgical adhesive disease, to me, could not cause incapacitating pain, and I certainly did not want to be referred to as a functioning addict, as one of my physicians termed patients like me." I wanted off the opioids, and I wanted to be well. I am not an attention-seeking person, and I certainly have always had better things to do than go to the doctor. Deep inside I knew there was a problem. I'm thankful that my pain management physician trusted in me and encouraged me to continue to examine my options.

My history of approximately 8 years ago led me to a specialist who diagnosed the endometriosis. I learned that endometriosis is again the source of my agony (there is no better term to describe it). It is this time in the retroperitoneal region, and I had all the classic symptoms: back pain, bladder dysfunction, pelvic pain, and abdominal tenderness. I did not respond to suppressive agents this time because of the position of the disease and the amount of adhesive tissue involved (hormones cannot penetrate scar tissue). Without the support of the pain center keeping me at a functional level while I continued to be evaluated and treated by my clinicians, I would have endured unbearable suffering. Physicians who typically see rare cases like mine would have two options: (*a*) treat the patient without a yet-proven diagnosis and feel very uneasy about the use of opioids, or (*b*) withdraw treatment because of lack of clinical evidence, rendering the suffering patient helpless and disabled emotionally and/or physically.

I did not know endometriosis could recur so quickly after pregnancy, but it can. I have never nor will I ever give up hope that pain can be kept under control. I had to be trained in a way to keep things in perspective and not to be afraid of opioid pain relief if that's what it takes to function. Because of my gastrointestinal condition, I cannot use nonsteriodal anti-inflammatory drugs. Many medical professionals would frown or raise their eyebrows if they read my medications, but this is not my choice for my life. I can accept it for now if it's what I have to do to function and raise my family. I understand the ethical difficulty a physician faces with a patient who has a difficult history; that is why I am very thankful for the pain management center. It has been an invaluable experience.

CASE 7

This is the history of a 43-year-old assembly line mechanic with failed back surgery syndrome. Prior to pain center treatment he was advised to curtail his activities, not pursue pain rehabilitation, and give up his job. He is now hopeful he will be returning to work.

My name is Ray. I am employed as a truck assembler for a company that builds over-the-road tractors. While working on the engine and transmission assembly line, on June 20, 1995, I injured my lower back. I was sent by the company nurse to a large clinic, where I was diagnosed as having a bulging degenerative disk that was pressing against the L5 nerve between L5 and S1.

The doctor chose a conservative treatment of physical therapy. This went on for 2 months without any relief. The doctor then ordered magnetic resonance imaging (MRI) and bone scan and issued a transcutaneous electrical nerve stimulation (TENS) unit to me for pain. After review of the MRI, the decision was made for surgery to remove part of the disk and to decompress the nerve. This surgery gave no relief from the pain in my lower back or left leg. Instead it left my left leg numb.

After 2 months of home recovery, the doctor ordered a nerve block, which also gave no relief from either pain or numbness. A month later, a second MRI revealed a growth of some kind in the L5 nerve root sac. This growth was determined by the radiologist to be either a cyst or a tumor. The decision was made to have the radiologist draw fluid from this growth. This was not something I was willing to do without a second opinion.

I set up an appointment with another doctor outside the realm of influence of the first doctor. This doctor put me into the hospital overnight for a myelogram and CT. After reviewing the results of these tests, this doctor set up an appointment for me at a neurosurgical clinic. Once I was examined and he studied the MRIs, CT, bone scan, and many radiographs, he requested still another MRI. The neurosurgeon, after studying these films and conferring with the other neurosurgeons in the office, concluded that there was a problem with scarring around the nerve. He ordered an EMG and nerve conduction velocity (NCV), which showed chronic nerve damage. After finding out the results of the nerve test, the neurosurgeon ordered another nerve block to try to reduce the scarring around the nerve and reduce the severe back and leg pain. This procedure also resulted in no relief of pain.

On my next visit, this doctor informed me there was nothing he could do for me and he would not operate on me a second time because of the possibility of making the condition worse. I refused to except this as the way I would remain, telling the doctor that with the technology available today, I could not believe there was nothing that could be done for me.

I wanted my back "fixed" and was determined to find someone who was willing to try.

At this time, the doctor referred me to the "main man" on backs in the state. This doctor, after reviewing all the studies done on me, gave me a thorough examination. He sat at his desk for a few minutes, then told me, "You have permanent nerve damage that is not reparable, and you will continue to fall down from time to time because the leg is not receiving the proper signals from the brain." He went on to tell me that the best thing for me to do would be to "take the workers compensation money you receive and retrain yourself for a job using your brain instead of your back. Your days of physical work are over."

This was the hardest blow delivered to me. I am a good mechanic. It's what I enjoy doing. After hearing this I began fighting back the tears, as did my wife. After a few moments, the doctor told me that the only thing he would do for me would be to refer me for placement of a neurostimulator in my spine to control the pain.

The next doctor reviewed all of the reports, films, and tests, examined me, looked at my wife and me, and said "I can fix your back. I may not remove the pain but I can get you off that cane and back to work." He then ordered a diskogram. This test was very painful, and after the results were received the doctor informed me that there was nothing he could do to fix my back. The only thing he felt would do me any good was the neurostimulator. I informed him that the company I worked for was not willing to pay for it. The doctor turned to me and said, "Okay, if they won't pay for that, we can try removing the scar tissue and some more of the disk and opening the area around the nerve by removing more of the bone next to it. If this doesn't work, we will install the neurostimulator for 6 weeks. If it works, we will go back in to install it permanently." If it did not relieve the pain, as a final procedure he would give me a fusion of the L5-S1 area.

The company said that because this doctor was suggesting so many surgeries, we should seek a second opinion with a doctor of its choosing. This angered me more than I can say. I had finally found someone who was willing to "do something" and at this point I really didn't care what. I just wanted relief from the pain and my life back.

I went to the next doctor, expecting him to verify the need for surgery, but that doctor claimed there was nothing wrong with me that could be helped by surgery. He told me he saw no reason I couldn't eventually work at my regular job. When I asked him about all the other doctors who had told me that this was permanent, he replied he didn't care what anyone else said, he was hired to review my case and give his opinion of surgery. He did, however, think I should be sent to a pain center and a work-hardening program because I had, in his words, "been lying around doing nothing for 16 months."

After leaving his office, my wife and I felt this was the end; the company had sought out a doctor whose recommendation they could control. We were about to be screwed over by the company. We were very frustrated, worried, and con-fused. Why were they doing this? I was trying to get better. What had I done to cause the company I enjoyed working for so much to do this to me?

It was at this time I began to see how much my condition had affected the woman I loved. She has had to take on the role of breadwinner and head of household. The daily suffering I endure is nothing when compared with what my wife is going through. From the very beginning, she has taken on all the responsibilities that were once mine. I felt guilty and frustrated for having let her down, emotionally, sexually, and financially. With our savings gone, all our plans were also gone. Our daughter will be starting college this fall, and this only adds to her worry.

My wife was aware of my progression to someone deeply depressed, withdrawing from life, and under a lot of stress. Chronic pain is a very private thing. Only another person who suffers with it can understand the effect it had on my life. I had changed from an outgoing, optimistic person who believed there was nothing I couldn't do to a person who could do nothing. I spent days watching television alone. Fighting the pain kept me physically and mentally exhausted. I felt worthless and on several occasions had thoughts of suicide; this was frightening. No one seems to understand the seriousness of my problems, and I don't know how to communicate what my pain feels like to either the medical profession or my family.

About a month later I received a letter from my case worker informing me that I had an appointment at the Center for Pain Medicine. I was outraged; I wanted surgery that would "fix" me. I contacted the State Industrial Commission in North Carolina to find out what I could do to stop my going to this center and get back to the doctor who could "fix" my back. They informed me that the company had the right to select which treatment I would receive as long as they were paying, and if I refused to go, they would no longer be held responsible for any medical treatment in my case.

I came into this program with the mind set that it would not work. I needed surgery first, and nothing these people said or did was going to change my mind. Pain centers were set up for one reason only: to teach people to learn to live with their pain. I didn't want to learn to live with this pain, I wanted to be pain free, the way I was before my injury. My attitude about this program was totally negative, and I intended to keep it that way. I have never been so wrong as I was about this program.

After the first week of rehabilitation, I could see a difference in the way I felt physically, mentally, and in my attitude concerning the program. I was still fighting it, but the physicians, therapists, psychologists, and my case worker at the center were beginning to make sense. I had finally found some people who understood what I was feeling and what it would take to change my situation from negative to positive. By using treatments of exercise, icing, and relaxation, I have learned to control my pain. I may not be able to return to life as it was prior to chronic pain, but I didn't give up on life because of chronic pain. It will require a change of lifestyles from being pain free to living with pain, but now I have control over the pain, not the pain having control over me.

Finally, let me say this: you cannot treat chronic pain as simply a physical condition. It must be treated as a physical, psychological, and social problem by professionals who understand how chronic pain can consume one's total life.

CASE 8

This is the history of a 35-year-old woman with fibromyalgia who learned not to let her myalgias disrupt her life.

When I think back, I really can't remember a time in my adult life that I was totally without pain. It was a living part of me that I accepted, fought, and learned to hate. It was a part of every decision I made and every contact with the people in my life. Each day my side nagged at me, stabbed me, or just whispered in my ear. I tried to hide from it, reason with it, and kill it. It never died. It fed on my fear of it and controlled my life. It made me cry, plead, and finally give up on life. You could say that my pain and I had a codependent relationship. We felt that neither of us could survive without the other. Every day for me was a bad hair day. I learned to hide. I removed all the mirrors in my house. I never voluntarily looked at my reflection. I hated to see the furrowed brow and pinched face. I never went out. I hurt, and I told everybody about it. I wanted somebody to tell me how to make it stop.

Prior to age 16, I was healthy, never having colds, headaches, or serious heartaches. Since age 16, I have had 12 surgeries and 3 very traumatic experiences, including rape. My teenage attempt at love ended with a severe beating. My first experience with pain began with migraines after my doctor told me I'd never have children as a result of the beating. I began to take pain medication at that time. In the following years, I lived, worked, hurt, and married. I was constantly having CT and minor surgeries and taking over-the-counter and prescription medications. I cried all the time and wallowed in depression. I added antidepressants to my pharmacopeia. It was the only way to cope with it all. Finally, after 7 years, my husband could not deal with me anymore. He left for greener pastures after informing me that I was "crazy and needed to grow up." I realized I was really alone but felt I deserved to be after whining and complaining all the time about how bad I felt. After talking to my friends and family, my next step was to see more doctors.

There have been many doctors in my life. Psychologists, psychiatrists, obstetrician-gynecologists (15!) surgeons, endocrinologists, cosmetic surgeons; the list goes on and on. My insurance company and I could have paid for a house in Beverly Hills. The sad part was that I only hurt more. Test after test came back negative for brain dysfunction, Crohn's disease, kidney failure, rheumatoid arthritis, tumors, and various forms of cancer. I remember one doctor telling me I was a hypochondriac, because every week I had a different ache or ailment. My family, sick of me and pills for everything under the sun, called me Dr. Welby and began to say things like, "If

you would just get up and do things, you would feel better" or "Nobody on God's green earth could be as sick as you." I listened and believed I'd found the answer when one psychiatrist said I had a bipolar disorder, another said I was a manic depressive, and still another said that depression and anger over the death of my mother was making me act out. The whole situation was out of control. Where did I go? I found other solutions: bulimia and anorexia nervosa. I found that I could control food. The eating disorder and pain medications almost killed me. All of this time, I was alone.

Of course my effectiveness on the job also suffered, but I hadn't a clue why. I was a teacher. At one time in my life, teaching was my biggest joy. I loved working with children. However, with the daily onslaught of pain and pills, I ended up isolating my inner self from everyone. I felt void of any feeling for any living thing. Children no longer had the power to make me smile. I was consumed with depression, pain, doctors, hospitals, and tests. I got help for my eating disorder. At one time I was seeing a different doctor for a different problem on a daily basis. To top the whole mess off, I gained 59 pounds after recovering from my eating disorder. The big picture? A 33-year-old fat woman, divorced, jobless, with chronic pain, diabetes, Grave's disease, and hating the world (especially skinny models) has to face reality. My prognosis was doom and gloom. I saw no end to my suffering. Why couldn't the doctors find the problem? cure me? understand me? *help me?* Truly, woe was me.

My story doesn't end with me throwing myself off a tower while raging at my fate or wasting away in a hospital psychiatric ward, a mere shadow of my former self while my helpless loved ones watched. Instead, after my divorce, I moved to Charlotte, North Carolina, got another teaching job, and took my pills. In the summer of 1990, I had a bone cyst removed from my leg. The happy part about that episode is that the surgeon told me, after looking at my chart (which rivals *War and Peace*), that she thought I might be suffering from a condition called chronic pain syndrome. I sat up, ignoring the wonderful haze of anesthesia and no pain, and asked for information. She gave me information, which I read, but I did nothing until I healed. Then I made an appointment at the pain center. After an examination, I was informed that I had 11 out of 18 areas involved in pain and that I had a condition called fibromyalgia. Joy and rapture! I could have kissed him. He believed I could be helped at the pain center. Afterward, I took a leave of absence from teaching to go into a month-long intensive physical rehabilitation and behavior modification program. I learned do much about myself and my pain behavior. I felt ashamed that I had been so weak. I participated in a vigorous exercise and behavior modification program, managed by a team to whom I will forever be indebted. They didn't allow frowns, furrowed brows, or whining. They taught me about pain behavior and how it affects everyone around you. They informed me that whining never solved problems and "Frankly, my dear, no one wants to hear it." They showed me how to relax and to breathe properly. They reminded me (often) about the importance of good posture. When the program ended, I had two tools to help me manage the rest of my life: exercise and the power of my own mind's ability to control pain. Now, when my old friend visits, I won't allow her to be in control of my behavior, my actions, or my relationship with people by cringing, being immobile, or hiding. The greatest gift from this whole experience has been knowledge that I was never crazy and that I never had a mysterious illness.

After leaving the program, I was afraid. What if going back into the real world made it all begin again? Working with the pain center's staff, an excellent endocrinologist, psychologist, and God, I ventured forth and conquered. I also attended the follow-up lectures offered by the center, which provided reinforcement and contact with new friends and those who were new to the program. I have had doctors say that fibromyalgia is a myth. I say to them that they have their opinions and I have mine. I don't take pills anymore. I have helped two other people who had similar problems to get help, and they are pleased with the results. I feel good that I have shared the knowledge. Today, I only take pills for Grave's disease and for premature menopausal symptoms due to surgery. My diabetes is controlled through exercise and diet. My weight is back to normal and I feel wonderful. I am outgoing, dating a wonderful man, enjoying people again, and attending college full time. The change in career has been a challenge, but I know I have made the best choice for myself. Getting my self-confidence back has caused me to take a good look at what I want for the future. The pain? It's not gone, but I can manage it. It's a great source of pride for me to say that. Sometimes when I have an especially bad episode, I get sad, but then I look at my lifestyle prior to the pain and I can always figure out what triggered the flare-up. Usually it's not enough exercise or being too stressed out about the unimportant. When these episodes occur, I know that I have to be careful not to regress into that other life. At times that means taking time for myself or making an appointment with my pain doc to reestablish communication and to reconnect with goals of the pain program. Whining and moaning are never an option. As a result, I have been virtually without serious pain for more than 2 years. I rejoice, smile, and tell myself every day, "Girl, you can do this. Take a deep breath and jump in!"

CASE 9

This is the history of a 34-year-old woman with chronic abdominal pain of undetermined origin.

My abdominal pain began when I was about 10 years old, and it was accompanied by a long series of misunderstandings and misdiagnoses. I was first hospitalized at age 12 with "acute gastroenteritis." The frequency and intensity grew as I reached my late teens. I underwent the complete range of testing for abdominal disorders, all of which were negative.

By the time I was 21, the pain was affecting my lifestyle in a profound way, severely limiting my ability to function on a daily basis. New doctors and new tests showed nothing, but the pain continued until I was again hospitalized. I was unable to sleep or eat, much less work. The crisis was exacerbated by a hemorrhage that resulted in a major blood loss over a 36-hour period. The cause again was undetermined. Once released, I was heavily medicated for pain, anxiety, and depression.

For 12 more years the pain would return intermittently, and medication had little or no effect. Not only did I attempt to tolerate and live with this pain, but I also endured the insulting, aggravating perception that as I was told, (a) my pain was all in my head, so therefore (b) my condition was not fully in the medical realm and warranted categorization into the "other," more nebulous group of abdominal pains called irritable bowel syndrome. I knew this diagnosis was far from accurate but was powerless to change it. At this point I was still unaware of my condition and relied on the expertise of my doctors for an explanation. As the symptoms began to validate my beliefs, my medication was changed and dosages increased. This had little to no effect on the level of pain, while leaving me drugged, disoriented, and depressed. This misunderstanding of my condition, symptoms, pain, and resulting emotional state continued for many years. They never believed me and considered they had no reason to. The test results were clear: no physical disorder; must be a mental problem.

The next crisis came at age 33, with another hospitalization and another series of tests. By this time, I truly wondered whether I was going to have to live like this for the rest of my life or even cared to do so. The abdominal pain was now a daily factor in my life. I tried to function as a normal person, but the condition was worsening. I lost time from work and subsequently lost my job because of absenteeism. My doctors grew increasingly frustrated at the crisis nature of my treatment and their inability to help my recovery to a fulfilling lifestyle. Clearly, the short-term approach inevitably resulted in a life-threatening situation devoid of prospects for improvement. Frustration, anger and depression became a daily part of my existence.

It was only at this time, after many years of unsuccessful treatment, that adhesions resulting from abdominal surgery I had had at age 2, growing for more than 30 years, wrapping around and attaching to my digestive organs, arose as a possible explanation for my condition. This hypothesis was based on case history and the personal experience of my doctor after conducting certain examinations and tests, not the results of a categorized test.

A year later, I was hospitalized again, unable to eat, drink, or sleep because of pain. It was at this time my doctor became aware of the Center for Pain Medicine and discussed this as a possible alternative to traditional therapies, which obviously were not working. I had never heard of a pain clinic before but was willing to try just about anything to improve the deteriorating quality of my life.

The program was the most comprehensive approach to debilitating pain I had ever seen. It included elements of medication, physical therapies, psychology, and relaxation training. In this format, all components were addressed in a structured and professional environment.

By the second week of the program, the segments had begun to come together. It was clear to me that this program had far more to offer than any other regimen I had encountered and would indeed address all of the contributing aspects of chronic pain while emphasizing management of the entire disorder.

I cannot fully describe the improvement in my condition and quality of life as a result of my involvement in this program. Through the combination of techniques and mild levels of medication, I am now in control of my pain for the first time ever. I have not lost time from work because of pain since I began treatment and have not needed increased dosages of pain medication. My outlook on the future is brighter and more positive than ever. I believe my pain will no longer dictate my future, restrict my involvement in life's activities, or influence my desire to live. The chronic pain has not disappeared, however. The primary difference lies in my newly acquired ability to *manage* my condition and in so doing, prevent pain from taking control of my body, mind and spirit ever again.

Despite numerous advances in the diagnosis and treatment of gastrointestinal disorders, they were essentially ineffective in this particular situation. Since a cause was unidentifiable, a cure was unattainable. Perhaps there are other scenarios that fall into a similar category. When all avenues of medical treatment were exhausted, my doctor went the extra mile in his attempts to help me find relief. He was open-minded enough to recommend investigating a program of this nature in an effort to help return my life to one that closely resembles normal. For this I am appreciative.

I implore members of the medical community to give pain management programs their earnest consideration when comprehensive attempts have proved ineffective and chronic pain remains a drastic impediment to a patient's daily existence. This type of program may be the patient's only opportunity for relief and a normal life. It is quite difficult to maintain a daily existence, much less be a nurturing, contributing member of a family or society while suffering with chronic pain. The Center for Pain Medicine bridges that gap through a variety of professionals with a common goal: assisting patients in methodically reducing their level of pain and regaining control of their lives.

More compelling for the professional faced with the frustrations of a chronic pain patient is the ability to provide a viable alternative when all other means have been systematically dismissed. A chronic pain sufferer, especially in the gastrointestinal area, typically endures the discomfort, indignity, and expense of multiple testing, all with the same result. Since public awareness of pain management clinics is practically nonexistent, a physician referral may be a successful course of action in an otherwise frustrating and disappointing physician-patient relationship.

Reference

1. Robey H. There's a dance in the old dame yet. Boston: Atlantic–Little, Brown, 1982.

CHAPTER 49

The Future of Pain Management

Daniel B. Carr and Gerald M. Aronoff

INTRODUCTION

In the second edition of this volume, the chapter bearing this title described two broad aspects of the future of pain management (1). The first concerned socioeconomics, and the second dealt with novel analgesics and delivery routes. These two areas continue to have great importance and in fact overlap in certian respects, such as in the emering field of pharmacoeconomics. Studies of home health care, for example to provide cost-effective spinal or patient-controlled analgesia, may blend considerations from both field. These and other newer trends warrant attention as harbingers of the next 5 years in clinical pain research and therapy. Such linked trends, well evident at the 1996 World Congress of the International Association for the Study of Pain (IASP) include the following (2):

1. Aggressive treatment (or prevention when possible) of acute pain on physiological grounds to avert a cascade of nociception-induced responses from gene expression to *N*-methyl-X-D-aspartate (NMDA) receptor activation to long-term neuronal remodeling (3, 4)
2. Refinement of analgesics and delivery modes (5) in a cost-conscious climate, with continued softening of distinctions between therapies deemed suitable for acute versus cancer or chronic pain or inpatient versus outpatient use
3. Growing interest by government and third-party payors in guidelines and standards based on outcomes data and evidence-based medicine, the latter embodied through Internet-based groups such as the Cochrane Collaboration (6)
4. Maturation, competition, and to some degree coalescence of pain-related organizations that are themselves issuing standards for training, education, and treatment to encourage patient-centered pain care

5. Active interest in all of these areas on the part of consumers of health care, who are becoming better and better informed and proactive, as the lay public at large recognizes the bond between pain control and quality of life, particularly at the end of life in an aging population

These trends have led us to a crossroads in pain medicine at which calls from many quarters to treat pain earlier and more effectively are balanced against pressures not to pay for specialist interventions such as for pain control. At the same time, pain medicine has matured to become a discipline with its own cohesive body of knowledge, clinical practice, and in the United States, diplomate status. This chapter begins by broadly surveying some of the clinical and administrative dimensions discussed in the first two editions, then briefly discusses each of these evolving trends and their implications (7).

ADMINISTRATIVE AND ECONOMIC DIMENSIONS

The future of pain medicine will no doubt parallel changes occurring in a variety of medical subspecialties at a time when the public's demands on the health care system are increasing. Health care providers are uncertain about what they will be "authorized" to provide; those subsidizing health care are uncertain about which services they should reimburse. We are all unclear as to how we should respond to these conflicting forces.

Each year consumers become more health conscious. They become more demanding but also more susceptible to confusion. The public is being informed about the relatively new areas of preventive and alternative medicine, exercise, nutrition, and substance use and abuse, as well as many unproven, potentially harmful "medical" treatments. Since the second edition of this text the Internet has become an increasingly popular information highway. Unfortunately, pain patients often are desperate and therefore extremely vulnerable to pseudo-experts who promise anything that patients want to hear.

Patients are becoming increasingly skeptical about traditional sources of medical information, as shown by the increasing frequency with which they question diagnoses or treatments and obtain multiple opinions before deciding on treatment. Indications of public discontent with traditional medicine are the rise in the number of malpractice suits in the last decade and the increasing frequency with which patients self-refer to chiropractors, faith healers, acupuncturists, herbalists, homeopaths, and other complementary approaches.

Regardless of our philosophical stance toward physicians who use the media to educate, they have grown in popularity as a result of the public's interest in learning more about health and illness. Public education has thus become a necessary aspect of medicine, and the media are an effective vehicle of delivery. The popular book market has been inundated with volumes on pain. Some of these are informative, factually accurate, and educational. Others are full of misinformation. If our goal is to have a well-informed patient who is actively involved in his or her own health care, we should attempt to demystify medicine. Aronoff estimates that more than half of his patients, when initially questioned about their pain, do not understand their diagnostic evaluation, their treatment, and the medications they are taking. He believes this lack of understanding contributes to poor compliance of patients with physicians' recommendations. There should be a concerted effort to improve public awareness of clinical and research advances.

Another important trend is the widening divergence between physicians' priorities and those of a continually expanding bureaucracy. Many physicians feel confused and oppressed by policies that determine which treatment will be reimbursed. For example, physicians in pain management have often found that diagnostic evaluations and invasive procedures are reimbursable, whereas conservative management and treatment by pain centers oriented toward wellness, functional restoration, and prevention of disability are not. This policy may account for some of the multiple surgical and nonsurgical procedures to which many pain patients are subjected and may act as a disincentive to multidisciplinary treatment with psychotherapy, physical therapy, and other noninvasive pain therapies. There has been a trend toward multispecialty group practice, such as health maintenance organizations (HMOs), as opposed to the traditional solo practice. For patients with chronic pain, this trend is a welcome one because it fosters multidisciplinary management. Attempts to delineate aspects of the chronic pain process that may predict responses individual to each treatment modality are under way. At pain centers, for instance, approximately one third of all pain patients do not show significant long-term gains. Likewise, a disturbing number of postsurgical patients continue to have

intractable pain syndromes and are classified as treatment failures. Our goal as pain physicians is to recognize these persons prospectively and to develop alternative treatments.

Patient selection, which certainly is important, raises several salient questions. As described elsewhere in this volume, a patient's attitudes and motivation, as well as support system, significantly affect treatment response, medication usage, and ultimately prognosis. What, then, do we do for the seemingly unmotivated patient? Examples include the obese patient with chronic low-back pain who refuses to diet, the emphysematous patient who refuses to stop smoking despite dyspnea or chest pains, or the industrial accident patient with pending litigation now receiving workers compensation who refuses to work. Studies suggest that patients with chronic pain who do not respond to treatment commonly have marginal motivation, negative attitudes, and a high incidence of secondary gain for their pain. Even with carefully developed admission criteria, is it better to be so restrictive that we exclude most treatment failures while rejecting some who would have been successful? Or should we be less restrictive and accept a higher rate of treatment failure but not deny treatment to those who may benefit from or desire our help? And what of the treatment process itself?

There are several major trends in treatment. There is more of a tendency toward subspecialization than ever before but also a blurring of boundaries between the specialties. We have witnessed a proliferation of advances in the clinical management of pain with a major effect on treatment of chronic pain syndromes. Much of this is in the area of behavioral medicine as a result of research by social scientists. In fact, it is rare to find a patient with chronic pain syndrome treated at a major pain center who has not had a psychological or psychiatric evaluation. There is every indication that this trend will continue. For many patients there is no definitive cure for their pain. Therefore it is hoped that treatment selection will encourage greater autonomy for the patient, minimizing perpetual dependence on the health care system.

The long-term use of sedative-hypnotics and barbiturates has been discouraged as a result of recognition that these drugs often complicate depression and have dysphoric effects. In the first and second editions of this text it was noted that opioids were being prescribed less frequently and monitored more closely. Certainly, the U.S. Food and Drug Administration (FDA) and the Drug Enforcement Administration guidelines have had their influence. However, it is now apparent that in carefully selected patients with chronic noncancer pain, maintenance opioids may be not only acceptable but desirable (8), as discussed in the chapter on pharmacological management. In a joint consensus statement, the American Academy of Pain Medicine (AAPM) and the American Pain Society (APS) last year issued a consensus statement on chronic opioid use in noncancer pain (9). These as well as various state guidelines and other reports issuing from an increasing number of state-level pain commissions are attempts to assist practicing physicians in providing analgesic treatment for complex patients with chronic pain. Clinicians must become more adept at recognizing this population, for whom undertreatment is as much a disservice as is overtreatment. It is also hoped that refinement and linkage between information systems will improve the ability of physicians to monitor difficult patients who may be getting prescriptions from more than one source.

Another concern to be expanded later in this chapter is third-party reimbursement. Economic pressures upon medical practice in every setting, particularly in hospital care, have increased beyond what could have been anticipated a decade ago. These pressures have in part allowed innovations in pain management to be viewed favorably by insurers and policy makers who see potential cost savings from rapid return to normal function after operation or from care at home rather than in hospital during chronic or terminal illness. Pain center programs are expensive, yet this cost should be weighed against the alternative, namely, repeated ineffective hospitalizations and evaluations. The health care system has finite resources. It has been estimated that given the trend of expenditures, Medicare is on its way to bankruptcy. State welfare funding is inadequate, and therefore many physicians do not accept welfare patients for treatment. The premiums of the private insurance carriers have been accelerating rapidly. Traditionally little attention has been given to preventive medicine in the reimbursement systems of most insurance carriers. This is slowly changing. HMOs now perform annual physical examinations, periodic blood pressure screening, and other attempts at preventive medicine, especially in the area of managed care. New agents proposed for inclusion in HMO formularies now must pass pharmacoeconomic muster.

Pharmacoeconomics connotes analysis of the incremental improvement in patient outcome that results from an incremental increase in resources expended upon drug therapy, including drug delivery (10). Australia, New Zealand, the United Kingdom, and parts of Canada now require pharmacoeconomic justification for approval of new drugs. In the United States, formulary committees of most health maintenance organizations base their decisions to include or reject new drugs upon such assessment (11). Clinical trials with a pharmacoeconomic orientation differ from traditional trials in that the former place greater emphasis on determining effectiveness (what happens under actual conditions of use) than efficacy (what occurs under ideal conditions). Outcomes examined in newer studies go beyond traditional biological or physiological measures to include measures of quality of life, productivity, and resource consumption. A variety of instruments have been developed to assess health-related quality of life generically and in specialized fashion for clinical trials, such as analgesic trials, in specific populations or health conditions (12). Pharmacoeconomics is an evolving discipline conducted by individuals with diverse perspectives and agendas. For example, cost analyses (13) can be conducted in terms of cost versus benefit, cost effectiveness (the latter defined with respect to a specific objective); cost utility, in which benefit is defined as quality of life, willingness to pay, and the patient's preference for one intervention over another; cost minimization; or cost of illness, which includes both direct and indirect measures such as workdays lost (14).

Much has been written about the complex interaction between psychosocial and organic factors contributing to intractable chronic pain syndromes and their associated disability. Nonetheless, Medicare guidelines for pain still find it preferable to admit such patients for more diagnostic evaluation, even if they already have had far too much, or for drug tapering if they are substance dependent. In this paradigm, the stoic pain patient who has resisted therapy with controlled substances, preferring to suffer quietly in severe pain, may be seen as less deserving than the acting-out substance abuser, for whom the medical system often legitimizes drug usage.

There is much concern about the physician's role in the health care system; our responsibility is not only to our patients but also to society at large. The following remarks concern a subgroup of patients with chronic pain syndromes. This is a small population notable for their multiple unsuccessful encounters with health care practitioners and their enmeshment within the health care system, often to the detriment of both the patient and the system.

We are concerned about the potential consequences of telling these patients what they need to hear and directly discussing with them and their significant others issues of their excessive use of the health care system and its entitlement programs and their often inappropriate request for disability status. We must continue to teach our patients about these issues. However, it is clear that pain clinicians spend much of their time documenting what they do for fear that an offended, manipulative, or sociopathic litigious patient whose "free ride" is threatened will seek retribution. Our goal must be to determine more carefully patients whose impairment, physical or psychological, warrants receiving disability and to assist those patients in any way we can to receive the assistance to which they are entitled. We should not, however, encourage anyone to remain unnecessarily disabled. The American health care system has long held a position of international preeminence, but this may be changing. Although technologically we are still at the forefront of medicine, ideologically, perhaps, we are not. Nowhere do physicians feel reprisal from patients as much as in the United States. Perhaps nowhere in the world is defensive medicine becoming the practice more rapidly than here, where needless diagnostic studies are often requested for purposes of documentation in case the patient later assumes an adversarial role.

It appears that some patients with chronic pain syndromes at a given time cannot be helped and may not want to be helped, those whose agenda of being enmeshed in the health care system has less to do with receiving health care than with receiving benefits. We must more efficiently identify this segment of the population and place appropriate limits upon their treatment. Regardless of the patients complaints, once we have established that the tools at our disposal are unlikely to ameliorate his or her symptoms, we should offer a series of recommendations, and if the patient is unable or unwilling to consider these, it may be that the system has adequately fulfilled its responsibility to that person and should go no further. We should not allow ourselves to be intimidated by patients who are inappropriately making demands on us and taxing the resources of the system (15).

We believe that in dealing with patients with chronic pain syndrome, physicians need to refine their clinical acumen in such a way as to reduce the tunnel vision that generally comes from specialty training in a given field. If one is trained as an anesthesiologist and referred a chronic pain patient, there is a good possibility that the recommended treatment will entail use of nerve blocks. A surgeon is more likely to consider surgical approaches, psychiatrists to offer a behavioral program, and so on. Most clinical medical specialties treat patients who have pain. Therefore, improved undergraduate medical courses should emphasize the complexity of the pain experience, the wide variation in pain expression, and the many factors that influence suffering, pain behaviors, and disability. At the graduate level, it would certainly seem advisable that the aspiring pain specialist have an extended fellowship at the conclusion of residency to rotate through approved multidisciplinary and interdisciplinary pain centers, being exposed to difficult clinical, administrative, and ethical problems (Appendix 49.1).

No single discipline has all of the answers for patients with intractable pain, although each may have much to offer. While there may be several useful treatments for a given patient, generally there is only one or at best a few that are clearly superior and are therefore considered treatments of choice. These should be the least invasive treatments capable of bringing about the desired effect. They should have a high benefit-to-morbidity ratio. In general, noninvasive should always be preferred over invasive therapy if the noninvasive therapy accomplishes the same result. We should be guided by the cardinal rule of medicine: first do no harm (16).

Any attempt at reconciling the divergent agendas affecting pain management and health care delivery should take into account the needs of the public consumer, the health care provider, and the cost to society. We can no longer approach medicine naively and idealistically, expecting that our recommendations will find acceptance and ultimate implementation. The health care system has reached such magnitude that technological and clinical resource allocations for pain treatment threaten to outstrip their economic support structure (17). Unfortunately, the consumer, provider, and bureaucrat have often taken adversarial positions, losing sight of why most of us chose our profession: to alleviate suffering and improve the health care of individuals and of our society.

It is anticipated that market forces will continue to drive health care. The public is increasingly dissatisfied with the effects of managed care on the health care system, and while clearly they are concerned about escalating costs, they also want to maintain our leadership in health care. We believe that

Table 49.1.   The New Specialty of Pain Medicine: Operational Criteria

A distinct and unique body of knowledge as evidenced by texts and journals
Clinical applicability sufficient to support a clinical practice
Ability to generate scholarly knowledge and support research
Ability to meet numerical standards for training programs, trainees, and practicing diplomates
De facto recognition as clear subject area by governmental bodies (e.g., NIH, NCI, AHCPR) and nongovernmental organizations (e.g., WHO, IASP, AAPM, APS)
Fills a recognized gap in health professional training

physicians must work within the organized structure of our pain societies (AAPM and APS) as well as the American Medical Association (AMA) to ensure the survival of our field. Doing so can meet our responsibility to our patients that we will ameliorate their pain and suffering in times of need. Since publication of the second edition of this text, the AMA has formally recognized pain medicine as a specialty. Operational criteria for recognizing pain medicine as a novel discipline are shown in Table 49.1. The AAPM has a seat in the AMA House of Delegates at a time when many other organizations have been unsuccessful in their petition for this status. In California, American Board of Pain Medicine (ABPM) certification is considered equivalent to American Board of Medical Specialties (ABMS) certification. It is anticipated that while pain medicine awaits ABMS status, other states will follow the lead taken by California. Also in California, the AAPM has been instrumental in introducing new codes that improved workers compensation reimbursement. It is hoped that this will establish a precedent for other states. For years the AAPM has advocated recognition of the complexity and time involved in pain assessment. The AAPM petitioned the AMA current procedural terminology (CPT) panel to revise the evaluation and management (E/M) codes for pain assessment and treatment, and while our needs are far from resolved, they are acknowledged. In the past several years several codes that should improve reimbursement for time-intensive pain evaluations have been added. The AAPM has also been involved with the AMA on another important project spearheaded by Dr. Philipp Lippe: the revision of the AMA *Guide to the Evaluation of Permanent Impairment,* which now has a separate chapter on pain. There is recognition that the evaluation of impairment from pain often requires special expertise and that some persons with chronic and intractable pain may not be at maximum medical improvement (MMI) until evaluated and treated at a multidisciplinary pain center (MPC).

One of the many criticisms leveled at MPCs has been the relative paucity of good outcome studies. We have been asked to adhere to a higher standard than is held for other treatments and procedures that are now considered acceptable medical practices. The AAPM Uniform Outcome Study, more than 3 years in development, is now in the clinical testing phase. It is hoped that this study will provide a vehicle to bring us closer to uniformity in nosology, diagnostic criteria, and treatment modalities and improve our clinical efficacy in the management of complex chronic pain problems. It will also provide a network in which pain clinicians may interact more successfully with one another and more easily pool our knowledge base.

One of the debates in which pain medicine is actively involved concerns physician-assisted suicide. Patients suffering from intractable pain related to terminal or incurable illness should not have to beg for assistance. As pain physicians we cannot remain silent when unfortunate patients are looking for ways to end their lives, seeking out a pathologist because he has had the courage to address needs unmet by conventional medicine. This is not to advocate for Kevorkian; however, he has at great personal risk championed a cause that needed a champion, and this sensitive and controversial matter is now being addressed openly. The driving force should have come from within pain medicine. Those of us involved in the secondary and tertiary care of patients who suffer with pain and lose their will to live must find better ways to ameliorate their suffering, assist them in maintaining their quality of life, and remain their advocates throughout their struggles with life and with death. Increasingly, pain medicine physicians will be brought into these crises. This is appropriate, and we must be prepared with an appropriate response (18). Both the AAPM and the APS have appointed task forces on end of life care to address the issues of euthanasia and physician-assisted suicide.

These socioeconomic reflections are an extension of the remarks that concluded the prior edition of this volume (1). As stated in the introduction, no consideration of the future of pain management can ignore several major scientific and cultural advances since then. We describe these and conclude by returning to areas of unsolved questions, controversy, or shortcomings in health care that must be addressed as the field of pain medicine continues to evolve.

THE ALGESIC CASCADE

More than 50 years ago Lorente de No made classic neurophysiological observations of amplification and reverberation within central neural networks (19). This and subsequent research on the ability of neurons to alter their interconnectedness, metabolism, and responsiveness to incoming stimuli have had comparatively little effect on clinical practice until recently. Two "new" motives now supplement traditional humane strivings for eradication of patients' pain. The first derives from recognition that pain is a malleable, evolving process in which intervention at an early stage or even in advance of tissue injury (as in the use of local anesthesia before surgical incision) may greatly simplify subsequent pain management (20). The second broad, physiologically based motive for providing aggressive analgesia reflects increasing awareness that pain perception is merely one aspect of a linked cascade of autonomic, metabolic, and neuroendocrine responses evoked by nociception that in aggregate influence clinical outcomes and costs of care (21).

Since the second edition of this volume there has occurred a pervasive but little-described paradigm shift in which spinal cord sensitization has supplanted pituitary-adrenal activation as the focus of research on pain-related stress (5). At the same time, hormone secretion into the bloodstream has also been supplanted as a marker of stress by intracellular changes within the dorsal horn of the spinal cord. Such responses include the expression of immediate-early genes such as *c-fos*, activation of enzymes such as protein kinase C (PKC) and nitric oxide synthase (NOS), internalization of membrane receptors (e.g., for substance P), secretion of nerve growth factors, and structural remodeling of the neurons themselves (3, 22). A rapid increase in understanding the chain of events precipitated in the spinal cord by painful peripheral stimuli has spurred novel drug discovery and also rekindled interest in spinal application of established drugs, alone or in combination.

During the past 5 years, the key role of spinal nociceptive processing and reorganization ("plasticity") in acute and chronic sequelae of tissue injury has been amply defined in preclinical models (4). Controversy clouds the generality of persuasive preclinical findings on preventing spinal sensitization by aggressive clinical analgesia, given that clinical testing of preemptive analgesia has led to mixed results. Dahl (23), Kissin (24), and others have clarified the shortcomings of clinical studies (incompleteness of afferent blockade, limits to drug dosing, prolonged versus brief nociceptive stimulation) that make demonstration of preemptive analgesic effects in such trials harder to achieve than in animal studies. They (and we) conclude that the principle of preemptive analgesia, like so many other concepts in medicine whose practical realization was delayed for technical reasons, remains logical and attractive. To harness it effectively in clinical practice, however, will require more complete blockade of single levels or concurrent blockade of several levels within algesic pathways than is now feasible in most clinical settings.

Because current approaches and future progress seek to achieve blockade of specific steps in the algesic cascade, a summary of this process is appropriate (Figure 49.1). The early-immediate proto-oncogene *c-fos* is rapidly expressed after calcium influx into postsynaptic dorsal horn neurons following afferent nociceptive stimuli provoked by inflammation or heating (25). Fos, the protein product of *c-fos*, after combining with Jun (the protein product of *c-jun*) to form a dimer, binds to the nuclear regulatory site AP-1, which is involved in transcription of many genes in many tissues, including enkephalins and dynorphin within the spinal cord (26). The presence of Ca^{++} is essential for the transcriptional activation of the *c-fos* proto-oncogene (27). Prolonged entry of Ca^{++} follows activation of the NMDA receptor Mg^{++}-gated Ca^{++} channel or voltage-gated Ca^{++} channels controlled by other receptors. Although *c-fos* is a nonspecific index of cellular depolarization and not a specific marker of nociceptive activity, there is good evidence that *c-fos* participates in regulation of opioid gene expression at the spinal level. Noxious thermal, chemical, or mechanical stimuli evoke *c-fos* expression

STIMULUS

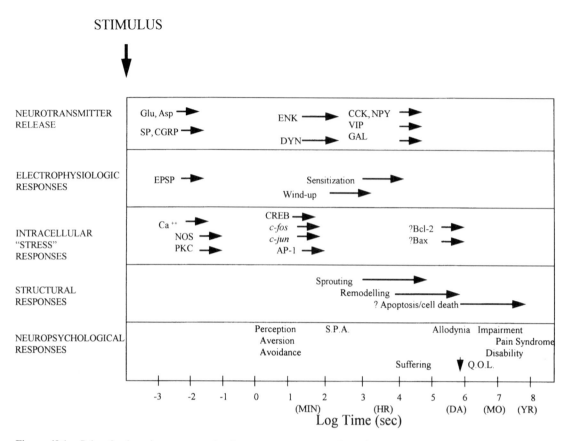

Figure 49.1. Pain stimulus triggers a cascade of events across many orders of magnitude of time and space (3, 74). S.P.A., stimulation-produced analgesia; Q.O.L., quality of life. (Reprinted with permission from Carr DB, Cousins MJ. Spinal route of analgesia: opioids and future options. In: Cousins MJ, Bridenbaugh PO, eds. Neural blockade in clinical anesthesia and management of pain. ed 3. Philadelphia: Lippincott-Raven, 1998.)

followed by enkephalin and then dynorphin expression in dorsal horn (29–31). Supraspinal morphine pretreatment in advance of a noxious stimulus produces dose-dependent inhibition of *c-fos* expression (32).

Biochemical events within cells of the dorsal horn that become sensitized and reorganized as a result of ongoing C fiber input are well described in acute models, and ongoing work has confirmed their involvement in subacute and chronic pain states. Intrathecal administration of substance P or neurokinin A produces hyperalgesia that is reversed by treatment with a substance P antagonist. There is strong evidence that other neuropeptides identified within C fibers (calcitonin gene-related peptides, vasoactive intestinal peptide, cholecystokinin) also provoke central hyperalgesia after peripheral injury, as do the excitatory amino acids aspartate and glutamate (33). Selective activation of the excitatory inotropic glutamate receptor by intrathecal administration of NMDA mimics the hyperalgesia that follows tissue trauma; this hyperalgesic response is reversed with an NMDA antagonist (34). Reinforcing interactions between distinct neuropeptide algesic transmitters, such as substance P and calcitonin gene-related peptide, and between excitatory amino acids and neuropeptides such as substance P and glutamate, take place

within the dorsal horn (35). About 90% of C fibers that contain substance P also contain glutamate. Indeed, corelease of substance P and glutamate to activate simultaneously the neurokinin-1 (NK-1) and NMDA receptors, respectively, appears necessary to induce postsynaptic depolarization sufficiently prolonged to overcome the basal, voltage-dependent magnesium block of the NMDA receptor, as application of glutamate by itself is unable to do so (36, 37). Antagonists at several sites on the NMDA receptor complex are under active investigation for use in reversing sensitized dorsal horn neurons to their basal state (38). The analgesic anesthetic ketamine, long applied in clinical anesthesiology and burn care because of its sympathomimetic and respiratory-sparing effects is now recognized to block the calcium channel of the NMDA receptor complex and in preclinical models prevents or reverses the temporal summation of C fiber afferent impulses (39). The NMDA antagonist MK-801, which acts upon the same (phencyclidine-binding) site within the calcium channel as ketamine, blocks the development of thermal hyperalgesia in a rat model of ligation-induced neuropathic pain (40).

Concurrent binding of glutamate to NMDA and non-NMDA (e.g., AMPA [α-amino-3 hydroxy-5-methyl-4 isoxazolepropionic acid]) receptors, substance P to the NK-1 receptor, and glycine to its receptor adjoining the NMDA receptor gives rise to sustained postsynaptic depolarization and an influx of calcium and sodium (41, 42). The inrush of calcium into the postsynaptic neuron causes activation of nitric oxide synthase (NOS) and PKC along with translocation of the latter enzyme from cytosol to cell membrane. PKC phosphorylates multiple proteins and thereby contributes to long-term changes in neuronal function and structure (e.g., dendritic sprouting) induced by persistent nociception (43). Calcium-induced NOS activation to generate NO also plays an important role in nociceptive processing (44). PKC and NO are involved not only in the generation of dorsal horn sensitization and hyperalgesia, but also in the development of morphine tolerance (45). Physiological adaptations in dorsal horn neurons common to both processes include NMDA receptor activation, calcium influx, and the activation of PKC and NOS. For example, rats made tolerant to morphine develop thermal hyperalgesia (42), and rats subject to an experimental ligation mononeuropathy have a diminished antinociceptive response to morphine (46). PKC in dorsal horn, activated either during morphine tolerance or hyperalgesia, phosphorylates the NMDA calcium channel and reduces magnesium-dependent channel blockade, thereby augmenting NMDA receptor activity and postsynaptic excitation. The actions of intracellular NO resemble those of PKC but are accomplished via somewhat different pathways, such as cyclic guanosine monophosphate (GMP) dependent protein kinases. Acute morphine antinociception is enhanced (47) and the development of morphine tolerance impeded (48) by concurrent administration of a NOS inhibitor.

In particular circumstances, one or another feature of this global response may be more prominent, yet they all lie within a larger continuum and share anatomical and physiological substrates. For this reason, interventions aimed at reducing acute or chronic pain may also enhance patients' rehabilitation through beneficial effects on pulmonary, cardiovascular, metabolic, or other key systems. Ongoing studies have begun to define patient populations or settings in which it is beneficial to uncouple these normal sequelae from the tissue damage or pain that normally evokes them. Defining precisely the safest and most effective analgesic techniques for distinct patient groups and assessing their effects on outcomes such as morbidity, mortality, patient satisfaction, length of hospital stay, and use of medical resources will take years. Nonetheless, early glimpses of the benefits that aggressive analgesia may offer have already been provided by studies in high-risk populations.

If aggressive pain control appears to be appropriate at the extremes of age or physiology, what about in between? As mentioned earlier in this chapter and elsewhere in this volume, many factors besides physiology or cost accounting enter clinical practice. Ethical concerns to reduce suffering and improve quality of life influence all health care professionals and are paramount in the feeling of patients and their families. Patients' preferences and satisfaction may motivate

an institution to offer a new technology, such as intravenous patient-controlled analgesia, to patients at home, even when such devices may offer only small reductions in morbidity or costs of care in such populations. In children, humane concerns are reinforced by awareness of the long-term neural sensitization or psychosocial scars that may follow undertreatment of their pain. For this reason a recent surge of textbooks, lectures, and research reports on children with pain will doubtless be followed by sustained diffusion of such knowledge into clinical care (49–51).

DRUGS, ROUTES, DEVICES

As scientists and clinicians become increasingly motivated to treat pain aggressively, improved pharmacotherapies make this easier to accomplish. Intriguingly, many "innovative" means of pain treatment may be traced back decades in the literature. Interference with tissue-derived inflammatory mediators as a means to inhibit pain and stress was suggested by Selye in the first half of this century (52). As cited earlier, Lorente de No's accounts of reverberation in neural circuits are likewise more than 50 years old. Bromage, in his 1954 monograph on epidural analgesia, emphasized its attractiveness for postoperative pain control (53). In the late 1960s Keeri-Szanto began to apply on-demand (i.e., patient-controlled) intravenous analgesia for clinical postoperative pain (54). Thus, if the future of pain control is like its past, "advances" in the next decade will largely consist of clinical applications of ideas now extant, in some cases already tested clinically. At the risk of oversimplification or neglect of behavioral approaches, these advances may be categorized as drugs or methods of delivery (55).

Nonsteroidal anti-inflammatory drugs (NSAIDs) were the first synthetic analgesics. Rediscovery of older observations that NSAIDs have a central as well as peripheral analgesic effect has rekindled interest in giving low doses of soluble NSAIDs centrally to provide nonopioid analgesia without systemic side effects (56). Two new observations hold promise for expanded use of NSAIDs to treat acute and chronic pain. First is the insight that cyclo-oxygenase has two forms, COX-1 and COX-2. The former is constitutively expressed, and its inhibition by traditional NSAIDs leads to their renal and gastrointestinal toxicity (57). COX-2 is expressed after tissue injury and mediates inflammation. Hence, clinical application of selective COX-2 inhibitors, now being reported in early clinical trials, is attractive. Second is the observation that some NSAIDs work not only by COX inhibition but also by inhibiting the nuclear transcription factor kB, which is critical for cytokine gene expression during inflammation, such as for interleukin-1 and interleukin-6 (58). Development of inhibitors to this and related transcription factors, or to cytokines themselves, could offer anti-inflammatory and analgesic benefits of NSAIDs without their well-recognized side effects.

Although morphine remains the reference standard for parenteral opioid analgesia, a continuing stream of new opioids or opioid-related agents (e.g., enkephalinase inhibitors) is under development. Two newer short-acting μ-opioids are phenylpiperidines related to fentanyl. These opioids, alfentanil and remifentanyl, are used as intraoperative infusions and have been given at a lower infusion rate postoperatively to secure continuing analgesia. Other than their short duration of action (not necessarily a practical advantage apart from facilitating quick emergence from anesthesia), they still evoke μ-opioid side effects such as nausea and respiratory depression. Fentanyl itself has been formulated in two distinct forms that as niche products have enjoyed growing sales in recent years. The transdermal fentanyl formulation is not intended for postoperative pain use but for chronic pain such as in cancer (the same target group as for time-release morphine). However, a new version of the fentanyl patch that incorporates a push-button and microchip to regulate iontophoretic drug delivery may soon find application for acute pain control as well as for chronic, recurring breakthrough pain. A grape-flavored fentanyl lozenge on a stick for buccal application has been introduced for use during brief painful procedures, to assist with induction of anesthesia (particularly in children), and for recurrent breakthrough pain during chronic illness such as cancer. Other phenylpiperidines have been administered by inhalation and pulmonary absorption, but this route is not yet employed clinically.

The motivation for use of non–μ-opioids is chiefly to avoid morphine-related side effects rather than to improve upon morphine analgesia. These side effects include sedation, respiratory depression, constipation, and other gastrointestinal effects such as nausea, urinary retention, and drug diversion. Approaches to overcome such effects include development or reformulation of agents that are partial agonists at the morphine (μ) receptor or that act upon other opioid receptors, such as κ-or δ-receptors (59). The FDA at present classifies neither butorphanol nor dezocine (both κ- and μ-antagonists) nor tramadol, which acts through μ-receptors and monoamine systems, as habit forming, although butorphanol is under consideration for rescheduling because of reports of substance abuse and drug dependence. Nonscheduled analgesics are attractive to clinicians who are concerned with diversion, who fear regulatory surveillance, and who treat chronic as well as acute pain. More than 80% of the total yearly U.S. sales of $50 million of butorphanol are in its nasal form, which is rapidly absorbed and targeted for migraineurs.

Since the prior edition of this volume, cloning of μ-, δ-, and κ-opioid receptor types has confirmed their separateness (60). Preclinical studies of the δ-opioid receptor as a target for selective analgesia show promise. δ-Agonists show less dependence liability and minimal prolongation of gastrointestinal transit time in animals. Few clinical reports involving minimal numbers of patients have been published, and they employed less selective compounds than available today. Given their likely expense, systemic application of δ-selective opioids in humans is unlikely, but they may find a role in spinal analgesia. Similarly, potent novel opioid peptide analogs and nonpeptidic analogs of opioid peptides have great analgesic potency but require additional testing in clinical trials before their role in acute pain control can be clarified.

Relevant to the future of enkephalin analgesia, although not to acute pain, is the strategy employed by several laboratories that have placed adrenal chromaffin cells into the spinal fluid. Such cells cosecrete enkephalins and catecholamines and can provide long-lasting analgesia, but in their present application are still restricted to trials for chronic, refractory cancer pain. Enkephalinase inhibitors were tested more than a decade ago for acute pain but are poorly tolerated and hence not released for that indication. The issue of selectivity is key, because such inhibitors run the risk of acting in unintended ways (e.g., to inhibit angiotensin-converting enzyme, another peptidase). Nonetheless, these agents are in clinical trials.

A wide variety of other agents are now also in clinical trials, chiefly for use in acute or cancer pain. Most of these, such as α₂-agonists, cholinergic agonists, calcium channel blockers, and NMDA receptor blockers, are for the most part administered spinally or in the case of novel local anesthetics such as ropivacaine or levobupivacaine also given by infiltration. Accordingly, the reader is referred to textbooks and reviews in the anesthesiology literature for detailed discussion of such agents.

Because of the enormous cost of thoroughly studying a new analgesic and carrying it from preclinical through clinical trials and the high attrition rate of test compounds before they ever reach clinical trials, an established trend is to seek analgesic synergy from combinations of commercially available agents that act through distinct, complementary mechanisms. The therapeutic benefits of employing combination, or in Kehlet's words, balanced analgesia (61) are considerable, and they are already a part of daily clinical practice. Opioids, for example, have been administered in the acute or chronic setting together with NSAIDs as recommended in Agency for Health Care Policy and Research (AHCPR) and World Health Organization (WHO) guidelines. Opioids have also been coadministered with local anesthetics, α₂-adrenergic agents, calcium channel blockers, antidepressants, or ketamine in preclinical and clinical trials that have demonstrated benefits from each of these combinations (5, 35). It will be some time before optimal combination therapy of two or more analgesics can be defined for all patient groups and for long- and short-term settings. As studies that address these combinations and methods to administer them unfold during the next decade, major factors defining what is "optimal" and how to achieve it in clinical practice will be cost and outcomes.

Until recently, the unwieldiness, cost, or frank unavailability of reliable pumps for use in delivering bedside infusions of intravenous or intraspinal medications has limited their application to the hospital setting. Now that we are entering the third or fourth generation of their design, microprocessors and pump motors are smaller and consume less power, software is nearly perfect, and batteries last longer. The possibility of preparing concentrated infusions of opioids such as hydromorphone (Dilaudid) now permits use of the subcutaneous route for systemic, low-volume opioid infusions of a potency suitable for clinical pain control. In such settings, intravenous access is not needed for pain control. Similarly, the excellent therapeutic ratio of effect to side effect for intraspinal infusions of local anesthetic and opioid mixtures (or morphine plus clonidine) renders this approach also appropriate for selected ambulatory outpatients with chronic cancer or noncancer pain (62). Increasing reliance on these technologies or other similar ones, such as continuous fentanyl administration via transdermal patch, has blurred the distinction between management options once thought suitable only for acute pain control in hospitalized patients or those in extremis and options deemed appropriate for chronic use in outpatients suffering from intractable pain, whether or not due to malignancy. If such new technologies offer, as they seem to in many instances, superior means of controlling clinical pain, the complexion of pain management, particularly at the end of life, will be significantly different at the beginning of the next millennium. Improved drugs, frequently administered in combinations and via previously unexploited routes, will offer effective pain relief to patients who, thanks to programable devices with preset safety limits, will respond to their own analgesic needs in the comfort of their homes.

EVIDENCE-BASED PAIN MEDICINE AND GUIDELINES

Sadly, it is quite possible that socioeconomic forces now in place may keep these advances from clinical practice, except for those few patients who are wealthy or lucky enough to escape from an ever-tightening net of bureaucracy. Calls to reduce health care costs now come from every quarter and are supported by institutional limits upon clinical practice, often at the behest of payors. Some restrictions are indirect, such as the need for prior approval of, say, a diagnostic sympathetic nerve block so as not to forfeit third-party reimbursement. Such "soft" limits may be quite effective: unreimbursed time is required to comply with them, and explaining the physiological rationale for a procedure to a claims reviewer with no background in pain may simply lead to a more articulate rechallenging of the plan. There is a continuum from reading a warning note by utilization reviewers in a patient's chart to mandatory written explanation if a "critical incident" is noted by a quality assurance committee to legal defense against a zealous state medical board if a patient's relative dupes one, say, into renewing a chronic opioid prescription after his or her unreported demise. Besides threats to autonomy that sometimes appear propelled by issues of control rather than patient well-being, financial restrictions increasingly deter practitioners from delivering their intended care (63). The effects of budget reductions at the state or federal level range from cutbacks in support staff to closure of entire health care institutions.

In this climate, reactions to recent significant federal initiatives to develop pain management guidelines have been understandably mixed (64). The Omnibus Budget Reconciliation Act of 1989 provided for "extensive research into what constitutes appropriate medical care, the effectiveness of current and future medical practices, and their benefit to Medicare patients" (65). To do so, a federal agency, the AHCPR "was established to enhance the quality, appropriateness, and effectiveness of health care services, and access to such services." Within this agency is the Office of the Forum for Quality and Effectiveness in Health Care, "whose general mission is the development, periodic review, and updating of clinical guidelines" and development of "standards of quality, performance measures, and medical review criteria by which providers and other appropriate entities may assess the quality of care" (King SH, personal communication [AHCPR], 1990).

The AHCPR has defined practice guidelines as "systematically developed statements to assist practitioner and patient decisions about appropriate health care for specific clinical circumstances" that describe "what is clearly appropriate or inappropriate care, and also describe care that the scientific evidence and consensus cannot definitively identify as appropriate or inappropriate" (King SH, personal communication [AHCPR], 1990). Eddy has discussed the distinctions between guidelines and standards that "are intended to be applied rigidly, and must be followed in virtually all cases," with the possibility of malpractice if they are violated (66). Guidelines "are intended to be more flexible. They *should* be followed in *most* cases [but] depending on the patient, setting, and other factors, guidelines *can and should* be tailored to fit individual needs. Deviation from a guideline does not by itself imply malpractice." Weaker than guidelines are options that "merely note that different interventions are available" but "leave practitioners free to choose any course." Specific attributes of such a guideline are given in Table 49.2. These attributes were published in the second edition of this volume, and we think it important to present these again because of interim shifts in usage of the term guideline toward a much less rigorous, even nebulous application.

While millions of copies of the AHCPR guidelines on acute and cancer pain were distributed, owing to political turbulence in AHCPR and controversy over its guideline on acute low-back pain funding, the entire guideline process was discontinued in 1995. In its place, AHCPR began to fund centers for evidence-based practice, through which systematic reviews of specific topics would be performed on a contract bid basis. At present it appears likely that funding of updates of the federal 1992 guidelines on acute and 1994 guidelines on cancer pain will at least be considered through this latter process. At the same time, though, the importance of systematic reviews of evidence as the basis for all of medical practice has gained considerable support. Indeed, evidence-based practice guidelines now appear to be the next step toward data-driven codification of medical practice. Strictly speaking, practice guidelines are not mandatory, but pressures to reduce costs and increase quality of care

Table 49.2.   Definition and Attributes of Pain Practice Guidelines

Definition
Practice guidelines are systematically developed statements to assist practitioners' and patients' decisions about appropriate health care for specific clinical circumstances. They describe what is clearly appropriate or inappropriate care and care that the scientific evidence and consensus cannot identify definitively as either appropriate or inappropriate. The guidelines pertain to specific clinical circumstances, which may include clinically relevant organizational factors, social considerations, and similar influences on health care delivery. They should be developed in a formal, systematic way that can be fully documented.

Attributes

Credibility
The degree to which guidelines are grounded in science, the qualifications and experience of those developing guidelines, and the degree of compatibility with factual real-world circumstances of practitioners and patients

Disclosure
The process of development outlined in detail, including the identities and biases of participants, procedures used for evaluation, and underlying assumptions

Validity
An explicit discussion of the way the evidence relates to the final product, assessments of the strength of scientific evidence and professional consensus, areas of conflict, and the relative weights given to consensus and science

Reliability and reproducibility
Proof that guidelines can be applied properly by a given practitioner in different situations and similarly by different practitioners in similar circumstances

Clinical adaptability
A clear description of population to which guidelines apply, including appropriate explanations of pathophysiology, demographic characteristics, social support systems, and so on

Flexibility
The extent to which exceptions are identified, foreseeable exceptions clearly identified, classification of idiosyncratic (unpredictable) exceptions, patients' preferences to be considered, any additional data to be collected as justification for exception

Clarity
Unambiguous language about appropriate populations and circumstances; all key terms defined

Scheduled review
A review date based on the pace and quality of relevant research

Applicability to health systems management
Applicable as a link between quality assurance and health systems management

Research relevance
Direct new research to provide information on patients' condition, improve treatments, reduce uncertainty about the appropriateness of alternative treatments, promote consensus

From the Department of Health and Human Services, Public Health Service, Agency Health Care Policy and Research, Rockville, Maryland.

have led health system administrators, insurers, and governmental agencies increasingly to encourage clinicians to follow such guidelines. The past 10 years have been termed a decade of guidelines in pain management because of numerous such documents issued by organizations and governments throughout the world (67). Some of these reports urge incorporation of pain assessment and treatment into quality assurance and improvement procedures so that inadequately treated pain is routinely identified and its cause corrected. In response to this lag, leading medical editors will soon require standardized performance and reporting of clinical trials (68). Jadad, McQuay, and many others around the world have also begun to apply established methods of meta-analysis to the area of pain control. However, this task is far from simple and will require sustained effort internationally, ideally through groups such as the International Association for the Study of Pain (IASP), AAPM, and APS, working though networks such as the Oxford-based Cochrane Collaboration for systematic reviews and clinical trials registries. The recent registration of a Cochrane Review Group specifically concerned with pain and palliative and supportive care bodes well for future efforts to consolidate and critique the present literature and to raise the quality of future clinical trials in these increasingly important fields.

STANDARDS FOR STANDARD BEARERS

The increase in guidelines and standards for pain treatment since the second edition of this book presumably reflects overlapping needs of primary care providers for guidance, patient advocates for better care, insurers for cost containment, and specialty societies to formulate coherent approaches to diagnosis and therapy. It is only natural amid the confluence of these needs that the question should arise as to who is best qualified to meet them. In other words, on what basis and under whose direction should a consultant or specialist in pain treatment be deemed such? Furthermore, what resources should be available at a facility that calls itself a pain treatment center? These questions are typical of the emergence of any medical or surgical specialty, although pain treatment is a problematic area in that many worthwhile forms of treatment are delivered by health professionals with diverse training in distinct disciplines.

If the 1980s witnessed a proliferation of pain-related organizations, in the 1990s a countertrend toward coalescence and standard setting may be dominant. This countertrend has been spearheaded globally by the IASP, task forces of which have just issued a pair of important standards and a related core curriculum. The first standard, laying the foundation for certification in pain management, defines requirements for a fellowship (69). As is evident from Appendix 49.1, its structure resembles others previously issued by varied subspecialty boards. The related core curriculum is available in pamphlet form from the IASP (70). These documents have engendered considerable debate, yet experience in other medical specialties suggests that persons not certified as consultants will always continue to provide key elements of care. In endocrinology, for example, the laboratory specialist who prepares a profile of exacting hormone measurements to aid in diagnosis; the nurse who delivers care ranging from titrated insulin doses to saline infusions for hypercalcemia; the radiology technologist who ensures a comfortable and technically acceptable series of magnetic resonance images to localize a pituitary or adrenal tumor; the radiologist who interprets these studies; and the operating room team of surgeons, anesthesiologists, nurses, and other personnel who carry out an operation to excise an adenoma have not found their livelihoods or professional status eroded by the existence of an accreditation process for specialists who coordinate their services. The process of accreditation in other spheres of health care has not always been seamless, as in intensive care, for which certification may be obtained through any of several boards. Yet in balance, uniformity within specialty accreditation is the rule, and pain practitioners will do well do stay abreast of evolving programs in this area. Confusingly at the moment, a non-APS, non-IASP organization (having the same initials as the AMA-affiliated American Academy of Pain Medicine) is offering certification with little or no screening process, initially for a $250 fee; how this accreditation will relate to those of the broader organizations remains to be decided. In contrast, the ABPM has addressed training and accreditation issues in pain medicine through rigorous procedures and has now, shepherded by its executive vice president, Philipp Lippe, and president, Peter Wilson, reached the point of formal application for full ABMS recognition. The equivalent of such recognition has, thanks to the efforts of Dr. Lippe, already been granted to ABPM in California.

The second set of recommendations issued by the IASP (69), which concerns pain treatment facilities, is presented in Appendix 49.2. The influence of the founder of the IASP, John Bonica, is very much in evidence, for the model of multidisciplinary pain care that it describes originated at the University of Washington under his direction (71). The IASP document does note that not every pain patient must routinely undergo multidisciplinary assessment and treatment, consistent with Carr's experience in most instances of pain after operation or with cancer. It fits, too, with the reality that the majority of pain diagnosis and treatment take place in primary care settings. Furthermore, its suggestion that outcomes be routinely monitored as a means to refine practice is very much in keeping with quality assurance trends described earlier and also accords with a monograph on program evaluation in chronic pain management programs prepared by the Commission on Accreditation of Rehabilitation Facilities (CARF) (72). The CARF report, however, has little to say about the nomenclature describing the scope of a chronic pain program or the mechanics of attaining its objectives but concentrates instead on setting forth goals for such programs, constructing measures for each goal, documenting collection of these measures, and ensuring that the data gathered improve program performance.

Precisely to whom pain management facilities and practitioners will report in a few years' time is unclear. From this brief account it is clear that forces embodied by the APS quality assurance subcommittee directed at the existing process of the Joint Commission for the Accreditation of Health Care Organizations (JCAHO) review of hospitals and other health organizations, the CARF report focusing on free-standing pain rehabilitation facilities, and the IASP guidelines relevant to either hospital-affiliated or free-standing contexts must all attain an equilibrium that it is hoped will be harmonious and well suited to the needs of pain physicians represented by the AAPM and ABPM.

CONCLUSION

This overview—from genome to pain clinic to Congress—has selected trends that will shape the practice of pain management and its organizational context during the next few years. In painting with broad strokes, this chapter has only mentioned in passing certain issues that are no less important—and possibly more so—for those who treat chronic pain. The appropriateness of opioid use for chronic nonmalignant pain is a focal point for clashing agendas of well-meaning legislatures determined to keep illicit drugs out of the hands of abusers and patients, whose long-term ability to function seems improved when so treated. Melzack has identified institutional and legal confusion between patients' needs for medication and the drug-seeking behavior of street addicts as one source of needless pain, but resolution of this conflict will not be speedy (73). Another unsolved aspect of pain practice is the appropriate timing of invasive therapies. Writing from the perspective of members of a tertiary care institution, it is not clear that patients are best served by deferring procedures such as cordotomy or celiac neurolysis until they are in extremis, if early application of such techniques might reduce or forever eliminate the need for escalating opioid doses and their side effects. The case for neurosurgical and related procedures in the management of chronic pain is presented in Chapter 38. Home health care has greatly expanded as an alternative to costly hospital stays. New technologies such as portable pumps and epidural catheters for ambulatory use permit home therapies that once were offered only to inpatients. Which patients are appropriate, how transitions are to be made smoothly from inpatient to outpatient care, how safety and effectiveness are to be ensured, and when readmission is desirable or mandatory are all open questions whose importance will grow in coming years. Finally, how to blend all of these elements, as well as to address psychosocial and spiritual needs to optimize care at the end of life, is a huge issue, as every developed country has proportionately greater numbers of the elderly.

The care of patients with pain has always been personally gratifying, and now it is intellectually rewarding as well. Once a narrow path traveled by few, it is now a high-speed superhighway with traffic exiting and entering through numerous interchanges and cloverleaves. Tremendously dynamic, it could be stopped by the funding equivalent of a fuel shortage, administrative traffic jams, or regulatory toll booths. Pain medicine is at the heart of 21st century health care. All pain practitioners should work together to ensure that it not only survives but prospers in the coming millennium.

Acknowledgment

We are grateful to our professional colleagues and trainees for their constant intellectual stimulation and dedication to the care of patients with pain. Support for Dr. Carr during the preparation of this manuscript was provided by the Richard Saltonstall Charitable Foundation, the Armington Foundation, and grants from the National Cancer Institute and the National Institute on Drug Abuse. Dr. Heinrich Wurm, Chairman of Anesthesia at Tufts University School of Medicine and New England Medical Center, has provided unstinting support and encouragement to those, including Dr. Carr, concerned with pain treatment at these institutions. Miss Evelyn Hall, Department of Anesthesia, New England Medical Center, provided expert secretarial assistance.

APPENDIX 49.1

STANDARDS FOR PHYSICIAN FELLOWSHIP IN PAIN MANAGEMENT

1. **Definition:** A physician fellowship in pain management is a period of specialized postgraduate training for physicians to enable the graduate of such a program to assess and manage patients with chronic pain of all types and to understand the sciences basic to the practice of pain management.
2. **Duration:** A fellowship in pain management should be a minimum of 1 year of full-time clinical training. Additional research training may be desirable, depending upon the fellow's career goals, but this should not erode the clinical training period.
3. **Prerequisites for fellowship in pain management:** To be eligible for a fellowship in pain management, the candidate must be board eligible or board certified in one of the recognized specialties of medicine; furthermore, the specialty area must involve experience with patient care. The fellow must be a graduate of an approved school of medicine. The fellow must provide at least three letters of reference and a curriculum vitae when applying for a fellowship position. The fellow must be licensed to practice medicine by the appropriate governmental agencies.
4. **Resources:** The fellowship must occur within a medical institution capable of providing a suitable educational environment. At least three recognized patient care specialty areas must be offered at the same institution. The institution must have a medical library with appropriate resources for this level of training. The clinical pain treatment program or its parent institution must be accredited by the appropriate governmental agencies. The pain treatment facility must have suitable space allocated for its clinical and educational activities. It must have a sufficient volume and variety of patients to provide the fellow or fellows with adequate educational opportunities. The pain treatment facility must see at least 100 new patients per year per fellow; there must be at least 500 patient visits per year per fellow. Pain treatment facilities that specialize in one region of the body or one type of disease are by themselves not adequate as a training resource.
5. **Director:** There must be a designated director of the pain management fellowship. The director shall be a physician who participates in the diagnosis and treatment of patients within the pain management facility offering the fellowship in pain management. The director of the fellowship need not be the administrative or medical chief of the pain treatment facility, but the fellowship director and the administrative and medical chiefs, if they are not the same, must demonstrate the ability to interact in such a way as to be conducive to the education of fellows. The director shall be responsible for the design and implementation of the fellowship; he or she shall be responsible for certifying that a fellow has successfully completed his or her training period and has mastered the requisite knowledge, skills, and attitudes. The director must be a member of the IASP and a national chapter. It is desirable that the director have extensive experience in the management of patients with the complaint of pain; it is also desirable that he or she have educational and administrative experience above and beyond the fellowship in pain management. The director shall be responsible for maintaining an up-to-date file on each fellow, documenting his or her educational progress and any deficiencies.
6. **Faculty:** There shall be at least three members of the pain treatment facility staff who are designated as faculty in addition to the director. Faculty members shall be appropriately certified in a patient care specialty. If one of the facility is not a psychiatrist, an additional faculty member must be a licensed clinical psychologist who has expertise in pain management. Faculty members shall also be members of the IASP and a national chapter. Faculty members of a fellowship in pain management shall represent at least three health care delivery specialties. Other types of health care providers in addition to physicians and psychologists may also be members of the faculty. Faculty members must spend a major part of their professional time working within the pain treatment facility.

Clinical Training Subjects

Although not every fellow will be fully trained in every area listed below, he or she should at least have had some exposure to patients whose care involves all of these areas.

I. Medical diagnosis and therapy
  A. History and physical examination
  B. Measurement of pain
  C. Physical therapies
  D. Vocational and rehabilitation assessment and management
  E. Participation in multidisciplinary assessment and treatment

F. Anesthesiological procedures (when appropriate for fellow's prior training)

G. Surgical procedures (when appropriate for fellow's prior training)

H. Other procedures appropriate to the fellow's prior specialty training

II. Psychologic diagnosis and therapy

A. Use of diagnostic tests

B. Collection of data from interview and standard forms

C. Comprehensive assessment

D. Treatment options

1. Individual, group, and family psychotherapy

2. Cognitive-behavioral therapies

3. Biofeedback and relaxation techniques

4. Hypnotherapy

III. Pharmacotherapy

A. Analgesics

1. Nonopioids

2. Opioids

3. Adjunctive drugs

B. Antidepressants

C. Sedative-hypnotics

D. Benzodiazepines

E. Others

IV. Specific types of painful conditions to be included in fellow's educational program

A. Pain associated with cancer, including issues of death and dying, palliative care, and hospice

B. Postoperative and posttrauma pain

C. Pain associated with nervous system injuries

D. Pain associated with chronic disease

E. Pain of unknown causation

F. Pain in children

G. Pain in the elderly

V. Regional pain syndromes to be included in fellow's educational program

A. Headache

B. Facial pain syndromes

C. Neck and upper back pain

D. Low-back pain

E. Extremity pain syndromes

G. Pelvic and perineal pain

APPENDIX 49.2.[1]

DESIRABLE CHARACTERISTICS FOR PAIN TREATMENT FACILITIES

DEFINITION OF TERMS

The following terms will be briefly defined in this section; a more complete description of the characteristics of each type of facility appears in subsequent portions of this report.

1. **Pain treatment facility:** A generic term used to describe all forms of pain treatment facilities without regard to personnel involved or types of patients served. Pain unit is a synonym for pain treatment facility.

2. **Multidisciplinary pain center:** An organization of health care professionals and basic scientists which includes research, teaching and patient care related to acute and chronic pain. This is the largest and most complex of the pain treatment facilities and ideally would exist as a component of a medical school or teaching hospital. Clinical programs must be supervised by an appropriately trained and licensed clinical director; a wide array of health care specialists is required, such as physicians, psychologists, nurses, physical therapists, occupational therapists, vocational counselors, social workers, and other specialized health care providers. The disciplines of health care providers required is a function of the varieties of patients seen and the health care resources of the community. The members of the treatment team must communicate with each other on a regular basis, both about specific patients and about overall development. Health care services in a multidisciplinary pain clinic must be integrated and based upon multidisciplinary assessment and management of the patient. Inpatient and outpatient programs are offered in such a facility.

3. **Multidisciplinary pain clinic:** A health care delivery facility staffed by physicians of different specialties and other nonphysician health care providers who specialize in the diagnosis and management of patients with chronic pain. This type of facility differs from a multidisciplinary pain center only because it does not include research and teaching activities in its regular programs. A multidisciplinary pain clinic may have diagnostic and treatment facilities which are outpatient, inpatient, or both.

4. **Pain clinic:** A health care delivery facility focusing upon the diagnosis and management of patients with chronic pain. A pain clinic may specialize in specific diagnoses or in pains related to a specific region of the body. A pain clinic may be large or small, but it should never be a label for an isolated solo practitioner. A single physician functioning within a complex health care institution that offers appropriate consultative and therapeutic services could qualify as a pain clinic if chronic pain patients were suitably assessed and managed. The absence of interdisciplinary assessment and management distinguishes this type of facility from a multidisciplinary pain center or clinic. Pain clinics can, and should be encouraged to, carry out research, but it is not a required characteristic of this type of facility.

5. **Modality-oriented clinic:** This is a health care facility that offers a specific type of treatment and does not provide comprehensive assessment or management. Examples include nerve block clinic, transcutaneous nerve stimulation clinic, acupuncture clinic, and biofeedback clinic. Such a facility may have one or

[1] Reprinted with permission from International Association for the Study of Pain. Task force guidelines for pain treatment facilities. Seattle: IASP, 1990.

more health care providers with different professional training; because of its limited treatment options and the lack of an integrated, comprehensive approach, it does not qualify for the term multidisciplinary.

DESIRABLE CHARACTERISTICS OF MULTIDISCIPLINARY PAIN CENTERS

1. A multidisciplinary pain center (MPC) should have on its staff a variety of health care providers capable of assessing and treating physical, psychosocial, medical, vocational and social aspects of chronic pain. These can include physicians, nurses, psychologists, physical therapists, occupational therapists, vocational counselors, social workers, and any other type of health care professional who can make a contribution to patient diagnosis or treatment.

2. At least three medical specialties should be represented on the staff of a multidisciplinary pain center. If one of the physicians is not a psychiatrist, physicians from two specialties and a clinical psychologist are the minimum required. An MPC must be able to assess and treat both the physical and the psychosocial aspects of a patients complaints. The need for other types of health care providers should be determined on the basis of the population served by the MPC.

3. The health care professionals should communicate with each other on a regular basis both about individual patients and the programs which are offered in the pain treatment facility.

4. There should be a director or coordinator of the MPC. He or she need not be a physician, but if not, there should be a director of medical services who will be responsible for monitoring of the medical services provided.

5. The MPC should offer diagnostic and therapeutic services which include medication management, referral for appropriate medical consultation, review of prior medical records and diagnostic tests, physical examination, psychological assessment and treatment, physical therapy vocational assessment and counseling, and other facilities as appropriate.

6. The MPC should have a designated space for its activities. The MPC should include facilities for inpatient services and outpatient services.

7. The MPC should maintain records on its patients so as to be able to assess individual treatment outcomes and to evaluate overall program effectiveness.

8. The MPC should have adequate support staff to carry out its activities.

9. Health care providers active in an MPC should have appropriate knowledge of both the basic sciences and clinical practices relevant to chronic pain patients.

10. The MPC should have a medically trained professional available to deal with patient referrals and emergencies.

11. All health care providers in an MPC should be appropriately licensed in the country or state in which they practice.

12. The MPC should be able to deal with a wide variety of chronic pain patients, including those with pain resulting from cancer and other diseases.

13. An MPC should establish protocols for patient management and assess their efficacy periodically.

14. An MPC should see an adequate number and variety of patients for its professional staff to maintain their skills in diagnosis and treatment.

15. Members of an MPC should carry out research on chronic pain. This does not mean that everyone should be doing both research and patient care. Some will only function in one arena, but the institution should have ongoing research activities.

16. The MPC should be active in educational programs for a wide variety of health care providers, including undergraduate, graduate, and postdoctoral levels.

17. The MPC should be part of or closely affiliated with a major health sciences educational or research institution.

DESIRABLE CHARACTERISTICS FOR A MULTIDISCIPLINARY PAIN CLINIC

The distinction between an MPC and a multidisciplinary pain clinic is that the former has research and teaching components that need not be present in the latter. Hence, items 15, 16, and 17 above are not required for a multidisciplinary pain clinic. All of the other items should be present.

DESIRABLE CHARACTERISTICS FOR A PAIN CLINIC

1. A pain clinic should have access to and regular interaction with at least three types of medical specialties or health care providers. If one of the physicians is not a psychiatrist, a clinical psychologist is essential.

2. The health care providers should communicate with each other on a regular basis both about individual patients and programs offered in the pain treatment facility.

3. There should be a director or coordinator of the pain clinic. If he or she is not a physician, there should be a director of medical services who is responsible for the monitoring of medical services which are provided to the patients.

4. The pain clinic should offer both diagnostic and therapeutic services.

5. The pain clinic should have designated space for its activities.

6. The pain clinic should maintain records on its patients so as to be able to assess individual treatment outcomes and to evaluate overall program effectiveness.

7. The pain clinic should have adequate support staff to carry out its activities.

8. Health care providers working in a pain clinic should have appropriate knowledge of both the basic sciences and clinical practices relevant to pain patients.

9. The pain clinic should have a trained health care professional available to deal with patient referrals and emergencies.

10. All health care providers in a pain clinic should be appropriately licensed in the country and state in which they practice.

References

1. Carr DB, Aronoff GM. The future of pain management. In: Aronoff GM, ed. Evaluation and treatment of chronic pain. 2nd ed. Baltimore: Williams & Wilkins, 1992.

2. Campbell JN, ed. Pain 1996: an updated review. Seattle: IASP Press, 1996.

3. Munglani R, Hunt SP. Molecular biology of pain. Br J Anaesth 1995;75:186–192.

4. Coderre TJ, Katz J, Vaccarino AL, Melzack R. Contribution of central neuroplasticity to pathological pain. Pain 1993;52:259–285.

5. Carr DB, Cousins MJ. Spinal route of analgesia: opioids and future options. In: Cousins MJ, Bridenbaugh PO, eds. Neural blockade in clinical anesthesia and management of pain. ed. 3. Philadelphia: Lippincott-Raven, 1998.

6. Bero L, Rennie D. The Cochrane collaboration: preparing, maintaining, and disseminating the results of systematic reviews of the effects of health care. JAMA 1995;274:1935–1938.

7. Carr DB, Cousins MJ. Trends in pain management 1987–1996: an evidence-based survey. Curr Opinion Anesthesiol 1997;10:xliii–xlvi.

8. Schug SA, Large R G. Opioids for chronic noncancer pain. Pain Clin Updates 1995;3:1–4.

9. Haddox JD, Joranson D, Angarola RT, et al. The use of opioids for the treatment of chronic pain. AAPM/APS, 1997:1–4.

10. Bootman LJ, Townsend RJ, McGhan WF, eds. Principles of pharmacoeconomics. 2nd ed. Cincinnati: Whitney, 1995.

11. Langley PC. Pharmacoeconomics and the quality of decision-making by pharmacy and therapeutics committees. Am J Health Syst Pharm 1995;52:S24.

12. Spilker B, ed. Quality of life in clinical trials. New York: Raven, 1990.

13. Jacox A, Carr DB, Mahrenholz D M, Ferrell. Cost considerations in patient-controlled analgesia. Pharmacoeconomics 1997;12:109–120.

14. Drummond M F. Cost-of-illness studies: a major headache. Pharmacoeconomics 1992;2:1–2.

15. Aronoff GM. What is happening to medicine? Clin J Pain 1988;4:65–66.

16. Aronoff GM. The future of pain management. Clin J Pain 1986;2:77.

17. Carr DB. Evidence, explanation—or "the power of myth." Curr Opin Anesthesiol 1996;9:415–420.

18. Aronoff GM. Where have we been? Where are we now? Where are we going? Clin J Pain 1997;13:3–5.

19. Lorente de No R. Analysis of the activity of the chains of internuncial neurons. J Neurophysiol 1938;1:207–244.

20. Dubner R. Neuronal basis of persistent pain: sensory specialization, sensory modulation, and neuronal plasticity. In: Jensen T S, Turner J A, Wiesenfeld-Hallin, eds. Seattle: IASP Press, 1997.

21. Carr DB. Opioids. In: Firestone L L, ed. Molecular basis of drug action in anesthesia. Int Anesth Clin 1988;26:273–287.

22. Mantyh PW, DeMaster E, Malhotra A, et al. Receptor endocytosis and dendrite reshaping in spinal neurons after somatosensory stimulation. Science 1995;268:1629–1632.

23. Dahl JB. The status of pre-emptive analgesia. Curr Opin Anesthesiol 1995;8:323–330.

24. Kissin I. Preemptive analgesia: why its effect is not always obvious. Anesthesiology 1996;84:1015–1019.

25. Hunt SP, Pini A, Evan G. Induction of c-fos-like protein in spinal cord neurones following sensory stimulation. Nature 1987;240:1328–1331.

26. Dubner R, Ruda MA. Activity-dependent neuronal plasticity following tissue injury and inflammation. Trends Neurosci 1992;15:96–103.

27. Morgan JI, Curran T. Role of ion flux in the control of c-fos expression. Nature 1986;322:552–555.

28. Reference deleted.

29. Draisci G, Iadorola MJ. Temporal analysis of increases in c-fos, preprodynorphin and preproenkephalin mRNAs in rat spinal cord. Mol Brain Res 1989;6:31–37.

30. Lima D, Esteves F, Coimbra A. C-fos activation by noxious input of spinal neurons projecting to the nucleus of the tractus solitarius in the rat. In: Gebhart GF, Hammond DL, Jensen TS, eds. Proceedings of the VII World Congress on Pain. Seattle: IASP Press, 1994.

31. Ruda MA, Iadorola MJ, Cohen LV, Young WS. In situ hybridization histochemistry and immunohistochemistry reveal an increase in spinal dynorphin biosynthesis in a rat model of inflammation and hyperalgesia. Proc Natl Acad Sci U S A 1988;85:622–626.

32. Gogas KR, Presley RW, Levine JD, Basbaum AI. The antinociceptive action of supraspinal opioids results from an increase in descending inhibitory control: correlation of nociceptive behavior and c-fos expression. Neuroscience 1991;42:617–628.

33. Coderre TJ, Melzack R. Central neural mediators of secondary hyperalgesia following heat injury to rats: neuropeptides and excitatory amino acids. Neurosci Lett 1991;131:71–74.

34. Dickenson AH. Spinal cord pharmacology of pain. Br J Anaesth 1995;75:193–200.

35. Yaksh TL, Malmberg AB. Interaction of spinal modulatory receptor systems. In: Fields H L, Liebeskind J C, eds. Pharmacological approaches to the treatment of chronic pain: new concepts and critical issues. Seattle: IASP Press, 1994.

36. Price DD, Mao J, Mayer DJ. Central neural mechanisms of normal and abnormal pain states. In: Fields H L, Liebeskind J C, eds. Pharmacological approaches to the treatment of chronic pain: new concepts and critical issues. Seattle: IASP Press, 1994.

37. Dougherty PM, Willis W D. Enhancement of spinothalamic neuron responses to chemical and mechanical stimuli following combined micro-iontophoretic application of N-methyl-D-aspartic acid and substance P. Pain 1991;47:85–93.

38. Klepstad P, Maurset A, Moberg ER, Oye I. Evidence of a role for NMDA receptors in pain perception. Eur J Pharmacol 1990;187:513–518.

39. Yaksh TL. Epidural ketamine: a useful, mechanistically novel adjuvant for epidural morphine? Reg Anesth 1996;21:508–13.

40. Davar G, Hama A, Deykin A, et al. MK-801 blocks the development of thermal hyperalgesia in a rat model of experimental painful neuropathy. Brain Res 1991;553:327–330.

41. Dickenson AH. NMDA receptor antagonists as analgesics. In: Fields HL, Liebeskind JC, eds. Pharmacological approaches to the treatment of chronic pain: new concepts and critical issues. Seattle: IASP Press, 1994.

42. Mao J, Price DD, Mayer DJ. Thermal hyperalgesia in association with the development of morphine tolerance in rats: roles of excitatory amino acid receptors and protein kinase C. J Neurosci 1994;14:2301–2312.

43. Dickenson AH. Pharmacology of pain transmission and control. In: Campbell JN, ed. Pain 1996: an updated review. Seattle: IASP Press, 1996:113–121.

44. Meller ST, Gebhart GF. Nitric oxide (NO) and nociceptive processing in the spinal cord. Pain 1993;52:127–136.

45. Basbaum AI. Insights into the development of morphine tolerance. Pain 1995;61:349–352.

46. Mao J, Price DD, Mayer DJ. Experimental mononeuropathy reduces the antinociceptive effects of morphine: implications for the common intracellular mechanisms involved in morphine tolerance and pain. Pain 1995;61:353–364.

47. Przewlocki R, Machelska H, Przewlocka B. Inhibition of nitric oxide synthase enhances morphine antinociception in the rat spinal cord. Life Sciences 1993;53:1–5.

48. Kolesnikov YA, Pick CG, Cisweska G, Pasternak GW. Blockade of tolerance to morphine but not kappa opioids by a nitric oxide synthase inhibitor. Proc Natl Acad U S A 1993;90:5162–5166.

49. Berde CB. The treatment of pain in children. Pain 1990;5(Suppl):S3.

50. Fitzgerald M. The developmental biology of pain. Pain 1990;5(Suppl):S1.

51. McGrath P. Assessment of pain in children. Pain 1990;5(suppl):S2.

52. Selye H. A syndrome produced by diverse nocuous agents. Nature 1936;138:32.

53. Bromage PR. Spinal epidural analgesia. Baltimore: Williams & Wilkins, 1954.

54. Keeri-Szanto M, Heaman S. Postoperative demand analgesia. Surg Gynecol Obstet 1972;134:647–651.

55. Payne R. Novel routes of opioid administration. In: Hill C S, Fields HL, eds. Advances in pain research and therapy, vol. 11. New York: Raven, 1989.

56. McCormack K. Non-steroidal anti-inflammatory drugs and spinal nociceptive processing. Pain 1994;59:9–43.

57. Mitchell JA, Akaraseenont P, Thiermann C, et al. Selectivity of nonsteroidal anti-inflammatory drugs as inactivators of constitutive and inducible cyclooxygenase. Proc Natl Acad Sci U S A 1994;90:11693–11697.

58. Kopp E, Ghosh S. Inhibition of NF-kB by sodium salicylate and aspirin. Science 1994;265:956–959.

59. Porreca F, Bilsky EJ, Lai J. Pharmacological characterization of opioid delta and kappa receptors. In: Tseng L F, ed. The pharmacology of opioid peptides. Langhorne, PA: Harwood, 1995.

60. Miotto K, Magendzo K, Evans CJ. Molecular characterization of opioid receptors. In: Tseng LF, ed. The pharmacology of opioid peptides. Langhorne, PA: Harwood, 1995.

61. Kehlet H. Postoperative pain relief (1994): a look from the other side. Reg Anesth 1994;19:369–377.

62. DuPen SL, Ramsey DH. Compounding local anesthetics and narcotics for epidural analgesia in cancer out-patients. Anesthesiology 1988;69:A405.

63. Aronoff GM. The disability epidemic. Clin J Pain 1989;5:203–204.

64. Kroussel-Wood MA. Winds of change. JAMA 1990;263:3085.

65. Brame JB. Federal practice guidelines and clinical autonomy. Texas Med 1990;86:65–67.

66. Eddy DM. Designing a practice policy: standards, guidelines, and options. JAMA 1990;263:3077–3084.

67. Miaskowski C. Effective cancer pain management: from guidelines to quality improvement. Pain: Clinical Updates 1994;2:1–4.

68. Begg C, Cho M, Eastwood S, et al. Improving the quality of reporting of randomized controlled trials: the CONSORT statement. JAMA 1996;276:637–9.

69. International Association for the Study of Pain: Desirable characteristics for pain treatment facilities and standards for physician fellowship in pain management. Seattle: IASP, 1990.

70. Fields HL, ed. Core curriculum for professional education in pain, ed. 2. Seattle: IASP, 1990.

71. Loeser JD, Egan KJ, eds. Managing the chronic pain patient: theory and practice at the University of Washington Multidisciplinary Pain Center. New York: Raven, 1989.

72. Commission on Accreditation of Rehabilitation Facilities: Program evaluation in chronic pain management programs. Tucson: CARF, 1987.

73. Melzack R. The tragedy of needless pain: a call for social action. In: Dubner R, Gebhart GF, Bond MR, eds. Proceedings of the V World Congress on Pain. New York: Elsevier, 1988.

74. Jones JG. The future of anesthesia. In: Keneally J P, Jones M R, eds. 150 years on: a selection of papers presented at the XI World Congress of Anaesthesiologists. London: World Federation of Societies of Anesthesiologists, 1996.

Suggested Reading

Aronoff GM, Sweet W. The future of pain management. In: Aronoff G M, ed. Evaluation and treatment of chronic pain. 1st ed. Baltimore: Urban & Schwarzenberg, 1985.

Cousins MJ. Prevention of postoperative pain. Pain 1990; 5(Suppl):S220–S221.

International Association for the Study of Pain. Task force guidelines for pain treatment facilities. Seattle: IASP, 1990.

CHAPTER 50

The Future of Pain Medicine

Philipp M. Lippe

THE CHALLENGE

"Dum loquimur, fugerit invida Aetas: carpe diem, quam minimum credula postero." (While we are talking, envious time is fleeting: seize the day, put no trust in the future.)

—Horace, *Odes.*

The preparation of a chapter on the future of the field of pain medicine has been a daunting and formidable challenge. Visions of the future are tenuous and illusory. Predictions are the domain of crystal gazers and prophets. Nevertheless, mindful of the dangers involved, I attempt to explore the future by a journey through the past and present. The focus will be on pain medicine as a specialty. No attempt will be made to predict scientific and technological advances in pain research or clinical practice.

Logically, the quest begins with a series of questions. What is the field of pain medicine? Is it a field in search of a disease process? What are the justifications and rationale for pain medicine as a specialty?

In its official policy statement the American Academy of Pain Medicine (AAPM) defines pain medicine:

The specialty of Pain Medicine is concerned with the prevention, evaluation, diagnosis, treatment, and rehabilitation of painful disorders. Such disorders may have pain and associated symptoms arising from a discrete cause, such as postoperative pain or pain associated with a malignancy, or may be syndromes in which pain constitutes the primary problem, such as neuropathic pains or headaches. The diagnosis of painful syndromes relies on interpretation of historical data; review of previous laboratory, imaging, and electrodiagnostic studies; behavioral, social, occupational, and avocational assessment; interview and examination by the pain specialist; and may require specialized diagnostic procedures, including central and peripheral neuro-blockade or monitored drug infusions. The special needs of the pediatric and geriatric populations are considered when formulating a comprehensive treatment plan for these patients.

The pain physician serves as a consultant to other physicians, but is often the principal treating physician and may provide care at various levels, such as direct treatment, prescribing medication, prescribing rehabilitative services, performing pain relieving procedures, counseling of patients and families, [directing a] multidisciplinary team, [coordinating] care with other health care providers, and [providing] consultative services to public and private agencies pursuant to optimal health care delivery to the patient suffering from a painful disorder. The pain physician may work in a variety of settings and is competent to treat the entire range of painful disorders encountered in the delivery of quality health care.

This definition is precise and comprehensive. But is it credible?

Other questions must be asked. What challenges, obstacles, and threats must be faced by pain medicine? What is its perceived value in the scientific, socioeconomic, and political arenas? Does pain medicine as a field have a future? And, most important, should it have a future? The answer to all of these questions is that it depends. While such an answer is simple and correct, it is, of course, useless. To seek a more meaningful answer it is necessary to explore the evolution of the field of pain medicine from the perspective of an emergent specialty.

THE PAST: LESSONS OF HISTORY

"I know no way of judging of the future but by the past."

—*Patrick Henry.*

Indeed, since the lessons of the past shape the realities of the future, it is appropriate to reflect on the management of painful disorders over the course of time. The intent is not to develop a detailed history of the field of pain medicine but rather to provide an adequate background to frame the discussion. In the most reductionistic sense, the management of painful disorders can be categorized as developing in three transitional epochs: pain as an unpleasant and undesirable consequence of bodily transgressions with connotations of wrongdoing and purification; pain as a manifestation of tissue pathology consistent with clinicopathological concepts of the traditional biomedical model; and pain as a unique human experience, a multifactorial entity with biopsychosocial components.

Since the beginning of time, pain and suffering have been ubiquitous and perpetual components of human nature. The word pain derives from Greek and Latin terms for penalty. Pain was often regarded as a punishment for transgressions. Not surprisingly, the treatment often was within the domain of priests, faith healers, witch doctors, and shamans, as well as practitioners of the learned healing arts. Pharmacological, physical, and spiritual remedies were employed to relieve suffering. Demons were exorcised. Compassion and passage of time became important allies. Emphasis clearly was on palliative relief. The healers of the time were mindful of an admonition later expressed by Voltaire: "The artful physician entertains the patient while nature effects a cure."

The age of enlightenment and the industrial revolution ushered in unprecedented advances in science and technology. The Renaissance saw the emergence of the biomedical model based on clinicopathological concepts. Pain was considered a nociceptive response to bodily injury consistent with cartesian thinking. Pain was considered more than mere punishment administered by the penal system for wrongdoing; it was also a means of deliverance and purgation in a theological sense. Pain was part of life. Pain built character and redeemed the soul.

During the early decades of the 20th century, aided in large measure by the Flexner report, traditional scientific medicine gained dominance in the healing arts. The biomedical model became the cornerstone of medical science. Pain was still regarded as a symptomatic response to a nociceptive generator in accordance with the cartesian paradigm. Medical specialties developed and flourished in response to rapid advances in physiology, pharmacology, neurosciences and surgical techniques. The battle injuries of World War I stimulated increasing interest in the understanding and management of pain problems. Physicians specializing in neurology and neurological surgery, recognizing the importance of the nervous system in pain transmission and perception, developed pain-alleviating procedures. Advances in anesthesiology ensured effective pharmacological pain relief and in turn permitted more advanced surgical techniques. Certain medical specialties became more involved in the treatment of disease-related pain. Emphasis had shifted to the neuroanatomical and neurophysiological substrate of pain. Sir William Osler cautioned, "It is not nearly so important as what disease a patient has, as what patient has the disease."

The neurosurgeon René Leriche became the godfather of the field of modern pain medicine when in 1937 he recognized pain as an illness rather than a symptom. His concept, however, was eclipsed by World War II. War casualties once again focused attention on injury- and disease-related pain. Scientific knowledge and technical progress advanced rapidly. In the mid-20th century John Bonica, an anesthesiologist, successfully bridged the conceptual chasm between pain as a symptom of disease or injury and pain as a complex human experience. He emphasized the psychosocial aspects of pain and pioneered the multispecialty interdisciplinary model of concurrent pain management. His pioneering efforts culminated in the publication of a textbook in 1953 and the establishment of the International Association for the Study of Pain (IASP) in 1975.

Recognition of the multidimensional elements of pain problems resulted in escalating interest in the field among certain specialties such as neurosurgery, anesthesiology, psychiatry, neurology, and physical medicine and rehabilitation. In large measure, these specialties were responsible for research, education, and clinical practice in pain management and the development of supporting organizational efforts. An expanding body of knowledge gave rise to subspecialization in pain management.

Certain specialties and subspecialties claimed ownership of pain management. Struggles of control and ownership within the profession raised hopes of enhanced status and employment opportunities. The increasing involvement of medical specialties and subspecialties in pain management resulted in fragmentation of the field and gave rise to unhealthy competition. The concurrent multispecialty approach to the management of pain disorders encouraged a "management by committee" approach with unpredictable results, unwarranted interventions, and escalating health care costs. Voltaire, in prophetic wisdom, stated: "Doctors pour drugs of which they know little to treat diseases of which they know less into human beings of which they know nothing." In the 1980s a group of physicians, reflecting on Osler's admonition, reaffirmed the concept of pain as a multifactorial entity with biopsychosocial components. The scene was set for the emergence of pain medicine as a specialty and the foundation of the American Academy of Pain Medicine (AAPM).

THE PRESENT: PAIN MEDICINE AS A SPECIALTY

"Those who talk about the future are scoundrels. It is the present that matters."

—*Louis Ferdinand Destouches,*
Journey to the End of the Night, *1932.*

Pain medicine is a unique medical field characterized by a distinct body of knowledge and a defined scope of practice, with an infrastructure based on scientific research and education. The specialty of pain medicine is acknowledged by medical organizations, regulatory agencies, and third party payors. It is founded on the basic concept that pain is a complex, multifactorial entity, an illness, with biopsychosocial components.

The Concepts and Dimensions of Pain Medicine

Recognition of the difference between pain as a symptom and pain as an illness is essential to the understanding of the field of pain medicine. Injury- or disease-related pain is predominantly a symptomatic response to a nociceptive stimulus, particularly in acute cases. Such "normal" or physiological pain, considered beneficial, can be described as *eudynia*. It serves as an early warning device, alerting the individual to potential tissue damage. Generally such pain is commensurate with the underlying somatic pathology. It responds to palliative measures and abates as the underlying somatic problem improves.

Persistent or intractable pain results in the development of "abnormal" pain. Such nonphysiological or pathological pain has no appreciable beneficial effect and can be described as *maldynia*. It is the result of a series of pathophysiological changes. Neuropathic, psychopathic, and musculoskeletal changes all become secondary pain generators. Aggravated by sociopathic changes, pain becomes a chronic, self-sustaining entity. Such nonphysiological pain cannot be directly correlated with any underlying somatic pathology, if indeed such pathology can be even delineated. Interventions focused on somatopathology are doomed to failure and are likely to aggravate the pain problem. Understanding this concept requires appreciation and acceptance of a paradigm shift from pain regarded as the consequence of a syndrome of disease-related comorbidities to pain regarded as an illness unique to human experience.

The historical transition of pain management over three epochs has been described. Similarly, medical management of pain problems can be categorized into three stages. Just as ontogeny recapitulates phylogeny, clinical practice recapitulates historical development.

Primary Stage

The physiological pain of nociception alerts the person to actual or potential tissue damage. It impels a patient to seek medical attention. The situation is usually acute, and the pain generally can be easily correlated with the somatopathology. Pain is relieved by palliative treatment of symptoms. Pain management at this stage is within the domain of most clinical practitioners.

Secondary Stage

Many chronic diseases, such as malignant disorders, acquired immunodeficiency syndrome, neurological disorders, progressive arthritic changes, and metabolic disorders are associated with persistent pain. Although the pain still correlates reasonably well with the underlying somatopathology, the nociceptive component is complicated by psychosocial and socioeconomic factors. Suffering compounds pain, and palliation is no longer adequate. Management at this stage focuses on illness-related pain and modality-focused treatment. This falls within the domain of physicians with specific subspecialty interests and expertise in pain management.

Tertiary Stage

Maldynia resulting from a cascade of pathophysiological changes becomes an entity no longer directly correlated to the precipitating or persistent somatopathology. When psychosocial components become predominant, pain and suffering become an all-encompassing phenomenon that often is self-perpetuating. The entity persists in the face of underlying pathological processes that have been adequately treated or are no longer demonstrable. Pain is no longer explained within the clinicopathological framework. Its evaluation and management at this stage are within the domain of specialists in pain medicine.

Criteria for a Medical Specialty

The American Board of Medical Specialties (ABMS) defines a medical specialty as "a defined area of medical practice which connotes special knowledge and ability resulting from specialized effort and training in the special field [which] may entail special concern with the problems of patients according to age, sex, organ systems or with the interaction between patients and their environment." A primary medical specialty may incorporate areas of knowledge of one or more other primary specialties; however, the specialty must include a core body of knowledge that is unique and distinct from other specialties. Pain medicine satisfies this definition of a primary medical specialty.

Pain medicine acknowledges its origins from contributions of many specialty fields such as neurosurgery, anesthesiology, psychiatry, and others. However, the specialty has a "soul," or essence, that is unique and distinct from all other specialties. The whole is greater than the sum of its parts.

The ABMS defines a medical subspecialty as "an identifiable component of a specialty to which a practicing physician may devote a significant proportion of time." A subspecialty focuses on a specific segment of the primary specialty. Additional training, education, and experience are required to gain competence in the subspecialty area. However, the subspecialty always must incorporate the totality of the core knowledge contained in the primary specialty, to which it is inexorably linked. The subspecialty of pain management within the field of anesthesiology is an example.

The delineation of a new primary medical specialty depends on common usage within the medical community and general societal acceptance using a new lexicon and terms of art. The criteria include the following:

- A title and definition of the medical specialty as established by common usage and as accepted by the medical, scientific, and lay communities
- A foundation of a scientifically validated information base including basic and clinical research published in indexed, peer-reviewed journals
- Consensus within the medical community that a period of additional specialized training and experience is necessary to become proficient in the specialty
- Professional organizations that promote research, training, continuing education, and scholarly activities within the specialty
- Administrative recognition of the specialty

Pain medicine as a specialty meets all of these criteria. Clinical practice in the field is supported by an understructure of research, education, and administrative organizations. Research in pain medicine is conducted at the basic and clinical levels, at academic centers, and at comprehensive pain centers. Education in the practice of pain medicine can be found at the undergraduate, graduate, and postgraduate levels. Continuing medical education is supported by numerous professional courses, awarding Category I Accreditation Council for Continuing Medical Education (ACCME) credits. The pain literature includes textbooks and journals.

The American Academy of Pain Medicine (AAPM), founded in 1983 as the American Academy of Algology, is the nation's only educational and professional organization of and for physicians specializing in pain medicine. The academy represents more than 1200 physician-members dedicated to relieving pain. Recognized by the American Medical Association (AMA) as the specialty society representing physicians in pain medicine, the academy has a seat in the House of Delegates of the AMA. Its mission is to provide for quality care to patients suffering with pain and to promote the advancement pain medicine as a specialty. *The Clinical Journal of Pain* is the official journal of the AAPM.

Societal Imperatives

It is widely recognized that societal needs for cost-effective relief of pain and suffering are not being adequately addressed by the medical profession. This is particularly relevant in the management of pain at the tertiary stage.

This problem has been addressed in a position paper by the AAPM. Tragically, pain, physiological and nonphysiological, frequently goes untreated, or worse, is mistreated, resulting in complications often more severe than the original condition. This has created a health care problem reaching epidemic proportions in this country. More than 50 million people in this country suffer from chronic pain to the extent that they are partially or totally disabled. Fully a third of the population reports pain of some degree on a chronic basis. Sometime during their lifetime 45% of the population will seek medical help for persistent pain problems. Productivity

losses to the national economy as a result of chronic pain are estimated in tens of billions of dollars. The annual cost of chronic pain is estimated at $100 billion. More than 70% of cancer patients have moderate to severe pain during their illness, but fewer than half of these receive adequate treatment for their pain. Improper care of pain becomes an assembly line of costly find-and-fix treatments, including unnecessary, ineffective, and harmful interventions.

Sequential, fragmented, ineffective services or "management by committee" often leads to dependence on the health care system, consumption of inordinate amounts of limited health care resources, and secondary health consequences for patients who already have unbearable pain. The properly trained specialist in pain medicine often first sees the patient when he or she has reached the end of the line. These unfortunate circumstances have been addressed in numerous studies and publications by the Institute of Medicine (IOM), the Health Care Financing Agency (HCFA), the Social Security Administration (SSA), the AMA, and the Agency for Health Care Policy and Research (AHCPR). Consistently all studies have concluded that chronic pain should be attended in a more thorough and systematic fashion. Physicians specializing in pain medicine are needed to advance research, education, and clinical practice in the field.

There is a rising public perception that traditional medicine has failed to provide effective and compassionate relief of pain. Undoubtedly this contributes to the multibillion-dollar alternative care industry largely supported by patients with unremitting pain who have failed to find satisfaction with contemporary traditional care. Articles in medical publications by the AMA and others have noted that physician-assisted suicide would be less of an issue if adequate and appropriate specialists in pain medicine were more numerous, more available, and more accessible.

There is a consensus among experts that an oversupply of physicians in the United States is imminent, at least with respect to certain specialties. The problem is compounded by maldistribution. Paradoxically, the field of pain medicine lacks adequate workforce resources to meet the needs of the public.

The American College of Surgeons recently noted in an editorial that as physicians in certain specialties increase in numbers, they tend to move into subspecialties to accommodate the burgeoning number of physicians and ensure a stronger economic base. Unfortunately, a fixed or decreasing patient base results in inadequate concentration of patients to support some of these subspecialties. As the frequency of patient visits decreases, subspecialty physicians are threatened by perceptions of decreasing experience, proficiency, and competency. Physicians unable to sustain an active practice in a subspecialty field will be driven to devote an increasing amount of time to their primary specialty field, thereby further eroding their proficiency in the subspecialty. The editorial notes that "one might ask whether additional subspecialization at this particular time will prove to be advantageous to the medical practitioner...to our changing health care system, or to the patient. . . .So far, the so called marketplace has not enthusiastically encouraged isolated subspecialists to practice only in their limited area of treatment. Indeed, many payors simply do not have a large enough volume of patients to support very narrowly defined subspecialties."

These reflections are relevant to the burgeoning rolls of physicians subspecializing in pain management in contrast to the paucity of physicians specializing in the primary field of pain medicine.

In addition to workforce issues, physicians practicing in pain medicine must cope with other trends in health care affecting the entire medical profession. These include a progressive downward pressure on reimbursement, professional liability issues, managed care and capitation, restricted patient access to physicians, micromanagement of practice, and restrictions on patient advocacy.

Medical Specialty Board Certification

Board certification in a medical specialty is regarded as a primary measure of competency, achieving the goals of public accountability and professional credibility. The ABMS is generally regarded as the standard for medical specialty board certification in this country. Founded in 1915 as the Advisory Board for Medical Specialties, it is composed of 24 primary specialties and more than 70 subspecialties. The ABMS maintains rigid standards for approval of new specialty boards.

In addition to the ABMS member boards, there are approximately 120 medical specialty boards not affiliated with the ABMS. These non-ABMS boards have requirements that range from minimal or no requirements to rigid requirements, emulating those by ABMS member boards.

The American Board of Pain Medicine (ABPM) was founded in 1991 as the American College of Pain Medicine. In 1994 the name was changed to be consistent with the nomenclature of other medical specialty boards. The mission of the ABPM is to serve the public by improving the quality of pain medicine as a specialty. Its goals are to evaluate candidates who voluntarily appear for examination and to certify as diplomates in pain medicine those who are qualified, to maintain and improve the quality of graduate medical education in pain medicine by collaborating with related organizations, and to provide information about the specialty of pain medicine to the public. From its inception the ABPM has maintained high standards for certification. These include the following:

- Possession of a current valid and unrestricted license to practice medicine
- Successful completion of a graduate residency training program accredited by the Accreditation Council for Graduate Medical Education (ACGME)
- Certification by an ABMS member board
- A minimum of 2 years of clinical practice in the field of pain medicine following completion of formal residency training

- Continuing medical education in the field of pain medicine, with a minimum requirement of 50 hours of ACCME-approved Category I credits that must be obtained within the 2 years preceding the examination.
- Two letters of reference
- Successful completion of an 8-hour psychometrically validated written examination

Since 1992 the ABPM has administered yearly examinations. It has enjoyed a robust growth during its tenure and has approximately 1000 diplomates. For a number of years the state of California has recognized potential problems related to medical specialty boards not affiliated with the ABMS. Recognizing the wide variation in eligibility requirements among non-ABMS boards, the state licensing agency, the Medical Board of California (MBC), has become increasingly concerned about its consumer protection mandate. Several years ago California enacted legislation having a direct bearing on medical specialty boards. Under California law, making a claim of board certification is allowed and considered appropriate, provided the certifying medical specialty board is recognized as "legitimate." A bona fide specialty board is defined by law as an ABMS member board or one approved by the MBC as "equivalent." In 1994 the American Board of Pain Medicine submitted its application to the MBC. After extensive and prolonged evaluation, the MBC found the ABPM to be a bona fide legitimate certifying body with legal status equivalent to that of ABMS member boards. To date the ABPM is only one of three medical specialty boards to gain such recognition. Confident of its strength and integrity, the ABPM is in the process of submitting its application to the ABMS for approval as a member board.

Competent accredited training in the specialty of pain medicine is essential to the viability of the specialty. Several years ago the ABPM, in cooperation with the AAPM, created a joint Graduate Medical Education Task Force (GMETF) for the purpose of reviewing graduate and postgraduate training programs in the specialty of pain medicine. The GMETF, in cooperation with the Training Program Review Committee (TPRC), has developed a comprehensive graduate program. The essentials of accredited training programs in graduate medical education can be found in *Institutional and Program Requirements for Pain Medicine Training Programs,* which has been approved and published by the ABPM. The proposed requirements envision a transition from a 1- or 2-year fellowship training program through a 2-year combined residency program and eventually to a fully developed 4-year intrinsic residency program.

THE FUTURE: WISHFUL THINKING OR WISH FULFILLMENT

"Who controls the past controls the future. Who controls the present controls the past."

—*George Orwell, 1984.*

Pain medicine as a specialty is proud of its rich heritage. It has enjoyed healthy growth. It anticipates a bright future. And yet a number of questions must be answered, a number of concerns must be addressed, and a number of problems must be resolved. Some of the many issues that must be pondered are the epidemiology of pain; predisposing factors; preventive measures; the neurophysiology and neuropathology of pain transmission, modulation and perception; the pathophysiology contributing to the transformation from eudynia to maldynia; the measurement, verification, and objective validation of pain; more effective pharmacological and nonpharmacological interventions; the proper use of opioids; the psychodynamics involved in pain; improved understanding of neurophysiology and the role of the autonomic nervous system; the role of alternative medicine; the development of cost-effective therapy protocols; the credible rating of impairment and disability related to pain. A national dialog, intramural and extramural, is necessary to address these various issues. Failure to do so may threaten the viability of pain medicine as a specialty. Its perceived bright future may be nothing more than the last flicker of a dying ember.

The Meaning of Pain

The development of a cogent, comprehensive, and consensual concept of pain is a matter of the highest priority. Success in this area will almost certainly ensure the future of pain medicine as a specialty. Failure, on the other hand, will weaken the specialty and may very well threaten its viability. Of the many definitions of pain, the one proposed by the IASP remains the most durable and popular. Inherent in the definition are the concepts that pain is a subjective, unpleasant, emotional experience generally associated with the perception of tissue damage. Despite such definitions, ambiguity and ambivalence about pain, prevalent in the past 2 centuries, persist.

Modern traditional medicine is rooted in scientific evidence-based methodology. The concept of pain has not found a comfortable niche in the biomedical or clinicopathological model. In this frame of reference, it is all too easy to dichotomize pain as either related to identifiable tissue pathology, hence real, or reflective of an emotional disorder, hence not real or at best, suspect. Pain is regarded by many as always psychological. Conversely, it is regarded by some as the result of afferent and efferent events within the nervous system. Neither reductionism encompasses the reality of pain as a human experience.

In clinical practice, pain is generally regarded as a syndrome resulting from disease-related comorbidities rather than a distinct multifactorial entity. The conceptual differences of eudynia and maldynia are generally not understood or accepted.

A medical field with an ill-defined understanding of its main object can demand neither respect nor recognition. Such a field will have difficulty legitimizing the claim of a true medical specialty. Consequently, it is necessary for the opinion leaders in the field of pain medicine to come together and develop an understanding and consensual agreement about pain. Only then can practitioners in the specialty of pain medicine hope to convince the medical profession and society of its legitimacy.

The concept of maldynia as a unique multifactorial entity is alien to traditional scientific medicine rooted in the clinicopathological model. Bridging the chasm requires a difficult paradigm shift. Fortunately, advances in basic science in the areas of immunology, neurophysiology, and neurochemistry are demonstrating identifiable indicators linked to pain. Perhaps the dichotomy between pain as a biopsychosocial entity and the clinicopathological model of scientific medicine is more apparent than real. Perhaps pain, particularly maldynia, can by justified in the context of the biomedical model.

Pain Medicine As a Specialty

Pain medicine meets all the criteria for a specialty. Its scope of practice and body of knowledge have been well defined. It is recognized as a specialty field by the AMA, by the medical profession at large, and by most sectors of society. Nevertheless, its vision and mission are not always well understood. If pain medicine as a specialty is to sustain its credibility and achieve wider acceptance, it will be necessary to mount increasing efforts of advocacy and representation. It is necessary to have interactive dialog with organized medicine at all levels, with allied health fields, with governmental and regulatory agencies, with employers and third party payors, with the academic community, and with all stakeholders in society.

Fragmentation of the specialty is a major threat. In part, this is a result of a lack of understanding of the specialty of pain medicine and its relation to the various subspecialties of pain management. However, it is difficult to ignore the perception that the claim of ownership of pain by many subspecialties is driven by visions of power and financial reward rather than allegiance to scientific accuracy. An undivided and united specialty of pain medicine is necessary to sustain research, education, and clinical practice in the field.

A medical specialty depends on a professional membership organization that represents the specialty and is devoted to advancing research, education, and clinical practice in the field on behalf of society at large and its members. The AAPM fulfills this need and obligation for physicians in the specialty and the patients they serve. Continued growth is a necessity to maintain human and financial resources and to avoid stagnation and indifference. The retention and recruitment of loyal, supportive, involved, and dedicated members are the lifeblood of a professional organization. The development of knowledgeable, energetic, committed and industrious physicians in leadership positions ensures the success of a volunteer member organization.

Research and Education

Ongoing research and education supporting clinical practice are essential to the viability of any medical specialty. This is an area of particular concern in the face of the diminishing availability of requisite funding.

Basic and clinical research in the field of pain medicine must be supported. The many areas to address include the epidemiology and genetics of pain; the pathophysiological changes associated with pain at all stages; and the immunological, neurophysiological, and neurochemical changes associated with persistent pain. Clinical studies are necessary to assess the psychodynamics of pain, to define reliable and objective measures validating pain, to develop effective pharmacological and nonpharmacological interventions, and to assess the efficacy and safety of surgical and nonsurgical procedures.

Only by actively supporting such research can one hope to advance the science of pain medicine. Success in this area will ensure acceptance of the specialty by a medical community that insists on scientifically validated, evidence-based methodology.

Education in the field of pain medicine at the undergraduate, graduate, and postgraduate levels is sadly wanting. Despite the fact that most practicing clinicians are confronted daily by patients suffering pain, medical students have virtually no exposure to the tenets of pain evaluation and management. Except for limited circumstances in certain specialties, physicians in residency programs receive virtually no training in the effective management of pain. Most postgraduate, postresidency programs maintain a subspecialty focus. Many of these programs have a disease-related, modality-oriented bias that emphasizes procedural intervention.

The specialty of pain medicine recognizes the need for comprehensive training in the field. Its vision is to create a comprehensive 4-year accredited residency program in the field of pain medicine. Given the present economic, bureaucratic, and political realities, this will not be an easy undertaking. It is anticipated that the goal can be reached only through the establishment of a graduated program that will make the transition through several phases. Initially, 1-and 2-year postresidency fellowship programs will be established. The next step will be to develop a 2-year residency program in pain medicine as a specialty preceded by 2 years of residency training in a related specialty. The final step will be the establishment of a full 4-year residency program in pain medicine.

Continuing competency in the field following formal training is essential. This can best be ensured by continuing medical education. Numerous conferences, seminars, and meetings offering ACCME-accredited Category I credits are already available. The AAPM provides a comprehensive review course in the field of pain medicine in conjunction with its annual meeting. Such educational opportunities are supplemented by a body of literature including books and journals devoted to the field of pain medicine. It is imperative that apathy and indifference not be allowed to erode existing educational facilities.

Board Certification

Medical specialty board certification is considered a primary indicator of public accountability and professional cred-

ibility. From a practical perspective, board certification is virtually essential for a successful medical practice. Academic and hospital appointments rely on board certification. Participation in workers compensation systems and managed care organizations depend on board certification. Clinical privileges are determined by board certification. The legal system generally inquires about board certification. Indeed, board certification has become a "medical passport" without which entry into clinical practice is difficult or impossible.

The ABPM is a medical specialty certifying board with rigorous requirements. At present it is not affiliated with the ABMS but is recognized by the state of California as being "legitimate" and "equivalent" to an ABMS-member board. Recognizing that the ABMS is generally accepted as the standard in medical board certification and that some members of the public and the profession have difficulty distinguishing between legitimate and nonlegitimate unaffiliated boards, the ABPM has submitted its application to the ABMS seeking approval. This is a lengthy and tedious process. Success is by no means a certainty. In the eyes of many, recognition and approval by the ABMS depends as much on bureaucratic and political considerations as on intrinsic merit.

The success of pain medicine as a specialty in large measure depends on recognition of its certifying board by the medical profession, by governmental agencies, and by other stakeholders. Consequently the ABPM must achieve acceptance and recognition either by approval by the ABMS or by other equally effective means.

Clinical Practice

The establishment and survival of a successful clinical practice in pain medicine in an economic and political climate considered by some as distinctly unfriendly depends on variables that merit further consideration. Recognition and acceptance of pain medicine as a specialty and its board certifying process are prerequisites already discussed. Other aspects deserve further comment.

The practice of medicine in a managed care environment brings with it many frustrations and challenges as well as opportunities for innovative practice. Many will find such incursions as micromanagement, restricted patient access, and limitations on patient advocacy virtually intolerable. Conflicts of interest, ethical dilemmas, and renewed threats of professional liability with unique causes of action will impose further burdens on the conscientious practitioner. Successful countermeasures depend on documentation of effective and cost-effective medical care predicated on explicit process and outcome criteria. The Uniform Outcome Measures Project of the AAPM is a unique and successful endeavor that will provide immeasurable help to the practicing pain physician in this regard.

An eroding economic base related to decreasing reimbursement is a considerable concern to many physicians. Many of the difficulties have been blamed on managed care with its emphasis on discounted fees, case payment rates, and capitation. Survival in the face of such economic threats will depend on a good business sense and financial acumen. Professional organizations should support physicians by offering comprehensive practice enhancement seminars. In the long run, the future of the field of pain medicine will depend on providing value and being able to prove it.

Alphanumeric coding of diagnostic impressions and professional services has become the requisite vehicle of communication between physicians and third-party payors, regulatory agencies, and epidemiologists. Current procedural terminology (CPT) by the AMA has become the standard in coding for professional procedures and services. Most of the surgical and nonsurgical procedures performed by pain physicians can be coded with reasonable facility by use of the CPT methodology. The coding of evaluation and management services, including consultations and office visits, is somewhat more cumbersome and arcane. The present coding system makes it difficult or impossible to reflect accurately the work, intensity, and time needed in the evaluation of a patient with a complex pain problem. Consequently it will become necessary to develop additional CPT codes for the purpose of adequate reimbursement as well as accurate data acquisition.

Diagnostic impressions must be encoded according to the International Classification of Diseases, Ninth Revision (ICD-9 CM). For a claim to be considered valid, the ICD-9 code must correlate with the CPT code. Any deviation from this may result in nonreimbursement or even charges of fraud and abuse. This is a unique problem for physicians in the field of pain medicine, inasmuch as there is no ICD-9 code that identifies maldynia, the unique multifactorial entity previously described. Pain physicians must use one of the numerous pain codes catalogued in three columns of the *Index to Diseases*. All of these refer to disease-related pain predicated on tissue pathology consistent with the clinicopathological model. Pain medicine is probably the only specialty that does not have a specific diagnostic code to describe the raison d' être for its specialty. It is inconceivable that the entity pain cannot find a place in a coding system that makes provisions for such events as accidents occurring while launching a spacecraft or as a result of falling from an aircraft without benefit of parachute.

Biomedical ethics pertaining to the field of pain medicine are in need of greater emphasis. These are relevant not only to animal laboratories but also to clinical practice. Principles of beneficence, autonomy, and distributive justice are particularly pertinent to relief of pain and suffering and end-of-life care. Participation in managed care adds another dimension for ethical concern. The specialty of pain medicine is in need of establishing guiding ethical principles over and above those in the AMA Code of Ethics.

The effective and humane management of painful disorders includes prevention, alleviation, and control of pain. The medical profession generally has been perceived as performing inadequately in discharging its obligation to relieve pain or suffering. Some organizations have established as a goal the eradication of the medical undertreatment of pain. Though laudable, this goal may be partially misdirected, since as much harm, if not more, may result from overtreatment. More properly, the profession should dedicate itself to the eradication of medical maltreatment by assuring safe and effective measures of pain relief.

To achieve this goal, the profession must undertake reliable outcome studies based on controlled, random, double-blind, cross-over methodology. Such studies must demonstrate the efficacy of not only pharmacological but also nonpharmacological interventions. Though it will be more difficult, the efficacy and safety of surgical and nonsurgical procedural interventions must also be determined.

The use of opioids in pain management are a case in point. There is little dispute that opioids should be used to alleviate and control pain that is disease related. However, there remains considerable controversy about the use of opioids in persistent, intractable pain of noncancerous origin. Polar passionate viewpoints have resulted in much heat but little light. A joint position paper released by the American Pain Society (APS) and the AAPM has been helpful but failed to achieve consensus. It seems that the debate is driven almost entirely by perceptions, factual and alleged, of misapplication of federal and state laws by overzealous enforcement officers. What is needed is less rhetoric and more research. Only then can the field of pain medicine achieve a balanced position based upon an intellectual foundation.

Concern over end-of-life care has stimulated considerable public and professional interest. This is an opportunity for pain medicine as a specialty to enter the debate and promulgate its vision and mission. End-of-life care includes such issues as adequate relief of pain and suffering and the specter of physician-assisted suicide. At the same time it is important for the field of pain medicine not to become exclusively identified with palliative and symptomatic relief of disease-related pain.

Pain that is persistent, intractable, and unremitting is a major source of functional impairment. Those with pain are frequently unable to enjoy activities of daily living or to participate in work-related tasks. The magnitude of this problem heavily affects the workers compensation system. Inasmuch as pain is subjective and cannot be measured or objectified, it is not surprising that most disability systems struggle with the issue of compensation. Many simply refuse to acknowledge the reality of pain that is not directly associated with tissue pathology. Many consider expressions of pain to be exaggerated or fabricated. Subconscious Renaissance convictions about the redemptive aspects of pain rise to the surface in the belief that pain is part of life, builds character, and always disappears eventually. Pain medicine as a specialty must rise to the challenge by devising an equitable and acceptable system of evaluating and rating impairment and disability related to pain, pain that is disease-related as well as pain that does not readily fall within the clinicopathological model.

Conclusion: Back to the Future

"The future is called 'perhaps' which is the only possible thing to call the future. And the important thing is not to allow that to scare you."

—*Tennessee Williams.*

Pain is a plural concept with many denotations and connotations. It is a unique human experience. Tissue damage is a frequent cause but not an absolute requirement. Many concepts of pain are difficult to reconcile with the clinicopathological model.

Although the field of pain medicine has roots in antiquity, it has emerged as a defined medical specialty during the past half century. It is a unique medical field characterized by a distinct body of knowledge and a defined scope of practice, with an infrastructure based on scientific research and education. It is supported and strengthened by medical organizations including the ABPM, a certifying body that has gained recognition and respectability.

To survive and thrive in the future, the field of pain medicine must rise to the challenge by addressing issues that confront it today. It must respond to these issues in the context of variables, attitudes, and values in many areas, including medical, psychological, social, societal, economic, and religious. Only by accepting and meeting these challenges can it assume its rightful place in the collegial community of medical specialties.

Physicians interested in the well-being of pain medicine as a specialty should always remember the past, shape the present, and create the future.

APPENDIX

RESOURCES FOR PAIN THERAPY AND MANAGEMENT

Professional Societies

American Pain Society (APS)
4700 W. Lake Ave.
Glenview, IL 60025
847-375-4715

U.S. Chapter, International Association for the Study of Pain (IASP)
L. E. Jones, BS
International Assoc. for the Study of Pain
N.E. 43rd St., Suite 306
Seattle, WA 98105

American Academy of Pain Medicine (AAPM)
4700 W. Lake Ave.
Glenview, IL 60025
847-375-4731

Journals

Pain. Journal of IASP; comes with membership. Dues on a sliding scale. Research journal. Published by Elsevier Science B.V., Amsterdam.
The Clinical Journal of Pain. Journal of the American Academy of Pain Medicine. Published by Lippincott, Philadelphia.
Pain Forum. Journal of the American Pain Society; comes with membership. Published by Churchill Livingstone, Secaucus, NJ.
Journal of Pain and Symptom Management. Published by Elsevier, New York.

Books

The IASP has a press that publishes medical and scientific research texts on the nuances of pain specialty problems, such as headaches, complex regional pain syndrome, and pharmacology.

Guilford Press, 72 Spring St., New York, NY 10012 has multiple publications on pain therapy from a psychosocial, behavioral medicine perspective.

Patients' Resources

Managing Pain Before It Manages You, by Margaret A. Caudill. Guilford Press, NY, 1995. Patient workbook for pain management. Audiotape available through ISHK Bookservice, Cambridge, MA; 800-222-4745. Spanish edition available through Guilford Press, New York.
Taking Control of Your Headache: How to Get the Treatment You Need, by Paul N. Duckro, William D. Richardson, and Janet E. Marshall. Guilford Press, New York, 1995. A self-management guide for headache treatment.
Learning to Master Your Pain, by Robert N. Jamison. Professional Resource Press, Sarasota, FL, 1996.
The Chronic Pain Control Workbook, by E.M. Catalano. New Harbinger Publications, Oakland, CA, 1987. Patient information book for pain treatment and management.
The Arthritis Help Book, by Kate Lorig and James Fries. Addison Wesley, Reading, MA, 1990. A tested self-management program for coping with arthritis.

Societies and support groups for specific diagnoses such as fibromyalgia, interstitial cystitis, scoliosis, and chronic pain in general

Endometriosis Association
8585 N. 76th Place
Milwaukee, WI 53223
414-355-2200

Interstitial Cystitis Association
P.O. Box 1553
Madison Square Station, New York, NY 10159
212-979-6057

National Chronic Pain Outreach Association, Inc.
7979 Old Georgetown Rd., Suite 100
Bethesda, MD 20814-2429
301-652-4948

American Chronic Pain Association
P.O. Box 850
Rocklin, CA 95677
916-632-0922

The American Fibromyalgia Syndrome Association, Inc.
6380 E. Tanque Verde Rd., Suite D
P.O. Box 31750
Tucson, AZ 85751-1750
520-733-1570
Also a resource for chronic fatigue syndrome and myofascial syndrome.

The Arthritis Foundation
1314 Spring St., N.W.
Atlanta, Georgia 30309
404-266-0795

National Scoliosis Foundation, Inc.
72 Mount Auburn St.
Watertown, MA 02172
617-926-0397

There is a growing number of Internet bulletin boards for fibromyalgia, cumulative trauma injury, and other chronic pain syndromes. Dr. Richard Chapman has linked many resources through the IASP website at http://weber.u.washington.edu/~cre/IASP.html.

Index